# CONCEPTS IN NONSURGICAL PERIODONTAL THERAPY

Kathleen O. Hodges, RDH, MS

*Associate Professor and Senior Clinic Coordinator*
*Department of Dental Hygiene*
*College of Health Professions*
*Idaho State University*
*Pocatello, Idaho*

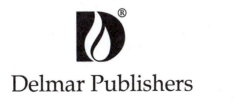

Delmar Publishers

*an International Thomson Publishing company* I(T)P®

Albany • Bonn • Boston • Cincinnati • Detroit • London • Madrid
Melbourne • Mexico City • New York • Pacific Grove • Paris • San Francisco
Singapore • Tokyo • Toronto • Washington

## NOTICE TO THE READER

Cover Design: Kathryn Sikule, Brownstone Graphics

**Delmar Staff**

Publisher: Susan Simpfenderfer
Acquisitions Editor: Dawn Gerrain
Project Development Editor: Coreen Filson
Production Coordinator: John Mickelbank
Art and Design Coordinator: Vincent S. Berger
Editorial Assistant: Donna L. Leto

COPYRIGHT © 1998
By Delmar Publishers
a division of International Thomson Publishing Inc.

The ITP logo is a trademark under license.

Printed in the United States of America

For more information, contact:

Delmar Publishers
3 Columbia Circle, Box 15015
Albany, New York 12212-5015

International Thomson Publishing Europe
Berkshire House
168–173 High Holborn
London, WC1V 7AA
England

Thomas Nelson Australia
102 Dodds Street
South Melbourne, 3205
Victoria, Australia

Nelson Canada
1120 Birchmount Road
Scarborough, Ontario
Canada, M1K 5G4

International Thomson Editores
Campos Eliseos 385, Piso 7
Col Polanco
11560 Mexico D F Mexico

International Thomson Publishing GmbH
Konigswinterer Strasse 418
53227 Bonn
Germany

International Thomson Publishing Asia
221 Henderson Road
#05-10 Henderson Building
Singapore 0315

International Thomson Publishing—Japan
Hirakawacho Kyowa Building, 3F
2-2-1 Hirakawacho
Chiyoda-ku, Tokyo 102
Japan

**Online Services**

**Delmar Online**
To access a wide variety of Delmar products and services on the World Wide Web, point your browser to:
    http://www.delmar.com
    or email: info@delmar.com

**thomson.com**
To access International Thomson Publishing's home site for information on more than 34 publishers and 20,000 products, point your browser to:
    http://www.thomson.com
    or email: findit@kiosk.thomson.com

A service of I(T)P®

 2   3   4   5   6   7   8   9   10   XXX   03   02   01   00   99   98   97

**Library of Congress Cataloging-in-Publication Data**

Concepts in nonsurgical periodontal therapy / Kathleen O. Hodges.
       p.      cm.
    Includes bibliographical references and index.
    ISBN 0-8273-6274-9 (alk. paper)
    1. Periodontics.   I. Hodges, Kathleen O.
    [DNLM: 1. Periodontal Diseases—therapy.   2. Periodontal Diseases—
    diagnosis.   3. Dental Instruments.   WU 240 C744 1997]
RK361.C585     1997
617.6'32—dc21
DNLM/DLC
for Library of Congress
                                                                        96–48459
                                                                           CIP

# CONTRIBUTORS

**Deborah Bailey Astroth, RDH, BS**

*Prevention and Maintenance of Occupational Hazards*

Clinical Instructor, Department of Dental Hygiene, University of Colorado School of Dentistry, Denver, Colorado; Director, Alliances

**Denise M. Bowen, RDH, MS**

*Introduction to Nonsurgical Periodontal Therapy and Use of Pain Control Modalities*

Professor and Chairperson, Department of Dental Hygiene, College of Health Professions, Idaho State University, Pocatello, Idaho

**Kimberly Krust Bray, RDH, MS**

*Supportive Treatment Procedures*

Associate Professor and Senior Clinic Coordinator, Division of Dental Hygiene, School of Dentistry, University of Missouri-Kansas City School of Dentistry, Kansas City, Missouri; Part-time Private Practitioner

**Kristin Hamman Calley, RDH, MS**

*Oral Self-Care Education and Case Presentation*

Assistant Professor, Department of Dental Hygiene, College of Health Professions, Idaho State University, Pocatello, Idaho; Part-time Private Practitioner

**Carole R. Christie, MCoun, LPC, NCC**

*Applying Communication Skills to Therapy*

Associate Professor, Department of Dental Hygiene, College of Health Professions, Idaho State University, Pocatello, Idaho; Licensed Professional Counselor and National Certified Counselor

**Steven W. Friedrichsen, DDS**

*Periodontal-Restorative Interactions*

Associate Professor and Chair of Idaho Dental Education Program, Affiliated with Creighton University School of Dentistry, Idaho State University, Pocatello, Idaho; Private Practitioner in General Dentistry, Pocatello, Idaho

**Kim Herremans, RDH, MS**

*Ultrasonic Periodontal Debridement*

Consultant, Advanced Ultrasonic Instrumentation; Full-time Private Practitioner, San Antonio, Texas

**Anita Herzog, RDH, MEd**

*Recommendations for Radiographs*

Associate Professor, Department of Dental Hygiene, College of Health Professions, Idaho State University, Pocatello, Idaho

**Gretchen G. Hess, RDH, BS**

*Implementing Nonsurgical Periodontal Therapy into General Practice*

Clinical Instructor, Department of Dental Hygiene, College of Health Professions, Idaho State University, Pocatello, Idaho; Part-time Private Practitioner

**Kathleen O. Hodges, RDH, MS**

*Instrument Selection: Philosophy and Strategies and Hand-Activated Instrumentation*

Associate Professor and Senior Clinic Coordinator, Department of Dental Hygiene, College of Health Professions, Idaho State University, Pocatello, Idaho; Part-time Private Practitioner

**Janet Ingrao, RDH, AS**

*Implementing Nonsurgical Periodontal Therapy into General Practice*

Full-time Private Practitioner, Boise, Idaho

**Carole Kawamura, RDH, MEd**

*Clinical Applications for Polishing*

Assistant Professor and Junior Clinic Coordinator, Department of Dental Hygiene, College of Health Professions, Idaho State University, Pocatello, Idaho

**Charla J. Lautar, RDH, PhD**

*Periodontal Diagnosis and Care Planning*

Assistant Professor, College of Technical Careers, Southern Illinois University, Carbondale, Illinois

**Salme E. Lavigne, RDH, MS**

*Periodontal Assessment* and contributed the Biological Basis for Periodontal Therapy Section in *Introduction to Nonsurgical Periodontal Therapy*

Associate Professor and Chairperson, Department of Dental Hygiene, Wichita State University, Wichita, Kansas

**John S. Mattson, DDS, MSD**

*Periodontal Maintenance Procedures*

Associate Professor and Chair, Department of Periodontics, Creighton University School of Dentistry, Omaha, Nebraska

**Deborah L. Miller, RDH, MS, MA**

*Medical History Evaluation and Alterations for Care*

Associate Professor, Department of Dental Hygiene, College of Health Professions, Idaho State University, Pocatello, Idaho

**Carlene S. Paarmann, RDH, MEd**

*Use of Pain Control Modalities*

Professor, Assistant Chairperson, and Expanded Functions Clinic Coordinator, Department of Dental Hygiene, College of Health Professions, Idaho State University, Pocatello, Idaho

**Janice F. L. Pimlott, DipDH, BScD(DH), MSc**

*Periodontal Diagnosis and Care Planning*

Professor; Acting Chair, Department of Dental Health Care; and Chair, Division of Dental Hygiene, Faculty of Dentistry, University of Alberta, Edmonton, Alberta

**Ellen J. Rogo, RDH, MEd**

*Career Development*

Associate Professor, Department of Dental Hygiene, College of Health Professions, Idaho State University, Pocatello, Idaho

**James Torosian, DMD**

*Surgical Intervention*

Clinical Assistant Professor, Department of Periodontics, Temple University School of Dentistry, Philadelphia, Pennsylvania; Private Practitioner in Periodontics and Implant Dentistry, Philadelphia, Pennsylvania

## Dedication

*Many people have enriched my life and it is to them that I dedicate this book.*

- *The biggest thank you goes to my husband Jim Cleary, and sons Gregory James and William Berkeley for their devotion, encouragement, patience, and love.*

- *To my parents, Kate and Berkeley, for lifetime personal and educational guidance.*

- *To my brother and sister-in-law, Rusty and Pam, for interest and concern in this seemingly endless project.*

- *To my past educators, this book is a product of your inspiration.*

- *To my former students, who sparked my enthusiasm for this book by asking "why."*

- *To my exceptional colleagues at Idaho State University for taking the time to teach, support, and believe in me. You are a special group of people. Your humor and friendship gave me the strength to continue.*

- *And finally, to those clinicians whose lives might be impacted as a result of the information presented in this book.*

*KOH*

# Table of Contents

*Preface* . . . . . . . . . . . . . . . . . . . . . . . . . . . . . . . . . . . . . . . . . . . . . . . . . . . . . . . . . . . . . . . . . . . . . . . . . . . . . . . . xi

SECTION I:     ASSESSMENT PHASE . . . . . . . . . . . . . . . . . . . . . . . . . . . . . . . . . . . . . . . . . . . . 1

*Chapter 1:*     **Introduction to Nonsurgical Periodontal Therapy** . . . . . . . . . . . . . . . . . 3
          Denise M. Bowen, RDH, MS

          *Introduction* . . . . . . . . . . . . . . . . . . . . . . . . . . . . . . . . . . . . . . . . . . . . . . 3
          *Definitions Associated with Nonsurgical Periodontal Therapy* . . . . . . . . . . . . 4
          *Review of the Periodontium* . . . . . . . . . . . . . . . . . . . . . . . . . . . . . . . . . . 6
          *Etiology and Associated Risk Factors in Periodontal Diseases* . . . . . . . . . . . . 10
          *Diseases of the Periodontium* . . . . . . . . . . . . . . . . . . . . . . . . . . . . . . . . 15
          *Biological Basis for Periodontal Therapy* . . . . . . . . . . . . . . . . . . . . . . . . . 19
          Summary . . . . . . . . . . . . . . . . . . . . . . . . . . . . . . . . . . . . . . . . . . . . . . 23
          Case Studies . . . . . . . . . . . . . . . . . . . . . . . . . . . . . . . . . . . . . . . . . . . . 23
          Case Study Discussions . . . . . . . . . . . . . . . . . . . . . . . . . . . . . . . . . . . . . 24
          References . . . . . . . . . . . . . . . . . . . . . . . . . . . . . . . . . . . . . . . . . . . . . 25

*Chapter 2:*     **Medical History Evaluation and Alterations for Care** . . . . . . . . . . . . . . . 29
          Deborah L. Miller, RDH, MS, MA

          *Introduction* . . . . . . . . . . . . . . . . . . . . . . . . . . . . . . . . . . . . . . . . . . . . 29
          *Medical History Evaluation* . . . . . . . . . . . . . . . . . . . . . . . . . . . . . . . . . 30
          *Pretreatment Alterations* . . . . . . . . . . . . . . . . . . . . . . . . . . . . . . . . . . . 36
          *Treatment Concerns* . . . . . . . . . . . . . . . . . . . . . . . . . . . . . . . . . . . . . . 43
          *Posttreatment Considerations* . . . . . . . . . . . . . . . . . . . . . . . . . . . . . . . . 47
          Summary . . . . . . . . . . . . . . . . . . . . . . . . . . . . . . . . . . . . . . . . . . . . . . 48
          Case Studies . . . . . . . . . . . . . . . . . . . . . . . . . . . . . . . . . . . . . . . . . . . . 48
          Case Study Discussions . . . . . . . . . . . . . . . . . . . . . . . . . . . . . . . . . . . . . 49
          References . . . . . . . . . . . . . . . . . . . . . . . . . . . . . . . . . . . . . . . . . . . . . 50

*Chapter 3:*     **Periodontal Assessment** . . . . . . . . . . . . . . . . . . . . . . . . . . . . . . . . . . . . 53
          Salme E. Lavigne, RDH, MS

          *Introduction* . . . . . . . . . . . . . . . . . . . . . . . . . . . . . . . . . . . . . . . . . . . . 53
          *Background Information* . . . . . . . . . . . . . . . . . . . . . . . . . . . . . . . . . . . . 53
          *Components of a Comprehensive Periodontal Assessment* . . . . . . . . . . . . . . 55
          *Appointment Planning and Scheduling* . . . . . . . . . . . . . . . . . . . . . . . . . . 55
          *Dental and Personal Histories* . . . . . . . . . . . . . . . . . . . . . . . . . . . . . . . . 56
          *Clinical Assessment* . . . . . . . . . . . . . . . . . . . . . . . . . . . . . . . . . . . . . . 56
          *Indices* . . . . . . . . . . . . . . . . . . . . . . . . . . . . . . . . . . . . . . . . . . . . . . 67
          *Supplemental Diagnostic Tests* . . . . . . . . . . . . . . . . . . . . . . . . . . . . . . . 73
          *Identification of Risk Factors* . . . . . . . . . . . . . . . . . . . . . . . . . . . . . . . . 78
          *Documentation* . . . . . . . . . . . . . . . . . . . . . . . . . . . . . . . . . . . . . . . . . 82
          Summary . . . . . . . . . . . . . . . . . . . . . . . . . . . . . . . . . . . . . . . . . . . . . . 82
          Case Studies . . . . . . . . . . . . . . . . . . . . . . . . . . . . . . . . . . . . . . . . . . . . 82

|  |  |  |
|---|---|---|
| Case Study Discussions | . . . . . . . . . . . . . . . . . . . . . . . . . . . . . . . . | 83 |
| References | . . . . . . . . . . . . . . . . . . . | 84 |

**Chapter 4:**   **Periodontal-Restorative Interactions** . . . . . . . . . . . . . . . . . . . . . . 88
Steven W. Friedrichsen, DDS

| | |
|---|---|
| *Introduction* . . . . . . . . . . . . . . . . . . . . | 88 |
| *Overview of Restorative Dentistry* . . . . . . . . . . . . . . . . . . . . | 88 |
| *Occlusion and Occlusal Traumatism* . . . . . . . . . . . . . . . . . . . . . . | 96 |
| *Care Planning* | 97 |
| *Periodontally Relevant Restorative Dentistry* . . . . . . . . . . . . . . . . . . . . | 98 |
| *Team Approach to Restorative Dentistry* . . . . . . . . . . . . . . . . . . . . | 110 |
| Summary . . . . . . . . . . . . . . . . . . . . | 113 |
| Case Studies . . . . . . . . . . . . . . . . . . . . | 113 |
| Case Study Discussions . . . . . . . . . . . . . . . . . . . . | 114 |
| References . . . . . . . . . . . . . . . . . . . . | 115 |

**Chapter 5:**   **Recommendations for Radiographs** . . . . . . . . . . . . . . . . . . . . 118
Anita Herzog, RDH, MEd

| | |
|---|---|
| *Introduction* . . . . . . . . . . . . . . . . . . . . | 118 |
| *Selection of Conventional Radiographs for Periodontal Evaluation* . . . . . . . . . | 118 |
| *Technical Factors Affecting Periodontal Interpretation* . . . . . . . . . . . . . . . . | 123 |
| *Interpretation of Periodontal Diseases* . . . . . . . . . . . . . . . . . . . . | 124 |
| *Correlating Radiographic and Clinical Findings* . . . . . . . . . . . . . . . . . . . . | 129 |
| *Predisposing Factors* . . . . . . . . . . . . . . . . . . . . | 135 |
| *Protocol for Exposure* . . . . . . . . . . . . . . . . . . . . | 137 |
| *Additional Images* . . . . . . . . . . . . . . . . . . . . | 140 |
| *Asepsis* . . . . . . . . . . . . . . . . . . . . | 143 |
| *Documentation* . . . . . . . . . . . . . . . . . . . . | 143 |
| Summary . . . . . . . . . . . . . . . . . . . . | 145 |
| Case Studies . . . . . . . . . . . . . . . . . . . . | 145 |
| Case Study Discussions . . . . . . . . . . . . . . . . . . . . | 146 |
| References . . . . . . . . . . . . . . . . . . . . | 148 |

**SECTION II:**   DIAGNOSIS AND PLANNING PHASES . . . . . . . . . . . . . . . . . 151

**Chapter 6:**   **Periodontal Diagnosis and Care Planning** . . . . . . . . . . . . . . . . . 153
Charla J. Lautar, RDH, PhD and Janice F. L. Pimlott, DipDH, BScD(DH), MSc

| | |
|---|---|
| *Introduction* . . . . . . . . . . . . . . . . . . . . | 153 |
| *Phases of Care* . . . . . . . . . . . . . . . . . . . . | 153 |
| *Decision-Making Process* . . . . . . . . . . . . . . . . . . . . | 154 |
| *Components of Care Planning* . . . . . . . . . . . . . . . . . . . . | 155 |
| *Selection of Mechanical Oral Self-Care Devices* . . . . . . . . . . . . . . . . . . . . | 163 |
| *Application of Planning to Nonsurgical Care* . . . . . . . . . . . . . . . . . . . . | 168 |
| Summary . . . . . . . . . . . . . . . . . . . . | 175 |
| Case Studies . . . . . . . . . . . . . . . . . . . . | 175 |
| Case Study Discussions . . . . . . . . . . . . . . . . . . . . | 176 |
| References . . . . . . . . . . . . . . . . . . . . | 178 |

SECTION III: IMPLEMENTATION PHASE ......................... 181

*Chapter 7:* **Applying Communication Skills to Therapy** .............. 183
Carole R. Christie, MCoun, LPC, NCC

*Introduction* ............................................. 183
*Principles of Communication* ............................... 183
*Forms of Communication* ................................... 185
*Documenting Communication* ............................... 190
*Improving Communication Skills* ............................ 193
Summary ................................................ 193
Case Studies ............................................. 193
Case Study Discussions .................................... 194
References .............................................. 195

*Chapter 8:* **Oral Self-Care Education and Case Presentation** ........ 196
Kristin Hamman Calley, RDH, MS

*Introduction* ............................................. 196
*Oral Self-Care* ........................................... 196
*Case Presentation* ........................................ 217
Summary ................................................ 223
Case Studies ............................................. 224
Case Study Discussions .................................... 224
References .............................................. 225

*Chapter 9:* **Use of Pain Control Modalities** ..................... 227
Denise M. Bowen, RDH, MS and Carlene S. Paarmann, RDH, MEd

*Introduction* ............................................. 227
*Use of Nitrous Oxide-Oxygen Analgesia for Conscious Sedation* ...... 228
*Use of Local Anesthesia in Nonsurgical Periodontal Therapy* ........ 235
*Use of Alternative Methods* ................................ 247
Summary ................................................ 249
Case Studies ............................................. 249
Case Study Discussions .................................... 250
References .............................................. 250

*Chapter 10:* **Instrument Selection: Philosophy and Strategies** ....... 253
Kathleen O. Hodges, RDH, MS

*Introduction* ............................................. 253
*Efficacy of Scaling and Root Planing* ........................ 253
*Nonsurgical and Surgical Interventions* ...................... 255
*Philosophy* .............................................. 255
*Anatomical Considerations* ................................. 256
*Deposit Characteristics* .................................... 264
*Instrument Selection Considerations* ......................... 268
*Selection Strategies* ....................................... 280
*Documentation* ........................................... 282
Summary ................................................ 282
Case Studies ............................................. 282

Case Study Discussions . . . . . . . . . . . . . . . . . . . . . . . . . . . . . .   283
References . . . . . . . . . . . . . . . . . . . . . . . . . . . . . . . . . . . . .   285

**Chapter 11:**     **Hand-Activated Instrumentation** . . . . . . . . . . . . . .   289
Kathleen O. Hodges, RDH, MS

*Introduction* . . . . . . . . . . . . . . . . . . . . . . . . . . . . . . . . .   289
*Geometric Terms* . . . . . . . . . . . . . . . . . . . . . . . . . . . .   289
*Instrument Sharpening* . . . . . . . . . . . . . . . . . . . . . . . . .   290
*Instrumentation Principles* . . . . . . . . . . . . . . . . . . . . . .   298
*Endpoint of Instrumentation* . . . . . . . . . . . . . . . . . . . . .   311
*Instrument Sequencing* . . . . . . . . . . . . . . . . . . . . . . . .   312
*Documentation* . . . . . . . . . . . . . . . . . . . . . . . . . . . . .   312
Summary . . . . . . . . . . . . . . . . . . . . . . . . . . . . . . . . . .   313
Case Studies . . . . . . . . . . . . . . . . . . . . . . . . . . . . . . . .   313
Case Study Discussions . . . . . . . . . . . . . . . . . . . . . . . . . .   313
References . . . . . . . . . . . . . . . . . . . . . . . . . . . . . . . . . .   318

**Chapter 12:**     **Ultrasonic Periodontal Debridement** . . . . . . . . . . . .   320
Kim Herremans, RDH, MS

*Introduction* . . . . . . . . . . . . . . . . . . . . . . . . . . . . . . . . .   320
*History of Ultrasonic Scaling Devices* . . . . . . . . . . . . . . . . .   320
*Principles of Ultrasonic Instruments* . . . . . . . . . . . . . . . . .   321
*Current Trends in Ultrasonic Equipment* . . . . . . . . . . . . . . .   322
*Background Information* . . . . . . . . . . . . . . . . . . . . . . . . .   327
*Case Selection* . . . . . . . . . . . . . . . . . . . . . . . . . . . . . . .   331
*Instrumentation Recommendations* . . . . . . . . . . . . . . . . . .   332
*Maintenance of Inserts* . . . . . . . . . . . . . . . . . . . . . . . . . .   339
Summary . . . . . . . . . . . . . . . . . . . . . . . . . . . . . . . . . .   339
Case Studies . . . . . . . . . . . . . . . . . . . . . . . . . . . . . . . .   339
Case Study Discussions . . . . . . . . . . . . . . . . . . . . . . . . . .   341
References . . . . . . . . . . . . . . . . . . . . . . . . . . . . . . . . . .   342

**Chapter 13:**     **Clinical Applications for Polishing** . . . . . . . . . . . . .   345
Carole Kawamura, RDH, MEd

*Introduction* . . . . . . . . . . . . . . . . . . . . . . . . . . . . . . . . .   345
*Philosophies* . . . . . . . . . . . . . . . . . . . . . . . . . . . . . . . . .   345
*Methods* . . . . . . . . . . . . . . . . . . . . . . . . . . . . . . . . . . .   349
*Abrasion* . . . . . . . . . . . . . . . . . . . . . . . . . . . . . . . . . . .   354
*Relationship of Polishing to Nonsurgical Periodontal Therapy* . . . . . . . . .   358
*Documentation* . . . . . . . . . . . . . . . . . . . . . . . . . . . . .   361
Summary . . . . . . . . . . . . . . . . . . . . . . . . . . . . . . . . . .   361
Case Studies . . . . . . . . . . . . . . . . . . . . . . . . . . . . . . . .   362
Case Study Discussions . . . . . . . . . . . . . . . . . . . . . . . . . .   363
References . . . . . . . . . . . . . . . . . . . . . . . . . . . . . . . . . .   364

**Chapter 14:**     **Supportive Treatment Procedures** . . . . . . . . . . . . . .   367
Kimberly Krust Bray, RDH, MS

*Introduction* . . . . . . . . . . . . . . . . . . . . . . . . . . . . . . . . .   367
*Overview of Chemotherapy* . . . . . . . . . . . . . . . . . . . . . . .   367
*Antimicrobial Rinses* . . . . . . . . . . . . . . . . . . . . . . . . . . .   369

*Irrigation* . . . . . . . . . . . . . . . . . . . . . . . . . . . . . . . . . . . . . . . . . . 376
*Controlled-Release Devices* . . . . . . . . . . . . . . . . . . . . . . . . . . . . . . 380
*Systemic Antibiotics* . . . . . . . . . . . . . . . . . . . . . . . . . . . . . . . . . . . 384
*Gingival Curettage* . . . . . . . . . . . . . . . . . . . . . . . . . . . . . . . . . . . . 386
*Overhang Removal* . . . . . . . . . . . . . . . . . . . . . . . . . . . . . . . . . . . . 387
*Dentinal Hypersensitivity* . . . . . . . . . . . . . . . . . . . . . . . . . . . . . . . 389
*Dental Implants* . . . . . . . . . . . . . . . . . . . . . . . . . . . . . . . . . . . . . . 394
*Documentation* . . . . . . . . . . . . . . . . . . . . . . . . . . . . . . . . . . . . . . 400
Summary . . . . . . . . . . . . . . . . . . . . . . . . . . . . . . . . . . . . . . . . . . . . 402
Case Studies . . . . . . . . . . . . . . . . . . . . . . . . . . . . . . . . . . . . . . . . . 402
Case Study Discussions . . . . . . . . . . . . . . . . . . . . . . . . . . . . . . . . . 403
References . . . . . . . . . . . . . . . . . . . . . . . . . . . . . . . . . . . . . . . . . . . 404

*Chapter 15:* **Prevention and Maintenance of Occupational Hazards** . . . . . . . . . . 412
Deborah Bailey Astroth, RDH, BS

*Introduction* . . . . . . . . . . . . . . . . . . . . . . . . . . . . . . . . . . . . . . . . . . 412
*Historical Perspective* . . . . . . . . . . . . . . . . . . . . . . . . . . . . . . . . . . . 412
*Ergonomic Hazards* . . . . . . . . . . . . . . . . . . . . . . . . . . . . . . . . . . . . 413
*Psychosocial Hazards* . . . . . . . . . . . . . . . . . . . . . . . . . . . . . . . . . . . 424
*Other Hazards* . . . . . . . . . . . . . . . . . . . . . . . . . . . . . . . . . . . . . . . . 428
*Federal Regulations Regarding Occupational Health* . . . . . . . . . . . . . . . 430
Summary . . . . . . . . . . . . . . . . . . . . . . . . . . . . . . . . . . . . . . . . . . . . 431
Case Studies . . . . . . . . . . . . . . . . . . . . . . . . . . . . . . . . . . . . . . . . . 432
Case Study Discussions . . . . . . . . . . . . . . . . . . . . . . . . . . . . . . . . . 432
References . . . . . . . . . . . . . . . . . . . . . . . . . . . . . . . . . . . . . . . . . . . 434

SECTION IV:    EVALUATION PHASE . . . . . . . . . . . . . . . . . . . . . . . . . . . . . . 437

*Chapter 16:* **Periodontal Maintenance Procedures** . . . . . . . . . . . . . . . . . . . . . 439
John S. Mattson, DDS, MSD

*Introduction* . . . . . . . . . . . . . . . . . . . . . . . . . . . . . . . . . . . . . . . . . . 439
*Objectives of Maintenance* . . . . . . . . . . . . . . . . . . . . . . . . . . . . . . . . 439
*Effectiveness of Maintenance* . . . . . . . . . . . . . . . . . . . . . . . . . . . . . . 440
*Components of a PMP Appointment* . . . . . . . . . . . . . . . . . . . . . . . . . 442
*Diagnosis* . . . . . . . . . . . . . . . . . . . . . . . . . . . . . . . . . . . . . . . . . . . 447
*Planning* . . . . . . . . . . . . . . . . . . . . . . . . . . . . . . . . . . . . . . . . . . . . 448
*Implementation* . . . . . . . . . . . . . . . . . . . . . . . . . . . . . . . . . . . . . . . 448
*Scheduling and Fees* . . . . . . . . . . . . . . . . . . . . . . . . . . . . . . . . . . . . 449
*Recare Intervals* . . . . . . . . . . . . . . . . . . . . . . . . . . . . . . . . . . . . . . . 450
*Client Compliance* . . . . . . . . . . . . . . . . . . . . . . . . . . . . . . . . . . . . . 450
*Referral to a Periodontist* . . . . . . . . . . . . . . . . . . . . . . . . . . . . . . . . 451
*Documentation* . . . . . . . . . . . . . . . . . . . . . . . . . . . . . . . . . . . . . . . 452
Summary . . . . . . . . . . . . . . . . . . . . . . . . . . . . . . . . . . . . . . . . . . . . 452
Case Studies . . . . . . . . . . . . . . . . . . . . . . . . . . . . . . . . . . . . . . . . . 452
Case Study Discussions . . . . . . . . . . . . . . . . . . . . . . . . . . . . . . . . . 454
References . . . . . . . . . . . . . . . . . . . . . . . . . . . . . . . . . . . . . . . . . . . 455

*Chapter 17:* **Surgical Intervention** . . . . . . . . . . . . . . . . . . . . . . . . . . . . . . . . 458
James Torosian, DMD

*Introduction* . . . . . . . . . . . . . . . . . . . . . . . . . . . . . . . . . . . . . . . . . . 458

*Principles of Surgery* .................................... 458
*Case Preparation* ....................................... 460
*Surgical Evaluation* ..................................... 461
*Surgical Case Management* ............................... 461
*Periodontal Flaps and Alveolar Bone Management* ......... 461
*Mucogingival Reconstruction* ............................ 466
Summary ................................................ 466
Case Studies ............................................ 466
Case Study Discussions .................................. 469
References .............................................. 474


SECTION V:    APPLICATION TO PRACTICE .................... 477

*Chapter 18:*    **Career Development** ...................... 479
     Ellen J. Rogo, RDH, MEd

*Introduction* ........................................... 479
*The Career Plan Description* ............................ 479
*The Employment Search* .................................. 487
*Compensation* ........................................... 495
*Future Career Development* .............................. 504
Summary ................................................ 504
Case Studies ............................................ 505
Case Study Discussions .................................. 505
References .............................................. 506

*Chapter 19:*    **Implementing Nonsurgical Periodontal Therapy
into General Practice** ................................. 507
     Gretchen G. Hess, RDH, BS and Janet Ingrao RDH, AS

*Introduction* ........................................... 507
*Development of a Nonsurgical Periodontal Therapy Program* .. 507
*Communication* .......................................... 510
*Implementation of Nonsurgical Periodontal Therapy* ...... 515
*Monitoring and Evaluation* .............................. 526
Summary ................................................ 527
Case Studies ............................................ 528
Case Study Discussions .................................. 528
References .............................................. 529

*Glossary* ......................................... 531

*Index* ............................................ 539

# Preface

## BACKGROUND

As knowledge of the etiology and classification of peri-odontal disease and its therapy rapidly advances, the demand for periodontal care grows. Consequently, dental hygienists and dentists are routinely challenged to keep informed of the latest treatment modalities in periodontics and clinical practice. Gingivitis and periodontitis, the two major forms of inflammatory diseases affecting the gingiva and periodontal attachment, both require appropriate assessment and periodontal diagnosis in order to provide timely, client-centered nonsurgical periodontal therapy (NSPT).

The principles of NSPT include suppression or elimination of pathogenic microorganisms through bacterial plaque and calculus removal, controlling infection, resolution or elimination of inflammation, and controlling systemic factors, if possible. These goals are accomplished by bacterial plaque removal involving the clinician and client, oral prophylaxis or periodontal debridement by the clinician as indicated, and other supportive therapy. Additional challenges presented to oral health care professionals include providing a thorough assessment in an efficient manner, greater decision making in care planning, and the need for enhanced communication to effectively discuss periodontal therapy with patients. Incorporation of contemporary therapeutic approaches and technology, development of maintenance programs for clients, and a greater need for a team approach in the practice setting are necessary to enhance the delivery of comprehensive periodontal care. While some of the concepts in nonsurgical periodontal therapy are not new, the means for achieving these goals are expanding. It has become evident that cotherapy between the client and oral health care provider is mandatory for nonsurgical periodontal therapy to be successful.

The rapid advancements in dental hygiene theory and periodontics have provided an impetus for change in professional terminology. For instance, *treatment planning* has been expanded to *care planning*, and *supportive periodontal therapy* (SPT) is referred to as *periodontal maintenance procedures (PMP)*. It is noticeable throughout the text that *client* and *patient* are used interchangeably. The Miller-Keane Encyclopedia and Dictionary of Medicine, Nursing, and Allied Health (O'Toole, 1992) defines *client* as "the term most often used as a synonym for a patient who receives health care in an ambulatory care setting, especially when health maintenance rather than illness care is the primary service provided," (p. 320). On the other hand, *patient* is defined as " a person who is ill or is undergoing treatment for disease" (O'Toole, 1992,

p. 1119). Generally, *client* refers to a group as well as an individual and connotes wellness rather than illness. The word *client*, however, is not embraced by all dental hygienists and dentists; therefore, both terms are incorporated.

## ORGANIZATION

The book is designed to provide the reader with current recommendations for nonsurgical periodontal care in a realistic and practical manner. It includes an overview of periodontology as well as detailed information about skills necessary to manage periodontal disease. The text is organized as if the reader is providing care for a patient, thus it is applicable to educational curriculums and practice settings. The book is divided into nineteen chapters and four sections based on the dental hygiene process of care: assessment, diagnosis and planning, implementation, and evaluation. A fifth section is incorporated discussing application of NSPT to the practice setting.

## AUDIENCE

An objective of this text is to blend periodontics and clinical dental hygiene while building upon the foundation knowledge and skill previously acquired by the dental hygiene student, dental student, or practitioner. The primary audience for this book includes second year or upper level dental hygiene students in periodontology or clinical dental hygiene classes. It is intended to help "close the gap" between the graduating dental hygiene student and the more seasoned dental hygienist. A concern when developing an upper level text is determining the amount of background material to incorporate. Review of material, however, will hopefully assist the student or practitioner in developing a solid and current knowledge base.

This text might also be useful for educating dental students in the nonsurgical periodontal phase of the curriculum. Additionally, its use is appropriate for continuing education programs, self-study for clinicians, and education of dental hygienists and dentists who wish to reenter the profession.

## FEATURES

Unique features of this book include the focus on NSPT, the combination of theory and practice recommendations, and examples of practical clinical forms to be used in recording components of periodontal therapy. Key words are found at the beginning of each chapter to aid the reader in locating significant terms, definitions, and concepts. Appropriate and thorough documentation of phases of therapy along with legal implications for practice are included within each chapter, when applicable. Self-evaluation exercises allow students and practitioners to review skills associated with certain phases of care. Each chapter concludes with five case studies to encourage application of knowledge, critical thinking, and decision making. Case study responses stimulate independent thinking and/or group discussion. Lastly, the comprehensive reference list at the end of each chapter will aid the reader in finding further information about theory, treatment options, and recommendations.

## ACKNOWLEDGMENTS

Editing and writing are very humbling experiences that cannot be accomplished without the help and guidance of others. I wish to acknowledge the dedication and expertise of all the contributors who helped make *Concepts in Nonsurgical Periodontal Therapy* possible. Your enthusiasm and initiative have made this project a reality. Particular recognition is given to the faculty, staff, and students at Idaho State University Department of Dental Hygiene for their untiring support and encouragement. Special thanks is given to Denise Bowen, Chairperson, Department of Dental Hygiene, Idaho State University, for sharing her knowledge in periodontology, and her brilliant critical thinking and writing skills. I am forever indebted to her kindness. Also, Darryl Bybee, DDS, is recognized for supporting NSPT in general practice to benefit our patients.

There are a great number of other people who have had a hand in this book and without whom it would not have been possible to finish. Invaluable technical assistance and camaraderie was provided by Terry Tetreault along with contributions from Chris Salstrom, Office Coordinator, Idaho State University Department of Dental Hygiene, and Dalene Tetreault. The individuals, authors, publishers, and manufacturers who gave permission to include concepts, tables, figures, photographs, and diagrams are also wholeheartedly acknowledged including, but not limited to, Hu-Friedy® Dental Manufacturing Co., Suter Dental Manufacturing Company, Inc, Oral-B Laboratories, Teledyne Water Pik, and Dentsply International Cavitron Division. Appreciation is extended to Dave Myers, former photographer at Idaho State University, for his expertise.

Thanks to the publishing team at Delmar Publishers, who exhibited foresight by recognizing the need for and taking the lead in publishing this book. Cori Filson, Project Development Editor, and the entire team have my gratitude. Appreciation is extended Pamela A. Lamb, Editorial & Communication Services, for professional editing, and to Gail Farrar, Publishers' Design and Production Services, Inc., for her publishing expertise. The professional reviewers are also acknowledged for their helpful and detailed suggestions: Marie Varley Gillis, Howard University; JoAnn Gurenlian, Gurenlian & Associates; Heather Mapp, Lanier Technical Institute; Sharon Pirk, University of Texas Health Science Center, San Antonio; and Trisha Moore Reid, Northern Arizona University; Michele Darby, BSDH, MS, Eminent Scholar and Graduate Program Director, Gene W. Hirschfeld, School of Dental Hygiene and Dental Assisting, Old Dominion University is also thanked for her mentorship and confidence in this project.

I am interested in readers' suggestions for revisions and additions as well as how the book is being used in educational and practice settings. Therefore, I would appreciate hearing readers' responses.

Kathleen O. Hodges

# SECTION I

# ASSESSMENT PHASE

# CHAPTER 1

# Introduction to Nonsurgical Periodontal Therapy

## Key Terms

active therapy
deplaquing
inflammation
initial therapy
nonsurgical periodontal therapy (NSPT)
oral prophylaxis

periodontal debridement
periodontal disease
periodontal disease activity
periodontal maintenance procedures (PMP)
root planing
scaling

## INTRODUCTION

The ultimate goal of periodontal therapy is to preserve or maintain the dentition in a state of health and comfort throughout life (Ramfjord, 1993). Ideally, periodontal therapy should eliminate inflammation, arrest progression of periodontal disease, improve aesthetics, and create an environment conducive to maintenance of health. When the ideal cannot be achieved, the pragmatic goal of therapy is to repair the damage resulting from disease (Consensus Report, 1989). Both surgical and nonsurgical treatment approaches are used to accomplish these goals (American Academy of Periodontology, 1993; Greenstein, 1992).

**Nonsurgical periodontal therapy (NSPT)** is defined as "plaque removal, plaque control, supra- and subgingival scaling, root planing, and the adjunctive use of chemical agents" (Ciancio, 1989, 1992). Nonsurgical periodontal therapy has historically been, and will continue to be, an integral and effective part of periodontal treatment. NSPT requires a thorough periodontal assessment and evaluation of risk factors prior to therapy and careful reevaluation following therapy. With scientific and technical advances related to instrumentation, development of improved chemotherapeutics and new assessment techniques, nonsurgical periodontal therapy promises to become even more efficacious. The clinician's ability to reach a specific therapeutic goal is determined by that individual's professional knowledge, skill, experience, and the availability of state-of-the-art equipment and supplies, as well as the host response and compliance of the client whose disease is being treated (Consensus Report, 1989). Development of new effective therapies for preventing and treating periodontal dis-

eases will augment the profession's capabilities, while challenging each practitioner to stay abreast of technological changes. An increasingly important challenge will be to apply new technologies in a cost-effective manner, so that essential periodontal care will be available to all who need it (O'Neil, Shugars, & Bader, 1991, 1993).

The demand for effective prevention and treatment of periodontal diseases is growing. Americans have become "prosumers" who want to play a more active role in self-treatment, and consumers are increasingly aware of the significance of periodontal disease. A 1991 national survey conducted by the Gallup Organization found that 76 percent of the respondents expressed concern about gingivitis and 49 percent about periodontitis. Additionally 76 percent of those surveyed indicated that their last dental visit was within the past year (American Dental Association, 1991). The aging American population also will have an impact on future demand for periodontal services. It has been estimated that, by the year 2030, 25 percent of all Americans will be over 60 years of age. Older Americans are not only keeping their teeth longer, but they are continuing to use dental services at rates comparable to middle-aged adults. In fact, only 4 percent of all Americans under the age of 65 are edentulous (Christersson, Grossi, Dunford, Machtel, & Genco, 1991).

Although periodontal diseases are prevalent in the United States, they are more limited in severity than previously thought. The National Survey of the Oral Health of United States Adults conducted by the National Institute of Dental Research in 1986 provided extensive data about the prevalence of periodontal disease (Miller, Brunelle, Carlos, Brown, & Löe, 1987). The populations studied included employed adults and ambulatory seniors. Prevalence in the subsample of 15,000 employed adults showed that at least one site of attachment loss (≥ 2 mm) was found in about 50 percent of 18- to 19-year-old subjects; about 80 percent of 35- to 39-year-old subjects; 87 percent for 45 to 49 years; and exceeded 90 percent for those 60 years and older. At least one area of severe periodontal destruction (≥ 6 mm) was found in only 8 percent of employed adults. In the subsample of 5,000 ambulatory older Americans, 34 percent of seniors had at least one area of severe periodontal destruction. These findings demonstrate that prevalence of attachment loss increases with age; however, the severity of periodontal diseases is limited. Most cases can be successfully treated by nonsurgical periodontal therapy. The vast majority of periodontal treatment needs are related to treating gingivitis and early periodontitis, preventing disease progression and maintaining periodontal health following therapy. Client assessment, treatment planning, individualized oral self-care instruction, preventive and nonsurgical periodontal therapy, supportive treatment for health maintenance, and reevaluation are all critical components of thorough periodontal care. A complete understanding of each of these clinical interventions and modalities is essential to the provision of quality preventive and nonsurgical periodontal services. Although this text is based upon current knowledge, understanding of the periodontium and various diseases which affect it is expanding rapidly. This knowledge is resulting in the evolution of new technologies and treatment approaches. Clinicians are continuously challenged to remain current in the practice of nonsurgical periodontal therapy.

## DEFINITIONS ASSOCIATED WITH NONSURGICAL PERIODONTAL THERAPY

The American Academy of Periodontology (AAP) (1995a) defines **scaling** as "instrumentation of the crown and root surfaces of the teeth to remove plaque and calculus." Most commonly scaling is employed only in areas where calculus deposits are detected, without intentional removal of tooth surface. When supragingival and subgingival scaling are combined with selective coronal polishing of the teeth, to remove plaque, calculus, and stains, an **oral prophylaxis** is performed. This procedure is preventive in nature and is indicated for healthy cases, or for treatment of gingivitis (Greenstein, 1992; Walsh & Robertson, 1985). **Root planing** is defined as "a definitive procedure designed for the removal of cementum and dentin that is rough, and/or permeated by calculus, or contaminated with toxins or microorganisms" (American Academy of Periodontology, 1995a). Therapeutic scaling and root planing is performed to treat established periodontal disease and to create conditions that are conducive to health. The procedure is technically demanding, time consuming and may require use of local anesthesia (AAP, 1993; Walsh & Robertson, 1985).

The question as to whether hand or traditional ultra-

sonic instruments are more effective in producing root smoothness has been studied extensively (Meyer & Lie, 1977; Oosterwaal, Matee, Mikx, van't Hof, & Renggli, 1987; Thornton & Garnick, 1982; Van Volkinburg, Green, & Armitage, 1976). Some authors report that the degree of root smoothness has no effect on clinical parameters (Khatiblou & Ghodossi, 1983; Rosenburg & Ash, 1974; Waerhaug, 1956). Numerous studies have, however, documented that scaling and root planing, whether performed with ultrasonic or hand instruments, is an effective treatment to improve periodontal status (Hughes & Caffesse, 1978; Morrison, Ramfjord, & Hill, 1980; Proye, Caton, & Polson, 1982; Sato, Yoneyama, Okamoto, Dehlen, & Lindhe, 1993; Slots, 1979). Gingival inflammation, bleeding, and probing depths are reduced following nonsurgical periodontal therapy. These clinical improvements have been shown to be significantly more effective than results obtained from supragingival plaque control alone (Baderstein, Nilvéus, & Egelberg, 1981, 1984; Caton, Bouwsma, Polson, & Epseland, 1989; Cercek, Kiger, Garret, & Egelberg, 1983; Corbet & Davies, 1993). Following scaling and root planing, a four- to six-week reevaluation of tissue and attachment levels is critical to determine success of nonsurgical therapy and to assess need for additional therapy (AAP, 1993; Consensus Report, 1989). This four- to six-week time interval is the minimum needed for healing following initial therapy; however, a longer period may be necessary if delayed healing is expected due to a compromised immune status.

A new perspective on nonsurgical periodontal therapy focuses on the importance of "periodontal debridement" as a suggested alternative to the traditional "scaling and root planing" approach. Stutsman-Young, O'Hehir, and Woodall (1993) define periodontal debridement as "the treatment of gingival and periodontal inflammation through mechanical removal of tooth and root surface irregularities to the extent that the adjacent soft tissues maintain or return to a healthy, noninflamed state." Removal of calculus is secondary; calculus is considered important only from the perspective of its plaque-retentive nature. Total debridement can involve supragingival debridement, subgingival debridement, and/or deplaquing. Supragingival debridement includes removal of all accessible plaque, plaque by-products and retentive factors (e.g., calculus) from the clinical crown of the tooth in order to foster the client's plaque control and gingival health. Subgingival debridement includes removal of all accessible plaque, plaque by-products, and retentive factors (such as calculus, overhangs, etc.), that may promote plaque formation and contribute to its retention in inflamed periodontal pockets and/or apical to the gingival margin. The purpose is to supplement the client's supragingival plaque control by removing or disrupting subgingival deposits which are inaccessible to the client. **Deplaquing** includes the removal or disruption of bacterial plaque and its toxins subgingivally, following the completion of supragingival and subgingival debridement. It is performed, using a curet or ultrasonic scaling instrument, at reevaluation and maintenance appointments. Deplaquing is a new concept, not well studied in the literature.

In the recent past, some authors have suggested that traditional scaling and root planing be replaced by periodontal debridement (Miller, 1995; Nield-Gehrig & Houseman, 1996; O'Hehir, 1995; Stutsman-Young, O'Hehir, and Woodall, 1993). Nield-Gehrig and Houseman (1996) define root surface debridement as the use of light, overlapping strokes covering every square millimeter of the root surface for deplaquing and removal of endotoxin. The basic difference between these two concepts is in the extent of periodontal instrumentation. Root planing may remove significant amounts of cementum and dentin in an effort to obtain a glassy smooth root surface which is free of all irregularities, contaminants, and calculus deposits. Periodontal debridement focuses primarily on removing bacterial plaque, its by-products and any plaque retentive factors such as calculus or overhanging restorations *only* to the extent that adjacent soft tissues maintain or return to a healthy state. Either technique can be performed with hand or mechanical instruments and both techniques require reevaluation to determine success of therapy based upon healing of the periodontal tissues; however, the periodontal debridement approach intensifies the need for reevaluation because of its emphasis on limiting periodontal instrumentation to the minimal extent required for healing. The trend is toward removal of as little tooth structure as possible.

It is important to note that the basic definition of supra- and subgingival debridement includes the removal of *all* plaque retentive factors (which includes removal of all detected calculus), and that the end point of both "debridement" and "root planing" is to foster periodontal health. Studies have found that complete calculus removal is possible on some root surfaces, but it is not 100 percent successful on all surfaces (Badersten, 1985; Brayer et al., 1989; Drisko and Killoy, 1991). Complete removal of cementum also is not usually accomplished, nor would it be a practical and realistic objective in practice. Although thorough subgingival debridement and planing are the desired treatment goals, complete removal of cementum and 100 percent calculus removal is probably not possible or even desirable at the expense of lost tooth structure and dentinal hypersensitivity. Thus the old notion of planing the root surfaces repeatedly, especially to the point of producing radiographic or explorer detectable alterations in root anatomy, can no longer be justified. On the other hand, the notion that periodontal debridement does not require complete removal of *clinically detectable* calculus deposits is a misconception that must be countered. Because calculus retains bacterial plaque, its removal is critical to successful periodontal therapy and, although root planing is not successful in removing 100 percent of the calculus, it has been shown to be effective in reducing inflammation

and preserving attachment levels in patients with periodontitis. The logical question that arises is, "How much calculus must be removed to allow for the reversal of inflammation and healing of the periodontal tissues?" The answer to this question is unknown because long-term clinical trials that have been conducted have employed traditional root planing techniques and no such data exists to document the effectiveness of periodontal debridement to a lesser extent. Without a doubt, all clinically detectable calculus deposits must be removed supragingivally and subgingivally or a clinician could be guilty of supervised neglect. Intentionally leaving detected deposits would constitute unethical and substandard care. Even the most skilled and experienced clinician, however, might unintentionally leave *clinically undetected* deposits. For this reason, a four- to six-week reevaluation of healing following nonsurgical periodontal therapy is an important component of successful treatment. Each individual's immune system may be capable of healing a periodontal lesion in the presence of different levels of microorganisms.

A practical approach to nonsurgical periodontal therapy would be to merge the goals of scaling and root planing procedures with those of periodontal debridement, as an intermediate endpoint. Based upon that philosophy, **periodontal debridement** is defined, for purposes of this text, as the removal of all subgingival plaque and its by-products (as evidenced by clinical signs of inflammation), clinically detectable plaque retentive factors (calculus, overhangs), and detectable calculus-embedded cementum to finish the root surface during periodontal instrumentation while preserving as much of the tooth surface as possible. This approach requires clinical judgement regarding the presence of inflammation as well as the presence or absence of calculus—embedded cementum. Removal of cementum and dentin solely for the purpose of smoothness, despite a clinical judgment that existing calculus has been removed, is unnecessary. But because nonsurgical periodontal therapy including subgingival scaling, root planing and/or periodontal debridement is performed using tactile skills rather than visually, it is impossible to ascertain that calculus deposits have been removed adequately at the time of initial treatment. Reevaluation of healing following periodontal debridement is the only mechanism for ascertaining efficacy by evaluating the periodontal tissues for elimination of inflammation, absence of bleeding, and level of attachment. If our ultimate therapeutic endpoints have been achieved, then an acceptable level of calculus and/or cementum removal has been attained for that patient's immune response. Long-term success then requires cooperative maintenance care by both the client and the clinician.

**Periodontal maintenance procedures (PMP)**, previously referred to as maintenance therapy or supportive periodontal treatment (SPT), is defined as an extension of periodontal therapy which involves continuing periodic assessment and preventive treatment of the periodontal structures to allow for early detection and treatment of new or recurring periodontal disease (McFall, 1989). It includes removal of bacterial flora from crevicular and pocket areas, scaling and polishing, and a review of the client's self-care efficiency (AAP, 1995a). PMP is performed at regular recall intervals following active nonsurgical and/or surgical periodontal therapy in order to arrest disease progression and maintain periodontal health. Typically, an interval of three months between appointments is an effective treatment schedule but this can vary (AAP, 1995a). Because neither initial periodontal therapy nor subsequent personal oral hygiene is likely to be perfect for every tooth, PMP will be indicated for all periodontitis cases. It is critical to the long-term success of periodontal therapy so compliance with recommended PMP intervals must be emphasized throughout active therapy (Cortellini et al., 1994; Demetriou et al., 1995). Because periodontitis is chronic in nature, PMP will be required for the rest of a client's life, or until new or recurring periodontal disease appears and additional diagnostic procedures and therapy must be considered (AAP 1995a; AAP 1995b). See Chapter 16 for a more detailed discussion of PMP.

Treatment planning approaches to periodontal therapy vary depending upon the type and severity of disease present and the philosophical approach of the clinician providing care. **Active therapy** can include nonsurgical periodontal therapy, periodontal surgery, or both. Nonsurgical periodontal therapy is the first phase of treatment in the majority of cases of periodontal disease (Ciancio, 1989); therefore, it also is sometimes referred to as **initial therapy**, or initial preparation or anti-infective therapy. Its goals are to eliminate or suppress infectious microorganisms and other etiologic factors, and to establish an environment which promotes health of the periodontal tissues and precludes further loss of attachment. The efficacy of NSPT as a total treatment, as stated previously, can only be determined by reevaluating the response to therapy at a four- to six-week interval following completion of initial therapy. The nonsurgical approach is most predictably successful in treating shallow to moderate pockets. The AAP has established a 5 mm probing depth as a benchmark or guide to the most predictable efficacious response; however, pockets deeper than 5 mm are felt to also respond successfully albeit with less predictability (Consensus Report, 1989).

Evaluation of the response to this first phase of periodontal therapy determines the next course of treatment. If inflammation and bleeding are resolved, attachment levels are stable and probing depths are maintainable by the client, periodontal maintenance procedures are planned. Frequent periodic appointments for observation, reevaluation, periodontal debridement and reinstruction in oral self-care practices are established for long-term maintenance. If reevaluation following initial, nonsurgical therapy indicates that inflammation and infection are not resolved and/or dis-

ease progression has occurred, a clinical decision must be made regarding the reason(s) for nonresponse and the need for further therapy, including surgery. It is important to determine the reason why response to NSPT was less than adequate. Problems with self-care, inflammation, or residual calculus may require reinstruction, redebridement or a chemotherapeutic approach, whereas progressive attachment loss may require more aggressive therapy. Surgical periodontal therapy is aimed at treatment of the unresolved periodontal pockets, advancing loss of attachment, or need for regenerative procedures. It represents the second phase of active periodontal therapy when the nonsurgical phase is not adequate as a sole treatment. Periodontal surgery also is followed by reevaluation and PMP to enhance long-term success. These two elements represent the third phase of periodontal therapy, the maintenance phase, which is an essential follow-up to active therapy whether it involves nonsurgical or surgical phases, or both. At any point during the maintenance phase that active disease is identified and/or attachment loss progresses significantly, active periodontal therapy can be reinstituted. In this case, treatment can involve active nonsurgical or surgical periodontal therapy depending, once again, on the type and severity of disease present.

## REVIEW OF THE PERIODONTIUM

A review of the clinical features and histology of each of the parts of the periodontium provides a basis for understanding periodontal disease progression and rationale for various therapeutic approaches. The periodontium is comprised of the gingiva, periodontal ligament, cementum, and alveolar bone (see Figure 1-1). The function of the tissues of the periodontium is to attach the tooth to the alveolar process.

### Gingiva

The gingiva is the part of the oral masticatory mucosa that covers the cervical and root portions of the teeth and the alveolar processes of the maxilla and the mandible. It extends from the mucogingival junction to the free gingival margin, except on the lingual of the

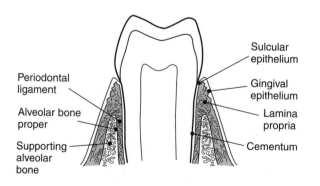

**Figure 1-1** Parts of the periodontium.

maxillary arch where it is continuous with the palatal mucosa. The gingiva is composed of the marginal gingiva (or free gingiva) and the attached gingiva (see Figure 1-2). The marginal gingiva surrounds the tooth on all surfaces forming a cufflike band of tissue. It includes the gingival margin as its most coronal portion on the facial and lingual surfaces. In health, the gingival margin is flat and scalloped, following the contour of the teeth, about 0.5 mm coronal to the cementoenamel junction (CEJ). The interdental gingiva also is a part of the marginal gingiva. It is comprised of two papilla: one facial and one lingual, connected beneath the tooth contact by a concave-shaped nonkeratinized tissue called the col. In health, the interdental gingiva fills the embrasure space between the teeth. The marginal gingiva attaches to the tooth at the base of the gingival sulcus, a space formed between the tooth and the free gingiva, by junctional epithelium and connective tissue fibers. In health, the gingival sulcus measures 1 to 2 mm facially and lingually and 1 to 3 mm interproximally. In disease, the marginal gingiva may become swollen (edematous), enlarged, red (erythematous), rolled, cratered, fibrotic, or it may recede apically. The depth of the sulcus may also increase beyond 3 mm by formation of a psuedo or true periodontal pocket. The gingival tissues may bleed upon provocation or spontaneously. These signs of periodontal disease affect the interdental gingiva first, followed by the marginal gingiva facially and lingually, and ultimately the attached gingiva.

The attached gingiva is that portion attached to the cementum of the tooth and to the underlying periosteum of the alveolar processes. It extends from the base of the gingival sulcus to the mucogingival junction. Width of attached gingiva varies throughout the mouth. It is generally widest in the anteriors of the maxilla and narrowest in the mandibular premolar areas. A mucogingival problem exists when no attached gingiva or too little (in the opinion of the individual practitioner) is present. Philosophies are changing regarding the need for a spe-

cific amount of attached gingiva. The need for treatment depends upon the cause and whether or not a loss of attached gingiva is progressing. An inadequate zone of attached gingiva most often occurs as a result of progressive recession of the gingival margin (Hall, 1989). Keratinized attached gingiva is important for withstanding mechanical stress in the oral cavity.

A brief review of the anatomical features of the normal periodontium is essential to understanding the periodontal disease process (see Figure 1-3). Refer to a basic histology or periodontology text for a more comprehensive review. The gingival epithelium is comprised of stratified squamous epithelium which is keratinized or parakeratinized on the outer surface of the marginal and attached gingiva, and nonkeratinized in the gingival sulcus and junctional epithelium. It is a continuous band of epithelial tissue made up of three areas: the oral epithelium, the sulcular epithelium and the junctional epithelium. The oral or outer epithelium, present on the outer surface of the gingiva, is continuous with the sulcular (or crevicular) epithelium which lines the sulcus (crevice). At the base of the sulcus, this epithelium attaches to the enamel and/or cementum of the root and is thus called the junctional epithelium. It is found within one millimeter of the cementoenamel junction. The length of the junctional epithelium ranges from 1.35 mm to 0.25 mm (Itoiz & Carranza, 1996). It joins onto the cementum by a hemidesmosomal, mucopolysaccharide attachment known as the epithelial attachment. This attachment consists of a basal lamina (basement membrane) that is comparable to that which attaches the epithelial tissue to connective tissue elsewhere in the body. Because the sulcular epithelium, col tissue, and junctional epithelium are nonkeratinized, they are more permeable to cells, fluids, and toxins than the outer gingival epithelium. The junctional epithelium, therefore, also serves as the preferred passageway for bac-

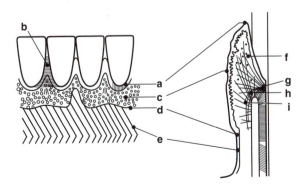

**Figure 1-2** Gingiva. *Key:* **a:** margin of gingiva; **b:** interdental papilla; **c:** attached gingiva; **d:** mucogingival junction; **e:** alveolar mucosa. In cross section (**f** through **i**): fibers of the lamina propria (connective tissue); **f:** circular fibers; **g:** dentogingival fibers; **h:** dentoperiosteal fibers; **i:** alveolo gingival fibers. (Public Domain, National Audiovisual Center)

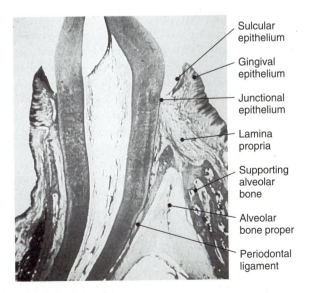

Sulcular epithelium

Gingival epithelium

Junctional epithelium

Lamina propria

Supporting alveolar bone

Alveolar bone proper

Periodontal ligament

**Figure 1-3** Cross section of the tooth and periodontium. (Public Domain, National Audiovisual Center)

teria and/or bacterial products to enter from the gingival sulcus into the connective tissue of the gingiva.

The connective tissue of the gingiva, called the lamina propria, is found underlying the epithelial portion of the gingiva. These two portions of the gingiva are connected by a basal lamina. The lamina propria is composed of gingival connective tissue fibers and intercellular ground substance. The gingival fibers are primarily collagen fibers (60 percent), but also include reticular fibers, oxytalan fibers, and elastic fibers, all arranged in fiber bundle groups that provide support for the marginal and interdental gingiva. The gingival fibers also provide support for the junctional epithelium reinforcing the attachment of the gingiva to the tooth (see Figure 1-2).

These five groups of gingival fibers also brace the gingiva firmly against the tooth and provide rigidity necessary for the gingiva to withstand mastication without being deflected away from the tooth surface (Bowen, 1994; Carranza & Perry, 1996). The circular or circumferential fibers encircle each tooth in a cuff within the marginal gingiva. The dentogingival fibers embed into the cementum apical to the junctional epithelium and fan out into the marginal and attached gingiva. These fibers coupled with the junctional epithelium comprise the dentogingival junction that attaches the gingiva to the tooth at the base of the sulcus. The dentoperiosteal fibers also are embedded into the same portion of the cementum, but extend apically over the alveolar crest and terminate in the alveolar bone after passing through the periosteum. The transeptal fibers embed in the same area of the cementum, but they run horizontally between the roots of adjacent teeth. The alveologingival fibers insert in the alveolar crest and splay out into the free gingiva. All of these connective tissue fibers serve as a unit to hold the gingiva firmly against the tooth and to attach the gingival tissue to the cementum. The intercellular ground substance, or matrix, of the connective tissue is a gel-like substance that surrounds connective tissue cells. It is essential for normal cell function and is composed of water, proteoglycans (mainly hyaluronic acid and chondroitin sulfate), and glycoproteins (mainly fibronectin). The predominant cell found in the gingival connective tissue is the fibroblast which synthesizes and secretes collagen fibers. Inflammatory infiltrate cells such as neutrophils, lymphocytes, and plasma cells also are found in small numbers in clinically normal gingiva. Although they are frequently found even in health, they are not a normal component of gingival tissue. As inflammation increases or persists in periodontal diseases, the number of these inflammatory cells in the gingival tissues and in the sulcus increases significantly as a result of the host response to bacterial and/or mechanical irritation.

## Periodontal Ligament

The periodontal ligament is a connective tissue structure that surrounds the root of the tooth and connects it with the alvelolar bone. It is continuous with the connective tissue fibers of the gingiva. Its collagen fibers embed into the cementum of the root on one side and into the alveolar bone on the other side. The terminal portions of these embedded fibers are known as Sharpey's fibers. The principal fibers of the periodontal ligament are arranged in bundles called principal fiber groups including oblique, alveolar crest, horizontal, apical, and interradicular fiber groups (see Figure 1-4). The oblique fiber group extends from the alveolar bone to the cementum in an oblique direction, allowing the tooth to bear masticatory stress in a vertical direction. It is the largest principal fiber group. The alveolar crest group extends from the cemetum, just apical to the junctional epithelium, obliquely to the alveolar crest. Horizontal fibers extend from cementum to bone at right angles to the long axis of the tooth. The apical group forms at the apex of the tooth after the root is completely formed. The final group, the interradicular fibers, extends from the alveolar bone to the cementum in the furcation areas of multirooted teeth.

The periodontal ligament is an integral part of the periodontium because it serves several important functions: physical, formative, nutritive, and sensory. Its physical function includes the aforementioned attachment of the tooth to the bone in the socket, and also the absorption of occlusal forces to protect the vessels, nerves, and bone from injury. The formative function includes the presence of cementoblasts, fibroblasts, and osteoblasts that are responsible for the continuous deposition of cementum, connective tissue, and alveolar bone. All structures of the periodontium, including the principle fibers, are constantly undergoing remodeling. The formative function of the periodontal ligament responds to physiologic tooth movement, occlusal forces, repair of injuries, and regeneration following periodontal therapy. The nutritive function of the periodontal ligament

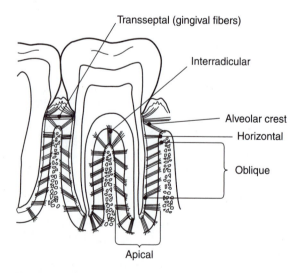

Transseptal (gingival fibers)

Interradicular

Alveolar crest

Horizontal

Oblique

Apical

**Figure 1-4** Principal fibers of the periodontal ligament. (Public Domain, National Audiovisual Center)

includes provision of nutrients to the bone and cementum via the blood vessels of the principal fiber groups. Similarly, its sensory function includes proprioceptive and tactile sensitivity to detect and localize external forces acting on each tooth. The periodontal ligament is supplied with nerve fibers capable of transmitting tactile, pressure, and pain sensations by the trigeminal nerve pathways (Carranza & Perry, 1996).

The thickness of the periodontal ligament varies from 0.05 to 0.25 mm depending on phases of eruption, age of the client, and function of the tooth. It is thicker in functioning teeth than in nonfunctioning teeth. Radiographic changes may occur in the size of the periodontal ligament space in relation to a tooth's function. It may appear wider when occlusal trauma is present and narrower when function is diminished or absent. The adjacent cementum may be unaltered or thickened by changes in tooth function.

## Cementum

Cementum is a calcified connective tissue covering the root of the tooth. Its main function is to connect the tooth to the periodontal ligament fibers. Cementum does not have its own blood vessels or nerves; it receives its nutrients from the periodontal ligament. It is similar to bone in structure except cementum has about 45 to 50 percent mineral content and bone has about 65 percent mineral content. Thickness of cementum varies. On the coronal half of the root it is thinner (16 to 60 microns or about .05 mm) and acellular. The apical half is thicker (up to 200 microns) and cellular. As teeth continuously erupt throughout life, cementum becomes thickest at the apex to compensate for the continuous eruption (Carranza & Ubios, 1996).

The relationship of the cementum to the enamel at the cementoenamel junction also varies. In 60 to 65 percent of the cases cementum will overlap enamel. In 30 percent of the cases cementum and enamel meet evenly at the junction, and in 5 to 10 percent of the cases, cementum and enamel do not meet. When gingival recession occurs, or during instrumentation, this latter group of teeth may have hypersensitivity due to the exposed dentin in the area of the cementoenamel junction.

The thickness of the cementum and its relationship to the enamel at the cementoenamel junction are of particular importance during root planing procedures. First, one must consider that cementum is only 16 to 60 microns thick in the coronal half of the root. If a clinician is overzealous in subgingival scaling and root planing, all of the cementum can be removed resulting in exposed dentin. This end result can also be caused by repeated root planing therapy over the course of many years. Caution should be taken to provide thorough debridement without excessive removal of tooth structure. Also, desensitization should be performed following therapy when recession is present and roots are exposed. The clinician also should consider the relationship of the cementum to

the enamel when performing periodontal instrumentation. In the majority of cases, when cementum overlaps the enamel, deposits can be removed with a few strokes to restore clinical smoothness in this area. However, if the cementum and enamel meet evenly, continuous vertical instrumentation strokes can cause ditching at the cementoenamel junction. Also, vigorous toothbrushing can cause abrasion in this area. Finally, if enamel and cementum do not join in this area, local anesthesia may be required for client comfort during root instrumentation.

## Alveolar Bone

The alveolar process is the part of the bone that supports the tooth in its socket (alveoli). It consists of two parts: the alveolar bone proper (cribiform plate) and the supporting alveolar bone (see Figure 1-3). The alveolar bone proper is the inner socket wall of compact bone that appears radiographically as the lamina dura. It contains the Sharpey's fibers from the periodontal ligament. The coronal rim of the alveolar bone proper is the alveolar crest which is normally located 1.5 to 2 mm apical to the cementoenamel junction. This 1.5 to 2 mm space is occupied by the junctional epithelium and connective tissue fibers of the gingiva that attach the gingiva to the root of the tooth. In health, the alveolar crest will run parallel between adjacent roots approximately 1.5 to 2 mm from each tooth's cementoenamel junction. This interdental septum consists of lamina dura and cancellous bone. The supporting bone has two parts: the cortical plate and the cancellous bone. The compact cortical plate covers the facial and lingual aspects of the alveolar bone. The cancellous, trabecular, or spongy bone is found between the cortical plates and the alveolar bone proper. Blood, lymph vessels, and nerves come from the periodontal ligament through the alveolar bone proper to provide nutrients and innervation to the cancellous bone.

The height and thickness of facial and lingual bone vary with tooth alignment, angulation of the root to the bone, and degree of occlusal forces (Carranza & Ubios, 1996). In teeth that are in labial version, the bone will be thinner and located more apically on the labial surface than on the lingual surface. In teeth that are in lingual version, the labial bone will be thicker than normal. These changes in contour often are reflected in the gingival tissues as well. Contour of the alveolar bone normally follows the contour of the cementoenamel junctions and the arrangement of the teeth. The shape of the alveolar crest generally parallels a line drawn between adjacent cementoenamel junctions (see Chapter 5). The cortical plate is thicker on the mandible than on the maxilla; therefore, it is easier to anesthetize the maxillary teeth by infiltration injections than it is on the mandible. The alveolar bone is thicker in the posterior regions than in the anterior regions, where the bone is thin with little or no cancellous bone between the cortical plates and the alveolar bone proper. Accordingly, radiographic appearance of bone will vary with interdental septa in the posterior regions being wider than in the anteriors, paralleling the adjacent cementoenamel junctions, and being covered by a dense white line. In the anterior area, trabecular bone may be little or nonexistent and alveolar crests will be thin and pointed. Clinicians should carefully evaluate the alveolar bone on radiographs (see Chapter 5), while being aware of the limitations of using radiographs alone, to detect periodontal disease.

The alveolar bone is the least stable of any of the periodontal tissues; it is in a constant state of change (Carranza & Ubios, 1996). In health, a sensitive physiologic balance is maintained between bone formation and resorption. This balance is easily affected, however, by local and systemic factors. Because the bone exists for the purpose of supporting the teeth during function, its preservation is dependent on stimulation from use. Osteoblasts and osteoclasts from the periodontal ligament remodel and redistribute bone to meet functional demands in response to occlusal forces.

In disease, local irritation from bacterial by-products can cause chronic inflammatory lesions that ultimately lead to bone resorption. The lesions constantly undergo processes of regeneration and repair; however, complete healing does not occur because of persistence of local irritants. These local irritants evoke a systemic response that, in turn, causes degeneration of new tissue elements formed. Prevention of progressive periodontal diseases and, failing that, treatment of periodontal diseases requires removal of local irritants so that the systemic response of the host will be able to regenerate tissue and repair the periodontal lesion. The goal is to attain a balance between local factors and the host response so that health can be maintained. An understanding of microbiology of bacterial plaque, risk factors associated with periodontal diseases, and the host response will provide essential background for the rationale for current nonsurgical periodontal therapy regimens.

## ETIOLOGY AND ASSOCIATED RISK FACTORS IN PERIODONTAL DISEASES

In common use, the term **periodontal disease** refers to a group of diseases that adversely affect the tissues of the periodontium. The majority of these diseases are inflammatory lesions caused by microorganisms that accumulate on the coronal tooth surface and subgingivally. In general, these diseases are classified as types of gingivitis when effects are confined to the gingiva and as periodontitis when destruction extends into the supporting structures of the teeth. While over 350 microbial species have been found in the oral cavity, less than 5 percent of these species have been identified as disease-producing periodontal pathogens. Periodontal infections appear to have some microbial specificity, and ongoing research continues to identify specific pathogens (AAP, 1992a; Wolff, Dahlen, Aeppli, 1994).

In periodontal diseases, microbial pathogens trigger inflammatory host responses which, along with direct irritation by the bacteria, cause most of the destruction (Genco, 1992). Although bacteria are essential etiologic agents, their presence alone is not sufficient to explain the periodontal disease process. The host must react to these bacterial irritants in order for disease to develop and progress. In any infection, the immune system localizes the invasion site and attempts to rapidly neutralize, destroy, or remove the bacterial agents. In chronic periodontal disease, the long-term presence of bacterial plaque causes a persistent and excessive host response. Rather than being protective, the host response contributes to the destruction. Successful periodontal therapy, therefore, not only depends upon altering the bacterial etiology, but also on consideration and evaluation of the host response to periodontal pathogens and to therapies targeted at their control. The goal of 100 percent plaque removal is unrealistic; however, when there is a balance between pathogens present and the host's ability to cope, health results. When plaque microbes or other local and systemic factors are sufficient to evoke a destructive host response, or when the host is compromised, periodontal disease can progress.

It also is now known that periodontal diseases are not infections to which everyone is equally susceptible. Current research is aimed at identifying sites, individuals and/or groups who are "at risk" more than others. Identification of specific risk factors will help clinicians target treatment efforts to those clients that are at risk for significant loss of attachment. Before discussing these risk factors and the host response in periodontal diseases, a review of historical and current perspectives of the microbiology of plaque will be presented.

## Historical Perspective of Bacterial Plaque

Background information regarding bacterial plaque as an etiologic factor in periodontal disease is helpful for understanding current knowledge as well as for evaluating the basis of present-day nonsurgical periodontal therapy modalities. Prior to the 1960s, the role of bacterial plaque in the initiation and progression of periodontal disease was not known. A causal relationship was first defined by Löe and others classic "Experimental Gingivitis in Man" study (Löe, Theilade, & Jensen, 1965). This landmark work demonstrated that gingivitis would result when plaque control was not performed, and that gingivitis would be reversed when plaque control was reinstituted. Based upon these findings, plaque became known as the primary etiologic factor in periodontal disease. At that time, a "nonspecific plaque hypothesis" emerged and progression of disease was associated with quantity of plaque present on the teeth. Little was known about bacterial species, and researchers observed changes in the morphology (shape) of plaque as it matured (e.g., predominant bacteria changed from cocci to rods to spirochetes). A single disease concept also was advanced in the 1960s. It was believed that periodontal disease evolved from health to gingivitis to periodontitis based upon the presence of bacterial plaque over an extended period of time. All individuals were considered to be equally susceptible to plaque and its effects on the periodontium; gingivitis was thought to always progress to periodontitis; so everyone received the same treatment (Kornman, 1986). Daily plaque control aimed at 100 percent plaque removal was considered essential for prevention of periodontal diseases in all clients. This theory was questioned because it was not upheld by clinical observations. For example, some clients with moderate plaque had little disease.

In the next decade, periodontal researchers built upon the knowledge gained in the late 1960s and further defined the nature of bacterial plaque and its relationship to periodontal diseases. Scientific technology also was improved and various bacterial species were identified within each group of morphotypes. The ability to culture bacteria allowed researchers to differentiate between certain types of organisms that could be associated with health and disease (Slots, 1977, 1979). This breakthrough led to the development of the "specific plaque hypothesis" that suggested that bacterial species found in healthy mouths differ from those found in cases of gingivitis and periodontitis. Quality of plaque became more important than quantity. That is, the specific types of bacteria and their pathogenic potential was determined to be more important than the amount of plaque present. The concept evolved that not all plaque is associated with disease. Researchers also began to study by-products of pathogenic plaque bacteria and their significance in periodontal disease. A lipopolysaccharide derived from gram negative bacterial cell walls and released upon cell death was found to be present on the roots of periodontally involved teeth (Hatfield & Baumhammers, 1971). Lipopolysaccharide (LPS) was recently renamed lipo-oligosaccharide (LOS); however, it is commonly referred to as endotoxin (Newman, Sanz, Nisengard, & Haake, 1996). This endotoxin was determined to be toxic to the cells of periodontal tissues, and its removal showed beneficial effects on healing (Aleo, DeRenzis, Farber, & Varboncoeur, 1974). Subsequent studies regarding scaling and root planing were conducted to evaluate the effects of endotoxin removal on the success of periodontal therapy. It was demonstrated that root planing and the use of ultrasonic devices decreased the amount of endotoxin found on periodontally-involved root surfaces (Jones & O'Leary, 1978). Consequently, nonsurgical periodontal therapy was directed at removing contaminated cementum to create a biologically acceptable root surface (Nishimine & O'Leary, 1979). In the latter part of the 1970s, researchers also identified differences between adherent (attached) plaque and loosely adherent (unattached) plaque as potential causative factors in periodontal disease (Fine, Tabak, Oshrain, Salkind, & Siegel, 1978a, 1978b). It was suggested that, although adherent plaque was present in greater quantities than loosely adherent plaque, the pathogenic potential of the loosely adherent plaque might be greater. These findings from the 1970s fostered efforts to further examine the complex interactions between specific periodontal pathogens and the resultant host response to further clarify their relationships.

In the 1980s, periodontal researchers continued to study the "specific plaque hypothesis" and periodontal diseases were reclassified to reflect several bacteriologically and immunologically distinct forms of periodontal disease. The focus of these efforts was to link specific bacterial species with various periodontal diseases: gingivitis, adult periodontitis, early-onset periodontitis, and refractory periodontitis. A closer examination of the destructive pathways of periodontal disease also focused research efforts on the significance of the host response in its initiation and progression. These results culminated in the theory that the presence of pathogens alone is not enough to produce disease. The host must be susceptible to the pathogens or disease will not result. Further research on the significance of endotoxin in periodontal disease during the 1980s indicates that endotoxin does evoke an inflammatory host response; however, it is routinely found on roots of teeth affected by periodontitis. Furthermore, after scaling and root planing, retoxification may occur. It also has been demonstrated that this lipopolysaccharide is weakly adherent and can be brushed away (Nakib, Bissada, Simmelink, & Golstine, 1982). Since endotoxin does not penetrate the cementum, excessive cementum removal to provide a glassy smooth root surface free of endotoxin appears to be unnecessary (Greenstein, 1992; Hughes, 1992; Miller, 1995).

Another important focus of periodontal research in the 1980s was with regard to similarities and differences in supragingival and subgingival plaque. It is now known that, in health and gingivitis, the growth, accumulation, and pathogenicity of subgingival plaque is strongly influenced by the presence of supragingival plaque. Inflammation of the gingiva caused by supragingival plaque results in an altered relationship between the gingival margin and the tooth. This change in the environment allows subgingival bacteria to colonize into bacterial plaque on the root surface, or adjacent to the epithelial tissue in the sulcus (Beltrami, Bickel, & Baehni, 1987; Corbet & Davies, 1993; Kornman, 1986). Anaerobic bacteria and other periodontal pathogens become organized subgingivally in adherent and loosely adherent plaque. These microbes produce toxins, enzymes, and metabolic products that cause direct injury to the periodontium, but more importantly, invoke an immune response that results in indirect toxicity. Subgingival bacteria act as antigens, and as the host responds to the irritant present, some destruction of the periodontal tissues occurs by a variety of immunopathologic reactions. Thus, elimination of supragingival plaque is critical to the prevention of periodontal diseases. Both supragingival and subgingival plaque control, however, are critical to successful periodontal therapy. If either is practiced independently, the outcome will be less beneficial than if both are practiced together. Because most patients with periodontal disease cannot achieve perfect control of plaque, particularly subgingivally, self-care without scaling and/or root planing results in less than desirable results (Caton et al., 1989; Cercek et al., 1983; Consensus Report, 1989; Smulow, Turesky, & Hill, 1983; Kho, Smales, & Hardie, 1985). The data from these trials indicate that supragingival control of plaque can reduce inflammation in gingivitis, but oral self-care alone is limited in altering parameters associated with periodontitis (e.g., probing depths and attachment levels). Professional subgingival mechanical instrumentation is needed to augment personal oral hygiene to achieve and maintain periodontal health (Greenstein, 1992). Patients with an inadequate immune response also have increased disease. They require more aggressive and frequent professional care and possibly microbiologic monitoring (see Chapter 3) and/or adjunctive antibiotic therapy (see Chapter 14, Systemic Antibiotics) to maintain health.

This knowledge from the 1980s supported the importance of routine performance of professional mechanical plaque control (i.e., oral prophylaxis, subgingival debridement and/or maintenance therapy) in conjunction with personal plaque control to prevent and treat periodontal diseases. Recommended approaches were expanded beyond daily mechanical plaque control by the client, to include professional preventive and periodontal care, use of chemotherapeutic agents, and frequent maintenance therapy. Advances also were made in improving periodontal assessment techniques. The present-day concept of bacterial plaque and its causal relationship to various forms of periodontal disease is quite complex. As a result, clinical approaches to nonsurgical periodontal therapy are expanding and oral self-care interventions are being continually improved.

## Current Perspective on the Role of Bacterial Plaque in Destructive Periodontal Diseases

Research efforts in the 1990s are being conducted to better understand the etiology of periodontal diseases and the relationship between bacterial plaque and host responses in the initiation and progression of various diseases. Socransky and Haffajee (1992) have identified several factors that must be present in order for periodontal disease to result from a pathogen. First, the periodontal pathogen must be present in a virulent form because there might be multiple (clonal) types of a periodontal pathogen and all of them may not be capable of producing disease. Second, because periodontal diseases are mixed infections, the right combination of bacteria must also be present in sufficient numbers to produce disease. Simple identification of a known pathogen will not predict disease activity or future attachment loss. The presence of beneficial or good bacteria may modify the effects of known pathogens, thereby reducing the likelihood of disease progression. These theories might explain why some "pathogens" are found in healthy sites

or subjects. Third, the host must be susceptible to the pathogen and the pathogens must be present in sufficient numbers to exceed the threshold of the host. A recent explosion of knowledge related to immunobiology has advanced understanding of the reactions between pathogenic microorganisms and the immune response of the host (Genco, 1992). Finally, the pathogen must be located in the right place and the local environment of the site must be one that is conducive to the virulence of the pathogens present. For example, as periodontal pockets become deeper, the environment fosters the disease-producing potential of periodontal pathogens.

In short, it is now known that presence of a specific periodontal pathogen does not necessarily mean instantaneous disease. The host is continuously impacted by various immunological states and by various risk factors associated with periodontal diseases. These risk factors can alter the balance between local factors and the host, resulting in an imbalance that allows for disease progression (Christersson et al., 1991). Socransky and Haffajee (1992) have defined concepts that interact to determine whether active periodontal disease will occur (see Figure 1-5).

## Risk Factors in Periodontal Diseases

Periodontal diseases are no longer regarded as infections to which everyone is equally susceptible. Because some clients are more "at risk" than others for destructive periodontal diseases, current research is rapidly identifying and determining the relative importance of these risk indicators. This trend has been followed in medicine, as well, in the past decade. For example, computer programs are available to analyze a variety of risk factors (family history, body weight, stress, diet, smoking, etc.) to predict an individual's risk for heart disease. Dental researchers are actively investigating such risk factors for periodontal diseases. Identification of these "at risk" clients or groups would help target treatment efforts to those in greatest need and to avoid overtreating persons who are not at risk. In practice, clinicians frequently observe that some clients have generalized plaque and calculus and little disease, while others have apparently good self-care with more rapidly advancing disease. To determine the need for more frequent professional periodontal therapy, it is important to be able to identify which individuals are at greatest risk for advancing attachment loss (Ramfjord, 1993).

Interest in identifying various risk indicators for periodontal disease stems from landmark longitudinal studies of the natural history of periodontal disease by Löe and coworkers (1978a, 1978b, 1978c, 1986, & 1992) in both Sri Lanka and Norway. This twenty-year study examined the course of periodontal disease in two cohorts: Sri Lankan teaworkers who were generally healthy, but had never received any dental care or been exposed to any preventive oral health education or treatment, and a group of students and academicians from

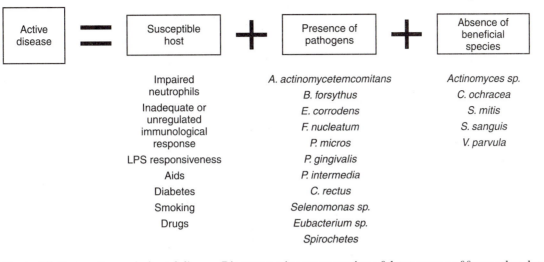

**Figure 1-5** Destructive periodontal disease. Diagrammatic representation of three groups of factors that determine whether active periodontal disease will occur in a subject or at a site. (Courtesy of S.S. Socransky & A.D. Haffajee, The bacterial etiology of destructive periodontal disease: Current concepts. *Journal of Periodontology,* American Academy of Periodontology, 1992)

Oslo, Norway, who had preschool, school, and postschool dental care (including preventive, restorative, and specialty services) on an annual basis. The Sri Lankan group had not only never received dental care, but toothbrushing was unknown to them. Monitoring periodontal disease progression in this group allowed researchers to avoid ethical dilemmas of withdrawing oral hygiene and professional care to examine disease progression over a twenty-year period. The findings of these studies showed that plaque, calculus, and gingivitis are common conditions in both Sri Lanka and Norway. These conditions lead to a slow loss of periodontal attachment with increasing age with approximately 0.1 mm of loss per year in Norway and 0.3 mm per year in Sri Lanka (see review, Ramfjord, 1993). In the Sri Lankan subgroup, which had received no periodontal therapy, the following disease progression patterns were identified: no progression beyond gingivitis (no attachment loss) in 11 percent of the cases, moderate progression (4 mm of attachment loss) in 81 percent of the cases, and rapid progression (9 mm of attachment loss) in 8 percent of the cases, at 35 years of age. It is interesting to note that no differences were found in oral hygiene or gingival inflammation between any of these three groups (Löe et al., 1986). Other risk factors must play a role in the progression of destructive periodontal diseases. In the Norwegian subgroup, which had high levels of professional and personal periodontal care, no rapid loss of attachment was observed. Only a very slowly progressing loss of periodontal attachment occurred with age. At 30 years of age the mean loss of attachment was less than 1 mm, and at 40 years of age the mean was slightly above 1.5 mm. In Sri Lankans, the mean loss of attachment at age 30 was 3.11 mm; and it increased to 4.50 mm by age 40. These results suggest that without interference of professional care and oral hygiene the periodontal

lesion will progress at a more rapid rate (Löe, Anerud, Boysen, & Smith, 1978c). Perhaps, even more importantly, the findings from the Sri Lankan subgroup identified that 10 percent of those individuals showed essentially no progress of periodontal disease beyond gingivitis between 14 and 46 years of age, despite the presence of plaque and calculus and absence of professional care. Research continues to identify those factors which affect the host and place an individual at risk for advancing periodontal destruction (Beck, 1994; Grossi et al., 1994; Grossi et al., 1995; Newman, Kornman, & Holtzman, 1994).

**Dentally-Related Risk Factors.** Perhaps the most significant dentally-related risk factor is the presence of established periodontal disease. Sites previously affected by periodontitis are at the greatest risk for future loss of attachment (Chrissterson et al., 1991; Grbic & Lamster, 1992; Grbic, Lamster, Celenti, & Fine, 1991). More frequent professional care has been shown to reduce risk; therefore, clients previously treated for periodontitis would require more frequent PMP at a maximum of three months for satisfactory maintenance of attachment levels (Axelsson, Lindhe, & Nystrom, 1991; Kaldahl, Kalkwarf, Patil, Dyer, Bates, 1988; Lindhe, Westfelt, Nyman, Socransky, & Haffajee, 1984; Pihlstrom, McHugh, & Oliphant, 1984; Ramjford et al., 1987). Missing teeth, mouthbreathing, mobile teeth, areas of food impaction and poor oral hygiene also have been shown to increase the risk of progressive periodontal disease. Of these factors, loss of attachment (2 mm or greater) which has already occurred is by far the most important and can be diagnosed only by regular professional examination at least once a year (Beck, Koch, Zambon, Genco, & Tudor, 1992; Ramfjord, 1993).

**Unchanging Subject-Related Risk Factors.** These risk indicators include genetics, gender, and race. A genetic predisposition to various forms of periodontal disease has been related to inherited systemic diseases, as well as to familial occurrence of specific periodontal diseases. Juvenile periodontitis seems to be genetically-related; thus, screening of relatives should always be undertaken when a case is diagnosed (Johnson, 1989). Genetic linkage to other forms of periodontal diseases may be related to immune responsiveness. A University of Minnesota study examined periodontal findings in twins who were reared together or apart. This study identified a significant genetic component for probing depth, attachment loss, and plaque that could not be explained by differences in family environment such as oral hygiene practices and frequency of dental visits (Michalowicz et al., 1991). Inherited or familial systemic diseases that result in defective tissue integrity and host defenses and that predispose to periodontal breakdown include: Papillon-Lefévre syndrome, Chediak-Higasi syndrome, Down syndrome, familial or cyclic neutropenia, and leukocyte adhesion deficiency (Johnson, 1989; Slots & Rams, 1991).

There is a commonly held misconception that females are more susceptible to periodontal diseases. Data from the National Institute of Dental Research Survey of Oral Health of Adults in the United States (Miller et al., 1987) dispels this myth. This study documents that males have greater incidence and severity of periodontal diseases, including both gingivitis and periodontitis. No firm evidence documents that race is a significant risk factor in destructive forms of periodontitis; other than as it may be related genetically (Johnson, 1989). In fact, when numerous risk factors are combined and weighted statistically, race is shown to be insignificant despite its significance as a single risk factor (Beck et al., 1992). Perhaps other environmentally related risk factors explain differences previously associated with race.

**Changing Subject-Related Risk Factors.** These risk factors include tobacco use, chronic alcoholism, age, stress, diet and nutrition, drugs (recreation and prescription), and systemic diseases affecting the immune system. Accumulating evidence indicates that both current and former smokers are at increased risk for periodontitis and that smoking is a major risk factor in destructive periodontal diseases (Bergstrom & Preber, 1994; Ismail, Morrison, Burt, Caffesse, & Kavanaugh, 1990; Preber & Bergstrom, 1990; Preber, Bergstrom, & Linder, 1992). Tobacco smoking may be the most important environmental factor associated with periodontal diseases in the United States and Europe (Haber & Kent, 1992). Smoking not only increases periodontal disease severity but loss of attachment increases with greater consumption (Martinez-Canut, Lorca, & Magan, 1995). Healing following nonsurgical periodontal therapy also is impaired in smokers (Preber, Linder, & Bergstrom, 1995). Effects seem to be related not only to the local effects in the oral cavity (heat, dryness, and increased

plaque and calculus), but also to a suppression of the immune system altering the host response to periodontal pathogens (McLaughlin, Lovat, MacGregor, & Kelly, 1993). Chronic alcoholism also is a risk factor for many chronic diseases because it affects the cardiovascular system, the nervous system, and the liver. An increased risk for periodontitis is suspected because of increased bleeding tendencies, poor oral hygiene due to overall neglect, and malnutrition that can accompany chronic alcoholism (Darby & Walsh, 1994).

While it is well-known that severity of periodontal destruction increases with age, it may only be that these increases are related to the cumulative effects of past breakdown (Gilbert & Heft, 1993; Grossi et al., 1994; Grossi et al., 1995; Miller et al., 1987). Data exist to document that the effect of age on the progression of periodontitis is minimal when good oral hygiene is maintained throughout life (Abdellatif & Burt, 1987; Christersson et al., 1991). Environmental factors affecting the aging population such as changes in diet and nutrition, frequency of prescribed medications, and increases in systemic diseases may also play a role.

Psychosocial factors also can influence immune functions. Although this relationship has not been shown to be causal, a linkage has been established between periodontal diseases and stress. Occurrence of necrotizing ulcerative gingivitis has long been associated with stress (Löesche, 1994; Shannon, Kilgore, & Leary, 1969). More recently, stressful life events such as divorce, joblessness, and lifestyle factors linked with stress have been correlated with advancing periodontal destruction (Clarke & Hirsh, 1995; Monteiro da Silva, Newman, & Oakley, 1995; Green et al., 1986). Stress variables also have been shown to be predictive of oral surgery complications based on self-reported and biological stress markers, indicating an effect on healing (Logan, Koorbusch, Hartwig, & Quinn, 1992).

The importance of diet and nutrition in maintaining tissue integrity and defense mechanisms is part of the dogma of the health sciences (Johnson, 1989). No direct linkages have been established between nutritional deficiencies and periodontal disease (apart from severe scurvy). Nonetheless, the relationship of nutrition to disease susceptibility in general cannot be ignored.

Prescription drugs also can affect the periodontium by causing gingival overgrowth. The most commonly cited medications include phenytoin, nifedipine, and cyclosporine. These drugs can cause a noninflammatory hyperplasia and/or result in gingival overgrowth that contributes to plaque accumulation and inflammation. They have little effect, however, on the alveolar bone or loss of attachment (Johnson, 1989; O'Valle et al., 1995). Immunosuppressive drugs such as steroids (prednisone) may also have an effect on host response such as a suppression of macrophage and leukocyte migration, inhibited phagocytosis and reduced capillary permeability (Gage & Pickett, 1994).

A discussion of systemic diseases associated with periodontal disease is presented in Chapter 2. Acquired defects in the immune system can exacerbate periodontal breakdown and/or affect healing following therapy. These diseases include: human immunodeficiency virus (HIV), leukemia (and associated myelosuppressive drugs), blood dyscrasias, diabetes mellitus (type 1 and 2), Crohn's disease, and sarcoidosis (Slots & Rams, 1991).

**Assessing Risk Factors and Predicting Periodontal Disease Progression.** At present, there is no exact formula for assessing risk factors and predicting periodontal disease progression. Research findings to date, however, do indicate that although bacterial plaque is the primary etiologic factor in periodontal disease, it is by no means the only factor. Studies of the natural history of periodontal disease indicate that other factors play an important role. Clinicians can use this information in practice by completing thorough health history reviews (see Chapter 2), considering oral habits, and correlating known risk factors with periodontal assessment findings (see Chapter 3). Treatment approaches can be individualized based upon this information. Those clients who are at high risk could be made aware of the impact of these factors and encouraged to seek more regular preventive and/or periodontal care. Self-care regimens can be expanded to include topical antimicrobials, oral irrigation, and/or antibiotics (see Chapter 14). Also, in failed cases of treatment, a reevaluation of associated risk factors and attention to addressing these concerns might lead to future success. Evaluation of local microbial factors, dentally-related risk factors, subject-related risk indicators, and signs and symptoms of disease will result in an accurate diagnosis and a logical course of therapy.

## DISEASES OF THE PERIODONTIUM

The diagnosis and classification of periodontal diseases is currently based on clinical assessments. To arrive at a diagnosis, the clinician depends upon the following factors: presence or absence of gingival inflammation, extent and pattern of alveolar bone loss, age of the client at the time of disease onset, rate of disease progression, and presence or absence of other signs and symptoms including pain, ulceration, and amount of plaque and calculus deposits present (AAP, 1992b; Armitage, 1987). Periodontal disease is not a single pathologic entity; it refers to a group of diseases that affect the tissues of the periodontium. The American Academy of Periodontology (1992a) recently presented a position paper modifying the general classification of periodontal diseases as represented in Table 1-1. This classification system focuses on types of disease based upon etiology and pathogenesis. It should not be confused with other classifications of periodontal diseases identified for purposes of insurance payments. Current insurance classifications include: Gingivitis (AAP Case Type I), Early Periodontitis (AAP Case Type II), Moderate Periodontitis (AAP Case Type III), Advanced Periodontitis (AAP

Case Type IV), and Refractory Periodontitis (AAP Case Type V). These are discussed further in Chapter 5.

## Gingivitis

The primary etiologic agent in gingivitis is bacterial plaque. As mentioned previously, early studies of plaque and gingivitis demonstrated that the inflammatory gingival lesion will not occur without plaque, develops after plaque is allowed to accumulate, and reverses itself when bacterial plaque is removed (Löe et al., 1965). Inflammation results not only from increases in quantity of plaque, but also due to qualitative changes in plaque microbes. There is a strong positive correlation between levels of oral cleanliness and both presence and severity of gingivitis (AAP, 1992a).

**Chronic Gingivitis.** Chronic gingivitis is the most common form of all periodontal diseases (Caton, 1989). It is characterized by redness, gingival bleeding, changes in contour, edema, enlargement, loss of tissue tone, and increase in gingival crevicular fluid (Carranza, 1996a; Greenstein, 1984; Suzuki, 1988). Inflammation and tissue destruction is confined to the gingiva without involvement of the deeper supporting structures. Therefore, no radiographic changes are detected in the periodontium in gingivitis. A gingival pocket, or pseudopocket, may occur due to changes in the junctional epithelium and enlargement of the marginal gingiva; however, the lesion has not extended into the alveolar bone. Gingivitis can persist for a long time without progressing into supporting tissues, depending on the presence of local factors and the host response. Gingival sensitivity may be present, although gingivitis is frequently asymptomatic. Plaque is the primary etiologic factor, so treatment involves control of plaque and correction or removal of any factors that favor its accumulation.

**Necrotizing Ulcerative Gingivitis.** Necrotizing ulcerative gingivitis is also known as NUG, acute necrotizing ulcerative gingivitis (ANUG), or Vincent's Infection. It is characterized by craterlike depressions at the crest of the interdental papilla, severe inflammation usually confined to the marginal gingiva, gingival bleeding, necrosis and ulceration of the interdental papilla, acute pain, and an apparent sudden onset with periods of remission and exacerbation. Other possible conditions that may or may not be present include: a grey or yellow pseudomembrane, fever, malaise, lymphadenopathy, and increased salivation. Foul breath (fetid odor) is a frequent manifestation. The median prevalence is estimated at 2 percent of the population (AAP, 1992a; Melnick, Roseman, Engel, & Cogen, 1988). NUG is believed to be related to poor oral hygiene and a systemically compromised host; however, the primary etiologic factor is unknown. Risk factors include stress, poor diet, and smoking. It also has been associated with impaired host defenses or immunosuppressive diseases. Treatment

**Table 1-1  Classification of Periodontal Disease and Predominant Microorganisms**

| Classification | Common Forms | Microorganisms |
|---|---|---|
| Gingivitis | Chronic gingivitis | *Actinomyces* (species)<br>*Fusobacterium nucleatum*<br>*Veillonella parvula*<br>*Prevotella intermedia*<br>*Treponema* (species) |
| | Necrotizing ulcerative gingivitis | *Spirochetes*<br>*Prevotella intermedia*<br>*Fusobacterium* (species) |
| | Gingivitis associated with systemic diseases<br>• Linear gingival erythema | • *Candida albicans*<br>  *Actinobacillus actinomycetemcomitans*<br>  *Fusobacterium nucleatum*<br>  *Camphylobacteria recta* |
| | • Scorbutic gingivitis<br>• Gingivitis associated with hormonal changes<br>• Gingival enlargement | • No change in composition of microflora<br>• *Prevotella intermedia*<br><br>• Increases in gingivitis-associated microorganisms increase the rate of overgrowth |
| Periodontitis | Adult periodontitis<br>• Early<br>• Moderate<br>• Advanced | *Actinobacillus actinomycetemcomitans*<br>*Porphoromonas gingivalis*<br>  *Prevotella intermedia*<br>  *Bacteriodes forsythus*<br>*Eikenella corrodens*<br>*Fusobacterium nucleatum*<br>*Camphylobacteria rectus*<br>*Treponema* (species) |
| | Early-onset periodontitis<br>• Prepubertal periodontitis | • *Prevotella intermedia*<br>  *Actinobacillus actinomycetemcomitans*<br>  *Eikenella corrodens*<br>  *Caphocytophaga sputigena* |
| | • Juvenile periodontitis (localized/generalized) or rapidly progressive periodontitis | • *Actinobacillus actinomycetemcomitans*<br>  *Prevotella* (species) |
| | Refractory periodontitis | Three microbial complexes identified:<br>• *Bacteriodes forsythus, Fusobacterium nucleatum, Camphylobacteria rectus*<br>• *Streptococcus intermedius, Porphoromonas gingivalis, Peptostreptococcus micros*<br>• *Streptococcus intermedius, Fusobacterium nucleatum* with and without *Porphoromonas gingivalis* |
| | Periodontitis associated with systemic diseases<br>• Periodontitis related with systemic disturbances<br>• Necrotizing ulcerative periodontitis | • Periodontitis associated pathogens<br><br>• Same as linear gingival erythema only or *Camphylobacteria recta* increases significantly |

includes removal of plaque, calculus, and pseudomembrane (if one is present) with adequate pain control. Antibiotics can be prescribed if systemic symptoms are present (fever, lymphadenopathy). This gingivitis tends to be recurrent and multiple episodes can lead to destruction of deeper supporting structures, a condition called necrotizing ulcerative gingivo-periodontitis (AAP, 1992a).

NUG is most commonly found in anterior teeth. It responds readily to local treatment. Necrotizing gingivitis in HIV-positive clients differs from NUG. It occurs, commonly with sloughing and necrosis, at any proximal site and it results in bone loss that is immediate if left untreated. Repeated infections are not necessary for alveolar bone involvement, as is the case with NUG. Treatment includes thorough local debridement including removal of necrotic tissue and twice daily antimicrobial (chlorhexidine) rinses. If improvement is not seen, antibiotics such as metronidazole should be prescribed. A client diagnosed with NUG should be suspected for possible HIV infection. Should routine treatment be unsuccessful or other symptoms are present, the client should be further tested for possible HIV-infection or another immunocompromising disease (Persson, 1993).

**Gingivitis Associated with Systemic Diseases.** A higher prevalence of gingivitis has been found in clients with systemic diseases that affect the host response and/or immunosuppressive conditions. The American Academy of Periodontology (1992a) identifies these diseases as: "acute leukemia, Addison's disease, diabetes, hemophilia, thrombocytopenia, Sturge-Weber syndrome, Wegener's granulomatosis, and combined immunodeficiency diseases." (see Chapter 2). These gingival diseases generally have characteristics like severe marginal erythema, necrosis, bleeding, and/or enlargement.

Linear gingival erythema, previously called HIV-associated gingivitis (HIV-G) is characterized by a distinct band of severe erythema (redness and inflammation) along the marginal gingiva. The attached gingiva may also be involved with a diffuse or punctuated erythema. There is no ulceration or loss of attachment, and it is usually generalized. HIV-G recently was renamed linear gingival erythema (LGE) as a result of recent worldwide meetings involving such groups as the World Health Organization Center on Oral Manifestations of Immunodeficiency Virus (Grbic et al., 1995; Persson, 1993). The diagnosis of LGE indicates HIV seropositive conversion, cyclic neutropenia, or other immunocompromised states. Treatment includes supragingival debridement in conjunction with antifungal agents because candidiasis commonly occurs with LGE (Grbic et al., 1995).

Scorbutic gingivitis is a classic feature of gingivitis associated with severe ascorbic acid deficiencies in patients with scurvy. It is uncommon in industrialized populations. Vitamin C deficiencies have not been otherwise associated with periodontal diseases (AAP 1992a).

Gingivitis associated with hormonal changes is seen primarily in pregnancy, but may also be associated with hormonal changes due to puberty, menstruation, steroid therapy, or birth control medication. It is characterized by gingival inflammation and/or enlargement, redness, edema, and bleeding that may be localized or generalized. Hormone-influenced gingivitis results from an exaggerated response to bacterial plaque. It may be related to the effect of elevated steroid levels on the gingival microvasculature and the subgingival microflora (AAP, 1992a; Kornman & Löesche, 1980; Lapp, Thomas, & Lewis, 1995).

Gingival enlargement or overgrowth is most frequently attributed to the effects of certain drugs leading to increased production of connective tissue matrix by fibroblasts. Many drugs can cause gingival overgrowth, or hyperplasia, but the three most commonly sited medications include phenytoin, cyclosporin, nifedipine (and other calcium channel blockers). The drug initially causes the enlargement, but the changes in size and contour lead to increased plaque accumulation in the affected area. This situation results in a combined enlargement as inflammation increases. The essential link between bacterial plaque and drug-induced gingival overgrowth is not clear; however, it is believed that poor oral hygiene will exaggerate the response (AAP, 1992a).

## Periodontitis

The characteristic feature of periodontitis is a loss of the connective tissue and alveolar structures, termed a loss of attachment. Gingival inflammation is a common concurrent feature. This loss of attachment will be evidenced by an apical migration of the junctional epithelium, which can result in a periodontal pocket (and/or gingival recession) that coincides with that apical migration. Gingivitis is usually a precursor to periodontitis, but not all gingivitis progresses to periodontitis. Periodontitis results from a host response to microbial plaque; however, mechanisms for its initiation and progression are still being studied.

Three models have been proposed to explain the progression of periodontitis. The term **periodontal disease activity** refers to the stage(s) of the disease characterized by loss of periodontal attachment. It implies that the natural history of periodontal disease has periods of active destruction and periods of relative inactivity, although chronic inflammation persists (Bowen, 1994). Caton (1989) summarizes the three theories of periodontal disease activity as: 1) the continuous paradigm that implies a slow, constant progression of periodontal degeneration; 2) the random burst theory that implies that short periods of destruction are followed by periods of no destruction, occurring randomly; and 3) the asynchronous multiple burst theory that implies that periodontal disease activity, and resultant destruction, occurs within a specific period of life and is followed by remission. Löe and coworkers (1986) assert that the rate of progress varies in different sites, at different ages, and between individuals and groups. The periodontitis lesion progresses steadily over time, even though there may be periods of slow progress and destructive processes. The fact remains, however, that in the absence of treatment or interference, the lesion will continue until the entire periodontium is involved and tooth loss results. Löe and coworkers (1986) emphasize that a steady, continuous progression does not rule out periods of exacerbation.

There are four major forms of periodontitis: adult, early-onset, refractory, and periodontitis associated with systemic diseases. Each of these major forms has subclassifications. Diagnosis is made on the basis of the clinical parameters documented in a thorough periodontal assessment, as well as consideration of the age of onset, rapidity of progression, and extent/pattern of alveolar bone loss.

**Adult Periodontitis.** Chronic adult periodontitis, or slowly progressive periodontitis, is usually not clinically evident until the mid-thirties; however actual onset may occur earlier in life (Caton, 1989; Suzuki, 1988). Progression of the disease is usually slow and the host response is generally normal. It is the most common form of periodontitis characterized by periodontal pockets, bone loss, and eventual tooth mobility. Clinical inflammation, recession and/or fibrosis may be present. The pattern of bone loss is generally bilateral with the interdental bone affected more severely than the buccal and lingual bone. Radiographically, evidence of bone loss can be detected as triangulation, loss of crestal bone, interproximal craters, horizontal or vertical defects and/or loss of interradicular bone (furcation involvement). Prevalence increases with age as a cumulative effect of disease progression. Adult periodontitis is commonly subclassified as early, moderate, or advanced depending on the degree of severity of bone loss.

Early adult periodontitis involves the alveolar bone crest, with slight bone loss and slight loss of connective tissue attachment. With normal gingival contour or inflammation, the usual probing depth is 3 to 4 mm, and average clinical attachment loss is 2 to 3 mm. Moderate adult periodontitis is a more advanced state of the disease, with increased destruction of the alveolar bone and usual probing depths of 5 to 7 mm when gingival contour is normal or inflammation is present. Probing depths would be less if recession had occurred. An average of 4 to 6 mm of clinical attachment loss would exist regardless of the position of the gingival margin because it is measured from the cementoenamel junction. Moderate adult periodontitis is sometimes accompanied by tooth mobility and partial furcation involvement in multirooted teeth. Advanced adult periodontitis is a further progression of the disease, with major loss of bone support, usual probing depths of 8 mm or greater, and an average of 6 mm or more clinical attachment loss (approximately one-half of the root length). Advanced periodontitis is often accompanied by increased tooth mobility, and likely furcation involvements. Treatment of adult periodontitis includes nonsurgical and/or surgical periodontal therapy depending on severity, followed by regular maintenance therapy.

**Early-Onset Periodontitis.** Forms of early-onset periodontitis include prepubertal periodontitis, juvenile periodontitis (localized or generalized), and rapidly progressive periodontitis. These aggressive forms of periodontitis have all been associated with rapid progression and abnormalities in neutrophil function, and the age of onset is younger than it is for adult periodontitis.

Prepubertal periodontitis is a rare periodontal disease that can be localized or generalized. It affects the primary or mixed dentition, and begins soon after eruption of the primary teeth. It is characterized by severe gingival inflammation, rapid loss of alveolar bone, mobility, and tooth loss. Prepubertal periodontitis has been associated with leukocyte defects. Treatment is experimental and cases should be referred to a specialist.

Juvenile periodontitis is a disease that affects the permanent dentition in otherwise healthy adolescents. It occurs around puberty and females are affected more than males. The disease may have a genetic basis and has a familial distribution. (Michalowicz, 1994). Characteristic features include severe, rapid bone loss that begins in the first molars and incisors; little gingival inflammation; and sparse plaque and calculus deposits that are incongruent with degree of destruction. Depressed neutrophil chemotaxis also has been shown in a majority of cases. The rate of attachment loss is three to five times faster than adult periodontitis (Caton, 1989). The localized form is confined to the first molars and/or incisors and the generalized form can affect the entire dentition. Defects are usually angular and bilaterally symmetrical (Suzuki, 1988). Treatment is similar to recommended therapy for adult periodontitis, except systemic antibiotics (tetracycline or metronidazole in combination with Amoxicillin) should be prescribed in conjunction with local therapy because pathogens seem to be more tissue invasive (Aa) (Artzi & Moses, 1995; Ciancio, 1989). Diligent and frequent maintenance therapy also is important. Use of diagnostic bacteriologic tests might be warranted to monitor endpoints of therapy.

Rapidly progressive periodontitis is similar to generalized juvenile periodontitis, and some authors believe it is a related disease (AAP, 1992c; Page et al., 1983). It shares many of the same features including age of onset (young adult), rapid loss of bone and neutrophil defects (AAP, 1992a, 1992c). Therefore, treatment recommendations are the same as for localized juvenile periodontitis.

**Refractory Periodontitis.** Refractory periodontitis, another aggressive form of periodontitis, occurs in multiple sites in patients who continue to demonstrate loss of attachment despite apparently appropriate treatment. These sites continue to be infected by periodontal pathogens even though home self-care seems adequate. Advancing bone destruction and tooth loss occur even with aggressive therapy. Treatment includes nonsurgical and/or surgical periodontal therapy with adjunctive use of antibiotics (Magnusson et al., 1994). Tetracycline, metronidazole, Clindamycin, Augmentin, and a combination of metronidazole and Amoxicillin have been shown to be effective (Gordon et al., 1985; Kornman & Karl, 1982; Slots, Mashimo, Levine, & Genco, 1979; Van Ness, Walker, Clark, & Magnusson, 1988; van Winkelhoff et al., 1989).

**Periodontitis Associated with Systemic Diseases.** Most of the early-onset and rapidly progressive forms of periodontitis are associated with systemic diseases, with the exception of localized juvenile periodontitis (LJP). Even LJP, however, has been associated with a neutrophil chemotaxis deficiency. Severe periodontitis has been observed in blood dyscrasias and in primary neutrophil disorders. Acquired immunodeficiency diseases also have been associated with rapidly advancing forms of periodontitis. These disease entities have been discussed earlier in this chapter. Treatment may include physician referral for coinciding diagnosis and/or treatment of the associated systemic disease.

Necrotizing ulcerative periodontitis, previously called HIV-associated periodontitis (HIV-P) is diagnosed when ulcerations and necrosis of the gingiva results in necrosis and exposure of the alveolar bone. It is accompanied by severe pain. Periodontal pockets do not form because gingival recession coincides with loss of bone. This form of periodontitis is extremely aggressive and can be localized or generalized. Loss of more than 90 percent of the alveolar bone has been observed in as little as three to six months (AAP, 1992a). HIV-P recently was renamed Necrotizing (Ulcerative) Periodontitis as a result of worldwide meetings concerning oral manifestations of the human immunodeficiency virus (Persson, 1993). No clear differences have been documented in microbes associated with HIV-associated periodontal diseases and those occurring in non-HIV positive clients. Treatment includes mechanical debridement and rinsing with providone iodine for control of pain and bleeding. Meticulous oral hygiene is essential. Antimicrobial (chlorhexidine) rinses are beneficial, and antifungal agents may be necessary if yeast infections are evident (AAP, 1994).

## BIOLOGICAL BASIS FOR PERIODONTAL THERAPY

Host responses play a major role in most forms of periodontal disease. Both gingivitis and periodontitis are chronic infections resulting from interactions between pathogenic microorganisms and the host response.

**Inflammation** is a defense reaction of the body that occurs in response to injury. Inflammatory cells migrate to an area of irritation through chemotaxis, a chemical process that causes them to become mobile and travel to the localized area of injury. These inflammatory cells (including mast cells, neutrophils, macrophages, lymphocytes, and plasma cells) phagocytize, or engulf, bacteria and bacterial components or remove injured tissue. Mast cells contain histamine within their cytoplasm; therefore, they are most important in hypersensitivity reactions of the anaphylactic type. Neutrophils, or polymorphonuclear leukocytes (PMNs), play a critical role in periodontal disease. They serve as the earliest responders, or the first line of defense, in inflammatory lesions of the periodontium. PMNs have many ingestive enzymes designed to ingest microorganisms and to neutralize toxic bacterial products. These enzymes are contained in lysosomes that can be destructive when released outside of the nucleus of the cell during phagocytosis. Thus, neutrophils may also cause tissue destruction (Trowbridge & Emling, 1993). Leukocytes are, nonetheless, critical to the initial host response. Abnormalities in leukocyte chemotaxis or response can lead to more

severe periodontal disease and are believed to occur in more aggressive forms of periodontitis (Nisengard, Newman, & Sanz, 1996).

In the initial phase of acute inflammation, vasodilation produces increased blood volume that can appear as erythema. Excess fluid in the blood vessels causes leakage of plasma into the tissues producing edema. Vascular permeability is mediated (increased) by the release of histamine and serotonin by mast cells in the connective tissue, as well as arachadonic acid metabolites (prostaglandins and leukotrienes), the kinin system, the fibrinolytic system, and various lysosomes produced by leukocytes (Trowbridge & Emling, 1993). As vasodilation is sustained, inflammatory cells leave the vessels, enter the connective tissues and move to the site of injury.

Macrophages are large mononuclear phagocytes that play a direct role in cell-mediated immunity, or delayed hypersensitivity. Cellular immunity does not involve circulating antibodies but rather involves an interaction of antigens with the surface of T lymphocytes, or T cells. There are actually two types of lymphocytes, T cells and B cells. T cells, are monocytes that migrate from the bone marrow to the thymus where they become immunocompetent. The helper T cells (CD4) join forces with macrophages to aid the response of B cells in differentiating into plasma cells and producing antibodies. B cells are mononuclear cells that are derived from the liver, spleen, and bone marrow and circulate in the blood and lymph. They are involved in humoral immune responses and are identified by their surface immunoglobulins, or amino acids. Human immunoglobulins are divided into five classes based upon structural differences including IgG, IgM, IgE, IgA, and IgD. IgG is the must abundant in the serum and is found equally in blood and in extravascular fluids. Its major role is to enhance phagocytosis by neutralizing toxins and binding to microorganisms, so it is important in host responses in periodontal disease. IgM is less numerous but antibodies of this class are the first to be released in the presence of an antigen. IgE is present in acute allergic reactions; IgA is principally found in exocrine secretions like tears and saliva; IgD is found in extremely low levels in serum; therefore, these three immunoglobulins are considered to be of lesser importance in periodontal diseases. The IgG and IgM classes of antibodies, which are glycoproteins, form antigen-antibody (Ag-Ab) complexes that activate complement. Complement consists of eleven proteins and glycoproteins that react with Ag-Ab complexes to lyse and alter cell membranes thereby promoting phagocytosis (Neisengard, Newman, & Sanz, 1996).

Again, macrophages and T cells play a major role in cell-mediated immunity that are the response of B cells. B cells and their surface immunoglobulins play a role in humoral immunity by forming Ag-Ab complexes after the antigen is prepared by the macrophages and T cells. B cells terminate as plasma cells, which produce immunoglobulins and antibodies. Complement is activated by Ag-Ab complexes and causes cell lysis and alteration thereby promoting phagocytosis. All of these immune reactions are protective in early stages of inflammation; however, phagocytosis of Ag-Ab complexes results in release of lysosomes in the tissues, and lymphocyte stimulation of Ag-Ab complexes produce lymphokines. Both of these substances can destroy tissue in the area of inflammation despite their intended protective mechanisms. Thus, the host response can be protective or destructive depending on the balance between bacterial products and bacterial invasion and the resultant host response. If the bacterial irritants are removed within a reasonable time period or controlled to a reasonable level, a healthy host may be able to combat tissue destruction. An altered host response or systemic disease, however, may cause more rapid destruction despite lower levels of bacterial irritation. The goal of therapy, therefore, is to maintain a proper balance between etiologic factors, such as bacterial plaque and its retentive factors, and the host response. As periodontal disease progresses, or the host is compromised, the challenge of maintaining that balance becomes greater. The progression of the periodontal lesion is controlled by both local and systemic factors. Disease activity is related to increased proportions of periodontal pathogens, changes in host response, and possibly bacterial invasion of the tissues. The exact mechanisms of disease perpetuation and pathogenicity are not known (Newman, Sanz, Nisengard, & Haake, 1996).

## Histopathology of Periodontal Disease

The current theories explaining the processes of pathologic changes in the periodontal lesion are founded upon the work of Page and Schroeder (1977). These authors described the histopathology of periodontal disease as a sequence of events divided into three different stages of gingivitis (initial, early, and established lesions) and an advanced lesion of periodontitis. Table 1-2 summarizes key features of each of these stages of inflammation in the periodontal lesion.

**Stages of Gingivitis.** Stage I gingivitis, or the initial lesion, is subclinical; therefore, changes are not evident upon clinical examination. Within two to four days after initial injury by bacterial plaque and its products, a brief period of vasoconstriction is soon followed by vasodilation and increased blood flow bringing large numbers of neutrophils (PMNs) into the area of irritation adjacent to the junctional epithelium at the base of the sulcus. In this cellular phase of inflammation, these neutrophils leave the axial stream and adhere to the endothelial walls (mar-

**Table 1-2  Stages of Inflammation in the Periodontal Lesion**

| Stages | Time Interval | Histological Changes | Clinical Changes |
|---|---|---|---|
| **I. Initial Lesion**<br>• Initial Response of Tissues to Bacterial Plaque<br>• Subclinical Gingivitis | 2 to 4 days | • brief vasoconstriction followed by vasodilation, margination, emigration, and migration of PMN's<br>• slight alteration of junctional epithelium (JE)<br>• increase in gingival crevicular fluid | none |
| **II. Early Lesion**<br>• Acute Gingivitis | 4 to 7 days | • continuation of initial lesion<br>• chronic inflammatory cells (macrophages and lymphocytes) appear<br>• JE invaginates with rete pegs<br>• ulcerations in sulcular epithelium<br>• destruction of connective tissue fibers | • redness<br>• swelling<br>• bleeding upon probing<br>• loss of tissue tone |
| **III. Established Lesion**<br>• Chronic Gingivitis | 14+ days | • continuation of changes in early lesion<br>• plasma cells predominate<br>• chronic inflammation; blood vessels are congested and blow flow is impaired; increases in collegenase and other enzymes<br>• elongated rete pegs in JE extending deep into connective tissue; breakdown of connective fibers | • moderate to severe inflammation<br>• an underlying bluish hue may occur<br><br>• in addition to color, changes in and consistency occur |
| **IV. Advanced Lesion**<br>• Transition from Gingivitis to Periodontitis | dependent upon host response | • continuation of changes in established lesion<br>• inflammation extends into the connective tissue attachment and alveolar bone<br>• repair manifests as fibrotic tissue<br>• bone resorption by osteoclasts and mononuclear cells; bone formation may also occur | • true periodontal pockets<br>• attachment loss<br>• bone loss |

gination). They then pass through the vessel walls (emigration or diapedesis) into the connective tissue and move to the area of injury (migration). Chemotaxis is the chemical response that produces a drawing effect attracting the neutrophils (PMNs) to the sulcular area so there is a slight alteration of the junctional epithelium and an increase in gingival crevicular fluid flow. The neutrophil is the primary cell type associated with acute inflammation and its main function is phagocytosis. The character and intensity of the host response, and the removal or continuation of bacterial insult, determine whether the periodontal lesion heals or progresses to the next stage (Carranza & Rapley, 1996).

Stage II gingivitis, or the early lesion, represents a continuation of the processes occurring in the initial lesion, or a persistence of the acute inflammatory response. Capillaries continue to engorge and proliferate, the junctional epithelium invaginates rete pegs into the connective tissue as collagen is destroyed in the area, and micro-ulcerations occur in the sulcular epithelium. The main fiber groups affected are the circular and dentogingival fibers. PMNs continue to respond but macrophages, T lymphocytes and B lymphocytes (mononuclear cells) become the most numerous inflammatory cells densely infiltrating within the connective tissue. Fibroblasts are altered by lysosomes released and thus, these reparative cells have less capacity for collagen production (Carranza & Rapley, 1996). Clinically, gingival inflammation is detected with redness due to the increased vascularity and vasodilation, bleeding upon probing due to microulceration and pathways established into the connective tissue, and loss of tissue tone due to collagen destruction. Because this lesion occurs four to seven days after presence of pathogenic microorganisms, it is diagnosed as acute gingivitis.

Stage III gingivitis, or the established lesion generally occurs after fourteen days. The blood vessels become engorged and venous return is slowed. The gingiva becomes increasingly inflamed and color changes from red to a bluish hue, become more evident. All inflammatory cells are responding; however, plasma cells, terminating from B lymphocytes found in the early lesion, predominate in the established lesion. Intact collagen bundles are replaced by increasing numbers of inflammatory cells. The junctional epithelium continues to invaginate into the lamina propria as connective tissue is destroyed by collagenase. Macrophages stimulate fibroblasts although irregular reparative tissue, or granulation tissue, is formed rather than collagen bundles. Clinically, the tissue may appear moderately to severely red (erythematous), swollen (edematous) and/or enlarged as time progresses. This stage is diagnosed as chronic gingivitis and may persist for weeks to years depending upon numbers and virulence of periodontal pathogens, elimination or suppression of those organisms, and the host response. Chronic gingivitis is a fluctuating disease with periods of exacerbation and remission, slow progression, and few symptoms (Carranza, 1996a).

**The Advanced Stage: Periodontitis.** Stage IV, periodontitis, results when gingival inflammation extends into the supporting periodontal tissues marking the transition from gingivitis to periodontitis. In cases of disease progression, gingival inflammation extends along collagen fiber bundles and blood vessels into the periodontal ligament and/or alveolar bone. Apical migration of the junctional epithelium, loss of connective tissue attachment, and bone resorption result in deepened pockets. Table 1-3 outlines the significant features of the histopathology of the periodontal pocket (Carranza, 1996b). Two cell types are involved in bone resorption: the osteoclast, which degenerates the mineral content, and the mononuclear cell, which degenerates the organic matrix. Inflammatory infiltrate is present in the advanced lesion (Carranza, 1996b).

The exact mechanisms of bone destruction in periodontitis are not fully understood. Destructive periods have been associated with: 1) subgingival ulceration and acute inflammatory reactions; 2) conversion from a predominately T cell-dominated lesion to one dominated by B-cell infiltrate; 3) increases in loosely attached, motile, gram-negative, anaerobic pocket flora; 4) tissue invasion by periodontal pathogens. Possible pathways by which bacterial plaque products may cause bone loss in periodontitis include: 1) direct action on the bone cells inducing osteoclasts, 2) direct action on the bone itself through noncellular mechanisms, 3) stimulation of gingival cells to release mediators, agents, cofactors, or chemicals that destroy bone with or without osteoclasts (Carranza 1996c).

The response of alveolar bone to inflammation includes bone formation as well as resorption; therefore bone loss in periodontitis is accompanied by both resorption and formation. The destructive process may parallel gingival inflammation with periods of exacerbation and remission. These varying periods of disease activity may coincide with previously mentioned changes in the extent of bleeding, amount of exudate, and composition of bacterial plaque. The basic aim of periodontal therapy is to control bacterial plaque, its retentive factors, and signs of inflammation thereby potentially removing the stimulus for bone resorption (Carranza, 1996c).

## Wound Healing in Periodontal Disease

Periodontal tissues are constantly undergoing renewal in the normal periodontium. The oral epithelium maintains its thickness by mitotic activity of epithelial cells in the basal layer and shedding of cells in the surface. Fibroblasts regenerate connective tissue fibers in the lamina propria of the gingiva. Cementoblasts form new cementum throughout continuous eruption patterns that occur over time. Cells of the periodontal ligament and bone (fibroblasts and osteoblasts) are continually involved in remodeling.

The effectiveness of periodontal therapy is made possible because of the exceptional healing capability of the

**Table 1-3 Histopathology of the Periodontal Pocket**

| Characteristic | Description | Microscopic Features |
|---|---|---|
| Soft Tissue Wall | connective tissue | • edematous<br>• infiltrated, with plasma cells, lymphocytes, and PMNs<br>• exhibits degeneration |
| | blood vessels | • increase in number<br>• dilated and engorged |
| | junctional epithelium | • shorter than that of a normal sulcus<br>• epithelial projections exist and extend into the adjacent inflammed connective tissue |
| | lateral wall | • represents proliferation and degenerative changes<br>• epithelial projections are infiltrated with leukocytes and edema<br>• cells degenerate and rupture causing vesicles<br>• ulceration<br>• exposure of the inflammed connective tissue and suppuration occur<br>• acute inflammation can be superimposed on chronic inflammation |
| | epithelium of the gingival crest | • intact<br>• thickened with prominent rete pegs |
| | bacteria | • filaments, rods, and coccoid organisms with gram negative cell walls invade lateral and apical walls in chronic periodontitis<br>• some transverse the basement membrane and basal lamina and invade the subepithelial connective tissue (the significance of bacterial invasion is not clear) |
| Microtopography of the Gingival Wall | flat surface with minor depressions | • represents periods of quiescence |
| | depressions | • areas of bacterial accumulation |
| | leukocytes are visible and numerous | • areas of emergence of leukocytes |
| | leukocytes are covered with bacteria representing phagocytosis | • areas of leukocytes—bacteria interaction |
| | semiattached and folded epithelial squames | • areas of intense epithelial desquamation |
| | exposed connective tissue with numerous leukocytes | • areas of ulceration<br>• areas of hemorrhage |
| As Healing Lesions | fluid and exudate | • destructive change; wall is bluish-red, spongy, soft, friable, and shiny |
| | formation of blood vessels to repair tissue damage | • constructive change; firm and pink |
| | presence of local irritants | • continues destruction; deceiving because can appear firm and pink on outside; inflammation occurs within tissue |
| Root Surface Wall | cementum | • structural changes—pathological granules, increased mineralization, demineralization (root caries) covered by calculus |
| | bacterial penetration of the dentinal tubules | • destruction of dentin |

periodontal tissues. The goals of periodontal therapy are to eliminate pain, inflammation, and bleeding; to reduce pocket depths and eliminate infection; to arrest tissue and bone destruction; to reduce pathologic mobility; to restore function and physiologic tissue contour; to prevent disease recurrence; and to reduce tooth loss. Local therapy is targeted at removing plaque and all factors that favor its retention, whereas systemic therapy is an adjunct to control systemic complications that aggravate the periodontal disease state. Healing can be delayed by failure to adequately control local factors, excessive tissue

manipulation during treatment, or inadequate consideration of systemic conditions (Carranza, 1996d). The basic healing processes are the same after all forms of periodontal therapy; however, specific aspects of periodontal healing have special bearing on the results obtained by various forms of treatment (Carranza, 1996d).

Regeneration is the "growth and differentiation of new cells and intercellular substances to form new tissues or parts. Regeneration takes place by growth from the same type of tissue that has been destroyed or from its precursor" (Carranza, 1996d). In the periodontium, it is a continuous process during health and it also occurs during disease to some extent. As mentioned previously, periodontal lesions are healing lesions; however, bacterial plaque and its by-products can retard healing. By removing bacterial plaque and creating an environment that reduces its new formation, nonsurgical or surgical periodontal therapy allows for regeneration.

Repair, also called healing by scar, simply restores tissue at the same level on the root as the base of the pre-existing pocket by a process of wound healing. It does not necessarily restore the original architecture or function of the part.

Epithelial adaptation is the close apposition of the gingival epithelium to the tooth without complete obliteration of the pocket. This close apposition does not allow passage of a periodontal probe; however, regeneration and repair have not resulted in a longer junctional epithelium. In some cases where epithelial adaptation is attained post therapy in a 4 to 5 mm pocket and no inflammation, bleeding, or further attachment loss is detected, epithelial adaptation is acceptable (Carranza, 1996d). Most often, however, the goal of nonsurgical periodontal therapy is to obtain both regeneration and repair resulting in the formation of a longer junctional epithelium. This outcome, coupled with shrinkage of the marginal gingiva, can result in reduced probing depths and healthy tissue in early to moderate periodontitis. Its success is more limited in cases of advanced destruction (Greenstein, 1992).

New attachment refers to the embedding of new periodontal ligament fibers into new cementum and formation of a new gingival attachment in an area previously degenerated by periodontitis (Carranza, 1996d). Although new attachment is the goal of surgery, often only regeneration and repair are attained, thereby producing similar results to NSPT. New attachment is most likely following periodontal surgical procedures that remove the existing periodontal attachment and provide for regeneration of the supporting structures (regeneration procedures such as autografts, allografts, and guided tissue regeneration) (Consensus Report, AAP, 1989) (see Chapter 17). Reattachment is not to be confused with new attachment. It refers to reattachment (to attach again) of periodontal tissues in an area not previously exposed to a pocket. Examples would be reattachment by repair after periodontal surgery following an injury or following a procedure to gain access to a periapical lesion (Carranza, 1996d).

Regardless of the periodontal therapy performed, healing of the periodontal pocket depends on certain conditions during the healing phase. If the epithelium proliferates apically on the root surface before the other supporting tissues reach the area, only a longer junctional epithelium will form. If connective tissue cells, periodontal ligament cells, or bone cells arrive first, regeneration of a new attachment is more likely following regenerative procedures. Healing also is improved by debridement (or removal of diseased tissue), immobilization of the healing area, and pressure on the wound (Carranza, 1996d). And, ultimately, sufficient elimination of bacteria is essential to wound healing in either nonsurgical or surgical periodontal therapy.

## Summary

Studies conducted over the past several decades have shown that nonsurgical periodontal therapy is an effective means of reducing clinical parameters of periodontal diseases and of arresting attachment loss in clients with periodontitis. If debridement, coupled with mechanical and/or chemotherapeutic oral self-care, can eliminate inflammation and arrest disease progression, then no further active treatment is necessary. On the other hand, surgical access may be necessary when nonsurgical periodontal therapy fails (Consensus Report, 1989). In early-onset forms of periodontitis and refractory periodontitis, adjunctive use of antibiotics in conjunction with local therapy may be indicated. Because periodontal diseases are known to be infections caused by a host response to bacterial plaque, a delicate balance must be achieved between local factors present and the competence of the host. Reevaluation of therapy, at four to six weeks post-treatment is a critical component of nonsurgical periodontal therapy to determine whether that balance has been achieved. Subsequent maintenance care, or PMP, also appears to be important to the long-term maintenance of periodontal health. Personal and professional plaque control can be combined for successful therapy. If either of these approaches is practiced independently, desirable outcomes are less likely. Thus, the ultimate goal of the clinician is to consider all etiologies and risk factors in planning treatment, and to work collaboratively with the client as a cotherapist, to achieve the goals of therapy.

## Case Studies

**Case Study One:** John Morris, a 15-year-old high school athlete, comes to the office for his scheduled visit with the dental hygienist. Health history findings are negative and plaque and calculus deposits are minimal. When viewing the radiographs, slight vertical alveolar bone loss is evident around the first molars and incisors. What classification of periodontal disease should be suspected in this case? What type of therapy should be considered?

**Case Study Two:** Mary Simmons, a 35-year-old executive who travels frequently, is appointed for a six-month recall visit. Examination findings include: generalized gingival inflammation, gingival bleeding, and probing depths on posterior proximal surfaces of 3 to 4 mm. Radiographs show involvement of the alveolar crest in these areas. Plaque and calculus deposits are detected on all proximal surfaces subgingivally, and supragingivally in the mandibular anteriors. Health history findings indicate that Mary is apparently healthy, although she has not had a recent physical exam. What classification of periodontal disease is suspected in this case? What is the apparent etiology and what other risk factors should be considered?

**Case Study Three:** Joe Valesco, a 25-year-old college student, presents a chief complaint of painful gingiva and foul breath. Examination reveals diffuse erythema, bleeding, and ulcerated interdental papilla throughout the mandible, a gray pseudomembrane and gingival recession in the mandibular anteriors, and coinciding bone loss around #24 and 25. Health history findings indicate that Joe has general malaise, and reports recent flulike symptoms. What classification of periodontal disease should be suspected in this case? What treatment should be considered?

**Case Study Four:** Susie Bennett, a 20-year-old licensed practical nurse, is a new client in your practice. She has not had her "teeth cleaned" for two years. Health history findings are negative; however, Susie takes birth control pills. Examination findings show localized erythema and edema around maxillary molars, mandibular incisors, and lingual to the mandibular molars. Plaque and calculus deposits also are found in these areas. Radiographic findings are normal with no alveolar bone loss detected. What is your preliminary diagnosis? What etiologic factors should be suspected in this case? What parts of the periodontium are involved?

**Case Study Five:** Rick Harbour, a 55-year-old building contractor, returns to your office for a reevaluation four weeks after nonsurgical periodontal therapy. His plaque control appears to be very thorough and no residual deposits are detected. Despite this fact, no gain in attachment is noted, probing depths remain about the same, and the gingiva bleeds upon provocation. What classification(s) of periodontal disease should be suspected, and how should treatment proceed from here?

## Case Study Discussions

**Discussion—Case Study One:** Localized juvenile periodontitis (LJP) should be suspected because of the age of onset, the absence of obvious local or systemic etiologic factors, and the areas of localized bone loss. LJP begins in the first molars and incisors around the age of puberty. It occurs in otherwise healthy adolescents, and destruction is not proportionate to plaque and calculus deposits. Treatment involves nonsurgical periodontal therapy with adjunctive antibiotics (such as tetracycline or metronidazole and Amoxicillin). Examination of John's siblings also should be performed due to the inherited nature of this disease. John should be placed on a frequent recall interval (initially one to two months extended to three to four months based upon reevaluation) for monitoring and maintenance therapy, as well.

**Discussion—Case Study Two:** Early adult periodontitis should be suspected due to the age of onset, probing depths, and radiographic findings. The apparent etiology is a host response to the plaque and calculus deposits present. Other risk factors that could be considered include: whether or not Mary smokes, job-related stress, diet and nutrition, and poor oral hygiene. Her recall interval for PMP also should be reduced to three to four months.

**Discussion—Case Study Three:** Periodontal disease associated with immunocompromising diseases such as human immunodeficiency virus (HIV), or necrotizing (ulcerative) periodontitis, should be suspected. It is accompanied by gingival necrosis, severe pain, and gingival recession coinciding loss of alveolar bone. Joe should be referred to a physician for HIV testing. Treatment includes mechanical debridement and rinsing with providone iodine. Meticulous oral hygiene with adjunctive chemotherapeutics also are essential.

**Discussion—Case Study Four:** Chronic marginal gingivitis and/or gingivitis associated with hormonal changes are two possible diagnoses. An oral prophylaxis should be performed and tissue should be evaluated for healing four to six weeks after treatment. If plaque control is adequate and inflammation does not subside, hormonal risk factors should be considered. The diagnosis of gingivitis, rather than periodontitis, is chosen due to the absence of bone loss and the presence of gingival inflammation. Only the gingiva and junctional epithelium are involved in gingivitis; periodontal ligament and alveolar bone are not affected.

**Discussion—Case Study Five:** Rick could have either refractory periodontitis or periodontitis associated with systemic disease. Reinstitution of nonsurgical periodontal therapy with adjunctive antibiotics and microbiologic monitoring may be indicated, or referral to a periodontist. A closer examination of Rick's health history, possible risk factors associated with periodontitis and, perhaps, a referral for a physical examination might also be considered.

# REFERENCES

Abdellatif, H. M. & Burt, B. A. (1987). An epidemiological investigation into the relative importance of age and oral hygiene status as determinants of periodontitis. *Journal of Dental Research, 66*, 13–18.

Aleo, J. J., DeRenzis, F. A., Farber, P. A., & Varboncoeur, A. P. (1974). The presence and biological activity of cementum-bound endotoxin. *Journal of Periodontology, 45*, 672–675.

American Academy of Periodontology. (1992a). *The etiology and pathogenesis of periodontal diseases.* Chicago: AAP Department of Scientific, Clinical and Educational Affairs, 1–9, November.

American Academy of Periodontology. (1992b). *Diagnosis of periodontal diseases.* Chicago: AAP Department of Scientific, Clinical and Educational Affairs, 1–8, November.

American Academy of Periodontology. (1992c). *Periodontal diseases in children and adolescents.* Chicago: AAP Department of Scientific, Clinical and Educational Affairs, 1–5, November.

American Academy of Periodontology. (1993). *Guidelines for periodontal therapy.* Chicago: AAP Department of Scientific, Clinical and Educational Affairs, 1–5, November.

American Academy of Periodontology. (1994). *Periodontal considerations in the HIV-positive patient.* Chicago: AAP Department of Scientific, Clinical and Educational Affairs, 1–9, April.

American Academy of Periodontology. (1995a). *1995 insurance coding update.* Chicago: AAP Department of Scientific, Clinical and Educational Affairs.

American Academy of Periodontology. (1995b). *Current procedural terminology and insurance reporting manual.* Chicago: AAP Department of Scientific, Clinical and Educational Affairs.

American Dental Association. (1991). *The dental IQ of the American public: Highlights of a national survey by the American Dental Association.* Morris Plains, NJ: Warner-Lambert.

Armitage, G. C. (1987). Diagnosing periodontal diseases and monitoring the response to periodontal therapy. In *Perspectives on oral antimicrobial therapeutics.* Littleton, MA: PSG Publishing.

Artzi, Z. & Moses, O. (1995). Juvenile periodontitis: Microbiology and the therapy approach. *Oral Health,* July: 23–28.

Axelsson, P., Lindhe, J., & Nystrom, B. (1991). On the prevention of caries and periodontal disease. Results of a 15-year longitudinal study in adults. *Journal of Clinical Periodontology, 18*, 182–189.

Badersten, A., Nilvéus, R., & Egelberg, J. (1981). Effect of nonsurgical periodontal therapy. I. Moderately advanced periodontitis. *Journal of Clinical Periodontology, 8*, 57–72.

Badersten, A., Nilvéus, R., & Egelberg, J. (1984). Effect of nonsurgical periodontal therapy. II. Severely advanced periodontitis. *Journal of Clinical Periodontology, 11*, 63–76.

Badersten, A., Nilvéus, R., & Egelberg, J. (1985). Effect of nonsurgical periodontal therapy. IV. Operator variability. *Journal of Clinical Periodontology, 12*, 190–213.

Beck, J. D. Methods of assessing risk for periodontitis and developing multifactorial models. (1994). *Journal of Periodontology, 65*, 468–478.

Beck, J. D., Koch, G. G., Zambon, J. J., Genco, R. J., & Tudor, G. E. (1992). Evaluation of oral bacteria as risk indicators for periodontitis in older adults. *Journal of Periodontology, 39*, 33–47.

Beltrami, M., Bickel, M., & Baehni, P. (1987). The effect of supragingival plaque control on the composition of the subgingival microflora in human periodontitis. *Journal of Clinical Periodontology, 14*, 161–164.

Bergstrom, J. & Preber, H. (1994). Tobacco use as a risk factor. *Journal of Periodontology, 65*, 545–550.

Bowen, D. M. (1994). Periodontics. In Darby and Bushee (Eds.), *Comprehensive review of dental hygiene* (3rd ed.). St. Louis: Mosby-Year Book, Inc.

Brayer, W. K., et al. (1989). Scaling and root planing effectiveness: The effect of root surface access and operator experience. *Journal of Periodontology, 60*, 67–73.

Carranza, F. A. (1996a). Clinical features of gingivitis. In F. A. Carranza & M. G. Newman (Eds.), *Clinical periodontology* (8th ed.). Philadelphia: W.B. Saunders Co.

Carranza, F. A. (1996b). The periodontal pocket. In F. A. Carranza & M. G. Newman (Eds.), *Clinical periodontology* (8th ed.). Philadelphia: W.B. Saunders Co.

Carranza, F. A. (1996c). Bone loss and patterns of bone destruction. In F. A. Carranza & M. G. Newman (Eds.), *Clinical periodontology* (8th ed.). Philadelphia: W.B. Saunders Co.

Carranza, F. A. (1996d). Rationale for periodontal treatment. In F. A. Carranza & M. G. Newman (Eds.), *Clinical periodontology* (8th ed.). Philadelphia: W.B. Saunders Co.

Carranza, F. A. & Perry, D. A. (1996). *Clinical periodontology for the dental hygienist* (2nd ed.). Philadelphia: W.B. Saunders Co.

Carranza, F. A. & Rapley, J. W. (1996). Gingival inflammation. In F. A. Carranza & M. G. Newman (Eds.), *Clinical periodontology* (8th ed.). Philadelphia: W.B. Saunders Co.

Carranza, F. A. & Ubios, A. M. (1996). The tooth supporting structures. In F. A. Carranza and M. G. Newman (Eds.), *Clinical periodontology* (8th ed.). Philadelphia: W.B. Saunders Co.

Caton, J. (1989). Periodontal diagnosis and diagnostic aids: In *Proceedings of the world workshop in clinical periodontics* (pp. I-1–I-22). Chicago: American Academy of Periodontology.

Caton, J., Bouwsma, O., Polson, A., & Epseland, M. (1989). Effect of personal oral hygiene and subgingival scaling on bleeding interdental gingiva. *Journal of Periodontology, 60*, 84–90.

Cercek, J. F., Kiger, R. D., Garret, S., & Egelberg, J. (1983). Relative effects of plaque control and instrumentation on the clinical parameters of human periodontal disease. *Journal of Periodontology, 10*, 46–56.

Christersson, L. A., Grossi, S. G., Dunford, R. G., Machtel, E. E., & Genco, R. J. (1991). Dental plaque and calculus: Risk indicators for their formation. *Journal of Dental Research, 71*(7), 1425–1430.

Ciancio, S. G. (1989). Non-surgical periodontal treatment. In *Proceedings of the world workshop in clinical periodontics* (Section II: II-1–II-12). Chicago: American Academy of Periodontology.

Ciancio, S. G. (1992). Agents for the management of plaque and gingivitis. *Journal of Dental Research, 71*(7), 1450–1456.

Clarke, N. G. & Hirsh, R. S. (1995). Personal risk factors for generalized periodontitis. *Journal of Clinical Periodontology, 22*, 136–145.

Consensus Report. (1989). *Proceedings of the world workshop in clinical periodontics* (Discussion Section II: II-13–II-20). Chicago: American Academy of Periodontology.

Corbet, E. F. & Davies, W. I. R. (1993). The role of supragingival plaque in the control of progressive periodontal disease: A review. *Journal of Periodontology, 20,* 307–313.

Cortellini, P., Pini-Prato, G., & Tonetti, M. (1994). Periodontal regeneration of human infrabony defects (V). Effect of oral hygiene on long-term stability. *Journal of Clinical Periodontology, 21,* 606–610.

Darby, M. L., & Walsh, M. M. (1994). *Dental hygiene theory and practice.* Philadelphia: W.B. Saunders Co.

Demetriou, N., Tsami-Pandi, A., & Parashis, A. (1995). Compliance with supportive periodontal treatment in private practice. *Journal of Periodontology, 66,* 145–149.

Drisko, C. & Killoy, W. (1991). Scaling and root planing: Removal of calculus and subgingival organisms. *Current Opinions in Dentistry, 1,* 74–79.

Fine, D. H., Tabak, L., Oshrain, H., Salkind, A., & Siegel, K. (1978a). Studies in plaque pathogenicity. Plaque collection limulus lysate screening of adherent and loosely adherent plaque. *Journal of Periodontal Research, 13,* 17–22.

Fine, D. H., Tabak, L., Oshrain, H., Salkind, A., & Siegel, K. (1978b). Studies in plaque pathogenicity. II. A technique for the specific detection of endotoxin in plaque samples using the limulus lysate assay. *Journal of Periodontal Research, 13,* 127–133.

Gage, T. W. & Pickett, F. A. (1994). *Mosby's dental drug reference.* Saint Louis: Mosby-Year Book, Inc.

Gartner, L. P. (1982). *Essentials of oral histology and embryology.* Reisterstown, MD: Jen House Publishing.

Genco, R. J. (1992). Host responses in periodontal diseases: Current concepts. *Journal of Periodontology, 63,* 338–355.

Gilbert, G. & Heft, M. (1993). Periodontal status of older Floridians attending senior activity centers. *Journal of Periodontology, 19,* 249–254.

Gordon, J., Walker, C., Lamster, I., West, T., Socransky, S., Seiger, M., & Fasciano, R. (1985). Efficacy of clindamycin hydrochloride in refractory periodontitis. 12 month results. *Journal of Periodontology, 56* (Suppl.), 75–81.

Grbic, J. T., Lamster, I. B., Celenti, R. S., & Fine, J. B. (1991). Risk indicators of future clinical attachment loss in adult periodontitis. Patient variables. *Journal of Periodontology, 62,* 322–329.

Grbic, J. T. & Lamster, I. B. (1992). Risk indicators for future attachment loss in adult periodontitis. Tooth and site variables. *Journal of Periodontology, 63,* 262–269.

Grbic, J. T. et al. (1995). The relationship of candidiasis to linear gingival erythema in HIV-infected homosexual men and parenteral drug users. *Journal of Periodontology, 66,* 30–37.

Green, L. W., Tryon, W. W., & Marks, B., et al. (1986). Periodontal disease as a function of life events stress. *Journal of Human Stress, 12,* 32–36.

Greenstein, G. (1984). The role of bleeding upon probing in the diagnosis of periodontal disease. A literature review. *Journal of Periodontology, 55,* 684–670.

Greenstein, G. (1992). Periodontal response to mechanical non-surgical therapy: A review. *Journal of Periodontology, 63,* 118–130.

Grossi, S. G. et al. (1994). Assessment of risk for periodontal disease. I. Risk indicators for attachment loss. *Journal of Periodontology, 65,* 260–267.

Grossi, S. G. et al. (1995). Assessment of risk for periodontal disease. II. Risk indicators for alveolar bone loss. *Journal of Periodontology, 66,* 23–29.

Haber, J., & Kent, R. L. (1992). Cigarette smoking in a periodontal practice. *Journal of Periodontology, 63,* 100–106.

Hall, W. B. (1989). Gingival Augmentation/Mucogingival Surgery. In *Proceedings of the world workshop in clinical periodontics* (pp. VII-1–VII-15). Chicago: American Academy of Periodontology.

Hatfield, C. G. & Baumhammers, A. (1971). Cytotoxic effects of periodontally involved surfaces of human teeth. *Archives of Oral Biology, 16,* 465.

Hughes, F. J. & Smales, F. C. (1992). Attachment and orientation of human periodontal ligament fibroblasts to lipopolysaccharide-coated and pathologically altered cementum in vitro. *European Journal of Prosthodontics and Restorative Dentistry, 2,* 63–68.

Hughes, T. P. & Caffesse, R. G. (1978). Gingival changes following scaling, root planing and oral hygiene. A biometric evaluation. *Journal of Periodontology, 49,* 245–252.

Ismail, A. J., Morrison, E. C., Burt, B. A., Caffesse, R. G., & Kavanaugh, M. T. (1990). Natural history of periodontal disease in adults: Findings from the Tecumseh periodontal disease study, 1959–1987. *Journal of Dental Research, 69,* 430–435.

Itoiz, M. A. & Carranza, F. A. (1996). The gingiva. In F. A. Carranza and M. G. Newman (Eds.), *Clinical periodontology* (8th ed.). Philadelphia: W.B. Saunders Co.

Johnson, N. K. (1989). Detection of high risk groups and individuals for periodontal diseases. *International Dental Journal, 39,* 33–47.

Jones, W. A. & O'Leary, T. J. (1978). The effectiveness of root planing in removing bacterial endotoxin from roots of periodontally involved teeth. *Journal of Periodontology, 49,* 337–342.

Kaldahl, W. B., Kalkwarf, K. L., Patil, K. D., Dyer, J. K., & Bates, R. E., Jr. (1988). Evaluation of four modalities of periodontal therapy: Mean probing depth, probing depth, probing attachment levels and recession changes. *Journal of Periodontology, 59,* 783–793.

Khatiblou, F. A. & Ghodossi, A. (1983). Root surface smoothness or roughness in periodontal treatment. A clinical study. *Journal of Periodontology, 54,* 365–367.

Kho, P., Smales, F., & Hardie, J. (1985). The effect of supragingival plaque control on subgingival microflora. *Journal of Clinical Periodontology, 12,* 676–686.

Kornman, K. S. (1986). The role of supragingival plaque in the prevention and treatment of periodontal diseases. *Journal of Periodontal Research, 21,* (Suppl.) 5-22.

Kornman, K. S. & Karl, E. H. (1982). The effect of long-term low dose tetracycline therapy on the subgingival microflora in refractory adult periodontitis. *Journal of Periodontology, 53,* 604–610.

Kornman, K. S. & Löesche, W. J. (1980). The subgingival microflora during pregnancy. *Journal of Periodontal Research, 15,* 111–115.

Lapp, C. A., Thomas, M. E., & Lewis, J. B. (1995). Modulation by progesterone of interleukin-6 production by gingival fibroblasts. *Journal of Periodontology, 66,* 279–284.

Lindhe, J., Westfelt, E., Nyman, S., Socransky, S. S., & Haffajee, A. D. (1984). Long-term effect of surgical/nonsurgical treatment of periodontal disease. *Journal of Clinical Periodontology, 11,* 448–458.

Löe, H., Ånerud, A., & Boysen, H. (1992). Natural history of periodontal disease in man: Prevalence, severity, and extent of gingival recession. *Journal of Periodontology, 63,* 489–495.

Löe, H., Ånerud, A., Boysen, H., & Morrison, E. (1986). Natural history of periodontal disease in man. Rapid, moderate and no loss of attachment in Sri Lankan laborers 14 to 46 years of age. *Journal of Clinical Periodontology, 13,* 431–440.

Löe, H., Ånerud, A., Boysen, H., & Smith, M. R. (1978a). The natural history of periodontal disease in man. Study design and baseline data. *Journal of Periodontal Research, 13,* 550–562.

Löe, H., Ånerud, A., Boysen, H., & Smith, M. R. (1978b). The natural history of periodontal disease in man. Tooth mortality rates before 40 years of age. *Journal of Periodontal Research, 13,* 563–573.

Löe, H. Ånerud, A., Boysen, H., & Smith, M. R. (1978c). Natural history of periodontal disease in man. The rate of periodontal destruction after 40 years of age. *Journal of Periodontology, 49,* 607–620.

Löe, H., Theilade, E., & Jensen, S. B. (1965). Experimental gingivitis in man. *Journal of Periodontology, 36,* 177–183.

Löesche, W. J. (1994). Periodontal disease as a risk factor for heart disease. *Compendium of Continuing Education in Dentistry, 15,* 976–991.

Logan, H., Koorbusch, G., Hartwig, A., & Quinn, J. (1992). Stress variables: Predictors of complications following oral surgery. (Abstr) *Journal of Dental Research, 71,* 185.

Magnusson, I., et al. (1994). Treatment of subjects with refractory periodontal disease. *Journal of Clinical Periodontology, 21,* 628–637.

Martinez-Canut, P., Lorca, A., & Magan, R. (1995). Smoking and periodontal disease severity. *Journal of Clinical Periodontology, 22,* 743–749.

McFall, W. T., Jr. (1989). Supportive treatment. In *Proceedings of the world workshop in clinical periodontics* (pp. IX-1–IX-23). Chicago: American Academy of Periodontology.

McLaughlin, W., Lovat, F., MacGregor, I., & Kelly, P. (1993). Immediate effects of smoking on gingival fluid flow. *Journal of Clinical Periodontology, 20,* 448–451.

Melnick, S. L., Roseman, J. M., Engel, D., & Cogen, R. B. (1988). Epidemiology of acute necrotizing ulcerative gingivitis. *Epidemiology Reviews, 10,* 191–211.

Meyer, K. & Lie, T. (1977). Root surface roughness in response to periodontal instrumentation by combined use of micro-roughness measurements and scanning electron microscopy. *Journal of Clinical Periodontology, 4,* 77–81.

Michalowicz, B. (1995). Genetic and heritable risk factors in periodontal disease. *Journal of Periodontology, 65,* 479–488.

Michalowicz, B., Aeppli, D., Virag, J., Klump, D., Hinrichs, J., Segal, N., Bouchard, T., & Pihlstrom, B. (1991). Periodontal findings in adult twins. *Journal of Periodontology, 62,* 293–299.

Miller, A. J., Brunelle, J. A., Carlos, J. P., Brown, L. J., & Löe, H. (1987). *Oral health of United States adults* (NIH Publication No. 97-2868). Bethesda, MD: National Institute of Dental Research.

Miller, N. L. (1995). Ultrasonic instrumentation and debridement: Current applications in dental hygiene therapy. *Journal of Practical Hygiene,* Jan.–Feb., 25–31.

Monteiro da Silva, A. M., Newman, H. N., & Oakley, D. A. (1995). Psychosocial factors in inflammatory periodontal diseases: A review. *Journal of Clinical Periodontology, 22,* 516–526.

Morrison, E. C., Ramfjord, S. P., & Hill, R. W. (1980). Short-term effects of initial nonsurgical periodontal treatment (hygiene phase). *Journal of Clinical Periodontology, 7,* 199–211.

Nakib, N. M., Bissada, N. F., Simmelink, J. W., & Golstine, S. (1982). Endotoxin penetration into the cementum of periodontally healthy and diseased human teeth. *Journal of Periodontology, 53,* 368–378.

Newman, M. G., Kornman, K. S., & Holtzman, S. (1994). Association of clinical risk factors with treatment outcomes. *Journal of Periodontology, 65,* 489–497.

Newman, M. G., Sanz, M., Nisengard, R. C., & Haake, S. K. (1996). Host-bacteria interactions. In F. A. Carranza & M. G. Newman (Eds.), *Clinical periodontology* (8th ed.). Philadelphia: W.B. Saunders Co.

Nield-Gehrig, J. S. & Houseman, G. A. (1996). *Fundamentals of periodontal instrumentation* (3rd ed.). Baltimore: Williams & Wilkins.

Nisengard, R. C., Newman, M. G., & Sanz, M. (1996). Host response: Basic concepts. In F. A. Carranza & M. G. Newman (Eds.), *Clinical periodontology* (8th ed.). Philadelphia: W.B. Saunders Co.

Nishimine, D. & O'Leary, T. J. (1979). Hand instrumentation versus ultrasonics in the removal of endotoxin from root surfaces. *Journal of Periodontology, 50,* 345–349.

O'Hehir, T. E. (1995). Effective mechanical instrumentation requires a light, controlled touch. *RDH, 15,* 32.

O'Neil, E., Shugars, D., & Bader, J. (Eds.). (1991). *Healthy America: Practitioners for the year 2005.* Durham, NC: Pew Health Professions Commission.

O'Neil, E., Shugars, D., & Bader, J. (Eds.). (1993). *Health professions for the future: Schools in service to the nation.* San Francisco: Pew Health Professions Commission.

O'Valle, F., et al. (1995). Gingival overgrowth by nifedipine and cyclosporin A. *Journal of Clinical Periodontology, 22,* 591–597.

Oosterwaal, P. J., Matee, M., Mikx, F., van't Hof, M., & Renggli, H. (1987). The effect of subgingival debridement with hand and ultrasonic instruments on the gingival microflora. *Journal of Clinical Periodontology, 14,* 528–533.

Page, R. C., & Schroeder, H.E. (1977). Pathogenic mechanisms. In Schluger, S., Youdelis, R., & Page, R. C. (Eds.), *Periodontal disease: Basic phenomena clinical management and restorative interrelationships.* Philadelphia: Lea & Febiger.

Page, R. C., Altman, L. C., Ebersole, J. L., Vandersteen, G. E., Dahlberg, W. H., Williams, B. L., & Osterberg, S. K. (1983). Rapidly progressive periodontitis. A distinct clinical condition. *Journal of Periodontology, 54,* 197–209.

Persson, R. G. (1993). Classification of periodontal diseases associated with HIV infection. *Dental Hygiene News, 5* (3), 14–17.

Pihlstrom, B. L., McHugh, R. B., & Oliphant, T. H. (1984). Molar and nonmolar teeth compared over 6 1/2 years following two methods of periodontal therapy. *Journal of Periodontology, 55,* 499–504.

Preber, H. & Bergstrom, J. (1990). Effect of cigarette smoking on periodontal healing following surgical therapy. *Journal of Clinical Periodontology, 17,* 324–328.

Preber, H., Bergstrom, J., & Linder, L. E. (1992). Occurrence of periodontal pathogens in smoker and nonsmoker patients. *Journal of Clinical Periodontology, 19,* 667–671.

Preber, H., Linder, L., & Bergstrom, J. (1995). Periodontal healing and periopathogenic microflora in smokers and non-smokers. *Journal of Clinical Periodontology, 22,* 946–952.

Proye, M., Caton, J., & Polson, A. (1982). Initial healing of periodontal pockets after a single episode of root planing monitored by controlled probing force. *Journal of Periodontology, 53,* 296–301.

Ramfjord, S. (1993). Maintenance care and supportive periodontal therapy. *Quintessence International, 24,* 465–471.

Ramfjord, S., Caffesse, R., Morrison, E., Hill, R., Kerry, G., Appleberry, E., Nissle, R., & Stults, D. (1987). Four modalities of periodontal treatment compared over 5 years. *Journal of Clinical Periodontology, 14,* 445–452.

Rosenburg, R. M. & Ash, M. M. (1974). The effect of root roughness on plaque accumulation and gingival inflammation. *Journal of Periodontology, 45,* 146–150.

Sato, K., Yoneyama, T., Okamoto, H., Dehlen, G., & Lindhe, J. (1993). The effect of subgingival debridement on periodontal disease parameters and the subgingival microbiota. *Journal of Clinical Periodontology, 20,* 359–365.

Shannon, I. L., Kilgore, W. G., & Leary, T. J. (1969). Stress as a predisposing factor in necrotizing ulcerative gingivitis. *Journal of Periodontology, 40,* 240–244.

Slots, J. (1977). Microflora in the healthy gingival sulcus in man. *Scandinavian Journal of Dental Research, 85,* 247–253.

Slots, J. (1979). The subgingival microflora and periodontal disease. *Journal of Clinical Periodontology, 6,* 351–357.

Slots, J. & Rams, T. E. (1991). New views on periodontal microbiota in special patient categories. *Journal of Clinical Periodontology, 18,* 411–420.

Slots, J., Mashimo, P. C., Levine, M. J., & Genco, R. J. (1979). Periodontal therapy in humans. I. Microbiological and clinical effects of a single course of periodontal scaling and root planing and of adjunctive tetracycline therapy. *Journal of Periodontology, 50,* 495–509.

Smulow, J., Turesky, S., & Hill, R. (1983). The effect of supragingival plaque removal on anaerobic bacteria in deep periodontal pockets. *Journal of the American Dental Association, 107,* 737–742.

Socransky, S. S. & Haffajee, A. D. (1992). The bacterial etiology of destructive periodontal disease: Current concepts. *Journal of Periodontology, 63,* 322–331.

Stutsman-Young, N., O'Hehir, T. E., & Woodall, I. (1993). Periodontal debridement. In I. Woodall (Ed.), *Comprehensive dental hygiene care* (4th ed.). St. Louis: Mosby-Year Book, Inc.

Suzuki, J. B. (1988). Diagnosis and classification of the periodontal diseases. *Dental Clinics of North America, 32,* 195–206.

Thornton, S. & Garnick, J. (1982). Comparison of ultrasonic to hand instruments in the removal of subgingival plaque. *Journal of Periodontology, 53,* 35–37.

Trowbridge, H. O. & Emling, R. C. (1993). *Inflammation: A review of the process* (4th ed.). Quintessence Publishing Co., Inc.: Chicago.

Van Ness, W., Walker, C. B., Clark, W. B., & Magnusson, N. I. (1988). Antibiotic susceptibilities associated with refractory periodontitis. *Journal of Dental Research, 67* (Special Issue), Abstract 1063.

Van Volkinburg, J. W., Green, E., & Armitage, G. C. (1976). The nature of root surfaces after curette, Cavitron, and alphasonic instrumentation. *Journal of Periodontal Research, 11,* 374–381.

van Winkelhoff, A. J., Rodenburg, J. P., Goené, R. J., Abbas, F., Winkel, E. G., & de Graaff, J. (1989). Metronidazole plus amoxycillin in the treatment of *Actinobacillus actinomycetemcomitans* associated periodontitis. *Journal of Clinical Periodontology, 16,* 128–131.

Waerhaug, J. (1956). Effect of rough surfaces upon gingival tissue. *Journal of Dental Research, 35,* 323–325.

Walsh, M. M. & Robertson, P. B. (1985). Professional mechanical oral hygiene practices in the prevention and control of periodontal diseases. *California Dental Association Journal,* 58–62.

Wolff, L., Dahlen, G., & Aeppli, D. (1994). Bacteria as risk markers for periodontitis. *Journal of Periodontology, 64* (Suppl.), 498–510.

CHAPTER 2

# Medical History Evaluation and Alterations for Care

## Key Terms

bacterial endocarditis
deductive reasoning
health history
medical history
organic heart murmur

osteoradionecrosis
rheumatic heart disease
self-administered written questionnaire
sensitivity
specificity

## INTRODUCTION

Taking a thorough **medical history** on every client is a necessary part of all dental hygiene care. In this chapter the terms medical history and **health history** are used interchangeably and refer to a set of questions, either written or verbal, used by oral health professionals to acquire information concerning their clients' health statuses. Although dental professionals have been evaluating their clients' physical health before rendering treatment for decades, the changes in dental client populations in the last 10 to 15 years have added greater significance to the procedure. The average dental client today is older. Although the majority of older Americans are healthy, four out of five people over the age of 65 have one or more chronic diseases (Niessen, Mash, & Gibson, 1993). Advances in medical technology have allowed medically compromised persons to live longer and lead more mobile lives thus enhancing the possibility of being treated in a dental office. An increase in the number of prosthetic devices, in the prevalence of heart murmurs, and in cardiac valvular disease have heightened the demand to assess antibiotic prophylactic need.

The rise in the use of medications by dental patient populations is also affecting the significance of complete medical history evaluation. Literature shows that between 42.4 to 47.6 percent of United States dental patients between 1979 and 1992 were taking some type of medication (Cottone & Kafrawy, 1979; Hart, Scianni, & Conklin, 1990; Miller, Kaplan, Guest, & Cottone, 1992; Moorthy, Coghlan, & O'Neil, 1984). Analgesics and cardiovascular agents were the most commonly used medications. Studies also show the elderly population uses more drugs and uses drugs more often than other pop-

ulations. Between 76 to 94 percent of persons 65 and older use medications with a average amount of 3 to 4.3 different medications taken daily (Miller et al., 1992).

The dental hygiene professional's ability to provide total oral health care requires the knowledge of the client's complete health status. Clients experiencing nonsurgical periodontal therapy (NSPT) are no exception. In fact, some of the factors that affect periodontal disease may be discovered and/or discussed during the medical history review process. In addition to providing for an individual's safety, the health history also serves as a medico-legal document should questions arise concerning the appropriateness of a treatment choice.

This chapter is organized around considerations related to NSPT and the client's health status. The first section discusses the medical history evaluation and emphasizes how to select a thoroughly written questionnaire. Also, verbal questions are reviewed to aid the reader in establishing reliable health information. The second section addresses pretreatment alterations including prophylactic antibiotics, bleeding disorders, cancer treatment, medications, infectious disease, and vital signs. Each of these categories have health ramifications for oral health care and must be addressed before invasive therapy is rendered. The middle portion of the chapter discusses conditions that affect the implementation of NSPT such as cardiovascular disease, diabetes, immunosuppression, and the use of local anesthesia. Posttreatment considerations to reduce the risk of secondary infection, delayed healing, or pain are also addressed. Although pretreatment, treatment, and posttreatment concerns apply to any invasive dental care, NSPT is a primary concern for the dental hygienist.

# MEDICAL HISTORY EVALUATION

There is no consensus as to the single best way to obtain an adequate health history. There is, however, no discrepancy in the purpose of a health history. The health history correlates the general health of a client, past and present, with current and future treatment for their oral needs. There are, however, variations in the method of collecting the health information. In the early 1980s there was much debate concerning the advantages of acquiring a history using a verbal technique. The verbal technique would aid in building rapport and ensuring the client understands the questions. Advantages of using a written format are that it saves time and ensures consistency and thoroughness (Brady & Martinoff, 1980; McCarthy, 1983). The **self-administered written questionnaire** is currently the most commonly used format because of the risk of dental malpractice claims and the need for written documentation (Bressman, 1993; deJong, Borgmeijer-Hoelen, & Abraham-Inpijn, 1991; McCarthy, 1983; McCarthy, 1985; Rieder, 1987).

Unfortunately, literature indicates that clients do not always provide valid data regarding their medical history using only the self-administered written questionnaire (Brady & Martinoff, 1980; Mohammad & Ruprecht, 1983). One explanation for client omission of information might be that elderly persons believe their signs and symptoms are a natural phenomenon of aging and, therefore, the omission is not important information. Other explanations for omissions are that clients do not have signs or symptoms of a disease or are unaware of their illnesses. Possible reasons for inaccuracy of information include not understanding the question asked on the form, the emotional state of clients in an anxious environment, or not understanding the need for dental personnel to know medical information (Brady & Martinoff, 1980; Halpern, 1975).

The inability of oral health care professionals to rely on either the questionnaire or verbal history alone indicates the necessity of using both methods to collect accurate health information. An excellent way to increase the reliability of results is to perform a concise verification of all affirmative replies made by the client on the written form and to cross check all answers by linking replies of different questions (deJong et al., 1991).

## Written Health History

There are certain administrative procedures that are considered standards of care after the self-administered written health history is completed, signed, and dated, in ink, by the client or client's guardian. The dentist or dental hygienist verbally addresses positive responses on the written history and makes notations on the form legibly in ink (Bressman, 1993; McCarthy, 1985). The initial review and documentation of pertinent health information will then take place as discussed in this chapter. At subsequent visits for NSPT (quadrant of periodontal instrumentation or a reevaluation visit) and restorative care, the clinician should ask about changes in the client's health, even if visits are scheduled at weekly intervals. It is best for the clinician to question the individual about the health changes in a very specific manner to elicit an accurate response. For example, asking "Are you taking any new medications, have you had any illnesses, have you visited a doctor, or have you been hospitalized since your last visit here?" should help the client to critically think about the issues and respond appropriately. Any changes in health status between visits reported by the client should be documented in the appropriate space on the medical history form (see the bottom of Figure 2-1). If this space is not available on the form, documentation in the record of services should suffice.

Because NSPT requires frequent maintenance appointments, usually at three-month intervals, a student clinician or practitioner is faced with choices about how to reassess the client's health. Questions arise about having the person complete a new health history form or updating the previous form. If the history is designed with spaces for documenting changes as the example in Figure 2-1 is, the client can be asked to review the previous form. If no changes or only minor changes have occurred in the three- to six-month interval then updating the history is warranted. Examples of minor changes include a visit to a physician for a blood pressure recheck that was within normal limits, or a change in the name of a medication. When significant health changes have occurred, completion of a new form is recommended. Examples of significant changes include heart attacks, strokes, cancer treatment, serious illnesses, or extended hospital stays. Some history forms do not have a space for recording changes. In this case, completion of a new form is the best option regardless of the type of health changes the client reports (none, minor, or significant). In summary, at maintenance visits a practitioner must make an informed decision about how to document health information.

Whenever a dental hygienist or dentist records information about a change in someone's health, the notation should be made in ink, dated, and signed by both the client and clinician. If a client's health has not changed "no changes" can be recorded (Bressman, 1993; McCarthy, 1983). For an individual's first visit to a practice, it is practical to suggest arriving fifteen minutes prior to the appointment time to complete personal information and medical history forms. At periodontal maintenance visits, team members other than the dentist or dental hygienist can aid in acquiring medical history information by identifying the appropriate use of the previous history form or a new form. This team member then facilitates completion of the form and forwards the information to the dental hygienist for review.

It is important to consider who should collect health data from clients. The professional who evaluates the health history information needs to be *licensed* and acutely aware of the signs and symptoms of disease. Also, this professional should be knowledgeable about clinical pharmacology including drug interactions, indications for antibiotic prophylactic coverage, questioning techniques to assess accuracy of information, and indications for a consultation with the client's physician. Literature indicates that in offices that employ a dental hygienist, 67 percent of "recall" patients have their medical history evaluated by the dental hygienist and 76 percent of new patients have their health status evaluated by hygienists and dentists collaboratively (Benicewicz & Metzger, 1989). Data also indicate that 73 percent of new patients are first scheduled with the dental hygienist (Campbell, Shuman, & Bauman, 1993).

If significant findings are noted on the medical history, a notation should be made on the outside of the chart with an identifying mark such as a sticker or colored label. The sticker indicates that a condition of vital importance is listed on the medical history, therefore it replaces the need to write out the medical condition of concern. Two examples of significant conditions are allergies to drugs and need for antibiotic prophylactic treatment. Increased confidentiality issues warrant discontinuing the identification of specific conditions on the outside of charts (Bressman, 1993).

Although most dental offices use a self-administered questionnaire, there is no consensus on the length, format, or content of the health history form (Minden & Fast, 1993; Thibodeau & Rossomando, 1992). What began in the 1950s and 1960s as asking the client "Are you in good health?" has expanded to include forms with as many as 88 questions. A study of health history forms from 50 United States and Canadian schools, commercial vendors, and the American Dental Association (ADA) reveals that the average number of questions per form is 58, with a range from 32 to 88 (Thibodeau & Rossomando, 1992). Table 2-1 lists a basic core of conditions which should be included in any written history. It would be advisable to evaluate the health history being used to ensure these elements are included. Also, professionals might find a need to add additional questions or conditions dependent on the needs of the practitioner and clients seeking care in the practice.

In summary, it is not the length of a health history that is the criteria for quality. In fact, the written medical history should not be cumbersome for either party. The medical history form should be thorough but not redundant and use simple language to facilitate understanding. The questions used on the medical history should also allow for a mix of sensitivity and specificity. **Sensitivity** (of the questions) refers to the need to be broad-based. A "history of hospitalization" is a broad based question that is necessary for a medical history. For example, if a client has a history of cancer the most vital information to the dental hygiene professional is the treatment, either radiation or chemotherapy. Questions asking about a past history of cancer give less information than questions concerning outpatient hospital treatment. **Specificity** (of the questions) on the other hand, refers to the ability to trigger another set of questions in the person conducting the interview. An affirmative reply to the question "Have you had a hip replacement?" should trigger more questions concerning antibiotic premedication to limit secondary infection. An example of a medical history showing both sensitivity and specificity is provided in Figure 2-1.

## Verbal Questioning

Once the client completes an adequate medical history, the clinician must employ quality verbal questioning techniques. Some questions such as "Who is your physician?" are asked to determine medical connections. In this day of multiple physicians, the identification of the appropriate physician for a consultation is necessary. The questionnaire can now be used as an information source for the next procedure, which is the verbal interview necessary to validate the written information. This process has often been referred to as the "art of history taking" (Trieger & Goldblatt, 1978). The interview consists of a programmed analysis comprised of pathways much like a computer program. Basic questions are asked and depending on the answers, further questions are asked. The pathway ultimately leads to identification and verification of valid medical data. The process can also be likened to **deductive reasoning**. Deductive reasoning involves the deriving of a conclusion by reasoning or inference in which the conclusion follows from the premise (Engel, 1991). A deductive inference relies on the truth of the premises to guarantee the truth of the

**Table 2-1  Basic Core of Conditions for a Written Health History**

| Condition | | |
|---|---|---|
| • Allergies | • Heart disease | • Pregnancy |
| • Arthritis | • Heart murmur | • Rheumatic fever |
| • Artificial joint/heart valve | • Hepatitis | • Seizures or epilepsy |
| • Asthma or hay fever | • High blood pressure | • Stroke |
| • Cancer therapy | • HIV/AIDS | • Tobacco use |
| • Changes in health in last year | • Hospitalization/operation | • Tuberculosis |
| • Diabetes | • Kidney disease | • Under care of physician |
| • Extensive bleeding/blood disorder | • List current medications | • Venereal disease |
| • Fainting spells | • Liver disease | |

**CLIENT NAME:** _____ **DATE:** _____

Directions: Please answer the following questions about your health by circling "yes" or "no". Your responses will be kept confidential and will be used to plan your dental care in our office.

| | | | |
|---|---|---|---|
| Yes | No | 1. | Do you have a current medical problem? |
| Yes | No | 2. | Are you currently under the care of a physician? Date of last visit. _____ |
| Yes | No | 3. | Have you been hospitalized or had a serious illness? |
| Yes | No | 4. | Do you have heart trouble or any form of cardiovascular disease? |

       _____ Angina (chest pains) Frequency _____     _____ Heart Surgery (date) _____
       _____ Congenital Heart Lesions                           _____ pacemaker
       _____ Heart Attack (date) _____             _____ bypass
       _____ Heart Murmur                                   _____ prosthetic heart valve
                                                                _____ High Blood Pressure
                                                                _____ Rheumatic Fever (date)_____
                                                                 _____ Stroke (date) _____

| | | | |
|---|---|---|---|
| Yes | No | 5. | Do you have diabetes? If YES, how is it controlled? _____ |
| Yes | No | 6. | Do you have kidney disease? (date) _____ |
| Yes | No | 7. | Have you ever had hepatitis? (date) _____ |

       _____ Type A infectious (Food)                    _____ Type B serum (Blood)
       _____ Unknown (explain) _____

| | | | |
|---|---|---|---|
| Yes | No | 8. | Have you ever had liver disease or jaundice? (date)_____ |
| Yes | No | 9. | Do you have any blood disease? |

       _____ Anemia       _____ AIDS or positive test      _____ Leukemia

| | | | |
|---|---|---|---|
| Yes | No | 10. | Do you have any problems with excessive bleeding? If YES, explain _____ |
| Yes | No | 11. | Have you ever had tuberculosis? (date) _____ |
| Yes | No | 12. | Have you ever had venereal disease? (date & type) _____ |
| Yes | No | 13. | Do you have emphysema, asthma or breathing problems? |
| Yes | No | 14. | Have you had a hip or other joint replacement? |
| Yes | No | 15. | Have you ever had any injury, pain or soreness from your jaw joint? (TMJ dysfunction) |
| Yes | No | 16. | Have you ever had any chronic head, neck or back pain problems? |
| Yes | No | 17. | Have you ever been diagnosed as having arthritis? |
| Yes | No | 18. | Do you have fainting spells, convulsions or epilepsy? |
| Yes | No | 19. | Have you had surgery, radiation or other treatment for a tumor, growth or cancer? |
| Yes | No | 20. | Is your diet medically prescribed? If YES, explain _____ |
| Yes | No | 21. | Are you pregnant? (Expected delivery date) _____ |
| Yes | No | 22. | Are you taking birth control pills? If YES, what pills are you taking? _____ |
| Yes | No | 23. | Have you reached menopause? If YES, what hormones are you taking? _____ |
| Yes | No | 24. | Are you allergic to or have you had any unusual reactions to any of the following?: |

       _____ Penicillin          _____ Local anesthetics       _____ Codeine
       _____ Erythromycin            _____ Novocaine             _____ Aspirin
       _____ Clindamycin            _____ Xylocaine           _____ Other pain medications
       _____ Keflex                 _____ Nitrous oxide (gas)      _____
       _____ Other antibiotics        _____ Epinephrine         _____ Any other drug allergies?
                                                                                       _____

| | | | |
|---|---|---|---|
| Yes | No | 25. | Have you ever been advised not to take a particular medication? |
| | | | If YES, please list _____ |
| Yes | No | 26. | Have you ever been advised to take antibiotic premedication before dental treatment? |
| Yes | No | 27. | Do you or have you had a substance abuse problem? |
| Yes | No | 28. | Do you regularly use tobacco or tobacco products? |
| Yes | No | 29. | Other conditions not listed. _____ |
| Yes | No | 30. | Please list medications you are currently taking and reasons for taking them. |

       _____ Reason: _____
       _____ Reason: _____

To the best of my knowledge, all the preceding answers are true and correct. If I have any change in my health or medications, I will inform the dentist/dental hygienist at my next appointment.

Client Signature _____ DDS or RDH Signature _____ Date_____
Current physician_____ Telephone_____

- - - - - - - - - - - - - - - - - - - - - - - - - - - - - - - - - - - - - - - - - - - - - - - - - - - - - - - - - - - - -

Changes in medical history:

1._____

| Change | Date | Client Signature | DDS or RDH Signature |
|---|---|---|---|

1._____

| Change | Date | Client Signature | DDS or RDH Signature |
|---|---|---|---|

1._____

| Change | Date | Client Signature | DDS or RDH Signature |
|---|---|---|---|

**Figure 2-1** Example of a quality health history. (Adapted from James W. Hodge, DDS, Inc.)

conclusion (Engel, 1991; Kearns, 1969). Organizing facts into a conclusion and then matching the information to the dental professional's knowledge of pathophysiology to check for errors aids in evaluating health history information. Relating the data to other pieces of information and correcting misunderstandings is the next step. The making of inferences or correcting inaccuracies can be accomplished throughout the process. Refer to Figure 2-2 for a diagram of a deductive reasoning model.

The following text provides an example of this deductive reasoning model. A client's written medical history indicates he has high blood pressure. When the clinician asks if he is on medication for the high blood pressure, the client replies "I stopped taking it six months ago and have not had any problems." The two premises are that the client has high blood pressure and the client takes no antihypertensive medication. The conclusion is that he does not need medication to control his high blood pressure. This conclusion is true only if both premises are true.

Pathophysiology reveals that hypertension does not have readily identifiable signs and symptoms; therefore, questions concerning monitoring of blood pressure and fluctuations in reading will help the clinician decide if the client truly "has not had any problems" without hypertensive medication. If the client is not monitoring his blood pressure, then the second premise might not be accurate. At this point the clinician should begin relating additional information, such as checking the date of his last visit to the physician. If this visit was six months ago or longer, the client could have discontinued the drug therapy without his physician's knowledge. The client's current blood pressure, taken and recorded at the time of the visit, is also correlated to the premise. Once all the data are collected, inaccuracies in the premise are altered and the clinician decides if a referral to, or consultation with the client's physician is necessary.

Only with the use of deductive reasoning and effective communication skills can health history informa-tion be considered accurate. The dental professional uses mental reasoning and knowledge of anatomy, phys-iology, and pathology, together with communication skills to form this "art of history taking." Attending and lis-tening skills are important to enhance communication. Conducting the interview while facing the client with a posture of involvement, (leaning forward with an open body posture) maintaining eye contact, and keeping environmental distractions to a minimum would be examples of using attending skills. These types of respons-es let the client know the information you seek is impor-tant. As you converse, observe the client, taking into account the eyes, facial expressions, posture, and ges-tures. These forms of nonverbal communication are all providing information to you (Bolton, 1979).

The types of questions chosen during the interview, affect the type of information each provides. Closed ques-tions usually require only a yes/no response. The use of open-ended questions is more appropriate, especially considering that the majority of written questions on the medical history are closed. Open-ended questions pro-vide space for the client to give information without being confined by the professional's categories. For example, "Do you have heart trouble?" can be misinter-preted or not answered affirmatively by those with heart murmurs, pacemakers, or cardiac arrhythmias. Using the question "Would you share with me any information your doctor has told you concerning you heart?" should allow for all ailments of the heart to be discussed. You might choose more open questions if the written form you use inadequately covers some physiological systems. If the client is unable to provide the essential information in a timely manner, "prompting" from the oral health care professional is acceptable. When responses from the clinician are required they should be nonjudgmental, concise, and demonstrate understanding and accep-tance. Further information about communication is pro-vided in Chapter 7.

As the practitioner questions the client concerning their disease status, there is specific information that must be determined such as:

1. The type and onset of disease.
2. The treatment received in the past.
3. The degree of severity of the disease or extent of damage.
4. The type of medical care the client is now receiv-ing; and
5. The results of follow-up testing.

Table 2-2 includes nine questions used to determine current disease status. Additional questions are necessary depending on the answers to these original questions. Another subset of questions is necessary if the client's dis-ease includes an "attack state" such as angina pectoris or stroke. "Attack states" will be addressed later in this chapter.

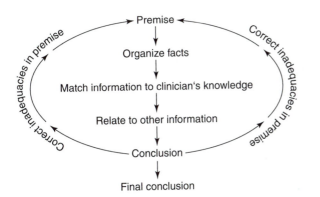

**Figure 2-2** A deductive reasoning model to evaluate health history information.

**Table 2-2  Questions to Determine Current Disease Status**

| Questions to Ask if "Disease State" Exists | Purpose for Asking the Question |
| --- | --- |
| 1. When was the condition diagnosed?<br>2. What type of disease or condition do you have? | • To determine type and onset of disease |
| 3. Were you treated by a physician for this condition? If so, what type of treatment? | • To determine treatment received in the past |
| 4. Do you have any limitations to your lifestyle as a result of this condition? If so, please describe them.<br>5. Were you hospitalized? If so, for how long? Were there any complications?<br>6. How extensive was the damage to the organ (e.g., heart, kidney, liver)? | • To determine degree of severity and/or extent of damage |
| 7. Are you taking any medications? What is the name and dosage of each prescription and nonprescription drug?<br>8. Are you currently seeking care from a physician for this condition? Are you currently receiving or are you scheduled to receive any treatment? | • To determine type of medical care currently receiving |
| 9. Have you had any follow-up testing? If so, what were the results? | • To determine results of follow-up testing |

Question 6 in Table 2-2 addresses the extent of damage to an organ to assess the need for treatment alterations. Depending on the client's responses, additional questions need to be asked by the clinician. For example, if the client answers affirmatively to liver disease on the medical history and if the extent of damage to the liver is significant, then the clinician must be alerted to potential bleeding problems due to liver dysfunction. If these questions confirm that bleeding is a problem, a physician consultation might be necessary before NSPT. If the treatment plan includes prescribing or administering drugs such as local anesthesia or erythromycin, this information should be discussed with the physician. Each different condition that results in extensive damage to an organ will have specific consequences that must be investigated prior to invasive treatment. Questions to determine bleeding potential may include:

1. Do you have abnormal bleeding?
2. Do you bleed after dental surgery or treatment?
3. Have you had any blood tests?
4. Do you know your prothrombin time?

In conclusion, the dental professional must possess effective listening skills including the ability to paraphrase, observe body language and verbal cues, stay present and not allow the mind to race ahead, and realize that words have different meanings for different people. Listening involves more than just hearing what the client is saying. The oral health professional who uses the written medical history, observes the client while performing verbal questioning, asks clear and concise questions, and uses deductive reasoning should feel confident that the information received is valid. Once this information is combined with the physical evaluation data,

including vital signs, adequate treatment plan alterations are made.

## Physician Consultations

If a consultation with the client's physician is necessary, the clinician should first obtain and document informed consent for the consultation in the record of services or via a specific document. The best alternative is to require written documentation before the request and release of information. Next, a document can be forwarded to the physician requesting specific health information including precautionary measures for dental/dental hygiene care (see Figure 2-3). This form can be faxed to the medical facility to expedite its return prior to the next dental hygiene visit. At times, a telephone conversation is needed to initiate or continue care during an appointment. In this case, the physician is the person of choice to speak to for this consultation. If a student is initiating the telephone call, it is viable to have a licensed professional confident with the procedure on the telephone during the professional discussion.

Information to be addressed during a physician's telephone consultation is outlined in Table 2-3. If the physician is not available, leave a time and phone number where you can be reached. If it is impossible to speak to the physician, then conversing with a licensed professional such as a Registered Nurse (RN) might be acceptable. After speaking to the physician or RN, notations are made in the client's record of services, including the date, name of the physician or RN, and information and treatment alterations. It is prudent to follow the telephone conversation with a written document requesting the physician's signature. Written documentation should always be filed in the client's chart for future reference.

**REQUEST FOR MEDICAL CONSULTATION**

Dental Hygiene Clinic
Department of Dental Hygiene
Idaho State University
Pocatello, ID 83209
(208) 236-3282 — FAX (208) 236-4071

TO:

_____
Physicians' Name

_____
Physician's Address

Date: _____

**CLIENT INFORMATION**

RE:

Name _____

_____

Address

Sex: _____ Birthdate: _____

---

**CLIENT CONSENT FOR RELEASE OF MEDICAL RECORDS**

I, _____ , consent to the release of my medical records to
               *(please print your name)*

_____ .
          *(office/clinic name here)*

_____     _____
Client Signature                          Date

---

**Request:** It is anticipated that dental hygiene treatment will extend over several months with appointments occurring weekly for 1-1/2- to 3-hour durations. Your client has reported the following:

_____ History of heart murmur, age _____
_____ History of rheumatic fever, age _____
_____ High blood pressure_____

_____ Anticoagulant therapy _____
_____ Diabetes, glucose level _____
_____ Other: _____

The treatment planned for your client includes:

    _____ Deep scaling and root planing/debridement (hemorrhage will occur)
    _____ Use of local anesthesia
    _____ Use of nitrous oxide analgesia
    _____ Other:_____

Our concerns for your client include the need for:

    _____ Antibiotic prophylactic premedication according to the AHA guidelines (1990)
    _____ Evaluation of high blood pressure prior to dental care
    _____ Evaluation of prothrombin time prior to dental care
    _____ Evaluation of glucose level prior to dental care
    _____ Other:_____

_____
Student Clinician Signature

_____
Registered Dental Hygienist Signature

_____
Supervising Dentist Signature

---

**Recommendations:** *Please indicate your recommendations/precautions for dental care in the space provided:*

_____    _____
Physician Signature                                 Date

**Figure 2-3** Sample medical consultation form. (Courtesy of Idaho State University, Department of Dental Hygiene, 1996)

**Table 2-3  Model for a Telephone Consultation**

| Information to Address | Example Dialogue |
|---|---|
| 1. Identify yourself to the receptionist. | "My name is _____ and I am a student dental hygienist/registered dental hygienist with _____ ." |
| 2. Identify the patient. | "Mr. M. J. Jones reports he is a patient of Dr. Blacks." |
| 3. Request to speak to the physician. | If the physician cannot be reached, leave a time when you can be contacted or request a convenient time to telephone the physician again. |
| 4. Identify your concerns. | "Mr. Jones reports a history of rheumatic fever, *or* a hip joint replacement in July 1994" *or* "Mr. Sellers blood pressure was recorded at 180/105 today prior to his dental treatment," or "Mr. Brown reports taking Coumadin." |
| 5. Share your treatment plan. | "I will be debriding Mr. Jones's teeth below the gumline. Hemorrhage will occur resulting in a bacteremia. Also, Mr. Jones will require local anesthesia." |
| 6. Ask specific questions. | "Should Mr. Jones be premedicated with antibiotics before therapy?" "Is Mr. Jones under your care for hypertension and is local anesthesia a risk?" *or* "What is the PT time or INR?" |

## PRETREATMENT ALTERATIONS

Aspects of a client's health that are significant to NSPT include antibiotic prophylactics, bleeding disorders, cancer treatment, medications, infectious disease, and vital signs. Safety of the client is the first concern of the dental hygienist and dentist. One criteria of an accurate medical history evaluation is the ability of the clinician to determine the need for pretreatment intervention. In other words, before the clinician uses an explorer or probes subgingivally to assess the client's periodontal condition, certain aspects of the client's health should be positively identified.

### Prophylactic Antibiotics

The American Heart Association (AHA) periodically publishes guidelines for antibiotic prophylactics to prevent **bacterial endocarditis**. The most recent guidelines were published in the Journal of the American Medical Association in 1990 and by the AHA in 1991 (Dajani et al., 1990; Dajani et al., 1991). Every dental professional needs to be aware of the current guidelines and have a copy readily available (see Table 2-4). These guidelines are published in medical and dental journals as well. Because consumers of oral health care are often not aware of the need for pretreatment antibiotic coverage, it is the responsibility of the clinician to establish that need (Dajani, Taubert, Millard, & Rahimtoola, 1991; Schlant, 1990).

The presence of rheumatic heart disease or an organic heart murmur are two indications for antibiotic prophylactic. **Rheumatic heart disease** is damage to the heart muscle and/or valves caused by the occurrence of rheumatic fever. Rheumatic fever is a group A beta-hemolytic streptococcal infection and in susceptible individuals results in permanent damage to the heart valve. Damage to the heart tissue might be evident during the acute stage of rheumatic fever or discovered long after the acute phase has subsided. A heart murmur is an abnormal sound heard during examination of the heart caused by altered blood flow into a chamber or through a valve. A murmur is classified by the time of its occurrence during the cardiac cycle, the duration, and the intensity of the sound. Systolic murmurs are graded by intensity on a scale from 1 to 6. The "grade" is determined by the physician or cardiologist who diagnoses and

**Table 2-4  Standard Adult Antibiotic Prophylaxis Regime for Dental Procedures for Patients Susceptible to Bacterial Endocarditis**

*For patients allowed to take amoxicillin/penicillin:*

Amoxicillin, 3.0 g orally 1 hour before procedure, then 1.5 g 6 hours after initial dose

*For amoxicillin/penicillin-allergic patients:*

Erythromycin ethylsuccinate, 800 mg, or erthromycin stearate, 1.0 g orally 2 hours before procedure, then half the dose 6 hours after original dose

OR

Clindamycin, 300 mg orally 1 hour before procedure and 150 mg 6 hours after initial dose

(Courtesy AMA. From American Medical Association "Prevention of Bacterial Endocarditis, Recommendations by the American Heart Association" by Adnan S. Dajani and others on the Committee on Rheumatic Fever, Endocarditis, and Kawasaki Disease of the Council on Cardiovascular Disease in the Young, 1990. *Journal of the American Medical Association, 264,* 2919–2922. © 1990 by the American Medical Association) rates the sound of the murmur from very faint (grade 1) to extremely loud (grade 6). An **organic heart murmur** is a pathologic murmur and needs antibiotic premedication. On the other hand, innocent, functional, or physiological heart murmurs often occur in childhood and are probably due to turbulence during the flow of blood through the heart. If these murmurs are innocent, they should disappear by adolescence. Functional murmurs can also occur during pregnancy due to the increased blood volume of the mother. A heart murmur caused by pregnancy will disappear soon after delivery. Therefore, clients with innocent, functional, or any nonorganic murmur do not have heart disease and do not require antibiotic prophylaxis. Functional heart murmurs can be correctly identified by the client's physician; however, referral to a cardiologist is sometimes necessary (Anderson, Anderson, & Glanze, 1994; Dajani et al., 1991).

A survey of commercially available health history forms in the United States and Canada reported 100 percent of the forms contained a question concerning rheumatic fever, but only 50 percent contained questions about a heart murmur (Thibodeau & Rossomando, 1992). If the health history form used does not specifically ask about the presence of a heart murmur, or any other condition specified by the AHA for antibiotic premedication, then these questions need to be added to the health history or included in the verbal dialogue. If a client responds "yes" to rheumatic fever or the presence of a heart murmur, the clinician should ask the client if a physician has recommended premedication for dental treatment or if he/she has been premedicated for previous oral health care. If either question is answered affirmatively, then the clinician knows antibiotic premedication is necessary for NSPT. However, if the client answers "no" to either of these questions, it is not automatically assumed that premedication with antibiotics is not needed. In this case, the oral health professional is legally responsible for determining the need for antibiotic premedication; not the client. It is advisable that the client's physician be consulted to ascertain the grade of heart murmur (grade 2 to 6 need antibiotic prophylactic) and/or the presence of rheumatic heart disease. Generally, clients are not able to determine need for antibiotic coverage; therefore, rheumatic heart disease or valvular dysfunction needs to be determined by their physician.

At times it is necessary for the client to visit the physician for a physical evaluation prior to care. If the attending physician is contacted for this evaluation, a letter similar to the one in Figure 2-3 might be used. This letter is either given to the client to be completed by the physician at the subsequent medical appointment or it is mailed directly to the physician. When a letter is used, a copy is retained in the client's chart. If a physician cannot be consulted to verify the need for antibiotic coverage or if the client is unable to see a physician for an evaluation, then antibiotic coverage should be initiated by the dentist for any invasive dental or dental hygiene procedures

included in the NSPT care plan. Invasive procedures include any dental treatment that causes bleeding such as exploring subgingivally, probing, scaling and root planing/debridement, or coronal polishing.

Other indications for antibiotic prophylactic determined by the AHA are listed in Table 2-5 (Dajani et al., 1990). A concise review of these conditions follows.

A prosthetic cardiac valve is an artificial heart valve and is considered at high risk for bacterial endocarditis. Anyone who has had bacterial endocarditis previously is also considered at high risk for bacterial endocarditis. Individuals currently receiving hemodialysis will have surgically constructed systemic-pulmonary shunts and require antibiotic premedication. The shunt or arteriovenous fistula allows the person to be "plugged in" to the hemodialysis machine at the fistula site. The individual's blood is passed through the hemodialysis machine, filtered, and returned to the individual. This surgically constructed shunt is potentially susceptible to infection

---

**Table 2-5  Cardiac Conditions\* for Which Endocarditis Prophylaxis May or May Not Be Indicated**

*Prophylaxis Recommended:*

- Prosthetic cardiac valves, including bioprosthetic and homograft valves
- Previous bacterial endocarditis, even in the absence of heart disease
- Surgically constructed systemic-pulmonary shunts
- Most congenital cardiac malformations
- Rheumatic and other acquired valvular dysfunction, even after valve surgery
- Hypertrophic cardiomyopathy
- Mitral valve prolapse with valvular regurgitation

*Prophylaxis Not Recommended:*

- Isolated secundum atrial septal defect
- Surgical repair without residual beyond six months of: secundum atrial septal defect, ventricular septal defect, patent ductus arteriosus
- Previous coronary artery bypass surgery
- Mitral valve prolapse without valvular regurgitation\*\*
- Physiological, functional, or innocent heart murmurs
- Previous Kawasaki disease without valvular dysfunction
- Previous rheumatic fever without valvular dysfunction
- Cardiac pacemakers and implanted defibrillators

\*This table lists selected conditions but is not meant to be all inclusive.
\*\*Persons who have mitral valve prolapse associated with thickening and/or redundancy of the valve leaflet may be at increased risk for bacterial endocarditis, particularly men who are 45 years of age or older.

(Courtesy AMA. From American Medical Association "Prevention of Bacterial Endocarditis, Recommendations by the American Heart Association" by Adnan S. Dajani and others on the Committee on Rheumatic Fever, Endocarditis, and Kawasaki Disease of the Council on Cardiovascular Disease in the Young, 1990. *Journal of the American Medical Association, 264* 2919–2922. © 1990 by the American Medical Association)

resulting from a bacteremia caused by dental procedures. The bacteremia also might be the source for infectious emboli that can cause endocarditis. Because of the use of heparin, a short-acting (four hours) anticoagulant used during dialysis therapy, clients should not be seen in the dental office the day of their dialysis treatment (Little & Falace, 1993). Clients with end-stage renal disease may require a consultation with a physician to discuss bleeding tendencies, healing problems, hypertension, hepatitis B surface antigen (HBsAG), or abnormal drug metabolism (Dajani et al., 1991; Little & Falace, 1993). Frequent recall intervals for maintenance of periodontal health are recommended for those on hemodialysis.

Congenital cardiac malformations that require antibiotic premedication include but are not limited to ventricular septal defect, pulmonary stenosis, patent ductus arteriosus, ventricular septal defect with pulmonary stenosis, aortic stenosis, and coarctation of the aorta. Septal defects refer to an opening in the wall separating the ventricular or atrial chambers of the heart. Stenosis refers to an abnormal condition characterized by a narrowing of an opening or passageway. Ductus arteriosus is a fetal connection between the pulmonary artery and aorta that allows fetal blood to bypass the lungs. If this passageway does not close within twenty-one days of birth, and remains patent (open), a cardiac condition results requiring antibiotic prophylaxis. Coarctation of the aorta is characterized by a narrowing of the aortic vessel. Hypertrophic cardiomyopathy is a condition characterized by gross hypertrophy of the ventricular septum and left ventricular free wall. This condition also affects the function of the heart causing reduced cardiac output and does require antibiotic prophylaxis before invasive dental procedures. If a patient reports a mitral valve prolapse, the presence of regurgitation must be determined. Mitral valve prolapse is a condition in which the leaflets or flaps of the valve are thickened. Consequently, the valve may not close tightly and regurgitation of blood may occur. If regurgitation is not present, antibiotic premedication is not required. A consultation with the client's physician will be necessary to determine the presence or absence of regurgitation.

Table 2-5 also includes conditions that do not require antibiotic prophylaxis. Congenital cardiac malformations not requiring antibiotic premedication include isolated secundum atrial septal defect and malformations that have been surgically repaired without residual beyond six months. Atrial septal defects are often the result of a patent foramen oval, an embryonic opening in the atrial septum between the atrial chambers, that does not close in 25 percent of the population. A small atrial septal defect does not require antibiotic prophylaxis. Generally, if a patient has had a surgical repair in which no synthetic materials were used and at least six months has elapsed since the surgery, antibiotic coverage is not necessary. However, patients are usually unaware of the type of material used in the surgical repair of a cardiac malformation; therefore, a consultation with the patient's physician is mandatory (Little & Falace, 1993). Previous coronary artery bypass graft surgery does not put the client at risk for endocarditis, therefore, it is not recommended to employ antibiotic premedication. It is, however, prudent to wait six months after the surgery before elective dental treatment is performed. Mitral valve prolapse without valvular regurgitation and physiological, functional, or innocent heart murmurs do not require premedication as previously discussed. Kawasaki disease or mucocutaneous lymph node syndrome is a disease primarily of young children characterized by inflamed mucous membranes of the mouth, strawberry tongue, cervical lymphadenopathy, and a rash on the trunk of the body. Other characteristics may include arthralgia, meningitis, or electrocardiographic changes. The signs and symptoms are similar to rheumatic fever and a previous Kawasaki disease without valvular dysfunction does not require antibiotic coverage.

Another condition that does not require premedication is rheumatic fever without valvular dysfunction. It should be remembered that it is not a history of rheumatic fever that is of concern for antibiotic premedication, but the existence of rheumatic heart disease. Studies indicate that between 30 percent and 80 percent of individuals with a history of rheumatic fever experience rheumatic heart disease characterized by valvular dysfunction (Little & Falace, 1993). Only a client's physician or cardiologist can determine if heart disease has occurred as a result of rheumatic fever. The final conditions listed in Table 2-5 that do not require antibiotic prophylaxis before invasive dental care include cardiac pacemakers and implanted defibrillators. There is insufficient data available to make a recommendation for individuals with cardiac transplants. The client's cardiologist and surgeon should be consulted. As with any organ transplant, the administration of powerful immunosuppressive drugs renders the person susceptible to infections.

There are instances when antibiotic prophylactic is necessary for conditions beyond endocarditis. An example is the risk of secondary infection for prosthetic implants. There is no evidence that intraocular lenses or breast implants are at risk from transient bacteremias produced by invasive dental procedures. Results of a recent survey indicate that there is little risk of infection from transient bacteremias with penile implants (Little & Rodus, 1992). Jaspers and Little (1985) conducted a nationwide survey of 1,600 orthopedic surgeons who reported that 57 percent of respondents believed a relationship existed between transient dental bacteremias and secondary infections of the prosthetic joint area. However, 93 percent of respondents recommended antibiotic prophylactic before invasive dental treatment. The drug of choice for the majority of respondents for joint prosthesis was cephalosporin (Jaspers & Little, 1985). There is currently a controversy regarding the need for antibiotic prophylactic of persons with joint replacements. This controversy involves the question of risk for the individual. Is the risk of secondary infection higher or lower than the risk of allergic reaction to the antibiotic? Some studies suggest a higher risk for allergic reactions to penicillin than risk of secondary infection (Jacobson, Schweizer, DePorter, & Lee, 1988). Until the time that specific guidelines are established for antibiotic prophylactic prior to NSPT, physician consultations are necessary for all clients with joint prostheses.

When a client is premedicated with antibiotics, specific information should be recorded in the record of oral health care services including the specific antibiotic prescribed, the route of administration, the dosage, the timing of leading dose, and the timing of following dose. Confirmation that the antibiotic was taken and statements concerning the posttreatment dose should be recorded for each appointment in which the antibiotic was taken by the client (Little, 1993). If the client you are premedicating with antibiotics is a female of childbearing age, information concerning the interaction of antibiotics and oral contraceptives needs to be given to her. Additional contraceptive devices must be considered during the entire month in which the antibiotic treatment is given (Zachariasen, 1991).

There should always be a seven- to fourteen-day hiatus of treatment between antibiotic premedications to allow the oral bacteria to return to its original state. If the client is already taking penicillin or any other antibiotic for any medical reasons, then the antibiotic used for dental prophylactic purposes must be a different antibiotic (Wahl & Wahl, 1993). For instance, if the client is taking a low dosage of penicillin to reduce the risk of a second occurrence of rheumatic heart disease, then the drug of choice for premedication is erythromycin. The purpose of switching the drug is to ensure that the oral cavity is not resistant to the prophylactic drug. If an adequate wait time is not feasible, rotating different antibiotics to minimize the possibility of resistance is also acceptable (Otomo-Corgel, 1990). Before erythromycin is prescribed it must be confirmed that the client is not taking terfenadine (Seldane) concurrently because of the potential for developing a life-threatening cardiotoxicity with that particular drug interaction (Wynn, 1993). Whatever the antibiotic prescribed, any allergies to the antibiotic to be used must be established prior to writing the prescription or dispensing the drug. There is a risk of allergic reaction every time an individual uses antibiotic medication; therefore, it is prudent of the oral health professional to explain the signs of allergy whenever a drug is dispensed.

The use of antibiotics is not the only way to help reduce the risk of endocarditis. Antimicrobial rinses should be used by the client prior to invasive procedures. Whenever possible, extensive procedures should be postponed until the maximum achievable health of the gingiva can be attained through thorough homecare techniques. Both antimicrobial rinses and optimal oral self-care can decrease the probability and magnitude of transient bacteremias; however, using these methods does not alleviate the need for antibiotic prophylactic. Frequent three- or four-month maintenance appointments and an emphasis on thorough oral hygiene is extremely important for clients susceptible to endocarditis because bacteremias can be caused by brushing or interdental cleaning. It is much easier for an individual to maintain oral health if the periodontal conditions are favorable; therefore, maintenance of periodontal health through NSPT is important (Tzukert, Leviner, & Sela, 1986).

## Bleeding Disorders

A second area of concern for the client that must be discussed and evaluated before any treatment is rendered involves bleeding disorders. Persons can experience bleeding tendencies as a result of vascular wall alterations, disorder of platelet function or number, or disorders of coagulation. Questions used to identify bleeding disorders include:

1. Have you ever experienced abnormal bleeding?
2. Do you bleed a long time after a cut?
3. Do you have a bleeding disorder?
4. Do you bruise easily?
5. Do bleeding disorders run in your family?
6. Are you taking anticoagulants, blood thinners, or aspirin?

Questions identifying family history of bleeding problems are aimed at identifying hereditary problems such as hemophilia, Christmas disease, and von Willebrand's disease. Questions concerning abnormal bleeding, bleeding disorders, or taking drugs might identify sources of acquired disorders of coagulation such as liver disease, or taking broad spectrum antibiotics or anticoagulants. Bleeding disorder questions might also identify sources of platelet dysfunction such as aspirin, nonsteroidal anti-inflammatory drugs, alcohol, or a reduction in platelet numbers caused by radiation therapy or leukemia.

Being aware of the causes for bleeding potential in clients and using multiple questioning techniques improve the clinician's ability to assess the need for alteration of treatment plans prior to therapy. For example, clients with disorders of platelet release often caused by recent use of acetylsalicylic acid (ASA) or ibuprofen do not need treatment alterations unless other platelet or coagulation disorders exist. The effects on platelets occur within hours of ingestion of aspirin or ibuprofen and last about nine days until "platelet reversal" occurs. "Platelet reversal" is the time needed for old platelets to be cleared from the body. In general, if clients are taking small doses of aspirin (less than 1,300 to 2,400 mg/day), then changes in homeostasis are not clinically significant. An Ivy bleeding time test is warranted if the dental professional is unsure of the client's ability to clot normally due to platelet or vascular phase dysfunction. Thrombocytopenia, or a reduction in platelet number, potentially caused by leukemia or radiation therapy does require physician consultation prior to treatment. Acquired disorders of coagulation such as liver disease or disruption in the intestinal flora that produces vitamin K also require a physician's consult before initiating oral health care.

If the client is taking oral anticoagulants (Coumadin), results of laboratory tests can indicate safety levels for providing treatment. Prothrombin time (PT), a test of extrinsic and common pathway function, is normally twelve to fifteen seconds. The test reflects the ability of blood lost from vessels in the area of the injury to effectively coagulate. The therapeutic range will be 1.2 to 1.5 times higher than the normal 12 to 15 seconds (Carr & Mason, 1992). The International Normalized Ratio (INR) expresses PT as a ratio of the patient's PT over the control PT and is now the preferred method of monitoring coagulation time. The INR numbers will be altered because the thromboplastins used for the PT test are obtained from a different source in an attempt to standardize oral coagulant control throughout the world. The therapeutic range for INR is generally between 2.0 and 3.0, which is equivalent to the North American PT time of 1.2 to 1.5 (Hirsh, Deydin, & Potter, 1986). Therefore, hemorrhage problems should not occur if the client's PT time is below 1.5 times normal or INR time is less than 3.0.

A client with a bleeding disorder, whether genetic or acquired, requires certain pretreatment procedures. Consultation with the attending physician ensures underlying conditions are identified and preparations made. Preparations might include alteration of anticoagulant drugs, use of local homeostatic agents, or avoidance of aspirin, aspirin-containing compounds and NSAIDs for pain or control of inflammation (Roda, 1992; Carr & Mason, 1992). The client's anticoagulant drug therapy should not be altered without consent from the appropriate physician. If PT or INR times are not within normal limits, no treatment that could result in bleeding should be undertaken without a physicians consultation.

## Cancer Treatment

Individuals who are scheduled to begin receiving cancer therapy (radiation or chemotherapy), those who are currently receiving it, or those who have received it in the past need to be identified via the health history. Pretreatment strategies, oral care during treatment, and frequent maintenance visits can minimize the oral complications from cancer therapy (Carl, 1981). If an individual is scheduled to begin head and neck radiation therapy, several pretreatment considerations exist. Teeth in the radiation field need a thorough periodontal evaluation prior to radiation therapy. All teeth, particularly the mandibular teeth due to decreased vascularity in the mandible, must be periodontally stable and healthy. Mandibular teeth with furcation involvement must be extracted fourteen to twenty-one days prior to radiation therapy (Barker, Barker, & Gier, 1992). There is evidence that a minimum delay of twenty-one days after tissue wounding should be recommended. If a surgical procedure must be performed in an area of irradiated tissue, a presurgical course of hyperbaric oxygen is necessary (Marx & Johnson, 1987).

Once the client is periodontally stable, maintenance of periodontal health is important. Ongoing periodontal disease is a contributing factor in **osteoradionecrosis** or bone necrosis due to irradiation. However, treatment for periodontal disease is a concern. Periodontal procedures, such as scaling and curettage in the area of radiation should be considered with caution, especially in the mandible (Beumer & Lewis, 1989). The longer the time since radiation treatment, the less vascularity and consequently the greater the risk for osteoradionecrosis (Marx & Johnson, 1987). NSPT using gentle hand instrumentation, without the use of ultrasonics, is indicated after completion of radiation treatment. If periodontal instrumentation is planned for an area that was in the direct field of radiation, there can be absolutely no loss of integrity of the epithelial attachment or the client is at risk for exposed bone. Subgingival scaling or root planing is contraindicated in mandibular areas that were in the direct field of radiation. Maxillary areas have better vascularity and can be successfully debrided with gentle hand scaling without extreme risk of osteoradionecrosis (Stauts, 1993; Yusof & Bakri, 1993).

Frequent recare is necessary for the individual after radiation treatment. Maintenance appointments should be scheduled at four- to six-week intervals for the first six months and then at three- to four-month intervals thereafter. Immaculate oral hygiene is important and must be reinforced by the periodontal therapist. If teeth become severely periodontally involved, a dilemma exists for the dentist because extraction of teeth even up to twenty-five years after radiation treatment can cause osteoradionecrosis. In addition to the client's periodontal needs, a fluoride tray should be prepared prior to radiation therapy because of salivary changes leading to radiation caries. A consultation with the client's oncologist is necessary prior to dental treatment to determine the location of radiation and boost fields, the dosages, and the dates of treatment (Barker et al., 1992; Marx & Johnson, 1987; Stauts, 1994; Yusof & Bakri, 1993). Oral complications resulting from radiation therapy of the head and neck might include salivary changes, xerostomia, mucositis, difficulty swallowing, loss of appetite, loss of taste, trismus, radiation caries, and osteoradionecrosis (Carl, 1993; Yusof & Bakri, 1993). Treatment for those with xerostomia after radiation therapy is dependent upon the residual salivary gland function. If salivary gland function remains, the use of a sialagogue, saliva production stimulator, should be considered. Research indicates Pilocarpine and Bethanechol may be successful in the relief of symptoms of xerostomia (Epstein, Burchill, Emerton, Le, & Silverman, 1994; Johnson, Ferretti, Nethery, Valdez, Fox, Ng, Muscoplat, & Gallagher, 1993; Ferguson, 1993). Additional treatment for xerostomia is covered in the following section on medications.

Forty to fifty percent of individuals receiving chemotherapy experience oral complications (Carl, 1993). These oral changes might include mucositis; decrease in platelet and leukocyte count; salivary changes with subsequent caries; and viral, bacterial and fungal infections. Pretreatment consultation with the attending oncologist is necessary after acquiring the medical history data and prior to planning oral health care. The presence of an indwelling catheter will determine if a periodontal assessment can be completed before the physicians consultation. The information that needs to be verified is white blood cell counts, platelet count, schedule and length of chemotherapy treatment, and presence of a catheter. If the person currently has a central indwelling venous catheter, antibiotic prophylactic according to the AHA guidelines is mandatory prior to invasive dental procedures (Spuller, 1988).

## Medications

A fourth pretreatment category that needs to be identified from the health history involves adverse pharmacological considerations of the medications taken by clients. As the body ages the incidence of periodontal disease increases. Although NSPT might be indicated for individuals of any age, the geriatric client is particularly susceptible to periodontal disease. When a geriatric client is in the dental office, the same adherence to in-depth medical history taking is necessary; however, even a greater concern for an accurate past and current history of medications is needed. Eighty-five percent of the elderly take at least three medications a day. Four out of five elderly people have at least one chronic disease and one out of two have more than two chronic diseases (Swapp, 1990; Terezhalmy, 1989). Over 150 frequently prescribed medications are known to cause approximately 46 oral and perioral side effects (Matthews, 1990). Data from a study of 3,217 non-institutionalized elderly showed that 51 percent were on medications causing xerostomia, 39 percent took medications affecting hemostasis, 28 percent were at risk of drug-induced soft tissue reactions, 22 percent reported taking medications that interact with drugs used in dentistry, 20 percent took medications requiring that a vasoconstrictor be minimized, and 16 percent took medications indicating reduced stress tolerance (Levy, Baker, Semla, & Kohout, 1988). Each of these side effects have the potential to alter the treatment; therefore, clinicians must be knowledgeable about their client's medications.

Chronic dry mouth, or xerostomia has been associated with dental disease. Although the presence of xerostomia does not increase the incidence of periodontal disease, it is associated with many clinical problems such as reduced denture retention, increased dental caries, and difficulties in mastication, swallowing, and talking. Drugs that can cause xerostomia include anticholinergics, antidepressants, antihypertensives, antipsychotics, diuretics, gastrointestinals, systemic antihistamines or decongestants, and systemic bronchodialators (Levy et al., 1988). If a client is experiencing xerostomia, the clinician can recommend using ice chips, sugarless candies, or frequent drinks of water for relief. The individual should refrain from eating spicy foods, eating dry and bulky foods, using tobacco or alcohol, or rinsing with commercial mouthwashes that contain alcohol. There are artificial saliva substitutes available for individuals who do not feel "relief" from previously mentioned techniques. A clinician could also suggest that the client consult with his physician to see about changing the medication to one without the side effects of xerostomia.

The most common ailments of the elderly are arthritis, neurological disorders, mental disorders, and cardiovascular disease (Swapp, 1990). A common medication for arthritis is nonsteroidal anti-inflammatory drugs (NSAIDs) such as acetylsalicylic acid (aspirin) or ibuprofen (Advil, Motrin, Lodine, Nalfon). NSAIDs are of special concern to dental professionals because naprosen (Naprosyn) and naproxen sodium (Anaprox), which are both NSAIDs, may be useful in the NSPT plan as an adjunct to periodontal instrumentation. Postoperative pain medication prescribed in dental offices often contains aspirin; therefore, a possible drug to drug interaction can occur. If a client takes a medication containing aspirin while on an NSAID, gastrointestinal effects and possible hemorrhage might occur (Roda, 1992).

Persons with compromised cardiovascular systems who may have suffered from a myocardial infarction (heart attack), angina pectoris, cerebral vascular accident (stroke), hypertension, cardiac arrhythmia, or congestive heart failure may be taking antihypertensives, angina pectoris medications, or antiarrhythmic medications. Any of these classifications of medications might require limiting the use of vasoconstrictors in local anesthesia. Desjardins (1992) published the twenty most common prescription drugs frequently encountered in dentistry. Seven out of twenty of these drugs were taken for cardiovascular disease and have adverse effects significant to dental professionals. The antihypertensive calcium channel blockers (Cardizem, Procardia, Calan) might cause taste changes and gingival hyperplasia. The gingival hyperplasia can be clinically indistinguishable from hyperplasia caused by phenytoin (Dilantin). The antihypertensive angiotesin converting enzyme (ACE) inhibitors (Vasotec, Capoten, Zestril) can cause taste impairment, oral ulcerations and angioedema of the lips, face, tongue, glottis, and larynx. If these side effects occur, the clinician must plan treatment accordingly. For example, oral ulcerations might be treated with sodium bicarbonate rinses, taste impairment might be relieved with zinc supplements, and gingival hyperplasia might be treated by surgical intervention. Benadryl elixir mixed with Kaopectate can be used as a topical anesthetic and coating agent for painful oral lesions (Little & Falace, 1993).

Medications that alter host resistance are of particular concern because of the potential for increased periodontal disease. Long-term antibiotics, insulin, oral hypoglycemics and systemic corticosteroids are all drugs that either cause immunosuppression or are taken by individuals with an altered response to infection. Oral candidiasis should be anticipated in immune compromised persons or in persons taking immunosuppressive drugs. Topical antifungal agents such as Nystatin oral suspension or Chlortrimazole should be used as rinses or allowed to dissolve in the mouth. Ketoconazole (Nizoral) and fluconazole (Difuican) are effective systemic drugs for mucocutaneous candidiasis (Little & Falace, 1993). In addition to increased susceptibility to infection, delayed healing may be a problem for clients taking insulin or corticosteroids. If oral health care is extremely stressful for the client, additional amounts of insulin or steroids may be indicated. Clients currently taking steroids may require doubling their normal dose on the day of the dental procedure. When an individual is in a stressful situation, cortisol must be available for the body to use. Individuals who have been taking corticosteroids might have suppressed adrenal production and, thus, will not be able to supply the body with the necessary cortisol. If this situation occurs, the individual may experience acute adrenal insufficiency that can result in death. Individuals who are extremely anxious about dental treatment and are taking corticosteroids or those who have just discontinued taking corticosteroids in the last two weeks are at greater risk for acute adrenal insufficiency. These individuals should have their steroid dosage doubled on the day of treatment. If significant posttreatment pain is anticipated, then doubling the normal steroid dose on the following day also might be necessary (Little & Falace, 1993).

Most clients taking medications will not experience the majority of the side effects discussed in this chapter. It is the responsibility of the dental hygienist to be aware of medication categories and possible adverse effects of medications associated with the length of time they are prescribed. In addition to asking the client which medications they have taken in the last year, the dental professional should inquire about indications for the medication, the dosage, who prescribed it, when it was prescribed, and when the drug was last taken. Resources should be available in the dental office that can provide information about adverse reactions, warnings, and contraindications for the drugs your clients take. The *Physicians' Desk Reference (PDR)* is a commonly used drug reference and is now available on computer or CD-ROM. Other reference books such as *Facts and Comparisons, USP DI and Advice for the Patient* are updated monthly and are, perhaps, more useful for oral health care professionals. Dental drug reference handbooks that identify specific dental considerations, such as *Mosby's Dental Drug Reference* (1996) are now available.

## Infectious Diseases

The presence of infectious disease in relation to asepsis is less problematic than in the past. The current standard of care is the application of universal precautions for all clients including the use of gloves, masks, and glasses. The use of disposable items and coverings, sterilization of all instruments including handpieces, and minimization of aerosol production are all prudent actions to take. The existence of an allergy to latex must be determined before entering the client's mouth with latex gloves. The proper use of the hepatitis B vaccination has significantly reduced the risk of contracting hepatitis B for dental hygienists and dentists, although the risk of hepatitis C still exists. If a client is in an active state of tuberculosis, hepatitis, measles, mumps, herpes, or sexually transmitted diseases, they should not receive oral health care until treatment, or time, has rendered them no longer infectious. The oral lesions of syphilis, gonorrhea, tuberculosis, herpes, and acquired immune deficiency syndrome (AIDS) are infectious. In addition, clients with a history of hepatitis should be evaluated for liver disease.

To date no dental professional using barrier techniques on a routine basis has contracted HIV within the confines of oral health care. The client who is seropositive to HIV does demand special consideration because of the oral symptoms involved and extreme immunosuppression. Increased frequency and duration of fungal, bacterial, and viral diseases of the oral cavity are common in the HIV-positive person. Increased severity of gingival and periodontal diseases creates the need to apply the principles of NSPT in the HIV seropositive individual including the use of antimicrobial treatment. The client's physician should be consulted prior to NSPT and meticulous aseptic technique should be practiced for the protection of both the client and oral health professional.

## Vital Signs

The final portion of pretreatment considerations involves the evaluation of the patient's vital signs including pulse rate and blood pressure. Vital signs should be taken on every new client for baseline data. Pulse rate greater than 100 or showing indications of irregular rhythm should be further investigated with the patient and then possibly with the physician. Routine monitoring of the pulse might be warranted depending on the reason for the irregularity. Systolic blood pressure readings of 140 to 160 and/or diastolic readings of 90 to 95 should be monitored for three consecutive appointments. Medical consultation is recommended if either the systolic or diastolic readings remains within these boundaries (Malamed, 1987). Blood pressure assessment should also be performed when therapy includes the use of nitrous oxide-oxygen analgesia and/or local anesthesia (see Chapter 9). Additionally, persons who have cardiovascular disease or who participate in hypertension therapy should have their blood pressure monitored each visit. Systolic pressure of 160 to 200 and/or diastolic pressure of 95 to 115 indicates a need for further evaluation (Malamed, 1987). Information such as age of the client, physician's monitoring of the blood pressure, and current or past use of antihypertensive medications should be taken into consideration. Depending on the situation, a consultation with the client's physician might be necessary. For example, an elderly patient with a blood pressure of 185/102 who is taking antihypertensives and being closely monitored by a physician, is at less risk for a cardiovascular emergency than a young person with the same blood pressure who is not under a physician's care or who is not taking antihypertensives. If systolic pressure is greater than 200 and/or diastolic pressure is greater than 115, NSPT should be postponed until clearance for treatment is obtained from the individual's physician (Malamed, 1987).

Client circumstances will dictate if blood pressure needs to be monitored at each three-, four-, or six-month interval for periodontal maintenance. For example, those with a past history of high blood pressure might be indicated for a recheck. Of course, clients whose blood pressure was monitored during the first series of appointments might also require monitoring at the maintenance visits. Malamed (1987) recommends those whose pressure is less than 140/90 be monitored yearly for new baseline data. In conclusion, a medical consultation should be considered for the safety of the client when vital signs, pulse, respiration, temperature, or blood pressure are not within "normal limits," and there is no reasonable explanation for this deviation.

## TREATMENT CONCERNS

In addition to pretreatment alterations, there is also information elicited from medical history or interview questions that indicate alterations in care during therapy. The conditions that may precipitate problems during therapy are stress, administration of local anesthesia, and client positioning.

### Stress

Information obtained from a health history that identifies cardiovascular disease, diabetes mellitus, or respiratory problems can be related to the stress of oral health care. If a client identifies a history of heart attack, angina pectoris, cardiac arrhythmia, congestive heart failure, hypertension, stroke, epilepsy, or asthma, special precautions of stress reduction protocol need to be implemented. Stress reduction protocol includes providing adequate pain control with local anesthesia and/or nitrous oxide, scheduling morning appointments, limiting the duration of the appointment, minimizing waiting time, talking to the patient about their fears and anxiety, and the use of pretreatment antianxiety medication (Malamed, 1987). When eliciting information from these clients during the health history interview, questions concerning the stability of the condition must be established. If a history of myocardial infarction, angina pectoris, cerebral vascular accident, asthma, epilepsy, or insulin-dependent diabetes is recorded, then the question strategy outlined in Table 2-6 is used to establish "risk of incident"

**Table 2-6 Questioning Strategy for "Attack" Conditions**

*A. Questions to ask the client to determine "risk."*

1. How often do you have attacks?
2. When was your last attack?
3. What brings on your attacks?
4. Are you under a physician's care?
5. Have you ever been hospitalized because of your attacks?
6. Are any of your normal activities limited?
7. Please describe a typical attack.

*B. Questions to ask to determine the client's management of the attack.*

1. How do you manage the episodes?
2. Do you use medications?
3. Do you have the medications with you?

*C. Clinician Choices after Questioning:*

1. Consult with physician.
2. Postpone treatment.
3. Continue with therapy.

during treatment. These initial seven questions (see Section A) should give the clinician enough information to know if more questions are necessary (see Section B). After questioning, the clinician has three choices: 1) to consult with the physician, 2) to postpone treatment, or 3) to continue with therapy (see Section C). Asking these questions should prepare the clinician for potential medical emergencies.

**Cardiovascular Disease.** If a patient has experienced a myocardial infarction, stroke, or cardiac bypass surgery within the last six months, it is suggested that treatment be postponed until after the six month point to decrease the risk of a second episode (Dajani et al., 1991; Perusse, Goulet, & Turcotte, 1992a). If a client reveals recent changes in the status of their disease, postponing treatment until the client visits the physician is prudent behavior. If the client reports the presence of a cardiac pacemaker inquire about its location, the type, and date of placement. In addition, the reason for the placement of the pacemaker is necessary to know because valvular disease is an indication for pacemakers and would require antibiotic premedication.

Because of the stress of a dental appointment, the clinician must be prepared for a medical emergency. The use of stress reduction protocol will reduce the risk of an emergency with a cardiovascularly compromised patient; however, three situations may manifest to elicit a medical emergency. First, the stress reduction may not be working. Secondly, the cardiovascular system may be more fragile than originally thought. Lastly, the procedure may be too involved for the client, because of the type of procedure or the length of the procedure. In the event of a medical emergency, specific procedures need to be followed depending on the specific problem encountered. Many textbooks and articles are dedicated to handling medical emergencies in the dental office (Malamed, 1993; Little & Falace, 1993).

**Diabetes Mellitus.** Diabetes mellitus is a chronic multifactorial disease that affects metabolism of carbohydrates, fats, and proteins. There are two types of diabetes mellitus. Type I, or insulin-dependent diabetes mellitus (IDDM), affects 10 to 15 percent of the population and was formerly known as juvenile diabetes. Type II, or non-insulin-dependent diabetes mellitus (NDDM), affects 85 to 90 percent of the population and was formerly known as adult-onset diabetes. The common factor in diabetes of both types is a relative or absolute lack of insulin or inadequate function of insulin in the body. Differences occur in the pattern of genetic inheritance, insulin responses, and origin of the disease (May, 1990).

A person with diabetes mellitus is of particular concern to dental professionals rendering NSPT. First, the diabetic is a "potential risk" for a medical emergency involving hypoglycemia. Once a client is determined to be diabetic, specific information needs to be collected to identify the risk potential. Information concerning age of onset, type of diabetes, and method of controlling the disease such as insulin, oral medication, diet, or exercise needs to be determined. In addition, the regularity of physician visits, the date of the last insulin reaction, the normal glucose level, the glucose level today, the insulin and eating schedule, and the time of last meal and insulin shot also need to be investigated. An awareness of cardiovascular and renal complications from diabetes should also be taken into account.

Secondly, there are numerous oral complications of diabetes mellitus, including xerostomia, cheilosis, reduced salivary flow, increased glucose in saliva, and increased fungal infections such as candidiasis. A controversy exists in the literature with regard to the prevalence, severity, and extent of periodontal disease in those with diabetes mellitus. This confusion and disagreement in the literature is due partially to researchers not differentiating between types of diabetes mellitus in their sample and the different measures and indices of periodontal disease. The variable nature of both diabetes and periodontal disease also makes comparing and contrasting results difficult. Another factor affecting the ability to generalize results of studies is that most clients have Type II diabetes mellitus, but most studies have been conducted using a sample of Type I diabetes or unknown types (Schossman, 1994). Beyond the controversy, there is general agreement that incidence and prevalence of gingivitis and periodontitis is higher in diabetic groups (Rees & Otomo-Corgel, 1992; Schossman, 1994). The extent of risk of periodontal disease might depend on the extent of control of the disease, therefore, treatment recommendations will be presented following that format.

NSPT is of particular importance to the diabetic not only due to reasons already discussed, but due to results of studies showing that the presence of plaque retentive calculus affects the severity of the periodontal disease (Sastrowijoto, Hillemans, van Steenbergen, Abraham-Inpijn, & deGraaff, 1989; Tervonen & Oliver, 1993). Therefore, regular maintenance appointments for periodontal debridement, motivation, and self-care instruction are essential components of nonsurgical care for diabetics. Well-controlled NIDDM individuals can be treated as healthy normal clients. NSPT is a valuable part of their total oral care plan due to increased incidence of periodontal disease. Eighty percent of NIDDM persons are overweight; therefore, nutritional counseling is appropriate. Confirmation of glucose level, medications, diet control, and physician visits should be documented. Medical complications of diabetes such as hypertension, cerebrovascular accident, coronary athererosclerotic heart disease, and renal disease should be monitored (Ross & Otomo-Corgel, 1992). Uncontrolled or questionably controlled NIDDM requires a referral to a physician prior to oral health care. Once control is achieved, aggressive therapy of periodontal disease is recommended because control of periodontal disease is an essential feature in establishing and maintaining metabolic control in diabetes (Sammalkorpi, 1989).

In controlled IDDM, NSPT can be performed with consideration given to previously mentioned precautions. Maintenance appointments should be scheduled at no more than three- to four-month intervals to permit close monitoring of periodontal disease. Appointments should be scheduled in the morning after breakfast and insulin administration. Confirmation and documentation that insulin was taken and of blood glucose level results is recommended. Epinephrine in local anesthesia should not exceed 1:100,000 and only a minimum amount should be used. Symptoms of an insulin reaction need to be monitored and recognized by the clinician (Bauman, 1989; May, 1990; Ross & Otomo-Corgel, 1992). In poor or questionably controlled IDDM clients, periodontal therapy including NSPT requires systemic support to enhance wound healing. Medical complications of diabetes tend to manifest during periods of poor control of blood glucose levels; therefore, a physician's referral and cooperation is necessary. If control is achieved and maintained, NSPT may be considered with close medical monitoring (Ross & Otomo-Corgel, 1992).

Management of oral complications of diabetes mellitus will include NSPT and treatment of dental caries as a result of reduced salivary flow and increased glucose in the saliva. Increased dental caries is seen primarily in poorly controlled diabetic patients (Murrah, 1985). A diabetic client can be an excellent candidate for NSPT once a health status has been established and the disease controlled. Posttreatment healing should always be closely monitored in diabetic patients (Bauman, 1989; Perusse, Goulet, & Turcotte, 1992b).

**Respiratory and Other Stress-Induced Problems.** Asthma is exacerbated by stress and often requires drug therapy. An individual should be asked the questions listed in Table 2-6 to ascertain the risk of a medical emergency in the dental environment. If an individual uses a bronchodilator, it should be available at each oral health care appointment and stress reduction protocol should be utilized during therapy.

Persons suffering from epilepsy may be taking phenytoin (Dilantin), which has a side effect of gingival hyperplasia. This type of gingival overgrowth will have consequences for the client undergoing NSPT. Dialogue questions similar to the ones listed in Table 2-6 will aid the clinician in risk assessment for a medical emergency in the dental office. Again, stress reduction protocol should be used.

## Immunosuppression

Oral health care for individuals who are infected with the human immunodeficiency virus (HIV) or who have advanced to the stage of acquired immunodeficiency syndrome (AIDS) presents a unique challenge for clinicians. The oral complications of HIV infection are of particular concern to dental hygienists and dentists alike. The dental hygienist may be the first health care professional to identify the HIV infection and is in a position to closely monitor the progression of the disease. The initial HIV infection manifests itself as a mononucleosis-like syndrome with a skin rash for two to four weeks. The infection then becomes asymptomatic for one to twenty years. The first of the later clinical stages is a persistent generalized lymphadenopathy with a low-grade fever. Lymphadenopathy is characterized by the presence of lymph nodes greater than one centimeter in diameter and present for more than three months (American Academy of Periodontology, 1994).

Individuals with either the asymptomatic infection or persistent generalized lymphadenopathy may show increased prevalence of candidiasis, herpetic stomatitis, angular cheilitis, and hairy leukoplakia (Phelan, Salzman, Friedland, & Klein, 1987; Silverman, Migliorati, Lozada-Nur, Greenspan, & Conant, 1986; Swango, Kleinman, & Konzelman, 1991). An increase in the prevalence of acute necrotizing ulcerative gingivitis (ANUG) in HIV-infected individuals has been noted also (Melnick et al., 1989; Swango et al., 1991). As the disease progresses, a client might present with persistent fever, diarrhea, weight loss, neurological disorders, secondary infectious diseases, and secondary cancers. Oral lesions such as hairy leukoplakia, Kaposi's sarcoma, ANUG, and HIV-associated periodontal diseases are seen with increasing frequency as the patient's immunocompetence declines (Laskaris, Hadjivassiliou, & Stratigos, 1992; Phelan et al., 1987; Silverman et al., 1986).

In an attempt to broaden the classification of HIV periodontal diseases to include other immunosuppressed persons, HIV-gingivitis is currently termed "linear gingival erythema" (LGE) as seen in HIV-infected individuals, and HIV-periodontitis is currently called "necrotizing ulcerative periodontitis" (NUP) as seen in HIV-infected individuals (American Academy of Periodontology, 1994). HIV-infected individuals with LGE demonstrate a 2 to 3 mm marginal band of intense gingival erythema with possible diffuse areas of erythema extending beyond the mucogingival line. The distinguishing clinical hallmark of LGE is that the condition does not respond to conventional scaling and root planing (Winkler, Murray, Grassi, & Hammerle, 1989). NUP seen in HIV-infected individuals manifests itself as marginal necrosis of the gingiva and rapid destruction of the alveolar bone (Winkler et al., 1989). Severe pain and spontaneous bleeding usually accompany NUP. Extensive destruction of the underlying alveolar bone can occur within three to six months (Williams, Winkler, Grassi, & Murray, 1990).

Management of LGE and/or NUP lesions in HIV-positive individuals involves NSPT. Scaling to remove plaque and calculus deposits is necessary and debridement of necrotic tissue when present is recommended (Porter, Luker, Scully, Glover, & Griffiths, 1989; Winkler et al., 1989; Winkler & Robertson, 1992). During debridement, povidone-iodine irrigation, such as a 10 percent oral suspension of Bentadine, should be used for its antiseptic, anesthetic, and coagulation properties (Winkler & Robertson, 1992). The povidone-iodine is administered as an intrasulcular lavage performed with a disposable syringe and blunt needle at each appointment. If an iodine allergy exists, a saline solution may be substituted. Antibiotics should be used with caution due to increased risk of *Candida albicans* in individuals who are HIV-infected. If antibiotics are necessary to control the disease process, a narrow spectrum antibiotic such as metronidazole is recommended. Metronidazole is effective in a short course, low dose (250 mg four times a day for four to five days), and helps reduce pain and promotes rapid healing (Williams et al., 1990; Winkler et al., 1989).

Following initial debridement in NSPT, frequent follow-up care is necessary to thoroughly remove deposits and encourage strict plaque control. The use of antimicrobial mouthrinses such as chlorhexidine is effective in reducing symptoms and preventing recurrence of LGE and NUP (Winkler et al., 1989). Regular long-term maintenance is necessary for HIV-positive clients. Once the oral conditions have become stabilized, three-month recall intervals for periodontal maintenance are recommended (Winkler & Robertson, 1992).

Oral lesions beyond LGE and NUP must also be managed by the oral health professional. Candidiasis should be treated with topical and systemic antifungal agents as discussed earlier. Viral infections, such as herpes simplex and herpes zoster can be treated with Acyclovir. Neoplasmas such as Kaposi's sarcoma and oral lymphoma are treated with frequent scaling and root planing and then radiation or chemotherapy (Little & Falace, 1993). The individual's response to NSPT depends upon conditions including the client's current HIV stage, intake of systemic medications to treat HIV infection, use of antibiotics, or current oral habits such as tobacco smoking (American Academy of Periodontology, 1994).

Clients with leukemia who are on myelosuppressive therapies show an increased risk of progressing periodontitis (Wright, 1987). It seems as though the use of immunosuppressive agents and broad spectrum antibiotics promote microbial shifts in the subgingival microflora. These shifts enable pocket colonization by opportunistic pathogens that may encourage destructive periodontal disease. The use of antimicrobial agents should be considered in treatment (Rams & Slots, 1990). If an individual is in the acute stage of leukemia, he or she should receive only conservative emergency care. Clients who are in a state of remission may receive NSPT if special considerations are taken. A consultation with the physician is necessary before any therapy is rendered. A bleeding time test should be obtained on the day of the appointment to establish that an adequate number of functional platelets is present. Prophylactic antibiotic therapy may be necessary to prevent postoperative infection if severe neutropenia is present. Special attention should be given to oral hygiene instruction to reduce the incidence of dental caries and periodontal disease (Little & Falace, 1993).

Other conditions that show progressive periodontitis are neutropenia, Papillon-Lefevre Syndrome, Crohn's disease, and Down syndrome. In each of these diseases the host response to periodontal disease is compromised and subgingival microorganisms may be difficult to eradicate with mechanical debridement alone. The use of supplemental systemic antimicrobial therapy may be necessary for effective treatment of periodontal disease (Slots & Rams, 1991).

## Tobacco Smoking

Tobacco smoking might be the most important environmental factor in the United States associated with periodontal disease (Haber & Kent, 1992). The effect of smoking on periodontal health has been discussed for decades. Recently, however, strong associations between cigarette smoking and alveolar bone loss, tooth loss, and the prevalence and severity of periodontitis have been documented (Haber, Crowley, Mandell, Josipura, & Kent, 1994; Horning, Hatch, & Cohen, 1992; Stoltenberg, Osborn, Pihlstrom, Herzberg, Aeppeli, Wolff, & Fisher, 1993; Thomson, Garito, & Brown, 1993). Horning et al. (1992) identified four factors that have a statistically significant relationship to the prevalence of periodontal disease. These factors were age, sex, smoking, and racial background. Smoking was the only significant risk factor identified of which the client has control. A study by Ismail, Burt, and Eklund (1983) showed greater severity of periodontal disease in smokers when age, race, sex, income, education level, and oral hygiene practices were held constant. Cigarette smokers are a high-risk group for periodontitis.

Diabetes mellitus was discussed earlier as a risk factor for periodontal disease. A study involving insulin dependent diabetes mellitus (IDDM) patients and nondiabetic patients showed smoking as a significant factor in the risk of periodontal disease for both groups. Among the 19- to 30-year-old nondiabetic group, 12 percent of the newer smokers, 36 percent of the former smokers, and 46 percent of the current smokers had signs of periodontal disease. In the 31- to 40-aged nondiabetic clients, 33 percent of the newer smokers, 50 percent of the former smokers, and 88 percent of the current smokers demonstrated clinical signs of periodontal disease. Within the IDDM patients, the pattern remained consistent. In the 19- to 30-aged IDDM patients, 13 percent of new smokers, 50 percent of former smokers and 56 percent of current smokers demonstrated clinical parameters consistent with periodontal disease. Likewise, in the 31 to 40 age group, 54 percent of new smokers, 56 percent of former smokers, and 87 percent of current smokers demonstrated signs of periodontal disease (Haber et al., 1993). In a recent study using a sample of medically healthy, middle-aged adults, it was concluded that the odds of having a mean probing depth greater than 3.5 mm was five times greater for smokers than for the nonsmoker subsample (Stoltenberg et al., 1993). These data imply that medical status does not change the effects of smoking on the periodontal health of an individual.

The exact mechanisms by which cigarette smoking influences periodontal health are unknown. There is evidence that smoking causes local effects such as less gingival bleeding and inflammation (Haber, 1994). The pattern of pocketing differs for smokers in that there are more periodontal pockets in the anterior segment of the mouth. There is also more recession on anterior teeth and the gingival margin is thickened and rolled (Haber, 1994). Evidence also exists for systemic effects of smoking. The effects include inhibition of peripheral blood and oral neutrophil function, reduced antibody production, and alteration of peripheral blood immunoregulatory T cell subset ratios (Haber, 1994). Subsequently, clients have a compromised blood supply, an inhibition of healing responses, and a decrease in their immune competence (Rivera-Hidalgo, 1986). There does not, however, appear to be a difference in prevalence or frequency of periodontal pathogens between smokers and nonsmokers (Preber, Bergström, & Linder, 1992; Stoltenberg et al., 1993). These local and systemic factors might affect how smokers react to NSPT.

Smokers tend to respond differently when treated for periodontal disease. Reduction of pocket depth is minimal in response to periodontal instrumentation, and repocketing often occurs. Clients who continue to smoke during maintenance therapy tend to exhibit attachment loss over time. Recent studies have shown 86 to 90 percent of clients with refractory periodontitis were current smokers. Based on these data, smoking might be a contraindication for surgery for clients with periodontitis (Haber, 1994).

Based on the evidence that cigarette smoking is a significant risk factor for periodontal diseases, smoking cessation should be considered an essential part of NSPT. The inclusion of a question on the medical history as to the client's status of tobacco use gives the clinician an opportunity to educate the client about the negative periodontal effects of smoking. Although there have been no longitudinal studies of the effects of smoking cessation on periodontal status, studies that included former smokers found the periodontal status of former smokers ranked between that of current smokers and those who have never smoked (Haber & Kent, 1992; Haber et al., 1993). In conclusion, smoking status should be considered in the diagnosis, prognosis, and care planning for clients with periodontal diseases.

### Local Anesthesia

The use of local anesthesia during NSPT is a medical concern to clients taking specific drugs or to those with dysfunctional liver, kidney, or cardiovascular systems. Many drugs taken by clients undergoing psychiatric treatment such as tricyclic antidepressants (TCA), monoamine oxidase inhibitors (MAOIs), antianxiety drugs, and antipsychotic drugs have an interaction with the epinephrine, norepinephrine, or levonordefrin. Limiting the amount of epinephrine for those taking antipsychotic or antianxiety drugs is a safe policy to adopt. Although some controversy exists with regard to epinephrine and MAOIs, the consensus is to avoid vasoconstrictors if at all possible. Evidence exists that the use of local anesthesia with norepinephrine or levonordefrin is dangerous in clients taking TCAs. The lowest dose of local anesthesia with epinephrine capable of effective pain control is advised (Bennett, 1984; Malamed, 1990).

Beta-blockers, usually prescribed for their antihypertensive, antiarrhythmic, or antianginal affects, are either cardioselective or nonselective. The use of local anesthesia with a vasoconstrictor is not a risk for individuals taking cardioselective beta-blockers; however, some literature indicates that a risk of potential complications exists for those taking nonselective beta-blocking agents. Goulet, Perusse, and Turcottee (1992) caution dental professionals to avoid the administration of local anesthesia with a vasoconstrictor to a client taking nonselective beta-blockers such as metoprolol (Lopressor), atenolol (Tenormin), acebutolo (Scetral), and betaxolol (Kerlone). Persons using digoxin (Lanoxin) for treatment of congestive heart failure or arrhythmias or persons taking a thyroid replacement (Synthroid) also warrant the limiting of vasoconstrictors (Desjardins, 1992). A person with a severely dysfunctional liver or kidney might be at risk for local anesthesia overdose due to the limiting of biotransformation or elimination of the drug. Other predisposing factors to a local anesthesia overdose include factors such as age and body weight, presence of pathology including liver disease, kidney disease, congestive heart failure, and genetic deficiencies that need to be discovered during the health history interview. Drug factors including vasoactivity, dosage, route of administration, rate of injection, vascularity of injection site, and presence of vasoconstrictors are all factors to be considered during treatment using local anesthesia (Bennett, 1984; Malamed, 1987; Malamed, 1990). Further information concerning the use of local anesthesia for NSPT is presented in Chapter 9.

### Positioning

Client positioning during treatment might be of concern for some clients. For example, individuals suffering from emphysema or congestive heart failure may not be able to sit in a supine position. Clients suffering from arthritis may need to frequently change positions and clients who are pregnant may require positioning alterations to be comfortable in a dental chair. These specific client needs are determined during the health history interview and used during treatment to ensure a positive experience.

## POSTTREATMENT CONSIDERATIONS

There are factors to be considered in the posttreatment phase of NSPT that are discovered during the health history evaluation. Any healing problems that clients may experience as a consequence of immune suppression need to be considered. The presence of diabetes, radiation or chemotherapy, leukemia, steroid use, or HIV enhances the risk for secondary infection or delayed healing. The use of posttreatment antibiotic coverage may be considered.

Posttreatment pain control is another factor to consider. The use of NSAIDs or aspirin needs to be limited in clients suffering from kidney disease or gastrointestinal discomfort. These drugs are also contraindicated for those with bleeding disorders or blood dyscrasias. As with the use or prescription of any medications, allergies to drugs must be established. If an allergy exists, substitution of the drug is required. As mentioned earlier in the chapter, if antibiotics are prescribed, the signs and symptoms suggestive of an allergic reaction should be discussed. The first indications of an allergic reaction will probably be a skin rash, urticarial swelling, itching, and burning. The reaction can continue and the signs and symptoms include nausea, vomiting, tightening in the chest, shortness of breath, laryngeal edema, bronchospasm, and cardiac collapse. Oral health care settings should always have injectable epinephrine in case of an anaphylactic reaction.

# Summary

Acquiring accurate medical information allows the oral health professional to provide NSPT without risking the client's safety. As the client population changes and dental professionals recommend NSPT for more medically compromised persons, superior skill in health history evaluation is essential. Using a written health history in conjunction with verbal questioning is the most thorough approach to "history taking." If a practitioner is skilled in verbal questioning techniques, compensation for any inadequacies in the written form can be accomplished.

Certain client conditions must be identified prior to initiating oral health care. Pretreatment considerations include antibiotic prophylactics, bleeding disorders, cancer therapy, medications, infectious diseases, and vital signs. The treatment modifications necessary depend on the client's specific conditions. Using questioning strategies to determine the extent of the problem or the risk to the client aids the practitioner in establishing treatment alterations based on the medical history. Treatment concerns are identified by the health history but manifest themselves during NSPT. Many of these conditions can result in medical emergencies in the dental office if the health history is not evaluated properly and if necessary precautions are not taken. Additionally, not knowing the relationship of some disease states to periodontal disease could negatively affect the outcome of the recommended care plan. Cardiovascular diseases, diabetes, immunosuppression, tobacco smoking, and the use of local anesthesia are primary concerns. Posttreatment considerations include pain medication and healing potential after NSPT.

It is the responsibility of dentists and dental hygienists to stay current in the field of health history evaluation. Numerous new medications are approved yearly for use in the United States so the potential for unknown or newly discovered drug-to-drug interactions exists. NSPT has the potential for increased use of NSAIDs and antibiotics as a part of treatment; therefore, the incidence of drug-to-drug interactions could increase. Because the host immune system affects the incidence of periodontal disease, clients indicated for NSPT have potentially more medical conditions of consequence. Therefore, appropriate training in the art of medical history evaluation, availability of drug reference texts including the AHA guidelines for preventing bacterial endocarditis, and the desire to provide a safe environment for clients are necessary for all oral health care professionals.

# Case Studies

**Case Study One:** Mary Bohn, a 28-year-old female, presents herself to your office for a dental hygiene appointment. She has not seen a dentist since she was a child. On the health history she indicated she was born with a heart murmur. Further questioning revealed she thought is was gone because she played college tennis and never had a problem. Her physician never said anything about premedication with antibiotics, but she has not seen him for about ten years. She has never been premedicated before and reports not being able to afford to see a doctor right now. Mary also reports she is allergic to penicillin, taking Seldane for her allergies and hayfever, and using Ortho-Novum as a birth control measure. Is it appropriate to render NSPT today? Discuss the rationale for your response.

**Case Study Two:** Chet Severe, a 70-year-old male, has made an appointment at your office because of your NSPT program. The medical history indicates that he had a myocardial infarction six years ago. He also had bypass surgery, without complications, two years ago. Chet currently carries nitroglycerin tablets because he has occasional angina pectoris attacks. He has chronic adult periodontitis with generalized moderate deposits and generalized 4 to 5 mm periodontal probing depths. Chet's pulse is 85 and blood pressure is 160/100. He is taking Isoptil as an antihypertensive. Debridement with anesthesia is treatment planned. How should this treatment be modified?

**Case Study Three:** Thelma Sutton, a 62-year-old female, is appointed for a three-month maintenance visit. Her severe arthritis in the last three months has made brushing nearly impossible. She does not feel well and her ulcer is bothering her. Thelma is taking 800 mg Anaprox three times daily for her arthritis. Her periodontal evaluation shows severe gingivitis and heavy bacterial plaque accumulation. During her treatment, it is discovered that her plaque retentive calculus is extremely tenacious and extensive manipulation is necessary to remove the calculus. Thelma is complaining that her gums hurt; therefore, posttreatment pain control is given. Acetylsalicylic acid 325 mg with Codeine 30 mg is dispensed to Thelma to take as needed. Ten days later Thelma is admitted into the hospital with a bleeding ulcer. Do you think her treatment was a contributing factor to her bleeding ulcer? Discuss your rationale for your response.

**Case Study Four:** Henry Paz, a 45-year-old male, presents with a chief complaint of "bleeding gums" and he wants his "teeth cleaned." The medical history reveals a history of hepatitis. Henry thinks it was hepatitis A because he contracted it while in the hospital for an appendectomy eight years ago. He reports having "a bit of bleeding" when he had his last extraction three years ago. He also reports frequent nosebleeds. Henry's health has not been evaluated by a physician for eight years. He is not taking any medications. Local anesthesia and ultrasonic scaling are treatment planned for the appointment. Should this care plan be altered? If so, what alterations are indicated?

**Case Study Five (Part one):** Paula Mitton, a 22-year-old college student, presents herself for her first visit to the office at 8 A.M. Paula is an insulin-dependent diabetic, under the care of a physician in her hometown 250 miles away, and has no other significant medical conditions. She takes 30 mg of Lenti and 10 mg of regular insulin subcutaneously at 7 A.M. She also takes 15 mg of Lenti at 8 P.M. What questions should you ask Paula?

**Case Study Five (Part two):** After asking the appropriate questions, it is determined that Paula is well controlled with blood glucose levels from 130 to 150. She was hospitalized for initial diagnosis and regulation at age fourteen. Paula understands the disease process and has been under control for ten years. She took her normal insulin this morning at 7 A.M. and brought her breakfast in the car, but she was late for her appointment so did not get a chance to eat. She thought that her appointment was for an examination only and that she would be back to the car by 9 A.M. Should the treatment planned for today be continued? Why or why not?

# Case Study Discussions

**Discussion—Case Study One:** No, therapy that could cause bleeding such as probing, exploring, and debridement should not be rendered without antibiotic coverage. Mary needs to be evaluated by a physician to see if the murmur is present. The fact that the heart murmur has not limited her physical activities does not indicate the murmur is functional. If Mary is unable to be evaluated by a physician, she needs to be covered by antibiotic premedication until the physician can establish an absence of an organic murmur. Premedication with amoxicillin is contraindicated due to the penicillin allergy. Premedication with erythromycin is contraindicated because Mary is taking Seldane and these two drugs can have a life-threatening interaction. Thus, Clindamycin is the drug of choice. Mary should be encouraged to use additional birth control measures this month because antibiotics interfere with the effectiveness of oral birth control methods.

**Discussion—Case Study Two:** Yes, treatment should be modified because Chet has a history of cardiovascular disease and his blood pressure is above normal limits. Ques-

tions about his normal blood pressure and compliance in taking his antihypertensive medication are necessary. If his answers indicate a recent increase in blood pressure, an evaluation by his physician is necessary. Stress reduction protocol is in order for Chet and he should bring his nitroglycerin to his appointments. The smallest amount of local anesthesia with 1:100,000 epinephrine necessary to attain anesthesia is indicated. Vital signs should be taken at each visit.

**Discussion—Case Study Three:** Yes, a drug-to-drug interaction will occur between the NSAIDs, Anaprox, and the aspirin containing pain medication. Both of these drugs have anticoagulant qualities and gastrointestinal effects. Not only should aspirin containing medications not have been dispensed to Thelma, but there should have been further investigation by the dental professional into the ulcers and the NSAIDs she was taking for her arthritis.

**Discussion—Case Study Four:** Yes, due to the bleeding problem Henry should be evaluated by a physician before treatment is rendered. Henry is sent to a physician to evaluate the bleeding problem. It is discovered that Henry actually contracted hepatitis B while in the hospital and is a carrier. Subsequently, a significant amount of liver damage has occurred in the last eight years and a bleeding potential exists. After Henry is under the care of a physician, treatment may be started with alterations depending upon his PT time. Local anesthesia is biotransformed in the liver, so limited amounts should be used.

**Discussion—Case Study Five (Part one):** The following questions should be asked:

1. When were you diagnosed as a diabetic?
2. What is your normal glucose level and what is your level today?
3. Do you consider yourself well controlled?
4. When was your last insulin reaction?
5. Were you hospitalized?
6. When did you last eat, what did you eat, and when are you due to eat again?
7. How are you feeling?
8. What are your first symptoms of hypoglycemia?

**Discussion—Case Study Five (Part two):** No, Paula took her insulin but did not eat; therefore, she is at risk for hypoglycemia. The dental professional should dismiss her to allow her to eat breakfast. If time permits in Paula's schedule and in your schedule, you can continue treatment once she has eaten. If treatment is rendered without allowing Paula to eat, you are placing her at risk. Vital signs should be taken on Paula at the first visit for baseline data and once a year because of the potential for cardiovascular complications. Posttreatment healing should also be evaluated. Paula should be placed on a three-month periodontal maintenance schedule.

# REFERENCES

American Academy of Periodontology. (1994). *Periodontal considerations in HIV-positive patient. Committee on Research, Science, and Therapy.* Chicago: American Academy of Periodontology.

Anderson, K. N., Anderson, L. E., & Glanze, W. D. (1994). *Mosby's medical, nursing, and allied health dictionary* (4th ed.). St. Louis: Mosby-Year Book, Inc.

Barker, G. J., Barker, B. F., & Gier, R. E. (1992). *Oral management of the cancer patient: A guide for the health care professional* (4th ed.). Kansas City: University of Missouri School of Dentistry.

Bauman, D. B. (1989). Controlling complications for the diabetic patient. *Dental Hygiene News, 2*(4), 1, 6-7.

Benicewicz, D. & Metzger, C. (1989). Supervision and practice of dental hygienists: Report of ADHA survey. *Journal of Dental Hygiene, 63,* 173–180.

Bennett, C. R. (1984). *Monheim's local anesthesia and pain control in dental practice* (7th ed.). St. Louis: Mosby-Year Book, Inc.

Beumer, J. & Lewis, S. (1989). Osteoradionecrosis. In R. A. Kagan & J. Miles (Eds.), *Head and neck oncology clinical management* (pp. 83–90). New York: Pergamon Press.

Bolton, R. (1979). *People skills.* New York: Simon & Schuster.

Brady, W. F. & Martinoff, J. T. (1980). Validity of health history data collected from dental patients and patient perception of health status. *Journal of the American Dental Association, 101,* 642–645.

Bressman, J. K. (1993). Risk management for the 90s. *Journal of the American Dental Association, 124*(3), 63–67.

Campbell, P. R., Shuman, D., & Bauman, D. B. (1993). ADHA graduate student/faculty research project: Health history. *Journal of Dental Hygiene, 67,* 378–386.

Carl, W. (1981). Oral and dental care of cancer patients receiving radiation and chemotherapy. *Quintessence International, 12,* 861–869.

Carl, W. (1993). Local radiation and systemic chemotherapy: Preventing and managing the oral complications. *Journal of the American Dental Association, 124,* 119–123.

Carr, M. M. & Mason, R. B. (1992). Dental management of anticoagulant patients. *Journal of the Canadian Dental Association, 58,* 838–844.

Cottone, J. A. & Kafrawy A. H. (1979). Medications and health histories: A survey of 4,365 dental patients. *Journal of the American Dental Association, 98,* 713–718.

Dajani, A. S., Bisno, A. L., Chung, K. T., Durack, D. T., Freed, M., Gerber, M. A., Karchmer, A. W., Millard, H. D., Rahimtoola, S., Shulman, S. T., Watanakunakorn, C., & Taubert, K. A. (1990). Prevention of bacterial endocarditis. Recommendations by the American Heart Association. *Journal of the American Medical Association, 264,* 2919–2922.

Dajani, A. S., Taubert, K. A., Millard, H. D., & Rahimtoola, S. (Eds.). (1991). *Cardiovascular disease in dental practice.* Dallas: American Heart Association.

deJong, K. J., Borgmeijer-Hoelen, A., & Abraham-Inpijn, L. (1991). Validity of a risk-related patient-administered medical questionnaire for dental patients. *Oral Surgery, Oral Medicine, Oral Pathology, 72,* 527–533.

Desjardins, P. J. (1992). The top 20 prescription drugs and how they affect your dental practice. *Compendium of Continuing Education in Dentistry, 13*(9), 740–754.

Engel, P. (1991). *The norm of truth.* Toronto: University of Toronto Press.

Epstein, J. B., Burchell, J. L., Emerton, S., Le, N. D., & Silverman, S. (1994). A clinical trial of bethanechol in patients with xerostomia after radiation therapy. *Oral Surgery, Oral Medicine, Oral Pathology, 77,* 610–614.

Ferguson, M. M. (1993). Pilocarpine and other cholinergic drugs in the management of salivary gland dysfunction. *Oral Surgery, Oral Medicine, Oral Pathology, 75,* 186–191.

Goulet, J. P., Perusse, R., & Turcotte, J. Y. (1992). Contraindications to vasoconstrictors in dentistry: Part III. *Oral Surgery, Oral Medicine, Oral Pathology, 74,* 692–697.

Haber, J. (1994). Cigarette smoking: A major risk factor for periodontitis. *Compendium for Continuing Education for Dentistry, 15*(8), 1002–1014.

Haber, J. & Kent, R. L. (1992). Cigarette smoking in a periodontal practice. *Journal of Periodontology, 63*(2), 100–106.

Haber, J., Wattles, J., Crowley, M., Mandell, R., Josipura, K., & Kent, R. L. (1993). Evidence for cigarette smoking as a major risk factor for periodontitis. *Journal of Periodontology, 64,* 16–23.

Halpern, I. L. (1975). Patient's medical status—A factor in dental treatment. *Oral Surgery, 9*(2), 216–226.

Hart, G. T., Scianni, R. A., & Conkin, J. E. (1990). Current medications of a dental patient population. *Journal of the Tennessee State Dental Association, 70,* 15–17.

Hirsh, J., Deykin, D., & Poller, L. (1986). Therapeutic range for oral anticoagulant therapy. *Chest, 89*(2) (Suppl.), 11s–15s.

Horning, G. M., Hatch, C. L., & Cohen, M. E. (1992). Risk indicators for periodontitis in a military treatment population. *Journal of Periodontology, 63,* 297–302.

Ismail, A. J., Burt, B. A., & Eklund, S. A. (1983). Epidemiologic patterns of smoking and periodontal disease in the United States. *Journal of the American Dental Association, 106,* 617–623.

Jacobson, J. J., Schweitzer, S., DePorter, D. J., & Lee, J. J. (1988). Chemoprophylaxis of dental patients with prosthetic joints: A simulation model. *Journal of Dental Education, 52,* 599–604.

Jaspers, M. T. & Little, J. W. (1985). Prophylactic antibiotic coverage in patients with total arthroplasty: Current practice. *Journal of the American Dental Association, 111,* 943–948.

Johnson, J., Ferretti, G. A., Nethery, W. J., Valdez, I. H., Fox, P. C., Ng, D., Muscoplat, C. C., & Gallagher, S. (1993). Oral pilocarpine for post-irradiation xerostomia in patients with head and neck cancer. *The New England Journal of Medicine, 329,* 390–395.

Kearns, J. T. (1969). *Deductive logic.* New York: Meredith Corporation.

Laskaris, G., Hadjivassiliou, M., & Stratigos, M. (1992). Oral signs and symptoms in 160 Greek HIV-infected patients. *Journal of Oral Pathology and Medicine, 21,* 120–123.

Levy, S. M., Baker, K. A., Semla, T. P., & Kohout, F. J. (1988). Use of medications with dental significance by a non-institutionalized elderly population. *Gerodontics, 4,* 119–125.

Little, J. W. (1993). Management of patients susceptible to bacterial endocarditis and related infections. *Journal of Dental Education, 57,* 811–814.

Little, J. W. & Falace, D. A. (1993). *Dental management of the medically compromised patient* (4th ed.). (Chapter 4, 11, 14, Appendix B). St. Louis: Mosby-Year Book, Inc.

Little, J. W. & Rhodus, N. L. (1992). The need for antibiotic prophylaxis of patients with penile implants during invasive dental procedures: A national survey of urologists. *Journal of Urology, 148,* 1801–1804.

Malamed, S. F. (1987). *Handbook of medical emergencies in the dental office* (3rd ed.). St. Louis: Mosby-Year Book, Inc.

Malamed, S. F. (1990). *Handbook of local anesthesia* (3rd ed.). St. Louis: Mosby-Year Book, Inc.

Malamed, S. F. (1993). Managing medical emergencies. *Journal of the American Dental Association, 124*(8), 40–53.

Marx, R. E. & Johnson, R. P. (1987). Studies in the radiobiology of osteoradionecrosis and their clinical significance. *Oral Surgery, Oral Medicine, Oral Pathology, 64,* 379–390.

Matthews, T. G. (1990). Medication side effects of dental interest. *Journal of Prosthetic Dentistry, 64,* 219–226.

May, O. A. (1990). Management of the diabetic dental patient. *Quintessence International, 21*(6), 491–494.

McCarthy, F. M. (1983). Medical history: The best insurance. *Journal of the California Dental Association, 11*(3), 61–64.

McCarthy, F. M. (1985). A new, patient-administered medical history developed for dentistry. *Journal of the American Dental Association, 111,* 595–597.

Melnick, S. L., Engel, D., Truelove, E., DeRoven, T., Morton, T., Schubert, M., Dunphy, C., & Wood, R. W. (1989). Oral mucosal lesions: Association with the presence of antibodies to the human immunodeficiency virus. *Oral Surgery, Oral Medicine, Oral Pathology, 68,* 37–43.

Miller, C. S., Kaplan, A. L., Guest, G. F., & Cottone, J. A. (1992). Documenting medication use in adult dental patients: 1987–1991. *Journal of the American Dental Association, 123*(11), 41–48.

Minden, N. J. & Fast, T. B. (1993). The patient's health history form: How healthy is it? *Journal of the American Dental Association, 124*(8), 95–100.

Mohammad, A. R. & Ruprecht, A. (1983). Assessment of dental patients' comprehension of health questionnaire. *Journal of Oral Medicine, 38*(2), 74–75.

Moorthy, A. P., Coghlan, K., & O'Neil, R. (1984). Drug therapy among dental out-patients. *British Dental Journal, 156*(7), 261.

Murray, V. A. (1985). Diabetes mellitus and associated oral manifestations: A review. *Journal of Oral Pathology, 14,* 271–281.

Niessen, L. C., Mash, L. K., & Gibson, G. (1993). Practice management considerations for an aging population. *Journal of the American Dental Association, 124,* 55–60.

Otomo-Corgel, J. (1990). Periodontal treatment for medically compromised patients. In F. A. Carranza (Ed.), *Glickman's clinical periodontology* (pp. 562-586). Philadelphia: W.B. Saunders Co.

Perusse, R., Goulet, J. P., & Turcotte, J. Y. (1992b). Contraindications to vasoconstrictors in dentistry: Part II. *Oral Surgery, Oral Medicine, Oral Pathology, 74,* 687–691.

Perusse, R., Goulet, J. P., & Turcotte, J. Y. (1992a). Contraindications to vasoconstrictors in dentistry: Part I. *Oral Surgery, Oral Medicine, Oral Pathology, 74,* 679–686.

Phelan, J. A., Salzman, B. R., Friedland, G. H., & Klein, R. S. (1987). Oral findings in patients with acquired immunodeficiency syndrome. *Oral Surgery, Oral Medicine, Oral Pathology, 64,* 50–56.

Porter, S. R., Luker, J., Scully, C., Glover, S., & Griffiths, M. J. (1989). Oral manifestations of a group of British patients infected with HIV-1. *Journal of Oral Pathology and Medicine, 18,* 47–48.

Preber, H., Bergström, J., & Linder, L. E. (1992). Occurrence of periopathogens in smoker and non-smoker patients. *Journal of Clinical Periodontology, 19,* 667–671.

Rams, T. E. & Slots, J. (1990). The subgingival microflora as a determinant on periodontal disease treatment planning. *PROBE, The Canadian Dental Hygienists' Association Journal, 24,* 89–92.

Rees, T. D. & Otomo-Corgel, J. (1992). The diabetic patient. In T. G. Wilson, K. S. Kornman, & M. G. Newman (Eds.), *Advances in periodontics* (pp. 278–295). Carol Stream, IL: Quintessence.

Rieder, C. E. (1987). Obtaining patient history. *Journal of the California Dental Association, 15*(12), 16–23.

Rivera-Hidalgo, F. (1986). Smoking and periodontal disease. A review of the literature. *Journal of Periodontology, 57,* 617–624.

Roda, R. S. (1992). Naproxen: Pharmacology and dental therapeutics. *Journal of the Canadian Dental Association, 58,* 401–404.

Sammalkorpi, K. (1989). Glucose intolerance in active infections. *Journal of Internal Medicine, 255,* 15.

Sastrowijoto, S. H., Hillemans, P., Van Steenberg, T. J. M., Abraham-Inpijn, L., & de Graaff, J. (1989). Periodontal conditions and microbiology of healthy and diseased periodontal pockets in type I diabetes mellitus patients. *Journal of Clinical Periodontology, 16,* 316–322.

Schlant, R. C. (1990). Prevention of bacterial endocarditis. *Journal of the American Medical Association, 264,* 2919–2921.

Schossman, M. 1994. Diabetes mellitus and periodontal disease—A current perspective. *Compendium of Continuing Education in Dentistry, 9*(8), 1018–1035.

Silverman, S., Migliorati, C. A., Lozada-Nur, F., Greenspan, D., & Conant, M. A. (1986). Oral findings in people with or at high risk for AIDS: A study of 375 homosexual males. *Journal of the American Dental Association, 112,* 187–192.

Slots, J. & Rams, T. E. (1991). New news on periodontal microbiota in special patient categories. *Journal of Clinical Periodontology, 18,* 411–420.

Spuller, R. L. (1988). The central indwelling venous catheter in the pediatric patient-dental treatment consideration. *Special Care in Dentistry,* March–April, 74–76.

Stauts, C. W. (1994). *Oncology patient information for clinical dentistry.* Available from the Mountain States Tumor Institute, Boise, Idaho.

Stoltenberg, J. L., Osborn, J. B., Pihlstrom, B. L., Herzberg, M. C., Aeppli, D. M., Wolff, L. F., & Fischer, G. E. (1993). Association between cigarette smoking, bacterial pathogens, and periodontal status. *Journal of Periodontology, 64,* 1225–1230.

Swango, P. A., Kleinman, D. V., & Konzelman, T. L. (1991). HIV and periodontal health: A study of military personnel with HIV. *Journal of the American Dental Association, 122,* 49–54.

Swapp, K. M. (1990). Drugs and the geriatric patient: A dental hygiene perspective. *Journal of Dental Hygiene, 64,* 326–331.

Terezhalmy, G. T. (1989). Rational pharmacotherapy for the elderly. *Dental Clinics of North America, 33*(1), 59–66.

Tervonen, T. & Oliver, R. C. (1993). Long-term control of diabetes mellitus and periodontitis. *Journal of Clinical Periodontology, 20,* 431–435.

Thibodeau, E. A. & Rossomando, K. J. (1992). Survey of the medical history questionnaire. *Oral Surgery, Oral Medicine, Oral Pathology, 74,* 400–403.

Thomson, M. R., Garito, M. L., & Brown, F. H. (1993). The role of smoking in periodontal diseases: A review of the literature. *Journal of Periodontal Abstracts, 41*(1), 5–9.

Trieger, N. & Goldblatt, L. (1978). The art of history taking. *Journal of Oral Surgery, 36*(2), 118–124.

Tzukert, A. A., Leviner, E., & Sela, M. (1986). Prevention of infective endocarditis: Not by antibiotics alone. *Oral Surgery, Oral Medicine, Oral Pathology, 62*, 385–388.

Wahl, M. J. & Wahl P. T. (1993). Prevention of infective endocarditis: An update for clinicians. *Quintessence International, 24*(3), 171–175.

Williams, C. A., Winkler, J. R., Grassi, M., & Murray, P. A. (1990). HIV-associated periodontitis complicated by necrotizing stomatitis. *Oral Surgery, Oral Medicine, Oral Pathology, 69*, 351–355.

Winkler, J. R., Murray, P. A., Grassi, M., & Hammerle, C. (1989). Diagnosis and management of HIV-associated periodontal lesions. *Journal of the American Dental Association, 119* (Suppl.), S25–S34.

Winkler, J. R. & Robertson, P. B. (1992). Periodontal disease associated with HIV infection. *Oral Surgery, Oral Medicine, Oral Pathology, 73*, 145–150.

Wright, W. E. (1987). Periodontium destruction associated with oncology therapy: Five case reports. *Journal of Periodontology, 58*, 559–563.

Wynn, R. L. (1993). Erythromycin and ketoconazole (Nizoral) associated with terfenadine (Seldane)-induced ventricular arrhythmias. *General Dentistry, 41*(2), 27–29.

Yusof, Z. W. & Bakri, M. M. (1993). Severe progressive periodontal destruction due to radiation tissue injury. *Journal of Periodontology, 64*, 1253–1258.

Zachariasen, R. D. (1991). Effect of antibiotics on oral contraceptive efficacy. *Journal of Dental Hygiene, 65*(9), 334–338.

CHAPTER 3

# Periodontal Assessment

## Key Terms

clinical attachment level
disease activity
disease severity
gingival crevicular fluid
predictive value

presumptive diagnosis
probing depth
sensitivity
specificity

## INTRODUCTION

The periodontal assessment is the foundation of excellence in client care. It is particularly significant in the dental hygiene process of care because the outcome of the assessment identifies if the client is in need of an oral prophylaxis or nonsurgical periodontal therapy (NSPT). In order to develop an acceptable diagnosis and care plan, the clinician must first identify all risk factors associated with periodontal disease that may affect the client's oral health status. These risk factors are multifold and may be grouped into three broad categories as mentioned in Chapter 1: dentally-related, unchanging subject-related, and changing subject-related.

Dentally-related risk factors include the presence of established periodontal disease, bacterial plaque, putative pathogens, stain and calculus, missing teeth, overhanging restorations, poor tooth arrangement, mobile teeth, mouthbreathing, areas of food impaction, and poor oral self-care. The clinical identification of the majority of these factors is accomplished by performing a thorough examination of the intraoral anatomical conditions and viewing updated radiographs. Unchanging subject-related risk indicators include factors a patient cannot control such as genetics, race, and gender. Genetic predisposition to a number of periodontal diseases has been suggested in the literature (Michalowicz, 1994; Marazita et al., 1994). When less common forms of periodontal diseases such as juvenile periodontitis, prepubertal periodontitis or rapidly progressive periodontitis are diagnosed, a genetic or familial source should be suspected. Unchanging subject variables are discovered through observation and medical or personal history information. Changing subject-related risk factors include those factors that have an impact on the host response of the individual. These risk factors include smoking, chronic alcoholism, age, stress, diet and nutrition, drugs, and

systemic disease. Several of these risk factors can be identified through a comprehensive health history as discussed in Chapter 2. Stress and nutrition, however, are difficult to identify through a health history questionnaire unless specific questions directed towards these factors are included. Further questioning of the client might be required to establish the presence of stress, and a detailed dietary analysis might be indicated if poor nutrition is suspected. These types of questions might also be included on the dental or personal history questionnaire.

A clinician identifies all risk factors by conducting a thorough periodontal assessment preceded by a comprehensive medical, dental, and personal history. Each examination will include a clinical assessment, analysis of appropriately updated radiographs, and possibly a microbiological, biochemical and/or immunological assessment. Although most periodontal examinations are limited to clinical assessments, recent development of rapid chairside and laboratory diagnostic tests have made it possible for the clinician to assess less traditional risk factors. This chapter focuses on dental and personal histories and the identification of dentally-related risk factors as determined by a thorough clinical examination. Use of supplemental diagnostic tests is also discussed in order to provide the reader with a better understanding of how these tests can be employed in clinical practice.

## BACKGROUND INFORMATION

The ultimate goal of the periodontal assessment is to identify and classify periodontal disease. The chances of detecting some type of periodontal disease are great as the majority of the population has some form of periodontal disease. The recognition of gingivitis only, although significant, involves a different therapeutic approach to care than when periodontitis is recognized.

## Gingivitis

Lesions confined to the gingiva alone that do not involve a loss of attachment are classified as "gingivitis". The classic methods for determining the presence of gingivitis include the assessment of gingival color, contour, texture, and consistency. These terms describe the external manifestations of the histological events of inflammation. The descriptors commonly associated with these terms describe *color* as coral pink, red (erythematous), blue (cyanotic) or pigmented; *contour* as marginally knife-edged or rolled and the papilla as being pointed, bulbous, blunted, or cratered; *texture* as stippled or smooth and shiny; and *consistency* as firm, edematous, or fibrotic. These descriptors give the clinician clues as to the presence or absence of inflammation or repair.

Additionally, more specific terms are employed delineating the *location* and *extent* of the disease. When the lesion is confined to one region of the mouth involving one to three teeth, it is said to be "localized." If the lesion occurs in an entire segment of the mouth (i.e., sextant, quadrant, arch), it is classified as being "generalized." Extent can be denoted in various ways, however, accepted terminology includes papillary, marginal, or diffuse gingivitis. Papillary gingivitis involves the interdental papilla and extends to the gingival margin. Marginal gingivitis involves the marginal gingiva and diffuse gingivitis extends into the attached gingiva. The most common variety of gingivitis is chronic marginal gingivitis, which is plaque-associated and may be localized or generalized. Other forms of chronic gingivitis include those associated with hormonal changes such as puberty, pregnancy, menopause; vitamin C deficiency; drugs that enlarge the gingiva such as phenytoin, nifedipene, cyclosporin, and diltiazem; HIV; and systemic diseases such as leukemia, Addison's disease, diabetes, hemophilia, thrombocytopenia, Sturge-Weber syndrome, and other immunodeficiency diseases. Acute conditions include primary herpetic gingivostomatitis; acute necrotizing ulcerative gingivitis (NUG); acute pericoronitis; acute gingival abscesses, and localized trauma-induced inflammation. Detailed descriptions of these conditions may be found in Chapter 1 of this text. It is important to recognize that gingivitis does not routinely progress to periodontitis although periodontitis is always preceded by gingivitis and gingivitis usually accompanies periodontitis (Maynard, 1994).

## Periodontitis

The establishment of a diagnosis of periodontitis is dictated by the presence of loss of attachment, which includes loss of both fibrous and bony connective tissue. The four major types of periodontitis as described in Chapter 1 include: adult, early-onset, refractory, and periodontitis associated with systemic diseases. The diagnosis of the type and severity of periodontal disease is based on parameters identified during the periodontal examination in conjunction with the radiographic evaluation. The extent of disease may be determined clinically by measuring periodontal pockets, attachment loss, furcations, recession, plaque, bleeding on probing. and suppuration. Radiographic evidence of bone loss will help to identify patterns of destruction that will assist in the diagnosis of the condition (see Chapter 5). Studies have shown that data collected during the clinical assessment have definite limitations, particularly in their ability to identify risk factors. It is hoped that further research in the area of supplemental diagnostic testing will enhance traditional assessment procedures.

Location and extent of periodontitis are also important. Location again refers to localized or generalized disease, and extent is described as either early, moderate, or advanced. Periodontitis can be localized to a certain area of the mouth or different areas can demonstrate different amounts of attachment and bone loss. The area with the greatest amount of destruction is used to describe the extent of disease and is combined with the appropriate form of the disease to arrive at a periodontal diagnosis. For instance, a client has loss of attachment and bone in both the maxillary and mandibular molar regions, but the maxillary disease severity is moderate and the mandibular area has early bone loss. As a result, the diagnosis is chronic adult periodontitis (form) with moderate bone loss (extent). While it is true that the moderate loss of bone is only localized, it still serves as the basis for the general periodontal diagnosis for the individual. Extent of periodontitis is discussed in detail in Chapter 5. For purposes of insurance reporting, different quadrants of periodontal instrumentation might be reported to the insurance company with different extents of disease. In this case, however, the periodontal disease diagnosis is still based on the area that involves the greatest extent of destruction.

## Existing Disease

The identification of existing disease must include both disease severity and disease activity (Jeffcoat, 1994). The **disease severity** is a measure of all the destruction and healing that has taken place prior to the examination. Severity can be established as an outcome of any clinical assessment no matter if the client is new to the practice or returning for care. Traditional tests for measuring periodontal disease severity include visual inspection, palpation, periodontal probing, and radiographs. When identifying disease severity, the clinician determines the disease classification (gingivitis or periodontitis) and the form of the disease as illustrated in the previous example. It is also valuable to recognize if the form of periodontitis is slowly progressing or aggressive because this differentiation is critical in planning the course of care and prognosis. The most commonly accepted classification system is presented in Chapter 1, Table 1-1. It must be remembered that multiple factors are necessary to classify disease and it might not be possible to determine each of these factors when treating a client who is new to a practice. For example, age of onset and rate of destruction might only be determined after periodic examinations are compared. Therefore, the diagnosis of a specific form of gingivitis or periodontitis might be altered once additional data is collected over time. For this reason, the clinical examination during initial therapy results in a preliminary or **presumptive diagnosis** (Kornman & Wilson, 1992). A final diagnosis is the result of clinical findings and evaluation of how the client responds to initial therapy (Kornman & Wilson, 1992).

**Disease activity** is more difficult to establish because it refers to bone or attachment loss that is ongoing at the time of the examination. Periodontal disease activity refers to the periods of quiescence and periods of exacerbation that are evident in active disease. Periods of quiescence (inactivity) are characterized by a reduced inflammatory response and little or no loss of bone and connective tissue attachment. On the other hand, periods of exacerbation (activity) are initialed by unattached plaque and anaerobic bacteria (gram-negative, motile), that result in loss of bone and connective tissue attachment creating deeper periodontal pockets. The exacerbation does not last for an exact period; the activity could continue for days, weeks, or months. Eventually, remission or quiescence will follow as a result of proliferation of gram-positive bacteria. This description of activity and nonactivity explains the episodic nature of periodontal disease. Clinically, this can only be measured retrospectively by comparing the current examination with previous ones (Jeffcoat, 1994). Thus, disease activity is routinely assessed at periodontal maintenance visits.

### Value of a Test

Clinical and supplemental diagnostic tests are evaluated according to their sensitivity, specificity and predictive value. The terms sensitivity and specificity are used to describe the diagnostic accuracy of the test in a population. **Sensitivity** refers to the ability of the test to detect disease when it is there, and **specificity** describes the ability of the test to rule out disease when it is absent (Jeffcoat, 1994). Most tests will be evaluated in terms of their degrees of sensitivity and specificity. If a test has both high sensitivity and specificity, it is said to have a high **predictive value**. In other words, the test can be used to accurately identify active disease and predict future disease. An ideal test would have a sensitivity and specificity of 100 percent and, thus, would have a perfect predictive value. In medicine and dentistry perfect diagnostic tests do not exist; however, a clinically useful test should have sensitivity and specificity values of 70 percent or greater (American Academy of Periodontology, 1995a). These terms are useful when discussing the value of measures of disease activity such as periodontal probing or when evaluating new supplemental tests. Bleeding on probing, suppuration, pocket depth, and attachment loss all have specificity of greater than 70 percent; however, the sensitivity value of each is well below 70 percent (Darby & Walsh, 1994).

## COMPONENTS OF A COMPREHENSIVE PERIODONTAL ASSESSMENT

A quality-oriented assessment is the foundation for the dental hygiene diagnosis, subsequent care plan, implementation of therapy, and evaluation of care. Without an accurate and thorough periodontal assessment, periodontal diseases are not detected or are misdiagnosed. Unfortunately, the periodontal examination is sometimes hastily performed or totally neglected. This can lead to very serious repercussions such as failure to diagnose periodontal disease, which is one of the most litigious areas of dental malpractice (Bailey, 1987). Examination of the periodontium occurs at each visit no matter how frequently the individual presents for care. It behooves each clinician to ensure that all clients receive a *comprehensive* periodontal assessment at least once a year including periodontal probing for bleeding, pocket depth, and measurements of loss of attachment, as well as examination of mobility, furcation involvement, recession, mucogingival problems, and radiographic bone loss (Jeffcoat, 1994). Comprehensive examination is also mandatory for all new clients to a practice and the scope of the assessment is, of course, dependent on the extent of disease that is recognized. For example, evaluation of mobility and furcation involvement are not conducted when the periodontal probing and radiographic examination reveal no loss of attachment or bone.

The completion of a comprehensive periodontal assessment involves six factors: ample time to conduct the assessment; current medical, dental, and personal histories; the clinical examination; supplemental testing, if indicated; a summary of risk factors; and appropriate recording forms. Each of these factors will be discussed in subsequent sections. Sharing of the findings with the client is a critical aspect of collaborative care that is discussed in Chapter 8.

## APPOINTMENT PLANNING AND SCHEDULING

Assessment for the client new to the practice typically involves more time than the evaluation performed at periodontal maintenance visits. While other components of the general assessment such as the extraoral, intraoral, and restorative examinations can involve a significant amount of time, it is often the periodontal assessment that is the most time-consuming for the dental hygienist. Comprehensive periodontal assessment on the first appointment involves a minimum of 30 minutes depending on the extent of conditions, equipment used, and available assistance from other staff members. For this reason, initial assessments warrant a higher fee than those conducted during periodontal maintenance procedures (PMP). A specific insurance code (00150) is offered for comprehensive oral evaluation which encompasses dental and medical history and general health assessment, as well as evaluation and recording of dental caries, missing or unerupted teeth, restorations, occlusal relationships, periodontal conditions and charting, hard and soft tissue anomalies, and other significant entities (AAP, 1995b).

Another insurance code exists, 00120, for periodic oral evaluation for a client of record. Its purpose is to determine any changes in the client's dental and medical status since the previous assessment. If additional diagnostic testing is indicated at the PMP appointment, it is reported separately to insurance companies using the 00415 code for bacteriological studies for determination of pathologic agents. This code may include, but is not limited to, tests for susceptibility to periodontal disease (AAP, 1995b). Time allocation and assessment information for PMP is covered in Chapter 16.

Acquiring ample time to conduct the periodontal assessment, along with the other assessment components, is challenging. The time allocation may differ from office to office depending on the factors previously mentioned as well as on which practitioner has the responsibility to collect the assessment information. If the dental hygienist is the first to see new clients, then the responsibility for complete assessment is usually hers. In this case, adequate time must be scheduled and the client must be informed of how the time for the first appointment will be used. This communication is significant because many new patients assume that they will complete care in one visit, especially if they have not participated in NSPT before. Frequently, dental offices will schedule the first appointment for a new client for at least 60 to 90 minutes to ensure the assessment is completed and client education is performed. Other offices might chose to schedule less time and perform screening procedures that indicate if further comprehensive assessment is indicated.

## DENTAL AND PERSONAL HISTORIES

Upon completion of the medical history (see Chapter 2), it is important to collect a dental and personal history. The dental history contributes information about the person's past dental experiences as well as why they are currently presenting for care. This information often provides the clinician with the client's chief complaint, whether they are experiencing pain, what previous care they have received, current oral hygiene habits, and valuable information about any adverse reactions to past treatment. Additionally, the clinician will gain insight into their clients' attitudes towards oral health by evaluating the frequency of dental visits and the reported daily self-care. Questions about the last exposures to dental radiation, nervousness about dental treatment, tooth sensitivity, chewing difficulty, or injuries to the head and

neck region should be included. Other questions might determine if clients are satisfied with the appearance of their teeth; if their gums bleed; if they have any sores in their mouth and if so, are they slow in healing. Answers to these questions provide clues about various preexisting conditions such as diabetes and periodontal disease.

In addition to a thorough dental history, a personal history should also be procured to assist in the identification of nondentally related risk factors such as smoking, diet, alcohol consumption, and stress. Knowledge of risk factors aids the clinician in developing the dental hygiene diagnosis and needs assessment in order to effectively provide holistic therapy to improve oral health status.

The dental and personal histories are collected in verbal or written format. Each format has advantages and drawbacks. Verbal questioning provides the practitioner with an opportunity to facilitate communication and encourage a collaborative relationship. Client responses must then be recorded by the clinician for current and future use. Commonly, dental and personal history data is collected through written format completed by the client at the same time as the medical history. The dental and personal history questions can be intermingled with the written health history questions, or appear as separate documents. The use of written dental and personal histories provides continuity from client to client and serves as a permanent record of information collected.

## CLINICAL ASSESSMENT

The AAP (Guidelines for Periodontal Therapy, 1993, pgs. 1 and 2), identifies the following procedures as essential components for the development of a periodontal diagnosis as well as for determining the health of tissues surrounding dental implants:

1. Updating and evaluating medical and dental histories.
2. General periodontal examination to evaluate the topography of the gingiva and related structures.
3. Presence and degree of gingival inflammation.
4. Periodontal probing to assess periodontal pocket depth and attachment level, and to provide information on the health of the subgingival area; e.g. presence of bleeding, purulent exudate, periodontal pockets, etc.
5. Presence and distribution of bacterial plaque and calculus.
6. Condition of tooth proximal contact relationships.
7. Degree of mobility of teeth and dental implants.
8. Presence and degree of clinical furcation involvements.
9. Presence of malocclusion or occlusal pathology.
10. Status of dental restorations and prosthetic appliances.
11. Interpretation of a satisfactory number of diagnostic quality periapical and bitewing radiographs.

Each of these components are assessed through clinical examination except the medical and dental histories that have been previously addressed. The following sections will focus strictly on the periodontal assessment components (2, 3, 4, 5, 7, and 8). Proximal contact relationships, malocclusion, occlusal pathology, dental restorations, and prosthetic appliances are discussed in Chapter 4. Implants are addressed in Chapter 14 and the role of radiographs in NSPT is discussed in Chapter 5. Chapter 5 also provides the reader with a summary of the correlation of clinical findings to radiographic findings for the purpose of formulating an accurate periodontal disease diagnosis in which to implement effective NSPT.

The following information relates to the periodontal assessment that is comprehensive in nature; therefore, it focuses on the client who is new to the practice or clinical situation, or who is being diagnosed with periodontal disease for the first time. The relationship of periodontal assessment to PMP is addressed in Chapter 16. Chapter 16 contains the information of interest to the therapist who is confirming a presumptive or preliminary diagnosis and who is making decisions about disease activity.

## Gingival Examination

The gingiva is the window to the periodontium. A clinician obtains many superficial clues about the health of the periodontium by observing the appearance of the gingival tissues. In order to interpret clinical observations from the gingival examination, the clinician must have an understanding of the underlying inflammatory response (see Chapter 1).

The clinical assessment of gingival inflammation may be assessed in a number of ways. Two of the classic signs of inflammation, redness and edema, are observed through visual inspection. Histological studies have verified that these two visual signs correspond to a significant gingival lesion ( Appelgren, Robinson, & Kaminski, 1979; Oliver, Holm-Pederssen, & Löe, 1969; Greenstein, Caton, & Polson, 1981). Research indicates that visual signs such as redness and swelling are late signs of inflammation exhibiting low predictive value for periodontal breakdown (Haffajee, Socransky, & Goodson, 1983). Bleeding, which will be discussed later, is the most widely accepted clinical sign of gingival inflammation. The visual signs of redness, swelling, and bleeding have been extensively investigated and are reliable signs for determining the presence or absence of inflammatory lesions within the periodontium, even though they are recognized as weak predictors of disease activity (American Academy of Periodontology, 1989). All signs of gingival inflammation must be considered in combination as none alone is indicative of disease.

The color of healthy gingival tissues, classically described as "coral pink," varies significantly, particularly when taking into account normal variations in skin tones or pigmentation. When redness is observed it commonly indicates that, histologically, there are engorged

blood vessels, escaped fluids, and vascular cellular elements present in the tissue spaces with thinning of the surface keratin layers. These changes are the result of the host inflammatory response. Redness, however, might occur in healthy tissue due to greater connective tissue to vascularity and/or thin epithelium. Because redness is not a reliable diagnostic sign of disease activity, it must not be forgotten that tissues appearing "normal" in color may have extensive attachment loss and bleeding on probing. Gingival color must be used in combination with other signs to be of any value.

Normal consistency of the marginal and papillary gingiva in health is usually "firm" and resilient. When inflammation occurs and excessive tissue fluid collects in the lamina propria, the gingiva will appear "flabby" or edematous. Often the attached gingiva appears very bulky and firm, or fibrotic, indicating an excessive amount of collagen or fibrosis (scar tissue) in the connective tissues due to repeated repair. The consistency of the gingival tissues is easily evaluated by gently placing the side of a periodontal probe against the gingival margins and papilla, and observing the amount of resistance created by the tissues.

The surface texture of the gingiva has been described as the least reliable indicator of gingival inflammation. Under healthy conditions, the free gingiva will not exhibit stippling while the attached gingiva may or may not exhibit varying degrees of stippling depending on location in the mouth. Stippling most frequently occurs on the attached gingiva on buccal surfaces; it rarely occurs on the lingual. In youth and old age little stippling can be found. Table 3-1 summarizes the terminology used to describe gingival inflammation.

The contour of healthy gingival tissues should follow the contour of the teeth. When teeth are normally positioned, the gingival margins will appear knife-edged and the papilla will appear pointed; thus, rolled or rounded marginal or papillary gingiva indicates inflammation. This appearance is indicative of the presence of excessive tissue fluid (edema) or tissue elements (enlargement) produced during the inflammatory and repair (processes) process. Changes in contour can also reveal past periodontal destruction. Blunted papilla or gingival clefts may coincide with periodontal attachment loss in periodontitis. Cratered papillae can indicate a history of necrotizing ulcerative gingivitis and marginal clefting may be a result of a poorly positioned labial frenum.

Position of the gingival tissues is another factor that is usually examined when evaluating inflammation. In health, the gingival margin is located about 1 to 2 mm coronal to the cementoenamel junction. Recession represents an apical shift in positioning of the gingival margin, usually accompanied by apical migration of the epithelial attachment. This loss of attachment indicates past periodontal destruction. Carranza (1996) identifies two terms associated with the position of the gingiva: actual and apparent. Actual position refers to the level of the epithelial attachment on the tooth and

**Table 3-1  Definitions of Descriptive Terms for Gingival Inflammation**

| Term | Definition |
|---|---|
| Color | 1. Normal/coral pink.<br>2. Erythematous (erythema): reddened area of variable size and shape due to increased vasodilation resulting from inflammation.<br>3. Cyanotic (cyanosis): a bluish discoloration of tissue due to excessive concentration of reduced hemoglobin in the blood.<br>4. Melanin pigmentation: a normal light brown to black pigmentation seen in Orientals, Blacks, Indians, and Caucasians of Mediterranean ancestry.<br>5. Amalgam tatoo: metals absorbed into the tissue may discolor the gingiva bluish-gray. |
| Consistency and Surface Texture | 1. Normal<br>2. Edematous (edema): an abnormal accumulation of fluid in the gingival tissues. Clinical appearance of edematous tissue may be bulbous, smooth, rolled, or rounded when fluid accumulation is present.<br>3. Fibrotic (fibrosis): a chronic condition resulting in scar tissue formation within the connective tissue. Clinical appearance may include an increase in density and stippling, and it is firm and nodular.<br>4. Hyperkeratinization: an abnormal increase in the thickness of the keratin layer of the epithelium. The gingiva will appear whiter in color and may exhibit increased density and/or firmness. Extrinsic etiology (smoking, tobacco chewing, etc.) should be considered. |
| Contour (Size) | 1. Normal<br>2. Enlarged (enlargement): an abnormal increase in size (or volume) of the tissue resulting from the proliferation of cells or development of additional tissue as a result of chronic inflammation. Clinical appearance of enlarged tissue may be rolled or rounded. Enlargement may or may not be accompanied by fluid accumulation (edema). Stippling or nodular appearance also is common.<br>3. Edematous (edema): an abnormal accumulation of fluid in the gingival tissue. Clinical appearance of edematous tissue may be bulbous, smooth, rolled, or rounded when fluid accumulation is present.<br>4. Hyperplastic (hyperplasia): an increase in size of tissue produced by increase in cells. Noninflammatory gingival hyperplasia is produced by factors other than local irritation. It is not common and occurs most often with phenytoin therapy. It appears as a beadlike or mulberry shaped, firm enlargement, usually pale pink and resilient. |
| Contour (Shape) | 1. Normal<br>2. McCall's festooning: semilunar enlargements of the free gingival margin resulting from compensatory hyperplasia and degeneration of gingival fibers. Clinically, McCall's festooning appears "lifesaver"-like and fibrotic in consistency.<br>3. Stillman's cleft: vertical clefts produced by atrophy of the labial gingiva, together with extension of adjacent hyperplastic tissue. The gingival clefting is associated. |
| Extent | In addition to noting whether a gingival change is localized or generalized, the extent of involvement also is included to fully describe distribution of erythema, cyanosis, enlargement, and/or edema.<br>1. Papillary: inflammation involving the papillary gingiva.<br>2. Marginal: inflammation involving the papillary gingiva and extending into the free (marginal) gingiva or encompassing the entire free (marginal) gingiva.<br>3. Diffuse: inflammation involving the papillary gingiva, marginal gingiva, and extending into any portion of the attached gingiva. |

it is used to determine severity of recession or attachment loss. Apparent position is the level of the crest of the gingival margin and it is used to easily assess recession when the CEJ is exposed. Recession is measured by placing the tip of the periodontal probe on the gingival margin and determining the distance (mm) to the CEJ. When the location of the gingival margin is equal to the CEJ, physiologic recession has occurred but this change is usually not recorded. Somewhere between the normal positioning of the gingival margin and clinically observable (apparent) recession, loss of attachment has

occurred. This enigma explains why early radiographic bone loss sometimes can be visible without corresponding recession and/or pocket depth. If radiographic bone loss is evident and the angulation of the x-ray is accurate, periodontitis associated with *early* bone loss is present.

Physiological (occurring with aging) and pathological (occurring with disease) recession are sometimes distinguished from one another; however, recent theory concludes that the increase in recession noticed with age is the result of minor pathological involvement and/or repeated trauma to the gingiva (Carranza, 1996). The etiology of recession can be inappropriate tooth-brushing that creates abrasion, malpositioning of teeth, gingival inflammation, and high frenum attachment. The two most significant outcomes of recession are root sensitivity and the potential for root caries.

The width of the attached gingiva will vary from one region of the mouth to another and from one person to another. The sulcus or pocket depth measurement can be subtracted from the width of the gingiva as measured from the gingival margin to the mucogingival junction. Care should be exercised to ensure the measurement is actually taken from the mucogingival junction instead of from an adjacent point. This point demarks the usual color change from pink to red that often occurs just coronal to the mucogingival junction. To accomplish this, the practitioner gently stretches the lips and moves the tissue to the right and left to identify the area where the movable and nonmovable mucosa meet. Insufficient width is evident when this stretching results in movement of the free gingival margin (Carranza, 1996).

The normal width of the attached tissue on the facial surfaces varies throughout the mouth. In the anteriors, width ranges from 3.5 mm to 4.5 mm in the maxilla and 3.3 mm to 3.9 mm in the mandible (Ainamo & Löe, 1966). The posterior and canine teeth have the least amount of attached gingiva and the maxillary anteriors have the most. In fact, the first premolar area has the least width (1.8 to 1.9 mm). Changes in the width are due to alterations in the tissue coronal to the mucogingival junction, because the position of the mucogingival junction never changes. Although it has been suggested that if less than two millimeters of attached gingiva exists the patient may require a referral to a periodontist for mucogingival surgery, there have been no significant findings reported to support this hypothesis (Greenstein, 1988). Decisions to refer to a specialist, to treat surgically, or to treat with NSPT are dependent on practitioner philosophy response to initial therapy, and causes of the narrow area of attached gingiva. An area that has a compromised width of attached gingiva less than 2 mm which is accompanied by severe recession, persistent inflammation, deep pocket depths, and/or progressive attachment loss is obviously indicative of further care and/or referral. Narrow bands of attached tissue not accompanied by these changes should be carefully monitored by both the clinician and client. Thus, the width of attached gingiva alone does not indicate a *mucogingival* problem. Nonetheless, widths of less than 2 mm should be recorded for historical purposes as possible risk factors, and clients can be educated regarding thorough, but gentle self-care practices.

Gingival inflammation can be monitored by clients at home. Self-evaluation is helpful in determining success and nonsuccess with oral care (see Chapter 8). Changes in color, consistency, contour, texture, and position are easily recognized when the dental hygienist includes this information in self-care education.

## Pocket Depths

Periodontal pockets are a direct result of the damage created late in the established lesion and throughout the advanced lesion as defined by Page and Schroeder (1977) (see Chapter 1). They are caused by destruction at the coronal end of the junctional epithelium and damage of the collagen fibers at the apical end of the junctional epithelium resulting in apical migration and deepened pockets (Caton, 1989). Pathologically, pockets are deepening of the gingival sulcus occurring in one of three ways: coronal enlargement of the gingival margin (gingival pocket/gingivitis), apical displacement of the gingival attachment (periodontal pocket/periodontitis), or a combination of the previous two means. Periodontal pockets can be further subdivided into two types: suprabony or infrabony (see Chapter 5). It was once believed that the depths of periodontal pockets were indicators and predictors of active disease. Recent research showing the episodic nature of periodontal destruction (Goodson, Tanner, Haffajee, Sornberger, & Socransky, 1982) questions the diagnostic significance of pockets. Although deep pockets are not necessarily indicative of active disease, they certainly are representative of the historical damage that has occurred in the tissues. Deep pockets are inaccessible to self-cleansing and less accessible to professional debridement; therefore, they become notable risk factors.

It is imperative that periodontal probing be routinely conducted to assess disease progression not only through increases in pocket depths, but most importantly through increases in attachment loss. Although diagnostically attachment loss is more significant than probing depth; therapeutically, probing depth becomes more important in the determination of treatment modalities. The depth of the pocket must be considered when selecting appropriate explorers, curets, and ultrasonic inserts because of the different instrument designs available to the therapist. Also, depth of the pocket combined with the topography of the embrasure space are considered when recommending the appropriate interproximal cleansing aid for the client's daily self-care.

**Manual Probing.** The measuring of periodontal pockets should be conducted at each treatment interval to assess deterioration or healing that may have occurred between visits. Although tedious, routine probing is the only available means to make comparative measurements. The most commonly used method of probing is the manual probe. **Probing depth** is the distance between the gingival margin and the location of the periodontal probe tip (Caton, 1989) against the epithelial attachment. Probing measurements are usually taken at six locations: mesiofacial, facial, distofacial, distolingual, lingual, and mesiolingual. It is important to remember that the probe must be "walked" around the entire circumference of the tooth to detect pockets in between these sites and placement at only these specific sites limits accurate results.

Manual probing has many limitations. The obvious limitations are the time it takes to complete the procedure, manual recording of the scores, and difficulty in maintaining asepsis. Another significant limitation is the inability to regulate the probing force not only between different examiners, but within one examiner. The accuracy of probing measurements has been questioned because most researchers agree that when probing inflamed tissues, a certain amount of penetration of the probe into ulcerated tissues will occur. Various studies have shown that the degree of probing force is directly related to the amount of penetration of the junctional epithelium (Robinson & Vitek, 1979; van der Velden, 1980). The issue of probing force led to the development of several automated pressure-sensitive probes available on the market today.

**Automated Probing.** Several automated probes have recently been developed and tested. The Florida Probe (Florida Probe Corp., Gainesville, FL) is capable of measuring both probing depths and attachment levels and has a reproducibility of 0.58 millimeters for probe depths and 0.28 mm for attachment level measures (Gibbs, Hirschfeld, & Lee, 1988). The Florida Probe interfaces with a computer that records and stores all measurements. Another automated probe, the Interprobe (Bausch & Lomb Oral Care Division, Tucker, GA) measures probing depths using an optical encoder. The encoder is attached to a disposable plastic fiber probe tip that retracts within a sleeve when paced into a sulcus or pocket. The depth is transmitted by fiber optics to a computer and stored on a memory card that allows for numerical and graphic displays to be printed. The reproducibility of this probe is approximately 0.8 mm (Goodson, 1992).

Due to the cost of automated probes, they are not routinely found in dental practice. A recent investigation by Perry and coworkers (1994) compared two electronic probes with a manual pressure-regulated probe and a conventional probe. Although results indicate significant differences between the conventional probe and the others in fractions of millimeter measurements, the authors concluded that these differences were not clinically significant. It was also noted that patients preferred the manual probes to the automated probes claiming more comfort with the manual probes. Some clinicians also are concerned about inability to maintain asepsis while manually charting probing depths. The solution to these limitations may be to use a manual probe and a voice-activated computerized charting system such as VICTOR™ (Pro-Dentec, Batesville, AR). This system charts, stores, and compares a variety of periodontal and restorative data including probing depths, gingival margin levels, attachment loss, bleeding points, suppuration, furcation involvement, tooth mobility, plaque, calculus, and stains. The clinician speaks into a small microphone held in position by a headband. The computer records all findings by voice command enabling the operator to complete a periodontal examination in approximately 8 minutes (McCullough, 1995).

**Periodontal Screening and Recording™ (PSR™).** In 1993, the American Academy of Periodontology (AAP), and the American Dental Association (ADA) with the corporate sponsorship of Proctor & Gamble, developed a screening mechanism called the Periodontal Screening and Recording (PSR) system. This system was designed in an attempt to encourage all practitioners to incorporate routine periodontal probing into client care. The PSR is not intended to replace a full mouth probing and recording of findings. Instead, it is intended to provide a rapid means of screening patients to determine if more extensive periodontal assessment is required. Even though it employs manual probing, it serves to alleviate some of the limitations previously mentioned.

The PSR system is a modification of the Community Periodontal Index of Treatment Needs (CPITN), developed in 1978 by the World Health Organization. Six sites on each tooth in a sextant are measured; however, only the highest score in a sextant is recorded. A special periodontal probe is used with a 0.5 mm ball at the tip and a color coded area 3.5 to 5.5 mm from the tip. A scoring form is provided that has a box for each sextant and scores are based on a 0 to 4 scale (see Figure 3-1). These scores consider the detection of calculus, defective margins, and bleeding on probing as well as other manifestations of periodontal disease such as furcation involvement, mobility, mucogingival problems, and recession. Once a score is determined in a sextant, that score is recorded in the appropriate box and the next sextant is examined. If any scores of 3 are noted, that particular sextant requires full examination. If two or more sextants have a score of 3 or any one sextant has a score of 4, a full mouth periodontal examination and recording of all findings are required (Charles & Charles, 1994).

Currently, the AAP and the ADA support use of the PSR (Diagnosis of Periodontal Diseases, 1995). The system can be purchased from the PSR Fulfillment Center (Fairfield, OH). The effectiveness of this screening system for identifying clients with previously undetected periodontal disease depends on future studies comparing the PSR to complete periodontal examinations (AAP, 1995a).

### Loss of Attachment

The assessment of loss of attachment is a definitive clinical indicator of disease progression. When the migration of the attachment mechanism between the tooth and the tissues is apical to the cementoenamel junction (CEJ), it is a relatively accurate indicator that bone loss also has occurred. The biological width of the gingival tissue attachment that extends from the cementoenamel junction to the crest of the alveolar bone was shown to remain constant at approximately 1.7 millimeters wide, even in the presence of disease (Ritchie & Orban, 1953). As the attachment migrates apically, the height of underlying

**PSR takes just three easy steps:**

1. Examine at least six sites on each tooth.
2. Walk probe around gingival crevice.
3. Record highest score in each sextant.
   - Go to next sextant whenever Code 4 is recorded.
   - Add * symbol whenever findings indicate clinical abnormalities.

Periodontal screening and recording

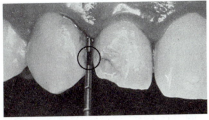

Sextant score    Month    Day    Year

## CODE 2

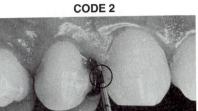

**Scoring System:**

Circled area of probe remains completely visible in the deepest probing depth in the sextant.

- Supra– or subgingival calculus detected, and/or
- Defective margins detected

**Treatment Implications:**

OHI.

Appropriate therapy, including:

- Subgingival plaque removal
- Removal of calculus
- Correction of plaque-retentive margins of restorations

Patients whose scores for all sextants are Codes 0, 1, and 2:

Should be screened in conjunction with every oral examination.

## CODE 1

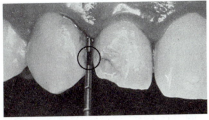

**Scoring System:**

Circled area of probe remains completely visible in the deepest probing depth in the sextant.

- No calculus or defective margins detected
- There <u>is</u> bleeding on probing

**Treatment Implications:**

Oral hygiene instructions (OHI).

Appropriate therapy, including subgingival plaque removal.

## CODE 0

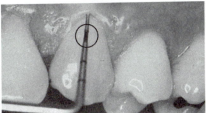

**Scoring System:**

Circled area of probe remains completely visible in the deepest crevice in the sextant.

- No calculus or defective margins detected
- Gingival tissues are healthy with no bleeding on probing

**Treatment Implications:**

Appropriate preventive care.

## CODE 3

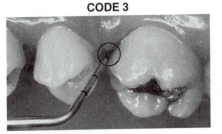

**Scoring System:**

Circled area of probe remains partly visible in the deepest probing depth in the sextant.

**Treatment Implications:**

**A comprehensive periodontal examination and charting of the affected sextant are necessary to determine an appropriate treatment plan.**

Examination and documentation should include:

- Identification of probing depths
- Mobility
- Gingival recession
- Mucogingival problems
- Furcation invasions
- Radiographs

If two or more sextants score Code 3: A comprehensive full mouth examination and charting are indicated.

If therapy is indicated and performed: A comprehensive examination is necessary to assess therapy and need for further treatment.

## CODE 4

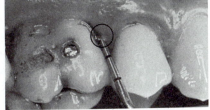

**Scoring System:**

Circled area of probe completely disappears, indicating probing depth greater than 5.5 mm.

**Treatment Implications:**

**A comprehensive full mouth periodontal examination and charting are necessary to determine an appropriate treatment plan.**

The examination and documentation should include:

- Identification of probing depths
- Mobility
- Gingival recession
- Mucogingival problems
- Furcation invasions
- Radiographs

It is probable that complex treatment will be required.

If therapy is indicated and performed: A comprehensive examination is necessary to assess the results of therapy and need for further treatment.

## CODE *

**Scoring System:**

The symbol * should be added to sextant score whenever findings indicate clinical abnormalities, such as:

- Furcation invasion
- Mobility
- Mucogingival problems
- Recession extending to the colored area of the probe (3.5 mm or greater)

**Treatment Implications:**

If an abnormality exists in the presence of Code 0, 1, or 2: Specific notation and/or treatment for that condition is warranted.

If an abnormality exists in the presence of Code 3 or 4:

**A comprehensive full mouth periodontal examination and charting are necessary to determine an appropriate treatment plan.**

LMP 7539   752-6083   Printed in U.S.A.   June 1992

©1992 by The American Dental Association and The American Academy of Periodontology

**Figure 3-1** Periodontal Screening and Recording™. (Reprinted with permission of the American Dental Association)

bone also is reduced. Therefore, the attachment measure can be used clinically to estimate the amount of bone loss; especially in the absence of radiographs.

It is also important to measure and record recession because it frequently occurs with attachment loss. This fact is often overlooked if the clinician only considers corresponding probe readings that can sometimes be 3 mm or "normal" sulcus depth. Clinicians must recognize that attachment loss is almost always present in a recessed area. The total attachment loss will be the determinant of the amount of periodontal degeneration that occurred prior to the time of the examination and will dictate the periodontal diagnosis. This historical data cannot be used alone to determine the presence or absence of active disease at the time of the examination. Other signs of inflammation such as bleeding on probing must also be considered as adjuncts in determining disease activity.

The "gold standard" for measurement of periodontal disease activity is clinical loss of attachment (Goodson, 1986). Epidemiological studies of United States populations and Kenyan populations respectively, showed similar results with respect to continued attachment loss throughout life without increasing pocket depths (Baelum, Fjerskov, & Manji, 1988; Carlos, Brunelle, & Wolfe, 1987). This occurrence was a result of concomitant recession accompanying the attachment loss. These studies have led researchers and clinicians to place new emphasis on attachment loss measures.

Attachment levels may be measured with either a manual probe or automated device with a stent. The **clinical attachment level** is the relative probing depth corresponding to the distance from the cementoenamel junction (CEJ) to the location of a periodontal probe tip (Consensus Report, Discussion Section I, 1989) against the epithelial attachment. This measurement is readily accomplished when recession is present; however, when the gingival margin is coronal to the CEJ, the CEJ to gingival margin measurement must be subtracted from the overall pocket depth (see Figure 3-2). It is important to consider total attachment loss when determining the periodontal diagnosis. In other words, diagnosis should not be based on pocket depths alone, but should include clinical attachment loss. For example, if a patient has generalized 3 mm probing depths but has an average total attachment loss of 6 mm due to coexisting recession of 3 mm, the determination of disease severity must focus on the 6 mm of attachment loss. This attachment level would result in a diagnosis of moderate periodontitis whereas the 3 mm probing depths alone would erroneously indicate periodontal health or gingivitis. Determination of the existence of active disease must then be established separately based upon signs of inflammation and/or bleeding.

## Bleeding on Probing

Because bleeding is one of the classic signs of inflammation, it was treated as the only true diagnostic sign of dis-

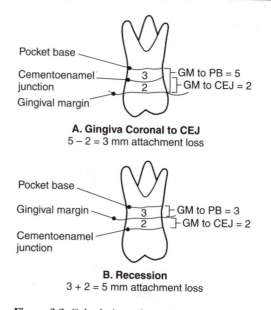

**A. Gingiva Coronal to CEJ**
5 – 2 = 3 mm attachment loss

**B. Recession**
3 + 2 = 5 mm attachment loss

**Figure 3-2** Calculation of attachment loss.

ease activity for many years. Recent research, however, has cast a shadow on this theory and bleeding is no longer considered the most reliable indicator of active disease (Galgut, 1988). When microbial invasion of the gingival sulcus occurs, concomitant ulceration of the epithelial attachment is a direct result of the inflammatory and immune responses. This ulceration exists because of a breakdown of the glycosaminoglycans that hold the epithelial cells together. This loss of epithelial integrity exposes the sulcus to the vascular lamina propria which, when provoked by routine probing, bleeds. However, due to multiple factors including operator probing force, one cannot always rely on bleeding as an indicator of active disease. It has been shown that probing of healthy intact epithelial attachments at forces greater than 0.25 N will result in bleeding in the absence of disease (Lang, Nyman, Senn, & Joss, 1991). Consistent absence of bleeding on probing, nonetheless, can be considered to be a fairly reliable indicator that disease is not present (Lang, Adler, Joss, & Nyman, 1990).

Historically, bleeding has been considered as an indicator of disease activity and has been used as a standard measure along with probing. Recent evidence suggests that bleeding has low sensitivity as an indicator of disease activity (Lang, Joss, Orsanic, Gusberti, & Siegrist, 1986; Galgut, 1988). The ability of any measure to be sensitive enough to consistently identify existing disease as well as specific enough to accurately rule out disease when it is absent results in high predictive value for disease progression. All clinicians and researchers agree that sites that bleed are not healthy. Most investigations show that bleeding has high specificity, suggesting that absence of bleeding may be a useful indicator of periodontal stability (Goodson, 1992). Bleeding, therefore, should be considered a consequence of disease rather than as a predictor of future disease (Haffajee et al., 1991).

Bleeding upon probing continues to be a valued portion of the periodontal examination. Many clinicians record sites that bleed by circling the probe readings in red or recording bleeding sites in red and nonbleeding pocket depths in blue. Others chart the sites that bleed on a separate chart similar to the one used for scoring plaque (see Figure 3-3). Numerous bleeding indices are available for epidemiological investigations and clinical application. A commonly used index is determined by adding the number of surfaces that bleed, and dividing this total by the number of available surfaces, and then multiplying by 100 to obtain a percentile measure (Ainamo & Bay, 1975). Obtaining a baseline bleeding score helps both the client and clinician establish measurable goals to assess at subsequent appointments and historical information for future comparison. Client evaluation of bleeding can also become a part of self-care (see Chapter 8).

## Exudate

Exudate from the gingival sulcus does not occur in healthy tissues. **Gingival crevicular fluid** is an exudate that flows from the gingival sulcus or the pocket. It is present in clinically normal sulci because these sulci invariably demonstrate inflammation at the microscopic level. In a strictly healthy gingiva, little or no fluid can be detected (Carranza & Bulkacz, 1996). GCF increases in quantity during inflammation and contains various by-products of the inflammatory response. Its presence reflects the nature of the inflammatory changes within the pocket wall (see Table 3-1). Purulent exudate (pus) consists of living, degenerated, and necrotic leukocytes, living and dead bacteria, serum, and fibrin (Carranza, 1996). It is sometimes observed during routine probing and may be "milked" from the tissues with a coronal finger stroke over the tissues. Isolated areas of deeper pockets should be checked for purulence as possible localized periodontal abscesses may exist. Additionally, sites with advanced periodontitis with extensive destruction and extreme mobility often reveal exudate on probing. Even though exudate is associated with advanced disease and secondary infection shallow pockets can divulge exudate and the majority of deep periodontal pockets do not reveal exudate.

Scarff, Walsh, and Darby (1994) differentiate exudate from suppuration. The GCF is suppuration when it is a clear serous liquid. Suppuration, however, is not always clinically evident. Because it is not readily visible, diagnostic paper strips are used to collect samples (see subsequent section describing diagnostic testing of GCF). Several studies have investigated various clinical parameters for the prediction of attachment loss and found the presence of suppuration increased the positive predictive value for disease progression (Badersten, Nilvéus, & Egelberg, 1990; Claffey, Nylund, Kiger, Garrett, & Egelberg, 1990). These authors did not distinguish between exudate and suppuration. Both exudate and suppuration should be added to the list of risk factors.

## Deposits

Assessment of the quantity of bacterial plaque, calculus, and stain routinely occur at each periodontal examination. Because calculus and stain are plaque-retentive factors, their identification and removal facilitate healing of the periodontal tissues.

**Bacterial Plaque.** Extensive research into the etiology of periodontal diseases has resulted in recognition of bacterial plaque as the prime etiological agent (Slots, 1986). Current thought has returned to the specific plaque hypothesis, thereby encouraging a multitude of research geared at the identification of specific periodontopathic pathogens. The mere presence of plaque, however, does not necessarily result in disease (Socransky & Haffajee, 1992). Bacterial plaque may be composed of microbes that are not harmful to, or even beneficial to, the periodontium. These concepts coupled with the concept of sequential colonization of bacterial plaque affect whether a critical mass of pathogens is present at a sufficient level to produce disease (Carranza & Newman, 1995). Disease can only occur when an imbalance of pathogens and host response exist (Socransky & Haffajee, 1992). However, because a clear relationship exists between bacterial plaque and periodontal disease, it is paramount that the presence or absence of plaque be evaluated during a periodontal assessment. Contributing factors such as overhanging restorations, poor tooth alignment, presence of stain and calculus, and poor oral hygiene must also be noted. Ideally, plaque should be measured at each visit in order to set goals with the client and to measure efficacy of self-care. Baseline plaque and bleeding scores can be used to identify and track inflammation that persists in the absence of plaque. If this occurs, the client may have removed all plaque within the past 24 hours more thoroughly than his/her normal routine; thus tissue inflammation is a more valid indicator. If, however, inflammation is generalized or severe in the absence of local etiologic factors, other risk factors such as the immune response, diet, drug intake, and smoking habits should be evaluated.

One of the most commonly used methods of scoring plaque is the Plaque Control Record (O'Leary, Drake, & Naylor, 1972) that calculates the percentage of surfaces with plaque. This scoring method utilizes a simple chart with either four or six surfaces per tooth and has several charts per form in order to make comparisons between appointments (see Figure 3-3). The total number of surfaces of plaque is divided by the total possible surfaces, and then multiplied by 100 in order to obtain a percentile measure. The ideal score is 10 percent (Wilkins, 1994); however, this percentile is relative to the client's clinical manifestations of disease. A score of 15 percent accompanied by no clinical inflammation, bleeding on probing, or other advanced condition (progressive disease) is acceptable. Bacterial plaque is identified by staining the teeth with either a red or purple

NAME _____

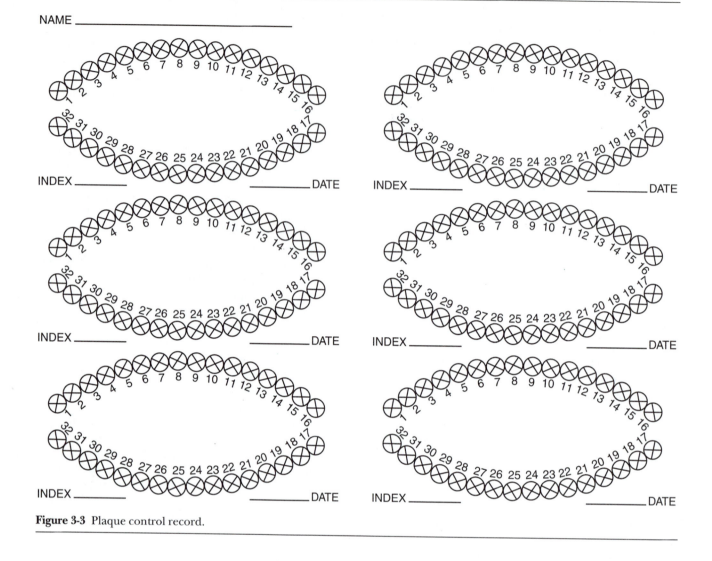

**Figure 3-3** Plaque control record.

disclosing dye or utilizing a yellow fluoricein dye visible only under an ultraviolet light. It is important not to deviate from the staining method used to identify plaque at baseline as inconsistencies in dyes will skew the results. There are several other methods to score plaque which quantify the plaque or assess specific pathogens present; however, they are more popular in research than in clinical practice.

In addition to amount of plaque, location is also significant. Bacterial plaque accumulation coinciding areas of bleeding on probing or pocket depth might be useful for client motivation for self-care. Plaque located on demineralized areas or on exposed root surfaces can also be related to the development of future carious lesions or sensitivity. Bacterial plaque formation and subgingival bacterial plaque are discussed in more detail in Chapter 10.

**Calculus.** Calculus has been defined as a tenacious material formed by the calcification of dental plaque (Woodall, 1993). Complex factors are involved in the calcification process of calculus involving minerals found in

both saliva and gingival crevicular fluid. Electron micrographs of calculus have repeatedly revealed a dense calcified matrix consisting of both living and nonliving microorganisms. The ability of calculus to harbor living organisms such as periodontal pathogens is of major concern. Repeated investigations have shown that the presence of living microorganisms is directly responsible for the initial insult that occurs to the gingival tissues when the endotoxins released by these microorganisms initiate the inflammatory response, which eventually leads to periodontal breakdown (Socransky & Haffajee, 1992; Slots, 1986). Calculus is considered a risk factor because of its rough surfaces that attract plaque formation and, thus, is capable of harboring living microorganisms. Prior to the conclusions of research revealing the role of microorganisms and the immune response in the initiation of periodontal disease, it was believed that calculus was the cause of periodontitis. Practitioners who still believe this limit their focus to calculus removal and polishing, even though there has been a major shift in the philosophy of periodontal care. It is now recognized that elimination of not just these risk factors, but addressing all risk factors present is the appropriate standard of care.

Because calculus deposits are found both supragingivally and subgingivally, it is necessary to locate these deposits and to include their removal in planning NSPT. Regardless of how meticulous the calculus removal, it has been repeatedly shown that not all deposits will be removed (Badersten, 1985; Brayer, Mellonig, Dunlap, Marinak, & Carson, 1989). Tissue response has been favorable in the majority of cases treated despite some calculus retention (Sherman, Hutchens, & Jewson, 1990). It is likely that enough calculus is removed to allow for a favorable host response. This premise, however, is not suggesting that attempts should be made to remove only easily accessible deposits; instead, it is merely an explanation of tissue response. The current standard of care still requires thorough calculus identification and removal of clinically detectable deposits and other plaque-retentive factors.

There are many systems for quantifying the amount of supragingival and subgingival calculus ranging from a simple scale describing the extent as light, moderate, or heavy to elaborate numerical systems. It is important to denote location, extent, and tenacity when incorporating any system into a periodontal examination. Identifying the tenacity and extent of the deposits will assist the clinician in appropriate treatment planning and instrument selection. Refer to Chapter 10 for a discussion of calculus formation and removal as it relates to periodontal instrumentation.

**Stain.** Stains are primarily an aesthetic problem rather than a periodontal one. They are the result of deposits by chromogenic bacteria, foods, and chemicals and are perceived to be more problematic by the patient rather than the clinician. If heavy stain such as tobacco stain accumulates, it could possibly be considered a risk factor as it can be plaque retentive.

## Mobility

Studies have shown mobility to be a predictor of attachment loss (Ismail, Morrison, & Burt, 1990; Wang, Burgett, Shyr, & Ramfjord, 1994). Mobility represents a function of the persisting height of the alveolar bone and width of the periodontal ligament. Mobility is a risk factor for periodontal disease that should be measured, especially when the extent of disease is moderate or advanced. It is essential to determine the cause of the mobility because it can be created by conditions other than periodontal destruction such as trauma or periapical pathology. Mobility can be measured in two ways: by bidigital evaluation when the teeth are not occluded, and by direct observation when the teeth are occluded (fremitus). Bidigital evaluation is the conventional way to measure mobility. Two handles of single-ended instruments are placed on the middle third of the tooth to secure a firm fulcrum for each hand, and an attempt is made to move the tooth buccolingually while visually observing it for movement. Movement is usually rated on a scale of 0 to 3, although the description of this numerical scale varies from system to system (see Table 3-2). No tooth has zero mobility unless it is ankylosed; therefore, normal physiologic movement is not graded.

Fremitus is measured by placing an index finger on the maxillary teeth when they are in function and requesting that the client grind in lateral and protrusive movements. Any movement seen or felt is considered fermitus (Magnusson & Wilson, 1992). Fremitus is often detected before bidigital tooth mobility and it is associated with increased attachment and bone loss. The degree of mobility is not always directly correlated to the amount of bone loss because trauma from occlusion, inflammation in the periodontal ligament, periodontal surgery, physiochemical changes (pregnancy and hormonal) in the periodontal tissues, and other pathological conditions (tumors) are all contributing factors. Minor mobility that does not impair oral function can usually be maintained by NSPT and PMP; however, a progressive increase in mobility over time might warrant a more frequent PMP interval and/or referral for surgery.

An automated device, the Periotest (Siemens, Germany), is a compact clinical instrument developed to measure tooth mobility (see Figure 3-4). This handheld probe consists of an impeller, or blunt ended pointer, which is held against the tooth at a 90-degree angle. When activated, the impeller taps against the tooth sixteen times and then averages out the return time providing the reading by both voice-synthesis and visual display. The probe uses a scale called Periotest units (PTU) that provide a reading ranging from 0 to 50 with the higher number indicating more severe mobility. Non-

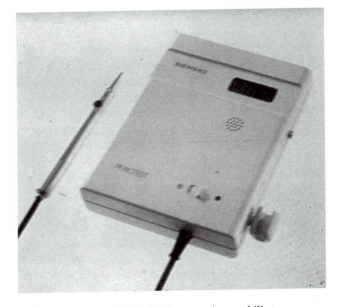

**Figure 3-4** Automated device for assessing mobility.

## Table 3-2 Systems for Classifying Mobility

| Source | Description |
|---|---|
| Darby & Walsh, 1994 | Class I°—Tooth can be moved up to 1 millimeter in any direction.<br>Class II°—Tooth can be moved more than 1 millimeter in any direction but is not depressible in the socket.<br>Class III°—Tooth can be moved in a buccolingual direction and is depressible in the socket. |
| Nield-Gehrig & Houseman, 1996 | N = normal physiologic mobility<br>Grade I = slight mobility, up to 1 millimeter of horizontal displacement in a facial-lingual direction.<br>Grade II = moderate mobility, greater than 1 millimeter of displacement in a facial-lingual direction.<br>Grade III = severe mobility, greater than 1 millimeter of displacement in all directions (vertical and horizontal). |
| Pattison & Pattison, 1992 | + mobility—Barely discernible movement. Anterior teeth because they usually have single, relatively short, conical roots normally display a + mobility.<br>I mobility—Combined facial-lingual movement totaling 1 mm.<br>II mobility—Combined facial-lingual movement totaling 2 mm.<br>III mobility—Combined facial-lingual movement totaling 3 mm or more and/or tooth depressible into socket. |
| Perry, Beemsterboer, & Taggart, 1996 | Grade 0: Physiologic mobility only.<br>Grade 1/2: Clinical mobility that is slightly greater than physiologic mobility, but less than 1 mm buccolingually.<br>Grade 1: Slight pathologic mobility; approximately 2 mm buccolingually, but no vertical displacement.<br>Grade 3: Severe pathologic mobility, greater than 2 mm buccolingually or mesiodistally, combined with vertical displacement. |
| Wilkins, 1994; Carranza, 1996 | N = normal, physiologic.<br>1 = slight mobility, greater than normal.<br>2 = moderate mobility, greater than 1 mm displacement.<br>3 = severe mobility, may move in all directions, vertical as well as horizontal. |

mobile teeth usually have values of less than 10 PTUs (Schulte, d'Hoedt, Lukas, Maunz, & Steppeler, 1988).

## Furcation Involvement

When loss of attachment extends into the bifurcation or trifurcation of multirooted teeth, it is referred to as a furcation involvement. Several studies have reported that teeth with furcation involvements are more likely to be lost than those without furcation involvements (Hirshfield & Wasserman, 1978; McFall, 1982; Wang, Burgett, Shyer, & Ramfjord, 1994). Additionally, a study by Grbic and Lamster (1992) revealed that molar teeth were more likely to exhibit attachment loss after treatment than any other teeth. Furcation involvement was identified as a risk factor in predicting periodontal breakdown during the World Workshop in Clinical Periodontics (McFall, 1989). A recent study investigating this relationship concluded that teeth with furcation involvements have significantly greater attachment loss than teeth without involved furcations and were 2.54 times more likely to be lost than teeth without furcation involvement (Wang, et al., 1994). Considerations in detecting furcations are that bone loss

frequently is angular not horizontal; cratering often develops in the interradicular area, and they are not always radiographically visible. Both horizontal and vertical probing need to occur to assess the extent for deposit removal, and probing might be the only means of detecting the defect. Considerations during assessment in preparation for treatment include root trunk length, the concavity of the inner surface of the exposed roots, the degree of separation of the roots, and presence of enamel projections that occur in about 15 percent of molars (Carranza & Takei, 1996).

The exact amount of furcation involvement is difficult to ascertain as vertical periodontal probes are not easily adapted to the curvatures of the furcation. A curved calibrated Naber's probe is commercially available for measuring furcations that readily adapt to these curvatures when gingival tissue does not occlude the furcation. These probes are available with color-coded markings and are usually calibrated in 3 mm intervals. Although more useful than the conventional straight probes, they still have their limitations as far as visibility in reading the measurements, particularly in maxillary distolingual furcations. Furcation involvement should be suspected whenever a periodontal pocket of 4 millimeters or more in depth is present on a multirooted tooth. Surprisingly, furcation roofs or entrances are relatively close to the gingival margin in health. Involvement is most frequently seen on the mandibular first molars. Chapter 10 provides the reader with an anatomical review of furcations and their relationship to instrument selection for detection and deposit removal.

Furcation involvements have been classified by Glickman (1953) as Grades I, II, III, and IV. The following is a summary of these grades: Grade I involves incipient bone loss in which the fluting between the roots can be felt but the roof of the furcation cannot be engaged; Grade II is partial bone loss where the probe can enter the furcation and the roof can be felt; Grade III is total bone loss with through and through opening of the furcation, and Grade IV is the same as Grade III except due to recession, the through and through furcation can be visibly detected. Table 3-3 offers characteristics of each grade and lists treatment options (Carranza & Takei, 1996). Chapter 17 discusses furcation involvements and surgery options.

## INDICES

Indices have been mentioned as a tool to measure and score periodontal assessment factors such as plaque, calculus, and bleeding for the benefit of both the clinician and client. An index score in clinical practice provides a reference point for change in the entity being measured from visit to visit. The clinician benefits because the score is easy to describe to the client and can be used to help motivate behavior change in oral self-care. The client benefits for the same reason, as a score or number is easier to comprehend than, for example, a description of gingival inflammation using erythema, edema, and bleeding. Limitations of indices in clinical practice are the time necessary to perform the index, the need to standardize all oral health care providers performing the index, and the fact that many indexes measure only a single few or few parameters of periodontal assessment.

For instance, even though an individual's plaque score is high, the score itself has relative meaning because the plaque accumulation might not be highly correlated to the degree of inflammation and disease. For this reason, multiple indexes are sometimes employed or an index selected that measures multiple factors such as the Periodontal Index that evaluates inflammation, pocketing, and mobility. Therefore, an index may be an asset in oral self-care, but never substitutes for essential periodontal assessment components and measurements.

Most indices were originally designed for research purposes to describe the prevalence, incidence, and severity of disease or deposits in large populations. In these cases, subsets of teeth are selected usually based on the six teeth (#3, 9, 12, 19, 25, and 28) selected for measurement in the Periodontal Disease Index (Ramfjord, 1967). A summary of indices measuring gingival and periodontal disease, bleeding, plaque, and oral hygiene is presented in Table 3-4.

**Table 3-3 Furcation Grades, Characteristics, and Treatment Options**

| Furcation | Characteristics | Treatment Options |
|---|---|---|
| Grade I | • early lesion<br>• suprabony pockets<br>• slight bone loss<br>• no radiographic changes | • scaling/root planing<br>• curettage<br>• gingivectomy<br>• odontoplasty |
| Grade II | • bone is destroyed on one or more aspects<br>• a portion of the alveolar bone and periodontal ligament remains intact<br>• partial penetration with a probe (termed "cul-de-sac")<br>• horizontal depth varies<br>• vertical loss might exist (interradicular crater)<br>• possible radiographic visibility; not absolute | • scaling/root planing<br>• osseous grafting<br>• guided tissue regeneration<br>• advanced lesions—root removal or resection |
| Grade III | • interradicular bone is absent<br>• facial/lingual entrances occluded by gingiva<br>• through and through tunnel exists<br>• probe passes through freely<br>• cratering in interradicular area<br>• radiographically visible | • scaling/root planing<br>• flap procedure<br>• removal or resection of a root |
| Grade IV | • interradicular bone is absent<br>• entrance is visible clinically<br>• through and through tunnel exists<br>• probe passes through freely<br>• radiographically visible | • scaling/root planing<br>• flap surgery |

**Table 3-4  Summary of Indices**

PLAQUE AND ORAL HYGIENE INDICES

| Index | Measures | Scoring Criteria | Calculations |
|---|---|---|---|
| Oral Hygiene Index (OHI) (Greene & Vermillion, 1960) | Debris and Calculus | **Debris Index**<br>0 = No debris or stain.<br>1 = Soft debris covering not more than one-third of tooth surface.<br>2 = Soft debris covering more than one-third but not more than two-thirds of tooth surfaces.<br>3 = Soft debris covering more than two-thirds of tooth surface.<br><br>**Calculus Index**<br>0 = No calculus<br>1 = Supragingival calculus covering not more than one-third of exposed tooth surface.<br>2 = Supragingival calculus covering one-third to two-thirds of exposed tooth surface and/or flecks of subgingival calculus.<br>3 = Supragingival calculus covering more than two-thirds of exposed tooth surfaces and/or a continuous band of subgingival calculus. | 1. Select the facial surface and the lingual surface in each sextant with highest debris index score.<br>2. Add the 12 Debris Index scores together and divide total by 12. This is the Debris Index Score.<br>3. Select the facial surface and the lingual surface in each sextant with the highest calculus index score.<br>4. Add the 12 Calculus Index Scores together, divide this total by 12. This is the calculus index score.<br>5. OH Index = Debris Index and Calculus Index. |
| OHI-S Simplified Oral Hygiene Index (Greene & Vermillion, 1964) | Debris and Calculus | Same as OHI. | 1. Measure only facial surfaces of #3, 8, 14 and 24 and the lingual surfaces of #19 and 30.<br>2. Add the debris scores for the six surfaces together and divide by 6. This is the Simplified Debris Index.<br>3. Add the calculus scores for the six surfaces together and divide by 6. This is the Simplified Calculus Index.<br>4. OHI-S = DI-S + CI-S. |
| Plaque Index (PI) (Silness & Löe, 1967) | Thickness of Plaque | 0 = No plaque.<br>1 = A film of plaque adhering to the free gingival margin and adjacent area of the tooth. The plaque may be recognized only after application of a disclosing agent or by running the explorer across the tooth surfaces.<br>2 = Moderate accumulation of soft deposits within the gingival pocket that can be seen with the naked eye or on the tooth and gingival margin.<br>3 = Abundance of soft matter within the gingival pocket and/or on the tooth and gingival margin. | 1. Four areas for each tooth are measured (mesial, facial, distal, lingual).<br>2. May do entire dentition or selected teeth.<br>3. Total the four scores and divide by 4 to obtain tooth score.<br>4. Add tooth scores together and divide by number of teeth to arrive at a PI score for the person. |
| Patient Hygiene Performance (PHP) (Podshadley & Haley, 1968) | Plaque and Debris | 0 = No deposit (or questionable).<br>1 = Debris definitely present. | 1. Apply disclosing agent.<br>2. Examine teeth 3, 8, 14, 19, 24, and 30. (Substitutions of adjacent molars and centrals may be used if teeth are missing).<br>3. Tooth surface divided into five areas.<br>4. One point is given for each area with plaque (maximum score per tooth = 5).<br>5. Add the six scores together and divide by 6. |

| Index | Measures | Scoring | Method |
|---|---|---|---|
| Turesky Modification of Quigley & Hein (1970) | Plaque | 0 = No plaque.<br>1 = Discontinuous band of plaque at gingival margin.<br>2 = Greater than 1 mm continuous band of plaque at gingival margin.<br>3 = Less than 1 mm band of plaque but covering greater than gingival one-third of tooth surface.<br>4 = Plaque covering less than one-third but greater than two-thirds of the tooth surface.<br>5 = Plaque covering two-thirds or more of tooth surface. | 1. Apply disclosing solution and rinse.<br>2. Examine all facial and lingual surfaces only.<br>3. Total all plaque scores and divide by the total number of surfaces examined. |
| Ramfjord Plaque Index (1967) | Plaque | 0 = No plaque.<br>1 = Plaque present on some but not all interproximal, facial, and lingual surfaces of the tooth.<br>2 = Plaque present on all interproximal, facial, and lingual surfaces, but covering less than one-half of these surfaces.<br>3 = Plaque extending over all interproximal, facial, and lingual surfaces, and covering more than one-half of these surfaces. | 1. Apply disclosing solution and have patient rinse.<br>2. Score teeth numbers 3, 9, 12, 19, 25, and 28 (four surfaces: facial, lingual, mesial, and distal).<br>3. Add the plaque scores for each tooth and divide by the number of teeth examined. |
| Plaque Control Record (O'Leary, Drake, & Naylor, 1972) | Plaque | Count the number of surfaces with plaque and calculate as percentage of plaque. | 1. Apply disclosing solution to teeth and rinse.<br>2. Record areas of plaque (may use four or six tooth surfaces).<br>3. Total number of teeth and multiply by either 4 or 6 (surfaces used).<br>4. Multiply the number of plaque-stained surfaces by 100 and divide by the total number of available surfaces:<br>$$\frac{\text{Total Number of Tooth Surfaces with Plaque}}{4\ (6) \times \text{Number of Teeth Present}} \times 100 = \%\ \text{Score}$$ |
| Plaque-Free Score (Grant, Stern, & Everett, 1979) | Surfaces with No Plaque | Plaque-free surfaces counted and converted to a percentage. | 1. Apply disclosing solution to teeth and rinse.<br>2. Examine four surfaces of all teeth for plaque and record.<br>3. Total the number of teeth present.<br>4. Multiply the number of teeth by 4 to determine number of surfaces available.<br>5. Subtract the number of surfaces with plaque from the total number of surfaces available to find the number of plaque-free surfaces:<br>$$\frac{\text{Number of Plaque-Free Surfaces}}{\text{Number of Available Surfaces}} \times 100 = \%\ \text{Plaque-Free Surfaces}$$ |
| Gingival Index (GI) (Löe & Sillness, 1963) | Gingival Inflammation | 0 = Normal gingiva.<br>1 = Mild inflammation slight change in color, slight edema. No bleeding on probing.<br>2 = Moderate inflammation, redness, edema, and glazing. Bleeding on probing.<br>3 = Severe inflammation, marked redness, edema, and ulceration. Tendency to spontaneous bleeding. | 1. Assign a score of 0 to 3 for mesial, distal, buccal, and lingual surfaces of teeth numbers 3, 9, 12, 19, 25, and 28.<br>2. Use a blunt instrument such as a periodontal probe to access bleeding.<br>3. Total scores per tooth and divide by 4.<br>4. Total all tooth scores and divide by the number of teeth examined. |

(continues)

**Table 3-4 (continued)**

## PLAQUE AND ORAL HYGIENE INDICES

| Index | Measures | Scoring Criteria | Calculations |
|---|---|---|---|
| | | | 5. Final score interpreted as follows:<br>0.1 to 1.0 = Mild Gingivitis<br>1.1 to 2.0 = Moderate Gingivitis<br>2.1 to 3.0 = Severe Gingivitis |
| Periodontal Index (PI) (Russell, 1967) | Gingival Inflammation Pocket presence, Mobility | 0 = Negative; no overt inflammation or loss of function resulting from destruction to supporting tissues.<br>1 = Mild gingivitis; overt area of inflammation in free gingiva but not circumscribing the tooth.<br>2 = Gingivitis; inflammation completely circumscribes the tooth, no apparent break in epithelial attachment.<br>4 = Used only when radiographs available. Early resorption of alveolar crest.<br>6 = Gingivitis with pocket formation; epithelial attachment broken (not merely a deepened crevice from swelling); normal masticatory function; no drifting or mobility.<br>8 = Advanced destruction; loss of masticatory function; teeth may be loose or drifted; may sound dull on percussion; may be depressible in socket. | 1. Assign a score of 0 to 8 for mesial, distal, buccal, and lingual surfaces of all the teeth in the mouth.<br>2. Interpret final score as follows:<br>0.0 to 0.2 = Clinically Normal<br>0.3 to 0.9 = Simple Gingivitis<br>1.5 to 5.0 = Established Destructive Periodontal Disease<br>3.8 to 8.0 = Terminal Periodontal Disease |
| Periodontal Disease Index (PDI) (Ramfjord, 1967) | Extent of Periodontal Disease | 0 = Absence of inflammation.<br>1 = Mild to moderate changes not extending around the tooth.<br>2 = Mild to moderately severe gingivitis extending around the tooth.<br>3 = Severe gingivitis, characterized by marked redness, tendency to bleed, and ulceration.<br>4 = Gingival crevice in any of four measured areas (mesial, distal, buccal, lingual) extending apically to cementoenamel junction, but not more than 3 mm.<br>5 = Gingival crevice in any measured areas extending apically to CEJ (3 to 6 mm).<br>6 = Gingival crevice in any of four measured areas extending apically more than 6 mm from CEJ. | 1. Assess gingivitis, gingival sulcus depth, calculus, plaque, occlusal and incisal attrition, mobility, and lack of contact for teeth numbers 3, 9, 12, 19, 25, and 28.<br>2. PDI score = $\dfrac{\text{Total Scores for All Teeth}}{\text{Number of Teeth Examined}}$<br>3. Group score of 3.5 = severe gingivitis.<br>4. Scores of 4 to 6 depict periodontitis. |
| Community Periodontal Index of Treatment Needs (COITN) (Ainamo, 1982) (WHO) | Periodontal Status and Treatment Needs | Code 0 = Healthy periodontal tissues.<br>Code 1 = Bleeding after gentle probing.<br>Code 2 = Supra- or subgingival calculus or defective margin of filling or crown.<br>Code 3 = 4 or 5 mm pocket.<br>Code 4 = 6 mm or deeper pathological pocket. | 1. Use a 0.5 mm ball tip WHO Periodontal Probe (Markings are .5 (ball), 3.5, 5.5, 8.5, 11.5 mm).<br>2. Mark the highest score per sextant.<br>3. Classify patients into treatment needs according to the higher code score.<br>0 = No need for treatment (Code 0).<br>I = Oral hygiene instruction (Code 1).<br>II = Oral hygiene instruction plus scaling and root planing, including elimination of plaque-retentive margins of fillings and crowns (Code 2 + 3). |

*The American Academy of Periodontology (AAP) and the American Dental Association (ADA) have modified this index to be used as a screening tool for individual patients. Periodontal screening and recording (PSR) for general practitioners is available through Proctor & Gamble Co., Cincinnati, OH.

| Index | Measures | Scoring Criteria | Calculations |
|---|---|---|---|
| Periodontal Screening Examination (O'Leary, 1967) | Gingival Inflammation, Pocket Depths | **Gingival Score**<br>0 = Normal gingiva.<br>1 = Slight to moderate inflammation not surrounding any teeth.<br>2 = Slight to moderate inflammation surrounding one or more teeth.<br>3 = Marked inflammation, ulceration, spontaneous bleeding, loss of surface continuity, and clefts of gingival tissue.<br><br>**Periodontal Index**<br>4 = Probe extends up to 3 mm apical to the CEJ of any tooth in the segment.<br>5 = Probe extends from 3 to 6 mm apical to the CEJ of any tooth in the segment.<br>6 = Probe extends 6 mm or more apical to the CEJ of any tooth in the segment. | 1. Probe the mesial line angles of all the teeth and record the highest score for each segment. |

## BLEEDING INDICES

| Index | Measures | Scoring Criteria | Calculations |
|---|---|---|---|
| Sulcus Bleeding (SBI) (Muhlemann & Son, 1971) | Sulcular Bleeding upon Probing | 0 = Healthy appearance of papilla (P) and margin (M), no bleeding on probing.<br>1 = Apparently healthy P and M with no swelling or color change; bleeding on probing present.<br>2 = Bleeding on probing and change of color caused by inflammation.<br>3 = Bleeding on probing and change in color and slight edematous swelling.<br>4 = (1) Bleeding on probing and change in color and obvious swelling.<br>    (2) Bleeding on probing and obvious swelling.<br>5 = Bleeding on probing and spontaneous bleeding and color changes and swelling with or without ulceration. | 1. Probe four areas for each tooth: marginal, gingival, labial, and lingual (m units) and interproximal mesial and distal.<br>2. Wait 30 seconds after probing before scoring.<br>3. Total scores per tooth and divide by 4.<br>4. SBI for individual: total individual tooth scores and divide by the number of teeth. |

*(continues)*

**Table 3-4 (continued)**

## BLEEDING INDICES (continued)

| Index | Measures | Scoring Criteria | Calculations |
|---|---|---|---|
| Gingival Bleeding Index (GBI) (Carter & Barnes, 1974) | Gingival Inflammation Determined by Interproximal Bleeding from Gingival Sulcus | Bleeding upon flossing after 30 seconds. | 1. Floss each area and wait for 30 seconds.<br>2. May score either 26 proximal areas (excluding 3rd molars) *or* two sulci per interproximal area.<br>3. Total number of areas that bleed are recorded. |
| Papillary-Marginal-Attached Gingival Index (P-M-A) (Shour & Massler, 1948) | Extent of Gingival Changes in Large Groups | **Papillary (P)**<br>0 = Normal; no inflammation.<br>1+ = Mild papillary engorgement; slight increase in size.<br>2+ = Obvious increase in size of gingival papilla; bleeding on pressure.<br>3+ = Excessive increase in size with spontaneous bleeding.<br>4+ = Necrotic papilla.<br>5+ = Atrophy and loss of papilla (through inflammation).<br><br>**Marginal (M)**<br>0 = Normal; no inflammation visible.<br>1+ = Engorgement; slight increase in size; no bleeding.<br>2+ = Obvious engorgement; bleeding upon pressure.<br>3+ = Swollen collar; spontaneous bleeding; beginning infiltration into attached gingiva.<br>4+ = Necrotic gingivitis.<br>5+ = Recession of the free marginal gingiva below the cementoenamel junction as a result of inflammatory changes.<br><br>**Attached (A)**<br>0 = Normal; pale rose; stippled.<br>1+ = Slight engorgement with loss of stippling; change in color may or may not be present.<br>2+ = Obvious engorgement of attached gingiva with marked increase in redness. Pocket formation present. Deep pockets evident.<br>3+ = Advanced periodontitis. | 1. Examine facial surfaces only from maxillary left second molar to right second molar; then mandibular right second molar and left second molar (third molars not included).<br>2. Press the side of periodontal probe against the gingiva in three areas: (P) papillary, (M) marginal, and (A) attached.<br>3. Count the number of P, M, and A units scored and record separately as follows: P-M-A = 6+1<br>4. May be translated to the following nominal scale:<br>1 to 4 papilla<br>0 to 2 margins } Mild Gingivitis<br>4 to 8 papilla<br>2 to 4 margins } Moderate Gingivitis<br>more than 8 papilla<br>more than 4 margins } Severe Gingivitis |
| Eastman Interdental Bleeding Index (Caton & Polson, 1985) | Interdental Gingival Bleeding | 0 = Absence of bleeding when a triangular toothpick is depressed 2 mm inserted interproximally four times, and checked 15 seconds later.<br>1 = Bleeding after above procedure. | Total the number of areas that bleed. |
| Gingival Bleeding Index (GBI) (Ainamo & Bay, 1975) | Bleeding on Probing | **Negative**<br>Absence of bleeding on probing after 10 seconds following probing.<br>**Positive**<br>Appearance of bleeding within 10 seconds following gentle probing. | Total the number of areas that bleed and divide by the number of gingival margins examined and multiply by 100 to get a percentage score. |

## SUPPLEMENTAL DIAGNOSTIC TESTS

Several supplemental diagnostic tests have been developed in an attempt to identify the presence of disease. Although none to date have been identified as an ideal diagnostic, several may have value as adjuncts to traditional tests in determining patients or sites that are at risk for periodontal breakdown. These tests are categorized under four general headings: physical, microbiological, biochemical, and immunological.

### Physical Assessment Tests

Measures of subgingival temperature and GCF flow are related to inflammation. The monitoring of subgingival temperature has recently been investigated based on the premise that "calor" or heat is one of the cardinal signs of inflammation. Because periodontitis is primarily a chronic inflammatory disease, researchers hypothesized that an increase in sulcular temperature at diseased sites would occur. Several studies have confirmed this hypothesis (Fedi & Killoy, 1992; Kung, Ochs, & Goodson, 1990; Ng, Compton, & Walder, 1978). Correlations between elevated sulcular temperature, presence of certain bacterial species, and bleeding on probing have been established, thus identifying sulcular temperature in conjunction with these other parameters as a predictor of future attachment loss (Haffajee, Socransky, & Goodson, (I), 1992a; Haffajee, Socransky, & Goodson, (II), 1992b; Haffajee, Socransky, Smith, Dibart, & Goodson, (III), 1992; Isogai, et al., 1994). Involved bacterial species include *P. gingivalis, A. actinomycetemcomitans,* and *P. intermedia.*

The PerioTemp System (Abiodent, Danvers, MA) (see Figure 3-5) consists of a temperature-sensitive thermocouple probe attached to a display panel with an internal computer that interfaces with a printer. The probe is designed to measure subgingival temperature relative to sublingual temperature. The probe internally computes the difference between the sublingual temperature and the sulcular temperature. Measurements are conducted in degrees Celsius, but are converted by the built-in computer to an ordinal scale of G(0), Y(1), R(2). This scale corresponds to a visual light-emitting diode (LED) panel with the green light translating to a normal temperature range (G), yellow to slightly warmer than normal (Y), and red indicating an elevated temperature (R). Upon completion of the examination, a printout of the ordinal scores provides a permanent record that may be filed in the patient's chart. Temperature measurements for six sites per tooth are activated by a foot-controlled rheostat, and the probe has standard millimeter calibrations allowing the probing depths and bleeding scores to be collected simultaneously. This system has been designed for use by the clinician, providing another physical measurement for inflammation that can be combined with bleeding on probing to determine the presence of disease activity. Because periodontal probing can be accomplished at the same time, it is easily incorporated into routine practice to establish a baseline record and for posttreatment reevaluation. Haffajee and coworkers (1992a & 1992b) discovered that sites recorded in the red temperature zone were two times as likely to have attachment loss as sites recorded in the green zone.

It has been well documented that the flow of GCF increases prior to the development of clinically evident gingivitis and has been closely related to periodontal status (Caton, 1989). Positive correlations have been found between increased GCF flow and clinical indices of inflammation (Brexc, Schlegel, Gehr, & Lang, 1987; Caton, 1989). The flow rate of gingival crevicular fluid has become a useful mechanism for monitoring the response to periodontal therapy. Actual decreases in GCF have been recorded following therapy (Löe & Holm-Pederson, 1965). As a predictor of future periodontitis, however, more refinement is required in the quantification of individual host normal flow values. It is not sufficient to measure the GCF flow, as normal flow varies from individual to individual. Current use of this technology is mostly limited to research. Gingival crevicular fluid flow is measured by an electronic instrument called the Periotron 6000. This instrument measures the area of a filter strip wetted with GCF and provides a digital readout of the volume of fluid collected.

### Microbiological Assessment

It has been widely accepted that more than one microorganism at any given time plays an active role in periodontal destruction. There are close to 300 bacterial species that have been isolated from the oral cavity, but only a dozen or so have been labeled periodontopathic or causative agents of periodontal disease (see Chapter 1, Table 1-1). Because periodontal diseases are mixed infections, no single microorganism can be specifically labeled as the sole causative agent. An exception of that is *A.*

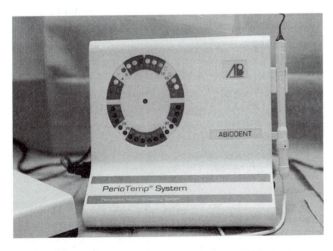

**Figure 3-5** PerioTemp™ system. (Courtesy of Abiodent, Danvers, MA)

*actinomycetemcomitans*, which has repeatedly been shown to be associated with forms of juvenile periodontitis (Moore et al., 1985; Zambon, 1985). A return to the specific plaque hypothesis has caused researchers to look more closely at combinations of specific bacterial phenotypes in an attempt to identify more specific patient protocols for treatment. Identification of specific microorganisms through microbial assessment techniques may be utilized to determine the causative agent, assess disease activity for treatment planning, select antibiotic regimes, monitor the effects of treatment, and to determine recall intervals (Genco, 1986).

Additionally, identification of the presence of any suspected periodontopathogens could be useful as risk indicators in the absence of disease. It is questionable as to whether the mere presence of the pathogens is predictive of active disease as these organisms may remain in periodontal pockets long after the disease activity has gone into remission (Socransky & Haffajee, 1992). It has also been well established that the pathogens must occur in sufficient numbers to cause disease. If a test is sensitive enough it may detect low numbers of these pathogens, but it may not be specific enough to rule out disease when it is not present. Therefore, it is important to pay close attention to the sensitivity, specificity, and subsequent predictive values of the particular test in question. If a future diagnostic test has high predictive value, it will be useful in determining not only future risk, but also the development of an appropriate course of treatment.

Culture techniques, until recently, were the only method of detecting and identifying putative periodontal pathogens and are still considered by most to be the "gold standard" or most accurate method for identifying and quantifying bacterial plaque components. Culturing techniques are time-intensive and expensive as they require specialized equipment and highly trained clinicians. Most university laboratories provide a culturing service for those clinicians who wish to utilize this method of microbial analysis. It is advisable for the clinician to identify the specific types of organisms present in a periodontal infection in order to prescribe the most effective antibiotic when aggressive forms of disease are present. The only means of determining antibiotic susceptibilities of suspected pathogens is by cultural analysis. The other microbial tests that can be rapidly administered are designed to detect a limited number of pathogens and they do not provide information about the antibiotic sensitivities of the infecting bacteria.

The phase contrast and darkfield microscopes were introduced into clinical practice in the early 1980s. Their use was based on the premise that increased numbers of motile bacteria, especially spirochetes, were present in the pockets of periodontally involved teeth while healthy sites had higher numbers of cocci and nonmotile bacteria (Listgarten & Hellden, 1978). This technology, however, is not capable of identifying specific bacterial species or genotypes, only bacterial morphotypes (shapes) (Greenstein & Polson, 1985). Additionally, many of the

periodontopathic species such as *A. actinomycetemcomitans* and *P. gingivalis* are neither spirochetes nor are they motile (Omar & Newman, 1986). Research results generally concur that microscopic monitoring does not appear to be a reliable predictor of periodontal disease nor is it a suitable system for monitoring disease activity (Greenstein, 1985). Many, however, appropriately use microscopy to motivate their clients and to monitor the phagocytic activity of the host cells. If host cells do not exhibit phagocytosis, which is generally visible in phase contrast microscopy, there is a possibility that the patient may be immunosuppressed and further medical tests may be required. In these cases, the person should be referred to a physician for further evaluation.

The use of enzymatic methods to identify bacteria associated with plaque has been researched since the mid 1980s (Löesche, 1986). These methods can distinguish *B. forsythus*, *P. gingivalis*, *T. denticola*, and the *Capnocytophaga* species because they have in common a small trypsin-like enzyme. The activity of this enzyme is measured by a test that utilizes a synthetic substrate, n-benzoyl-DL-arginine-B-naphthylamide (BANA). All of these pathogens have been associated with periodontal disease. Löesche (1986) reported that periodontal pockets that are 7 mm deep or greater demonstrated 80 to 90 percent positive BANA reactions whereas shallow pockets only demonstrated positive testing 10 percent of the time. A new BANA test that can be used inexpensively at chairside during an assessment or maintenance appointment is being marketed in Canada as the BANA™ Test by Nowell Pharmaceuticals (see Figure 3-6).

The presence of various microorganisms may be identified by antigen-antibody reactions. Immunological assays that measure these reactions include latex agglutination, flow cytometry, immunofluorescent microscopy, and enzyme-linked immunosorbant assays (ELISA) (Greenstein, 1988). These techniques depend on the availability of specific antibodies that will bind to selected bacterial antigens that are then detected by either fluorescent markers or through a colorimetric reaction (Listgarten, 1992). As such, they measure an antibody reaction to a specific antigen rather than simply detecting its presence. These tests are available for research purposes only at this time.

A rapid chairside ELISA test was recently introduced in Canada and Europe (Evalusite™; Eastman Kodak Co., Rochester, NY). This test individually identifies three periodontopathic microorganisms: *P. gingivalis*, *P. intermedia*, and *A. actinomycetemcomitans* and is an easy step-directed process taking approximately 10 minutes to perform. This test shows a great deal of promise not only for its ease of use and rapid results, but for its reported sensitivity and specificity levels of higher than 90 percent (Zambon, Reynolds, Chen, & Genco, 1985). FDA approval is required for use of this product in the United States and it may be available for clinical use in the near future. If approved, this accurate and easy to use chairside test could be used by the clinician to ascertain

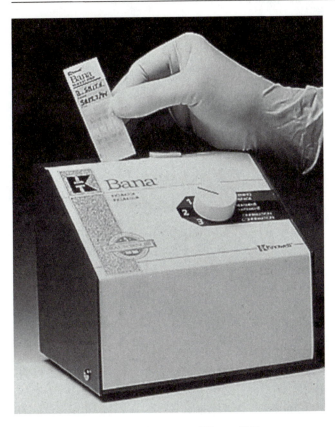

**Figure 3-6** BANA™ test. (Courtesy of Knowell Pharmaceuticals, Toronto, Ontario, Canada)

whether antibiotic therapy for these three common pathogens is indicated and, if so, which antibiotic(s) would be appropriate. It would not, however, assess all possible pathogens and opportunistic microorganisms like the full ELISA assay or culturing techniques performed in laboratory settings.

DNA probes are used to identify periodontal pathogens by identifying the presence of bacterial DNA fragments within a sample. This technique involves the preparation of pieces of single-stranded DNA from the bacterial species under investigation. The pieces are tested until a segment is found to be unique for only that species and does not cross-react with any other species. The pieces of DNA can be derived either directly from the bacteria (genomic probes) or from isolated sequences of either DNA unique to the species or from shorter sequences of ribosomal RNA (oligonucleotide probes) (Löesche, 1992). The advantages of this technology include the stability of the DNA, which allows for identification even after bacterial death, and the ability of the probes to detect as few as 1,000 bacterial cells per plaque sample (French et al., 1986). Additionally, sensitivity and specificity levels have been reported at levels higher than 90 percent when compared with culture techniques (Moncla, Braham, Dix, Watanabe, & Schwartz, 1990; Savitt, Strempko, Vaccarro, Peros, & French, 1988).

Two separate diagnostic tests have been developed utilizing DNA technology. The DMDX™ test (Omnigene, Inc., Cambridge, MA) utilizes both genomes and oligonucleotide probes that require laboratory processing. This offers the clinician the option of identifying up to six periodontal pathogens. The most commonly identified pathogens are *P. gingivalis*, *P. intermedia*, and *A. actinomycetemcomitans*. The clinician collects the plaque samples with paper points that are placed in a sterile vial and sent by mail to the laboratory for analysis (see Figure 3.9). Results are reported in approximately ten to fourteen days. The second test (Affirm™ DP; Microprobe Corporation, Bothell, WA) employs oligonucleotide DNA probes to ribosomal RNA utilizing a nonradioactive enzymatic reporter system that does not require laboratory processing. This chairside test is not commercially available.

**Biochemical Assessments**

Biochemical assessments were developed to study the nature of the host response in GCF. Biochemical markers found in GCF have been studied extensively and have been related to gingivitis and periodontitis (Caton, 1989). In contrast to the measurement of the rate of GCF flow discussed previously, biochemical markers are extracted from the GCF and studied. Most recently, GCF has been related to disease activity and certain markers may be capable of predicting future risk for periodontal breakdown (Fine & Mandel, 1986). There are over forty components of gingival crevicular fluid that can be divided into three main groups: host-derived enzymes, tissue breakdown products, and inflammatory mediators (Newman & Sanz, 1996). Tests for the components collagenase, prostaglandin E2, beta-glucuronidase, and aspartate aminotransferase will be discussed because they are the most applicable.

Collagenase is the enzyme that breaks down collagen, which is the main structural protein of the gingival connective tissues. Collagenase is produced by fibroblasts and the breakdown of collagen is part of the normal remodeling process. Studies have shown that collagenase found in GCF of patients with chronic adult periodontitis originated in the polymorphonuclear leukocyte (PMN) cells of the host (Sorsa, Uitto, Suomalainen, Vauhkonen, & Lindy, 1988). Several experimental gingivitis studies in both dogs and humans have demonstrated elevated levels of collagenase during diseased states (Caton, 1989). Additionally, studies have shown strong correlations with clinical attachment loss in patients having elevated levels of collagenase and other neutral proteases such as alkaline phosphatase and PMN elastase (Lamster, 1992). Although these tests show promise, most are not yet commercially available.

A neutral protease test was recently made commercially available by Pro-Dentec, Incorporated (Batesville, AR). Periocheck™ is a simple rapid chairside test that detects and measures matrix metalloproteinases or neutral proteinase enzymes including collagenase (see Figure

3-7). The test employs the collection of GCF utilizing a paper strip that is inserted 1 to 2 mm under the gingival margin for 3 minutes, incubated for 12 minutes, and then compared with a color chart for measurement of enzyme activity (Pro-Dentec, 1995). The manufacturer suggests that this test be used to monitor the response to nonsurgical periodontal therapy, monitor recurrent active disease, and as a monitoring device for implant breakdown. A five-week study comparing clinical measurements with Periocheck™ scores in nonsurgical periodontal therapy patients, found a strong association (p < 0.001) between assay scores and calculus, bleeding, and gingival indices (Dreher, Shelburne, & Wolff, 1993). Although the predictive value of this test has yet to be established, it may be useful as an adjunctive monitoring system to traditional clinical measures. Periocheck™ could be used both pre and post initial therapy, as well as at maintenance visits.

Prostaglandin E2 (PGE2) is an arachadonic acid metabolite produced by the cycloxygenase pathway. It is a strong inflammatory mediator found to be associated with inflammation and bone loss. PGE2 has been found in a longitudinal study to be five times greater in sites of clinical attachment loss than in healthy sites (Offenbacher, Odle, & Van Dyke, 1986). In the same study, PGE2 elevations were detectable in GCF six months prior to the detection of periodontal disease activity. The sensitivity and specificity of PGE2 as a screening test to identify patients experiencing clinical attachment loss was 76 percent and 96 percent respectively (Lamster, 1992). This test to date is not commercially available.

Beta-Glucuronidase(Bg) is a lysosomal enzyme released by polymorphonuclear leukocytes (PMNs) during the inflammatory process that can be identified and quantified in GCF. Extensive testing of Bg by Lamster and coworkers has revealed promising results. In a year-long study, a relationship between Bg in GCF to clinical attachment loss showed that persistently high levels of Bg were associated with disease activity and that this disease activity could be predicted three to six months in advance

(Lamster, Oshrain, Celenti, Fine, & Grbic, 1991). In this study, the sensitivity and specificity of lysosomal Bg as a screening tool to detect disease activity were 92 percent and 86 percent respectively. These results were also confirmed in a multisite clinical trial in which 140 patients were evaluated for six months. Results revealed high levels for both sensitivity and specificity yielding a total predictive value of 90 percent (Lamster et al., 1991). A diagnostic kit for assessing Bg activity in GCF is currently being developed by Abbott Laboratories (Abbott Laboratories, North Chicago, IL).

Aspartate aminotransferase (AST), is a cytoplasmic enzyme that is released only upon cell death. Because cell death is an integral part of the inflammatory process, this chemical marker is found in elevated quantities during the inflammatory process. Several studies have revealed promising results showing elevated levels of AST at associated disease active sites (Page, 1992). A colorimetric test is currently under development for chairside in-office use for the identification of AST (PerioGard™ Xytronyx, Inc., San Diego, CA).

## Immunological Assessments

Immunological methods to assess periodontal disease activity have revolved around the identification of antibodies to specific periodontal pathogens in either the blood serum or the gingival crevicular fluid. Research has focused more on developing the serum tests. Serum antibody titers to *A. actinomycetemcomitans* were found to be elevated in patients with localized juvenile periodontitis. Similar findings were reported for *P. intermedia* for acute necrotizing ulcerative gingivitis and for *P. gingivalis* for adult and rapidly progressive periodontitis (Caton, 1989). Although correlations were found between elevated antibody levels and active disease, the relationship to disease progression has not been established. A chairside test for the identification of serum antibody levels of several periodontal pathogens has recently been introduced for in-office use (PerioAlert™; Avitar, Inc., Canton, MA). The usefulness of the test results, however, remains to be established.

## Decision Making

Table 3-5 summarizes supplemental diagnostic testing. With all the available adjunctive diagnostic tests, it is difficult to identify which ones to use, when to use them, and with whom to use them. It has been suggested that three categories of cases be considered for diagnostic testing: previously untreated cases, cases treated and on maintenance, and those diagnosed with refractory or rapidly progressive periodontitis (Lamster, Celenti, Jans, Fine, & Grbic, 1993). Clients who have not been previously treated might benefit from diagnostic testing in order to establish a baseline for monitoring disease progression at subsequent visits, although these tests are time-consuming and expensive so they are not commonly used at

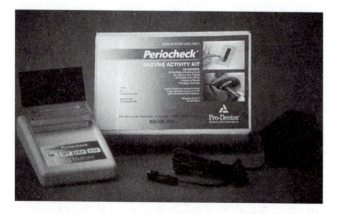

**Figure 3-7** Periocheck™. (Courtesy of ProDentec, Inc., Batesville, AR)

**Table 3-5  Summary of Supplemental Diagnostic Tests**

| Categories | Risk Factor | Rationale | Examples of Test/Instrument | Used in Clinical Practice |
|---|---|---|---|---|
| Physical Assessment | • Subgingival temperature | • heat is a cardinal sign of inflammation | • PerioTemp™ System, Abiodent | • Yes |
| | • GCF flow | • increases prior to development of gingivitis; however, flow rate normally differs from person to person | • Periotron 6000 Instrument | • No |
| Microbiological Assessment | • Culturing of putative periodontal pathogens | • accurate method for identification and quantification of bacterial species; however, time-intensive and expensive | • Culture by university/clinical laboratories | • Limited |
| | • Enzymatic methods to identify periodontopathic microorganisms | • identify *T. denticola*, *P. gingivalis*, and *B. forsythus*, which are associated with attachment loss | • BANA™, Knowell Pharmaceuticals | • Yes (Canada) |
| | • Immunological assays to identify microorganisms | • specific antibodies bind to selected bacterial antigens that can then be detected by fluorescent markers or colorimetric reaction; Evalusite™ identifies *P. gingivalis*, *P. intermedia*, and *A. actinomycetemcomitans* | • Latex agglutination<br>• Flow cytometry<br>• Immunofluorescent microscopy<br>• ELISA (Evalusite™, Eastman Kodak) | • No |
| | • DNA probing to identify periodontal pathogens | • the presence of bacterial DNA fragments within a sample are identified; DNA is stable even after bacterial death | • DMDX™, Omnigene (identifies up to six periodontal pathogens including *P. gingivalis*, *P. intermedia*, and *A. actinomycetemcomitans*)<br>• Affirm™ DP, Microprobe Corporation | • Limited<br><br><br><br><br>• No |
| Biological Assessment | • Collegenase | • elevated levels of collegenase show strong correlations to attachment loss | • Periocheck™, Pro-Dentec | • Yes |
| | • Prostaglandin E2 (PGE2) | • elevated levels of PGE2 exist in sites with clinical attachment loss | • NA | • No |
| | • Beta-Glucuronidase (Bg) | • high levels of Bg are associated with disease activity | • Diagnostic kit being developed by Abbot Laboratories | • No |
| | • Aspartate aminotransferase (AST) | • high levels of AST are associated with disease activity | • PerioGuard™ Xytronyx, Inc. is being developed | • No |
| Immunological Assessment | • Serum antibody titers are evaluated for periodontal pathogens | • correlations were found between elevated antibody levels and active disease | • PerioAlert™, Avitar, Inc. | • Limited |
| | • GCF antibody levels | • GCF antibodies increase in diseased sites | • NA | • No |

baseline. Periodontal maintenance therapy outcomes could be monitored more closely in order to assess stability or periods of exacerbation early enough to provide interceptive therapy, especially in more aggressive forms of periodontal disease. In the future, as these tests become more "user friendly," they might also help to identify appropriate recall intervals. At this time, however, they have the most benefit in cases of refractory or rapidly progressive periodontitis to identify specific microorganisms that can help confirm the diagnosis and aid in determining appropriate antibiotic therapy and other supportive therapies. Clues to the cause of the poor response may also be identified.

## IDENTIFICATION OF RISK FACTORS

It is important to recognize that the periodontal assessment serves as an historical record, enabling the clinician to clearly see trends in disease progression from appointment to appointment. Forms such as the one shown in Figure 3-8, are excellent for summarizing risk factors and enabling the clinician to track factors that have been addressed and eliminated over time. There is no real limitation or score that can predict an individual's periodontal disease susceptibility or progression; however, the higher the number of risk factors, the greater the chances of the client having some form of periodontal disease. Prior to arriving at a diagnosis and developing a care plan, it is essential that as many risk factors as possible be identified and discussed with the patient in order to prevent future breakdown.

### Recording Forms

An essential component of a thorough examination is having a comprehensive recording form. Examples of recording forms are provided in Figures 3-9, 3-10 and 3-11. The recording form must always include a place or manner for recording probing depths, clinical attachment loss, plaque description and/or scores, bleeding on probing, suppuration, recession, mobility, furcation involvement, calculus description or location, and other

---

**DENTALLY-RELATED RISK FACTORS**

PERIODONTAL DISEASE:    CLASS: _____ Gingivitis      _____ Periodontitis

                         FORM: _____ Slowly progressing      _____ Aggressive

                         EXTENT: _____ Early     _____ Moderate     _____ Advanced

BACTERIAL PLAQUE:    Percent Present _____      Pathogens/DNA Test

                                              ___ pG ___ pI ___ aA

CALCULUS:             Class 1 _____ 2 _____ 3 _____ 4 _____ 5 _____

STAIN:               Light _____ Moderate _____ Heavy _____

TEETH:               Missing: _____        Malposed: _____

MOBILITIES: _____

OVERHANGING RESTORATIONS: _____

FOOD IMPACTION: _____ SELF-CARE: _____        TOTAL: _____

**UNCHANGING SUBJECT-RELATED RISK FACTORS**

RACE: _____

FAMILY HISTORY OF EARLY TOOTH LOSS: _____

GENDER:                     M _____ F _____        TOTAL: _____

**CHANGING SUBJECT-RELATED RISK FACTORS**

AGE: _____    SMOKING:          YES _____     NO _____

               ALCOHOL CONSUMPTION:    YES _____     NO _____

DIET/NUTRITION: _____

DRUGS: _____

STRESS: _____        TOTAL: _____

SYSTEMIC DISEASE: _____      FINAL TOTAL: _____

**Figure 3-8** Risk factor summary.

| Date | Maxillary | 1 | 2 | 3 | 4 | 5 | 6 | 7 | 8 | 9 | 10 | 11 | 12 | 13 | 14 | 15 | 16 |
|---|---|---|---|---|---|---|---|---|---|---|---|---|---|---|---|---|---|
| | Maintenance appt. 2 | | | | | | | | | | | | | | | | |
| | Maintenance appt. 1 | | | | | | | | | | | | | | | | |
| | Re-eval probing depth | | | | | | | | | | | | | | | | |
| | Total loss of attachment | | | | | | | | | | | | | | | | |
| | Recession/tissue-CEJ height | | | | | | | | | | | | | | | | |
| | Baseline probing depth | | | | | | | | | | | | | | | | |

**Occlusal examination:**

Molar – Right I  II  III
        Left  I  II  III
Canine – Right I  II  III
         Left  I  II  III
Overbite_____ mm
Overjet_____ mm
Midline shift_____ mm to  R  L
Open bite #_____
Cross bite #_____
Other _____

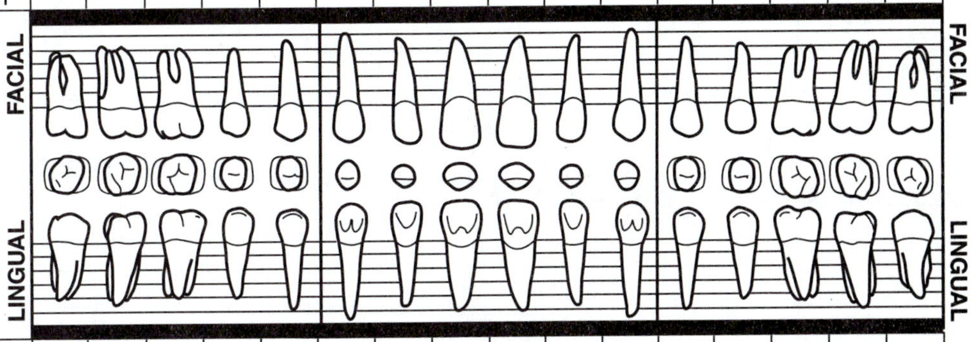

FACIAL — LINGUAL — FACIAL — LINGUAL

| | Baseline probing depth | | | | | | | | | | | | | | | | |
|---|---|---|---|---|---|---|---|---|---|---|---|---|---|---|---|---|---|
| | Recession/tissue-CEJ height | | | | | | | | | | | | | | | | |
| | Total loss of attachment | | | | | | | | | | | | | | | | |
| | Re-eval probing depth | | | | | | | | | | | | | | | | |
| | Maintenance appt. 1 | | | | | | | | | | | | | | | | |
| | Maintenance appt. 2 | | | | | | | | | | | | | | | | |
| Date | Maxillary | 1 | 2 | 3 | 4 | 5 | 6 | 7 | 8 | 9 | 10 | 11 | 12 | 13 | 14 | 15 | 16 |

| Date | Mandibular | 32 | 31 | 30 | 29 | 28 | 27 | 26 | 25 | 24 | 23 | 22 | 21 | 20 | 19 | 18 | 17 |
|---|---|---|---|---|---|---|---|---|---|---|---|---|---|---|---|---|---|
| | Maintenance appt. 2 | | | | | | | | | | | | | | | | |
| | Maintenance appt. 1 | | | | | | | | | | | | | | | | |
| | Re-eval probing depth | | | | | | | | | | | | | | | | |
| | Total loss of attachment | | | | | | | | | | | | | | | | |
| | Recession/tissue-CEJ height | | | | | | | | | | | | | | | | |
| | Baseline probing depth | | | | | | | | | | | | | | | | |

**The Ramfjord teeth**
**Maxilla:**
#3 - right 1st molar
#9 - left central incisor
#12 - left 1st premolar
**Mandible:**
#19 - left 1st molar
#25 - right lateral incisor
#28 - right 1st premolar

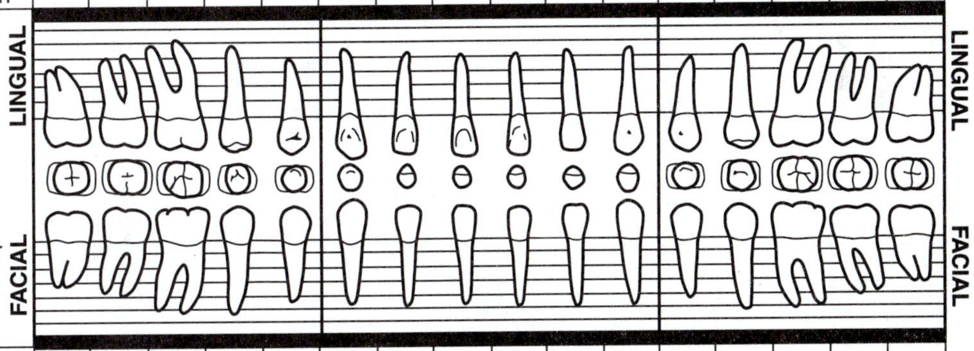

LINGUAL — FACIAL — LINGUAL — FACIAL

| | Baseline probing depth | | | | | | | | | | | | | | | | |
|---|---|---|---|---|---|---|---|---|---|---|---|---|---|---|---|---|---|
| | Recession/tissue-CEJ height | | | | | | | | | | | | | | | | |
| | Total loss of attachment | | | | | | | | | | | | | | | | |
| | Re-eval probing depth | | | | | | | | | | | | | | | | |
| | Maintenance appt. 1 | | | | | | | | | | | | | | | | |
| | Maintenance appt. 2 | | | | | | | | | | | | | | | | |
| Date | Mandibular | 32 | 31 | 30 | 29 | 28 | 27 | 26 | 25 | 24 | 23 | 22 | 21 | 20 | 19 | 18 | 17 |

**Figure 3-9** Periodontal assessment and calculus charting. (Courtesy of Wichita State University, Wichita, KS, 1995)

CLIENT________________________ HYGIENIST________________________

**Bleeding Points** = dot above number **Suppuration** = circle number **Recession** = measure each surface with probe **Mobility** = record on crown, I, II, III **Furcation** = record at tooth apex, designate furca, I, II, III (Ex: B-I, DL-II) **Probe** = probe score **T.A.L.** = Total Attachment Loss

**CASE TYPE _____**

Facial
Date_____

Upper Right | Upper Anterior | Upper Left

| | | | | | | | | | | | | | | | | |
|---|---|---|---|---|---|---|---|---|---|---|---|---|---|---|---|---|
| Probe | | | | | | | | | | | | | | | | |
| Rec. | | | | | | | | | | | | | | | | |
| T.A.L. | | | | | | | | | | | | | | | | |

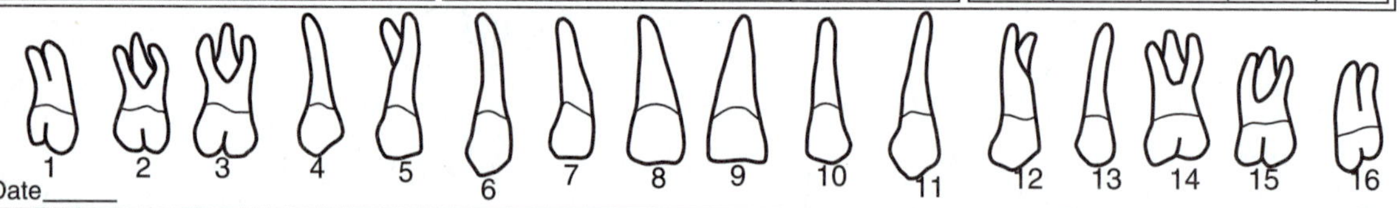

1
2
3
4
5
6
7
8
9
10
11
12
13
14
15
16


Lingual Date_____

| | | | | | | | | | | | | | | | | |
|---|---|---|---|---|---|---|---|---|---|---|---|---|---|---|---|---|
| Probe | | | | | | | | | | | | | | | | |
| Rec. | | | | | | | | | | | | | | | | |
| T.A.L. | | | | | | | | | | | | | | | | |

Lingual Date_____

| | | | | | | | | | | | | | | | | |
|---|---|---|---|---|---|---|---|---|---|---|---|---|---|---|---|---|
| Probe | | | | | | | | | | | | | | | | |
| Rec. | | | | | | | | | | | | | | | | |
| T.A.L. | | | | | | | | | | | | | | | | |

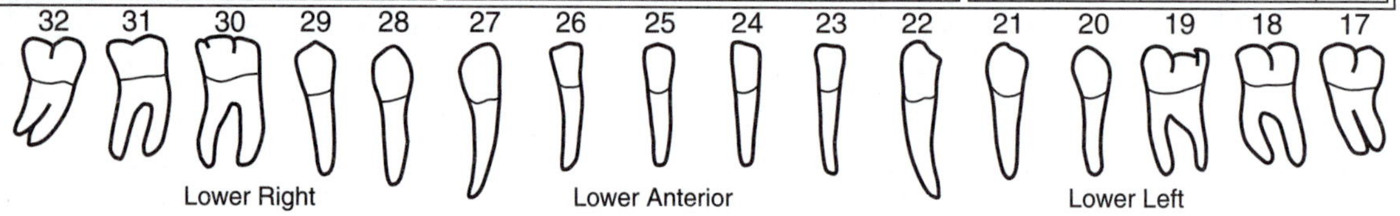

32
31
30
29
28
27
26
25
24
23
22
21
20
19
18
17


Facial
Date_____

Lower Right | Lower Anterior | Lower Left

| | | | | | | | | | | | | | | | | |
|---|---|---|---|---|---|---|---|---|---|---|---|---|---|---|---|---|
| Probe | | | | | | | | | | | | | | | | |
| Rec. | | | | | | | | | | | | | | | | |
| T.A.L. | | | | | | | | | | | | | | | | |

Probing/Bleeding/Plaque Summary

| | 4 | 5-7 | 8> | B | P |
|---|---|---|---|---|---|
| UR | | | | | |
| UA | | | | | |
| UL | | | | | |
| LL | | | | | |
| LA | | | | | |
| LR | | | | | |
| TOTAL | | | | | |

Plaque Record % Plaque _____

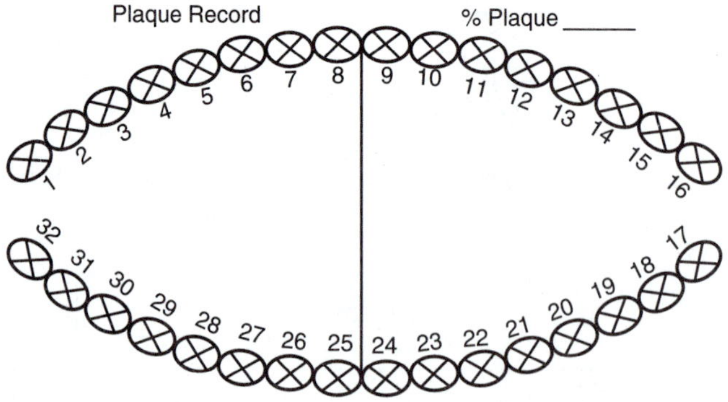

1
2
3
4
5
6
7
8
9
10
11
12
13
14
15
16
32
31
30
29
28
27
26
25
24
23
22
21
20
19
18
17


Gingival Description ____________________________________________

____________________________________________

Revised 12-91

**Figure 3-10** Periodontal assessment. (Courtesy of Northern Arizona University, Department of Dental Hygiene, Flagstaff, AZ, 1995)

| Name | | | | | | | Date | |
|---|---|---|---|---|---|---|---|---|

**FUNCTIONAL ASSESSMENT (CR = CO)**

| Classification | | Crossbite | | Midline Shift | Edge to Edge | End to End | Open Bite | Overbite | Overjet |
|---|---|---|---|---|---|---|---|---|---|
| R | L | A | P | | | | | | |
| | | | | | | | | | |

| Prematurities: | |
|---|---|

**INTERFERENCES**

| Right Working Side | Balancing | Left Working Side | Balancing |
|---|---|---|---|
| | | | |

**HABITS**

| Mouthbreather | | Thumb Sucking | | Bruxism | |
|---|---|---|---|---|---|
| Clenching | | Deviant Swallowing | | Other: | |

| Abrasion | Attrition | Erosion |
|---|---|---|
| | | |

**STAIN**

| Intrinsic | L  M  H | |
|---|---|---|
| Extrinsic | L  M  H | |

**CONTRIBUTING FACTORS TO GINGIVAL CONDITION**

| Plaque | Supra Calc | Sub Calc | Prognosis |
|---|---|---|---|
| L  M  H | L  M  H | L  M  H | Good   Fair   Poor |

| Restorations | | Habits | | Diet | |
|---|---|---|---|---|---|
| Hormonal Imbalance | | Trauma | | Other | |
| Medical/Systemic | | Chemical Abuse | | | |

| Explain the relationship to periodontal disease: | |
|---|---|
| Client goals and method for evaluating success of attaining goals: | |
| Client desires the following treatment: | |

PATIENT ASSESSMENT IV PG. ____

**Figure 3-11** Patient assessment. (Courtesy of Northern Arizona University, Department of Dental Hygiene, Flagstaff, AZ, 1995)

risk factors. It is ideal if the recording form has available space to rerecord these entities at subsequent maintenance appointments, thus allowing the dental hygienist to evaluate disease severity and potential disease activity by reviewing only one form (see Figure 3-9). If rerecording involves documentation on a new form at each main-

tenance visit, it is both time-consuming and cumbersome to make comparisons of the data.

Charts with summary sections for probing depths, total attachment loss, bleeding on probing, and plaque scores are excellent for tracking historical data, making comparisons at subsequent appointments, and for patient motivation (see the bottom of Figure 3-10). Ideally, the checklist format for risk factors (see Figure 3-8) could be included in a summary section on the assessment form. Categories can be grouped according to the type of risk: dental, unchanging subject, and changing subject.

## DOCUMENTATION

Accurate documentation of all findings is every clinician's obligation. Literature suggests that poor record keeping is one of the most common causes of loss in litigation (Bailey, 1987; Comer, 1990; Dunne & Brown, 1991). It is imperative that all assessment findings be clearly recorded on appropriate forms. It would also be wise to have an area on both the dental and medical histories for the patient signature indicating that the information they provided is accurate to the best of their knowledge. All pocket recordings and assessment findings must be clearly dated to avoid any doubt should these records be entered as exhibits in a court of law.

Although a thorough recording form will accurately represent clinical data, it will not indicate that the findings and associated risk factors were discussed with the client. Therefore, recording of essential elements of the periodontal assessment and the corresponding discussion is indicated (Dunne & Brown, 1991; Ebersold, 1989; Reifeis, 1990). For example, the record of services for a client presenting for care for the first time should reflect the results of the periodontal assessment as follows:

> Periodontal assessment: generalized 4 to 5 mm pocket depth discussed along with critical probe depth, attachment loss, bleeding points, generalized chronic marginal inflammation, and presumptive diagnosis of chronic adult periodontitis in the early stage. Expected healing outcomes discussed and educated about clinical signs of disease. Self-evaluation of gingival inflammation was taught. Commented "I was aware of pockets, but never knew I had a disease."

In the above example the client's reaction to the discussion was added in the form of a quotation. Documentation of client responses helps assess needs and fosters effective communication.

## Summary

Effective client care is highly dependent upon a thorough and accurate periodontal assessment resulting in a diagnosis and comprehensive care plan. So often the assessment phase of care is short-changed resulting in inadequate treatment planning or a lack of diagnosis of periodontal disease. This form of care is unacceptable and may result in litigation. The comprehensive assessment, regardless of the type of recording form utilized, must always include the key components of the clinical assessment: gingival inflammation, periodontal probing depths, attachment loss, bleeding, plaque, calculus, mobility, furcations, and radiographic bone loss. Other adjunctive tests such as sulcular temperature, GCF flow, and various microbial assessments may also be utilized when additional information regarding risk factors is required. These tests, particularly the microbial identification tests, may provide the clinician with valuable information required for the formulation of a treatment plan as the presence of certain microorganisms may warrant either systemic or local antibiotic therapy.

Inherent in the thorough assessment is the identification of all risk factors. Some risk factors such as the presence of plaque and calculus are revealed through the clinical examination, while other risk factors such as diabetes, systemic drug intake, and immunosuppressive diseases are identified through the comprehensive medical history review. Other risk factors, however, are not as readily identified unless the clinician purposely takes the time to question the patient regarding personal habits, lifestyles, exposure to stress, and other factors that may contribute to lowering the host response. A personal history may also reveal some of these risk factors. Once a lowered immune response is suspected, the patient may be referred for further testing.

Taking the time to monitor risk factors and disease progression each time the client presents for care will keep clients informed, goal-oriented, and hopefully motivated enough to take ownership of their oral health. It will also provide a comprehensive means for tracking the success or failure of therapy and may signal the clinician to alter treatment approaches. Ongoing risk factor identification provides not only a more comprehensive approach to NSPT, but encourages a more holistic approach to the delivery of oral health care.

## Case Studies

**Case Study One:** Annette Miles, a 32-year-old single mother of three small children, presents for an examination for the first time in ten years. She indicates that she has no dental insurance and is struggling financially. Her medical history reveals a persistent cough, a history of repeated upper respiratory tract infections, and generalized fatigue. She smokes two packs of cigarettes daily and currently takes Ortho-Novum 1/50 once daily. Her assessment reveals generalized recession and probing depths of 5 to 7 mm in most molar regions with attachment loss of up to 7 mm. Her bleeding index is over 60 percent, however, her plaque score is only 10 percent revealing a relatively plaque-free mouth despite the nicotine staining. How would you classify Annette's condition? How would you explain the presence of disease in the absence of significant amounts of plaque?

**Case Study Two:** George Parker, a 52-year-old architect has been under your care for the past three months. Initially, he was diagnosed with early chronic adult periodontitis with probing depths of 4 and 5 mm and generalized attachment loss of 1 to 2 mm. George's self-care was only fair with moderate amounts of plaque and gingival bleeding upon probing. You completed four quadrants of thorough debridement. During the course of therapy, George was very responsive to your home care instructions and reduced both plaque and bleeding scores significantly. He has returned for his six week post therapy reevaluation appointment. You find that his pockets have either improved by 1 mm or remained stable, however, the distal buccal surface of tooth #3 has a significant increase in pocket depth from the original 5 mm to 7 mm. Bleeding on probing is also present at this site while overall bleeding on probing and plaque scores are less that 10 percent. How would you explain the breakdown at tooth #3? What diagnostic tests could you recommend for Mr. Parker in order to deal with this problem?

**Case Study Three:** Jennifer Radtke, a 15-year-old high school sophomore is seen in your office for the first time. She complains that her two front teeth have moved as they now have a space between them that they never had before. Periodontal probing reveals pockets of 6 and 7 mm in all the maxillary anterior teeth and radiographs reveal an arch-shaped area of vertical bone loss. Prior to making a final diagnosis, you decide to take a microbiological sample with a commercially available DNA probe that you will send away for analysis. What condition do you suspect? What microorganism are you expecting the test to identify?

**Case Study Four:** A sales representative has just brought in a PerioTemp™ temperature probe for you to try out. You decide to incorporate it into Sara Transtrum's periodontal assessment. She is a 45-year-old new patient who has no significant medical history. She has been on Premarin 0. 625 mg daily since having a hysterectomy a year ago. Several areas in the upper right quadrant reveal elevated temperatures. The other areas of the mouth have normal readings. Generalized pocket depths of 3 mm are recorded throughout the mouth, however, bleeding on probing is only detected on two teeth in the upper right quadrant. Very few signs of gingival inflammation are present, the plaque score is 22 percent, and her oral care is generally good. How would you correlate these findings? What information would you provide for Sarah?

**Case Study Five:** Mrs. Smith, a 58-year-old widow, who is extremely overweight, presents with a history of non-insulin dependent diabetes mellitus (NIDDM), hypertension, and depression. She is currently on the following medications: Procardia, Lasix, Orinase, and Prozac. She indicates that she has been smoking more heavily than normal since her husband passed away last year as it "calms her nerves." She reveals how depressed she has been since her husband's death and how she finds it difficult to prepare meals for herself. Your clinical examination reveals major periodontal breakdown with probe depths ranging between 5 and 8 mm with attachment losses of up to 6 mm. How many risk factors for periodontal disease does Mrs. Smith have? What other conditions would you expect to see in the oral cavity?

## Case Study Discussions

**Discussion—Case Study One:** Annette has a preliminary or presumptive diagnosis of rapidly progressive periodontitis based on the amount of attachment loss and bleeding on probing. Despite the small amounts of plaque, this patient is at significant risk for periodontal breakdown based on her history of heavy smoking and high stress due to her personal and financial state. Stress has been shown through research to suppress the immune system to the extent that it lowers the patient's host resistance as evidenced by her numerous respiratory tract infections and periodontal condition. Annette will require extensive nonsurgical periodontal therapy, a smoking cessation program, and possible professional counseling.

**Discussion—Case Study Two:** The breakdown at the distal of tooth #3 could be caused by an isolated deficiency in cleansing as Mr. Parker appears to have influenced the healing in the other areas of the mouth. Given the site-specific nature of periodontal disease, however, it is also possible that this particular area may have putative periodontal pathogens in sufficient numbers to cause disease. A microbial assay such as Omnigiene's DMDX™ DNA test could be used at this site to identify the pathogens present. If positive test results are revealed, local drug delivery with tetracycline fibers might be considered.

**Discussion—Case Study Three:** The age of the patient, the drifted teeth, and the vertical pattern of bone loss are all signs of juvenile periodontitis. This diagnosis will be confirmed if test results reveal the presence of *Actinobacillus actinomycetemcomitans* in numbers higher than $10^4$. Appropriate treatment for juvenile periodontitis consists of systemic tetracycline and nonsurgical periodontal therapy.

**Discussion—Case Study Four:** Although the general oral health appears good, the combination of bleeding and elevated sulcular temperatures present in the upper right quadrant are indicators of disease. The pocket depth and appearance of the gingival tissues in this region have not yet been affected by the pathology, however, Mrs. Transtrum should be informed that disease activity in the upper right region is present and that she is at risk for periodontal breakdown. She should also be informed that the Premarin she is taking is an additional risk factor for hormonally-related gingivitis. Nonsurgical periodontal therapy should be treatment planned immediately to help prevent further disease in the upper right region.

**Discussion—Case Study Five:** Mrs. Smith is at high risk for periodontal disease based on several risk factors including: NIDDM, age, smoking, stress, depression, diet, and systemic medication. All of these conditions have been shown to place her at higher risk for periodontal breakdown and when a combination exists, the risk increases considerably. The other conditions that one would expect to see in Mrs. Smith's mouth would be xerostomia related to the intake of Prozac and possibly gingival enlargement related to the Procardia.

## REFERENCES

Ainamo, J. & Bay, I. (1975). Problems and proposals for recording gingivitis and plaque. *International Dental Journal, 25,* 229.

Ainamo, J., Barnes, D., Beagrie, G., Cutress, T., Martin, J., & Sardo-Infirri, J. (1982). Development of the World Health Organization (WHO) Community Periodontal Index of Treatment Needs (CPITN). *International Dental Journal, 32,* 281.

Ainamo, J. & Löe, H. 1966. Anatomical characteristics of the gingiva. A clinical and microscopic study of the free and attached gingiva. *Journal of Periodontology, 37,* 5.

American Academy of Periodontology. (1989). *Proceedings of the world workshop in clinical periodontics.* Chicago: American Academy of Periodontology.

American Academy of Periodontology. (1995a). *Diagnosis of periodontal diseases.* Chicago: AAP Department of Scientific, Clinical, and Educational Affairs, November.

American Academy of Periodontology. (1993). *Guidelines for periodontal therapy.* Chicago: AAP Department of Scientific, Clinical, and Educational Affairs.

American Academy of Periodontology. (1995b). *Current procedural terminology and insurance reporting manual.* Chicago: AAP Department of Scientific, Clinical, and Educational Affairs.

American Dental Association and The American Academy of Periodontology. (1992). *Periodontal screening and recording™.* Sponsored by Procter & Gamble.

Appelgren, R., Robinson, P. J., & Kaminski, E. J. (1979). Clinical and histologic correlation of gingivitis. *Journal of Periodontology, 50,* 540.

Badersten, A., Nilvéus, R., & Egelberg, J. (1985). Effect of nonsurgical periodontal therapy. IV. Operator variability. *Journal of Clinical Periodontology, 12*(3), 190–200.

Badersten, A., Nilvéus, R., & Egelberg, J. (1990). Scores of plaque, bleeding, suppuration, and probing depth to predict probing attachment loss. 5 years of observation following nonsurgical periodontal therapy. *Journal of Clinical Periodontology, 17,* 102–107.

Baelum, V., Fjerskov, O., & Manji, F. (1988). Periodontal diseases in adult Kenyans. *Journal of Clinical Periodontology, 15,* 445–452.

Bailey, B. L. (1987). Malpractice and periodontal disease. *Journal of the American Dental Association, 115,* 845.

Bergstrom, J., Eliasson, S., & Preber, H. (1991). Cigarette smoking and periodontal bone loss. *Journal of Periodontology, 62,* 242–246.

Brayer, W. K., Mellonig, J. T., Dunlap, R. M., Marinak, K. W., &

Carson, R. E. (1989). Scaling and root planing effectiveness: The effect of root surface access and operator experience. *Journal of Periodontology, 60*(1), 67.

Brecx, M. C., Schlegel, K., Gehr, P., & Lang, N. P. (1987). Comparison between histologic and clinical parameters during experimental gingivitis. *Journal of Periodontal Research, 22,* 50.

Bretz, W. A., Ecklund, S. A., Radicchi, R., Schork, M. A., Schork, N., Schottenfeld, D., Lopatin, D. E., & Löesche, W. J. (1993). The use of a rapid enzymatic assay in the field for the detection of infections associated with adult periodontitis. *Journal of Public Health Dentistry, 53*(4), 235–240.

Carlos, J. P., Brunelle, J. A., & Wolfe, M. D. (1987). Attachment loss vs. pocket depth as indicators of periodontal disease: A methodologic note. *Journal of Periodontal Research, 22,* 524–525.

Carter, H. G. & Barnes, G. P. (1974). The gingival bleeding index. *Journal of Periodontology, 45,* 801.

Carranza, F. A. & Bulkacz, I. (1996). Defense mechanisms of the gingiva. In F. A. Carranza and M. G. Newman (Eds.), *Clinical periodontology* (8th ed.). Philadelphia: W.B. Saunders Co.

Carranza, F. A. (1996). Clinical features of gingivitis. In F. A. Carranza and M. G. Newman (Eds.), *Clinical periodontology* (8th ed.). Philadelphia: W.B. Saunders Co.

Carranza, F. A. & Rapley, J. W. (1996). Gingival inflammation. In F. A. Carranza and M. G. Newman (Eds.), *Clinical periodontology* (8th ed.). Philadelphia: W.B. Saunders Co.

Carranza, F. A. & Newman, M. G. (1995). *Clinical periodontology* (8th ed.). Philadelphia: W.B. Saunders Co.

Carranza, F. A. & Takei, H. H. (1996). Treatment of furcation involvement and combined periodontal-endodontic therapy. In F. A. Carranza and M. G. Newman (Eds.), *Clinical periodontology* (8th ed.). Philadelphia: W.B. Saunders Co.

Caton, J. (1989). Periodontal diagnosis and diagnostic aids. In *Proceedings of the world workshop in clinical periodontics.* Chicago: The American Academy of Periodontology.

Caton, J. & Polson, A. (1985). The interdental bleeding index: A simplified procedure for monitoring gingival health. *Compendium of Continuing Education in Dentistry, 6,* 88.

Cerda, J. G., Vazquez de la Torre, C., Malacara, J. M., & Nava, L. E. (1994). Periodontal disease in non-insulin dependent diabetes mellitus (NIDDM). The effect of age and time since diagnosis. *Journal of Periodontology, 65,* 991–995.

Charles, C. J. & Charles, A. H. (1994). Periodontal Screening and Recording. *Journal of the Canadian Dental Association, 22*(2), 43–46.

Claffey, N., Nylund, K., Kiger, R., Garrett, S., & Egelberg, J. (1990). Diagnostic predictability of scores of plaque, bleeding, suppuration, and probing depth for probing attachment loss. 3½ years of observation following initial periodontal therapy. *Journal of Clinical Periodontology, 17,* 108–114.

Cohen-Cole, S., Cogen, R., & Stevens, A. (1981). Psychosocial, endocrine, and immune factors in acute necrotizing ulcerative gingivitis (trenchmouth). *Psychosomatic Medicine, 43,* 91.

Comer, L. (1990). Referral to periodontists: The need to document. *Compendium of Periodontics (COP), 11*(3), 182–184.

Darby, M. L. & Walsh, M. N. (1994). *Dental hygiene theory and practice.* Philadelphia: W.B. Saunders Co.

Dreher, K., Schelburne, C., Wolff, L. (1993). Clinical indices and proteolytic enzymes measured by (Periocheck) periodontal care monitoring system. *Journal of Dental Research, 72:* Abst. #2408.

Dunne, M. & Brown, J. L. (1991). Risk management in dentistry. *Current Opinion in Dentistry, 1*(5), 668–671.

Ebersold, L. A. (1989). Periodontal malpractice: Current standards and record keeping requirements. *Journal of the Michigan Dental Association, 71*(9), 483–486.

Fedi, P. F. & Killoy, W. J. (1992). Temperature differences at periodontal sites in health and disease. *Journal of Periodontology, 63,* 24–27.

Fine, D. H. & Mandel, I. D. (1986). Indicators of periodontal disease activity: An evaluation. *Journal of Clinical Periodontology, 13,* 533.

French, C. K., Savitt, E. D., Simon, S. L., Lippke, L. A., Raia, F. F., & Vaccaro, K. K. (1986). DNA probe detection of periodontal pathogens. *Oral Microbiology and Immunology, 1,* 58–62.

Galgut, P. M. (1988). The bleeding/plaque ratio in the treatment of periodontal disease. *Journal of Clinical Periodontology, 15,* 606–611.

Genco, R. J., Zambon, J. J., & Christersson, L. A. (1986). Use and interpretation of microbiological assays in periodontal disease. *Oral Microbiology and Immunology, 1,* 73.

Genco, R. J. (1992). Host responses in periodontal diseases: Current concepts. *Journal of Periodontology, 63,* 338–355.

Gibbs, C. H., Hirshfeld, J. W., & Lee, J. G. (1988). Description and clinical evaluation of a new computerized periodontal probe—the Florida Probe. *Journal of Clinical Periodontology, 15,* 137–144.

Glickman, I. (1953). *Clinical periodontology* (1st ed.). Philadelphia: W.B. Saunders Co.

Goodson, J. M., Tanner, A. C. R., Haffajee, A. D., Sornberger, G. C., & Socransky, S. S. (1982). Patterns of progression and regression of advanced destructive periodontal disease. *Journal of Clinical Periodontology, 9,* 479.

Goodson, J. M. (1986). *Periodontal screening and recording.* Cincinnati: Proctor & Gamble.

Goodson, J. M. (1992). Diagnosis of periodontitis by physical measurement: Interpretation from episodic disease hypothesis. *Journal of Periodontology, 63,* 373–382.

Grant, D. A., Stern, I. B., & Everett, F. G. (1979). *Periodontics* (5th ed.). St. Louis: Mosby-Year Book, Inc., 529–531.

Grbic, J. T. & Lamster, I. B. (1992). Risk indicators for future clinical attachment loss in adult periodontitis. Tooth and site variables. *Journal of Periodontology, 63,* 262–269.

Greene, J. C. & Vermillion, J. R. (1960). The oral hygiene index: A method for classifying oral hygiene status. *Journal of the American Dental Association, 61,* 172.

Greene, J. C. & Vermillion, J. R. (1964). The simplified oral hygiene index. *Journal of the American Dental Association, 68,* 7.

Greenstein, G., Caton, J. G., & Polson, A. M. (1981). Histologic characteristics associated with bleeding after probing and visual signs of inflammation. *Journal of Periodontology, 52,* 420.

Greenstein, G. (1985). Changing periodontal concepts. Part 1. Etiology and Diagnosis. *Compendium of Continuing Education in Dentistry, 6*(4), 242–252.

Greenstein, G. & Polson, A. (1985). Microscopic monitoring of pathogens associated with periodontal diseases. A review. *Journal of Periodontology, 56,* 740.

Greenstein, G. (1988). Microbiological assessments to enhance periodontal diagnosis. *Journal of Periodontology, 59,* 508–515.

Greenstein, G. (1994). Assessment of periodontal disease activity: Diagnostic and therapeutic implications. *Periodontal disease management.* Chicago: The American Academy of Periodontology.

Haffajee, A. D., Socransky, S. S., & Goodson, J. M. (1983). Clinical parameters as predictors of destructive periodontal disease activity. *Journal of Clinical Periodontology, 10,* 257.

Haffajee, A. D., Socransky, S. S., Lindhe, J., Kent, R. L., Okamoto, H., & Yoneyama, T. (1991). Clinical risk indicators for periodontal attachment loss. *Journal of Clinical Periodontology, 18,* 117–125.

Haffajee, A. D., Socransky, S. S., & Goodson, J. M. (1992a). Subgingival temperature (I). Relation to baseline clinical parameters. *Journal of Clinical Periodontology, 19,* 401–408.

Haffajee, A.D., Socransky, S. S., & Goodson, J. M. (1992b). Subgingival temperature (II). Relation to future periodontal attachment loss. *Journal of Clinical Periodontology, 19,* 409–416.

Haffajee, A. D., Socransky, S. S., Smith, C., Dibart, S., & Goodson, J. M. (1992). Subgingival temperature (III). Relation to microbial counts. *Journal of Clinical Periodontology, 19,* 417–422.

Hirshfield, L. & Wasserman, B. (1978). A long-term survey of tooth loss in 600 treated periodontal patients. *Journal of Periodontology, 49,* 225–237.

Holm, G. (1994). Smoking as an additional risk for tooth loss. *Journal of Periodontology, 65,* 996–1001.

Ismail, A. L., Morrison, E. C., & Burt, B. A. (1990). Natural history of periodontal disease in adults; findings from the Tecumseh study periodontal disease study, 1959–87. *Journal of Dental Research, 69,* 430–435.

Isogai, E., Isogai, H., Hirose, K., Kimura, K., Fujii, N., Shibahara, N. (1994). Subgingival temperature in rats with natural gingivitis. *Journal of Periodontology, 65,* 710–712.

Jeffcoat, M. K. (1992). Radiographic methods for the detection of progressive alveolar bone loss. *Journal of Periodontology, 63,* 367–372.

Jeffcoat, M. K. (1994). Diagnosis of periodontal disease: Building a bridge from today's methods to tomorrow's technology. *Journal of Dental Education, 58*(8), 613–619.

Kornman, K. S. & Wilson, T. G. (1992). Treatment planning for patients with inflammatory periodontal diseases. In T. G. Wilson, K. S. Kornman, M. G. Newman (Eds.), *Advances in periodontics.* Chicago: Quintessence Publishing Co., Inc.

Kung, T. V. R., Ochs, B., & Goodson, J. M. (1990). Temperature as a periodontal diagnostic. *Journal of Clinical Periodontology, 17,* 557–563.

Lamster, I. B. (1992). The host response in gingival crevicular fluid: Potential applications in periodontitis clinical trials. *Journal of Periodontology, 63,* 1117–1123.

Lamster, I. B., Celenti, R. S., Jans, H. H., Fine, J. B., & Grbic, J. T. (1993). Current status of tests for periodontal disease. *Advances in Dental Research, 7*(2), 182–190.

Lamster, I. B., Holmes, L., Gross, K., Oshrain, R., Rose, L., & Cohen, D. W. (1991). The relationship of clinical attachment loss to B-Glucoronidase in crevicular fluid. *Journal of Dental Research, 70,* 354 (Abstract 707).

Lamster, I. B., Oshrain, R. L., Celenti, R. S., Fine, J. B., & Grbic, J. T. (1991). Indicators of the acute inflammatory and humoral immune responses in gingival crevicular fluid: Relationship to active periodontal disease. *Journal of Periodontal Research, 26,* 261–263.

Lang, N. P., Adler, R., Joss, A., & Nyman, S. (1990). Absence of bleeding on probing—an indicator of periodontal stability. *Journal of Clinical Periodontology, 17,* 714–721.

Lang, N. P., Joss, A., Orsanic, T., Gusberti, F. A., & Siegrist, B. E. (1986). Bleeding on probing. A predictor for the progression of periodontal disease? *Journal of Clinical Periodontology, 13,* 590–596.

Lang, N. P., Nyman, S., Senn, C., & Joss, A. (1991). Bleeding on probing as it relates to probing pressure and gingival health. *Journal of Clinical Periodontology, 18,* 257–261.

Lang, N. P. & Corbet, E. F. (1995). Periodontal diagnosis in daily practice, *FDI/World Dental Press.*

Lavine, W. S., Maderago, E. G., & Stolman, J. (1979). Impaired neutrophil chemotaxis in patients with juvenile and rapidly progressing periodontitis. *Journal of Periodontal Research, 14,* 10–19.

Linden, G. J. & Mullally, B. H. (1994). Cigarette smoking and periodontal destruction in young adults. *Journal of Periodontology, 65,* 718–723.

Listgarten, M. A. (1992). Microbiological testing in the diagnosis of periodontal disease. *Journal of Periodontology, 63,* 332–337.

Listgarten, M. A. & Hellden, L. (1978). Relative distribution of bacteria at clinically healthy and periodontally diseased sites in humans. *Journal of Clinical Periodontology, 5,* 115–121.

Löe, H. (1967). The gingival index, the plaque index and the retention index system. *Journal of Periodontology, 38,* 610.

Löe, H. & Holm-Pederson, P. (1965). Absence and presence of fluid from normal and inflamed gingivae. *Periodontics, 3,* 171.

Löesche, W. J. (1986). The identification of bacteria associated with periodontal disease and dental caries by enzymatic methods. *Oral Microbiology and Immunology, 1,* 65–70.

Löesche, W. J. (1992). DNA probe and enzyme analysis in periodontal diagnostics. *Journal of Periodontology, 63,* 1102–1109.

Löesche, W. J., Bretz, W. A., & Kerschensteiner, D. (1990). Development of a diagnostic test for anaerobic periodontal infections based on plaque hydrolysis of benzoyl-DL-arginine-naphthylamide. *Journal of Clinical Microbiology, 28,* 1551–1559.

Marazita, M. L., Burmeister, J. A., Gunsolley, J. C., Koertge, T. E., Lake, K., & Schenkein, H. A. (1994). Evidence for autosomal dominant inheritance and race-specific heterogeneity in early-onset periodontitis. *Journal of Periodontology, 65*(6), 623–630.

Massler, M. (1967). The P-M-A Index for the assessment of gingivitis. Part II. *Journal of Periodontology, 38,* 592.

Maynard, J. G. (1994). Eras in periodontics. *Periodontal disease management.* Chicago: The American Academy of Periodontology.

McCullough, C. (1995). Clinical applications of voice chart computer technology in the practice of dental hygiene. *The Journal of Practical Dental Hygiene, 4*(6), 29–31.

McFall, W. T., Jr. (1982). Tooth loss in 100 treated patients with periodontal disease: A long-term study. *Journal of Periodontology, 53,* 539–549.

McFall, W. T. (1989). Supportive Periodontal Therapy. In *Proceedings of the world workshop in clinical periodontics.* Chicago: AAP, 1x/9.

Michalowicz, B. S. (1994). Genetic and heritable risk factors in periodontal disease. *Journal of Periodontology, 65*(5), 479–488.

Moncla, B. J., Braham, P., Dix, K., Watanabe, S., & Schwartz, D. (1990). Use of synthetic oligonucleotide DNA probes for the identification of *bacteroides gingivalis. Journal of Clinical Microbiology, 28*(2), 324–327.

Moore, W. E. C., Holdeman, L. V., Cato, E. P., et al. (1985). Comparative bacteriology of juvenile periodontitis. *Infection and Immunology, 48,* 507.

Newman, N. G. & Sanz, M. (1996). Advanced diagnostic techniques. In F. A. Carranza and M. G. Newman (Eds.), *Clinical periodontology,* (8th ed.). Philadelphia: W.B. Saunders Co.

Ng, G. C., Comptom, F. I. I., & Walder, T. W. (1978). Measurement of human gingival sulcus temperature. *Journal of Periodontal Research, 13,* 295–303.

Muhlemann, H. R. & Son, S. (1971). Gingival sulcus bleeding—A leading symptom in initial gingivitis. *Helv. Odontol. Acta, 15,* 107.

Offenbacher, S., Odle, B. M., & Van Dyke, T. E. (1986). The use of crevicular fluid prostaglandin E2 lends as a predictor of periodontal attachment loss. *Journal of Periodontal Research, 21,* 101–112.

O'Leary, T. J. (1967). The periodontal screening examination. *Journal of Periodontology, 38,* 617.

O'Leary, T. J., Drake, R. B., & Naylor, J. E. (1972). The plaque control record. *Journal of Periodontology, 43,* 38.

Oliver, R. C., Holm-Pederssen, P., & Löe, H. (1969). The correlation between clinical scoring, exudate measurements, and microscopic evaluation of inflammation of the gingiva. *Journal of Periodontology 40,* 201.

Omar, A. A. & Newman, H. N. (1986). False results associated with darkfield microscopy of subgingival plaque. *Journal of Clinical Periodontology, 13,* 814–817.

Page, R. C. (1992). Host response tests for diagnosing periodontal disease. *Journal of Periodontology, 63,* 356–366.

Page, R. C. & Schroeder, H. E. (1977). Pathogenic mechanisms. In R. C. Page, S. Schluger, & R. Youdelis, (Eds.), *Periodontal disease: Basic phenomena, clinical management, and restorative interrelationships.* Philadelphia: Lea & Febiger.

Perry, D. A., Taggart, E. J., Leung, A., & Newbrun, E. (1994). Comparison of a conventional probe with electronic and manual pressure-regulated probes. *Journal of Periodontology, 65*(60), 908–913.

Podshadley, A. G. & Haley, J. V. A. (1968). A method for evaluating oral hygiene performance. *Public Health Report, 83,* 259.

Ramfjord, S. P. (1967). The Periodontal Disease Index (PDI). *Journal of Periodontology, 38,* 602.

Reifeis, P. E. (1990). Periodontal diseases: Failure to diagnose and treat. *Journal of the Indiana Dental Association, SE;69*(5), 31–32.

Ritchie, B. & Orban, B. (1953). The crests of the interdental alveolar septa. *Journal of Periodontology, 24,* 75–87.

Robinson, P. J. & Vitek, R. M. (1979). The relationship between gingival inflammation and resistance to probe penetration. *Journal of Periodontal Research, 14,* 239.

Russell, A. L. (1967). Epidemiology of periodontal disease. *International Dental Journal, 17,* 282.

Savitt, E. D., Strempko, M. N., Vaccarro, K. K., Peros, W. J., & French, C. K. (1988). Comparison of cultural methods and DNA probe analysis for the detection of *Actinobacillus actinomycetemcomitans, bacteroides gingivalis,* and *bacteroides intermedius* in subgingival plaque samples. *Journal of Periodontology, 59,* 431–438.

Scarff, A. F., Walsh, M. M., & Darby, M. L. (1994). Periodontal and oral hygiene assessment. In M. L. Darby and M. M. Walsh (Eds.), *Dental hygiene theory and practice.* Philadelphia: W.B. Saunders Co.

Schour, I. & Massler, M. (1948). Survey of gingival disease using the P-M-A Index. *Journal of Dental Research, 27,* 733.

Schulte, W., d'Hoedt, B., Lukas, D., Maunz, M., & Steppeler, M. (1992). Periotest for measuring periodontal characteristics—correlation with periodontal bone loss. *Journal of Periodontal Research, 27,* 184–190.

Sherman, P. R., Hutchens, L. H., Jr., & Jewson, L. G. (1990). The effectiveness of subgingival scaling and root planing: II. Clinical responses related to residual calculus. *Journal of Periodontology, 61,* 9–15.

Sherwood, L. (1989). *Human physiology, from cells to systems.* St. Paul, MN: West Publishing Company.

Slots, J. (1986). Bacterial specificity in adult periodontitis. A summary of recent work. *Journal of Clinical Periodontology, 13,* 912–917.

Socransky, S. S. & Haffajee, A. D. (1992). The bacterial etiology of destructive periodontal disease: Current concepts. *Journal of Periodontology, 63*(4), 322–331.

Sorsa, T., Uitto, V. J., Suomalainen, K., Vauhkonen, M., & Lindy, S. (1988). Comparison of interstitial collagenase from human gingiva, sulcular fluid, and polymorphonu-clear leukocytes. *Journal of Periodontal Research, 23,* 386–393.

Suzuki, J. B., Park, S. K., & Falker, W. A. (1984). Immunologic profile of juvenile periodontitis I. Lymphocyte blastogenesis and the autologous mixed lymphocyte response. *Journal of Periodontology, 55,* 453–460.

Taubman, M. A., Ebersole, J. L., & Smith, D. J. (1982). Association between systemic and local antibody and periodontal diseases. In R. J. Genco & S. E. Mergenbagen (Eds.), *Host parasite interactions in periodontal diseases* (pp. 282–298). Washington, DC: American Society for Microbiology.

Trowbridge, H. O. & Emling, R. C. (1993). *Inflammation. A review of the process* (4th ed.). Chicago: Quintessence Publishing Co., Inc.

Turesky, A., Gilmore, N., & Glickman, I. (1970). Reduced plaque formation by the chloromethyl analogue of Vitamin C formation. *Journal of Periodontology, 41,* 41.

Van der Velden, U. (1980). Influence of periodontal health on probing depth and bleeding tendency. *Journal of Clinical Periodontology, 7,* 129.

Wang, H. L., Burgett, F. G., Shyr, Y., & Ramfjord, S. (1994). The influence of molar furcation involvement and mobility on future clinical periodontal attachment loss. *Journal of Periodontology, 65,* 25–29.

Wilkins, E. M. (1994). *Clinical practice of the dental hygienist* (7th ed.) Baltimore: Williams & Wilkins.

Woodall, I. R. (1993). *Comprehensive dental hygiene care* (4th ed.). St. Louis: Mosby-Year Book, Inc.

Zambon, J. J. (1985). *Actinobacillus actinomycetemcomitans* in human periodontal disease. *Journal of Clinical Periodontology, 12,* 1–20.

Zambon, J. J., Reynolds, H. S., Chen, P., & Genco, R. J. (1985). Rapid identification of periodontal pathogens in subgingival dental plaque. *Journal of Periodontology, 56* (Suppl.), 32–40.

# CHAPTER 4

# Periodontal-Restorative Interactions

## Key Terms

bruxism
cavity preparation
dental restoration
dentinopulpal complex
direct restorations
emergence angle or profile

extracoronal restorations
indirect restorations
intracoronal restorations
microleakage
primary occlusal traumatism

## INTRODUCTION

The proximity of dental restorations to the soft tissues of the oral cavity mandates that oral health care professionals recognize the effects of the restorative process on the periodontium. After this recognition, the effects should receive consideration in the treatment planning and implementation of periodontal therapy. Evaluation and treatment of a client's periodontal status apart from their existing restorative situation and future needs can be a futile endeavor. A similarly narrow perspective of restorative dentistry can be equally futile. The goal of dental therapy is to develop a treatment plan where the client's restorative treatment is closely coordinated with the periodontal therapy. Careful interaction and communication among the treating clinicians is an important component of the success of both restorative dentistry and nonsurgical periodontal therapy.

Restorative dentistry has been positively influenced by the evaluation of the effects of restorations on soft tissue health reported in the periodontal literature. An emphasis of this research has been to continue to refine restorative materials and techniques available, including their interaction with the surrounding periodontal tissues. The concepts of marginal quality, margin location, anatomic contours, biocompatibility and occlusal harmony are all integral to both restorative dentistry and to periodontal health. This chapter will provide the reader with an overview of restorative dentistry, a brief discussion of occlusion and occlusal traumatism, and a unique treatment planning philosophy. Periodontally relevant restorative dentistry, such as root surface caries; excessive root exposure and furcation involvement; maintenance of restorative materials, and marginations will also be reviewed. The last section of the chapter focuses on the team approach to restorative dentistry and highlights the role of the dental hygienist.

## OVERVIEW OF RESTORATIVE DENTISTRY

Following eruption, the hard tissues of the teeth—enamel, dentin, and cementum—are continuously affected by the oral environment. Unlike other tissues in the body and the oral cavity, the hard tissues of the teeth are unable to repair themselves. Tooth structure can be lost due to fracture, wear, or dental caries. Dental caries remains the most frequent reason for loss of tooth structure. The greatest successes in eradication of this disease have come from preventive efforts. Despite great strides in reducing its incidence, dental caries is a disease that affects the majority of the populace (Caplan & Weintraub, 1993). Dental caries is a posteruptive pathological process of external origin that results in destruction of the hard tissues of the tooth. Dental caries, like periodontal disease, is a disease mediated by bacteria in the oral cavity. It is a progressive disease, with several definable stages involving the enamel and dentin of the tooth (see Figure 4-1A through H).

In the early stages of the disease process, the effects on tooth enamel are reversible with appropriate therapy targeted at altering the bacterial plaque and microenvironment that precipitated the carious lesion. Once the caries process progresses beyond reversibility, cavitation and irreversible changes make the removal and replacement of tooth structure a necessary intervention. Tooth fracture, missing teeth, teeth with a hopeless restorative or periodontal prognosis are also needs that will continue the demand for restorative and prosthetic dentistry.

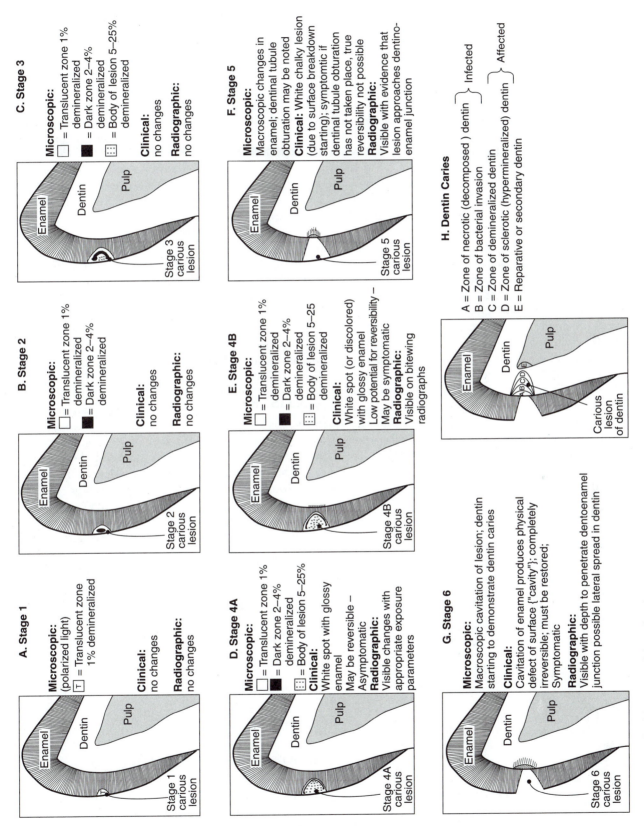

**C. Stage 3**

**Microscopic:**
☐ = Translucent zone 1% demineralized
■ = Dark zone 2–4% demineralized
▦ = Body of lesion 5–25% demineralized

**Clinical:**
no changes

**Radiographic:**
no changes

**F. Stage 5**

**Microscopic:**
Macroscopic changes in enamel; dentinal tubule obturation may be noted
**Clinical:** White chalky lesion (due to surface breakdown starting); symptomtic if dentinal tubule obturation has not taken place, true reversibility not possible

**Radiographic:**
Visible with evidence that lesion approaches dentino-enamel junction

**H. Dentin Caries**

A = Zone of necrotic (decomposed ) dentin ⎱ Infected
B = Zone of bacterial invasion ⎰
C = Zone of demineralized dentin ⎱
D = Zone of sclerotic (hypermineralized) dentin ⎰ Affected
E = Reparative or secondary dentin

**B. Stage 2**

**Microscopic:**
☐ = Translucent zone 1% demineralized
■ = Dark zone 2–4% demineralized

**Clinical:**
no changes

**Radiographic:**
no changes

**E. Stage 4B**

**Microscopic:**
☐ = Translucent zone 1% demineralized
■ = Dark zone 2–4% demineralized
▦ = Body of lesion 5–25 demineralized

**Clinical:**
White spot (or discolored with glossy enamel
Low potential for reversibility – May be symptomatic

**Radiographic:**
Visible on bitewing radiographs

**A. Stage 1**

**Microscopic:**
(polarized light)
⊤ = Translucent zone 1% demineralized

**Clinical:**
no changes

**Radiographic:**
no changes

**D. Stage 4A**

**Microscopic:**
☐ = Translucent zone 1% demineralized
■ = Dark zone 2–4% demineralized
▦ = Body of lesion 5–25%

**Clinical:**
White spot with glossy enamel
May be reversible – Asymptomatic

**Radiographic:**
Visible changes with appropriate exposure parameters

**G. Stage 6**

**Microscopic:**
Macroscopic cavitation of lesion; dentin starting to demonstrate dentin caries

**Clinical:**
Cavitation of enamel produces physical defect of surface ("cavity"); completely irreversible; must be restored; Symptomatic

**Radiographic:**
Visible with depth to penetrate dentoenamel junction possible lateral spread in dentin

**Figure 4-1** Definable stages of dental caries.

The following sections include terminology and background information to facilitate understanding of subsequent discussions in this chapter.

## Background Information

The removal of caries-altered tooth structure to render it capable of receiving a dental restoration is commonly referred to as tooth or **cavity preparation**. The replacement of the missing tooth structure with appropriate dental materials is termed *restoration*. The branch of dentistry that concerns itself with the preparation and restoration of teeth is called *restorative dentistry*. The **dental restoration** itself is defined in the Glossary of Prosthodontic Terms (1987) as "a broad term applied to any material or prosthesis that restores or replaces lost tooth structure, teeth or oral tissues." A basic understanding of the different classification systems for dental restorations is a prerequisite to discussion about the dental materials and their interaction with the periodontium.

Dental restorations can be classified as either intracoronal or extracoronal. **Intracoronal restorations** (see Figure 4-2A) are located within the confines of the cusps and normal proximal axial contour. Intracoronal restorations can be classified by the surfaces involved in the cavity preparation (see Table 4-1). Classic examples of intracoronal restorations include silver amalgam alloys, gold or other metallic inlays, porcelain inlays, and composites. **Extracoronal restorations** (see Figure 4-2B) are outside or external to the crown portion of a natural tooth. Extracoronal restorations include artificial crowns made of porcelain, porcelain fused to metal, gold or other metal alloys, and veneers for facial surfaces of teeth made of porcelain or composite.

The additional classification of restorations into indirect and direct is relevant to the discussion on restorative materials. **Indirect restorations** are those which are formed partially or wholly outside the tooth preparation, often from an impression and subsequent cast of the preparation. Indirect restorations can represent intracoronal metallic inlays, porcelain inlays and processed resin inlays, or extracoronal artificial crowns and porcelain veneers. Indirect restorations are usually cemented or luted to the remaining tooth structure for retention in the mouth. **Direct restorations** are fabricated within the confines of the preparation and are typically composed of materials that harden or polymerize after placement in the preparation. Direct restorative materials include silver amalgam alloy, composite resins, and glass ionomers. Direct restorative materials are utilized primarily in intracoronal restorations.

Direct and indirect restorations represent different attributes and deficiencies relative to their acceptance by the periodontium. It is procedurally more difficult to replicate extensive axial and cusp contours with direct restorative materials. Direct restorative materials offer a single tooth to dental material interface. This interface or margin is often a microscopically imperfect junction which allows for leakage of oral fluids referred to as **microleakage**. Radioisotope tracers, dyes, scanning electron microscopic evaluation, and other techniques can demonstrate the extent of microleakage. In clinical practice, the extent of microleakage is a combination of both the material's physical characteristics and the operator's technique. Indirect restorative materials are usually formed outside of the oral cavity on a dental stone replica of the preparation called a die. Most extracoronal restorations are also indirect restorations. Since indirect restorations are fabricated extra orally, they can replicate the entire contours of the tooth's crown more readily. Indirect restorative materials have a luting material inter-

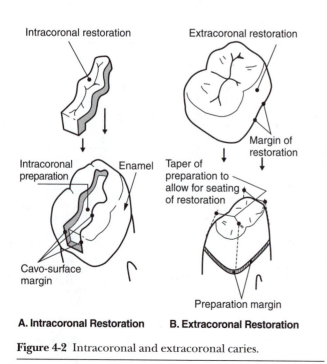

**A. Intracoronal Restoration        B. Extracoronal Restoration**

**Figure 4-2** Intracoronal and extracoronal caries.

**Table 4-1  Caries Classification**

| Class | Description |
| --- | --- |
| Class I | Decay in the pits and fissures of occlusal surfaces. |
| Class II | Decay on the interproximal surfaces of posterior teeth. |
| Class III | Decay on the interproximal surfaces of anterior teeth. |
| Class IV | Decay involving the incisal angle(s) of anterior teeth. |
| Class V | Decay involving the facial or lingual surfaces in the cervical one-third of the teeth. |
| Class VI | Decay involving the cusp tips or other normally self-cleansing regions of occlusal one-third of the tooth. |

posed between the tooth and the restoration and thus have a more complex interface or margin than direct restorations. Most indirect restorative techniques also involve the effects on the periodontium of impression taking and temporization.

Ideal margins on both direct and indirect restorations represent an imperfect seal of the restoration against the tooth structure (see Figure 4-3A). Deviation from the ideal margins produces a variety of defects in the marginal integrity of a restoration. When present, marginal defects can include deficient or open margins (see Figure 4-3C and D) which result from the dimensional changes involved with the various materials or from errors in placing the material in the cavity preparation. Another common defect in margins involves an excess of material, most frequently found at the gingival cavosurface margin. An overhang (see Figure 4-3B) is an excess of restorative material located at the gingival margin of the restoration. Because they represent a detrimental aspect of restorative dentistry, overhangs should be carefully evaluated to determine how to reduce the overhang or replace the restoration.

### The Restoration to Tissue Interface

All dental materials are foreign to the oral environment and have the potential for effects on the pulp, hard tissues of the teeth, and the adjacent soft tissue. In considering the various tissues of the individual tooth, the dentin and pulp can be thought of as separate tissues or as the dentinopulpal complex. The **dentinopulpal complex** integrates the concepts that dentin is the mature

end-product of the odontoblast cells of the pulp and the dentin contains protoplasmic extensions of the odontoblasts called odontoblastic processes. Because of this intimate and inseparable relationship, the dentin and pulp should be considered as one compound tissue. Involvement of the dentin from wear, fracture, caries, or restorative dentistry immediately involves the pulp through the protoplasmic extensions and elicits a response from the cells housed in the pulp chamber. The dentinopulpal complex and tissues of the periodontium are capable of physiologic reactions to dental materials as well as the physical and structural interactions characterized by restoring the enamel and dentin of the teeth.

Classically accepted elements of interaction at the tooth/tissue interface are described differently by different authors, but can be reduced to morphology or contour of the restoration, quality of the marginal adaptation, and location of the margin (Wilson, 1992). In addition, the increasing number of restorative procedures that involve multiple materials and increased understanding of the effects dental materials have on other tissues has added the issue of biocompatibility to the list of factors which must be considered in any assessment of restorative dentistry's effect upon periodontal health.

**Restoration Morphology.** The morphology of a restoration includes the location and magnitude of contour of the restoration replacing the natural tooth structure. Proximally, contours provide for appropriate interproximal contact with adjacent teeth and delineate the embrasure space available for the soft tissue. The facial and lingual contours can also influence the gingival health on those surfaces. The shape of a restoration should also include consideration of the **emergence angle** or **profile**. The emergence angle or profile is indicated by the angle or outline between the natural tooth structure and the restoration at their juncture (see Figure 4-4A and B).

Although the concept of self-cleansing contours has been abandoned, the ability of a restoration's shape to positively or negatively influence the periodontal status should not be abandoned. An appropriately shaped proximal contour, provides for a contact area with the adjacent tooth rather than a contact point. Appropriate tooth contours create both a faciolingual and an occlusocervical dimension for the interproximal contact area. These dimensions provide for protection of the papilla of marginal tissue and assist in maintaining the tooth contacts during normal tooth movements found in occlusal contact (Trott & Sherkat, 1964). The appropriate occlusocervical dimensions also create gingival embrasure spaces that allow the soft tissue to occupy the space appropriately. The development of contact area dimensions should be related to the tooth's existing crown length to facilitate the projected ideal soft tissue contours (Kay, 1982). Restorations that do not display an appropriate contour have been shown to not only hinder oral hygiene (Campbell, 1989), but may even promote the evolution

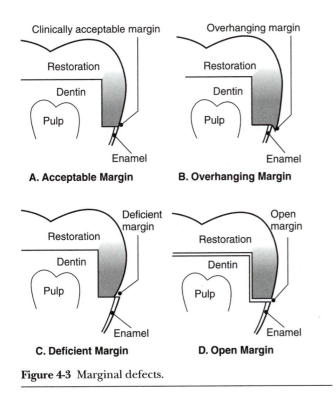

**Figure 4-3** Marginal defects.

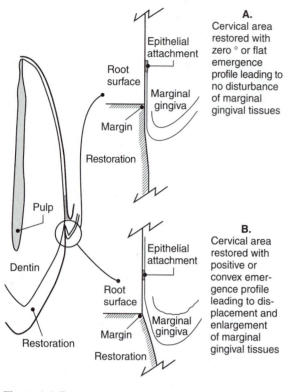

**A.**
Cervical area restored with zero ° or flat emergence profile leading to no disturbance of marginal gingival tissues

**B.**
Cervical area restored with positive or convex emergence profile leading to displacement and enlargement of marginal gingival tissues

**Figure 4-4** Emergence angle or profile.

of a destructive subgingival flora (Brunsvold & Lane, 1990).

Excessive tooth contours on restorations are common (Parkinson, 1976) and can result in soft tissue distensions and displacements (Wilson & Maynard, 1983). The tissue's reaction to the inappropriate contours are inflammation and capillary stasis. Clinically, the tissue appears edematous, enlarged, and changes in color from light pink to a darker reddish-blue. A flat to concave emergence profile becomes integral to the periodontal success of a restoration (Stein & Kuwata, 1977). The therapeutic goal of a restoration's morphology is to replicate or improve upon the existing tooth's contours by exhibiting a flat or concave emergence profile, facial and lingual heights of contour which are neither over or undercontoured, and proximal contours which allow adequate dimensions and strength to the interproximal contacts while permitting an appropriate embrasure space for needed interproximal tissue contour.

**Margin Quality.** Because it is dually significant to both periodontal and pulpal health, marginal quality is an issue that is at the forefront of most evaluations of dental materials (Löe, 1968). A usable dental material must be able to adequately seal the hard tissues of the tooth from oral fluid ingress, without damaging the soft tissues. No material in use is able to adapt perfectly to the tooth structure; therefore, there is always a measurable interface or marginal gap between the tooth and restorative material. It is important that materials be able to produce a

marginal gap that does not exceed 10 µm to 50 µm. The addition of a bonding agent or luting agent will create two interfaces, tooth–luting agent, and luting agent–restorative material. The dual interface results in a more complex marginal gap.

In addition to the microscopic marginal gaps that are intrinsic to the physical properties of the restorative material, macroscopic defects can occur, adversely affecting margin quality. From a periodontal perspective, the overhang is one of the least desirable situations. It is well documented that overhangs are detrimental to the health of the periodontium. In clinical studies, the presence of overhangs results in increased inflammation and periodontal probing depths (Vale & Caffesse, 1979; Spinks, Carson, Hancock, & Pelleu, 1986). Even though overhangs are not desirable, they appear to be a frequent result of restorative care (Pack, Coxhead, & McDonald, 1990). The location of the restoration influences the frequency of overhangs. The more difficult a location is to instrument, the more likely there will be an overhang. The overhang's simple mechanical blockage of complete plaque removal (Waerhaug, 1956), the consequent increased plaque (Highfield & Powell, 1978; Jeffcoat & Howell, 1980), and even a change in the subgingival microflora (Lang, Kiel, & Anderhalden, 1983) contribute to the deleterious effects. The removal of overhangs in otherwise serviceable restorations improves the health of the periodontium (Hodges & Bowen, 1985).

Deficient and open margins can create areas that are not readily cleansable and contribute to both periodontal problems and caries. Open margins on indirect restorations permit exposure of excessive amounts of cementing or luting agents, which are the weakest link in the indirect restorative process. Indirect restorative materials rely upon luting agents of various types that present their own marginal problems (Abbate, Tjan & Fox, 1989). Traditional dental cements are soluble, leading to marginal defects over the course of time, resin based cements demonstrate increased plaque retention (Thomas & Wickens, 1989) and the glass ionomer-based cements exhibit structural cracks and breakdown, resulting in a lessened ability to keep the margins plaque free (Van Zeghbroeck, Feilzer, & Davidson, 1989; Van Zeghbroeck, Davidson, & DeClerq, 1989). The drive to create esthetic restorations increases the intracrevicular placement of margins, which have a higher potential to be rough and overcontoured (Wilson, 1988).

Clinical evaluation of margin quality is conducted with tactile and visual procedures. Visual inspection of supragingival margins and explorer evaluation of both supragingival and subgingival margins is needed. Tactile evaluation is less discriminatory in locations that are difficult to access. Access is inhibited in margins that are located deep within the gingival sulcus and in the posterior areas of the oral cavity. Radiographic evaluation can serve as a visual aid to tactile exploration in specific situations, but is not indicated as a routine postrestorative evaluation.

Improvement of margin quality is best accomplished at the time of placement for direct restorative materials and upon insertion for indirect restorations. Defects in existing restorations should be evaluated for clinical effects. Those restorations presenting with inadequate margin quality that display clinical effects must be treatment planned for correction or replacement. Those restorations presenting with minimal marginal quality defects that are without clinical effects of caries, periodontal disease, or esthetics should be evaluated on a benefit to risk basis. Planned correction may be treatment planned if there is a sufficient preventive or therapeutic basis to justify the time and expense. The therapeutic goal relative to marginal quality is to produce a tooth to restoration interface that has minimal microleakage and does not exhibit an overhang, deficiency, or open margin.

**Margin Location.** Margin location is the third leg of the classical triad of restorative factors that influence periodontal health. The healthy gingival sulcus is shallow and narrow. From a purely periodontal perspective, the ideal location for a restoration's margin is supragingival or coronal to the free gingival margin (Newcomb, 1974). To compliment efforts aimed at periodontal health, dental restorations that must be placed subgingivally must remain intracrevicular. Removal of caries, previous restorations, a need for additional preparation length to increase a restoration's retention, and esthetic demands may all force the restorative dentist to invade the biologic width (Wilson, 1985). For optimum periodontal health, the attachment tissues must interface with healthy, smooth tooth structure and not with restorative material. If invasion of the biologic width is expected, crown lengthening or forced eruption should be considered in the periodontal portion of the treatment plan. Margin location in the biologic width will result in the physiologic establishment of a new attachment, often of diminished quality over one that is purposefully obtained.

The majority of margins are located between the two extremes of clearly supragingival and clearly invasive of the biologic width. Within this range, it is evident that margin quality and location influence the gingival health. When compared with matched, nonrestored teeth, cast restorations increase gingival inflammation when located subgingivally (Bader, Rozier, McFall, & Ramsey, 1991). Depth of location within the sulcus is meaningful as well. Deeper placement results in increased periodontal problems (Flores-de-Jacoby, Zafiropoulos, & Ciancio, 1989). Shallow (up to one millimeter) placement of the margin combined with adequate margin quality can result in minimal adverse effects, while deeper placement is associated with significant increases in periodontal probing depth (Frielich, Niekrash, Katz, & Simonsen, 1992). Deeper margin location also adversely affects the ability to achieve and evaluate margin quality, a situation that is dually destructive (Reeves, 1991). The therapeutic goal of margin location is to place a restorative margin that allows for removal of caries and existing restorations, is supragingival or shallowly placed in the gingival crevice, and is esthetically acceptable.

**Biocompatibility.** All dental materials represent a foreign substance to the tissues in the oral cavity. Each tooth to soft tissue interface is unique and elicits a response to foreign materials necessary for restorative dentistry. Biocompatibility can be considered the cellular or tissue response to a material. Side effects from dental restorative materials are unintentional injuries caused by the materials. Side effects can be toxic, irritative, or allergic in nature (Munksgaard, 1992). Even though the side effects attributable to dental materials are infrequent and usually benign (Kallus & Mjor, 1991), there is a continuing need for evaluation of the biocompatibility of dental materials (Christensen, 1994).

As dentistry has continued to advance, restorative material biocompatibility has become decidedly more complex. The issue of suitable evaluation of the biocompatibility of various restorative materials has also become complicated. With increasing frequency, dental materials are utilized in combination to produce a restoration. The multiple materials and their individual properties form a complex restorative system more difficult to evaluate from both a theoretical and practical standpoint. The other problem involves the speed at which dental materials are being developed and modified. A poignant quote from Ralph W. Phillips, a dentist and foremost authority in dental materials, states, "Every year, clinical studies are published that present 2, 3, or even 4 year results on materials no longer available or so significantly altered as to render much of the data of questionable value" (Phillips et al., 1990, p. 74). In addition to the biological considerations of dental materials themselves, the techniques and medicaments utilized in the production of the restorative dentistry are of importance to the health of the gingival tissues.

Restorative material biocompatibility is a function of not just the material itself, but also the application with which it is being used and its combination with ancillary items such as bioactive luting agents and bases. As an example, porcelain can exhibit significantly different tissue responses when it is fired versus cast; that is, when it is used without metal versus a metal/porcelain margin. Even all porcelain margins differ in their response depending upon the use as a butt margin in a porcelain crown, versus a knife-edge margin with a laminate veneer. Similarly, a porcelain butt margin will produce differing levels of response depending upon the use of a resin cement, a glass ionomer, or a polycarboxylate cement. All dental materials are tested for cellular level compatibility. Higher biocompatibility is associated with a diminished potential for reactive or rejective phenomena. In the current environment, it is necessary to consider that the factor of cellular biocompatibility translates to a mere prerequisite for use of a material intraorally. The process and technique of use is of fundamental importance from a periodontal perspective.

Periodontal compatibility of a particular material includes not just cellular biocompatibility (assessed readily in vitro) but also ion exchanges that can occur between the metal alloys and gingival tissues. Surface reactivity of various restorative materials relate to plaque formation and inhibition. Complicating this need for increased evaluation is the understanding that the various formulations of alloys are complex, so complex that even extrapolation of results to groups of alloys is inappropriate, and each alloy should be considered individually (Jendresen, Allen, Bayne, Hansson, Klooster, & Preston, 1992). In addition, the concept of application of multiple materials needs further exploration within the profession. The properties of the various material when used in concert with one another or utilized in variable techniques may significantly alter the known effects of a single material.

The factors of physical surface characteristics and reactivity are of paramount importance to the periodontal tissues. Both the physical characteristics of a particular material and its biochemical properties affect the development and retention of the primary etiologic agents of periodontal disease, plaque, and calculus. Numerous studies have been conducted throughout the years characterizing the various materials and their smoothness. All materials in use are capable of producing adequate initial smoothness for plaque removal. The maintenance of appropriate surface characteristics is an area that is receiving increasing evaluation and is discussed later in this chapter.

An additional factor more recently brought to light is that of surface reactivity. A dental material that is highly ionic in nature tends to be more appealing to bacterial colonization. The attachment mechanisms for the bacteria are apparently enhanced under those conditions. The insight into this finding was related to the dual discovery of agents that could reduce the reactivity of all materials and tissues and the discovery that certain cast porcelains were less susceptible than tooth enamel to plaque formation, even with similar levels of smoothness. The therapeutic goal relative to biocompatibility is to use materials with acceptable cellular and tissue compatibility as well as surface reactivity and physical surface characteristics that are free of side effects to the surrounding tissue.

## Characteristics of Restorative Materials

Each of the various restorative materials have unique characteristics relative to their acceptance by the periodontal tissues. From a marginal quality standpoint, the highest standard of adaptation in the past has been the pure gold (mat, foil, or powdered) to tooth junction. The high malleability of pure gold produced the least microleakage among the restorative materials that were not chemically or micromechanically bonded to the tooth's enamel or dentin. The direct gold materials, however, are no longer widely utilized because they are significantly limited in appropriate use and technically difficult beyond their applicability.

**Silver Amalgam Alloys.** A dental amalgam alloy is the result of a combination of liquid mercury with a solid silver-tin alloy that also usually contains small amounts of copper and zinc. The mixing of liquid and solid metals by trituration produces a plastic mass of metal that is placed into a cavity preparation by a technique called condensation. The metals undergo chemical reaction changing metallurgically into new phases or structures that are solid at intraoral temperatures. Once the solidification process begins, the alloy can be shaped or carved, until it suitably restores the lost tooth structure. The use of a mercury containing alloy has periodically been the subject of significant controversy (Corbin & Kohn, 1994). To date, this material is the most commonly used restorative material without widespread deleterious effects. The research literature and special evaluations have demonstrated few problems from use of this material. Periodontal biocompatibility studies have produced mixed results on the inflammatory potential of the amalgam alloys. Similar to other materials, the biocompatibility will continue to be the subject of scrutiny and research. Investigation also continues on developing an ideal restorative material that is completely acceptable in the oral environment.

Stepping down from the pure gold standard, the silver amalgam restorations present with the next ideal marginal interface. Amalgam alloys, when properly handled, will result in a restoration that can actually display decreasing marginal leakage as the restoration ages (Elderton & Mjor, 1992). Clinical researchers in controlled longitudinal studies produce amalgam alloy restorations with survival rates so long that prediction of half lives is extremely difficult (Smales, Webster, & Leppard, 1992). Despite those findings, it is noted that inadequate handling and inappropriate use lead to much higher replacement rates (Mjor, 1992). Estimates have been made that 56 percent of studied amalgam failures are due to errors in cavity preparation and 40 percent are due to material manipulation errors (Phillips, 1973). If validated, these findings would result in an actual material failure rate of 4 percent—a level of failure that would likely be considered acceptable by most evaluation criteria.

**Composite Resins.** The composite materials are composed of two primary constituents. They have a resin matrix, usually a BIS-GMA resin and an inorganic filler material. The composites are a heterogeneous group and attempts to easily classify them usually center on the size or sizes of inorganic fillers used in them. The inorganic fillers are present in a number of sizes from several microns to fractions of a micron. The fillers are designed to help strengthen the material, reduce wear, and reduce the setting shrinkage and coefficient of thermal expansion. The resin matrix and inorganic fillers are bound together by silane coupling agents. The polymerization or cure of the matrix material is usually completed by way of a visible light-activated agent. In use, the composite resins are now almost exclusively acid etch retained to enamel and are increasingly also used with dentin bonding agents that are rapidly becoming contributors to reduced microleakage and restoration retention (Swift, Perdigao, & Heymann, 1995).

In use, the enamel is microscopically etched with an acid solution and a dentin bonding agent may be used with or without etching the dentin depending upon the system involved. Once the enamel has microscopic tags, unfilled resin is flowed over the tags and cured. The composite resin is then incrementally placed, semishaped and cured. The resin matrix material from the unfilled and filled portions polymerize together, thus binding the restoration into the micromechanical undercuts created by the etching process. This micro-mechanical retention is highly effective at retaining the restoration in or on the tooth and assists in reducing the microleakage.

Unlike amalgam alloys, all other materials tend to display marginal integrities that are either static or deteriorating over time. Composites characteristically shrink on setting because of the polymerization of the matrix material and produce contraction gaps at the cavosurface margins. In the past these marginal discrepancies have been considered especially problematic to proximal posterior restorations (Ferracane, 1992). More recent studies utilizing currently available materials have demonstrated less of the antecedent strains that lead to the opening of margins (Sakaguchi, Peters, Nelson, Douglas, & Poort, 1992). Recent reports of 1 to 3 µm gaps (Reeves, Lentz, O'Hara, McDaniel, & Tolbert, 1992) are indicative, that under closely controlled conditions, the phenomenon may be less detrimental than previously suspicioned.

The utilization of composites can take two different forms, direct and indirect. Direct composites are less complicated to place than indirect composites. Direct composites offer the operator less control over some attributes such as interproximal form, contour, and contact formation. The indirect composites along with composite luted porcelain systems offer more controlled cure and embrasure space replication as well as enhanced cervical adaptation, but can result in excess luting agent in the interproximal region (Douvitsas, 1991). When well placed, the amount of plaque and degree of inflammation adjacent to composites was not significantly greater than glass ionomer restorations or enamel (van Dijken & Sjostrom, 1991).

**Glass Ionomers.** The original glass ionomers were developed combining the chemistry of polycarboxylate cements with that of the silicate cements. Although the glass ionomer cements were adhesive to tooth structure and released fluoride, they were slow to set, had relatively poor tensile strength, were not as esthetic as competing composites and were adversely affected by the wet oral environment until completely set. The addition of photo initiators and resin to the glass ionomers has greatly

expanded the utilization of the materials, especially in the treatment of cervical lesions.

The resin glass ionomers as restorative materials have retained significant benefits and deserve to be included in the modern restorative armamentarium. The development and refinement of light cure or dual cure hybrid resin glass ionomers has increased the ability to produce an adequate restoration as a one appointment procedure. Correct application results in an adequate surface smoothness and marginal adaptation with the added benefit of fluoride release (Van Dijken & Sjostrom, 1991). The attendant time savings have helped to make glass ionomers a relevant product for everyday use. In addition to use as a restorative, the resin ionomers have been gaining as basing agents and cements used in conjunction with other restorative materials.

**Ceramics.** Dental porcelains belong to a class of ceramics that are primarily glasses. Despite significant differences depending upon how they are formed and utilized, ceramic materials share important physical properties. They are extremely stable materials and are brittle to the point of exhibiting no ductility at environmental temperatures. They have low thermal expansion, high strength, and stiffness. Ceramics are utilized in an indirect fashion and consist of all ceramic inlays, crowns and veneers, porcelain fused to metal crowns, and acid-retained prostheses. For those restorations with ceramic margins, the marginal adaptation varies by the method utilized. Platinum foil, direct lift, wax replacement, various liquid investments, and support for the porcelain margin have all been studied (Koidis, Schroeder, Johnston, & Campagni, 1991). All ceramic margins do tend to distort more when fired than those supported by metal. All ceramic marginal gaps exceed those found in a porcelain fused to metal crowns (Castellani, Clauser, & Bernadini, 1994). Plaque accumulation potential is greatest, however, on areas of metal and the middle third of the porcelain. Plaque accumulation is related to characteristics other than surface roughness.

**Cast Metal Alloys.** The cast metal alloys are used as indirect restorative materials both by themselves and in combination with dental porcelain. The cast alloys are usually classified by their nobility, with gold and palladium serving as the two most frequent noble metals used. Even within the categories of high, medium, and low nobility, the diversity among formulations is phenomenal. Because of the extreme variety, extrapolation of the results of research is unsuitable within the prevalent groups and each alloy must be considered individually (Jendresen, Allen, Bayne, Hansson, Klooster, & Preston, 1992).

The desire for decreasing the cost of casting alloys has generally focused on development of materials with higher base metal content. These low-noble alloys and even some of the nongold noble metals have been recognized as potential sources for biocompatibility problems of local irritation and hypersensitivity. Clinical presentation of metal sensitivity may range from gingival inflammation surrounding the restoration to other intraoral and extraoral lesions. A higher percentage of the reactions are noted in females. Although frequencies of reported side effects are low, questionnaire-based studies would indicate that the incidence may be higher than that indicated strictly by voluntary self-reporting (Hensten-Petterson & Jacobsen, 1991).

The indirectly formed castings are suitable for replication of extensive tooth contours and occlusal surfaces, but the variety of materials and multiple procedures used in the production of the restorations leads to greater potential for marginal discrepancies. Margin quality, tooth morphology changes, biocompatibility problems, and location of margins may all be present in cast crowns and are all deleterious to the gingival health.

**Impressions and Temporization.** Restorations that are formed from cast alloys and ceramics require an impression of the prepared tooth from which the restoration is fabricated. Although optical impressions are utilized in computer assisted design and manufactured restorations (CAD-CAM) physical impressions are far more frequently utilized. The taking of an impression usually involves the use of a method or agent to retract the gingival tissues away from the margins of the preparation. The retraction process can damage the gingival tissues both physically and chemically. In most cases, judicious planning and careful techniques can minimize the irreversible damage that takes place.

Most indirect restorations also involve the temporization of the tooth in the interim while the restoration is being constructed. Interim restorations often display less than satisfactory marginal integrity and morphology. Poorly constructed temporaries can cause periodontal tissue damage that may result in the need for repreparation and new impressions of the involved teeth. Minimally, poor temporization results in acutely inflamed and friable tissue that increases the difficulty of assessing the quality of the restoration and maintaining an adequate environment for cementation.

## OCCLUSION AND OCCLUSAL TRAUMATISM

The restoration to tissue interface is a well defined and important contribution that restorative dentistry can make to periodontal health. The relationship between an appropriate occlusal scheme and periodontal health is also important yet somewhat less well defined. When considered from the classic static morphologic classification system rather than functional standpoint, malposition of the teeth or malocclusion does not correlate to periodontal disease as it is currently understood (Geiger, Wassermann, Thompson, & Turgeon, 1972). Although there have been reports of the increased coexistence of

malocclusion and periodontal disease (McCombie & Stothard, 1964) with appropriate oral hygiene, malocclusion of the teeth is of little periodontal significance (Ainamo, 1972).

Independent of the class of occlusion, in the presence of both normal and malocclusion, teeth are subjected to pressures and forces while in function. The types and directions of forces applied to the teeth directly bear upon the periodontium, hard tissues of the teeth, pulp, temporomandibular joints, and the entire stomatognathic neuromuscular system. Of primary concern to periodontics are the effects that the occlusion has on the periodontium. The principles of pathology apply to the domain of occlusion. Once the magnitude, frequency, or direction of force exceeds the periodontium's capacity for physiological accommodation, pathosis is considered to be in play. There is incomplete agreement as to a clear and precise role that occlusal pathosis plays in periodontal diseases.

### Occlusal Traumatism

Occlusal traumatism is one of several terms utilized in the literature to describe the pathological injury to the attachment apparatus as a result of occlusal forces (Caffesse, 1980). The injury encompasses all of the tissues involved in the attachment. Aseptic inflammatory changes occur resulting in degeneration and necrosis of the collagen fibers and resorption of both bone and cementum. Changes in quality, quantity, and orientation of the periodontal ligament fibers, coupled with osseous resorption allow for increased mobility. The change from physiologic mobility to pathologic mobility (see Chapter 3) is one of the key indicators of occlusal trauma.

Occlusal trauma may be classified as either primary or secondary. **Primary occlusal traumatism** is applied to those situations where abnormal forces (either in direction or quantity) acting on relatively sound periodontal structures produce signs or symptoms of pathosis. Secondary occlusal traumatism refers to the condition of a weakened or absent supporting bone and attachment system that is unable to sustain normal (or abnormal) physiologic forces without signs or symptoms of pathosis. In addition to effects on the periodontium such as advanced mobility, occlusal trauma may also be associated with wear facets, chipping or fracturing of involved teeth, pulpal sensitivity, and possibly even necrosis.

Occlusal traumatism is not associated with the initiation of periodontal disease nor has it been demonstrated to be a factor in gingivitis (Svanberg, 1974). Resolution of existing periodontal disease cannot be accomplished solely by treatment of the occlusal trauma (Lindhe & Ericsson, 1982). In the presence of other inciting factors for periodontal disease, the coexistence of occlusal trauma can increase the amount of bone loss that occurs (Meitner, 1975). While occlusal trauma may not play a direct role in the development of periodontal disease, the role in therapy and healing is less distinct. Studies in the past have indicated that mobility was not related to healing (Glickman, Smulow, Voger, & Pasamonti, 1966). More recent studies have indicated an inverse relationship between tooth mobility and long-term results of several treatment modalities (Fleszar et al., 1980), and two-year results demonstrate a greater gain in attachment when coupled with a reduction in occlusal trauma by occlusal adjustment (Burgett et al., 1988).

## Functional and Parafunctional Occlusal Forces

The occlusal forces found in humans can be divided into those stemming from activities that are termed functional and parafunctional. Functional occlusal forces would be considered as those necessary for mastication, deglutition, articulation, emotive responses, and other normal and necessary purposes. The stresses or force levels produced for most functional activities can be supported by teeth that display significant bone resorption and loss of attachment. Parafunctional occlusal forces result from activities that are performed on a subconscious or reflex-controlled level. Parafunctional activities include clenching and grinding of teeth, biting on objects, and repetitive abnormal movements of the mouth. The parafunctional activities that result in interarch tooth contact usually produce an abnormal direction or amount of force. In an intact dentition with normal or adequate periodontal support, occlusal traumatism is usually the result of parafunctional rather than functional forces.

**Bruxism** is a term that is often applied to the contacting parafunctional activities and is the most destructive to the dentition and surrounding periodontium. Bruxism is frequently defined as the repetitive grinding of maxillary and mandibular teeth against each other. The teeth involved may be as few as one from each arch or all teeth in both arches. Bruxism is also considered to include clenching of the teeth (sometimes called centric bruxing) and may be more destructive than the commonly associated grinding because of the wider distribution of teeth involved and the more occult nature of this activity. There are two factors that are often identified as contributing to the etiology of bruxism. Emotional factors such as tension, anger, fear, and neuroses in general have been implicated as contributing to the development of bruxism. Occlusal factors such as centric prematurities and eccentric interferences have also been cited as stimuli for the development of a bruxing habit. There is no established hierarchy or certainty as to the relative importance of the two factors and their independence or interdependence. In some cases, bruxism appears to result from significant occlusal disharmony and minimal emotional overlay and in other cases the opposite pattern exists. Irrespective of the balance or interplay of the two factors, if occlusal traumatism is a result of the clenching or grinding, bruxism becomes an important etiologic factor in the diagnosis and treatment planning of periodontal therapy.

## Occlusal Therapy

When the diagnosis of occlusal traumatism is made, treatment is often justified based upon factors that may include the influence of the periodontal status. Therapy for occlusal traumatism is varied and may include reversible treatments such as removable splints, extracoronal splinting of teeth, and habit control. Therapy may also include irreversible modalities such as occlusal equilibration or restorations with an altered occlusal morphology. More involved irreversible modalities include orthodontics and restorative therapy that involves alteration in the occlusal vertical dimension.

From a periodontal perspective, a conservative approach to occlusal therapy that is closely aligned with specific signs and symptoms indicating that occlusal traumatism is a factor in a particular case is advised. Application of occlusal therapy, especially involved therapy, for the exclusive treatment of periodontal disease is certainly not indicated by the literature or by clinical experience. The World Workshop in Clinical Periodontics (American Academy of Periodontology, 1989) developed the following indications for occlusal therapy: 1) to reduce traumatic forces to teeth exhibiting increasing mobility or discomfort during function; 2) to achieve functional relationships and efficiency associated with restorative treatment, including orthodontics or orthognathic surgery when indicated; 3) as adjunctive therapy that may reduce the damage from habits; 4) to reshape teeth that produce soft tissue trauma; and 5) to adjust marginal ridge relationships and cusps that contribute to food impaction.

## CARE PLANNING

Restorative dentistry can not only be noninjurious to the periodontal situation, but can be beneficial if well planned and integrated with the proposed periodontal care plan. As it relates to periodontal disease, restorative dentistry is designed to achieve two goals. First, the restorative phase of care should eliminate pain and infection and provide adequate temporization or initial restorative care that will support the treatment plan for establishing periodontal health. Second, after achieving periodontal health, restorative therapy should be designed to be central to maintaining the pulpal and periodontal health of the teeth and to fulfill the requirements of esthetics and longevity needed for the individual client.

Achieving the goals begins with an assessment of the individual's restorative needs. The needs are then interfaced with the periodontal needs of the client. Because periodontal disease can demonstrate clinical signs without significant symptoms, the precipitating reason for seeking care will often involve a perceived restorative need rather than a periodontal need. If the need for periodontal therapy and adequate healing times is not related effectively to the client, periodontal therapy can be viewed as a roadblock to the restorative work that the person desires. Two elements will help the patient understand the necessary role of both periodontal and restorative care. First, adequate client education about the goals of both the periodontal and restorative therapy is vital. The ability to provide adequate education means that all involved practitioners and ancillary staff must have a substantial understanding of the goals and therapies designed to achieve those goals. The desired level of understanding is primarily achieved by communication among those involved. It is especially important that information is accurately communicated if the periodontal and restorative therapies are being provided by different individuals and if treatment is being performed in different locations. Second, the client must be provided with suitable restorative temporization or stabilization so that the pressure for restorative therapy is alleviated during active periodontal therapy and healing. A client who is provided with a temporary crown that is comfortable, functional, and esthetic will be far more compliant with needed periodontal therapy. The individual's ability to improve self-care will be enhanced when their restorative condition does not serve as a hindrance to adequate home care.

### Considerations in Care Planning

Factors that should be assessed in the restorative evaluation include the following:

1. Restorability of existing teeth.
2. Acute caries that threaten the pulpal health of involved teeth.
3. Existing restoration suitability.
4. Extension of existing restoration and the likely extension of proposed restorations.
5. Esthetics of needed restorations.
6. Functional requirements of needed restorations.

In addition to the pure restorative evaluation, it is necessary that the restorative dentist be aware of the following periodontal considerations:

1. Periodontal prognosis for the individual teeth and for the entire case.
2. Occlusal relationships, including the presence and extent of occlusal traumatism.
3. Adequacy of existing attached gingival tissues.
4. Location of the attachment level in relation to the proposed restoration's margin as indicated by the existing restoration, caries location, esthetic considerations, and retentive features of the restoration.
5. Proposed periodontal and other treatment including oral surgery and endodontic therapy.

Attempting to rehabilitate a dentition that is still in an active disease state becomes an exercise in futility. Active periodontal disease both complicates and com-

promises the restorative process. Chapter 6 addresses care planning for NSPT.

## PERIODONTALLY RELEVANT RESTORATIVE DENTISTRY

There are several keys to producing clinical restorative dentistry that are compatible with periodontal health. Each of the keys should be thought of as a series of building blocks with the ultimate goal being successful restorative dentistry surrounded by a healthy periodontium. Like a series of building blocks, each step builds upon the previous foundation. An error early in the procedure cannot easily be corrected later. Any building block that is weak or missing can cause the whole process to fail. An exquisite preparation without adequate diagnosis to support it may lead to failure of the entire case. Similarly, adequate interproximal contact is impossible without appropriate wedging. The ability to condense and carve a restoration may be impossible without a cavity preparation designed to sustain those activities. Each step in the restorative process becomes integrally linked to the steps that have preceded and those that will follow.

It should also be recognized early, that in the practice of restorative dentistry, there are sometimes periodontal compromises that must be considered to achieve successful restoration of the tooth. The most frequent among the compromises would be margin placement. Existing restoration margins and recurrent caries or fracture will often result in the necessity of an intracrevicular margin. In some cases, especially of recurrent caries, the margin will be located within the existing area of the biologic width. It will sometimes be necessary to allow for or facilitate establishment of a new attachment level to accommodate the restorative dentistry.

The first key to success with both restorative dentistry and periodontal therapy involves an accurate diagnosis. Critical to the diagnostic process is recording of the appropriate information. Careful attention should be paid to the issue of crevicular depth, location of the free gingival margin in relation to the cementoenamel junction, zone of attached gingiva, and location of any existing margins in relation to the attachment level. At the time of initial diagnosis, planning for additional restorative evaluation following periodontal therapy may be necessary. It must be recognized that periodontal therapy and the client's response can modify the proposed restorative treatment plan.

If it can be determined in advance that the location of the restorative margin will involve reducing the zone of attached tissue in an area that already displays minimal attached tissue (see Figure 4-5), then it will be necessary to consider a plastic periodontal surgical procedure to compliment the other periodontal therapy and establish a sufficient zone of attached tissue in preparation for the restorative procedure. Likewise, if the attachment level will need to be located further apically to accommodate an adequate restoration, it is best to prepare the

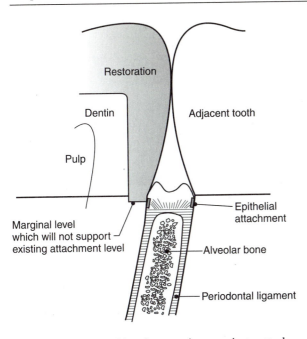

**Figure 4-5** Relationship of restorative margin to attachment level.

gival wall of proximal box preparations. This clearance is often difficult to achieve with the broad contacts created by the interproximal surfaces of adjacent maxillary molars. In creating adequate extension, margination, recontouring and repolishing of adjacent, sound restorations can be considered for the benefits it may provide for the proximal contours of both teeth.

Adequate clearance of the margins should be complimented by adequately supported enamel of the gingival floor on proximal box areas of the preparation. There is a tendency to produce an unsupported enamel margin because of the natural spread of caries laterally at the dentinoenamel junction (see Figure 4-6A). The gingival margin's enamel should be supported by sound dentin (see Figure 4-6B) or by a base material that has sufficient

tissues in advance. It must also be recognized in the treatment plan that there are significant healing periods that must be accommodated so that the soft tissue is not additionally compromised by the restorative process.

## Direct Restorative Materials

With direct restorative materials, the challenges center on the ability to reproduce the necessary tooth anatomy intraorally and maintain adequate contour, contact, and marginal integrity. Each of the various restorative materials present with common and unique characteristics that dictate the need for modifications in techniques to produce superior results.

**Silver Amalgam Alloy.** Silver amalgam alloy restorations are among the easiest materials to use restoratively. Amalgams also are relatively forgiving of minor technique errors. However, those errors do produce a restoration that is of lesser quality than one that is placed with careful attention to all aspects of technique. Along with the internal anatomy of a preparation necessary for the retention and resistance of the restoration, the cavosurface margin that is near the gingival tissues must exhibit certain characteristics. The extension of the cavity preparation must be adequate to allow for access for carving and finishing procedures preventing gingival excess and to permit evaluation of the marginal integrity. Although the concept of extension of the cavity preparation for immunity against caries is no longer valid, adequate extension for appropriate finishing remains necessary. A cavosurface margin that will allow the distal one-third of a sharp explorer tip to pass between the preparation and the adjacent tooth is usually sufficient. It is of special importance that this clearance be provided on the gin-

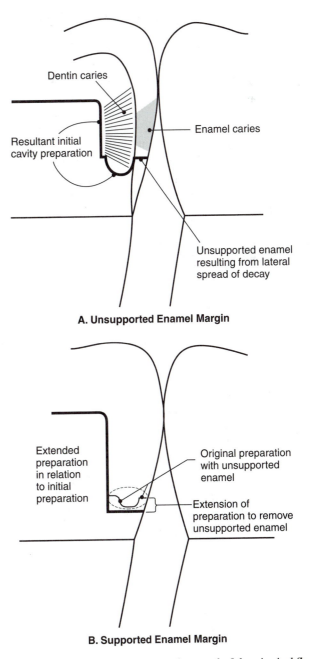

**A. Unsupported Enamel Margin**

**B. Supported Enamel Margin**

**Figure 4-6** Adequately supported enamel of the gingival floor.

strength to support the enamel. A slight cervical slope will often assure that a sound enamel margin can be maintained in the condensation and carving of the amalgam alloy restoration. The gingival margin should be checked carefully after wedging to assure that there has not been an occult fracture of the enamel that would provide an avenue for plaque accumulation and eventual caries and periodontal pathosis (see Figure 4-7).

Once an adequate gingival margin has been achieved, adequate sealing with the amalgam alloy is necessary. Use of the matrix band and a wedge are indicated to assist with containing the amalgam during the pressures of condensation and carving. The matrix band should be cut and contoured to follow the attachment and to seal the gingival margin. For adequate closure of the margin, a minimum of 0.5 mm of matrix band material beyond the margin is necessary. The wedge should reinforce the closure by applying force beyond the margin of the matrix band in cases where there is minimal clearance. A useful guideline would suggest that interproximal direct restorative margins should not be placed closer than 1 mm from the beginning of the attachment apparatus (see Figure 4-8A).

Use of wooden wedges against the previously contoured matrix band serves multiple purposes. Correct wedging (see Figure 4-8B) provides pressure against the band to help seal the gingival margin, preventing an excess of alloy, which could form an overhang. Figure 4-8C illustrates incorrect wedge placement resulting in abnormal contour. Wedging separates the teeth slightly to provide for an appropriate interproximal contact and aids in establishing the final contours of the gingival por-

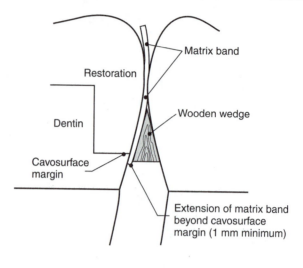

**A. Proper Placement of Wooden Wedge and Matrix Band**

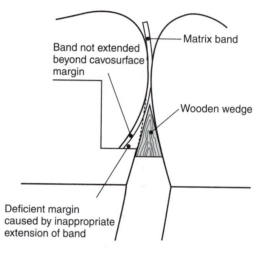

**B. Proper Wooden Wedge Placement; Improper Extension of Matrix Band**

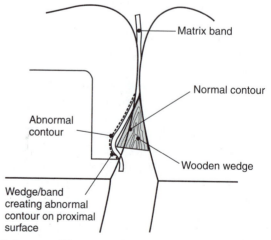

**C. Improper Placement of Wooden Wedge and Matrix Band**

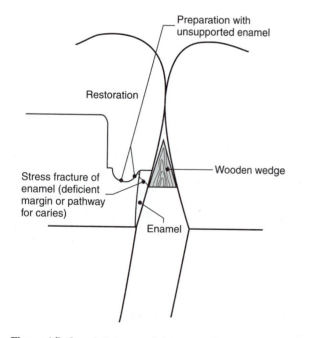

**Figure 4-7** Occult fracture of the enamel.

**Figure 4-8** Wooden wedge and matrix band relationship.

tion of the restoration. Wooden wedges can also aid the rubber dam in retraction of the soft tissues. To achieve these goals, wedges, like matrix bands, must be utilized correctly. Wedges should be trimmed with a sharp scalpel when necessary and used after being wet with water to help form the appropriate contours of both the gingival cavosurface margin and the gingival portion of the restoration. The wedge should be placed so that it provides a transmission of pressure from the hard tissue of the adjacent tooth to the tooth being restored and not just from the surrounding soft tissues. The pressure that the wedge exerts against the restored tooth should be enough to displace the tooth by the thickness of the matrix material. Although the lingual embrasure is usually wider than the facial, at the gingival level of the restoration there is significant variety. Wedging from the facial and using two wedges are methods commonly utilized to achieve the goal of adequately wedging the matrix band.

Once the matrix band is secured, the gingival box portion of the preparation should be reevaluated to assure that there is no soft tissue or rubber dam impingement between the band and the cavosurface margin. The gingival floor and adjacent areas of the facial and lingual margins must be adequately closed to prevent excess alloy. Closure is extremely important with the spherical amalgam alloys, because of their increased ability to flow under the condensation pressures and produce an excess of material. If there are any areas where gingival closure is incomplete or weak and the area cannot be wedged differently or adequately, the area should be noted mentally and careful attention should be directed to the area in the carving process so that any excess material is not left as an overhang. Once wedging is completed, the matrix band may need to be released to allow for adequate bowing of the band against the adjacent tooth if the facial and lingual extensions are significant (see Figure 4-9).

If there is any reason to suspect that an enamel fracture has occurred during the wedging process, the area(s) need exploration to assure that a fracture has not occurred. Even in cases where the enamel appears to be well supported, small fractures can exist after wedging. Those fractures, even if not displaced, provide an avenue for bacterial ingress which can lead to both recurrent caries and periodontal disease. If displaced after completion of the restoration, the fractures provide for an immediately defective margin that may escape detection until the next periodic examination or until irreversible changes have taken place.

During the condensation of the alloy, the convenience form and technique must allow for the condenser to provide pressure on the gingival floor as well as the facial and lingual walls so that the alloy seals adequately against all margins. The flow of the amalgam during appropriate condensation, should create a slight excess of alloy at the margins that must be removed during the carving process to prevent producing an overhang. Following condensation and removal of the wedges, the

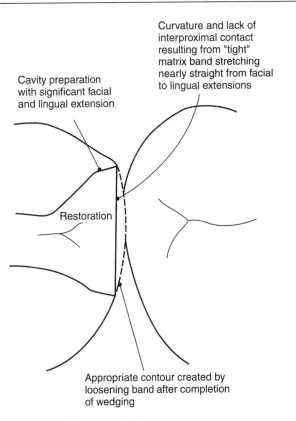

**Figure 4-9** Matrix band release.

matrix band is removed occlusofacially while supporting the marginal ridge to prevent fracture. The interproximal region is carved utilizing various hand instruments to remove excess amalgam and contour this area of the restoration. If inadequate extension has been provided in the preparation phase, it will be nearly impossible for the operator to access, carve, and finish the margins appropriately. The use of a thin, sharp interproximal carver can greatly aid in the operator's ability to carve the area as needed. Depressions on the surface of the root or crown may be more adequately carved with a small discoid cleoid carver.

Following completion of the gingival area of the restoration, the rest of the surfaces of the tooth are carved. Careful attention to the occlusal and morphological features of the tooth will greatly aid in providing a service that enhances both the tooth and periodontium. The use of floss to evaluate the dimensions and strength of the interproximal contact as well as to smooth the interproximal amalgam immediately following the carving procedure is useful. Once the carving is complete, the restoration should be evaluated to assure the following criteria are achieved:

1. The restorative material is well condensed with no voids
2. The restorative adaptation to the margins is complete and no excess or openings exist.
3. The restoration represents contours that replicate or improve upon the original tooth structure.

4. The restoration has interproximal contacts that are of adequate dimensions and strength to prevent food impaction.
5. Occlusal contacts that permit force transmission along the long axis of the tooth, do not include excursive interferences, and do not include plunger cusp contacts on marginal ridges.
6. The restorative material has a smooth surface that aids in plaque removal.

**Composite Restorations.** Composite resin restorations are the second most frequently used direct restorative material. The composites are used in areas of esthetic importance because of their enhanced ability to replicate the tooth's natural color. Composites have become increasingly utilized for both anterior and posterior restorations. The physical and chemical properties of composites require significant differences in technique to produce clinically serviceable restorations. The primary obstacle with composites involves incomplete polymerization and wear, which is related to fatigue and subsequent fracture of microparticles (Oilo, 1992). Estimates for polymerization of visible light-cured composites range from 60 to 75 percent polymerization. The unpolymerized material permits leaching and more rapid degradation of the unpolymerized components. Composites also display a polymerization shrinkage that increases proportionally with the mass of the material cured.

Clinically, composite resins flow under significantly less pressure than alloys. The condensation pressure used in placing silver amalgams aids in producing well-sealed margins and adequate interproximal contact. Composites require increased separation in the wedging process and additional support of the matrix band to produce adequate contact dimensions and adequate pressure on the adjacent tooth. Composite contraction on polymerization can produce significant tensile forces of up to 7 MPa on the perimeter of the material. To counteract this contraction force, bonding of the restoration to the enamel and dentin is necessary. Bonding of the composite restorations to dentin is constantly improving, yet is more technique sensitive and not as predictable as enamel bonding. Composite restorations are also extremely sensitive to moisture and contamination (Jendresen et al., 1992). Careful isolation becomes a strict prerequisite for composite placement. Excess material at the cavosurface margin (flash) is more difficult to detect because of the tooth color of the composite material. In addition, the lack of a partially set stage for the materials and the extension of the acid-etched retentive area beyond the cavosurface margin makes flash more difficult to remove especially in the critical interproximal region. A careful prerestorative evaluation of the cavity preparation can help critically evaluate the marginal extension following placement of composites.

The following technique modifications are necessary for excellent composite resins. Case selection becomes increasingly important with the increase in technique

sensitivity. Enamel margins are preferred due to the greater ease in obtaining a restoration with minimal microleakage. Lack of an enamel margin on the gingival cavosurface of posterior interproximal surfaces remains a relative contraindication for composites. Future studies that demonstrate the adequacy of dentinal bonding in clinical settings may remove this contraindication. Along with enamel margins, the presence of occlusal contacts on unrestored areas of the tooth so that the composite restoration is not the sole support of occlusal contact is considered important. The inability to isolate the tooth adequately with posterior restorations should lead to reconsideration of the use of the material.

Once the case selection process has determined the suitability of a particular restoration, the tooth should be isolated with a rubber dam. Use of a wedge to gently separate the teeth during the preparation process (prewedging) has proven useful to obtaining adequate interproximal contact. Once the preparation is complete, any areas notably deeper than ideal may be lined with a glass ionomer. Any areas of dentin not coated with glass ionomer should be treated with a dentin bonding agent or should be treated with a combined dentin and enamel bonding agent.

In providing for interproximal restoration, the same criteria are relative to the gingival attachment as were considered for amalgam restorations. The wedging and matrix material of either clear mylar material or thin dead soft metal should assist in separating the teeth, preventing gingival excess and developing interproximal contour. Use of matrix material on only the interproximal surface being restored and sequential rather than concurrent restoration of multiple teeth increases the ability to produce adequate interproximal contact. Insertion of the composite should be completed on an incremental basis. The use of multiple thin layers to build up composite restorations recognizes the physical properties of the material. Curing of layers that are 1 to 2 mm thick promotes adequate curing and minimizes the shrinkage effects that occur with the material. Insertion of a single large mass or thick layers will not allow for adequate curing of the material that is deeply placed and will result in shrinkage that may exceed the bonding strength of the enamel or dentin bonding agents. Incremental addition also will allow for more accurate placement around the cavosurface margins minimizing the finishing necessary to produce an adequate restoration.

The placement of material should be directed toward adequate material to produce a restoration that can be produced with minimal finishing. When finished appropriately, the amount of plaque retention and degree of gingival inflammation adjacent to composites is not significantly greater than glass ionomers or enamel (Van Dijken & Sjostrom, 1991). Finished composites should have the same lack of flash, overhangs, and ditching of margins and should display the adequate contours and occlusal and interproximal contacts expected of all restorations (see Figure 4-10).

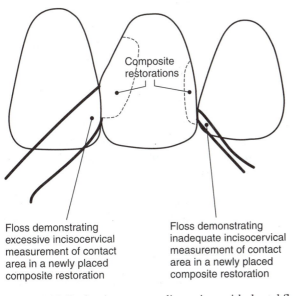

Floss demonstrating
excessive incisocervical
measurement of contact
area in a newly placed
composite restoration

Floss demonstrating
inadequate incisocervical
measurement of contact
area in a newly placed
composite restoration

**Figure 4-10** Evaluating contact dimensions with dental floss.

**Glass Ionomers.** Glass ionomer and hybrid ionomer restorations are currently best utilized in very conservative Class I restorations on occlusal surfaces and Class V restorations in cervical regions. As an occlusal restorative, glass ionomers should be used for conservative restoration of minimally involved pits and fissures. No occlusal contact should be supported solely by the glass ionomer. Increased size of the preparation beyond that prescribed should be an indication for use of another material.

Use of glass ionomer to restore cervical lesions is well accepted. The use of glass ionomer materials should be indicated for root surface caries. Their ability to release fluoride and adhere to dentin are desirable qualities for restorative materials in this region. The adequate isolation of the restorative material during placement and curing is paramount. The location of cervical lesions at, near, or below the crest of the gingival tissue frequently works in opposition to the ability to isolate the tooth for restoration. Use of retraction cord and preformed plastic matrices can assist in the needed isolation in those situations. The least amount of finishing needed to produce an adequately sealed and contoured restoration is best. Even though the resin components of the VLC hybrid ionomers set up immediately, it has been reported that the glass ionomer components continue to cure in a manner similar to the original self-cure glass ionomers. Having a softer component makes achieving a finer finish more difficult in the promoted one appointment use. The finish does appear to be adequate and holds up well on examination following complete curing.

### Indirect Restorations

The use of cast metal, porcelain, and porcelain fused to metal restorations requires attention to preparation detail to assure an adequate restoration. As an indirect material, laboratory constructed restorations involve the use of an impression technique. Impression techniques involve significantly more manipulation of the gingival tissues and can therefore cause more periodontal problems. Indirect restorations also involve several additional dental materials (impression materials, die stone, investment, casting metals, etc.) and therefore, have a higher potential for problems of "fit" of the restorative material into or onto the cavity preparation. Constructed in wax or porcelain before they are cast or fired, these restorations have a greater ability to replicate natural tooth contours and to more accurately reproduce or improve the occlusal pattern and other morphological features of the tooth.

The laboratory constructed indirect restorations also require an interim restoration that occupies the cavity preparation while the restoration is being constructed. The ideal interim restoration (temporary) has virtually all the same morphological features of contact, contour, and occlusion as the final restoration, but is made of a material that is not as durable. The use of light- or self-curing acrylic resins is popular. The highly exothermic nature of self-curing acrylic resins should be mitigated in the construction phase to prevent both pulpal and gingival damage. Self-curing resins also have a high percentage of residual monomer, which can be an irritant to both pulp tissue and gingival tissue. The shrinkage of self-curing monomers can result in contraction gaps between the temporary material, and tooth preparation may necessitate a thick intermediate luting agent. Temporary luting agents can be rough and are more readily soluble in the oral environment. Gingival health can be compromised either temporarily or permanently by poor fitting temporary restorations. Temporary changes in gingival health or architecture are usually reversible upon insertion of the permanent restoration and the patient's ability to perform adequate self-care is no longer compromised.

Permanent changes in gingival level secondary to poor preparation, impression technique, or temporization can be problematic from both esthetic and functional aspects. In some cases, retemporization, or repreparation, reimpression, and retemporization are necessary. In a few cases it may even be necessary to redevelop an appropriate attachment through gingival grafting before the restoration can be completed. It is obvious that careful attention to all facets of the restorative process is necessary to preserve the gingival health.

Preparation techniques that promote gingival health throughout the indirect restorative process begin with adequate gingival health. Direct restorations can be constructed as part of the initial periodontal therapy to serve as a cotherapeutic measure, i.e., removing overhangs, areas of caries, establishing interproximal contact, etc. Indirect restorations on the other hand should be reserved for the stage of treatment after periodontal health has been achieved. If existing indirect restorations must be replaced to improve gingival health, intermediate term temporization should be utilized until gingival health is achieved and gingival architecture is stabilized. Complete healing, stabilization, and maturation of gingival levels may require up to eight months if surgical intervention has occurred. This may involve almost three recall periods for the client who is on a three-month periodontal maintenance schedule. Although the restorative care is ongoing over this period, it is important that clients realize the need to continue the recommended periodontal maintenance regime.

After beginning with healthy tissues, the next key is to utilize an atraumatic technique for preparation. The goal of an atraumatic preparation is to develop a gingival margin on the restoration that is supragingival where possible and within the confines of the sulcus when the margin must be subgingival. For subgingival preparation regions, a single strand of thin unimpregnated retraction cord can be placed near the base of the crevice. The preparation margin is created coronal to the cord insuring the integrity of the gingival attachment. A second method involves the development of the initial preparation at the crest of the free gingival tissues. The initial preparation level is then marginated by adding a bevel for metal margins or is turned into a shoulder with a sharp hand instrument such as a hoe or margin trimmer. The second method develops a subgingival margin that is uniformly placed below the gingival crest in an intra-crevicular location and does not compromise the gingival attachment. The initial preparation can be completed with relatively aggressive and course diamond burrs without fear of damage to the internal surface of the crevice. The margination component of the preparation is completed with fine diamonds and or hand instruments and does little or no damage to the soft tissues of the crevice.

A relatively atraumatic preparation will lead rather naturally into a similarly atraumatic impression. If the sulcular cord is utilized, it can remain in place for the impression while a second cord is placed to retract the tissues from the margin of the preparation. If a single cord is used, it should be relatively easy to pack the retraction cord so that the margin is exposed following removal of the cord. With the use of modern impression materials such as polyvinylsiloxane and polyether impression materials, very little tooth structure beyond the margin needs to be exposed. The impression materials are extremely stable and accurate, but their ability to flow into a deep thin crevice is less than earlier impression materials such as the polysulfides (Hondrum, 1994). To recognize the difference in the newer materials, the objective of the packing procedure is to produce a widened sulcus that extends just beyond the well-defined margin.

A significant portion of the restorative literature deals with utilization of medicaments for hemostatic control to help achieve an environment suitable for the relatively hydrophobic impression materials. With gingival health and an atraumatic technique there should be a diminished need for hemostatic agents. If not medically contraindicated, the use of an epinephrine impregnated cord to achieve rapid and effective hemostasis under these conditions should not be contraindicated. If the

preparation process has damaged enough soft tissue or if the tissue is so highly inflamed that the projected systemic absorption of epinephrine in the impression process is questioned, the impression should not be attempted.

Temporization is an important component of overall success of the indirect laboratory restorative procedures. The goal of temporization is to achieve appropriate tooth contours, interproximal contact of adequate dimensions, and strength and positive occlusal contact that is atraumatic, nonirritating to the pulp or gingival tissues and marginal adaptation so that the temporary luting material can seal the temporary adequately. Once the goals are understood, the selection of one of the many materials available becomes secondary. Lined temporary metal or polycarbonate crowns, custom-fabricated acrylic temporary crowns with either self-cured or light-cured materials are acceptable.

In most cases of single unit and uncomplicated multiple tooth restoration, the impression should be treatment planned for the same appointment as the tooth is prepared. With complex multiple unit restorations or multiple single units, it is sometimes advantageous to prepare and temporize at one appointment and make an impression at another appointment. Replacement of existing crowns or bridges that have a detrimental effect on the tissue should be planned for intermediate to long-term temporization following preparation. Adequate temporization of teeth will allow for periodontal therapy to proceed and gingival health to be attained before finalization of the preparations and impressions.

Once constructed, the indirect restoration will need to be luted to the tooth; often referred to as cementing or seating the restoration. Prior to insertion, an inspection of the restoration's fit and suitability on the laboratory dies is usually indicated. Areas of misfit, inappropriate contours, and poor interproximal contacts or occlusal discrepancies should be noted for careful intraoral evaluation and potential modification. In those cases where a soft-tissue model has been constructed, the emergence profile, surface contours, and margin development relative to the shape and location of the soft tissues can be evaluated. With a critical preappointment evaluation, obvious problems or areas needing laboratory correction can be made prior to the appointment. Any corrections that are made in advance of the appointment permit more efficient use of the chair time and generally provide the patient with a better service.

The procedure for the seat appointment involves removal of the temporary restoration, and cleaning any retained cement from the tooth and tissues. In most cases anesthesia is not needed for the seating appointment. If anesthesia is needed, the obtunded sensations need to be carefully considered when evaluating the interproximal and occlusal contacts. The initial evaluation of the restoration involves interproximal contact and contour. The contacts should be adjusted so they do not prevent the restoration from seating completely. The interproximal contact should be a positive, passive force with the adjacent tooth or teeth. The "strength" of the contact is usually judged by the force required to pass floss between the adjacent teeth. It is usually desirable that the strength of the contact be equivalent to that of other teeth in the quadrant or equal to that of the contralateral teeth. In addition to judging the strength of the contact, the dimensions occluso-gingivally and facio-lingually should be evaluated for suitability. Floss can be utilized for this evaluation as well. Once the contact is evaluated and modified to be appropriate in strength and dimensions, the interproximal contour is evaluated. With adequate temporization, the gingival architecture should be reestablished and it should be relatively easy to evaluate if the contour will allow for the tissue to form a normal interproximal contour. The most frequent contour problem involves overcontouring of the full coverage restoration.

Removal of excess restorative material is accomplished so the embrasure space for the tissue is adequate.

The next stage of the seating appointment involves evaluation of marginal integrity. The restoration must have appropriate interproximal contact and contours to assure that it does not interfere with the restoration's complete seating before an accurate evaluation of marginal integrity can take place. All margins of the restoration should be flush with the margin of the preparation. Visual evaluation with an operatory light and magnification, if available, and tactile evaluation with a sharp explorer tip should be completed. An appropriate margin is "closed" to visual and tactile evaluations (see Figure 4-11A through D) and does not demonstrate an overhang. The emergence profile of the restoration's anatomy should follow that of the natural tooth structure at that

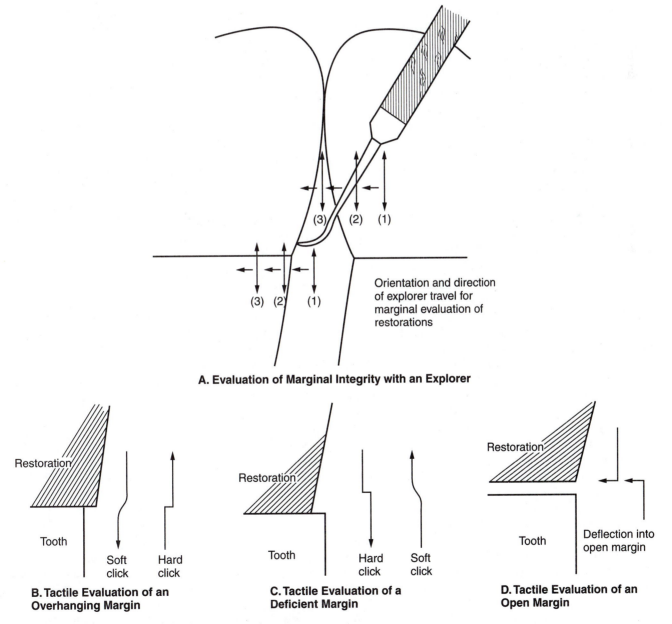

**A. Evaluation of Marginal Integrity with an Explorer**

**B. Tactile Evaluation of an Overhanging Margin**

**C. Tactile Evaluation of a Deficient Margin**

**D. Tactile Evaluation of an Open Margin**

**Figure 4-11** Tactile evaluation of improper margins.

point. For subgingival restorations, a zero degree emergence angle is usually advocated. With current impression techniques, materials available, and laboratory techniques there is also a diminished need for adjustments.

## Special Restorative Situations

There are several situations where restorative modifications are required as a result of the sequela of periodontal disease. Additionally, there are significant periodontal alterations that can occur as a result of restorative procedures. The most frequent restorative modification results from apical location of the periodontal tissues.

**Root Surface Caries.** Advanced recession of the periodontal tissues involves exposure of the cementoenamel junction. Exposure of the tissues beyond the cementoenamel junction results in exposure of the root surface to the oral environment. Along with recession, significant pocket depth exposes the root surface to the unique environment of the gingival sulcus. Root surface caries can occur with either frank exposure of the root or in the tissue blanketed surface of the periodontal pocket. Exposed root surface caries are more readily detected and treated than those covertly developing in the gingival sulcus. Treatment of intracrevicular caries should involve periodontal treatment for both disease reduction and exposure of the carious root surface.

Restorative therapy for root surface caries requires an understanding of the significant characteristics that the root surface lesion displays. The carious lesion on the root surface develops in the cementum and dentin, tissues that differ significantly from the tooth's enamel. The well-demarcated process and stages of the carious lesion are not readily apparent in root surface caries. As the least mineralized tissue of teeth, cementum presents little resistance to the initial acidogenic attack. Relatively quickly, the carious process involves the dentin, which is more susceptible to rapid progression of the carious lesion. The bacterial microculture of the root surface lesion displays colonies of proteolytic organisms which are more capable of destruction of the inorganic dentin.

Clinically, the root surface lesion appears as an unchanged to mildly discolored area that is soft to exploration. Classically, the lesion is fairly broad both at the surface and in the depths of the progressing decay. The parallelism of the progressing lesion contrasts with the classic enamel lesion and the dentinal spread of coronal caries. The unique pattern of decay results from the dentinal architecture in the root. There is usually not a definitive margin to the root surface lesion, making it difficult to develop a cavosurface margin that adequately removes all the carious dentin. The relatively restricted amount of dentin between the tooth surface and the pulp in the root can contribute to the rapid pulpal involvement of this type of lesion.

Direct restoration of the carious lesion of the root surface should be accomplished with a material that requires minimal preparation beyond removal of the lesion. Direct restorative materials that can be bonded to dentin have a significant advantage in this situation. Restorative materials or base/lining materials that are cariostatic or release fluoride are beneficial in reduction of the recurrent caries, which tend to occur at the cavosurface margins. Glass ionomer restorations, especially the visible light-cured hybrid ionomers, can be advantageous in restoration of the root surface lesion. The ability of the glass ionomers to bond to tooth structure, release fluoride, and fulfill esthetic requirements in most situations are positive characteristics. Composites bonded to glass ionomer bases, the "sandwich" restorations, also display many of the positive characteristics desired for the root surface lesion. Amalgam alloy restorations are suitable for use in cases where the disease process is no longer active, the margins of the lesion are readily discerned, and where esthetics is of lesser importance.

Use of indirect restorations such as crowns in the presence of root surface caries are sometimes indicated by extensive loss of coronal tooth structure, previous use of indirect restorations, or as retainers for prostheses. Caution should be exercised to assure that the complete extent of the root surface caries is removed. Complete removal will often leave a deficit of tooth structure near the cervical extent of the restoration. Use of a glass ionomer for basing out this region should be considered as optimal. Cementation with a fluoride releasing cement should be considered as a bioactive measure to enhance the success of this restoration.

Margin placement is a critical element in treatment of root surface caries. Periodontal therapy necessary to provide for supragingival margin placement should be treatment planned to prevent both gingival inflammation and continuation of the carious process. It is well established that subgingival placement of restorations can lead to gingival inflammation. Equally important, the environmental conditions that permitted the subgingival carious process to occur on the root surface may not be adequately addressed if the restoration is placed subgingivally. The subgingival restoration placed for active root surface caries has heightened the potential for recurrent caries at the gingival cavosurface margin.

Intracrevicular placement is possible if sufficient change in the conditions that predisposed the tooth to root surface caries has occurred. Adequate tissue displacement without compromise of the periodontal attachment must be achieved to permit finishing and polishing of the restoration. Appropriate tissue displacement is frequently difficult because the soft tissue lost in the process of recession or pocketing that permitted the root surface caries to occur often compromises the width of the attached tissue. Packing of the tissue to attain the necessary access for the preparation and finishing of the restoration can cause an iatrogenic mucogingival defect. Preventive measures to prevent recurrence of root surface caries and careful reevaluation of the restoration and adjacent tooth surface must be completed at each recare visit.

**Excessive Root Exposure and Furcation Involvement.**
Apical migration of the epithelial attachment can expose significant portions of the root surface. The root surface is often involved in restoration with both direct and indirect restorations. The restorative process on the root surface embodies some unique characteristics. The morphology of the root can complicate the restorative process. The structure of the tooth in the root region and the proximity of the unattached gingiva to the zone of attached gingiva can also provide challenges to the adequate restoration of the root surface of the tooth.

Exposure of the root surface results in a lengthened clinical crown. The elongated crown requires modification of the indirect restorative process. Ensuring that the restoration has the ability to "draw" from the preparation is an important component of achieving marginal integrity. The increased length of the clinical crown can sustain an increase in the taper to assure that the path of withdrawal is adequate. With extension of the preparation onto the root surface, the ability to develop sufficient thickness for some restorations may be compromised. There may not be 1.5 to 2.0 mm of tooth structure between the surface of the root and the pulpal tissue to place a porcelain fused to metal or all ceramic restoration. Invasion of the pulp to provide for adequate thickness may result in devitalization of the tooth and endodontic therapy.

As with crowns that involve the coronal surface of the tooth, supragingival margins are optimal. The diminished zone of attached tissue present with most teeth exhibiting significant recession provides additional impetus to achieve supragingival margins. Intracrevicular margins require an atraumatic technique to prevent mucogingival involvement. In the event that a mucogingival defect is present or created in the impression process, gingival grafting procedures (see Chapter 17) to produce a zone of attached gingiva will be needed.

On multi-rooted teeth, exposure of part or all of the furcation region can be seen with loss of very little periodontal attachment. On mandibular molars, the furcation is located as little as 3 to 4 mm from the facial or lingual cementoenamel junction. On the distal of maxillary molars and mesial of maxillary premolars, the furcation is located further from the cementoenamel junction, but those furcations are contiguous with developmental depressions on the surfaces of the roots and even crowns. The coherent nature of the depression and furcation complicate both the periodontal and restorative outcome. The restorative preparation for teeth with exposed furcations and developmental depressions involves fluting the preparation into the involved area. The fluting will allow for adequate material and for an alteration in contour in the facial and lingual furcation areas. In facial and lingual furcations, the normal tooth anatomy should be altered so that the fluting is carried down to the margin of the preparation with a slight supramarginal height of contour (see Figure 4-12). Gingival health is readily maintained in furcation-involved teeth that are restored in this manner.

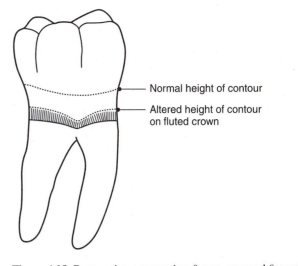

Normal height of contour

Altered height of contour on fluted crown

**Figure 4-12** Restorative preparation for an exposed furcation.

Mesial and distal furcations and developmental depressions should be restored with maximum consideration for cleansability. When possible, restorative morphology that is cleansable with the appropriate dental aid is most desirable. Often the anatomy of the original tooth has contributed to the problem, and with mesial and distal furcations an alteration is beneficial. Interproximally, a long fluted region leading to the furcation is undesirable because it will readily harbor plaque. A slightly convex to flat proximal surface that has a minimal lead-in to the fluted or furcation area is desired. The lead-in should swiftly, but smoothly become concave to match the furcation. The contour change should be supragingivally placed and have a magnitude that is cleansable by an interproximal brush, or wooden toothpick. Preparation design can help diminish the magnitude of the furcation or depression so that it ameliorates the defect somewhat (see Figure 4-13).

## Maintenance of Restorative Materials

In the past, most restorative materials were subject to only minor changes with normal prophylaxis procedures. The increased variety of restorative materials, continued emphasis on nonsurgical periodontal therapy, and advances in technology and therapeutics mandate that careful consideration be given as to how restorative materials are maintained. The esthetic procedure of extracoronal vital bleaching has the potential for changes in restorative materials as well.

A major advance in periodontal therapy has been the increased use of ultrasonic and sonic instruments for tooth debridement and gross calculus removal. Longer and thinner instrument inserts, or microultrasonics, as well as a philosophical change in the goals for root surface preparation have been instrumental in bringing about this change. Ultrasonic scaling instruments operate at a frequency of 25 to 45 kHz (kilohertz) while the sonic instruments operate at lower frequencies of 2 to 6

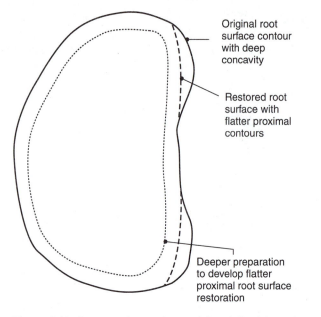

Original root surface contour with deep concavity

Restored root surface with flatter proximal contours

Deeper preparation to develop flatter proximal root surface restoration

**Figure 4-13** Contour change for mesial and distal furcations.

kHz. Reports of the effects of use of power instruments on various dental restoratives are generally not favorable. Damage and increased marginal leakage are reported around margins of composite restorations (Arcoria, Gonzalez, & Vitasek, 1992) and porcelain veneers and porcelain crowns (Miller, 1992; Vermilyea, Prasanna, & Agar, 1994). Effects on the margins of alloy restorations is equivocal (Rajstein & Tal, 1984). The effects on cast restorations with adequate margins is potentially disruptive of the luting agent, especially if a brittle cement such as resin or glass ionomer has been used. Although the same marginal damage can occur with sharp curets, the damage is magnified with the increased intensity and decreased tactile sensitivity which accompanies mechanized scaling.

Avoidance of the direct marginal contact with the working tip of these instruments is recommended. Maintaining a 1 mm distance between the working tip and the margins will maintain some of the advantages such as irrigation or lavage, cavitation, and acoustic microstreaming while minimizing the potential for actual margin damage. Use of correct tip adaptation, lowest effective power setting, and minimal lateral pressure will also produce less chance for damage of the restorative materials as well as the adjacent root surface (Young, 1995). Chapter 12 is devoted to ultrasonic debridement and elaborates on some of the concepts mentioned herein.

Air-abrasive polishing of tooth surfaces is a valuable addition for the removal of stains. Air polishing effectively cleans pits, fissures, and other areas inaccessible by conventional rubber cup, brush, and prophylaxis pastes. Along with increased access, air-abrasive polishing increases the potential for problems to restorative materials. Most affected is the surface condition of composites (Nash, 1993). Composites can be adversely affected by

conventional polishing (Serio, Strassler, Litkowski, Moffitt, & Krupa, 1988), toothbrushing (Garber, 1989), and especially by air-abrasive polishing (Tjan, Dunn, & Sanderson, 1989). Based upon these studies, avoidance of composites with air-abrasive techniques is strongly advised. Air polishing has also been implicated as potentially damaging to cement interfaces, especially at all porcelain facial margins. Chapter 13 provides the reader with a thorough review of the literature on air polishing.

Along with significant changes in technology, advances in therapeutic and other chemical agents have increased the potential for problems with maintenance of restorative materials. Use of chlorhexidine rinses for microbial control of certain aspects of periodontal disease along with caries and other uses has increased the potential for problems. Tooth-colored restorative agents such as composites and glass ionomers can be permanently stained requiring replacement for esthetics. See Chapter 14 for more information on antimicrobials. Fluorides with APF formulations can damage both composites and porcelain restorations (Wozniak, Naleway, Gonzalez, Schemehorn, & Stookey, 1991) and should be substituted with neutral sodium fluorides.

The use of 35 percent hydrogen peroxide and 8 to 12 percent carbamide peroxide for extracoronal bleaching of vital teeth has been advocated as a relatively safe procedure, but has not been extensively studied for effects it may have. There have been indications that it alters the tooth enamel rendering it less able to accept bonded resin restorations. Other studies have indicated that there are no notable color changes in composite resin restorations subjected to bleaching, but those same restorations exhibited significant changes when evaluated at the SEM level. The best approach to such situations will likely involve bleaching prior to restoration and utilization of additional bonding materials beyond those designed for enamel bonding only. As with any area undergoing rapid change, a constant review of the literature on the subject is also advised.

## Margination

As has been previously discussed in this chapter, excess restorative material at the cervical cavosurface margins or overhangs are a frequent outcome of restorative dentistry. Overhangs can result from inadequate matrix band adaptation, insufficient carving of the cavosurface margin, or expansion of the alloy. The predilection for overhangs is increased in areas that demonstrate difficult access and tooth anatomy such as coronal depressions. *Margination* is a term used to describe the process of removing the excess restorative material at the cavosurface margin. Margination can be a valuable adjunct to conventional restorative dentistry and has been shown to positively influence gingival health (Hodges & Bowen, 1985). Margination is indicated when the following conditions exist:

1. No recurrent caries or other marginal discrepancies such as voids, deficiencies, or open margins exist.

2. There is sufficient access to the margins when both interproximal space and tissue level are considered.
3. The morphology of the tooth is conducive to correction.
4. The restoration is not indicated for replacement due to other caries, inadequate contact, or contour.

Effective margination requires attention to the indications and careful technique. Caution should be exercised in selecting restorations for margination because the same conditions of access and tooth anatomy that may have contributed to the overhang can confound the ability to adequately marginate the restoration. Margination can be effected with hand, ultrasonic, rotary, and reciprocating instruments. Hand instruments include files, hoes, gold knives, and other interproximal carving instruments. Margination with hand-activated instruments takes considerable time and is suitable only for minimal overhangs where tactile sense is important. Ultrasonic tips can be used for margination, but their potential for problems such as a rough surface post-treatment and the lack of tactile sense make this a less desirable choice. Rotary instruments are fast and effective, but access to the margin can be a problem. Mar-

gination with rotary instruments is best accomplished if the neighboring proximal surface is missing as in an edentulous segment or while a restoration on an adjacent tooth is being completed. Reciprocating instruments are designed for margination and can give ideal results if the indications are observed.

Detection of overhangs involves clinical observation, tactile sensation, and radiographic findings. Clinically, using an adequate light source, compressed air, and both direct and indirect vision, the cavosurface margins should be examined for location of overhangs, for open or deficient margins that would contraindicate treatment, and for tissue condition and location of the overhang relative to the epithelial attachment. Tactilely, explorers and floss can help determine the presence and magnitude of the overhang and help to rule out recurrent caries. Radiographic evaluation will assist in determining the size of overhang, location in relation to cementoenamel junction and osseous crest as well as the presence of recurrent caries or other defects or problems with the restoration. Once evaluated, overhangs can be classified (see Table 4-2) and a determination of whether the margination should be attempted or if the restoration should be replaced. Type I overhangs can be routinely marginated,

## Table 4-2  Overhang Treatment Planning

|  | Type I Characteristics | Type II Characteristics | Type III Characteristics |
|---|---|---|---|
| *Size* | Less than one-third of interproximal embrasure space | One-third to one-half of interproximal embrasure space | More than one-half of interproximal embrasure space |
| *Location* | Supragingival to minimally intracrevicular | Intracrevicular, more than 1 mm from attachment, more than 2 mm from bone | Intracrevicular, less than 1 mm from attachment, less than 2 mm from bone |
| *Restoration Type* | Direct—alloy, composite, glass ionomer | Indirect—cast malleable metal and well sealed porcelain margin | Indirect—nonmalleable metal |
| *Tissue Condition* | Inflammation soft tissues only—adequate zone of attachment | Inflammation soft tissue and evidence of past osseous effects | Evidence of ongoing osseous tissue reaction to overhang |
| *Tooth Morphology* | Flat to convex surface on interproximal surface | Slightly concave surface of tooth with overhang | Deeply concave surface or overhang in furcation area |
| *Condition of Restoration* | No other defects, evidence of good marginal integrity except overhang | Restoration has other correctable defects and is serviceable after correction | Restoration is fractured; has uncorrectable margin defects or demonstrated decay |
| *Access* | Overhang accessible to all correction modalities | Not all modalities usable because of location in mouth or adjacent tooth position | Modalities severely limited by location and/or adjacent tooth surfaces |
| *Treatment** | Treat by margination and repolishing restoration | Treat by margination or replacement depending upon predicated final result, prognosis of tooth, complexity, and cost of replacement versus margination | Treat by replacement of restoration |

*Classification of treatment indicated by Type I to III depending upon the finding in the highest category.

Type II overhangs may be marginated or replaced, and Type III overhangs should be treated with replacement of the restoration.

Margination is accomplished in an orderly sequence with extreme care to preserve the integrity of the existing restoration and prevent damage to the adjacent tooth structure (Rogo, 1995). The bulk of excess restorative material is removed from the proximal area (and other involved surfaces) first. Once the bulk is removed, a smooth continuous marginal relationship is established. Next, the embrasures and line angles are smoothed and blended while preserving adequate contact and contour. Finally, the restoration is polished and appropriate post care instructions and hygiene measures are provided to the client. Margination can be a time-consuming and methodical procedure that has the potential to significantly improve the client's periodontal health. The reader can find specific procedural information about overhang removal in Chapter 14: Treatment Procedures.

## TEAM APPROACH TO RESTORATIVE DENTISTRY

Changes in the epidemiology of dental disease will bring significant changes to the practice of dentistry in the future. Many of the changes are already impacting the practice of dentistry. Reductions of tooth loss approaching 15 percent and decreases in the rate of edentulism by almost one half from 1971 to 1985 (Brown, 1994) have already changed the needs of clients. Decreases in needs for complete denture construction, surgical periodontal treatment, and noncomplex restorative care have already been seen as a clinical outcome of the research findings (DiAngelis, 1994). The needs of clients have changed not only from shifts in predominate age cohorts, changes in disease patterns, and increased retention of already restored teeth, but also as a result of the individual's expectations of care. The profession of dentistry must be flexible enough to adapt the delivery of care to meet the changing needs and expectations of clients. The respective roles of the dental hygienist, dentist, and dental specialist treating periodontal disease is well illucidated throughout this text. The roles of these team members in restorative care are equally important to assure that periodontally relevant restorative dentistry is provided. The dental team working in concert can provide for the client what no individual team member can accomplish. Maximizing the effectiveness of the dental team's efforts requires prior planning of individual roles, a system of uniform data collection for patient assessment, and a common philosophy of treatment. The role of the dental hygienist is emphasized in the following sections.

### Assessment

Practice appointment patterns often place the hygienist in the role of primary assessor of existing oral condi-

tions. The hygienist is usually well prepared to complete the initial periodontal assessment, but is less likely to feel comfortable assessing the restorative conditions. The initial assessment should include an evaluation of the suitability of existing restorations, their potential role in the eitiology of periodontal problems, a limited assay of occlusal interactions, and potential options for restorative treatment. A practicable system involves the use of an internally standardized routine initial examination for all clients. The routine examination is designed to identify and record key indicators of the various different parameters. This examination should be completed in a like manner each time with findings recorded in a consistent method. Figure 4-14 provides an example of a complete charting format where both periodontal and restorative findings are recorded. Completion of the examination in this manner will assure that all areas are completely assessed and that no critical area is forgotten or deferred because of extensive findings in another area. The obvious example would involve finding abnormal periodontal probe readings and being sidetracked into a complete periodontal evaluation without completing the intraoral and extraoral soft tissue assessment. Potential oversight of these areas could lead to disastrous consequences if a potential malignant lesion was not detected, while a complete periodontal assessment was recorded. Positive responses in any area may indicate the need for more extensive and focused evaluations of the area(s) in order to make an adequate diagnosis and treatment plan. These focused evaluations may be termed subroutine exams and one or several of these may be needed to adequately evaluate the client's needs. Table 4-3 provides an example of routine and subroutine examinations. Evaluation criteria and methodology for determining the suitability of existing restorations should be approached collaboratively by the dental team members involved in the examination procedures. Periodically, all the team members should jointly evaluate common clients to assure that each member is consistently applying the criteria selected. Use of intraoral photography can greatly aid in standardizing the office examination process. Such extra effort will reward the practice with a team of professionals who are well prepared to evaluate the needs of their clients.

Appropriate examination of existing restorations can best be carried out on teeth that are free of calculus and stain, and dried and observed under magnification with adequate illumination. Evaluation of existing restorations should include the following areas of consideration. First, the restoration and surrounding tooth structure should be evaluated for evidence of caries and extent of caries, if present. A recurrent carious lesion, or new caries on another surface of the same tooth will usually indicate the need for a new restoration. Second, the restoration should be evaluated for marginal and structural integrity. Gradation of marginal integrity can be accomplished by using one of the published standards or by internal office depiction. Structural integrity should be

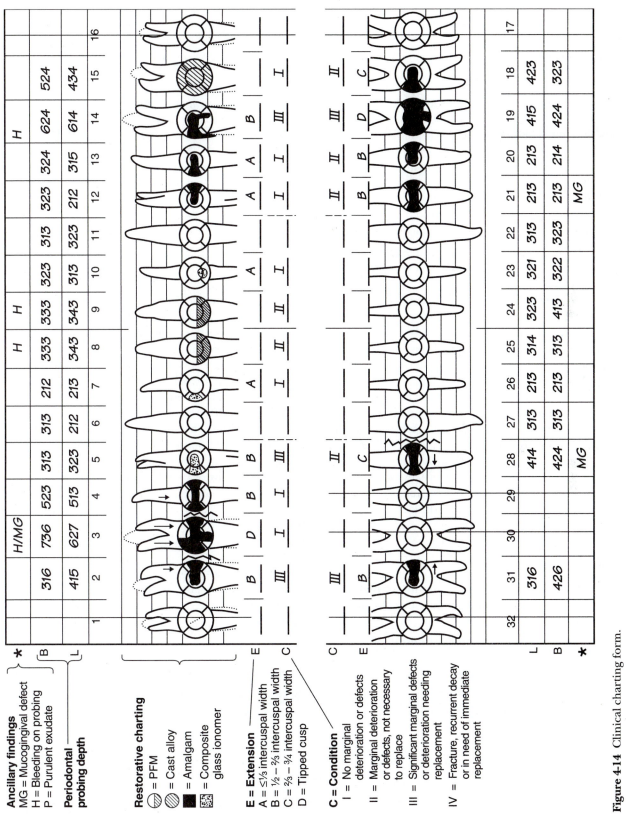

**Figure 4-14** Clinical charting form.

111

**Table 4-3  Example of Routine and Subroutine Examination Components**

| Routine Examination* | Subroutine Examination |
| --- | --- |
| Extraoral Tissues | Comprehensive evaluation of lesions, masses. |
| Intraoral Tissues | Findings up to and including biopsy/referral. |
| Existing Restorations<br>• Extension<br>• Quality | Extensive restorative evaluation, study models (mounted), diagnostic wax up |
| Periodontal Tissues<br>• Pocketing/Exudate<br>• Gingival Tone, Color, Size<br>• Attached Gingiva | Complete periodontal evaluation: gingival examination, full-mouth probing, zone of attached tissue, mobility recording, furcations, new diagnostic testing (see Chapter 3) |
| Occlusal Traumatization<br>• Mobility<br>• Fracture/Faceting | Occlusal evaluation, mounted study models with facebow, centric relationship bites, evaluation of parafunctional activities |
| Temporomandibular Joint<br>• Dysfunction<br>• Movements | TMJ evaluation, extensive history, dual axis, depression analysis (potential psychological-medical consult) |

*Positive findings in the routine examination indicate the need for subroutine examinations.

evaluated to determine that the material itself has not fatigued and fractured under normal or abnormal use patterns. Third, the restoration should be evaluated for appropriate contour, interproximal and occlusal contact, tissue biocompatibility, and its role in periodontal etiology. Fourth, the restoration should be evaluated for surface finish and its ability to meet the functional and esthetic requirements of the client. Evaluation of a particular restoration in those four parameters will provide direction for any planned replacement or modification of the restoration. The findings in these four areas will help influence the treatment planning process for replacement of the restoration if necessary. Table 4-4 provides the reader with related questions to consider when examining restorations for these four considerations.

## Education

Identifying and recording the initial findings from client assessment is an important function of the dental hygien-

ist. Educating the person, relative to restorative dentistry, involves two components. The hygienist is in a key position to: 1) advise the client about preliminary findings regarding the condition of existing restorations, and 2) recommend preventive measures that help maintain the current restorative work and prevent the need for future restorative care. Communication of the initial findings to the client will often generate questions regarding treatment. The ability to effectively communicate available options without committing to a specific procedure or therapy will help educate the clients and aid in their ability to make informed decisions. Clinically acceptable margins on dental restorations still tend to accumulate plaque and generally are the first location for carious breakdown on a tooth. Advising clients of the potential for problems in the marginal areas where plaque accumulation is noted is of paramount importance. Preventive measures should be recommended such as increased plaque control, dietary modifications, and home fluoride administration, etc.

**Table 4-4  Examination of Existing Restorations**

| Areas to Consider | Questions to Analyze |
| --- | --- |
| Restoration and Surrounding Tooth Structure | • Are there new caries or recurrent caries? |
| Marginal and Structural Integrity | • Is the margin defective? If so, is it open, deficient, or an overhang?<br>• Is the structure functional, or is it fatigued or fractured? |
| Appropriate Contour, Interproximal and Occlusal Contact, Tissue Biocompatibility | • Is the faciolingual and occlusocervical dimension appropriate?<br>• Is the emergence angle appropriate?<br>• Is the ideal soft tissue contour enhanced?<br>• What is the tissue response to the restorative material? |
| Surface Finish | • Does the surface finish meet the functional requirements of the individual?<br>• Does the surface finish meet the aesthetic requirements of the individual? |

## Maintenance of Dental Restorations

Along with the evaluation of existing restorations and self-care education, dental hygienists can assist in the maintenance of restorative dentistry. Appropriate selection of techniques employed during the nonsurgical care can help prevent iatrogenic damage of the clients already completed restorative therapy. Proper use of ultrasonic and sonic scaling devices around porcelain and composite margins is essential. Direct contact of the activated tip on the margins must be avoided. Restricting airpolishing around composite restorations and pit and fissue sealants is also imperative. Some medium to coarse prophylaxis pastes will also remove the gloss from composite restorations and may remove a high polish from gold and alloy restorations. Acidulated phosphate fluoride preparations should not be utilized with composite and porcelain restorations and some home bleaching agents should be carefully evaluated before use in the same conditions. From a positive perspective, the hygienist and dentist should establish some conditions whereby the hygienist may actively improve the quality of restorations. Simple marginations as indicated, superficial stain removal, and repolishing both composite and amalgam restorations can all be accomplished in a routine recare appointment if time allows. Those services will help the hygienist aid the client in maintaining a high level of periodontal and restorative health.

## Restorative Placement

In some jurisdictions, dental hygienists are legally permitted to place, carve, and polish some direct restorative materials. In those states, the right to place the restorations must be balanced with the obligation to develop and maintain a high level of competency. A situation where the hygienist only occasionally places restorative materials or is called upon on an ad hoc basis to avert a scheduling crisis does a distinct disservice to both the individual practice and the involved practitioners. Only through continued utilization of the restorative materials and updating of skills is the dental hygienist able to maintain the level of skill necessary to provide high-quality restorative dentistry.

## Combining Restorative and Periodontal Treatment Appointments

In some selected circumstances, there may be an advantage to combining the planned restorative care with periodontal therapy. Indications for accomplishing both types of therapy at the same appointment are: 1) limited periodontal problems with good to excellent prognosis, 2) neither the periodontal therapy nor restorative therapy will be compromised by joint treatment, or 3) a distinct benefit to be derived by joint treatment. The usual circumstances involve pocket depths of 4 to 6 mm around maxillary or mandibular molars that need a direct restorative. The direct vision and straight line access to root surfaces once the old restoration is removed is often beneficial to the scaling and root planing process. The existing restoration often had an overhang or other anatomy that complicated the ability to thoroughly clean the root surfaces involved. Care must be taken to assure that bleeding from the pocket is controlled before placement of the new restoration. Other situations involve removal of an existing indirect restoration, temporization, and treatment of the periodontal conditions with an adequately contoured and sealed temporary.

---

# Summary

The provision of restorative dentistry can and indeed must be coordinated with periodontal therapy. Without coordination and consideration of the often diverse therapies, neither the periodontal health nor the restorative dentistry can achieve the level of care needed for today's dental consumer. A thorough understanding of the materials involved and their utilization in an appropriate manner will ultimately benefit periodontal therapists in their quest for periodontal health. Likewise, a keen understanding of the periodontal tissues along with the proposed therapeutic goals can aid the restorative dentist in design and implementation of the restorative treatment. Understanding and communication can help clients receive the level of care needed to provide them with comprehensive dental health.

---

# Case Studies

**Case Study One:** Kathy Hep is a 42-year-old female who presents with a complaint of "irritated gums" around the crown on her maxillary right central incisor. A detailed history reveals that the tissue has been "red and puffy" from the date of placement. The tissue has been treated by soft tissue curettage in the past without success. Her medical history is significant for allergic reactions to multiple medications, some foods, and metals. Clinical examination demonstrates a porcelain fused to metal crown with good, but not excellent, marginal integrity. The gingival tissue surrounding the tooth displays erythema of the marginal tissues along with enlargement. Periodontal probing depths are a consistent 3 mm on the proximal surfaces and at the straight facial and lingual, while the adjacent unrestored central incisor has 2 mm interproximal probings and 1 mm facial and lingual probings. The client demonstrates good plaque control and is desirous of correcting the situation. The treatment plan involves replacement of the existing crown.

At what point in the treatment would you want to consider periodontal reevaluation and nonsurgical intervention? Would you want to consider a different material in the construction of the new crown? If so, what would be an alternative?

**Case Study Two:** Fred Davis is a 56-year-old male who presents for initial exam with no particular problem or major complaint. His medical history is uncomplicated except for mild hypertension, which he makes no attempts to control even though his physician keeps encouraging him. Clinically, Fred presents with multiple crowns and bridges. The crowns and bridges which were finished about four years ago, do not display caries or gross marginal discrepancies, but they are overcontoured and have inadequate gingival embrasure spaces in many cases. Periodontal findings involve generalized gingival inflammation with a significant edematous component. The average periodontal probing depth is 4 mm and several sites exhibit bleeding on probing. The patient expresses a desire to complete his treatment in one appointment because of his busy schedule.

What challenges does the dental hygienist face in: 1) planning and execution of treatment, and 2) nonsurgical treatment of the tissues and stain removal (relative to the existing restorations)?

**Case Study Three:** Phyllis Jensen is a 34-year-old female who presents at initial exam with a complaint of shredding floss and food trapping on the upper left side. Her medical history is insignificant. Clinical examination demonstrates the maxillary left first molar to have a Type II overhang on the distal surface and a deficient contact on the same surface. The periodontal condition involves 5 mm probing on the distal surface, subgingival calculus, and bleeding upon probing. The rest of her periodontal examination is within normal limits except for some marginal gingivitis noted on the linguals of her mandibular molars. Should the treatment plan involve replacement or margination of the Type II overhang? Can the margination or restoration be treatment planned for the same appointment as the nonsurgical periodontal therapy?

**Case Study Four:** Jill Deter is a 62-year-old female who presents because her "physician wants her to get a dental checkup." Her medical history is significant for advanced rheumatoid arthritis. Significant medications include intermittent high dose prednisone therapy for the past six years with the last round ending six months ago. She currently takes methotrexate 10 mg per week as a single dose. Since her last recare visit two years ago, she displays evidence of several recurrent carious lesions around the margins of existing Class V composite restorations. Periodontally, she displays generalized gingivitis with maximum periodontal probing depths of 4 mm around the molars. Her plaque control is inadequate especially in the gingival third. What aids and adjuncts would be beneficial to help this client maintain plaque control and what recare schedule would you prescribe? What restorative material might be considered for replacement of the involved Class V composites?

**Case Study Five:** Merlin Butler is a 55-year-old male who presents at initial exam stating he is "certain there are problems in there" because he has a couple of teeth that have had "holes" in them and they are now symptomatic. His medical history is significant for past "bouts" with alcoholism, hypertension (which he would like to control but he takes his medicine irregularly), and smoking (one-pack-a-day smoker for the past forty years). Clinically, Mr. Butler demonstrates large carious lesions on seven teeth (including two teeth with permanent crowns) and significant overhangs or marginal discrepancies on three other teeth. Two of the molars are transiently symptomatic with cold and hot foods and beverages. Periodontally, Mr. Butler has moderate bone loss in localized areas and advanced bone loss around his maxillary incisors and the mandibular molar on the left side. The prognosis for the teeth with advanced bone loss is poor, but not hopeless. He is unaware of the periodontal disease and is desirous of keeping his teeth if possible. The treatment plan will involve coordinated therapy with a dental hygienist, restorative dentist, and periodontist. Using the treatment planning protocol presented in this chapter, develop a general treatment plan outlining which phases of treatment involve the: 1) restorative components of therapy and, 2) nonsurgical periodontal components of therapy.

## Case Study Discussions

**Discussion—Case Study One:** The lack of success with the previous nonsurgical therapy would indicate that the local factors influencing gingival health need to be corrected before additional nonsurgical therapy is initiated. Because nonsurgical therapy has the potential to alter the level of the gingival margin and thus the esthetics of the case, it would be best to treatment plan nonsurgical therapy during the time when the client is wearing a temporary. The treatment plan should allow for an intermediate term of temporization so that periodontal healing and tissue response can be assessed before the final restoration is seated.

With Ms. Hep's medical history and lack of response to previous therapy, it would be wise to consider a non-metallic crown. If an all-ceramic crown was not feasible from a restorative perspective, the highest noble metal available should be used to increase the potential biocompatibility.

**Discussion—Case Study Two:** As indicated from his medical history and desire for expedited therapy, the most significant challenges will center on self-care education and compliance. Mr. Davis must be educated about the need for therapy and his role in control of the periodontal conditions present in his mouth. The dental hygienist will need to nicely, but yet firmly, establish that the best care will result from a collaboration between Mr. Davis and the dental hygienist with each being aware of their responsibilities. Although it is possible to accommodate reasonable requests, it is the dental professional's role to determine length and number of appointments, as well as healing times between procedures and reevaluation. If therapy is desired, it is the client's responsibility to comply with the necessary home care instructions and recare/return visits planned.

The excessive contours and inadequate embrasure spaces will hinder the hygienist's ability to instrument the tooth surfaces and tissues. In some areas this hindrance may prevent adequate instrumentation of the involved surfaces. It would be wise to point this out to Mr. Davis in advance of therapy. The porcelain material may inhibit the hygienist's ability to use powered scaling and polishing instruments so that marginal integrity is maintained and the glaze of the porcelain is preserved.

**Discussion—Case Study Three:** Although the overhang is a Type II overhang and could be treatment planned for margination, the lack of adequate proximal contact increases the overhang to a Type III and thus replacement of the restoration is indicated. When the periodontal findings can be related to the morphology of the restoration and the periodontal disease is localized, joint treatment of the restorative and periodontal problems can be accomplished at the same appointment. An acceptable technique involves removal of the existing restoration, scaling and root planing of the distal surface, bleeding control, and then placement of a direct restorative.

**Discussion—Case Study Four:** The dental hygienist's efforts should be aimed toward increasing the client's ability to maintain plaque control along with mitigating the effects of unremoved plaque, which will persist. Use of an efficacious mechanical toothbrush, floss holder (possibly with a custom handle), oral irrigation device, and home fluoride rinse would all be possible suggestions for this client. In addition, if Ms. Deter has a home care nurse or aide, it would be beneficial to instruct that person in assisting with daily plaque removal. Ms. Deter would also benefit from an accelerated recare visit schedule of once every three months. The probability of incomplete plaque control, advanced disease, and medications can work in combination to produce rapid changes in her oral health. To help reduce the likelihood of future recurrent caries, utilization of a glass ionomer or resin modified ionomer should be considered. The adhesive nature of the restorative material and fluoride release would be beneficial at reducing the rate of recurrent caries.

**Discussion—Case Study Five:** The restorative therapy will consist of both direct and indirect restorations. The restorative therapy will likely be involved with the symptomatic, disease reduction, rehabilitative, and maintenance phases. Reduction of thermal sensitivity will enhance Mr. Butler's comfort level and ability to comply with self-care recommendations and treatment. The disease reduction phase will involve removal of the overhangs, marginal discrepancies, and cavitated areas that harbor plaque and calculus. Indirect restoratives will be delayed until the rehabilitation phase when stable and healthy periodontal tissues have been realized. The nonsurgical periodontal procedures will be encompassed in the disease reduction, rehabilitative, and maintenance phases. Prior to surgical intervention in the disease reduction phase and as an adjunct to any planned surgical rehabilitation, nonsurgical periodontal procedures will be needed. With a poor prognosis, those teeth with advanced disease will likely need continued nonsurgical intervention to maintain tissue health and prevent future disease.

## REFERENCES

Abbate, M. F., Tjan, A. H., & Fox, W. (1989). Comparison of the marginal fit of various ceramic crown systems. *Journal of Prosthetic Dentistry, 61,* 527–531.

Ainamo, J. (1972). Relationship between malalignment of teeth and periodontal disease. *Scandinavian Journal of Dental Research, 80,* 104.

American Academy of Periodontology. (1989). *Proceedings of the world workshop in clinical periodontics,* Section III (p. III-15–19). Chicago: The American Academy of Periodontology.

Arcoria, C. J., Gonzalez, J. P., & Vitasek, B. A. (1992). Effects of ultrasonic instrumentation on microleakage in composite restorations with glass ionomer liners. *Journal of Oral Rehabilitation, 19,* 21.

Bader, J. D., Rozier, R. G., McFall, W. T., & Ramsey, D. L.

(1991). Effect of crown margins on periodontal conditions in regularly attending patients. *Journal of Prosthetic Dentistry, 65,* 75–79.

Brown, L. J. (1994). Trends in tooth loss among U.S. employed adults from 1971 to 1985. *Journal of the American Dental Association, 125,* 533–540.

Brunsvold, M. A. & Lane, J. J (1990). The prevalence of overhanging dental restorations and their relationship to periodontal disease. *Journal of Clinical Periodontology, 17,* 67–72.

Burgett, F., Charbeneau, T., Nissle, R., Morrison, E., Ramfjord, S., & Caffesse, R. (1988). A randomized occlusal adjustment in periodontitis patients (Abstract). *Journal of Dental Research, 67,* 124.

Caffesse, R. G. (1980). Management of periodontal disease in patients with occlusal abnormalities. *Dental Clinics of North America, 24,* 215.

Campbell, S. D. (1989). Evaluation of surface roughness and polishing techniques for new ceramic materials. *Journal of Prosthetic Dentistry, 61,* 563–568.

Caplan, D. J. & Weintraub, J. A. (1993).The oral health burden in the United States: A summary of recent epidemiologic studies. *Journal of Dental Education, 57*(12), 853–862.

Castellani, D., Clauser, C., & Bernadini, U. (1994). Thermal distortion of different materials in crown construction. *Journal of Prosthetic Dentistry, 72,* 360–366.

Christensen, G. J. (1994). Aesthetic dentistry. *Mirage Dental Systems 1994 Conference,* December 1, 1994: Kansas City.

Corbin, S. B. & Kohn, W. G. (1994). The benefits and risks of dental amalgam: Current findings reviewed. *Journal of the American Dental Association, 125,* 381–388.

DiAngelis, A. J. (1994). The good news of oral health. *Journal of the American Dental Association, 125,* 531–532.

Douvitsas, G. (1991). Effect of cavity design on gap formation in class II composite resin restorations. *Journal of Prosthetic Dentistry, 65,* 475–479.

Elderton, R. J. & Mjor, I. A. (1992). Changing scene in cariology and operative dentistry. *International Journal of Dentistry, 42,* 165–169.

Ferracane, J. L. (1992). Using posterior composites appropriately. *Journal of the American Dental Association, 123,* 53–58.

Fleszar, T. J., Knowles, J. W., Morrison, E. C., Burgett, F. G., Nissle, R. R., & Ramfjord, S. P. (1980). *Journal of Clinical Periodontology, 7,* 495.

Flores-de-Jacoby, L., Zafiropoulos, G. G., & Ciancio, S. (1989). The effect of crown margin location on plaque and periodontal health. *International Journal of Periodonal Restorative Dentistry, 9,* 197–205.

Frielich, M. A., Niekrash, C. E., Katz, R. V., & Simonsen, R. J. (1992). Periodontal effects of fixed partial denture retainer margins: Configuration and location. *Journal of Prosthetic Dentistry, 67,* 184–190.

Garber, D. A. (1989). Direct composite veneers versus etched porcelain laminate veneers. *Dental Clinics of North America, 33,* 301–304.

Geiger, A. M., Wasserman, B. H., Thompson, R. H., & Turgeon, L. R. (1972). Relationship of occlusion and periodontal disease. V. Relation of classification of occlusion to periodontal status and gingival inflammation. *Journal of Periodontology, 43,* 554.

Glickman, I., Smulow, J., Voger, B., & Pasamonti, G. (1966). The effect of occlusal forces on healing following mucogingival surgery. *Journal of Periodontology, 37,* 319.

Glossary of Prosthodontic Terms. (1987). *Journal of Prosthetic Dentistry 58*(6), 713–762.

Hensten-Pettersen, A. & Jacobsen, N. (1991). Perceived side effects of biomaterials in prosthetic dentistry. *Journal of Prosthetic Dentistry, 65,* 138–144.

Highfield, J. E. & Powell, R. N. (1978). Effects of removal of posterior overhanging metallic margins of restorations upon the periodontal tissues. *Journal of Clinical Periodontology, 5,* 169–181.

Hodges, K. O. & Bowen, D. M. (1985). Effectiveness of margination procedures in relation to periodontal status. *Journal of Dental Hygiene, 57,* 320–324.

Hondrum, S. (1994). Tear and energy properties of three impression materials. *International Journal of Prosthodontics, 7,* 517–521.

Jeffcoat, M. K. & Howell, T. H. (1980). Alveolar bone destruction due to overhanging amalgam in periodontal disease. *Journal of Periodontology, 51,* 599–602.

Jendresen, M. D., Allen, E. P., Bayne, S. C., Hansson, T. L., Klooster, J., & Preston, J. D. (1992). Report of the committee on scientific investigation of the American Academy of Restorative Dentistry. *Journal of Prosthetic Dentistry, 68,* 137–190.

Kallus, T. & Mjor, I.A. (1991). Incidence of adverse effects of dental materials. *Scandinavian Journal of Dental Research, 99,* 236–240.

Kay, H. B. (1982). Esthetic considerations in the definitive periodontal prosthetic management of the maxillary anterior segment. *International Journal of Periodontal Restorative Dentistry, 2*(3), 44.

Koidis, P. T., Schroeder, K., Johnston, W., & Campagni, W. (1991). Color consistency, plaque accumulation and external marginal surface characteristics of the collarless metal-ceramic restoration. *Journal of Prosthetic Dentistry, 65,* 391–400.

Lang, N. P., Kiel, R. A., & Anderhalden, K. (1983). Clinical and microbiological effects of subgingival restorations with overhanging and clinically perfect margins. *Journal of Clinical Periodontology, 10,* 563–578.

Lindhe, J. & Ericsson, I. (1982). Effect of elimination of jiggling forces on periodontally exposed teeth in the dog. *Journal of Periodontology, 53,* 562.

Löe, H. (1968). Reactions of marginal periodontal tissues to restorative procedures. *International Journal of Dentistry, 18,* 759–778.

McCombie, F. & Stothard, O. L. (1964). Relationship between gingivitis and other dental conditions. *Journal of the Canadian Dental Association, 30,* 506.

Meitner, S. (1975). Co-destructive factors of marginal periodontitis and repetitive mechanical injury. *Journal of Dental Research, Special Issue C,* 78.

Miller, L. M. (1992). Porcelain veneer protection plan: Maintenance procedures for all porcelain restorations. *Journal of Esthetic Dentistry, 2*(3), 63.

Mjor, I. A. (1992). Placement and replacement of amalgam restorations in Italy. *Journal of Operative Dentistry, 17,* 70–73.

Munksgaard, E. C. (1992). Toxicology versus allergy in restorative dentistry. *Advances in Dental Research, 6,* 17–21.

Nash, L. B. (1993). The hygienist's role in posterior restorations. *Journal of Practical Hygiene, May/June,* 11–15.

Newcomb, G. M. (1974). The relationship between the location of subgingival crown margins and gingival inflammation. *Journal of Periodontology, 45,* 151–154.

Oilo, G. (1992). Biodegradation of dental composites/glass-ionomer cements. *Advances in Dental Research, 6,* 50–54.

Pack, A. R. C., Coxhead, L. J., & McDonald, B. W. (1990). The prevalence of overhanging margins in posterior amalgam restorations and periodontal consequences. *Journal of Clinical Periodontology, 17,* 145–152.

Parkinson, C. F. (1976). Excessive crown contours facilitate endemic plaque niches. *Journal of Prosthetic Dentistry, 35,* 424.

Phillips, R. W. (1973). *Skinner's science of dental materials.* Philadelphia: W.B. Saunders Co.

Phillips, R. W., Jendresen, M. D., Klooster, J., McNeil, C., Preston, J. D., & Schallhorn, R. G. (1990). Report of the committee on scientific investigation of the American Academy of Restorative Dentistry. *Journal of Prosthetic Dentistry, 64,* 74–110.

Rajstein, J. & Tal, M. (1984). The effect of ultrasonic scaling on the surface of class V amalgam restorations—a scanning electron microscopy study. *Journal of Oral Rehabilitation, 11*, 299.

Reeves, W. G. (1991). Restorative margin placement and periodontal health. *Journal of Prosthetic Dentistry, 66*, 733–736.

Reeves, W. G., Lentz, D. L., O'Hara, J. W., McDaniel, M. D., & Tolbert, W. E. (1992). Comparison of marginal adaptation between direct and indirect composites. *Journal of Operative Dentistry, 17*, 210–214.

Rogo, E. J. (1995). Overhang removal: Improving periodontal health adjacent to class II amalgam restorations. *Journal of Practical Hygiene, 4*(3), 15–23.

Sakaguchi, R. L., Peters, M. C. R. B., Nelson, S. R., Douglas, W. H., & Poort, H. W. (1992). Effects of polymerization contraction in composite restorations. *Journal of Dentistry, 20*, 178–182.

Serio, F. G., Strassler, H. E., Litkowski, L. J., Moffitt, W. C., & Krupa, C. M. (1988). The effect of polishing pastes on composite resin surfaces. *Journal of Periodontology, 59*, 837–840.

Smales, R. J., Webster, D. A., & Leppard, P. I. (1992). Predictions of restoration deterioration. *Journal of Dentistry, 20*, 215–220.

Spinks, G. C., Carson, R. E., Hancock, E. B., & Pelleu, G. B. (1986). An SEM study of overhang removal methods. *Journal of Periodontology, 57*, 632–636.

Stein, R. S. & Kuwata, M. (1977). A dentist and a dental technologist analyze current ceramo-metal procedures. *Dental Clinics of North America, 21*, 729.

Svanberg, G. (1974). Influence of trauma from occlusion on the periodontium of dogs with normal or inflamed gingivae. *Odontological Review, 25*, 165.

Swift, E. J., Perdigao, J., & Heymann, H. O. (1985). Bonding to enamel and dentin: A brief history and state of the art, 1995. *Quintessence International, 26*, 95.

Thomas, M. & Wickens, J. (1989). Microleakage of resin-retained porcelain veneers (Abstract). *Journal of Dental Research, 68*, 590.

Tjan, A. H., Dunn, J. R., & Sanderson, I. R. (1989). Microleakage patterns of porcelain and castable ceramic laminate veneers. *Journal of Prosthetic Dentistry, 61*, 276–282.

Trott, J. R. & Sherkat, A. (1964). Effect of Class II amalgam restorations on health of the gingiva: A clinical survey. *Journal of the Canadian Dental Association, 30*, 766–770.

Vale, J. D. F. & Caffesse, R. G. (1979). Removal of amalgam overhangs. *Journal of Periodontology, 50*, 245–249.

van Dijken, J. W. V. & Sjostrom, S. (1991). The effect of glass ionomer cement and composite resin fillings on marginal gingiva. *Journal of Clinical Periodontology, 18*, 200–203.

Van Zeghbroeck, L. M., Davidson, C. L., & DeClercq, M. (1989). Cohesive failure due to contraction stress in glass ionomer luting cements (Abstract). *Journal of Dental Research, 68*, 1014.

Van Zeghbroeck, L.M., Feilzer, A. J., & Davidson, C. L. (1989). Spontaneous failure of glass ionomer cements (Abstract). *Journal of Dental Research, 68*, 613.

Vermilyea, S. G., Prasanna, M. K., & Agar, J. R. (1994). Effect of ultrasonic cleaning and airpolishing on porcelain labial margin restorations. *Journal of Prosthetic Dentistry, 71*, 447.

Waerhaug, J. (1956). Effect of rough surfaces upon gingival tissue. *Journal of Dental Research, 35*, 323–325.

Wilson, R. D. (1985). Restorative dentistry and total oral health, advances in tissue management. ADA "Emphasis" Series. *Journal of the American Dental Association, 111*, 550–564.

Wilson, R. D. (1988). Fundamental restorative dentistry. *Tennessee Journal of Dentistry, 68*(2), 35–38.

Wilson, R. D. (1992). Restorative dentistry. In T. G. Wilson, K. S. Kornman, & M. G. Newman (Eds.), *Advances in periodontics* (pp. 226–244). Chicago: Quintessence Publishing Co., Inc.

Wilson, R. D. & Maynard, J. G. (1983). The relationship of restorative dentistry and periodontics. In J. W. Clark et al. (Eds.), *Clinical dentistry*. New York: Harper and Row.

Wozniak, W. T., Naleway, C. A., Gonzalez, E., Schemehorn, B. R., & Stookey, G. K. (1991). Use of an in vitro model to assess the effects of APF gel treatment on the staining potential of dental porcelain. *Dental Materials, 7*, 263–267.

Young, N. A. (1995). Periodontal debridement: Re-examining nonsurgical instrumentation. *Seminars in Dental Hygiene, 5*(1), 1–7.

# CHAPTER 5

# Recommendations for Radiographs

## Key Terms

categories of disease progression, "Case Types"
digital radiography
digital subtraction radiography
horizontal bone loss
horizontal angulation
kilovolt peak (kVp)

paralleling technique
transmission radiographs
triangulation
vertical angulation
vertical bitewing radiographs
vertical (angular) bone loss

## INTRODUCTION

Dental radiographs play an important role in the evaluation and treatment of periodontal diseases. Use of radiographs is essential because they are an integral part of the practice of modern dentistry and provide the clinician with information that may not be clinically apparent. Radiographs disclose information about the periodontal ligament, the alveolar bone, and the teeth within the bone. In a state of disease the remaining bone support indicates the type of loss that has occurred, the distribution of that loss, and the severity of loss. Predisposing factors related to periodontitis, such as overhanging restorations or calculus, might also be observed in the radiograph. Thorough evaluation and prognosis of disease cannot be determined without the use of adequate radiographs. Additionally, radiographs serve as a permanent record to be used to compare changes in the periodontium that occur over time.

Although radiographs are vital for accurate diagnosis and treatment of periodontal diseases, there are limitations to their use. A thorough clinical evaluation is essential before viewing radiographs. Clinicians will recall that by the time the most incipient changes are radiographically visible, significantly greater destruction has occurred clinically. Radiographs are not sufficient to demonstrate early bone loss, the presence or absence of pockets, exact morphology of bone deformities, buccal and lingual bone status, tooth mobility, level of epithelial attachment, nor early furcation involvement (Carranza, 1990; Williamson, 1993). Therefore, the radiograph is always used as an adjunct to, never a substitute for, a clinical periodontal examination. The periodontal examination routinely includes the chief complaint or concern, medical and dental histories, clinical examination, and analysis of the appropriately updated radiographs (American Academy of Periodontology, 1993).

Radiographs for clients should be selected on a case by case basis. Both clinical symptoms and the history of disease (periodontal deterioration) are considered when making decisions about which radiographs to expose. Time intervals between exposures are based on need and expected diagnostic yield. This chapter will address selection of conventional radiographs for the periodontal assessment as well as technical factors, interpretation, and protocol for exposure. Additional images are covered including recent developments such as computer-assisted radiography, the relationship of radiographic and clinical findings, and computed tomography. Information included within this chapter is intended to review or enhance the clinician's knowledge about radiographs used in the diagnosis and treatment of periodontal diseases. The reader is referred to various textbooks to enhance background information in oral radiology, if needed, (Haring & Lind, 1993; Goaz & White, 1994). These texts cover physics of ionizing radiation, the biological effects of radiation safety, imaging techniques, dental caries, dental anomalies, and other lesions not discussed in this chapter.

## SELECTION OF CONVENTIONAL RADIOGRAPHS FOR PERIODONTAL EVALUATION

Various types of intraoral and extraoral radiographs have been used and studied over the years to determine which will produce the best reproduction of the periodontium for interpretation and diagnosis of periodontal diseases. Among those most extensively studied are periapical, bitewing, and panoramic radiographs as well as the grid and ruler method, xeroradiography, and the newer methods of digital imaging. Results of these studies are as diverse as the number of researchers who conducted the studies (Akesson, Hakansson, & Rohlin, 1992; Benn, 1990; Hausmann, Allen, & Piedmonte, 1991; Kantor, Zeichner, Valachovic, & Reiskin, 1989; Molander, Ahlqwist, Grondahl, & Hollender, 1991; Osborne & Hemmings, 1992; Shrout, Powell, Hildebolt, Vannier, & Ahmed, 1993). Currently, conventional intraoral radiographs such as periapicals and/or bitewings appear to be superior to other systems for evaluating periodontal structures. The American Academy of Periodontology (1993) states that interpretation of a satisfactory number of diagnostic quality periapical and bitewing radiographs is essential for development of a periodontal diagnosis. The periodic exposure of full sets of radiographs is encouraged because this survey yields the most information. Conventional interpretive radiology represents a test of relatively high specificity meaning that radiographs have the ability to help the clinician exclude disease progression if it is truly not present (American Academy of Periodontology, 1989a). Conventional radiographs are, therefore, useful in confirming the presence of disease. Future predictions suggest that a non-conventional method of radiology, computer assisted digital enhancement, will play a major role in the interpretation of dental diseases including periodontitis. Table 5-1 summarizes the recommendations for periapical, bitewing, and panoramic films discussed in the following sections.

## Periapical Radiographs

The periapical view in the full mouth series is designed to gain a maximum amount of information because it is an image of the entire tooth. It is best used to evaluate root length, shape, and position alveolar bone near the apex; and pathology. All dental radiographs represent a two-dimensional recording of three-dimensional objects where the objects overlay one another. Because of this, even with excellent radiographs it is difficult for clinicians to interpret slight changes in structures that might indicate disease. The major problem influencing the sensitivity of periapical films in diagnosis is **vertical angulation** where elongation or foreshortening can appear to either increase or decrease bony support when no actual change has occurred. This is especially true in the maxillary molar region (see Figure 5-1). The foreshortening apparent in the periapical film (see Figure 5-1A) makes the bone level appear to be close to the cementoenamel junction. With this type of distortion it is difficult to accurately assess bone height. In order to determine the amount of distortion that occurred from vertical angulation error, the clinician measures the distance between buccal and lingual cusp tips. Ideally, buccal and lingual cusps should be approximately the same height on the radiograph. Measuring the distance between these cusps gives an approximation of the amount of vertical error that has occurred. This same measurement is then applied to the interproximal bone to assess the crestal level. For example, the distance between the buccal and

## Table 5-1 Selection of Conventional Radiographs for Periodontal Examination

| Type | Indications | Limitations | Technique Recommendations |
|---|---|---|---|
| Periapical | • to assess root length, shape, and position <br> • estimate severity and pattern of bone loss <br> • to detect pathological lesions | • accurate assessment of bone height and density | • paralleling technique is the method of choice <br> • use aiming devices <br> • use a long, 16-inch PID <br> • consider the use of 14 to 20 films |
| Bitewing | • to accurately assess bone height and density <br> • horizontally positioned films are indicated when early bone loss or gingivitis is suspected <br> • vertically positioned films are indicated for moderate to advanced bone loss | • assessment of root length, shape, and position <br> • detection of apical pathological lesions | • a +8 degrees vertical angulation is recommended for posterior bitewings <br> • use a +10 degrees vertical angulation for anterior vertical films <br> • use aiming devices <br> • use a long, 16-inch PID <br> • horizontal bitewings: use 2 to 4 no. 2 films depending on the age and dentition <br> • vertical bitewings: use 4 to 6 no. 2 films in the posterior depending on the dentition and 1 to 3 anterior films |
| Panoramic | • to view a large area of the maxilla and mandible | • not indicated for diagnosing periodontal diseases or caries | • follow the manufacturer's recommendations |

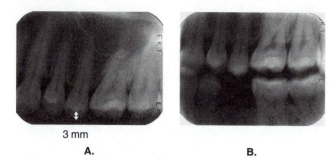

3 mm

**A.**                                    **B.**

**Figure 5-1** Improper vertical angulation. **A.** Improper vertical angulation in the periapical film illustrates how incorrect interpretation of bone loss can occur. The foreshortening makes the bone level appear close to the cementoenamel junction. **B.** The bitewing film demonstrates the correct angulation and true interproximal bone level.

lingual cusps of the maxillary second premolar in the periapical film on the left (see Figure 5-1A) measures just under 3 mm. This 3 mm measurement indicates approximately a 3 mm "bone gain" in the periapical view. The "bone gain" makes the bone appear to be within 2 to 3 millimeters of the cementoenamel junction, which would indicate early bone loss. If the clinician does not take the vertical angulation error into account, the degree of bone loss would be inaccurately assessed. When one uses the bitewing radiograph (Figure 5-1B) to assess height it is apparent that more bone loss is present.

It is accepted that standardized reproducible techniques are required in order to obtain high-quality radiographs. When periapical films are taken, the **paralleling technique**, also called the right-angle technique or long-cone technique, is the method of choice (Williamson, 1993). Clinicians will remember that the basis for this technique is that the x-ray film is placed parallel to the long axis of the teeth and the central ray of the x-ray beam is directed at right angles to both the film and the teeth. The relationship of the teeth, film, and central ray to one another minimizes geometric distortion. When the paralleling technique began to gain in popularity many years ago, studies were conducted comparing the parallel and bisection techniques. Results indicated that use of the paralleling technique reduced the number of undiagnostic radiographs by more than half (Bean, 1969; Weissman & Longhurst, 1971). The assistance of aiming devices is suggested to help provide consistently adequate diagnostic radiographs. Examples of these beam-guiding, film-holding devices are the X-C-P (Xtension Cone Paralleling distributed by Rinn Corporation) the Precision Instruments (distributed by Precision X-ray Company), and V.I.P. (Versatile Intraoral Positioner distributed by UP-RAD Corporation). These devices are helpful because subsequent films can be taken in as similar a position as possible to the initial film for comparative purposes. An additional principle advises use of a

long sixteen-inch cone, or Position Indicating Device (PID), in order to minimize magnification and distortion. The long PID also results in a decrease in patient exposure. Typically, fourteen to twenty periapical films are required for a full mouth survey depending on the dentition and the size of film utilized.

**Bitewing Surveys**

Later in this chapter, computer-assisted digital enhancement will be discussed in relation to periodontal diagnosis. Until this technique is made easily usable and affordable for the average dental office, the best alternative for interpreting bone loss is to use the conventional technique that produces the least amount of distortion. The bitewing film appears to be the radiograph of choice for periodontal assessment because it minimizes distortion by achieving the principles required for accurate photographic reproduction (Hausmann, Allen, Christersson, & Genco, 1989; Jeffcoat, 1992a; Reddy, 1992). The principles of photographic reproduction that affect the ability to evaluate the radiograph and to which the bitewing technique adheres are: 1) the distance between the film and oral structure is minimal, 2) the tooth and the film are positioned parallel to one another, and thus 3) the central beam is directed perpendicular to both. The result is a minimum of elongation, foreshortening, and erroneous projection of structures that might occur with use of periapical films even when employing the paralleling technique.

Although conventional horizontal bitewings are better than periapical films for interpreting bone loss, they limit the amount of alveolar bone that is visible in both arches at one time. For this reason, **vertical bitewing radiographs** are a more appropriate choice when disease has progressed beyond the early stages. Use of the vertical bitewing allows the clinician to view a maximum of osseous tissue in both arches simultaneously (Hausmann et al., 1989; Jeffcoat, 1992a; Thomson-Lakey & Tolle-Watts, 1994a; Williamson, 1993). When exposing this type of bitewing, the film is placed in either the posterior or anterior region of the mouth with the long axis of the film positioned vertically. Two posterior vertical bitewings on each side of the mouth will generally provide adequate coverage of the posterior region. On occasion a third film is required. Vertical bitewings may also be exposed in the anterior region. Depending on the size of the arch in the anterior region, two or three such films are usually sufficient. It is suggested that the clinician use two bitewing tabs placed end to end to provide an extra extension for better positioning of the anterior bitewing film.

Posterior horizontal and vertical bitewing films are exposed using a +8° vertical angulation on the tube head angle guide. A +10° vertical angulation is used for exposing anterior vertical bitewings. The horizontal and vertical posterior bitewings in Figure 5-2A and B illustrate the

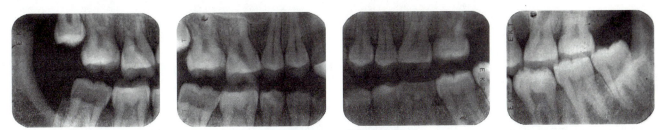

**A. Horizontal Posterior Bitewings**

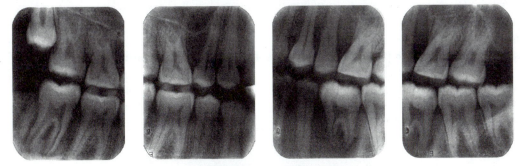

**B. Vertical Posterior Bitewings**

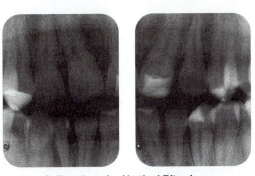

**C. Two Anterior Vertical Bitewings**

**Figure 5-2** Comparative bitewings.

additional information exhibited in the vertical bitewing when compared to the horizontally positioned film. Figure 5-2C demonstrates use of two anterior vertical bitewings. Vertical films are recommended to assess bone height when the clinician clinically assesses 4 mm of attachment loss is present indicating that periodontitis has reached the moderate or advanced stage. Some practitioners routinely expose vertical bitewings when they suspect periodontitis, even in its earliest stage. Use of vertical bitewings with early bone loss helps the clinician compare vertical bitewings exposed at subsequent maintenance appointments to the baseline vertically positioned films.

Another important factor affecting accurate interpretation of any type of bitewing is the **horizontal angulation**. The horizontal angulation must be directed perpendicular to the contact areas of the teeth in order to prevent overlapping the crowns of the teeth and surrounding tissues. Figure 5-3 illustrates that horizontal

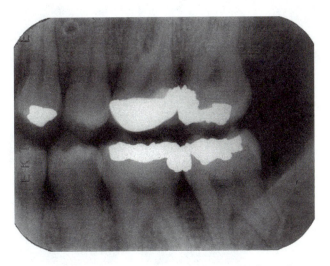

**Figure 5-3** Improper horizontal angulation. Horizontal overlapping occurs between the maxillary first and second molar and the mandibular first molar and second premolar.

overlapping decreases the ability to view interproximal carious lesions, and that it repositions interproximal bone so as to distort the position of that bone to the teeth. Additionally, the width of both the periodontal ligament space and lamina dura are distorted when horizontal overlapping occurs.

A single radiograph or set of radiographs yields information only on past activity of disease and healing; therefore, it is critical that comparisons of radiographic examinations be made over time (Hollender, 1992; Jeffcoat & Reddy, 1991; Thompson-Lakey & Tolle-Watts, 1994b). Radiographs used in this manner are referred to as **transmission radiographs**. Comparative or transmission radiographs should always be correlated with corresponding clinical evaluations. Figure 5-4 represents transmission bitewing radiographs over a six-year period of time. Viewing several sets of films such as these demonstrates progression of disease. Film mounts are available that allow several sets of bitewings to be mounted in the same holder to facilitate viewing.

## Panoramic Films

Panoramic radiography has been used in dentistry for many years (see Figure 5-5). This single film produces an image of both maxillary and mandibular arches and all the supporting facial structures, and takes only about twenty seconds to expose. It is a simple and convenient radiograph to expose and results in significantly less client radiation than a full set of periapical films. The main disadvantage of panoramic radiographs is poor resolution. The anatomic detail is not as clear as the detail produced in intraoral radiographs. This lack of detail coupled with magnification, distortion, and overlapping of teeth make diagnosis of caries and periodontal diseases extremely difficult on the panoramic film. For these reasons, panoramic films are not recommended as a component of the periodontal examination. When panoramic images are compared with images using the long cone paralleling technique, there is a tendency to underestimate early marginal bone destruction and overestimate

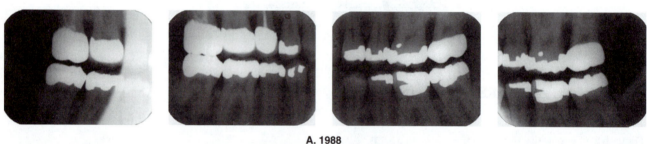

**A. 1988**

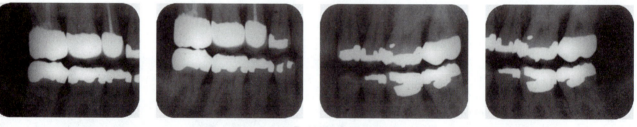

**B. 1990**

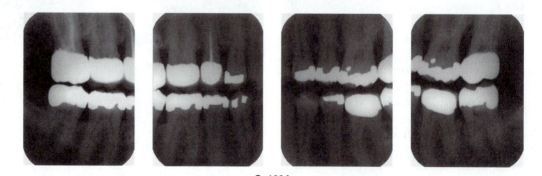

**C. 1994**

**Figure 5-4** Transmission radiographs.

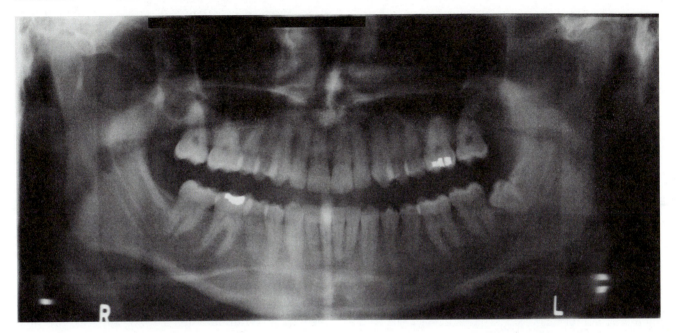

**Figure 5-5** Panoramic radiograph. A panoramic radiograph is adequate to demonstrate a general impression of tissue health. Poor resolution makes it inappropriate for use as a diagnostic tool for detecting the early stages of periodontal disease.

major destruction (Gröndahl, Gröndahl, & Webber, 1984). Refer to Table 5-6 on page 138 for the recommended protocol for exposure of panoramic radiographs.

## TECHNICAL FACTORS AFFECTING PERIODONTAL INTERPRETATION

There are a number of technical factors such as film speed, machine settings, and quality assurance which may affect the processed radiograph. The operator has complete control over these factors and should follow prescribed procedure closely in order to produce a quality radiograph. Each of these factors combined with appropriate selection and exposure of radiographs aids the clinician in enhancing interpretation and diagnosis of periodontal diseases.

### Film Speed

The most commonly used types of intraoral film are: 1) the newer Ektaspeed (E-speed) and, 2) the older Ultraspeed (D-speed) film. The size of the silver halide grains in the film is what controls the film speed. Ektaspeed (E) has a larger crystal size when compared to Ultraspeed (D). As a result, E-speed film is twice as fast as D-speed film. As film speed increases, exposure time is decreased. E-speed film requires less radiation for film exposure and, therefore, decreases patient exposure by approximately 50 percent when compared to D-speed (Frederiksen, 1994; Goaz & White, 1994; Kantor et al., 1989; Thomson-Lakey & Tolle-Watts, 1994a). For this reason, the use of E-speed film has gained popularity in dental

practices. Because of the larger grain in E-speed film, loss of detail occurs. The resulting radiograph may appear slightly fuzzy to the practitioner who has traditionally used D-speed film. Although the contrast is slightly compromised when using E-speed film, both E-speed and D-speed films have approximately the same density. A thorough review of the literature reveals that image resolution or the clarity of the image with the finished E-speed film is equal to the D-speed and the ability to diagnose disease is also equal (Kantor et al., 1989).

Ektaspeed Plus, introduced into dentistry by Eastman Kodak in 1994, has virtually overcome the problem of decreased detail. Crystals in the E-Plus emulsion have been flattened to a tabular grain shape in order to increase the surface area to receive more radiation so that the radiation is used more effectively. The flat surface produces a film with more consistent image quality. The film is extremely stable and is very forgiving of the day-to-day variances in film processing. As a result, it effectively eliminates the trade-off between image quality and radiation reduction to the patient that was apparent between D-speed and E-speed film. Dental practitioners using E-Plus can now obtain excellent diagnostic images and still maintain the 50 percent reduction of radiation exposure.

### Control Factors

The image quality and radiation dose are also influenced by the machine settings selected. Dental radiographs are generally taken at either a low **kilovolt peak (kVp)** setting (65–70 kVp), or at a high kVp setting (90 kVp). The kilovoltage is related to the energy of the x-ray beam. The higher the kVp, the greater the energy or penetrating power of the beam. High energy beams are more likely to pass through the object being radiographed rather than being absorbed by it. The client's tissue dose is decreased by using high energy beams or 90 kVp. Some studies have estimated that when 90 kVp is used instead of 65 to 70 kVp, the amount of radiation an individual receives is reduced between 30 and 40 percent (Frederiksen, 1994). The combination of using high (90) kVp in conjunction with E- or E-Plus speed film is an effective means of decreasing total patient exposure.

The 90 kVp machine setting also provides the advantage of long-scale contrast on the radiograph. Long-scale contrast produces an image with small differences in density within the objects being radiographed. As a result, there are many shades of gray on the processed film. When evaluating less dense tissues to discern slight changes in the periodontium, it is necessary to have the slightly lighter image produced by the high kVp machine setting. This type of contrast allows the clinician to view more finite structures in the periodontium whereas when lower kVp settings are used, the finer structures tend to become "burned out" by the radiation (see Figure 5-6). For clinicians accustomed to seeing a high contrast of mostly black and white or short-scale, this type of radiograph will appear to be light and slightly fuzzy. Nonetheless, the diagnostic quality of long-scale contrast is best for evaluating periodontal disease even though it may not be aesthetically pleasing (Frommer, 1992; Goaz & White, 1994; Williamson, 1993). With practice, interpretation of caries and other pathological conditions can also be accomplished using this higher kVp technique. When possible, practitioners should try to incorporate the use of high kVp into their practices to eliminate duplication of exposures or having to use one setting for viewing caries and another for viewing the periodontium. E-Plus film has greatly improved the diagnostic quality of the radiograph to the extent that viewing all pathologic conditions on a single machine setting is now easy to achieve.

## Quality Assurance

Oral health care professionals are aware that a system of quality control must be implemented in the practice setting in order to produce films of consistently high quality. This quality control system is divided into three main components: 1) processing in the darkroom, 2) the features of the darkroom, and 3) the x-ray machine. Processing involves the use and maintenance of chemicals; and, the processing unit itself. First, care should be taken to maintain an optimum concentration level of chemicals used. Regular replenishment with fresh chemicals is essential for processing. A schedule for complete cleaning of the processing system and replacement of chemicals should also be developed and employed. If weak chemicals are used, poor quality radiographs will result,

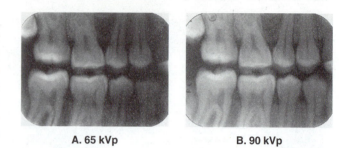

**A. 65 kVp**                    **B. 90 kVp**

**Figure 5-6** Kilovolt settings affect image quality. The high kilovoltage setting yields significantly more periodontal information.

which may lead to retaking films and doubling client exposure in the area.

The darkroom itself is also frequently evaluated. Countertops and equipment must be kept scrupulously clean. Test for light leaks by allowing the eyes to adjust to the dark for 5 minutes then marking any areas of visible light with chalk. Those areas of light leakage must be sealed by using heavy-duty tape or weather stripping. Check the manufacturer's recommendations for correct safe lights and filters based on the fastest type of film being processed in the darkroom. A simple method for evaluating the darkroom safelight for potential film fogging is the "coin test." Under darkroom conditions, open an unexposed film, place a coin on the film, and leave it on the countertop in close proximity to the safelight area for approximately three minutes. After this three-minute interval, process the film as usual. Upon examination, if the outline of the coin appears on the film, the safelight conditions in the darkroom are inadequate. It must be determined whether the fogging is a result of the safelight being too bright, having the wrong filter, or the result of light leaking into the darkroom. Daily comparison of processed films with a test film (one processed in a clean tank with fresh chemicals at optimum exposure setting) is necessary.

The x-ray machine should be tested every two years to assure the correct operation and output of the unit. A variety of means exists to complete this task, but it is best to have the equipment examined and calibrated by individual state departments of health. There is either a minimal charge or no charge for this service. Commercial laboratory services are also available for this purpose.

## INTERPRETATION OF PERIODONTAL DISEASES

Thorough interpretation of radiographs requires careful evaluation and experience. Interpretation refers to the ability of the clinician to read or distinguish what is present on the radiograph. On the other hand, diagnosis is actually a conclusion the practitioner makes by correlating clinical data with the radiographic findings. Before the interpretation begins, adequate viewing conditions should be established (see Table 5-2) (Farman, Christoffel,

**Table 5-2 A Review of Adequate Viewing Conditions for Radiographs**

| Condition | Rationale |
|---|---|
| • View in a darkened room | • fine details are easily visible |
| • Use a viewbox with bright, even illumination | • fine details are indistinct when radiographs are held up to room light |
| | • lack of detail could lead to inaccurate diagnosis |
| • Place in mounts with an opaque background | • clear backgrounds allow extraneous light from the viewbox to be transmitted to the viewer's eye |
| | • extraneous light from any source makes it difficult for the eyes to accommodate the entire range of light |
| • Use a magnifying glass | • focusing on specific areas of significance is enhanced |

& Wood, 1994). Next, the interpretation is conducted systematically. It is best to view a set of radiographs film by film and evaluate one feature at a time. For example, the clinician assesses the alveolar crest in each film and then assesses the lamina dura in each film. Another technique used to enhance evaluation is to view the radiographic survey bilaterally. The clinician notes 1) if: the changes identified on one side of the mouth are also present on the opposite side and 2) if the changes are generalized throughout the posterior or anterior region. Viewing the survey bilaterally allows the clinician to identify if the changes noted are normal or abnormal for the particular individual. Viewing a specific tooth or support structure in more than one film is also a good habit to develop. Structures and disease processes, especially caries or slight periodontal changes, may appear different in various films because of angulation.

Table 5-3 is an evaluation form for radiographic assessment. Interpretation is divided into sextants of the mouth knowing that different stages of disease can be visible in any single client's oral cavity. This format can be used to evaluate bitewing, periapical, or full mouth series of films. It is recognized that many of these entities are charted or documented elsewhere in the client's permanent record; however, this form is useful for educating or standardizing oral health care professionals.

## Normal Alveolar Bone

The first step in assessing any disease process is to be able to recognize normal anatomic appearance in the area of interest. Once baseline is determined, disease can be recognized and evaluated. Periodontally this recognition includes evaluation of the supporting structures of the periodontium. The periodontium consists of four components: the gingiva, periodontal ligament, cementum, and alveolar bone which are reviewed in Chapter 1. For purposes of this chapter, only the features of the alveolar bone that have radiographic relevance are discussed. Radiographically visible components include the periodontal ligament space and portions of the alveolar bone. The normal appearance of periodontal structures is presented in Figure 5-7.

The alveolar crest is the most coronal portion of the alveolar bone. It is composed of dense cortical bone and appears as a thin, radiopaque line that is continuous with the lamina dura. In health, it is typically located approximately 1.5 to 2.0 mm apical to the cementoenamel junction (Haring & Lind, 1993). In the posterior regions, the shape of the alveolar crest is dependent upon the proximity and position of adjacent teeth. The crest of the alveolar bone appears smooth and flat in

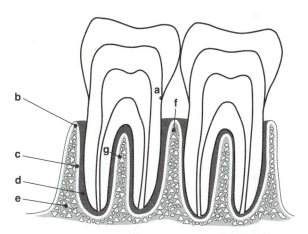

**A. Diagram of the Radiographically Visible Features**

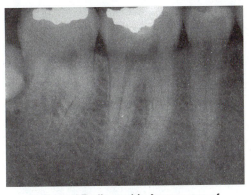

**B. Normal Radiographic Appearance of Periodontal Structures**

**Figure 5-7** Appearance of normal periodontal structures. *Diagram Key:* **a:** cementoenamel junction (CEJ); **b:** alveolar crest located 1 to 2 mm apical to the CEJ; **c:** lamina dura (alveolar bone proper); **d:** periodontal ligament (PDL) space; **e:** supporting bone; **f:** interproximal bone; **g.** interradicular bone.

**Table 5-3  Periodontal Interpretation of Radiographs**

| QUESTION | R MAX POST Y | R MAX POST N | MAX ANT Y | MAX ANT N | L MAX POST Y | L MAX POST N | R MAND POST Y | R MAND POST N | MAND ANT Y | MAND ANT N | L MAND POST Y | L MAND POST N |
|---|---|---|---|---|---|---|---|---|---|---|---|---|
| 1. Does the alveolar bone appear normal as evidenced by the alveolar crest (located within 2 mm from the CEJ), lamina dura, and the PDL space of the supporting bone? | | | | | | | | | | | | |
| 2. Does the alveolar bone appear diseased as evidenced by the alveolar crest (located over 2 mm from the CEJ), lamina dura, and the PDL space of the supporting bone? If yes, continue the interpretation. | | | | | | | | | | | | |
| 3. Is the percentage of bone loss: | | | | | | | | | | | | |
| • less than 30% = early | | | | | | | | | | | | |
| • 30 to 50% = moderate | | | | | | | | | | | | |
| • greater than 50% = advanced | | | | | | | | | | | | |
| 4. Is the bone loss pattern: | | | | | | | | | | | | |
| • horizontal | | | | | | | | | | | | |
| • vertical | | | | | | | | | | | | |
| 5. Is there evidence of: | | | | | | | | | | | | |
| • furcation involvement | | | | | | | | | | | | |
| • interproximal cratering | | | | | | | | | | | | |
| • interproximal hemisepta | | | | | | | | | | | | |
| • alveolar dehiscence | | | | | | | | | | | | |
| • a periodontal abscess | | | | | | | | | | | | |
| 6. Are there predisposing factors such as: | | | | | | | | | | | | |
| • calculus | | | | | | | | | | | | |
| • overhanging restorations | | | | | | | | | | | | |
| • defective crowns | | | | | | | | | | | | |
| • traumatic occlusion | | | | | | | | | | | | |
| • root resorption | | | | | | | | | | | | |
| • open contacts | | | | | | | | | | | | |
| • marginal ridge discrepancies | | | | | | | | | | | | |

7. What is the appropriate description of the disease progression?
☐ Case Type I—Gingivitis
☐ Case Type II—EP
☐ Case Type III—MP
☐ Case Type IV—AP
☐ Case Type V—RP

8. Is the periodontal disease:
☐ stable
☐ progressing

posterior regions and sharp and pointed in the anterior due to the size and proximity of adjacent teeth. In health, the crest should be parallel to an imaginary line drawn between adjacent cementoenamel junctions.

The lamina dura, an apical continuation of the alveolar crest, is the thin plate of cortical bone forming the wall of the tooth socket. This plate of bone is perforated by numerous microscopic foramina providing access for various types of blood vessels and nerves to the periodontal ligament. Radiographically, the lamina dura appears as a continuous radiopaque line surrounding the root of the tooth adjacent to the periodontal ligament (PDL) space. This space contains connective tissue fibers, blood vessels, nerves, and lymphatics. In health, the PDL space appears as a thin radiolucent line between the root and the lamina dura. This line completely surrounds the root and should remain uniform in width.

The supporting bone has a radiographic appearance that varies among individuals. Figure 5-8 illustrates the normal and subtle differences in appearance between anterior and posterior trabecular patterns. In general, the radiopaque trabeculae in maxillary anterior bone are thin and numerous making the radiolucent marrow spaces very small and this pattern extends in a vertical direction. Posterior patterns in the maxillary arch are very similar except that the marrow spaces are usually larger. In contrast to the maxilla, mandibular marrow spaces are large and few in number due to the thicker trabeculae. The mandibular anterior spaces appear in a horizontal pattern. The mandibular posterior pattern is much the same as the mandibular anterior with the exception of the apical areas of the molars where there is an apparent decrease or absence of trabeculae. The density of the interproximal supporting bone will increase or decrease depending on the root proximity of adjacent teeth. Likewise the form and position of multirooted teeth affect the bone between the roots or the interradicular bone. If there is a wide space between the roots, the interradicular bone will be very dense and provide strong support for the teeth (see Figure 5-9).

### Diseased Alveolar Bone

Clinically, assessment of bone loss is achieved by correlating attachment loss, tissue inflammation, and the radiographic evaluation of the periodontium. A margin of clinician error can occur in each of these procedures, but the radiograph is particularly difficult to assess. It contains visual images of the teeth, cortical and trabecular bone, and anatomical structures as well as restorative materials and/or disease processes. All of these entities make it challenging for the human eye to process the multitude of information present on the radiograph. Because of these extraneous forces, documentation shows that before changes in the bone can be seen radiographically, even to the most experienced clinicians, a 30 to 50 percent loss of mineralization must occur (Jeffcoat, 1992a; Jeffcoat & Reddy, 1991). It is, therefore,

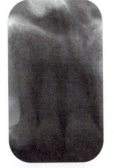
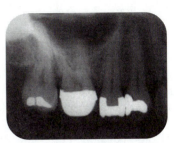

**A. Maxillary Anterior Bone**

**B. Maxillary Posterior Bone**

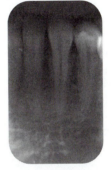

**C. Mandibular Anterior Bone**

**D. Mandibular Posterior Bone**

**Figure 5-8** Normal anterior and posterior trabecular patterns.

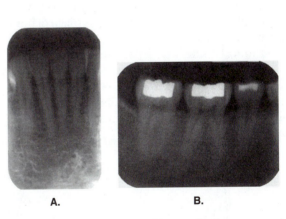

**A.**

**B.**

**Figure 5-9** Interproximal and interradicular root proximity. **A.** The density of interproximal bone increases or decreases as the proximity of the roots increase or decrease. **B.** Notice how the formation of the roots on the first molar increases the density of the interradicular bone.

essential that the proper type and quality of dental radiographs be used in conjunction with the clinical examination to diagnose and treat periodontal disease. Even though radiographs are valuable in assessing periodontal status, they are but one form of data and must not be used as the sole source for diagnosis. Remember, any given examination does not show disease activity. In fact, a client might have undergone successful periodontal therapy evidenced by elimination/reduction of pockets and inflammation and stabilization of attachment level. In this case, the radiographs reveal moderate bone loss but the condition is stable. Another client's radiographs might also reveal moderate bone loss, but inflammation and 4 mm of attachment loss are apparent. For purposes of this text, the general characteristics of diseased alveolar bone are divided into two subheadings: 1) quantification of bone loss and 2) patterns and distribution of bone loss.

**Quantification of Bone Loss.** The severity of bone loss is determined by the amount of bony destruction which has taken place. Quantification of this loss is determined in two ways: 1) by measuring the distance from the cementoenamel junction to the alveolar crest and/or 2) by determining the percentage of bone support that has been lost. Assessing the distance from the cementoenamel junction to the alveolar crest estimates the difference between the physiologic bone level and the height of remaining bone. In health, this measurement should approximate 1.5 to 2.0 mm; therefore, when a measurement greater than 2.0 mm is calculated, it is indicative of disease. Obviously, the greatest implication for this test is in determining if the client has gingivitis or periodontitis.

Once it is established that periodontitis exists, the clinician will want to quantify the amount of bone loss as a percentage. To calculate the percentage, first examine the overall root length from the cementoenamel junction to the root tip (12 mm). Next, identify the height of the alveolar crest and its distance from the cementoenamel junction (4 mm). Third, estimate the percentage of bone loss as a ratio of this distance as compared to the root length (4 mm/12 mm = 33%). Usually, practitioners visually estimate this percentage; however, rulers, the periodontal probe, or a template can be used to measure the length of the root in millimeters and to measure the millimeters of bone loss from the cementoenamel junc-

tion to the alveolar crest. This percentage is then equated to the severity of bone loss: early, moderate, or advanced. Generally, a loss of less than 30 percent indicates early disease. A loss of 30 to 50 percent represents moderate periodontitis. Advanced bone loss is indicated by a greater than 50 percent loss of supportive bone. The determination of bone loss by *percentage* of loss rather than the millimeter measurement is critical. For example, a 4-millimeter loss on a canine or molar where the root or roots are long, is much less serious than the same 4-millimeter loss on a mandibular incisor where the root is significantly shorter.

**Patterns and Distribution of Bone Loss.** Bony pockets, as measured clinically with a periodontal probe, may be either suprabony or infrabony (intrabony) as illustrated in Figure 5-10. The differences between these types of pockets is in the relationship of the soft tissue to the bone, the direction or pattern of bone loss, and the direction of the transseptal periodontal fibers. Suprabony pockets have their base *coronal* to the level of the alveolar bone so that the pattern of bone loss is in a horizontal direction, and the transseptal periodontal fibers are also connected horizontally between the base of the pocket and the alveolar bone. Suprabony pockets are characterized by **horizontal bone loss** as seen in Figure 5-11. Horizontal bone loss is the term used to describe the uniform loss of interproximal bone. As the bone loss progresses in an apical direction, the crest of the bone is still evident in a horizontal plane parallel with an imaginary line extending between the cementoenamel junctions of adjacent teeth, and perpendicular to the long axes of those teeth. An infrabony (intrabony) pocket, on the other hand, is evidenced by a **vertical (angular) bone** loss. Vertical loss occurs because the base of this type of pocket is apical to the crest of the alveolar bone. Figure 5-11 also demonstrates vertical loss where the bone is

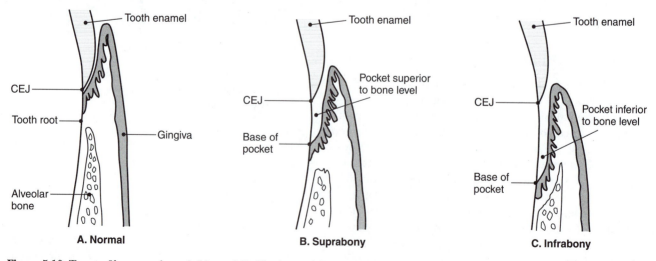

**Figure 5-10** Types of bony pockets. **A.** Normal. **B.** The base of the *suprabony* pocket is coronal to the level of the alveolar bone. Suprabony pockets are characterized by horizontal bone loss. **C.** The base of the *infrabony* (intrabony) pocket is apical to the crest of the alveolar bone. This type of pocket is evidenced by vertical or angular bone loss.

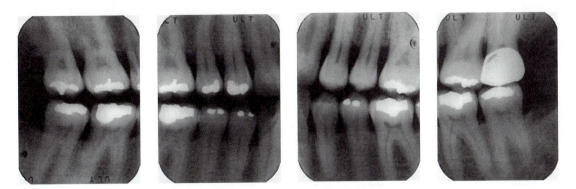

**Figure 5-11** Bone loss. Vertical bone loss is evident on the distals of #4, #12, #20, #22, #27, and #30 as well as the mesial of #12; horizontal bone loss is present in all other areas.

reduced on one side of the proximal crest between adjacent teeth at a greater degree than on the other. Vertical loss of bone appears as a V-shaped defect along the proximal side of the root. The transseptal fibers are, therefore, also connected obliquely rather than horizontally. No longer is the bone parallel to the two corresponding cementoenamel junctions, nor perpendicular to the long axes of those teeth. When looking for angular bone loss, the clinician must take care to evaluate the levels of adjacent cementoenamel junctions. If the client's occlusion places the teeth at uneven levels, the cementoenamel junctions will also be uneven. Therefore, the appearance may be one of angular or vertical bone loss when in fact, no loss has occurred (see Figure 5-12).

Alveolar bone loss may be further classified by distribution and is described as being either localized or generalized. Localized bone loss occurs in isolated areas of the mouth, generally bilateral, whereas generalized bone loss occurs in a fairly uniform pattern throughout. Horizontal bone loss can be localized or generalized. As disease progresses, it is commonly seen as generalized loss. Vertical or angular bone loss, however, is most often localized, even when disease is advanced. The most common location for an angular infrabony pocket is on the mesial surface of second and third molars. Other common sites relate to areas of traumatic occlusion.

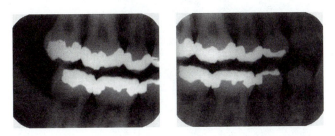

**Figure 5-12** Uneven cementoenamel junctions. Malocclusion demonstrates uneven bone level, which parallels uneven cementoenamel junctions. Observe the areas between #3 and #4 as well as between #29 and #30. The bone level is actually normal in these areas.

## CORRELATING RADIOGRAPHIC AND CLINICAL FINDINGS

There is a generally accepted sequence of radiographic changes associated with periodontitis. After practitioners determine the quantity of bone loss as early, moderate, or advanced; and recognize patterns and distribution of loss, the appropriate **category of disease progression** or **"Case Type"** is determined for insurance reporting (see Table 5-4). The categories or "case types" are based on the disease progression at the time of the examination and evaluation (Current Procedural Terminology for Periodontics and Insurance Reporting Manual, 1995). The following discussion will elaborate on these descriptions to help the dental hygienist correlate clinical and radiographic findings, and select the appropriate case type.

It is customary for clinicians to categorize periodontal diseases after radiographs are interpreted because the radiographs are usually the final piece of data collected in the periodontal assessment. Although clinical and radiographic information must be correlated to categorize disease, the radiographs usually serve to confirm the clinical data. When clinical and radiographic findings do not correlate, reexamination of attachment loss and other assessment data alone is in the best interest of the client. When exposure of radiographs is not indicated, clinical data must be used to estimate the category of disease. Previous radiographs should also be incorporated into the decision-making process.

Case Type I, or gingivitis, is an inflammatory gingival lesion involving only soft tissue; therefore, it cannot be seen radiographically. All other periodontal disease classifications have radiographic implications. In making decisions about the descriptions of disease progression, consider that if even one area of the mouth exhibits conditions falling in a higher category, the client is classified as having the most advanced category of disease. For instance, if the maxillary molars exhibit 30 percent bone loss and other regions of the mouth exhibit 20 percent or less, the condition is classified as moderate periodontitis.

Bony changes in early periodontitis (Case Type II) are the incipient stages of disease and are limited to only

**Table 5-4  Descriptions of Disease Progression**

| Category | Description |
| --- | --- |
| Case Type I—Gingival Disease | Inflammation of the gingiva characterized clinically by changes in color, gingival form, position, surface appearance, and presence of bleeding and/or exudate. |
| Case Type II—Early Periodontitis | Progression of the gingival inflammation into the deeper periodontal structures and alveolar bone crest, with slight bone loss. There is usually a slight loss of connective tissue attachment and alveolar bone. |
| Case Type III—Moderate Periodontitis | A more advanced stage of the above condition, with increased destruction of the periodontal structures and noticeable loss of bone support, possibly accompanied by an increase in tooth mobility. There may be furcation involvement in multirooted teeth. |
| Case Type IV—Advanced Periodontitis | Further progression of periodontitis with major loss of alveolar bone support usually accompanied by increased tooth mobility. Furcation involvement in multirooted teeth is likely. |
| Case Type V—Refractory Periodontitis | Includes those patients with multiple disease sites that continue to demonstrate attachment loss after appropriate therapy. These sites presumably continue to be infected by periodontal pathogens no matter how thorough or frequent the treatment provided. |

the crestal bone (see Figure 5-13). Slight bone loss may be exhibited with a usual probing depth of 3 to 4 mm, an average of 3 mm of clinical attachment loss, and a slight loss of both connective tissue attachment and bone. In the early stages of radiographically evident disease, the lamina dura becomes unclear and it no longer appears continuous at the interproximal aspect of the alveolar crest. Because the inflammation has progressed to the crestal bone, the result is widened vessel channels and an associated reduction in calcified tissue in the area. The crest itself also begins to break down. The normally flat interdental crest in the posterior areas loses its cortical

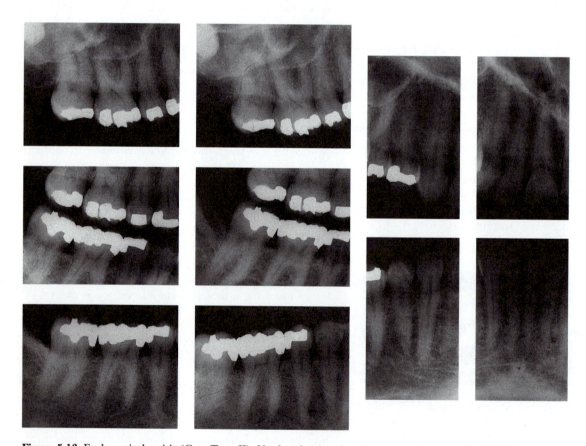

**Figure 5-13**  Early periodontitis (Case Type II). Unclear lamina dura is seen on the mesial of #30. Triangulation is visible on the distals of #5 and #29. Generalized loss of bone height is less than 30 percent.

density and appears fuzzy. Figure 5-13 also demonstrates wedge-shaped radiolucent areas formed between the crestal proximal bone and the tooth surface. These radiolucent areas are called **triangulation** because of the triangular appearance, which appears as an inverted triangle with the apex pointing apically. Triangulation is a result of bone resorption of the interdental septum creating a widened periodontal ligament space. In the anterior region the usual sharp crest undergoes erosion and becomes rounded instead of pointed, along with the occurrence of corresponding triangulation. This type of breakdown at the alveolar crest is generally seen in only isolated areas of the mouth. Care must be taken when evaluating triangulation because the periodontal ligament (PDL) space is slightly widened in the crestal region in health.

The destructive process continues as the inflammatory cells and fluids proliferate deeper into the connective tissue resulting in increased bone resorption. Although the alveolar bone begins to degenerate during this stage of disease, the topography of the bone remains fairly normal. As the disease progresses beyond the triangulation stage, the PDL space continues to widen apically beyond the crest and may involve the entire root. As the erosion of the alveolar crest continues, a bony pocket develops. The depth of the pocket is no longer confined to the gingival tissue and destruction of the supporting periodontal structures occurs. As previously stated, the loss of bone in early periodontitis is less than 30 percent of the root length and there is generally no tooth mobility evident.

Moderate periodontitis (Case Type III) is a more advanced state of disease, with increased destruction of the alveolar bone (see Figure 5-14). Usual probing depth is between 5 and 7 mm with an average of 4 mm clinical attachment loss. Radiographically, moderate periodontitis (MP) is evidenced by a loss of 30 to 50 percent of the supporting bone. When the alveolar loss has progressed to this extent the topography or shape of the bone is no longer satisfactory. Horizontal and/or vertical bone loss can be seen radiographically. Because of the amount of loss of interradicular bone, furcation involvement in the posterior areas occurs and tooth mobility of individual teeth or groups of teeth can exist. Early furcation involvement is sometimes difficult to observe radiographically. As previously stated, actual clinical bone loss is usually greater than what is radiographically visible to the clinician. This is especially true in the maxillary molar region where the opaque palatal root may mask bone loss in the trifurcation. The angulation at which the radiograph is taken may also interfere with diagnosis. It is, therefore, critical that a true paralleling technique be employed if periapical radiographs are selected for periodontal assessment instead of bitewings. To assist in the detection of radiographic furcations the clinician should consider three factors: 1) look for any decreased density in the furcation area, especially when there appears to be an increase of bone density across the root area, 2) be alert

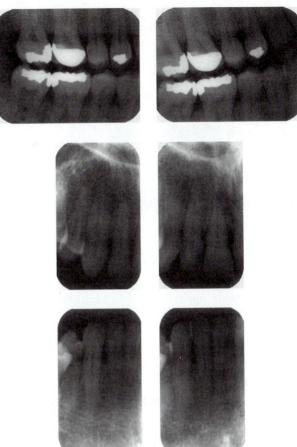

**Figure 5-14** Moderate periodontitis (Case Type III). Horizontal bone loss is generalized except on the mesials of #3 and #30 that illustrate vertical bone loss. Furcation involvement is seen on #31. An interproximal crater is seen between #28 and #29. Generalized loss of bone height approximates 30 percent but is less than 50 percent.

to the fact that when there is substantial bone loss on a single root of a multirooted tooth, there is likely to be furcation involvement (see Figure 5-15), and 3) most importantly, investigate clinically any radiographic change in the furcation area. The previous factor number (2) referred to as the single root rule, is important because if therapy is limited to the diseased root only, as the healing of that root progresses, the furcation area might become closed or sealed. If this situation occurs, drainage in the area would become impossible and the development of a periodontal abscess would be a certainty.

In addition to horizontal and vertical bone loss, there are other alveolar defects that may be evident. Because of the three-dimensional overlapping of structures it is not always possible to see all of these lesions radiographically. In some cases, only slight increases in radiolucency may be apparent. Thus, it becomes essential to reiterate the importance of careful probing. Troughlike depressions called interproximal craters can occur (see Figure 5-14). These defects are bordered on two sides by the

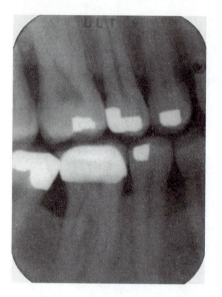

**Figure 5-15** Single root rule. Significant bone loss is seen on the distal root of #30. (Courtesy of Richard E. Ferguson, DDS, MS, Boise, ID)

roots of adjacent teeth and on two sides by facial and lingual cortical plates. Images of the proximal side walls of bone will be evidenced on the radiograph, but the extent of depression between the facial and lingual plates is less apparent. The individual walls may be seen in some cases when one wall (the one more apically projected) appears more dense and the other is reduced in density. If the two walls are perfectly superimposed, the crater may simply appear as a linear area of decreased density between the two teeth (Goaz & White, 1994). Interproximal craters might exist and not be visible radiographically. Cratering is more prevalent in posterior segments of the mouth. An interproximal hemisepta exists when one interproximal wall is missing as well as one or both of the facial or lingual walls (see Figure 5-16). It appears as a vertical V-shaped radiolucent defect. When both facial and lingual plates are gone, it is radiographically impossible to

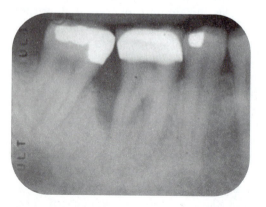

**Figure 5-16** Interproximal hemisepta. This osseous defect is seen on the distal of #30. (Courtesy of Richard E. Ferguson, DDS, MS, Boise, ID)

tell the difference between the interproximal hemisepta and vertical or angular bone loss.

Advanced periodontitis (Case Type IV) is a further progression of the disease. Usual probing depths of 8 mm or greater are present, with an average of 5 mm or more clinical attachment loss. Radiographically there is a greater than 50 percent loss of supporting bone around the root (see Figure 5-17). Interradicular bone loss or furcation involvement will occur to a much greater extent than the barely discernible radiolucency evidenced in moderate periodontitis. In addition there will be definite mobility of remaining teeth, and usually some missing teeth. In cases where the entire facial or lingual cortical plate has been almost completely destroyed, there may appear to be a horizontal line of demarcation running across the roots. Care must be taken to not confuse this line with one caused by superimposition of heavy lips, or the nose in the maxillary anterior region. These two structures may appear on the radiograph when high kVp technique is used.

There are two other conditions that are associated with advanced disease: an alveolar dehiscence and a periodontal abscess. An alveolar dehiscence is a condition where the marginal bone dips apically to expose a length of root surface. Dehiscences appear most often on labial surfaces of anterior teeth and are frequently bilateral. Because these defects occur on the facial surface and less frequently on the lingual surface, they are difficult to observe radiographically because of superimposition over the root (Goaz & White, 1994). A periodontal abscess occurs deep in a soft tissue pocket. However, it is a rapidly progressive destructive lesion which, if left untreated, can cause extensive bone destruction (see Figure 5-18). This type of abscess originates in one of two ways: 1) complication from infection in an existing periodontal pocket or 2) infection caused by trauma from foreign objects such as popcorn husks being forced into the sulcus. The coronal portion of the pocket often becomes occluded so the purulent matter cannot escape. When this situation occurs a fistula develops and, many times, a drainage passage is formed. This abnormal passage progresses through the bone to the surface of the gingiva or mucosa (Wilkins, 1994).

Refractory periodontitis (RP), or Case Type V, can be determined by assessing attachment loss at periodontal maintenance visits and comparing current readings to baseline readings. RP is characterized by continued attachment loss after appropriate therapy. It is presumed that probing attachment level measurements correlate with interproximal bone height; therefore, the clinician should see subsequent loss of proximal bone depth when viewing transmission radiographs. Generally, loss of attachment proceeds at a rate of 0.25 mm per year with Adult Periodontitis and 1 to 2 mm per year with other more progressive forms (Scarff, Walsh, & Darby, 1995).

Juvenile periodontitis, a form of early-onset periodontitis, affects the permanent dentition in otherwise healthy adolescents. The localized form generally affects

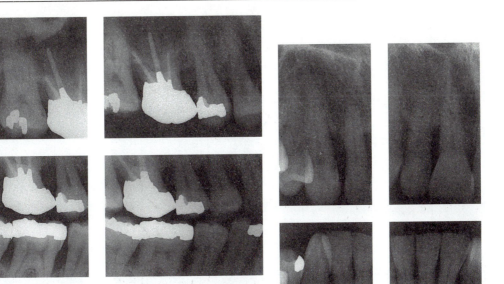

**Figure 5-17** Advanced periodontitis (Case Type IV). Furcation involvement is seen on #3, #30, and #31. Examples of vertical bone loss are seen on the distals of #29 and #4. Loss of bone height is greater than 50 percent on the distals of #7 and #8 and on the mesials of #6 and #7.

the first molars and incisors, and advances very rapidly. The generalized form of juvenile periodontitis involves most of the dentition. This form is also a very rapidly advancing and destructive disease. It is important to review the patient history as well as the transmission radiographs to assess these uncommon types of periodontal diseases. The rate of progression is of great importance in the evaluation both clinically and radiographically

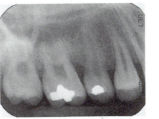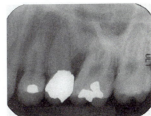

**Figure 5-19** Juvenile periodontitis.

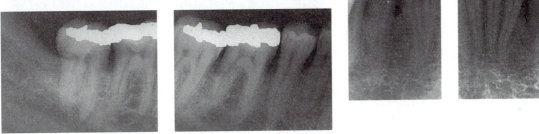

**Figure 5-18** A periodontal abscess appears on the mesial root of #30. Although the density on the mesial of #29 is similar, it does not involve the periodontal ligament. (Courtesy of Richard E. Ferguson, DDS, MS, Boise, ID)

(see Figure 5-19). Juvenile periodontitis is not recognized in insurance reporting; therefore, the practitioner must assess the severity of bone loss and select a case type. Generally, Case Type III (moderate) or Case Type IV (advanced) periodontitis will be appropriate.

In summary, the amount of bone loss is usually categorized by evaluating the height of the alveolar crest in relation to the length of the root. This comparison provides the clinician with a percentage of bone loss which, in turn, can be transferred to severity (early, moderate, or advanced) of bone loss. At this point, radiographic and clinical findings can be correlated to identify the case type or description of disease. Table 5-5 represents a summary of the radiographic implications for disease progression. It should be remembered that the descrip-

**Table 5-5 Summary of Radiographic Implications for Disease Progression**

| Category | Description | % of Bone Loss | Measurement from CEJ to Alveolar Crest* | Characteristics of Bone** |
|---|---|---|---|---|
| Case Type I—Gingival Disease | Inflammation of the gingiva characterized clinically by changes in color, gingival form, position, surface appearance, and presence of bleeding and/or exudate. | NA | 1.5 to 2.0 mm | NA |
| Case Type II—Early Periodontitis | Progression of the gingival inflammation into the deeper periodontal structures and alveolar bone crest, with slight bone loss. There is usually a slight loss of connective tissue attachment and alveolar bone. | less than 30% | >2.0 mm (range 3 to 4 mm) | • unclear lamina dura<br>• triangulation<br>• horizontal bone loss |
| Case Type III—Moderate Periodontitis | A more advanced stage of the above condition, with increased destruction of the periodontal structures and noticeable loss of bone support, possibly accompanied by an increase in tooth mobility. There may be furcation involvement in multirooted teeth. | between 30% and 50% | >2.0 mm (range 5 to 7 mm) | • bony pockets<br>• horizontal and/or vertical bone loss<br>• furcation involvement<br>• interproximal craters<br>• interproximal hemisepta |
| Case Type IV—Advanced Periodontitis | Further progression of periodontitis with major loss of alveolar bone support usually accompanied by increased tooth mobility. Furcation involvement in multirooted teeth is likely. | greater than 50% | >2.0 mm (range 8 mm or more) | • characteristics of MP<br>• alveolar dehiscenses<br>• periodontal abscesses |
| Case Type V—Refractory Periodontitis | Includes those patients with multiple disease sites that continue to demonstrate attachment loss after appropriate therapy. These sites presumably continue to be infected by periodontal pathogens no matter how thorough or frequent the treatment provided. | usually >30% | >2.0 mm | • very rapid bone loss<br>• multiple sites |

*Figures are approximates based on average root lengths. Note that canine measurements would be greater due to increased root length.

**Not all characteristics need to be present to characterize a disease state.

tions of disease progression are only for insurance purposes and the actual diagnostic periodontal disease classification is based on additional factors such as age of the client, systemic health, rate of attachment loss and bone loss, location of bone loss, amount of gingival inflammation, etc. (Current Procedural Terminology for Periodontics and Insurance Reporting Manual, 1995).

## PREDISPOSING FACTORS

There are a number of factors that contribute to the advancement of periodontal disease. By themselves these factors do not directly cause disease, but instead they indirectly contribute to disease. These factors need to be considered in planning therapy for the individual. Contributing factors are addressed in some manner by removal, restoration, and/or monitoring. The most obvious of the predisposing factors are calculus and overhanging restorations (see Figures 5-20 and 5-21 respectively). Both of these local irritants are important because of their plaque-retentive nature. Calculus and overhangs both promote bacterial plaque formation and contribute to its retention in inflamed periodontal pockets. The clinician should not depend on radiographs alone for determining the extent of calculus present. The density of the deposit is the determining factor as to whether the calculus will be visible on the radiograph. As the deposit increases in density, it slows and absorbs the beam of radiation before it reaches the film. This is the same principle that is found when viewing other oral structures. More dense materials and structures such as amalgam and enamel slow and absorb the x-ray beam. Thus, no radiation reaches the film to expose it so it remains clear or white upon processing. Because of this, a patient could have generalized moderate calculus that might not be visible on the radiograph. Likewise, small dense spicules of calculus might be easily visible. Defective crowns that fail to have adequate contour might also cause trauma to the gingival tissue resulting in a state of disease.

"Traumatic occlusion does not cause periodontitis, affect the epithelial attachment, or lead to pocket formation. It does, however, cause traumatic lesions, which develop in response to occlusal pressures that are greater than the physiologic tolerances of the tooth's supporting tissues. These lesions occur as the result of malfunction" (Goaz & White, 1994, p. 336). Trauma from occlusion may produce radiographic evidence suggesting increased tooth mobility. As evidenced in Figure 5-22, these changes may include widening of the PDL space, decreased definition of the lamina dura (or increased width and density in the case of occlusal stress), changes in the morphology of the alveolar crest, and/or altered trabeculation or changes in density of the surrounding bone. Marginal ridge discrepancies should alert the clinician to the possibility of occlusal trauma. The advanced bony defect associated with occlusal trauma appears as areas of vertical or "cupped out" destruction (Fleszar, 1992). Root resorption, hypercementosis, and root fractures can also be radiographic evidence of traumatic occlusion.

Orthodontic treatment is another factor that may contribute indirectly to disease. If tooth movement has occurred too quickly or client response to movement has been inadequate, root resorption can occur (see Figure 5-23). This in itself is not a problem unless the client's periodontal condition progresses to moderate or advanced disease status. Because the root length is shortened from the resorption, the effects of bone loss become clinically significant earlier than on a root of normal length. Open contacts may contribute to periodontal disease because of the potential for food entrapment (see Figure 5-24). When food is trapped between teeth an inflammatory response takes place and subsequent progression of disease may occur which could result in bone loss. A similar process occurs when marginal ridge discrepancies exist. Clinical evidence of either of these conditions should alert the clinician to carefully observe and probe the periodontal tissues, and evaluate the radiographs for signs of bone loss.

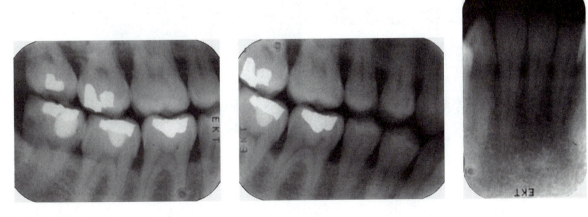

**Figure 5-20** Generalized calculus.

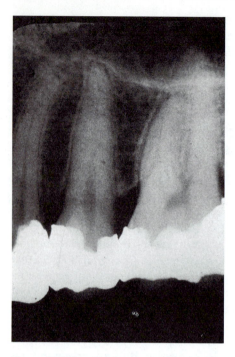

**Figure 5-21** Inadequate restorative contour. The overhanging margins on the mesial and distal of #13, and mesial of #14 relate to the bone loss in the adjacent interproximal areas.

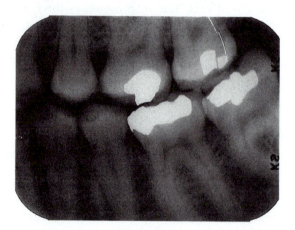

**Figure 5-22** Occlusal trauma. Marginal ridge discrepancies may contribute to changes in the surrounding periodontium. In this example, the lamina dura is thickened around the root of #19 and sclerotic bone formation is present on the mesial of #20.

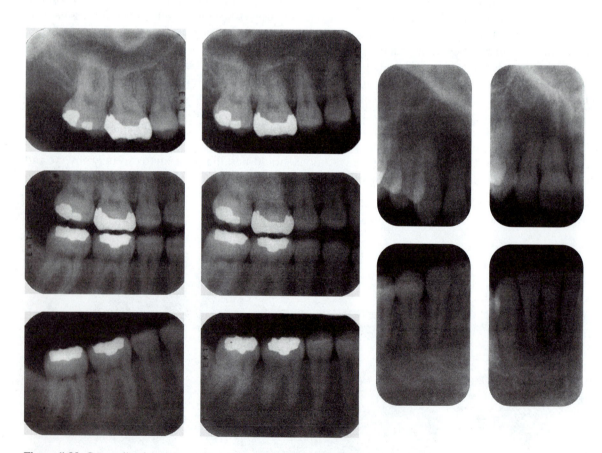

**Figure 5-23** Generalized root resorption from orthodontic movement.

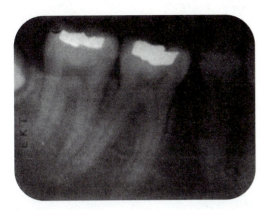

**Figure 5-24** Open contact. Triangulation is present on the mesial of #30.

## PROTOCOL FOR EXPOSURE

Sound professional judgment is required in exposing dental radiographs. An essential component of making discreet judgments is the collection of data including a complete client history. Knowledge of past medical and dental exposure, updated at each periodontal maintenance appointment, is essential in order to determine the risk versus benefit factor. In the decision-making process, the goal to keep in mind is to use the least amount of radiation necessary to yield the best diagnostic results. The dental hygienist has the responsibility of educating the client about the rationale for exposure and the appropriate selection of numbers and types of radiographs. The rationale or need for x-ray films sometimes creates "fear" for the client. Information concerning the role radiographs play in diagnosis, therapy, and monitoring of periodontal disease helps to allay this apprehension. Many clients are unaware of the fact that without radiographs, a clinician's ability to care for the client is compromised. Discussing limitations of performing only a clinical examination would be beneficial. Also fear is sometimes reduced if it is communicated that the most current safety standards are followed. The following dialogue is an example of how "need" can be explained to a client.

*Clinician:* Jean, I understand that you are not interested in receiving x-ray films today?

*Client:* Yes, I don't think it is necessary.

*Clinician:* Could I explain, in a little more detail, why I recommended radiographs to you? Perhaps I did not thoroughly discuss their benefits.

*Client:* Okay, go ahead.

*Clinician:* While I was probing, I recorded some pocket depths of 4 mm. As we previously discussed, even though these measurements are not extremely deep,

they indicate that periodontitis, or bone loss, could be present. I cannot see the bone support for your teeth because gum tissue is covering the root. With the x-ray films, I would be able to see if bone loss is present.

*Client:* So it would help you see what is happening below the gums?

*Clinician:* Yes. If bone loss is discovered, then I will recommend nonsurgical periodontal care for you, which involves various types of therapy. Another advantage of the radiographs is finding tooth decay. Touching the tops of your teeth with this instrument is one way of checking for decay on the chewing surfaces. x-ray films, however, allow us to see if decay has occurred between your teeth where they touch. Without x-ray films, decay in this area can not be detected. Also, when I take the radiographs, I will use the least number of films possible and follow all recommended safety precautions for your protection.

*Client:* Okay, I guess you better take the films. I didn't know they would be so helpful in planning my care.

Education about radiographs does not stop with the need for exposure. Additionally, most clients will be interested in viewing the radiographs with the clinician. During this viewing, the dental hygienist can share with the client what conditions are present on the radiograph. The addition of this visual aid helps the individual understand bone loss and its significance to long-term health or disease. With the aid of the clinician, it is fairly easy for most clients to recognize an area of bone that is not diseased versus an area where bone loss has occurred. If both normal and abnormal bone contour is not apparent on the client's own radiographs, another survey can be incorporated into the education.

It is imperative that dental hygiene professionals, as well as other team members who expose x-ray films, be familiar with the guidelines for prescribing dental radiographs as outlined by the *Dental Patient Selection Criteria Panel.* (U.S. Department of Health and Human Services, 1987). Table 5-6 presents the essentials of this report. The chart is presented in a three-way matrix format: 1) Patient Category in a horizontal dimension by age: child, adolescent, or adult. 2) Patient Category in a vertical dimension by patient type: new or recall, and 3) Risk factors identified beneath the new or recall category: caries; history of, or active periodontal disease; growth and development. These guidelines are meant to be flexible because of the uniqueness of each person receiving oral health care.

### Other Considerations

There are other conditions, such as previous radiation exposure, biological conditions, and psychological concerns that must be considered when prescribing radiographs. Determining the history of previous radiation

**Table 5-6  Guidelines for Prescribing Dental Radiographs**

| Patient Category | Child | |
| --- | --- | --- |
| | Primary dentition (*prior to eruption of first permanent tooth*) | Transitional dentition (*following eruption of first permanent tooth*) |
| ***New Patient\**** | | |
| All New Patients to Assess Dental Diseases and Growth and Development | Posterior bitewing examination if proximal surfaces of primary teeth cannot be visualized or probed | Individualized radiographic examination consisting of periapical/occlusal views and posterior bitewings or panoramic examination and posterior bitewings |
| ***Recall Patient\**** | | |
| Clinical Caries or High-Risk Factors for Caries\*\* | Posterior bitewing examination at 6-month intervals or until no carious lesions are evident | |
| No Clinical Caries and No High-Risk Factors for Caries\*\* | Posterior bitewing examination at 12- to 24-month intervals if proximal surfaces of primary teeth cannot be visualized or probed | Posterior bitewing examination at 12- to 24-month intervals |
| Periodontal Disease or a History of Periodontal Treatment | Individualized radiographic examination consisting of selected periapical and/or bitewing radiographs for areas where periodontal disease (other than nonspecific gingivitis) can be demonstrated clinically | |
| Growth and Development Assessment | Usually not indicated | Individualized radiographic examination consisting of a periapical/occlusal or panoramic examination |

The recommendations in this chart are subject to clinical judgment and may not apply to every patient. *They are to be used by dentists only after reviewing the patient's health history and completing a clinical examination. The recommendations do not need to be altered because of pregnancy.*

\* Clinical situations for which radiographs may be indicated include:

A.  Positive Historical Findings
   1. Previous periodontal or endodontic therapy
   2. History of pain or trauma
   3. Familial history of dental anomalies
   4. Postoperative evaluation of healing
   5. Presence of implants

B.  Positive Clinical Signs/Symptoms
   1. Clinical evidence of periodontal disease
   2. Large or deep restorations
   3. Deep carious lesions

   4. Malposed or clinically impacted teeth
   5. Swelling
   6. Evidence of facial trauma
   7. Mobility of teeth
   8. Fistula or sinus tract infection
   9. Clinically suspected sinus pathology
   10. Growth abnormalities
   11. Oral involvement in known or suspected systemic disease
   12. Positive neurologic findings in the head and neck
   13. Evidence of foreign objects
   14. Pain and/or dysfunction of the temporomandibular joint

exposure is mandatory and should include both medical and dental experiences. Dental radiographs should be requested from previous offices if the client is new to the practice. Prior to exposing new films, the previous radiographs should be evaluated for viewing quality and to determine whether they are current enough to be used. Other historical information also needs to be obtained. This data includes relevant biological conditions, such as radiation therapy, traumatic incidence, and evaluation of chronic disease. Any recommendation from personal physicians must be considered. Pregnancy always gives rise to the question of whether or not radiographs should be taken. According to the guidelines in Table 5-6, the state of pregnancy should not alter the normal recom-

mendation. The pregnant patient is exposed to higher doses of naturally occurring background radiation during the nine months of pregnancy than from one full mouth set of radiographs. All patients including the pregnant patient, should be provided the use of lead aprons and thyroid collars when being exposed to radiation in order to reduce scatter radiation to the gonadal region and other radiosensitive tissues. Psychological concerns such as fear and stress are also considerations. The previous client and clinician dialogue addressed an element of client fear. In cases of extreme fear or stress, further discussion will be necessary.

According to the Dental Radiographic Patient Selection Criteria Panel (U.S. Department of Health and

| Adolescent | Adult | |
|---|---|---|
| Permanent dentition *(prior to eruption of third molars)* | Dentulous | Edentulous |

| | | |
|---|---|---|
| Individualized radiographic examination consisting of posterior bitewings and selected periapicals. A full mouth intraoral radiographic examination is appropriate when the patient presents with clinical evidence of generalized dental disease or a history of extensive dental treatment. | | Full mouth intraoral radiographic examination *or* panoramic examination |
| Posterior bitewing examination at 6- to 12-month intervals *or* until no carious lesions are evident | Posterior bitewing examination at 12- to 18-month intervals | Not applicable |
| Posterior bitewing examination at 18- to 36-month intervals | Posterior bitewing examination at 24- to 36-month intervals | Not applicable |
| Individualized radiographic examination consisting of selected periapical and/or bitewing radiographs for areas where periodontal disease (other than nonspecific gingivitis) can be demonstrated clinically | | Not applicable |
| Periapical *or* panoramic examination to assess developing third molars | Usually not indicated | Usually not indicated |

15. Facial asymmetry
16. Abutment teeth fixed or removable partial prosthesis
17. Unexplained bleeding
18. Unexplained sensitivity of teeth
19. Unusual eruption, spacing, or migration of teeth
20. Unusual tooth morphology, calcification, or color
21. Missing teeth with unknown reason

** Patients at high risk for caries may demonstrate any of the following:
1. High level of caries experience
2. History of recurrent caries
3. Existing restoration of poor quality
4. Poor oral hygiene
5. Inadequate fluoride exposure
6. Prolonged nursing (bottle or breast)
7. Diet with high sucrose frequency
8. Poor family dental health
9. Developmental enamel defects
10. Developmental disability
11. Xerostomia
12. Genetic abnormality of teeth
13. Many multisurface restorations
14. Chemo/radiation therapy

Human Services, 1987), there is no preferred frequency or number of exposures suggested. Keeping in mind the goal of minimizing exposure, it is recommended here that a complete full mouth set of periapical films plus appropriate bitewings be taken for initial evaluation of periodontal conditions. Thereafter, a series of four to six posterior vertical bitewings and one to two anterior bitewings should be utilized between exposures of complete mouth surveys. The Panel recommends bitewings be exposed at intervals of twelve to eighteen months for high-risk individuals. In this case, "high-risk" refers to detecting caries; however, it is noted that care should be taken to examine for evidence of periodontal or occult disease. Selected periapical radiographs may be taken as a supplement when indicated. It has been suggested that in advancing periodontal disease, full mouth series should be taken approximately every two years (Wilson, 1992).

Duplication of films or use of double film packets is strongly recommended to satisfy the needs of insurance companies or examining boards. Additional exposure to radiation for such administrative purposes is unsatisfactory and discouraged. Duplicated films will also be needed to send to other dental or specialty offices. The Panel also discourages the use of radiographs for detection of infrequent lesions presenting no clinical signs or symptoms (occult lesions). Occult lesions could include impacted teeth, apical pathology, retained roots, foreign material, or intrabony cysts. Their review of the literature revealed that when radiographs were used as a screening device, no more hidden or unsuspected lesions were discovered than if radiographs were not used. On the other hand, radiographs *are* recommended for patients with a history of radiation therapy to the head and neck region.

## Implants

Presurgical radiographic examination of the implant site is required to assess height, width, and quality of available bone. Generally, a combination of intraoral films, a panoramic survey, and a lateral cephalometric view are recommended. Assessment of the site also must include its proximity to other teeth and structures such as the sinuses, mandibular canal, and foramina. Periapical films have limited diagnostic usefulness. If periapicals are used to evaluate single implant sites, a precise paralleling technique and a radiopaque stent are necessary. This technique can provide an accurate assessment of bone height in the mandibular posterior area. Panoramic films provide a general overview allowing the clinician to get an overall sense of all anatomic structures in relation to the implant site. Again a limitation of the panoramic survey is that the images within this type of radiograph can be magnified and the true relationship of structures slightly distorted. If sites in the anterior regions are being considered, lateral cephalometric films are suggested to assess height and width of the anterior areas of bone, anterior palate, and maxillary sinuses (Iacono & Livers, 1992).

Postsurgical evaluation involves both dental and radiographic evaluation. Generally, periapical films are used at three-year intervals to assess mesial and distal marginal bone as measured using predetermined fixture threads as a reference point. This method allows the clinician to compare the bone level in current radiographs to previous films. A successful osseous integration will be represented by distinct bone margins and apical migration of the alveolar bone (Gratt & Shetty, 1994). Figure 5-25

represents a successful and nonsuccessful endosteal implant. Research findings reveal the mean crestal bone height of preimplant bone structures adjacent to initially submerged implants decreased by 0.9 to 1.6 mm during the one-year healing phase and 0.05 to 0.13 mm thereafter during the maintenance phase (Hämmerle & Lang, 1994). Panoramic radiographs are also useful in the maintenance phase of evaluation. They may be used to check the adaptation of the abutment to the fixture, assess the system for fracture, and to evaluate the bone for absence of disease (Gratt & Shetty, 1994).

There are six general criteria for implant success supported by the American Academy of Periodontology (American Academy of Periodontology, 1989b). Criteria number two states that there should be no significant or progressive loss of supporting bone. Specific criteria addressing crestal bone loss are also established for both root forms, and blade implants. With root forms, crestal bone loss should be measured by periapical radiographs using the paralleling technique. The accepted standard for bone loss is 0.2 mm/year after the first year. Also, absence of peri-implant radiolucency is a criteria for success. With blade implants, crestal bone loss is evaluated in the same manner and after the first year bone loss should not exceed 1 mm during the next five years. Again, absence of peri-implant radiolucency is a requirement for success. In conclusion, periapical x-ray films are used with the paralleling technique to evaluate the success of implant modalities. Panoramic films are also employed for posttreatment assessment. Chapter 14 covers further information about implants.

## ADDITIONAL IMAGES

There are a variety of radiographic techniques available in dentistry today. Not all have proven to be effective in their diagnostic value, especially in the diagnosis of periodontal disease. Some are still in their infancy as tools in dentistry. Others have value in the assessment of some types of oral diseases, but not in others. A brief description of some of these techniques and their indications for use is presented to enhance the reader's understanding, although it is not intended to be a comprehensive review.

### Computer-Assisted Radiography

The advances in computer technology over the last decade have contributed to the use of a variety of new techniques in dentistry. One of those new techniques is that of **digital radiography** (see Figure 5-26). This "film-less" method of recording images uses charged sensors about the size of an x-ray film. These sensors are solid-state electronic devices which store and transfer energy. The sensor is placed in the patient's mouth and a cord attaches it to a computer. A low voltage x-ray beam is then

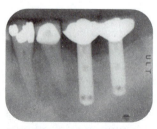
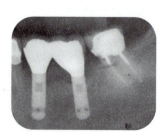

**A. Healthy Implants; 4 Years in Place**    **B. Early Failing Implants**

**Figure 5-25** Endosteal implants. (Courtesy of Richard E. Ferguson, DDS, MS, Boise, ID)

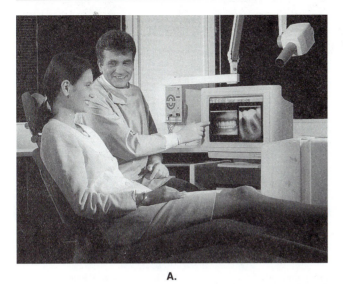

**A.**

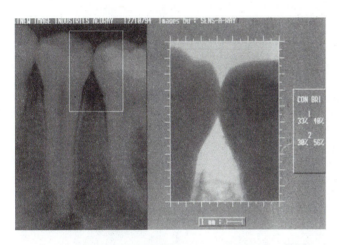

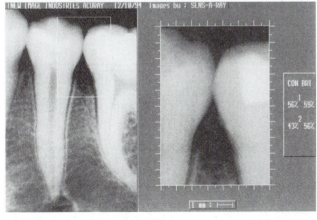

**B.**

**Figure 5-26** Digital radiography. **A.** An example of a typical imaging station. (Courtesy of Trophy Radiology, Inc., Marietta, GA) **B.** The digitized radiographs demonstrate the ability to adjust density and magnify any part of the image that is of interest. (Courtesy of Dr. Alan Farman, University of Kentucky, Louisville, KY)

produced and the sensor produces and stores the image. Also, traditional radiographs can be scanned using light, laser energy, or a video camera and stored on a computer disc. Storage of this type of radiographic image on discs has the advantages of reducing the number of misplaced films, improving speed and efficiency of reproduction of films, and makes filing, retrieval, and transmittal of radiographs all very easy. Another advantage of digital imaging is that because it is stored digitally, it can be manipulated electronically to improve contrast, remove information irrelevant to the image, change density, and magnify specific objects or areas of the radiograph. Furkart, Dove, McDavid, Nummikoski, and Matteson (1992) found when studying simulated periodontal lesions that the direct digital radiography system offered comparable results with the conventional dental x-ray film. Currently, the widespread use of digital imaging has been impeded by such factors as cost, standardization of the video display, and learning to interpret the computer image.

**Digital subtraction radiography** is used for longitudinal assessment of slight changes in periodontal structures. Digital subtraction radiography makes it possible to quantify and objectively assess an area. Data from two films taken at initial and recall appointments are stored digitally. These two radiographs must be taken from exactly the same vertical and horizontal angles and have very similar density and contrast. The stored information on the films can then be manipulated to subtract all unchanging structures, such as teeth, that the two films have in common. The remainder is an image of the difference. Increased radiolucency indicates progressive bone loss, while increased density indicates bone deposition (Jeffcoat, 1992b). The process involves taking a picture of the two radiographs to be compared using a black and white video camera. A computer then superimposes a grid over the picture and converts the various levels of gray in each of the grid boxes to a numerical value. This value varies from zero, which is totally black, to 255, which is totally clear or white. This computer-assisted image analysis methodology is technically known as computer-aided densitometric image analysis, generally abbreviated as CADIA. Once the information is in the computer and each grid has been assigned a numerical value, the computer then subtracts the gray value in each grid on the first radiograph from the same grid on the second radiograph. Wherever no change occurs, the value becomes zero. The numerical value of areas where change has occurred is displayed by the computer as white for bone gain, and dark for bone loss (see Figure 5-27). This is a highly sophisticated method of assessing change in the alveolar bone and is extremely difficult to achieve. It requires a method of exact repeatable film alignment and film density, and a precise method of measuring changes in that density. To date, digital subtraction radiography has not been practical or employed

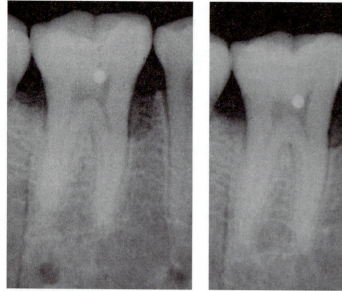

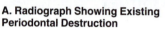

**A. Radiograph Showing Existing Periodontal Destruction**

**B. Subsequent Radiograph of Same Region**

**C. Subtraction Image Showing Additional Loss of Crestal Bone as Dark Patches**

**Figure 5-27** Digital subtraction. (Courtesy of Dr. Richard Webber, Bowman-Gray Medical School, Salem, NC)

in private clinical practice because of the difficulty in achieving these two dependent variables.

## Computed Tomography, Magnetic Resonance Imaging, and Nuclear Medicine Bone Scanning

Computed tomography, also known as CT scanning; magnetic resonance imaging (MRI); and nuclear medicine bone scanning are all established procedures used in medicine and have only recently begun to be selectively utilized in dentistry. CT scanning and MRI have little relativity to periodontal disease diagnosis as discussed within the context of this chapter. To date the most useful CT application to dentistry has been in relation to identifying lesions in the maxillofacial region and determining available space above the mandibular canal for implants. Figure 5-28 is an example of a tomography system used in dentistry along with a radiograph of the temporomandibular joint region.

At present MRI is not well suited to answering questions relevant to alveolar bone support, however, it can provide information in relation to temporomandibular joint problems. Nuclear medicine bone scans show more promise in the assessment of periodontitis. Bone scans have been successfully used and tested in the evaluation of bone loss due to the periodontal disease process. Studies are preliminary, but results indicate a diagnosis of active disease with over 90 percent accuracy in cases which were subsequently verified radiographically (Jeffcoat & Capilouto, 1990). In bone scan technique, radi-

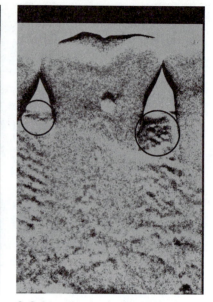

**A.**

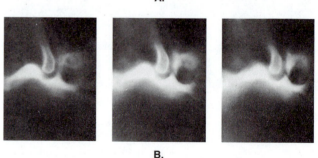

**B.**

**Figure 5-28** Computed tomography. **A.** Tomographic unit and computer system. **B.** A series of tomographs showing various views of the temporomandibular joint. (Courtesy of Incubation Industries, Warrington, PA)

olabeled pharmaceuticals are specifically designed to be taken up selectively by the tissue of interest, in this case the alveolar bone. The bone scan detects areas of alteration or change in bony metabolism. Because the scan is not disease-specific, it must be performed in conjunction with a clinical periodontal examination. The radiopharmaceutical 99m-Tc-methylene diphosphonate is injected intravenously and after allowing time for bony absorption, the area of interest is either measured by an intraoral detector or imaged using a gamma camera. Of the current medical imaging techniques, nuclear bone scans appear to show the most promise in relation to the potential for use in prognosticating bone loss due to periodontitis (Jeffcoat & Capilouto, 1990). Figure 5-29 is an example of a nuclear bone scan of the entire skull. The computer can then focus on any portion of the skull, section the area of interest, and enlarge it for closer evaluation.

## ASEPSIS

Not all potentially infectious patients can be identified even when meticulous care is given to obtaining a thorough medical history and clinical examination. As a result, radiographic infection control policies must be all-inclusive. However, as stated by Brand et al. (1992) in the *Infection Control Guidelines for Dental Radiographic Procedures*, "over-concern as well as under-concern can be a

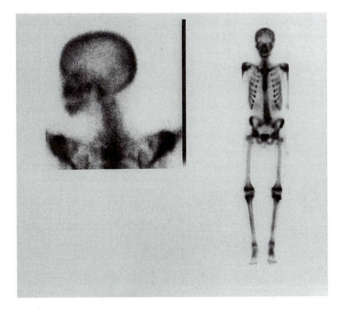

**Figure 5-29** Nuclear bone scan. (Courtesy of Incubation Industries, Warrington, PA)

problem if patients forego necessary treatment as a result of undue fear. Risk-benefit analysis is as appropriate to infection control as it is to radiation use. Guidelines should lead to practices that protect sufficiently, yet they should be practical enough to permit one standard of care to be used with all patients" (p. 248). Specific guidelines for infection control were developed by a select committee of dental radiologists and approved by the American Academy of Oral and Maxillofacial Radiology (Brand et al., 1992). Table 5-7 provides a brief synopsis of these recommendations.

## DOCUMENTATION

Recording information about radiographic interpretation and exposure is recommended. Interpretation aspects usually are included in a charting form, while significant findings such as a periodontal abscess or the degree of disease progression might also be recorded in the client's record of services. Table 5-8 represents a format for recording the results of the clinician's interpretation. This chart could be added to a client's periodontal examination form. When recording radiographic exposure, the clinician must ensure records are complete enough so that if required in a court of law, computation of exposure could be calculated. It is best to record all exposures, including unacceptable films in sequential order in the record of services. The number and type of films exposed, including a separate listing for retakes; and the machine settings are documented. The machine setting should include the mA, kVp, and exposure time. Additionally, if target-to-film distance or image receptor systems (film speed or film screen) changes from the norm, those data are recorded as well. It is suggested that the radiographic recording be listed in a client's record of services in an area separated from the written notations. Such a requirement is beneficial for locating the radiographic history of the client at subsequent appointments without having to read the entire record. Table 5-9 provides a historical recording of chart entries.

Documentation of patient refusal of radiographic services should also be recorded. The patient must be informed of the procedure to be completed, possible risks involved, protection procedures employed, and diagnostic information expected. If the patient refuses service after the explanation, he should sign a refusal-for-radiographic services release form, or sign the record of services after this notation (Lowdrey & Drew, 1995; Morris, 1995). If a separate form is used, it would be filed in the patient's permanent dental record. Refer to Chapter 8 for information about informed refusal. Additional documentation should be included when radiographs are sent to another dental office or given to the patient for any reason.

**Table 5-7  Infection Control Guidelines**

| Administration | Physical Facilities and Equipment | Operative Procedures | Darkroom Procedures |
|---|---|---|---|
| • Each practice or facility shall develop a written infection control policy.<br><br>• All patients should be treated as potentially infectious (patient-to-operator, operator-to-patient, patient-to-patient).<br><br>• In any setting a supervisor should be designated to be responsible for establishing, implementing, and monitoring guidelines and policies on infection control.<br><br>• A supervisor shall also provide for education of all personnel regarding potential hazards and how to minimize the hazards. | • Operators shall avoid touching any environmental surfaces with contaminated gloves. If this occurs, disinfection procedures shall be accomplished.<br><br>• Items used with patients should be kept on either a covered or disinfected surface.<br><br>• All nondisposable items that come in patient contact must be heat or gas sterilized. Cold sterilization is unacceptable.<br><br>• All stationary items coming in patient contact must be disinfected.<br><br>• Disposable contaminated items shall be sealed in plastic bags and disposed of in a manner that minimizes risk to patients, employees, and the community. | • Charts shall be kept away from sources of contamination.<br><br>• Gloves shall be worn during all procedures while handling contaminated film packets, supplies, instruments, and during cleanup procedures. Hands must be washed before and after glove use.<br><br>• Surfaces likely to be contaminated should be covered including exposure switches, PID, and chair controls.<br><br>• Film packets and supplies should be obtained prior to seating the patient. If additional supplies are required during the appointment, overgloves can be worn or work gloves removed and new ones put on before continuing the procedure. | • All contaminated surfaces shall be disinfected after use.<br><br>• Contaminated film packets shall be wiped dry in the x-ray room and transported.<br><br>• Gloves shall be worn when unwrapping contaminated packets and the film dropped onto a covered surface, then processed with ungloved hands.<br><br>• Gloves shall not be worn when handling processed film or paperwork.<br><br>• Daylight loaders are discouraged because contamination is difficult to avoid. If such a loader must be used, the following protocol is recommended:<br>1. Remove gloves and wash hands.<br>2. Pass the contaminated film (in a cup or towel) along with clean gloves, through the cover of the loader.<br>3. Put gloves on inside the loader to unwrap the film, then remove gloves, wash hands, and process film. |

**Table 5-8  Format for Recording the Results of Periodontal Interpretation**

Periodontal Interpretation

| Alveolar Bone | Normal _____ Diseased _____ | Disease Progression: | Case Type I _____ |
|---|---|---|---|
| Percentage of Bone Loss | Less than 30%  _____<br>30 to 50%  _____<br>Greater than 50%  _____ | | Case Type II _____<br>Case Type III _____<br>Case Type IV _____<br>Case Type V _____ |
| Bone Loss Pattern | Horizontal  _____<br>Vertical  _____ | Periodontal Maintenance Procedures | Conditions stable _____<br>Conditions progressing _____ |
| Distribution of Loss | localized  _____<br>where _____<br>generalized  _____ | | Explain _____<br>_____<br>_____ |

**Table 5-9. Historical Recording of Chart Entries**

| Record of Services | | |
|---|---|---|
| Date | Radiographic Services | Treatment Notes |
| 6/2/92 | 2 Occ, 2 BW, 4 PA 10/70 .4 sec. | |
| | 1 PA retake at same setting | |
| | | |
| 12/14/94 | 4 BW, 16 PA 15/90 12 imp. | |
| | | |
| 7/10/96 | 4 BW, 15/90 10 imp, | |
| | 1 pano, 15/88* | |

*A time recording is not necessary for panoramic films because each individual machine exposes every film for the same length of time.

## Summary

The competent clinician who is proficient in radiographic technique and interpretation is an asset in any dental practice. Selection of the type of radiographs that will yield the most information for each individual case is important for assessment and for protection of the patient. Periapical films permit the clinician to view more of the periodontium than bitewings, however, their use is limited in assessing bone height due to the possibility of vertical angulation error. Periapicals are necessary for determining the total root length, shape, and position, and to detect pathological lesions. Bitewing radiographs, especially when positioned vertically, adhere to the principles of photographic reproduction and are more useful than periapicals in determining bone height. The bone height helps the practitioner evaluate the severity of periodontitis and the category of disease progression for insurance purposes. Panoramic radiographs are not used for the interpretation and diagnosis of periodontal diseases. When appropriate, a full-mouth survey of x-ray films including periapical films and bitewings should be considered in planning nonsurgical periodontal care.

Once the radiograph has been exposed, the clinician must be thoroughly prepared to evaluate normal conditions as well as the disease processes. To accurately plan periodontal maintenance procedures for nonsurgical care, the clinician needs to evaluate the progress of these disease processes. Transmission radiographs provide a means to accomplish this. It is essential that past radiographs be available and used in the appraisal process. The proper use of radiographs is an integral part of the assessment and treatment of periodontal disease. Their importance in this process cannot be overstated, because without radiographs, the underlying periodontal tissues and remaining bone are not adequately evaluated. In addition, it is essential that a thorough clinical examination be conducted. Assessment of oral soft tissues and periodontal probe readings lay the foundation for treatment. However, if this clinical data is not correlated with radiographic findings, a less than complete client evaluation would result.

## Case Studies

**Case Study One:** Jennifer Alexander, a 37-year-old telephone solicitor, arrives for an initial visit in your office. She has not had any dental hygiene care for seven years. She has a noncontributory medical history and no physical symptoms of dental disease. Clinical examination reveals 4 to 5 millimeter pockets throughout the mouth, no recession, and bleeding upon probing. What radiographs should be recommended and why?

**Case Study Two:** Don Hansen is a 42-year-old entrepreneur who arrives in your office for an appointment with the dental hygienist. Don's last appointment was twelve months ago at which time four horizontal bitewing radiographs were taken. His history indicates that he has two occlusal "watch" areas for caries in the mandibular molar region. He also has probe readings of 3 mm on those same molars with no accompanying recession. These conditions have remained unchanged for his last several appointments. Upon clinical examination, there is no further evidence of any dental disease, and the patient reports no noticeable symptoms that would indicate otherwise. What radiographs would you recommended in this case and why?

**Case Study Three:** Kim Webster, a 19-year-old college student presents for care. Her last dental visit was eighteen months ago at which time minimal restorative work was required, and three areas of bleeding upon probing were recorded around a single crown. The bleeding areas measured 2 to 3 mm with a periodontal probe and no recession is present. Current clinical findings include a complaint of erupting wisdom teeth, 4 mm pockets with bleeding without concurrent recession around the crown on #12, poor oral hygiene, and a deep restoration with intermittent pain on #30. What type of radiographs would you recommend and why? What principles would you need to remember when documenting the exposures?

**Case Study Four:** Observe the radiographs of 28-year-old Mike Dixon and determine the category of periodontitis present (see Figure 5-30). Keep in mind these findings are only preliminary and need to be verified with a clinical examination. Present rationale for your decision. Include in this rationale the pattern and type of bone loss and if the area between #13 and #14 is vertical or horizontal bone loss.

**Case Study Five:** Observe the radiographs of 61-year-old Donna Thompson (see Figure 5-31). Determine Donna's category of periodontal disease progression and present rationale for your decision.

## Case Study Discussions

**Discussion—Case Study One:** The recommendation would be a full mouth intraoral radiographic survey. The New Patient-Adult matrix in the *Guidelines for Radiographic Selection* (see Table 5-6) prescribes a full periapical survey

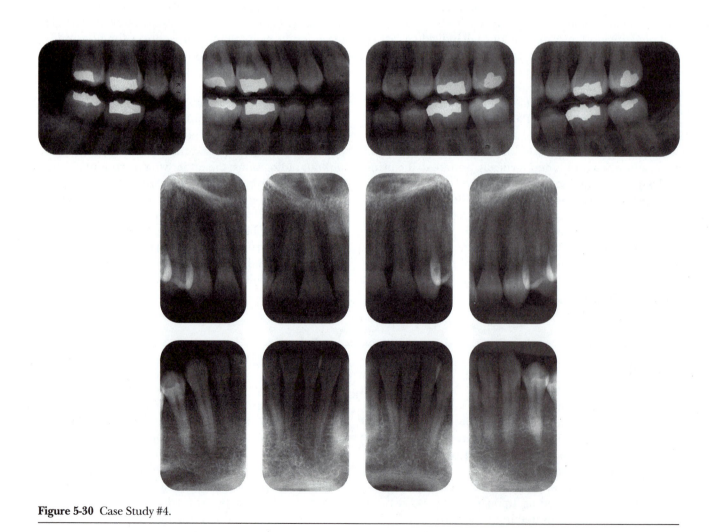

**Figure 5-30** Case Study #4.

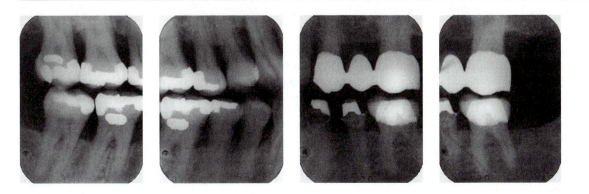

**Figure 5-31** Case Study #5.

plus bitewings because the patient is new to the practice and previous x-rays are not available. In addition, the patient's clinical examination is indicative of periodontitis. Vertical bitewings would be appropriate because of the pocket depth. A panoramic film would not be recommended because close evaluation of the entire periodontium is required, and the definition on the panoramic film is not adequate for that purpose.

**Discussion—Case Study Two:** Careful examination of transmission radiographs would be required to assess the areas of potential problems. If no change has occurred, further radiographic examination is not indicated at this time. The Recall Patient-Adult matrix (see Table 5-6) indicates that with no evidence of current disease, only posterior bitewings, would be prescribed and those would only be recommended every two to three years. Because there is no clinical evidence of disease or change, the three-year time span should be considered.

**Discussion—Case Study Three:** The recommendation would be a panoramic film, four posterior bitewings, and a periapical film of #30. The Recall Patient-Adolescent matrix (see Table 5-6) with positive clinical symptoms prescribes: 1) a panoramic examination to assess third molars, 2) bitewings to assess bone level and caries activity due to bleeding of the gingival tissue with associated pockets and poor oral hygiene, and 3) a periapical to assess the soundness of the deep restoration and to assure the area is free of infection because of the associated pain. Horizontally positioned bitewings are appropriate. The exposures would be recorded on Kim's record of services keeping these principles in mind.

1. Exposures should be recorded in the order in which they were taken.
2. Any retakes should be listed separately from the initial exposure.

3. The number and type of films need to be identified. In this case, 4 horizontal BW, 1 pano, 1 PA.
4. The mA, kVp, and exposure time will be included. The panoramic survey does not need to have an exposure time recorded.
5. If either the speed or film screen changed from the normal exposure used in the office, then this should also be documented.

**Discussion—Case Study Four: Early periodontitis (Case Type II). Rationale:**

1. Bone loss is less than 30 percent in all areas.
2. Generalized loss of pointed crestal alveolar bone leading to triangulation is evident in anterior interproximal areas.
3. Triangulation appears on the mesial of #3.
4. Decreased density appears in posterior areas, especially in the maxilla.
5. Unclear lamina dura is present in the premolar regions.
6. Generalized horizontal bone loss is evident.
7. Bone loss between #13 and #14 is horizontal because the pattern is parallel with a line drawn between the adjacent cementoenamel junctions.

**Discussion—Case Study Five: Advanced periodontitis (Case Type IV). Rationale:**

1. Even though the general bone level is between 30% to 50%, teeth #2, #3, #4, #5 have a greater than 50% loss. The category, therefore, is based on the area where the most extensive bone loss is present.
2. Cratering is evident throughout.
3. Furcation involvement of molars is clearly evident even though the density of the bone somewhat obscures the maxillary region.

# REFERENCES

Akesson, L., Hakansson, H., & Rohlin, M. (1992). Comparison of panoramic and intraoral radiography and pocket probing for the measurement of the marginal bone level. *Journal of Clinical Periodontology, 19,* 326.

American Academy of Periodontology. (1989a). *Proceedings of the world workshop in clinical periodontics.* Consensus Report. Discussion Section I. Periodontal diagnosis and diagnostic aids (pp. I-23–31). Chicago: The American Academy of Periodontology.

American Academy of Periodontology. (1989b). *Proceedings of the world workshop in clinical periodontics.* Discussion Section VIII. Implant therapy. (VIII-11–18). Chicago: The American Academy of Periodontology.

American Academy of Periodontology. (1993). *Guidelines for periodontal therapy.* Research, Science, and Therapy Committee. Chicago: American Academy of Periodontology.

Bean, L. R. (1969). Comparison of bisecting angle and paralleling methods of intraoral radiology. *Journal of Dental Education, 33,* 441.

Benn, D. K. (1990). Limitations of the digital image subtraction technique in assessing alveolar bone crest changes due to misalignment errors during image capture. *Dentomaxillofacial Radiology, 19,* 97–104.

Brand, J., Benson, B., Ciola, B., Glass, B., Katz, J., Otis, L., Parks, E., & Pettigrew, J. (1992). Infection control guidelines for dental radiographic procedures. *Oral Surgery, Oral Medicine, Oral Pathology, 73,* 248–249.

Carranza, F. A. (1990). Radiographic and other aids in the diagnosis of periodontal disease. In F. A. Carranza & M. G. Newman (Eds.), *Clinical periodontology* (8th ed.). Philadelphia: W.B. Saunders Co.

Cowdrey, M. L. & Drew, M. (1995). *Basic law for the allied health professions* (2nd ed.). Boston: Jones and Bartlett Publishers.

*Current procedural terminology for periodontics and insurance reporting manual* (1995) (7th ed.). Chicago: American Academy of Periodontology.

Farman, A. G., Christoffel, J. N., and Wood, R. E. (1994). Principles of image interpretation. In P. W. Goaz & S. C. White (Eds.), *Oral radiology: Principles and interpretation* (3rd ed.) (pp. 291–305). St. Louis: Mosby-Year Book, Inc.

Fleszar, T. J. (1992). Occlusal trauma: Clinical application. In T. J. Wilson, K. S. Kornman, & M. G. Newman (Eds.), *Advances in periodontics* (p. 217). Chicago: Quintessence Publishing Co., Inc.

Frederiksen, N. L. (1994). Health physics. In P. W. Goaz & S. C. White (Eds.), *Oral radiology: Principles and interpretation* (3rd ed.) (pp. 47–65). St. Louis: Mosby-Year Book, Inc.

Frommer, H. H. (1987). A comparative clinical study of group D and E dental film. *Oral Surgery, 63,* 738–742.

Frommer, H. H. (1992). *Radiology for dental auxiliaries* (5th ed.). St. Louis: Mosby-Year Book, Inc.

Furkart, A. J., Dove, S. B., McDavid, W. D., Nummikoski, P., & Matteson, S. (1992). Direct digital radiography for the detection of periodontal bone lesions. *Oral Surgery, Oral Medicine, and Oral Pathology, 73,* 652–660.

Goaz, P. W. & White, S. C. (1994). *Oral radiology: Principles and interpretations* (3rd ed.). St. Louis: Mosby-Year Book, Inc.

Gratt, B. M. & Shetty, V. (1994). Implant radiology. In P. W. Goaz & S. C. White (Eds.), *Oral radiology: Principles and Interpretation* (3rd ed.) (pp. 703–715). St. Louis: Mosby-Year Book, Inc.

Gröndahl, K., Gröndahl, H. G., & Webber, R. L. (1984). Influence of variations in projection geometry on the detectability of periodontal bone lesions: A comparison between subtraction radiography and conventional radiographic technique. *Journal of Clinical Periodontology, 11,* 411–420.

Hämmerle, C. H. F. & Lang, N. P. (1994). Tissue: Integration of oral implants. In N. P. Lang & T. Karring (Eds.), *Proceedings of the 1st European workshop on periodontology* (pp. 297–316). London: Quintessence Books.

Haring, P. J. & Lind, L. J. (1993). *Radiographic interpretation for the dental hygienist.* Philadelphia: W.B. Saunders Co.

Hausmann, E. A., Allen, K. M., Christersson, L., & Genco, R. (1989). Effects of x-ray beam vertical angulation on radiographic alveolar crest level measurement. *Journal of Periodontal Research, 24,* 8–19.

Hausmann, E. A., Allen, K. M., & Piedmonte, M. R. (1991). Influence of variations in projection geometry and lesion size on detection of computer-simulated crestal alveolar bone lesions by subtraction radiography. *Journal of Periodontal Research, 26,* 48–51.

Hollender, L. (1992). Decision making in radiographic imaging. *Journal of Dental Education, 56,* 834–843.

Iacono, V. J. & Livers, H. N. (1992). Special radiographic techniques for implant dentistry. In T. J. Wilson, K. S. Kornman, & M. G. Newman (Eds.), *Advances in periodontics* (pp. 341–342). Chicago: Quintessence Publishing Co., Inc.

Jeffcoat, M. K. (1992a). Imaging techniques for the periodontium. In T. J. Wilson, K. S. Kornman, & M. G. Newman (Eds.), *Advances in periodontics* (pp. 47–57). Chicago: Quintessence Publishing Co., Inc.

Jeffcoat, M. K. (1992b). Radiographic methods for the detection of progressive alveolar bone loss. *Journal of Periodontology, 63,* 367–372.

Jeffcoat, M. K. & Capilouto, M. L. (1990). Problems in risk assessment in periodontal disease-use of clinical indicators. In J. D. Bader (Ed.), *Risk assessment in dentistry* (pp. 109–113). Chapel Hill: University of North Carolina Dental Ecology.

Jeffcoat, M. K. & Reddy, M. S. (1991). A comparison of probing and radiographic methods for detection of periodontal disease progression. *Current Opinions in Dentistry, 1,* 45–51.

Kantor, M. L., Zeichner, S. J., Valachovic, R. W., & Reiskin, A. B. (1989). Efficacy of dental radiographic practices: Options for image receptors, examination selection, and patient selection. *Journal of the American Dental Association, 119,* 259–268.

Kleier, D. J., Hicks, M. J., & Flaitz, C. M. (1987). A comparison of ultraspeed and ektaspeed dental film: In vitro study of the radiographic appearance of interproximal lesions. *Oral Surgery, 63,* 381–385.

Matteson, S. R., Phillips, C., Kantar, M. L., & Leinedecker, T. (1989). The effect of lesion size, restorative material, and film speed on the detection of recurrent caries. *Oral Surgery, 68,* 232–237.

Molander, B., Ahlqwist, M., Gröndahl, H. G., & Hollender, L. (1991). Agreement between panoramic and intraoral radiography in the assessment of marginal bone height. *Dentomaxillofacial Radiology, 20,* 155–100.

Morris, W. O. (1995). *The dentist's legal advisor.* St. Louis: Mosby-Year Book, Inc.

Osborne, G. E. & Hemmings, K. W. (1992). A survey of disease changes observed on dental panoramic tomographs taken of patients attending a periodontology clinic. *British Dental Journal, 173,* 166–168.

Reddy, M. (1992). Radiographic methods in the evaluation of periodontal therapy. *Journal of Periodontology, 63,* 1078–1084.

Scarff, A. F., Walsh, M. M., & Darby, M. L. (1995). Periodontal and oral hygiene assessment. In M. L. Darby & M. M. Walsh (Eds.), *Dental hygiene theory & practice* (p. 364). Philadelphia: W.B. Saunders Co.

Shrout, M. K., Powell, B. J., Hildebolt, C. F., Vannier, M. W., & Ahmed, N. M. (1993). Digital radiographic image based bone level measurement: Effect of film density. *Journal of Clinical Periodontology, 20,* 595–600.

Thomson-Lakey, E. & Tolle-Watts, L. (1994a). A practical guide for using radiographs in the assessment of periodontal diseases, Part I: Technique. *Journal of Practical Hygiene, 3*(1), 11–16.

Thomson-Lakey, E. & Tolle-Watts, L. (1994b). A practical guide for using radiographs in the assessment of periodontal diseases, Part II: Interpretation and future advances, *Journal of Practical Hygiene, 3*(2), 11–14.

U.S. Department of Health and Human Services. (1987). *The selection of patients for x-ray examinations: Dental radiographic examinations.* (HHS Publication FDA 88-8273). Washington, D.C.: U.S. Government Printing Office.

Weissman, D. D. & Longhurst, G. E. (1971). Clinical evaluation of a rectangular field collimating device for peripheral radiography. *Journal of the American Dental Association, 82,* 580.

Wilkins, E. J. (1994). *Clinical practice of the dental hygienist* (7th ed.). Lea & Febiger.

Williamson, G. F. (1993). Radiographic assessment. In I. R. Woodall (Ed.), *Comprehensive dental hygiene care* (4th ed.) (pp. 96–230). St. Louis: Mosby-Year Book, Inc.

Wilson, T. G. (1992). Examination of patients with periodontal disease. In T. J. Wilson, K. S. Kornman, & M. G. Newman (Eds.), *Advances in periodontics* (pp. 26–27). Chicago: Quintessence Publishing Co., Inc.

# DIAGNOSIS AND PLANNING PHASES

# CHAPTER 6

# Periodontal Diagnosis and Care Planning

## Key Terms

care plan
clinical or objective factors
contributing or subjective factors
decision making

dental hygiene diagnosis
interventions
powered toothbrush
reevaluation

## INTRODUCTION

Planning the client's care involves more than a treatment plan or plan of treatment, it also encompasses the broad range of preventive, educational, therapeutic, and support services within the scope of dental hygiene practice (Darby & Walsh, 1994, pg. 417). The dental hygiene care planning process focuses on this expanded approach to client care that is required and requested by today's sophisticated dental consumer. This shift in philosophy has lead to the change in terminology from treatment planning to care planning.

Dental hygiene care plans are based on two sets of criteria. The first set of criteria are **clinical** or **objective factors**; while the second set are **contributing** or **subjective factors.** Current dental hygiene theory places emphasis on individual client's needs (Darby & Walsh, 1994) and dental hygiene care plans must take into consideration not only the physical need of health, but also the need for self-determination and active participation in treatment. These considerations are subjective in nature; therefore, if the client is to become a partner in care it is important to provide a full explanation regarding the plan for care. This communication offers the client the opportunity to collaborate with the dental hygienist and the dentist. The client's role in the design of the dental hygiene care plan is based on both informed consent and expressed consent (see Chapter 8) and other contributing factors such as motivation and financial resources. The dental hygienist's role in the design of the dental hygiene care plan is based not only on the needs, wants, and desires of the client, but also on the professional's clinical abilities, experience, and philosophy.

This chapter provides an introduction to dental hygiene care plans as an integral element of nonsurgical

periodontal therapy (NSPT). The relationship of care planning to traditional phases of care, components of the care planning, therapeutic options for those with periodontal disease, and selection of oral self-care devices are discussed. Additionally, cases are enclosed that illustrate planning strategies and their written documentation.

## PHASES OF CARE

The **care plan** is a "blueprint" or guide to determine how many appointments are needed and what procedures will be performed at each appointment session. The written care plan is the result of the planning phase of the dental hygiene process of care. The primary goal of the plan is to coordinate all treatment procedures and to estimate the treatment length with the aim to establish a well functioning dentition in a healthy periodontal environment (Carranza, 1996). Table 6-1 outlines the traditional phases of care that comprise general dental treatment planning (Carranza, 1996). The Preliminary Phase focuses on treating the emergency needs. Phase I therapy includes self-care education, diet control, removal or correction of plaque-retentive factors, antimicrobial therapy, and dental caries management. Phase I therapy is an essential phase because it focuses on controlling the etiologic influences responsible for the dental diseases. Initial dental hygiene care is the primary focus of Phase I, and it is essential that these services are well integrated with the other Phase I therapies.

Phase II therapy focuses on periodontal surgery including placement of implants and endodontic therapy. Phase III therapy consists of prosthetic treatment and the final management of dental caries along with periodontal examination to re-evaluate response to

## Table 6-1  Phases of Care Planning

| Phase | Examples of Services |
|---|---|
| ***Preliminary Phase***<br>• Emergency Needs | • treatment of emergency (periodontal/periapical abscess) |
| ***Phase I***<br>• Initial or Active Therapy | • self-care education<br>• diet control<br>• removal of plaque-retentive calculus (debridement)<br>• removal/correction of other plaque-retentive factors (overhanging margins)<br>• antimicrobial therapy<br>• dental caries management (restorations)<br>• occlusal therapy |
| ***Phase II***<br>• Surgical Care | • periodontal surgery<br>• endodontic therapy<br>• implants |
| ***Phase III***<br>• Prosthetic Treatment | • final management of dental caries (final restorations)<br>• reevaluation of periodontal assessment |
| ***Phase IV***<br>• Maintenance | • periodontal maintenance procedures<br>  • assessment<br>  • self-care education<br>  • deposit removal<br>  • evaluation of recare interval |

## Table 6-2  Clinical Components of Dental Hygiene Care

| | |
|---|---|
| 1. General Assessment | • Health history (personal history)<br>• Dental history<br>• Head and neck exam (soft tissue)<br>• Radiographs<br>• Risk assessment |
| 2. Periodontal Assessment | • Mobility<br>• Furcations<br>• Probing depth<br>• Loss of attachment<br>• Recession<br>• Gingival conditions |
| 3. Restorative Assessment | • Existing restorations<br>• Quality of restorations<br>• Need for caries management<br>• Occlusion |
| 4. Instrumentation | • Local anesthesia/nitrous oxide-oxygen analgesia<br>• Plaque removal (hand or ultrasonic)<br>• Calculus removal (hand or ultrasonic)<br>• Overhang removal (hand or mechanized method) |
| 5. Polishing Procedures | • Selective polishing<br>• Polishing restorations |
| 6. Oral Self-Care Education | • Needs assessment<br>• Disease theory education<br>• Skill enhancement (aids)<br>• Nutrition education<br>• Smoking cessation |
| 7. Supportive | • Fluoride application<br>• Dental sealant application<br>• Mouthguard fabrication<br>• Subgingival irrigation<br>• Desensitization<br>• Local/systemic antibiotics<br>• Implant maintenance |
| 8. Referrals | • Restorative treatment<br>• Periodontal surgery<br>• Orthodontics<br>• Endodontics<br>• Oral surgery<br>• Oral pathology diagnosis |

restorative procedures. In Phase IV therapy, the long-term maintenance or follow-up is provided. This phase, similar to Phase I, is primarily the dental hygienist's responsibility and consists of preventive therapy including oral self-care education, deposit removal, supportive therapy, and recare/maintenance interval evaluation. Chapter 16 reviews periodontal maintenance procedures (PMP). It must be remembered that the dental hygiene care plan is part of the total dental treatment plan for an individual client.

Although not a fully inclusive list, Table 6-2 outlines the many components of dental hygiene care that are delivered during Phase I or Phase IV therapy. Services will vary according to client needs making each care plan unique to that individual. Services will also vary according to legal requirements and practice guidelines for the dental hygienist. Even if clients receive the same services the care plan will reflect variances in the manner in which the services were delivered.

## DECISION-MAKING PROCESS

Dental hygiene care planning is one of the many decision-making processes dental hygienists are responsible for. **Decision making** is the judgment or conclusion made as a result of the critical thinking process. This procedure is a crucial and integral part of the dental hygiene process for without it implementation and evaluation of care can be haphazard and unsuccessful. In the last five years, the concepts of the dental hygiene diagnostic process and individualized approach to dental hygiene treatment have been advanced by several authors (Darby & Walsh,

1994; Woodall, 1993). Historically, care planning was not always considered part of the dental hygiene process because diagnosis of periodontal disease was not considered within the scope of dental hygiene practice. Dental hygienists generally relied on a standardized routine approach to care and made treatment decisions intuitively rather than objectively. This approach contributed to the variability in the decision-making process. Decision making is now considered the most important factor in the development of a care plan. In the treatment of clients, dental hygienists continually make decisions according to the specific situations they encounter. For example, dental hygienists assess indications for and contraindications to treatment and they determine if health or active disease exists.

Treatment decisions are influenced not only by clinical findings, but also by the contributing factors that define the subjective nature of care. Figure 6-1 illustrates many factors that influence dental hygiene decision making. Examples of clinical factors influencing periodontal care planning include a health history reporting a systemic disease (such as poorly controlled diabetes or AIDS) or deep pockets and attachment loss. These factors indicate a need for multiple appointments for nonsurgical dental hygiene therapy. Two examples of contributing factors influencing planning are clients' present and future ability to maintain effective self-care and their financial resources including the availability of third-party payments. It is the latter group of findings, the subjective component, that provides the therapist with the greatest challenge because effective communication and collaboration are necessary to identify and incorporate these factors into care. Experience and self-evaluation both aid the clinician in enhancing this aspect of NSPT. The professional must have a desire to care for each client in a unique manner or care plans, like treatment plans, will appear similar and routine. While the clinical assessment regime may be somewhat standardized for the majority of clients, the discovery of and attention to con-

tributing factors is enhanced with professional experience and desire.

The establishment of an appropriate care plan can be developed only after a complete health history, comprehensive clinical examination, and thorough understanding of the client's goals are accomplished. Risk factors associated with periodontal disease such as age, systemic diseases, smoking, bacterial plaque, calculus, poor oral care, and periodontal pathogens also need to be identified (Staff, 1994) as addressed in Chapters 1 and 3. The individualized approach emphasizes the need for dental hygienists to assess and to diagnose the periodontal condition treated as well as to address the goals, wants, and desires of the client. Several examples of questions that the dental hygienist can internally analyze in order to arrive at a suitable plan are as follows:

1. What is the best treatment to achieve the desired clinical outcomes?
2. What are the client's priorities?
3. What are the client's preferences?
4. What is the motivation level of the client?
5. Are there any financial limitations?
6. Do I or another practitioner have the skill to provide the necessary services?
7. Are there any legal/ethical dilemmas?
8. Do I have all the information I need to develop the care plan?
9. Do I need to use other diagnostic tools or consultations to further clarify the diagnosis?

Many questions arise that require decision making, for example, choice of polishing agent, need and type of fluoride therapy, or recommendations for effective oral self-care aids. It is incumbent upon the professional to develop the optimal care plan for the client, regardless of the time or monetary constraints.

## COMPONENTS OF CARE PLANNING

Darby and Walsh (1994) suggest there are four components of planning. These include: 1) establishing priorities that require a team approach with the client, dental hygienist, and dentist(s) (general and specialists); 2) setting goals and evaluation measures; 3) identifying **interventions,** which is the individual client's treatment regimen for meeting the assessed needs; and finally 4) writing or documenting the care plan. The written plan, together with informed consent (see Chapter 8), becomes a contract between the dental hygienist and the client while also providing the necessary medicolegal documentation.

### Priorities

Client assessment is the basis for identifying the priorities of the care plan. The assessment phase of treatment includes data collection (see Chapters 2 through 5),

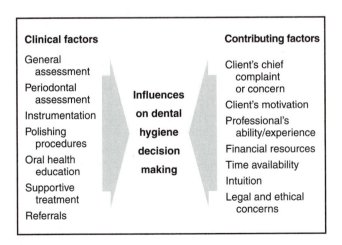

| Clinical factors | Contributing factors |
|---|---|
| General assessment | Client's chief complaint or concern |
| Periodontal assessment | Client's motivation |
| Instrumentation | Professional's ability/experience |
| Polishing procedures | Financial resources |
| Oral health education | Time availability |
| Supportive treatment | Intuition |
| Referrals | Legal and ethical concerns |

*Influences on dental hygiene decision making*

**Figure 6-1** Influences on decision making.

questioning the client, assessing risk factors, developing perceptions, and other forms of interaction with the client. Refer to Chapter 3 for a detailed discussion of periodontal assessment. During the assessment phase the dental hygienist begins to synthesize oral health problems and the outcome results in the dental hygiene diagnosis. The dental hygiene diagnosis focuses on problems or potential problems that are related to oral health and disease, rather than on the disease itself. Gurenlian (1993) maintains that dental hygienists diagnose within the concepts of their knowledge and practice standards. More specifically, a definition of **dental hygiene diagnosis** is "a formal statement of the dental hygienist's decision regarding the actual or potential problems of a patient that are amenable to treatment through the dental hygiene process of care" (Gurenlian, 1993, p. 364). Notice that the diagnosis is usually referred to in a singular manner, however, dental hygiene diagnosis can actually be a combination of statements or conclusions about oral health problems of the client. Darby and Walsh (1994) further enhanced this concept by developing the *Human Needs Conceptual Model for Dental Hygiene.* Needs of the client are identified through a concrete process and written format. The dental hygiene diagnosis is then derived from the needs assessment by evaluating deficits in client needs. Needs assessment is further discussed in Chapter 8 and the reader is referred to *Dental Hygiene Theory and Practice* (Darby and Walsh, 1994) for further clarification.

## Goals

Goals can be either general or specific, stated orally or written, and established by the client or clinician. No matter how goals are determined in clinical practice they are always client-oriented. Written goals provide a means of evaluation for treatment because they reflect expected and desired outcomes of dental hygiene care.

## Interventions for NSPT

To this point, the discussion has centered around the priorities, goals, and evaluation for general care planning based on the dental hygiene diagnosis. Chapter 3 discusses the presumptive or preliminary diagnosis and the final diagnosis which are both specific to the periodontal disease diagnosis. These diagnostic terms, while only relevant to the status of the periodontal disease, are critical factors in determining the therapeutic regimes that are best suited to the client undergoing NSPT. It is recognized that comprehensive care planning involves more than NSPT; however, a synopsis of therapy recommendations follows based on only the classification and form of periodontal disease (see Table 6-3) (Wilson, Kornman, & Newman, 1992). This table is not intended to be all inclusive. Instead, it is a guide to possible treatment interventions for NSPT with recognition of where surgical intervention might be needed. Each of the thera-

peutic options is discussed in subsequent chapters (oral self-care, Chapter 8; supportive care such as chemotherapy and implants in Chapter 14; and periodontal instrumentation in Chapters 10, 11 and 12).

**Chronic Disease States.** Generally, chronic gingivitis and chronic adult periodontitis progress slowly and respond in a predictable manner to quality NSPT directed at reducing the disease-causing bacteria. Therapy for chronic disease states is comprised of active therapy and periodontal maintenance procedures (PMP). Initial NSPT is the dental hygienist's responsibility and, at times, surgery is an element of initial therapy. The main focus of NSPT with chronic forms of disease is oral self-care education and mechanical removal of deposits by both the client and professional. Client involvement occurs with plaque removal at the professional visit. The professional's responsibilities include removal of subgingival plaque, calculus, and plaque-retentive factors. Debridement is indicated in areas of inflammation, pocketing, and/or where plaque-retentive factors are present. Either hand-activated or ultrasonic instrumentation or a combination of the two is acceptable. Ultrasonic scaling is advantageous when treating acute conditions. Selective polishing should be considered for areas of stain.

Use of antimicrobial mouthrinses or irrigation is useful when treating periodontitis when gingivitis coexists. Literature, however, does not support the use of antimicrobial mouthrinses or irrigation for treatment of periodontitis only (see Chapter 14). Implant therapy can be initiated during the initial phase of care or is considered part of Phase II care. Periodontal surgery might be indicated for advanced sites or cases of chronic periodontitis (see Chapter 17). Most cases of early and moderate extent can be treated nonsurgically if access to subgingival deposits is attainable. As with any form of periodontal disease, client compliance with self-care practices is critical to successful NSPT. This compliance is particularly effective with chronic forms because of the major role bacterial plaque plays in disease initiation.

**Aggressive Disease States.** Aggressive forms of periodontitis and some noncommon forms of gingivitis will not respond to NSPT in a predictable manner. Aggressive forms of periodontitis also progress rapidly. For these reasons, detection of these forms of disease at the earliest point in dental hygiene care is imperative for the individuals well-being. Traditional NSPT is recommended although vast bacterial plaque and calculus deposits are not present because the host response and specific periodontal pathogens are more responsible for the disease than the critical mass of bacterial plaque. Additionally, systemic and local chemotherapy (see Chapter 14), microbiological testing (see Chapter 3), and physician consultation or referral (see Chapter 2) are considered. Generalized and localized forms of prepubertal periodontitis are treated with the same therapy; however, referral and treatment by a physician might not be indi-

**Table 6-3 Interventions for Different Forms of Periodontal Disease**

| Classification | Form | Etiology | Treatment Recommendations |
|---|---|---|---|
| Chronic Gingivitis | Plaque Alone | • bacterial plaque | • self-care education<br>• client removal of plaque<br>• professional debridement/scaling<br>• antimicrobial mouthrinses<br>• irrigation with antimicrobial |
| | Trauma | • local injury or tooth eruption | • relieve pain<br>• topical antimicrobials to prevent secondary infection<br>• self-care education |
| | Steroid Hormone Influenced | • pregnancy<br>• menstruation (prior)<br>• puberty<br>• oral contraceptive<br>• increase in *P.* [*Bacteriodes*] *intermedia* | • consult with endocrinologist or gynecologist (birth control)<br>• self-care education<br>• scaling/debridement<br>• possible surgical correction |
| | Medication Influenced Overgrowth | • phenytoin<br>• cyclosporin<br>• nifedipine | • physician consultation for an alternative medication<br>• self-care education |
| | Other | • blood dyscrasia | • referral to physician to correct hemotologic disorder<br>• self-care education |
| | Desquamative Gingivitis | • dermatoses<br>  – erosive lichen planus<br>  – phemphigoid<br>  – pemphigus<br>• allergic reactions | • consult with physician about topical or systemic corticosteroids for dermatoses<br>• discontinue if cause allergy |
| Acute Gingivitis | Plaque Alone | • bacterial plaque | • self-care education |
| | Acute Necrotizing Ulcerative Gingivitis | • spirochetes<br>• fusiform bacilli | • immediate scaling/debridement<br>• immediate self care education<br>• systemic antibiotics if associated with fever, sore throat, lymphadenopathy or if mechanical debridement does not resolve infection<br>• non-antibiotic topical antimicrobials |
| | AIDs Associated | • immunosuppression<br>• bacterial plaque | • topical antimicrobials (povidone iodine or chlorhexidine)<br>• debridement |
| Periodontitis | Chronic Adult (CAP) | • bacterial plaque accumulation | • self-care education<br>• debridement<br>• reevaluation for surgery needs |
| | Localized Juvenile (LJP) | • systemic host defense defect<br>• primary causative microorganism is *A. actinomycetemcomitans* | • self-care education/debridement<br>• systemic antibiotics (tetracyclines)<br>• locally delivered antibiotics (site-specific areas)<br>• microbial diagnostic testing (DNA probe analysis)<br>• chlorhexidine rinses<br>• surgery |
| | Generalized Juvenile (GJP) | • systemic host defense defect | • same therapy as LJP but surgery not advisable until periodontal stability exists |
| | Rapidly Progressive (RPP) | • microbial<br>• host response (undiagnosed systemic disease) | • same as LJP<br>• referral to physician to consider undiagnosed systemic disease |
| | Refractory (RP) | • might be a single disease or several diseases | • self-care education<br>• scaling/debridement<br>• systemic antibiotics<br>• locally delivered antibiotics<br>• microbial diagnostic testing<br>• surgery considered only if stability achieved |
| | Generalized Prepubertal (GPP) | • defects of neutrophils and monocytes | • referral to physician for evaluation and treatment of systemic conditions<br>• self-care education<br>• scaling/debridement<br>• systemic antibiotics may or may not be helpful (Amoxicillin, Augmentin®)<br>• extractions of primary teeth might be indicated based on disease severity |
| | Localized Prepubertal (LPP) | • defects of neutrophils and monocytes | • self-care education<br>• scaling/debridement<br>• systemic antibiotics |

cated with the localized form because the host defect is thought to be less severe than with the generalized form (Wilson, Kornman, & Newman, 1992). Rapidly progressive periodontitis treatment modalities encompass traditional NSPT and strengthening of the host response by controlling systemic conditions, reducing stress, achieving rest, maintaining adequate nutrition, and eliminating periodontal pathogens. The latter is accomplished via microbial testing and chemotherapy. This form of disease, encountered from puberty to thirty-five years of age, is frequently associated with depression, malaise, and a lowered immune response (Wilson, Kornman, & Newman, 1992). Refractory periodontitis is suspected when disease progression occurs even in sites of early and moderate bone loss, not just where severely diseased sites are seen. Disease progression occurs despite quality NSPT and routine PMP. Therapy recommendations are similar to those for rapidly progressive periodontitis. Aggressive forms of disease, except localized juvenile periodontitis, often do not benefit from surgery. In fact, it is detrimental to perform surgery before a chronic state of periodontal stability is reached (Kornman & Wilson, 1992), thus NSPT is the primary means of care.

All aggressive cases need close reevaluation and monitoring with PMP. Periodontists and their dental hygienists most often treat clients with aggressive disease, but with increased knowledge and diagnostic testing more cases are being identified and treated in the general practitioner's office. Initial therapy might well be the responsibility of the dental hygienist in the general practice not only because of improved recognition of these disease states, but also because identification and confirmation of these forms is not always accomplished during initial therapy. Many times reevaluation or subsequent maintenance visits are needed to recognize these diseases. As a result, knowledge about the recommended therapy for aggressive periodontal disease is every dental hygienist's responsibility. Misdiagnosis of this form is somewhat common and although the majority of the population does not have aggressive disease, for those who do, this is devastating.

## Evaluation

There are two forms of evaluation to consider when planning care: 1) evaluation that occurs continually throughout the implementation phase of care, and 2) evaluation that occurs after initial therapy is completed (reevaluation). The dental hygiene diagnosis dictates what procedures or therapies are needed at the present time and what alternate procedures may be recommended in the future. This diagnosis may be altered as new assessment criteria become available during the dental hygiene care phase of treatment. Examples of altered or new assessment criteria are improved client self-care, an increase in healing response time, or results from diagnostic microbiological or medical screening tests. Each of these additional pieces of information will

impact the care plan and the final outcome of treatment. Because evaluation is ongoing throughout all phases of care, plans are not static.

**Reevaluation** in NSPT is a formal process of care planning that occurs four to six weeks after the completion of initial or active therapy. The purposes of reevaluation are to evaluate response to initial care and recommend additional therapy as needed. An outcome of reevaluation is a final diagnosis made by confirming or modifying the presumptive diagnosis. Elements of a reevaluation appointment are as follows:

1. reassess to evaluate healing,
2. evaluate self-care practices,
3. reeducate the client when necessary,
4. remove residual deposit or debride nonresponsive sites,
5. perform supportive treatment (desensitization or antimicrobial mouthrinse),
6. reassess the maintenance interval and adjust if indicated.

The necessary appointment time depends on the client needs and if any additional therapy is planned such as amalgam polishing or selective polishing. A thirty-minute appointment period is usually ample and if not, reappointment for retreatment can occur. For example, a quadrant or area is not responding to debridement therapy. This nonresponse is identified as a new problem because the outcome of NSPT—healing—is not occurring. Hypotheses are generated focusing on potential reasons for the lack of healing. Possible causes could range from incomplete removal of deposits, systemic factors, or an abundance of specific periodontal disease-causing microorganisms. More than one course of action could be taken, such as:

1. perform deposit removal again and reevaluate,
2. review the client's oral self-care techniques in this area and make necessary recommendations,
3. perform a microbiological screening test to determine if antibiotic therapy would be needed,
4. use an antimicrobial agent in this area, or
5. consult with or refer the client to a physician and/or periodontist.

These alternative choices of action or additional therapies would demand more data; therefore, further internal questioning is reviewed such as:

1. What information needs to be explained to the client in regard to this problem area?
2. Is there a dexterity or motivation problem?
3. Is another oral hygiene adjunct more appropriate than what is presently used to clean and deplaque the area?
4. Does the client have an allergy or sensitivity to antibiotics? If so, which ones?
5. How does the person feel about referral?

Expected outcomes of those with a presumptive diagnosis of chronic periodontitis are a reduction of probe depths by 1 to 2 mm and of disease activity as reduction or resolution of inflammation and bleeding on probing. Evaluation for surgery is indicated when advanced bone loss and attachment loss are present. If nonresponse is discovered, evaluation of the site/case is imperative. Nonresponse in sites that were difficult to treat does not necessarily indicate an aggressive form of disease. The final diagnosis can be determined by retreating the area and scheduling another reevaluation visit or PMP appointment. If signs of disease activity exist around a tooth with Class 1+ mobility or fremitus (see Chapter 3), occlusal adjustment is indicated (Kornman & Wilson, 1992). If mobility continues to advance at subsequent visits further occlusal adjustment, habit appliances, splinting, or a combination are considered. When reevaluation reveals a more aggressive form of the disease, microbial analysis is a diagnostic consideration.

The inclusion of reevaluation in a care plan is dependent on the following factors assessed during initial therapy:

1. gingival inflammation,
2. bleeding on probing,
3. depth, number, and location of periodontal pockets,
4. expected client response to oral self-care, recommendations, and
5. the presumptive diagnosis.

Clients with suspected or confirmed aggressive forms will always need reevaluation. Those with early chronic periodontitis with localized pockets of 4 mm might not be indicated for reevaluation if other risk factors are not identified. If poor compliance with self-care or PMP is expected, however, the reevaluation visit may serve to motivate the client toward continuing care. The addition of any risk factors such as smoking or diabetes increases the need for reevaluation for further education and motivation. If a reevaluation visit is not scheduled, the outcome of NSPT must be measured against the treatment goals at the final visit of initial therapy. This is not ideal because an appropriate four to six week interval for healing is not considered. Evaluation of goals creates a need for the clinician to revisit the decision-making process related to dental hygiene care. The reader is referred to *Dental Hygiene Process: Diagnosis and Care Planning* (Mueller-Joseph & Petersen, 1995) for further information about dental hygiene diagnosis.

## Care Plan Documentation

There are many variations of planning forms; those that are a brief document or very detailed ones. Some forms provide areas to write and describe the planned treatment, and others employ a checklist form (see Figures 6-2, 6-3, and 6-4). The plan, regardless of the format, should include: 1) the procedures or course of action to be rendered, 2) the appointment sequence or the order in which the treatment will be given, 3) the approximate time for each procedure or total time for each appointment, and 4) the key factors to consider when developing the care plan (Wood, 1985; Woodall, 1993). Forms need to be easy to use and understand. Practicing dental hygienists will likely work with forms provided by the private dental office or other practice facilities, however, they may develop their own forms suitable to the practice philosophies and setting.

Darby & Walsh (1994) suggest that the care plan format "should provide the dental hygienist with an opportunity to document assessment findings, dental hygiene diagnoses, client-centered goals, dental hygiene interventions, evaluative outcomes anticipated from treatment, and the expected date of goal attainment" (p. 423). The actual planning and time allotment for the appointment sessions are similar between dental hygiene students and practicing dental hygienists. The only real difference may be that dental hygiene students, due to their lack of experience, will take longer to complete treatment procedures and may have unrealistic expectations about the amount of time needed.

Care plans should be written to provide permanent documentation and are considered an integral part of the client's file. As discussed in Chapter 19 of this text, recordings should be clear, concise, legible, and able to withstand legal scrutiny. Failing to plan treatment can potentially become a legal quality assurance problem (Ursu, 1992). Any changes to the initial dental hygiene care plan presented to the client should be documented; and should clearly and objectively reflect facts, not clinician biases or subjective interpretation of clients' motives (Betta, 1993; Greenlaw, 1992; Iyer, 1991). Client input into the design of the plan is essential. The importance of motivation, communication (see Chapter 7), and client compliance in NSPT (see Chapter 8), are crucial for success. The client's autonomy should be respected and clients should be partners or cotherapists in treatment (Barrows & Pickell, 1991; Canadian Dental Association, 1989; Wood, 1985). Examples of questions that need to be discussed with clients during development of the plan and before initiation of dental hygiene therapy are as follows:

1. How does the client feel about returning for several appointments?
2. Does the client prefer long or short appointments?
3. Should the appointments be close together or a week or two apart?
4. What are the scheduling concerns of both the client and the dental hygienist?
5. What is the expense?
6. What are the discomforts or side effects of treatment?

Some of these questions will also be reviewed with the client again during case presentation and acquiring of informed consent (see Chapter 8).

CLIENT NAME _____  DATE _____  CLINICIAN NAME _____

| ASSESSMENT | Minutes Per Appointment | | | | | | | |
|---|---|---|---|---|---|---|---|---|
| | Appt. 1 | Appt. 2 | Appt. 3 | Appt. 4 | Appt. 5 | Appt. 6 | Appt. 7 | Appt. 8 |
| Health History | | | | | | | | |
| Intra- and Extraoral Exam | | | | | | | | |
| Dental Charting | | | | | | | | |
| Perio Exam and Charting | | | | | | | | |
| Indices | | | | | | | | |
| Radiographs, Type | | | | | | | | |
| **DISEASE PREVENTION** | | | | | | | | |
| Brushing Techniques | | | | | | | | |
| Interdental Aids | | | | | | | | |
| Periodontal Disease | | | | | | | | |
| Dental Decay | | | | | | | | |
| Tobacco Use | | | | | | | | |
| Nutritional Education | | | | | | | | |
| Fluoride Therapy | | | | | | | | |
| Blood Pressure | | | | | | | | |
| Other | | | | | | | | |
| **TREATMENT PROCEDURES** | | | | | | | | |
| Anesthesia | | | | | | | | |
| Ultrasonic Debridement Quadrant (Q) | | | | | | | | |
| Sextant (S) | | | | | | | | |
| Hand-Activated Debridement Quadrant (Q) | | | | | | | | |
| Sextant (S) | | | | | | | | |
| Subgingival Irrigation | | | | | | | | |
| Selective Polishing | | | | | | | | |
| Fluoride Treatment | | | | | | | | |
| Desensitization | | | | | | | | |
| Margination | | | | | | | | |
| Amalgam Polishing | | | | | | | | |
| Other | | | | | | | | |
| Total Appointment Time | | | | | | | | |
| Recare Interval | | | | | | | | |
| Referral(s) | | | | | | | | |

Q1 = Quadrant    Q2 = Quadrant    Q3 = Quadrant    Q4 = Quadrant

## GOALS

Treatment goals
1
2
3

Client Goals
1
2
3

## ORAL SELF-CARE

CURRENT ORAL SELF-CARE METHODS

| Recommendations | Variable Diameter Floss | Mounted Toothpick |
|---|---|---|
| Brush | | Wooden Wedge |
| Specialty Brush | Dental Tape/Floss | Rubber Tip |
| Interdental Brush | Floss Threader/Aid | Other |

REAPPOINTMENT UPDATES

| 2 Updated: | Changes: |
|---|---|
| 3 Updated: | Changes: |
| 4 Updated: | Changes: |
| 5 Updated: | Changes: |
| 6 Updated: | Changes: |
| 7 Updated: | Changes: |
| 8 Updated: | Changes: |

**Figure 6-2** Care planning: Checklist format. (Adapted with permission from Idaho State University, Department of Dental Hygiene, Pocatello, Idaho, 1995)

**PROBLEM ORIENTED CARE PLAN FOR DENTAL HYGIENE SERVICES**

Periodontal Classification: _____

Instructor Signature: _____

APPROVAL TO PROCEED:

[     ]   D.D.S./D.M.D. Examination

[     ]   Radiographs – Specify_____

[     ]   Dental Hygiene Problem Oriented
          Treatment Plan and Services

DDS/DMD: _____

Date: _____

Patient's Name: _____

Patient's Number: _____

Student's Name: _____

Date: _____

Treatment Plan Phase I:

Approval: _____

**OVERALL GOAL FOR PATIENT:**

| PROBLEM OR GOAL | APPT # | TIME | COURSE OF ACTION | REVISIONS | Patient Initials | Instr. Initials |
|---|---|---|---|---|---|---|
|  |  |  |  |  |  |  |

SUGGESTED REFERRALS
TO DDS/DMD OR SPECIALIST

TO BE MONITORED BY DH

ENTIRE PREVENTIVE TREATMENT PLAN DISCUSSED AND APPROVED BY PATIENT

DATE: _____   PATIENT'S SIGNATURE: _____

**Figure 6-3** Care planning: Descriptive format. (Adapted with permission from Camosum College, Dental Hygiene Program, Victoria, British Columbia, 1996)

Needless to say, the client's participation in the development of the plan is an essential element in meeting treatment goals. Clients are selective in their choice and frequency of dental services (Edgington, 1994), which also includes dental hygiene care; therefore, they must understand the nature of periodontal disease, what causes it, how it can be treated, and how recurrence can be prevented (Pattison & Pattison, 1992). In addition, third-party payers (e.g., insurance companies, government programs) are becoming increasingly involved, exercis-

Client_____　Student _____

| A. ASSESSMENT | DATE | DDS | RDH |
|---|---|---|---|
| Medical and Dental History | | | |
| Soft Tissue Inspection (STI) | | | |
| Dentogram | | | |
| Indices (at onset of care) | | | |
| Radiographic Interpretation | | | |
| Impressions | | | |
| **B. PLANNING** | **DATE** | **DDS** | **RDH** |
| Identifying Goals | | | |
| Oral Self-Care Plan | | | |
| Treatment Plan | | | |
| **C. IMPLEMENTATION** | **DATE** | **DDS** | **RDH** |
| Initial Oral Self-Care Delivery | | | |
| Debridement Completed | | | |
| Selective Polish | | | |
| Fluoride Treatment | | | |
| Amalgam Polish | | | |
| Pit and Fissure Sealants | | | |
| Desensitizing | | | |
| Subgingival Irrigation | | | |
| **D. EVALUATION** | **DATE** | **DDS** | **RDH** |
| Follow up Oral Self-Care | | | |
| Indices (Post Care) | | | |
| Pockets (Post Care) | | | |
| Evaluation of Care | | | |

**Figure 6-4** Care planning: Combination format. (Adapted with permission from George Brown College, Dental Department, Toronto, Ontario, 1995)

ing control over care rendered to clients, and can be considered as making treatment decisions (Hogue, 1990). Insurance coverage and financial issues are presently an economic concern, as those procedures not covered by third parties become the responsibility of the client. Thus, it is unfortunate that insurance coverage may dictate the treatment choices of the client. It is incumbent upon the dental hygiene professional to recommend necessary care and to explain consequences of less than ideal treatment.

# SELECTION OF MECHANICAL ORAL SELF-CARE DEVICES

A central theme of any NSPT care plan is control of bacterial plaque. Inherent in its control is the clinician's ability to recommend the best aids, and client compliance with self-care practices. The dental hygienist assumes the responsibility of selecting the best self-care aids based on three factors: 1) client needs and desires, 2) oral conditions, and 3) dexterity. This approach allows dental hygienists to choose devices and techniques that will maximize client compliance and that are appropriate for the periodontal condition. This section will include the most important plaque control device, the toothbrush, as well as various interdental aids including dental floss, flossholders, toothpicks, rubber tip stimulators, and interdental brushes. Compliance with an aid that is not effective for that particular person is of little value in reaching the established goals of NSPT.

## Toothbrushes

The toothbrush serves to improve gingival health; however, it has limited therapeutic effects on other aspects of periodontal health (AAP, 1991). The type of toothbrush recommended should be based on the client's individual requirements. Three factors should be taken into consideration when recommending a toothbrush: type, size, and bristle features (Grant, Stern, & Listgarten, 1988). Brushes are available in manual or powered designs. There is a multitude of manual toothbrushes available to the consumer. As with toothbrushing methods, there is a lack of long-term scientific studies to substantiate the selection of one manual brush over another. In the majority of situations the manual brush will be adequate for the needs of the client, although there may be instances where a **powered toothbrush** is recommended. Powered brushes are particularly useful for cases where the manual brush is not achieving the desired result. Recent designs have different brushing motions than the traditional powered models. A counter-rotational brush (Interplak) has tufts that rotate independently and it is used with its own brand of dentifrice. The reciprocal rotating brush (Braun Oral-B Plaque Remover) has cup-shaped bristles and a round head that can be used with commercial toothpastes. An electronic toothbrush (Sonicare) operates by low-frequency acoustic energy targeted at altering bacterial adherence to help control periodontal diseases. Studies evaluating mechanical toothbrush devices have demonstrated improvement in plaque control, deeper subgingival cleansing, less gingival bleeding, and delivery of antimicrobials further subgingivally when compared to manual toothbrushing (AAP, 1991). Some of the newer powered brush designs are recommended for the client with periodontal disease or other special periodontal needs such as Class II or Class III furcations, fixed appliances, or delayed post-surgical healing (Bowen, 1994). Other situations where a powered brush may be chosen are for the noncompli-

ant and gadget-oriented individual, or the client with physical or mental disabilities. Several recent powered toothbrush designs have a built-in timer which informs the users (by a flashing light or automatic turnoff) when the appropriate brushing time has been completed. This is particularly useful to guide the client to brush for the desired length of time.

An important factor to keep in mind is the size and shape of the head of the brush. The brush should be small enough to be accessible to all areas of the mouth but at the same time large enough to cover several teeth (Grant, Stern, & Listgarten, 1988). A client with a small dental arch may require a compact or petite size adult brush or even a child-sized toothbrush. Therefore, the dental hygienist should have a variety of sizes of toothbrushes available to select the type best suited for each client. Currently, the most common toothbrush design is a flat-bristled brush. However, there is a growing number of toothbrushes on the market that advertise improved and advanced plaque removing ability with a ripple design intended to increase interproximal cleaning. Although several short-term studies show improved plaque removal results with this design, there is limited long-term data to substantiate these findings.

Currently, the majority of dental hygienists recommend a soft toothbrush bristle texture for their clients (Woodall, 1993). Many toothbrush manufacturers are providing consumers with the choice of soft and ultra soft bristle firmness. The ultrasoft bristles are frequently recommended for: 1) fragile gingival tissue and embrasure sensitivity, 2) the interim healing period following surgery (Grant, Stern, & Listgarten, 1988), or 3) limiting the amount of gingival trauma due to aggressive toothbrushing.

Recent research indicates that there are no significant differences between toothbrushing methods (Perry & Schmid, 1996). Although most clinicians have their preferred methods, what must be taken into consideration is the extent of disease (or health) and the present brushing technique and habits of the client. Clients often experience frustration and confusion when they perceive mixed messages by different clinicians regarding appropriate techniques. Therefore, standardization of philosophy within a practice is beneficial for clients. An important concept to remember is not to change a toothbrushing method if the client is performing one of the acceptable brushing techniques, is thoroughly cleaning all tooth surfaces, and is not causing tissue trauma. Additionally, the relationship of plaque accumulation to gingival inflammation and periodontal pocketing should be considered. If plaque is present with no clinical signs of disease than perhaps the method is effective enough to reduce the critical mass of plaque to the level that compliments the host response. The method most commonly taught and favored by dental hygienists is the Modified Bass technique. The roll method seems to be the least effective. For any method to be effective the sequence and duration of brushing must be satisfactory. Table 6-4

**Table 6-4  Mechanical Oral Hygiene Aids**

| Aid | Designed for Clients With | Directions for Use |
|---|---|---|
| Toothbrushing<br>Modified Bass<br>Technique | • excellent plaque control and gingival stimulation<br>• sulcular removal of bacterial plaque<br>• periodontal health or disease | ***Posterior and Anterior Facial***<br>1. Place the bristles against the gingival margin at a 45° angle to the long axis of the tooth.<br>2. Press gently so the bristles enter the gingival sulcus, and the gingiva blanches.<br>3. Vibrate the brush with a short back and forth motion for 10 seconds (strokes).<br>4. Activate a rolling stroke over the teeth toward the occlusal surface.<br>5. Replace by overlapping the previous area, and repeat steps.<br>***Anterior Lingual Surfaces***<br>1. Place the toothbrush with the handle parallel to the long axis of the tooth (vertically).<br>2. The vibratory motion is changed to a short up and down stroke with the toe (or heel) of the brush bristles.<br>***Occlusal Surfaces***<br>1. Place enough pressure on the brush bristles to penetrate into the pits and fissures. |
| Dental Floss/Tape<br>• waxed<br>• unwaxed<br>• polyetrafluoroethylene floss/tape (PTFE) | • Type I embrasures<br>• gingivitis with minimal gingival recession or evidence of periodontal pockets (floss becomes less effective as interproximal recession progresses) | 1. Select a piece of floss 12 to 18 inches in length.<br>2. Hold floss securely between fingers, tie the ends together in a loop, or wrap around fingers.<br>3. Hold taut and use 1/2-inch segment.<br>4. Insert floss between contacts, ease it through in a "seesaw" motion.<br>5. Wrap floss around tooth (in "C" shape), move it down to the base of the sulcus.<br>6. Repeat the step up and down movement six times.<br>7. Clean adjacent tooth in same manner.<br>8. Gently remove from contact.<br>9. Change segment used periodically. |
| Variable Diameter Floss<br>(Superfloss, Johnson & Johnson) | • large interproximal spaces or Types II embrasures<br>• distal surfaces of most posterior teeth<br>• mesial and distal abutments and pontics of fixed and removal; prosthesis (implants)<br>• orthodontic appliances | Variable diameter floss has three sections:<br>1. A stiffened end to be used as a floss threader between tight contacts or under fixed bridges.<br>2. Tufted area to use around pontics or abutments and orthodontic bands.<br>3. Section of regular floss to use in interproximal areas. |
| Floss Holder<br>(Butler, E-Z Floss) | • lack of manual dexterity<br>• large hands/small mouth<br>• need for motivation<br>• caregivers | 1. Place floss in holder.<br>2. Ease through the contact and pull mesially or push distally to wrap the floss (in a "C" shape) around the tooth.<br>3. Move down to the base of the sulcus (up and down six times).<br>4. Ease from the contact area. |
| Mounted toothpick or Toothpick in a Holder (Interdental Handle, Oral-B Laboratories; Perio-Aid, Marquis Dental Manufacturing) | • interproximal spaces with Type II embrasures<br>• periodontal pockets<br>• accessible furcation areas<br>• poor compliance/refusal to use floss<br>• current use of toothpicks | 1. Insert a tapered rounded toothpick in the toothpick handle and fasten securely.<br>2. Moisten the end with saliva.<br>3. Place the toothpick at a 45° angle with the tooth surface and insert subgingivally.<br>4. Angle into root concavities and around convex surfaces.<br>5. Do not point into the epithelial attachment. |

**Table 6-4 (continued)**

| Aid | Designed for Clients with | Directions for Use |
|---|---|---|
| Interdental Toothpicks or Wooden Wedges (Stim-u-dent Wedge, Johnson & Johnson; Orapik and Dental Pik, Dental Concepts, Inc.) | *Thin Variation (circular toothpick)*<br>• interproximal spaces with Type II embrasures<br>• shallow periodontal pocket/normal sulcus depth<br>• furcation areas<br>• poor compliance/refusal to floss<br>*Triangular Wedge*<br>• areas of moderate papillary recession (Type II embrasures)<br>• gingival stimulation<br>• who prefer over floss<br>• supragingival removal only | *Thin Variation Toothpick*<br>1. Technique is similar for the use of the toothpick in a holder.<br>*Wedge Variation Toothpick*<br>1. Base of wedge is placed interproximally and tipped slightly occlusally or incisely to follow the contours of the embrasure space.<br>2. Move gently back and forth from facial to lingual in short motions. |
| Interdental Brushes (conical or tapered) (John O. Butler, Oral-B Laboratories) | • large interproximal areas with moderate papillary recession or Type II or III embrasures<br>• exposed furcation areas<br>• difficult access areas<br>• post periodontal surgery<br>• fixed dental appliances | 1. Select brush size that is larger than the focus areas.<br>2. Place the brush interproximally.<br>3. Angle the brush to follow the contour of the gingival form.<br>4. Short back and forth strokes (3 to 4 times). |
| End Tuft Brush (available in tapered or flat head) (John O. Butler, Oral-B Laboratories) | • hard to reach posterior areas<br>• malaligned teeth<br>• areas with Type III embrasure spaces<br>• lingual areas (often these areas are less thoroughly brushed by clients)<br>• fixed dental appliances | 1. Place the brush along the gingival margin.<br>2. Activate the brush by using small rotating motions or sulcular brushing stroke. |
| Rubber Tip Stimulator (John O. Butler, Oral-B Laboratories) | • the need of reshaping and massaging the soft tissue:<br>  – following periodontal surgery<br>  – edematous and bulbous areas<br>  – sensitive areas<br>  – hard to reach areas<br>• moderate to severe gingivitis | 1. Place the tip interproximally, directed occlusally or incisally to follow the contours of the interproximal gingiva.<br>2. Press gently against the gingiva and move the tip in small rotary or back and forth motions.<br>3. For marginal gingiva, direct slightly apically and follow the contour of the gingiva. |

reviews the procedure for performing the Modified Bass technique and summarizes appropriate use of interdental aids.

## Interdental Cleaning Devices

Toothbrushes are not able to reach the proximal surfaces of teeth; therefore, it is necessary to use interdental cleaning devices. The most popular and most frequently recommended interdental cleaning device is dental floss, despite the fact that client compliance with this aid is low and it is only effective in areas with normal gingival contour and embrasures (see Table 6-4). When clients who have previously received periodontal treatment used various aids, it was found that an interdental brush used with a toothbrush is more effective in removing plaque from proximal surfaces than a toothbrush used alone or with dental floss (Kiger, Nylund, & Feller, 1991). Figure 6-5 illustrates the use of floss and an interdental brush on proximal surfaces. The Consensus of the Discussion Session on Nonsurgical Periodontal Treatment (AAP, 1989) stated that interproximal brushes are the superior interdental aid when space exists for their use and that mounted toothpicks are effective at specific sites.

Types of embrasure spaces (Perry & Schmid, 1996) are critical to analyze because they provide the clinician with the best information about potential effectiveness of an interdental aid. Type I embrasures are occupied by the interdental papilla, therefore, floss is recommended. Type II embrasures display slight to moderate degrees of recession where the interdental brush (see Figure 6-6) or wooden toothpicks are effective. Wooden mechanical plaque removal devices include toothpicks and balsa wedges. Wooden toothpicks have been shown to perform subgingival plaque removal 2 to 3 millimeters subgingivally (Morch & Waerhang, 1956). Balsa wedges are useful for supragingival plaque removal (see Figure 6-7). Type III embrasures have extensive recession or complete

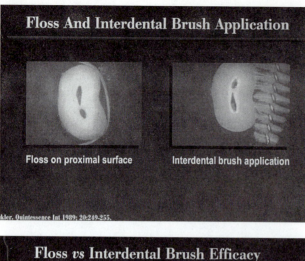

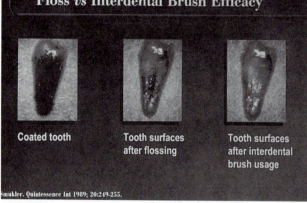

**Figure 6-5** The use of floss versus interdental brushes. (Courtesy of Smukler, H., et al. *Interproximal tooth morphology and its affect on plaque removal.* Chicago: Quintessence Publishing Co., Inc., 20:249–255, 1989)

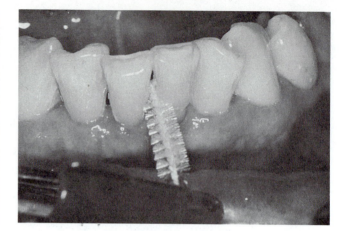

**Figure 6-6** Interdental brush adapted to a Type II embrasure space. (Courtesy of Oral-B Laboratories)

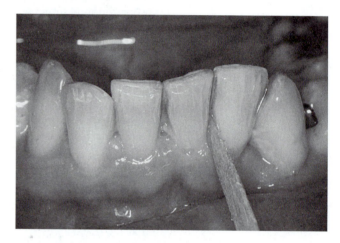

**Figure 6-7** Wooden wedge adapted to a Type II embrasure space. (Courtesy of Oral-B Laboratories)

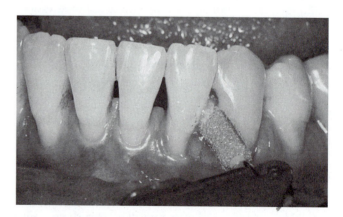

**Figure 6-8** Soft tip interdental brush adapted to a Type III embrasure space. The soft tip is recommended for clients with root sensitivity or for site-specific delivery of antimicrobials. (Courtesy of Oral-B Laboratories)

loss of papilla and the unitufted brush or other interdental brushes are recommended (see Figure 6-8). Interdental brushes are also useful for root concavities and furcations as are mounted toothpicks (see Figure 6-9).

Floss adjuncts or aids include floss holders, floss handles, and flexible (variation in diameter) filament floss (see Figure 6-10). The latter is effective in Type II embrasures due to the large diameter of a portion of the floss. The end-tuft toothbrushes, because of their small head, are effective devices not only for Type II and III embrasure spaces, but also for hard to reach and hard to clean areas (see Figure 6-11). These difficult areas include malaligned or crowded teeth, lingual areas especially the mandibular anterior teeth, the distals of the last teeth in each arch, furcations, crown and bridge areas (pontics), and around fixed orthodontic appliances. Rubber tips, sometimes referred to as rubber tip stimulators, can be used for limited plaque removal, but are generally used for gingival contouring after periodontal surgery and gingival massage (see Figure 6-12). In fact, they are contraindicated for use when tissues are healthy and when contour is normal.

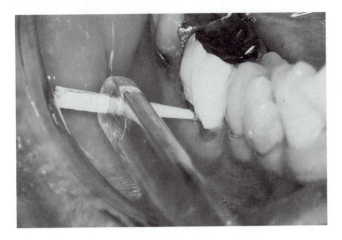

**Figure 6-9** Mounted toothpick in an exposed furcation. (Courtesy of Oral-B Laboratories)

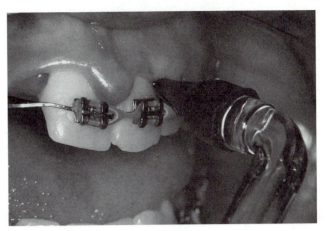

**Figure 6-12** A rubber tip stimulator for gingival massage around fixed orthodontic appliances. (Courtesy of Oral-B Laboratories)

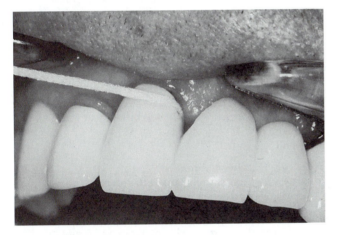

**Figure 6-10** Variable diameter floss in a Type II embrasure space. (Courtesy of Oral-B Laboratories)

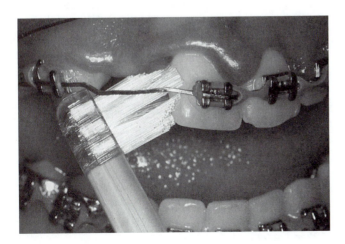

**Figure 6-11** End-tuft brush for an inaccessible area around fixed orthodontic appliances. (Courtesy of Oral-B Laboratories)

Due to the fact that clients have individual needs based on dexterity, their ability to remove plaque, and their oral conditions that may inhibit plaque removal (e.g., furcations, fixed orthodontic appliances, pontics, embrasure spaces, etc.), it is necessary for the dental hygienist to be knowledgeable of oral self-care adjuncts available for meeting the client's oral care needs. A practice philosophy about recommending interdental aids is useful for enhancing practitioner knowledge and reducing client frustration with aids. Factors to consider when developing a philosophy include the indications and contraindications for use of various interproximal aids as well as the following:

1. If the interproximal aid being used is effective in plaque reduction and maintaining health, modification is not necessary.
2. One aid used well is preferred over two aids, even if the same effectiveness could be achieved.
3. If two aids are equally effective for the periodontal conditions, then rely on the client to choose the one that will best fit into the daily care routine.
4. When different conditions in the mouth ideally warrant more than one aid, make choices based on client preference and adherence. If the client is noncompliant, one aid must be selected first to reach the majority of areas or to treat the most involved sites. When the client complies with use of the first aid, consider whether to introduce a second aid remembering that the more aids one uses the less likely the follow through.
5. If a client will not use the most appropriate aid, select the next best aid or the one he will use. Any aid used routinely is better than no aid at all, unless it is harmful to the tissues.
6. If a client is using an aid routinely but it is not effective for the conditions, discuss with the client the rationale for another aid based on its design

and recent research findings. Recommending a different aid is necessary if the client's chosen aid is ineffective. Most of the time the person is unaware that another aid is more appropriate.

7. Neither floss nor the toothpick are effective in removing subgingival plaque from deep periodontal pockets. The client needs to be aware that frequent NSPT and PMP, and/or possibly surgical correction, are necessary for maintenance of the periodontal health.

## APPLICATION OF PLANNING TO NONSURGICAL CARE

Three case scenarios follow accompanied by sample care plans. The format of each case will consider the client's goal(s), assessment findings, courses of actions, sequencing, timing, and other factors associated with dental hygiene therapy. Alterations in the suggested plans would be indicated if the profile of the client changed. For example, the need for antibiotic prophylaxis may warrant an adjustment in the length of appointments and maintenance interval. Another example is a history of high blood pressure requiring monitoring at each appointment. In this case, the professional allocates a few extra minutes per appointment for this procedure. Selection of a local anesthetic and chair positioning would also be considerations. The client who smokes will require time for discussion of the relationship of smoking to oral health and for instructions in oral cancer self-examination.

Encountering more difficulty than originally anticipated due to tenacious calculus or other hindrances with instrumentation may require further changes in care plans. Tissues not responding to dental hygiene therapy demand additional treatment beyond what was anticipated during the assessment phase of care. Clients' nonclinical needs are important as dental hygienists encounter individuals who are talkative, require more verbal explanations, and require reassurance about their dental hygiene therapy. It must be remembered that the plan is a guide that changes or alters from appointment to appointment. The appointment time necessary for care varies based on intraoral conditions, client nonclinical needs, phase of care (active or maintenance), degree of difficulty of periodontal debridement, and indicated supportive care. Typically, sixty- or ninety-minute intervals are scheduled depending on if the client is new to the practice or a client of record and the number, extent, and types of services included in the care plan.

### Case One

Mrs. Johnson, age 55, has a past history of seeking dental care only when she needs immediate attention for pain. In her words "it has been a while since she has been to the dentist." Mrs. Johnson is now experiencing pain from a fractured restoration. During the dental appointment for replacement of the restoration, the dentist discusses the need for dental hygiene treatment with Mrs. Johnson. It is explained to her that the dental hygiene care cannot be accomplished in one appointment, but instead may take several sessions with the dental hygienist. Mrs. Johnson agrees to commence dental hygiene care. How would you proceed if you were the dental hygienist?

**Assessment and Diagnosis.** Philosophies of dental offices vary as to whether the dental hygienist or dentist sees the client on the initial visit for the periodontal assessment. In this scenario, it is the dental hygienist who will assess the periodontal condition and formulate the dental hygiene diagnosis. Table 6-5 outlines the assessment findings. The first appointment for assessment is usually scheduled for 60 to 90 minutes. During this appointment, periodontal charting including full mouth probing and bleeding points are recorded with or without the assistance of a dental assistant. In this case, the client has not been maintained in a dental office for a considerable

---

**Table 6-5  Case One: Assessment Findings**

*Health History*
- no contraindications to treatment
- digital arthritis
- high blood pressure controlled by medication
- smoker
- age 55

*Intra- and Extraoral Exam*
- oral cancer screening exam performed: no abnormalities detected

*Periodontal and Gingival Assessment*
- probe depths are generalized, 4 mm and 5 mm in quadrants 2 and 3
- slight recession is generalized, client has moderate sensitivity to cold air in quadrant 1
- Type II embrasure spaces
- clinical attachment level ranges from 4 to 6 mm
- vertical bitewings show horizontal bone loss and overhanging restorations on #14 distal, #19 mesial
- bleeding points are generalized
- tissue is shiny, spongy, swollen, red
- heavy cervical plaque
- heavy supragingival calculus is found on buccal surfaces of maxillary molars and on lingual and facial surfaces of mandibular anteriors, subgingival moderate calculus and plaque are generalized

*Oral Care Habits/Compliance History*
- client brushes twice a day with a soft tooth brush using the horizontal scrub technique
- flosses infrequently, when "something gets caught"
- client has limited dexterity due to arthritis
- Oral Hygiene Index-Simplified (OHI-S) score = 4

*Other Factors*
- motivation: perceives treatment as something she must do
- financial concerns: covered by dental insurance (80%)

length of time, and therefore, diagnostic radiographs are probably indicated. Radiographs will be valuable for providing comprehensive assessment for NSPT as well as for formulating the periodontal disease diagnosis. The decision to expose a full-mouth series or vertical bite-wings depends on the individual needs of the client.

Other assessment procedures that should be considered are plaque, bleeding, or gingival indices. Additional factors such as dexterity, motivation, financial status, and time concerns should also be evaluated in this phase. After the priorities and dental hygiene diagnosis are established the treatment goals are determined. The periodontal disease diagnosis is based on the classification system presented in Chapter 1. Based on the case description and assessment findings, the presumptive diagnosis is chronic adult periodontitis. The extent of the condition appears to be "moderate" based on the clinical attachment level measurements. The dental hygiene diagnosis is dependent on the needs assessment which has not been formally conducted in this example. The goals are outlined in the following list.

1. To reduce pocket depth.
2. To eliminate signs of inflammation.
3. To remove plaque and calculus deposit.
4. To remove overhanging restorations.
5. To evaluate client's oral care techniques.
   – reinforce proper techniques
   – determine need of other oral care adjuncts
6. To reduce or stop client's smoking.
7. To motivate client to maintain dental/dental hygiene care

**Selection of Self-Care Devices.** During all appointments, reinforcement of oral care was provided through the use of Oral Hygiene Index-Simplified (OHI-S) plaque index and through the review of toothbrushing technique. The utilization of a mounted toothpick was recommended and demonstrated during appointment three. Mrs. Johnson will try to incorporate this aid into her daily routine despite her arthritis. She commented that it should be easier than flossing and appreciated being informed of the alternative aid. At the last appointment the client was asked if she had any questions or concerns regarding the oral self-care devices. Fluoride therapy and the process of decay were explained during appointment two and three as several areas with recession were sensitive and the exposed cementum may be more susceptible to root caries. Throughout the series of appointments gingivitis and periodontitis are discussed. It is also important that the client is acknowledged for her attempt to quit smoking and for the improved index score.

**Approach to Debridement.** In the past, a variety of sequences for periodontal instrumentation have been advocated such as: 1) ultrasonic scaling or gross scaling the entire mouth to remove ledges of calculus followed with fine scaling and root planing on subsequent appoint-

ments; 2) treating one side of the mouth, either left or right, on the first appointment and then the other side on the second appointment; and 3) arch treatment, that is, treating either the maxillary or mandibular before proceeding to the other arch. Polishing and fluoride were often reserved for the final appointment after scaling and root planing were completed. Each of these sequences have their advantages and disadvantages. For example, the advantage of "gross" scaling either with hand or ultrasonic/sonic instruments is to remove heavy supragingival ledges of calculus that may interfere with probing assessment, client oral self-care, or esthetics (Pattison & Pattison, 1992). The disadvantages are thought to outweigh the advantages, as three major problems may occur. First, incomplete calculus removal may cause an abscess. Second, complete calculus removal may not be attained due to tissue shrinkage. And third, clients may feel that their teeth were "cleaned" and there is no need for further treatment (Nield-Gehrig & Houseman, 1996; Pattison & Pattison, 1992).

The accepted approach is a therapy regime that includes segmental NSPT where each quadrant or sextant is completed before progressing to other areas (Pattison & Pattison, 1992; Woodall, 1993; Wilkins, 1994). Thoroughness, accomplished by scaling and root planing (debridement) is considered a determinant of successful nonsurgical dental hygiene therapy (Page, 1993). Anesthesia is indicated in deep periodontal pockets that harbor plaque-retentive calculus (see Chapter 9). It is through the use of local anesthesia that the dental hygienist is able to render high-quality treatment with less patient discomfort (Woodall, 1993). Other benefits of segmental debridement is the ability to compare treated with untreated areas and to evaluate the clients self-care effectiveness. Furthermore, the client is able to condition the areas not yet treated, through improved self-care techniques. Also the localization of discomfort or sensitivity to one area permits the client to chew adequately on the other side of the mouth. For further information regarding implementation of dental hygiene therapy refer to Chapters 9 through 14 of this text. The decision as to where to begin the segmental approach should be a mutual decision between the client and the dental hygienist. The area with the most destruction or sensitivity may be treated first, or this area may be treated at a subsequent appointment or even at the last visit to permit the client to ease into treatment and to build confidence in the treatment.

As outlined in Figure 6-13, Mrs. Johnson's dental hygiene therapy was planned for a series of ninety-minute appointments to ensure thoroughness. Time was allocated for evaluation of previously treated areas through periodontal assessment. The OHI-S index was chosen due to its ease and efficiency. This index was used at each appointment to reinforce plaque control and motivate the client. The use of subgingival irrigation and other adjunctive chemotherapeutic procedures were not considered in this case.

CLIENT NAME _____  DATE _____  CLINICIAN NAME _____

| ASSESSMENT | Appt. 1 | Appt. 2 | Appt. 3 | Appt. 4 | Appt. 5 | Appt. 6 | Appt. 7 | Appt. 8 |
|---|---|---|---|---|---|---|---|---|
| | | | | Minutes Per Appointment | | | | |
| Health History | 5 | 2 | 2 | 2 | 2 | 2 | | |
| Intra- and Extraoral Exam | 5 | 2 | 2 | 2 | 2 | 2 | | |
| Dental Charting | 10 | | | | | | | |
| Perio Exam and Charting | 20 | 3 | 2 | 2 | 2 | 10 | | |
| Indices | 5 | 5 | 5 | 5 | 5 | 5 | | |
| Radiographs, Type *Vert. BWX* | 10 | | | | | | | |
| **DISEASE PREVENTION** | | | | | | | | |
| Brushing Techniques | 5 | 3 | 1 | 1 | 2 | 2 | | |
| Interdental Aids | | | 5 | 3 | 2 | 2 | | |
| Periodontal Disease | 5 | 4 | 2 | 2 | 2 | 2 | | |
| Dental Decay | | 3 | 5 | | | 1 | | |
| Tobacco Use | 5 | 3 | 2 | 1 | | | | |
| Nutritional Education | | | | | | | | |
| Fluoride Therapy | | 2 | 1 | | | | | |
| Blood Pressure | 5 | | | | | | | |
| Other | | | | | | | | |
| **TREATMENT PROCEDURES** | | | | | | | | |
| Anesthesia | | Q1 15 | Q2 15 | Q3 8 | Q4 8 | | | |
| Ultrasonic Debridement Quadrant (Q) | Q1 30 | Q2 30 | Q3 35 | Q4 35 | 10 | | | |
| Sextant (S) | | | | | | | | |
| Hand-Activated Debridement Quadrant (Q) | Q1 10 | Q2 10 | Q3 10 | Q4 10 | | | | |
| Sextant (S) | | | | | | | | |
| Subgingival Irrigation | | | | | | | | |
| Selective Polishing | | | | | 5 | | | |
| Fluoride Treatment | | | | | 3 | | | |
| Desensitization | | 3 | 3 | 3 | 3 | 3 | | |
| Margination | | | #14-10 | #19-10 | | | | |
| Amalgam Polishing | | | | | | | | |
| Other | | | | | | | | |
| Total Appointment Time | 75 | 85 | 93 | 85 | 82 | 37 | | |
| Recare Interval | 3 months | | | | | | | |
| Referral(s) | none | | | | | | | |

Q1 = Quadrant   Q2 = Quadrant   Q3 = Quadrant   Q4 = Quadrant

---

**GOALS**

Treatment goals
1 Reduce pocket depth/Reduce bleeding
2 Improve interproximal care and brushing technique
3 Reduce smoking

Client Goals
1 Quit smoking
2 Repair broken and rough fillings
3 Reduce bleeding

**ORAL SELF-CARE**

CURRENT ORAL SELF-CARE METHODS
toothbrushing 2x/day, soft brush, horizontal scrub
flosses infrequently

| Recommendations | | Variable Diameter Floss | |
|---|---|---|---|
| Brush (Powered) | ✓ | Dental Tape/Floss | |
| Specialty Brush | | Floss Threader/Aid | |
| Interdental Brush | | Mounted Toothpick | ✓ |
| | | Wooden Wedge | |
| | | Rubber Tip | |
| | | Other | |

**REAPPOINTMENT UPDATES**

2 Updated: *September 1/95*   Changes: *OHI-S 3.5*
*bleeding less in mandibular anterior*

3 Updated: *September 8/95*   Changes: *OHI-S 2.9*
*client reports difficulty with mounted toothpick*

4 Updated: *September 15/95*   Changes: *OHI-S 2.7*
*gingiva less red and edematous, client reports smoking reduced, client reports toothpick is helpful*

5 Updated: *October 5/95*   Changes: *OHI-S 3.7*
*Client away on vacation, interdental plaque removal is not regular, smoking increased*

6 Updated: *November 5/95*   Changes: *OHI-S 2.5*
*gingival color and contour improved, reduced bleeding, slight bleeding in posteriors, using toothpick daily, smoking reduced*

7 Updated:   Changes:

8 Updated:   Changes:

**Figure 6-13** Case One: Care plan example.

**Reevaluation.** Reevaluation (Appointment #6) is planned four to six weeks after all debridement has been completed. The purposes of this appointment are to detect and remove any remaining deposit, to evaluate the client's plaque control efforts, and to assess the periodontal and gingival condition. Because selective polishing (stain removal) and fluoride therapy were completed four weeks earlier, these two procedures are not indicated at this appointment. Completing stain removal and fluoride at the reevaluation visit can motivate the client to return for this evaluation.

**Periodontal Maintainance Procedures.** Maintenance treatment has three purposes: to evaluate the previous dental hygiene care and improvement in periodontal health; to establish a maintenance or recall phase of treatment; and to provide periodontal debridement (Woodall, 1993). This last purpose is perhaps the most important as the three-month maintenance interval for professional scaling and root planing has been showed to significantly enhance periodontal health (Greenwell, Bissada, & Wuttwer, 1990). Maintenance will be provided three months after the last debridement visit. If healing had not been adequate at the reevaluation visit and debridement was completed, then the recare interval would be determined from the date of the reevaluation visit. This maintenance appointment requires assessment of probing depths and bleeding points. It is suggested that this appointment be scheduled for 60 to 90 minutes using a periodontal dental assistant to chart recordings. The need for local anesthesia is dependent on the individual needs (probing depth or client sensitivity). PMP is discussed further in Chapter 16.

## Case Two

Mrs. Brown, age 49, is a nonsmoker who has a congenital heart murmur that requires antibiotic prophylaxis for dental and dental hygiene appointments. This need was addressed over the telephone and a prescription procured. As a result, Mrs. Brown was premedicated with the appropriate antibiotic regime upon arrival.

**Assessment and Diagnosis.** The assessment phase included completing a thorough health history, an intra- and extraoral examination, dental charting, a full periodontal examination, vertical bitewings, and recording of a plaque score (see Table 6-6). The presumptive diagnosis is chronic adult periodontitis with early bone loss. It is expected that disease progression will be slow and that results of care will be predictable.

**Selection of Oral Self-Care Devices.** Self-care education consisted of refining the brushing method, emphasizing frequency and choice of toothbrush, and reviewing dental flossing technique. Self-care education focused on gingivitis and periodontitis and the causative roles of bacterial plaque and the host response.

### Table 6.6 Case Two: Assessment Findings

*Health History*
- heart murmur requiring antibiotic premedication
- high blood pressure controlled by antihypertensive medication
- nonsmoker
- age 49

*Intra- and Extraoral Exam*
- oral cancer screening exam performed: no abnormalities detected

*Periodontal and Gingival Assessment*
- periodontal pockets 4 mm
- slight horizontal bone loss, triangulation, and unclear lamina dura
- gingiva-marginal redness, slight edema, interdental papilla slightly swollen, mild bleeding
- slight supragingival plaque, 30% plaque present
- minimal subgingival calculus
- supragingival calculus lingual and facial of mandibular anterior and maxillary molars
- moderate staining (tea and coffee consumption)
- Type I embrasure spaces

*Oral Care Habits/Compliance History*
- brushes twice a day
- flosses 2 to 3 times/week

**Approach to Debridement.** Due to relatively few deposits of calculus and plaque, a general full-mouth debridement was scheduled for 30 minutes employing ultrasonic instrumentation. Extrinsic stains were removed with the ultrasonic, therefore, selective polishing was not indicated. Topical fluoride gel was applied. With the assessment phase, the entire treatment was scheduled for 90 minutes (see Figure 6-14).

**PMP.** A four-month appointment interval was jointly established with Mrs. Brown. It was determined that a one-month reevaluation visit would not be scheduled due to the oral conditions and the need for antibiotic premedication for reprobing. Her past compliance with care was also considered.

## Case Three

Mr. Smith, age 63, is a heavy smoker and has high blood pressure that is controlled by medication.

**Assessment and Diagnosis.** Assessment findings are outlined in Table 6-7. The intra- and extraoral examination reveals a leukoplakia-type lesion on the buccal mucosa adjacent to tooth #3 and #4. Radiographic examination involved seven vertical bitewing films. The periodontal examination determined deep probing depths in the posterior regions of all quadrants (7 to 8 mm) with generalized spontaneous bleeding. A Class III furcation was found on tooth #15 with Class II mobility on #8 and #9. Poor gingival health was evident by generalized redness, edema, bulbous contours and shiny texture, as well as several areas

CLIENT NAME _____  DATE _____

| ASSESSMENT | Appt. 1 | Appt. 2 | Appt. 3 | Appt. 4 | Appt. 5 | Appt. 6 | Appt. 7 | Appt. 8 |
|---|---|---|---|---|---|---|---|---|
| | Minutes Per Appointment | | | | | | | |
| Health History | 5 | | | | | | | |
| Intra- and Extraoral Exam | 5 | | | | | | | |
| Dental Charting | 5 | | | | | | | |
| Perio Exam and Charting | 10 | | | | | | | |
| Indices | 3 | | | | | | | |
| Radiographs, Type *Vert. BWX* | 10 | | | | | | | |
| **DISEASE PREVENTION** | | | | | | | | |
| Brushing Techniques | 3 | | | | | | | |
| Interdental Aids | 3 | | | | | | | |
| Periodontal Disease | 5 | | | | | | | |
| Dental Decay | | | | | | | | |
| Tobacco Use | | | | | | | | |
| Nutritional Education | | | | | | | | |
| Fluoride Therapy | 2 | | | | | | | |
| Blood Pressure | 5 | | | | | | | |
| Other | | | | | | | | |
| **TREATMENT PROCEDURES** | | | | | | | | |
| Anesthesia | | | | | | | | |
| Ultrasonic Debridement Quadrant (Q) | 30 | | | | | | | |
| Sextant (S) | | | | | | | | |
| Hand-Activated Debridement Quadrant (Q) | | | | | | | | |
| Sextant (S) | | | | | | | | |
| Subgingival Irrigation | | | | | | | | |
| Selective Polishing | | | | | | | | |
| Fluoride Treatment | 3 | | | | | | | |
| Desensitization | | | | | | | | |
| Margination | | | | | | | | |
| Amalgam Polishing | | | | | | | | |
| Other | | | | | | | | |
| Total Appointment Time | 89 | | | | | | | |
| Recare Interval | *4 months* | | | | | | | |
| Referral(s) | *none* | | | | | | | |

Q1 = Quadrant   Q2 = Quadrant   Q3 = Quadrant   Q4 = Quadrant

CLINICIAN NAME _____

**GOALS**

Treatment goals  *"Antibiotic Premedication Required"*
1 *Eliminate bleeding*
2 *Reduce plaque 10–15%*
3 *Improve floss use and refine brushing technique*

Client Goals
1 *Stop bleeding*
2 *Floss daily*
3

**ORAL SELF-CARE**

CURRENT ORAL SELF-CARE METHODS
*brushes 2x daily*
*flossing 2–3x/week*

| Recommendations | | |
|---|---|---|
| Brush | Variable Diameter Floss | ✓ |
| Specialty Brush | Dental Tape/Floss | |
| Interdental Brush | Floss Threader/Aid | |
| | Mounted Toothpick | |
| | Wooden Wedge | |
| | Rubber Tip | ✓ |
| | Other | |

**REAPPOINTMENT UPDATES**

2 Updated:  Changes:
3 Updated:  Changes:
4 Updated:  Changes:
5 Updated:  Changes:
6 Updated:  Changes:
7 Updated:  Changes:
8 Updated:  Changes:

**Figure 6-14** Case Two: Care plan example.

## Table 6.7  Case Three: Assessment Findings

### Health History

- high blood pressure controlled by antihypertensive medication
- smoker, two packs/day
- 63 years old

### Intra- and Extra-Oral Exam

- oral cancer screening exam performed: leukoplakia detected on buccal mucosa adjacent to tooth #3 and #4

### Periodontal and Gingival Assessment

- probe depths, generalized to posterior regions 7 to 8 mm
- generalized spontaneous bleeding
- poor gingival health: generalized redness, bluish (cyanotic) red gingiva adjacent to #8, #9, #14, #15, #19; diffuse gingivitis
- generalized edematous, shiny bulbous gingiva
- recession 2 to 3 mm generalized in anterior
- clinical attachment level 8 mm or less
- Class II furcation on #15, #30, #31
- Class II mobility on maxillary centrals #8 and #9
- plaque score 93%
- generalized tenacious subgingival deposits, moderate banding of supragingival calculus-mandibular anteriors

### Oral Care Habits/Compliance History

- brushes once/day in morning
- no flossing
- uses toothpicks occasionally

---

of cyanosis. Generalized ledges of calculus were found interproximally supra- and subgingivally. Plaque was present on almost all surfaces (plaque score 93%). There is poor compliance with oral self-care. Mr. Smith brushes a maximum of once per day for 45 seconds and uses wooden toothpicks occasionally. The presumptive diagnosis is chronic adult periodontitis with advanced bone loss.

**Referrals.** Referrals are indicated for this client. First the leukoplakia type lesion needs further assessment by a dentist, or surgeon, and/or oral pathologist. Follow-up on this referral would be in the best interest of the client. Second, an occlusal adjustment by a dentist may be required to reduce tooth mobility related to occlusal trauma. Third, the advanced stage of periodontitis warrants the consultation of a periodontist. Fourth, a smoking cessation treatment program may be prescribed by the dental hygienist or a physician.

**Selection of Oral Self-Care Devices.** The disease theory presented in Appointment #1 focused on prevention and oral care. To monitor progress and provide client education and motivation, a plaque index was taken and repeated at each subsequent appointment. The oral care emphasis during appointment #1 was on improved brushing technique. The disease processes of periodontitis was discussed concentrating on smoking cessation. During appointment #2 chlorhexidine mouthrinse was prescribed for a two-week period. A review of the toothbrushing technique taught during appointment #1 was conducted. The

use of the mounted toothpick was introduced during appointment #3 because of the furcation involvement which was partially occluded by gingiva and the contour of the embrasure spaces (Class II and III), and familiarity with the aid. During appointments #4 to #6, a thorough review of the use of the interdental aid was completed. An end-tufted brush would have been an option.

**Approach to NSPT.** Treating this case required seven appointments (see Figure 6-15). The following is a brief outline of the appointment sequence determined in the care plan.

Appointment #1 is designated as an assessment appointment. This appointment, scheduled for 90 minutes, included health history documentation, periodontal assessment, and restorative assessment. However, due to the heavy deposits of subgingival calculus, periodontal probing for pocket depth and attachment loss was not performed on the first appointment, but was completed immediately after debridement in each quadrant during appointments 2 through 5.

Because of the history of high blood pressure and administration of local anesthesia, blood pressure monitoring was conducted at each visit with the health history update. During the remaining time scheduled for this appointment, ultrasonic scaling was initiated in the mandibular anterior because this was a visible area for the client to recognize improvements in gingival status. At this appointment, referral to an oral pathologist was made for evaluation of the leukoplakia.

Appointments #2 through #6 were devoted to instrumentation and supportive interventions. Prior to beginning the instrumentation during each appointment, the health history and intra- and extra-oral exam were reviewed. The active implementation of dental hygiene procedures was performed in five sixty- to ninety-minute appointments. In these appointments, ultrasonic debridement in conjunction with hand-activated instrumentation was employed in segmental quadrant approach. After each quadrant of debridement, subgingival irrigation was provided to promote gingival healing. Localized selective polishing and fluoride application were completed at appointment #6. Selective polishing occurred even after ultrasonic scaling due to reaccumulation of stain in previously debrided quadrants. Another option would be to remove the reaccumulated stain with ultrasonic instrumentation.

**Reevaluation and PMP.** One month after the completion of care, a reevaluation appointment was scheduled (appointment #7). This sixty-minute appointment involved a reassessment of the health history including blood pressure and the intraoral examination focusing on gingival inflammation (healing) and reevaluation of the lesion. Complete recording of periodontal probe readings and the plaque index occurred to provide data to compare to previous measurements. Thirty minutes were scheduled to debride subgingival plaque, stain, and

CLIENT NAME _____  DATE _____

CLINICIAN NAME _____

| ASSESSMENT | Appt. 1 | Appt. 2 | Appt. 3 | Appt. 4 | Appt. 5 | Appt. 6 | Appt. 7 | Appt. 8 |
|---|---|---|---|---|---|---|---|---|
| Health History | 5 | 2 | 2 | 2 | 2 | 2 | 2 | |
| Intra- and Extraoral Exam | 5 | 2 | 2 | 2 | 2 | 2 | 2 | |
| Dental Charting | 5 | | | | | | | |
| Perio Exam and Charting | 15 | Q3 8 | Q4 8 | Q1 8 | Q2 8 | | 15 | |
| Indices | 5 | 5 | 5 | 5 | 5 | 5 | 5 | |
| Radiographs, Type: Vert. BWS | 10 | | | | | | | |
| **DISEASE PREVENTION** | | | | | | | | |
| Brushing Techniques | 5 | 3 | 2 | 1 | 1 | 1 | 1 | |
| Interdental Aids | | | 5 | 2 | 2 | 5 | 3 | |
| Periodontal Disease | 5 | 3 | 3 | 1 | 1 | | | |
| Dental Decay | | | | | | | | |
| Tobacco Use | 3 | 3 | | 1 | | 5 | | |
| Nutritional Education | | | | | | | | |
| Fluoride Therapy | | | | | | 2 | | |
| Blood Pressure | 3 | | | | | | | |
| Other CHX Rinse | | 3 | | | | | | |
| **TREATMENT PROCEDURES** | | | | | | | | |
| Anesthesia | | Q3 8 | Q4 8 | Q1 15 | Q2 15 | | | |
| Ultrasonic Debridement Quadrant (Q) | | Q3 35 | Q4 35 | Q1 40 | Q2 40 | Q2 15 | 30 | |
| Sextant (S) | 20 | | | | | | | |
| Hand-Activated Debridement Quadrant (Q) | | Q3 15 | Q4 15 | Q1 10 | Q2 10 | | | |
| Sextant (S) | | | | | | | | |
| Subgingival Irrigation | | 5 | 5 | 5 | 5 | 5 | | |
| Selective Polishing | | | | | | 5 | | |
| Fluoride Treatment | | | | | | 3 | | |
| Desensitization | | | | | | | | |
| Margination | | | | | | | | |
| Amalgam Polishing | | | | | | | | |
| Other | | | | | | | | |
| Total Appointment Time | 81 | 92 | 90 | 92 | 91 | 50 | 58 | |
| Recare Interval | 3 month | | | | | | | |
| Referral(s) | 1) Physician for smoking cessation 2) Oral Pathologist for evaluation of leukoplakia 3) Referral to periodontist | | | | | | | |

*Minutes Per Appointment*

Q1 = Quadrant  Q2 = Quadrant  Q3 = Quadrant  Q4 = Quadrant

## GOALS

**Treatment goals**

1 Reduce pocket depths, maintain attachment level, improve gingival health
2 Daily compliance w/aids
3 Encourage smoking cessation – consider referral

**Client Goals**

1 Client wants to improve look of gums and teeth
2 Client wants to stop smoking
3 Client wishes to rectify lost teeth

### ORAL SELF-CARE

CURRENT ORAL SELF-CARE METHODS

brushes 1x/day, AM
toothpicks occasionally

| Recommendations | | | |
|---|---|---|---|
| ✓ Variable Diameter Floss | | Mounted Toothpick ✓ | |
| Brush | | Wooden Wedge | |
| Specialty Brush | Dental Tape/Floss | Rubber Tip | |
| Interdental Brush | Floss Threader/Aid | Other CHX Rinse ✓ | |

### REAPPOINTMENT UPDATES

2 Updated: *January 6, 1996*  Changes: *Plaque 75%*
*Improved brushing technique (2x daily) and gingival condition, Chlorhexidine rinse initiated gingiva mandibular anterior less inflammation*

3 Updated: *January 13, 1996*  Changes: *Plaque 60%*
*Chlorhexidine rinse used daily for 1 wk, bleeding reduced, gingival contour improved Gingiva Q3 less inflammation and bleeding*

4 Updated: *January 20, 1996*  Changes: *Plaque 35%*
*Chlorhexidine rinse used for 2 weeks, quit smoking, Q4 less inflammation and bleeding*

5 Updated: *January 27, 1996*  Changes: *Plaque 30% CHX discontinued*
*Brushing daily, using mounted toothpick  Q1-less inflammation & bleeding*

6 Updated: *February 3, 1996*  Changes: *Plaque 25%*
*Brushing daily, smoking cessation continuing Q2-gingiva appears to be healthy except for furcation areas*

7 Updated: *February 10, 1996*  Changes: *Plaque 15%*
*Reviewed all oral care strategies, localized bleeding, improved color, contour, and texture*

**Figure 6-15**  Case Three: Care plan example.

calculus deposits that were residual or forming. This amount of time might not be necessary, but it was planned due to the advanced periodontitis and self-care practices. At this appointment the maintenance period will jointly be determined. A three-month interval is recommended.

## Summary

The main objectives of dental hygiene therapy are to preserve or reestablish periodontal health to prevent the reoccurrence or onset of periodontal diseases. In order to achieve these objectives, the establishment of a dental hygiene care plan is essential in mapping out the appointment or series of appointments in a logical and efficient manner. There is no longer the concept of dental hygienists "cleaning teeth"; but providing treatment for a periodontal infection, that is periodontal disease. In providing treatment, it is necessary to plan time in the appointment sessions to thoroughly assess, treat, and reevaluate the client's condition (Galvis, 1993; O'Hehir, 1984).

In collaborative practices, dental hygienists, as cotherapists with dentists, make decisions regarding not only the needs of clients, but also plan and implement treatment plans specific to dental hygiene care (Darby & Walsh, 1994). Dental hygiene treatment (care) plans should be the responsibility of dental hygienists as specialists with expertise and a distinct body of knowledge (Canadian Dental Association, 1989; Nielsen, 1983).

## Case Studies

**Case Study One:** Christine Roelen, a 45-year-old teacher, returns for care in your office six months after her previous NSPT. The health history indicates a history of asthma, but Christine has not had an attack in several months; nevertheless, she carries an inhaler in her purse. The soft tissue examination is negative and the periodontal assessment reveals marginal gingivitis due to redness, edema, slight stippling, and blunted papillae. Recession of 1 mm is charted in localized areas. There is generalized bleeding on probing. Probe readings are 4 to 5 mm in the interproximal areas of molars in all four quadrants. Clinical attachment loss measures from 4 to 5 mm. Radiographs, taken six months ago at the previous visit, showed caries that have been restored, and generalized early bone loss with localized moderate bone loss. Oral self-care seems almost adequate based on a 20% plaque score and client report of flossing four times per week. Moderate calculus is present in the lingual and interproximal areas of the mandibular anterior teeth and light calculus is located subgingivally in the posteriors. Identify the presumptive diagnosis. Discuss a care plan for Christine using one-hour appointment periods. Discuss the maintenance interval.

**Case Study Two:** Anne, a 25-year-old woman, has been faithful to her recare appointments since she was a child. However, in the past two years, she has had a very busy life and her dental hygiene has not been a priority. During the assessment phase, the only two changes in her health history have been the birth of a child within the last year, and the taking of oral contraceptives. Anne reports that she has not been feeling well lately, has a fever, has lost weight, and has noticed movement and bleeding of several teeth. She accounts this to the lifestyle changes that she has encountered due to the recent birth of her child. Her mouth is relatively deposit-free with only areas of localized supragingival and subgingival calculus and a plaque score of 15%. Upon probing, generalized pockets are found in the 7 mm range with bleeding and heavy subgingival plaque. Radiographs show both vertical and horizontal bone loss. Microbial screening shows the presence of *porphyromonas gingivalis.* What is the presumptive diagnosis? What assessment criteria are used to determine this diagnosis? What would be an acceptable care plan for this client?

**Case Study Three:** Jack Brenn seeks oral health care on a regular basis for treatment of periodontal disease related to acquired immunodeficiency syndrome (AIDS). The health history indicates no changes since his last appointment three months ago. The intra- extraoral examination reveals the classic AIDS lesions of oral hairy leukoplakia, candidiasis, and Kaposi's sarcoma. Cervical soft tissue necrosis is occurring. Design a treatment plan taking into consideration debridement, polishing, fluoride, and the oral care needs of Jack's treatment.

**Case Study Four:** Tom Clear has had regular dental hygiene treatment. He has recently changed dentists and this is the first time this particular dental hygienist has treated him. There are a few areas where his toothbrushing and flossing are not adequate and these areas warrant more of Tom's effort in oral care. Tom's major concern is a Class II furcation on the maxillary left first molar that has been restored many times and recently has had endodontic treatment and a porcelain fused to metal crown. Tom reports that food still "gets caught in this area," that there has always been bleeding in this area, and that previous dental hygienists have spent extra time instrumenting this furcation. The gingiva does not occlude the furcation entrance. Tom spends a lot of time away from home due to his employment situation and his interest in camping and hiking. He packs lightly when he travels and does not want to be bothered with any device that needs electricity or batteries. List three possible self-care devices that would be suitable for Tom. Select one of the three that would be most appropriate and explain why.

**Case Study Five:** Three months ago, Mary Higgins sought dental hygiene care because of bleeding gingiva associated with pregnancy. She was in her first trimester. At that time, the dental hygienist discussed with Mary the influence of hormonal levels on her existing gingival inflammation caused by inadequate self-care. Both the dental hygienist and Mary decided to reevaluate Mary's gingival tissue and plaque control in a few months during the second trimester. What presumptive diagnosis would you assume was made three months ago? Briefly discuss the plan for Mary's future appointment(s).

## Case Study Discussions

**Discussion—Case Study One:** The presumptive diagnosis relies on recognizing these significant factors; the client's age, extent of disease, systemic health, compliance with oral self-care, and extent of deposits. She appears to have periodontitis that is chronic or slowly progressing based on these factors.

A notation is made in the health history about asthma and the bronchodialator for breathing assistance. Because radiographs were taken within the year, there is no need for x-rays unless the visual exam indicates any suspicious areas of new or recurrent decay or progressive periodontal problems. It is important that the probe readings and clinical attachment level be recorded at this appointment to provide comparison recordings for subsequent visits. Instrumentation should be performed not only to remove the calculus, but also to disrupt any subgingival plaque. She is to be commended for her plaque score. Although there is little supragingival bacterial plaque accumulation, there is a concern about the gingival inflammation, bleeding, and the amount of calculus. Further questioning is needed to determine her compliance with *daily* self-care, hormonal tolerances, and length of maintenance interval. Most likely her NSPT will take 3 to 4 one-hour appointments depending on the gingival healing, self-care, and professional's choice of instruments for debridement. A reevaluation visit is essential to assess the periodontal status.

A three-month interval would be ideal to monitor the gingival tissues, probing depths, and oral self-care. Also, vertical bitewings would be indicated to detect not only caries but also to detect further bone loss in the interproximal areas.

**Discussion—Case Study Two:** The presumptive diagnosis of this condition would be rapid progressive periodontitis. The diagnosis is made based on the following assessment criteria: the apparent episodic nature of the periodontal attacks; the bone loss; her age; the recent

hormonal change; the general discomfort, fever, and loss of weight; the subgingival plaque, probe depths, and bleeding on probing. The first consideration in this care plan would be to refer Anne to a periodontist.

Figure 6-16 shows a flow chart for the treatment of rapid progressive periodontitis. The assessment phase of this client's treatment reveals criteria that would indicate a specific type of periodontal disease; however, results of microbial analysis would aid in determining this diagnosis. The initial dental hygiene therapy would be thorough debridement and plaque control similar to the treatment of other periodontal diseases. Furthermore, in conjunction with instrumentation, an antibiotic(s) would be utilized to reduce the levels of the specific pathogenic microorganisms. After completion of initial therapy, a second microbial analysis would be conducted to verify a decrease of the periodontal disease-causing microorganisms. At this time it would be necessary to outline treatment options including continuation of active therapy or maintenance. Surgical intervention would only be considered if and when periodontal stability, comparable to that of chronic periodontitis, is achieved.

Initial therapy would include quadrant debridement; however, chemotherapy would likely be included. Oral care would include a review of present techniques with additional emphasis on the use of mounted toothpick for the pocket areas. Anne would be cautioned that there is a possibility that the periodontal condition may not respond to the treatment even with proper care and maintenance. Further information regarding treatment planning for rapid progressive periodontitis can be found in Page, et al., 1983, and Kornman and Wilson, 1992.

**Discussion—Case Study Three:** Before care is initiated (see Figure 6-17), it will be necessary to contact the physi-

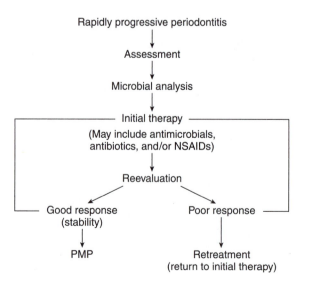

**Figure 6-16** Rapidly progressive periodontitis. (Adapted with permission from Wilson, Kornman, and Newman, *Advances in periodontics,* pg. 89. Quintessence Publishing Co., Inc., Chicago, 1992)

CLIENT NAME _____  DATE _____

CLINICIAN NAME _____

| ASSESSMENT | Appt. 1 | Appt. 2 | Appt. 3 | Appt. 4 | Appt. 5 | Appt. 6 | Appt. 7 | Appt. 8 |
|---|---|---|---|---|---|---|---|---|
| | Minutes Per Appointment | | | | | | | |
| Health History | 5 | | | | | | | |
| Intra- and Extraoral Exam | 5 | | | | | | | |
| Dental Charting | 5 | | | | | | | |
| Perio Exam and Charting | 10 | | | | | | | |
| Indices | 5 | | | | | | | |
| Radiographs, Type | | | | | | | | |
| **DISEASE PREVENTION** | | | | | | | | |
| Brushing Techniques | 5 | | | | | | | |
| Interdental Aids | 5 | | | | | | | |
| Periodontal Disease | | | | | | | | |
| Dental Decay | | | | | | | | |
| Tobacco Use | | | | | | | | |
| Nutritional Education | | | | | | | | |
| Fluoride Therapy | | | | | | | | |
| Blood Pressure | | | | | | | | |
| Other *CHX/desen. toothpaste* | 5 | | | | | | | |
| **TREATMENT PROCEDURES** | | | | | | | | |
| Anesthesia | | | | | | | | |
| Ultrasonic Debridement Quadrant (Q) | | | | | | | | |
| Sextant (S) | | | | | | | | |
| Hand-Activated Debridement Quadrant (Q) | Q1–Q4=30 | | | | | | | |
| Sextant (S) | | | | | | | | |
| Subgingival Irrigation | | | | | | | | |
| Selective Polishing | 8 | | | | | | | |
| Fluoride Treatment | | | | | | | | |
| Desensitization | 5 | | | | | | | |
| Margination | | | | | | | | |
| Amalgam Polishing | | | | | | | | |
| Other | | | | | | | | |
| Total Appointment Time | 88 | | | | | | | |
| Recare Interval | 3 months | | | | | | | |
| Referral(s) | none | | | | | | | |

Q1 = Quadrant    Q2 = Quadrant    Q3 = Quadrant    Q4 = Quadrant

## GOALS

Treatment goals
1  *Consult physician regarding antibiotic coverage and possible bleeding problem*
2  *To make client as comfortable as possible*
3

Client Goals
1  *To maintain oral health*
2  *To prevent oral infections*
3

### ORAL SELF-CARE

CURRENT ORAL SELF-CARE METHODS

*Brushes 2–3 x daily*

| Recommendations | | | | |
|---|---|---|---|---|
| Brush | ✓ | Variable Diameter Floss | | Mounted Toothpick |
| | | | | Wooden Wedge |
| Specialty Brush | | Dental Tape/Floss | ✓ | Rubber Tip |
| Interdental Brush | | Floss Threader/Aid | | Other *CHX Rinse* ✓ |

### REAPPOINTMENT UPDATES

2 Updated: _____  Changes: _____

3 Updated: _____  Changes: _____

4 Updated: _____  Changes: _____

5 Updated: _____  Changes: _____

6 Updated: _____  Changes: _____

7 Updated: _____  Changes: _____

8 Updated: _____  Changes: _____

**Figure 6-17** Case Study Three: Care plan.

cian regarding the need for antibiotic prophylaxis and a potential bleeding problem because of severe thrombocytopenia (the decrease in number of blood platelets). Utmost care is needed during any instrumentation and examination procedure to prevent postoperative infections and to alleviate further discomfort. With the utilization of universal precautions, there is no need to schedule Jack any differently than other clients.

The assessment phase of care includes an updated review of any significant changes in the health history or oral conditions. Oral self-care education focuses on the use of soft toothbrushing (due to the sensitivity of the gingival tissue), and gentle flossing (assisted by caregiver if necessary). A fluoride desensitizing toothpaste, compatible with chlorhexidine could also be recommended, not only to prevent root and enamel caries, but to help with tooth sensitivity that may occur as a result of tissue necrosis. Treatment procedures causing aerosols, such as ultrasonic scaling and rubber cup polishing are kept at a minimal and, therefore, are not recommended in this treatment plan. Full-mouth debridement is completed by hand-activated instruments followed by a toothbrushing and a fluoridated desensitization varnish application. Assuming no difficulties arise during treatment, a continuation of the three-month maintenance would be planned. Further information regarding treatment planning for AIDS can be found in Cohen and Wilkins, 1992; Friedman, 1987; and Wooley, 1992.

**Discussion—Case Study Four:** Three possible adjuncts would be: a mounted toothpick, a rubber tip stimulator, a specialty tapered end tuft toothbrush. The best choice for this client's oral care of the Class II furcation would be a mounted toothpick or interdental brush. Either aid would not only deplaque the furcation, but also may help with the dislodging of food, as Tom reports, that gets caught in this area. Because the Class II furcation is exposed, access with an interdental brush is possible. A rubber tip stimulator may not be as effective as the toothpick or interdental brush in adapting around the molar root surface and into the furcation area. Additional consideration in recommending an aid include his preference, access to the furcation, corresponding pocket depth and gingival inflammation, contour of the embrasure spaces, and dexterity.

**Discussion Case Study Five:** The presumptive diagnosis is hormone-influenced gingivitis. Time is allowed in the care planning for interruptions (e.g., client's frequent urination, changing client's position) while maintaining a short appointment. The assessment phase consists of review of health history, intra- and extraoral exam, and gingival and periodontal examination with emphasis on the changes in the gingival tissues. The dental hygienist inquires if Mary notices less bleeding with brushing; this was her major concern three months ago. A plaque index reinforces the need for immaculate bacterial plaque control especially during pregnancy. Nutritional counseling provides the opportunity to inform Mary about caries prevention and prenatal care as they relate to her present eating habits. Treatment procedures include full-mouth debridement. Assuming that rubber cup polishing and fluoride therapy was completed three months earlier, only a toothbrush "polishing" is indicated for this appointment. A future appointment is scheduled postpartum. Radiographs would be exposed and a discussion of bottle caries and oral care for the infant will be incorporated in this postnatal session.

## REFERENCES

American Academy of Periodontology. (1989). *Non-surgical periodontal treatment.* Consensus Report Discussion Section II. (pp. II 13–II 17). *Proceedings of the world workshop in clinical periodontics.* Chicago: American Academy of Periodontology.

American Academy of Periodontology. (1991). *Local delivery of antimicrobials: Adjuncts to periodontal therapy?* Chicago: American Academy of Periodontology, Department of Scientific and Educational Affairs.

Axelsson, P. (1994). Mechanical plaque control. In N. P. Lang & T. Karring (Eds.), *Proceedings of the 1st European workshop in periodontology.* London: Quintessence Publishing Company.

Barrows, H. S. & Pickell, G. C. (1991). *Developing clinical problem-solving skills: A guide to more effective diagnosis and treatment.* New York: W.W. Norton & Company.

Betta, P. A. (1993). Documenting to stay out of the courtroom. *Imprint, 38*(2), 39–40.

Bowen, D. (1994). Personal mechanical oral hygiene care and chemotherapeutic plaque control. In M. L. Darby & N. M. Walsh (Eds.), *Dental hygiene theory and practice.* Philadelphia: W.B. Saunders Co.

Canadian Dental Association. (1989). *Report of the CFDE/CDA: Conference on ethics in Canadian dentistry and dental education.* Ottawa, Ontario: Canadian Dental Association.

Carranza, F. A. The treatment plan. In F. A. Carranza and M. G. Newman (Eds.), *Clinical periodontology,* (8th Ed.) Philadelphia: W.B. Saunders Co.

Carranza, F. A. & Rapley, J. W. (1996). Gingival inflammation. In F. A. Carranza & M. G. Newman (Eds.), *Clinical periodontology* (8th ed.). Philadelphia: W.B. Saunders Co.

Cohen, P. A. & Wilkins, E. M. (1992). A hospital-based dental clinic for patients with HIV infection in the United States. *Canadian Dental Hygienists' Association Journal/PROBE, 26*(2), 65–68.

Darby, M. L. & Walsh, M. M. (1994). *Dental hygiene theory and practice.* Philadelphia: W.B. Saunders Co.

Edgington, E. M. (1994). The communication imperative: A critical thinking paradigm. *The Canadian Dental Hygienists' Association Journal/PROBE, 28*(2), 65–68.

Friedman, P. R. (1987). The patient with AIDS: Management procedures. *Oral Health, 77*(8), 27–31.

Galvis, D. L. (1993). Patients deserve more than a generic dental appointment. *RDH, 13*(4), 38–40.

Grant, D. A., Stern, I. B., & Listgarten, M. A. (1988). *Periodontics: In the tradition of Gottlieb and Orban* (6th ed.). St. Louis: Mosby-Year Book, Inc.

Greenlaw, J. (1992). Documentation of patient care: An often underestimated responsibility. *Law, Medicine & Health Care, 10*(4), 172–174.

Greenwell, H., Bissada, N. F., & Wuttwer, J. W. (1990). Periodontics in general practice: Professional plaque control. *Journal of the American Dental Association, 121*(5), 642–646.

Gurenlian, J. R. (1993). Diagnostic decision making. In I. R. Woodall (Ed.), *Comprehensive dental hygiene care* (7th ed.). St. Louis: Mosby-Year Book, Inc.

Hogue, E. E. (1990). The liability of payers and providers in health care treatment decisions. *Pediatric Nursing, 16*(3), 317.

Iyer, P. W. (1991). Six more charting rules: To keep you legally safe. *Nursing,* July, 34–49.

Kiger, R. D., Nylund, K., & Feller, R. P. (1991). A comparison of proximal plaque removal using floss and interdental brushes. *Journal of Clinical Periodontology, 18,* 681–684.

Kornman, K. S. & Wilson, T. G. (1992). Treatment planning for patients with inflammatory periodontal diseases. In T. G. Wilson, K. S. Kornman, & M. G. Newman (Eds.), *Advances in periodontics.* Chicago: Quintessence Publishing Co., Inc.

Meuller-Joseph, L. & Petersen, M. (1995). *Dental hygiene process: Diagnosis and care planning.* Albany: Delmar Publishers.

Morch, T. & Waerhang, J. (1956). Quantitative evaluation of the effect of toothbrushing and toothpicking. *Journal of Periodontology, 27,* 183.

Nield-Gehrig, J. S. & Houseman, G. A. (1996). *Fundamentals of periodontal instrumentation* (3rd ed.). Baltimore: Williams & Wilkins.

Nielsen, N. J. (1983). Decision making associated with dental hygiene practice. *Dental Hygiene, 57*(12), 24–31.

O'Hehir, T. (1984). Planning treatment. *RDH,* July/August, 18–21.

Page, R. C., Altman, L. C., Ebersole, J. L., Vandesteen, G. E. Dahlberg, W. H., Williams, B. L., & Ostberg, S. K. (1983). Rapidly progressive periodontitis: A distinct clinical concern. *Journal of Periodontology, 54*(4), 197–209.

Page, R. C. (1993). Periodontal therapy: Prospects for the future. *Journal of Periodontology, 64*(8), 744–753.

Pattison, A. & Pattison, G. L. (1992). *Periodontal instrumentation* (2nd ed.) Norwalk, Connecticut: Appleton & Lange.

Perry, D. A. & Schmid, M. O. (1996). Plaque control. In F. A. Carranza, & M. G. Newman (Eds.), *Clinical periodontology* (8th ed.) Philadelphia: W.B. Saunders Co.

Staff. (1994). Coming up with a profile of patients most likely to harbour periodontal disease. *The Oral Care Report, 4*(2), 1–4.

Ursu, S. C. (1992). Legal considerations in clinical decision making. *Journal of Dental Education, 56*(12), 808–811.

Wilkins, E. M. (1994). *The clinical practice of dental hygiene* (7th ed.). Philadelphia: Lea & Febiger.

Wilson, Kornman, & Newman (1992). Diagnosis of periodontal diseases and conditions using a traditional approach. In T. G. Wilson, K. S. Kornman, & M. G. Newman (Eds.), *Advances in periodontics.* Chicago: Quintessence Publishing Co., Inc.

Woodall, I. R. (1993). *Comprehensive dental hygiene care* (4th ed.). St. Louis: Mosby-Year Book, Inc.

Wood, N. K. (1985). *Treatment Planning: A pragmatic approach.* River Forest, Illinois: The Woodline Publishing Company.

Wooley, C. (1992). Canada's first hospital dental clinic for patients with HIV infection. *Canadian Dental Hygienists' Association Journal/PROBE, 26*(2), 59–64.

# IMPLEMENTATION PHASE

CHAPTER 7

# Applying Communication Skills to Therapy

## Key Terms

active listening skills
communication
expression of body
tone of voice

facilitative communication
language
paraphrasing
self-exploration

## INTRODUCTION

When implementing NSPT, effective communication is essential, particularly when one considers the fact that multiple visits and interactions are usually required to provide the client with adequate care. NSPT is challenging to discuss with and obtain commitment from the individual, especially compared to the traditional prophylaxis completed in one short appointment. Dental hygienists have extensive education in the prevention of dental disease, and through multiple appointments for NSPT, greatly affect the client/provider relationship (Sisty-LePeau, 1995).

**Communication** can be defined as a giving or exchanging of information, signals, or messages by talk, gesture, or writing (Guranik, 1976). It can also be information or a message itself. Effective communication has always been an important factor in dental therapy for both the clinician and client. Unfortunately, communication might be an often overlooked component of dental care. Clients know very little about a dental professional's skill level. In fact, according to David (1987), "Most patients are not interested in understanding all the technical skills and procedures that go into producing quality dentistry, but they are very interested in how they feel about you and the treatment received. Patients use how they feel as the main criteria for evaluating the quality of service" (p. 6).

Dental professionals are not to be viewed as technicians, but as helping professionals involved holistically with their clients. Not only are clinicians competent in performing technical skills, such as deposit removal or the administration of local anesthesia; they are also skilled in assessing human feelings and behaviors such as fear and motivation. Unfortunately, in the past, an over-

crowded professional curriculum prevented thorough exploration of these important areas of human behavior leaving dental professionals to learn these skills the hard way—through experience (Egan, 1982). It is hoped that modern professional curriculums stress the role of communication in effective health care delivery.

Communication is highlighted as an essential component of NSPT because it affects the success of every aspect of therapy. This chapter discusses elements of effective communication that lead to cooperative treatment between clients and the dental professional. The examples enclosed center on the verbal and nonverbal exchanges that occur between the client and clinician during NSPT self-care education. Oral self-care was chosen as the focus of this chapter because this is the phase of care where the initial communication process begins to encourage client compliance. These examples are incorporated to enhance the reader's utilization of the theoretical concepts.

## PRINCIPLES OF COMMUNICATION

Communication never has a starting point or an ending point; it is continuous. Theoretically, we could never speak another word yet messages are still conveyed to others. Geboy (1985) classifies the continuing nature of communication into four important principles: communication is *inevitable, irreversible, conducted on several levels,* and *influenced by the physical setting* (see Table 7-1). An experienced clinician is aware of these concepts, but it can be helpful to periodically review basic principles and apply them to NSPT.

From the moment clients step into the dental office until the time they leave the office, some type of com-

**Table 7-1 The Four Principles of the Continuing Nature of Communication**

| Principle | Explanation |
| --- | --- |
| Inevitable | Mannerisms and spoken words are continually relaying a message. |
| Irreversible | What is said cannot be reversed or erased and needs to be dealt with before continuing to communicate. |
| Conducted on Several Levels | The individuals communicating are on unequal levels or status. The clinician is the center of knowledge and skill and the client receives the knowledge/skill. |
| Influenced by the Physical Setting | The physical setting makes silent statements to the client and in turn influences the clinician/client interaction. |

munication has surfaced or is surfacing. Even the way the dental professional greets the clients in the reception room and asks them back to the operatory, makes a statement about how pleased the dental professional is to see the clients. The following examples are presented to clarify Geboy's (1985) principles on the continuous nature of communication.

The clinician's mannerisms and/or spoken words relay some type of message to the client; therefore, communication is inevitable. The message being received by the client might not actually be the one the dental professional intended to send. The meaning of the dental hygienist's mannerisms and spoken words are always being processed by those within viewing and listening distance.

*Example 1: Communication is inevitable*

*RDH:* The dental hygienist presents herself and asks the client to come to the operatory. Rather than standing in the doorway to the reception room and calling her name, the hygienist smiles, walks over slowly in a relaxed fashion to where she is seated, and calmly greets her.

The dental hygienist walking over to greet the client and extending her hand would exhibit to the client that a calm and friendly atmosphere is present in this office.

The principle of communication being irreversible is sometimes the one that causes trouble for the dental professional. For example, have you ever made a statement while providing self-care education that you wish you had not made?

*Example 2: Communication is irreversible*

*RDH:* "If you would floss regularly as we discussed your gums would not bleed."

*Client:* "I don't understand how that could be because I do floss at least once a day."

This type of statement tends to stop communication and leads the hygienist into explaining what she was trying to say. What the hygienist has said cannot be erased in the client's mind. Cherry (1974) states "What you say, you cannot unsay. You can, of course, apologize, withdraw, or want to sink through the floor—but it is irreversible; you are committed . . ." (p. 24). The client then must mentally process information the clinician has presented and come to some conclusion about his feelings regarding the message.

Communication often is conducted on different levels in dentistry. Many times the dental hygienist/client relationship is developed on unequal levels or status. Usually the clinician is the center of knowledge and skill and the client is the receiver of the knowledge and skill. In order for the transfer of knowledge and skill to facilitate change in the person's oral self-care practices, a feeling of cooperation must exist between the dental hygienist and client.

*Example 3: Communication is conducted on different levels*

*RDH:* Susan, I know you are busy with your work and family responsibilities, so in order for us to design a workable periodontal self-care plan, let's consider the best times of day for you to brush and use a periodontal aid. Also let's consider how often each day it is reasonable for you to use these aids.

*Client:* I'm so busy in the morning getting the kids ready for school that I really only have time to brush in the morning. You know how uncoordinated I am with other aids; it would take me forever.

*RDH:* I agree, using a periodontal aid is awkward when you are first learning. Actually, you might find it easier to use than dental floss. Maybe evenings after the children are in bed would be a better time?

*Client:* It's worth a try.

*RDH:* I'm glad you're willing to make an effort. Now let's take a minute to review the techniques you have been using, and hopefully we can decrease the time it takes you to perform your self-care.

The clinician must learn from the client the methods which will be most successful and then use that knowledge and skill to design an individualized self-care plan.

Communication also is influenced by the physical setting. The reception room, the operatory design, the organization of the armamentarium, and the arrangement of the equipment within the operatory and the general office decor, all make silent statements to the client and influence interaction.

*Example 4: The physical setting has a bearing on communication*

Ms. Mentor sits in the dental chair within a small operatory with a front-end entry instrument tray covered with aseptic barrier material. Cords from the handpieces are twisted and hanging in her lap. Naturally, she might feel somewhat confined and ill at ease. Communication does not flow as freely in this environment if the client is not comfortable and relaxed.

## FORMS OF COMMUNICATION

While communication is always occurring, the form of communication and the manner in which the message is expressed varies. There are two forms of communication: intrapersonal and interpersonal. The manner in which the message is expressed can be further categorized as being nonverbal and/or verbal. Nonverbal and verbal responses are expressed both intrapersonally and interpersonally. An explanation of these concepts is presented in the following sections.

### Intrapersonal Communication

This form of communication means the conveying of a message within oneself and to oneself (Carr, 1979; Geboy, 1985; Klinzing & Klinzing, 1985). One example of intrapersonal communication with which you might identify is taken from personal experience. This experience deals with scheduling an appointment at a dental office. Intrapersonal communication (within oneself) occurred even before telephoning the dental office. The client began with an internal discussion of the pros and cons of the dental appointment while considering whether to schedule an appointment or to continue to make excuses for not doing so, whether to wait another month, or even whether to return to this particular dental office. The client mentally reviewed the last visit of one year ago and decided to call and make the appointment. This person did not need another person to assist in the discussion; he communicated with himself through intrapersonal communication. Self-talk does not end here; it continues with our clients as they wait in the reception room the day of their appointment.

*Example of reception room intrapersonal communication*

A client observes the organization of the magazines in the reception room, the types of the magazine issues available, and most likely the date of the magazines. Something as simple as magazines in a reception room can tell a person much about the dental practice he is visiting. The organized matter in which the magazines are placed in the reception room might tell a person that the treatment received in the dental office will be orderly and well thought out. Also, the types of magazines might express the outside interests of the office staff, and the dates of the magazines might trigger a thought in the client's mind about how current and up-to-date the staff remains in their own professional education.

Notice with intrapersonal communication that a client can develop preconceived ideas about the office organization, staff interests, and staff continuing education practices that might be accurate or inaccurate. These ideas come from the client's own personal life experiences, beliefs, and values. There is a good chance that after speaking to the office staff these preconceived ideas about the office will change. Also, health professionals might have preconceived opinions about the thoughts of their clients. Therefore, it is important to incorporate effective interpersonal communication to validate preconceived notions or change thinking.

### Interpersonal Communication

This form of communication is a message shared between two or more people (Carr, 1979; Geboy, 1985). Interpersonal communication focuses on the interaction and interpretation of a conversation with nonverbal behaviors and spoken words. The dental hygienist needs to be able to focus on the client's feelings and thoughts in order to be effective in communicating. When the clinician states what is seen (nonverbal) and heard (verbal), it helps to verify the intended messages. This serves to involve the client and enhance accuracy of communication. Interpersonal communication includes all of the actions in the following discussion of nonverbal and verbal behaviors. Examples of both forms of interpersonal communication will be presented throughout the following two sections.

**Nonverbal Behavior.** This type of behavior includes **expressions of body** and **tone of voice** (Carr, 1979; Drafke, 1994; Geboy, 1985). Specifically nonverbal skills include body orientation, posture, facial expressions, gestures, touch, distance/space, and voice tone and hesitation (Bolton, 1979; Davies, 1994; Garza, Childers, & Walters, 1982). Researchers find that nonverbal behaviors provide 90 to 93 percent of the meaning to a message (Covey, 1989; Drafke, 1994). This type of behavior is displayed by both the speaker and the listener. Whether the clinician is listening or speaking, nonverbal behavior is being read by the clients and vice versa. It is critical that nonverbal behaviors are not overlooked.

Body orientation and posture are crucial to the interpretation of a message. An example of a positive body position connoting interest and involvement in the other person can be demonstrated by sitting in a relaxed position, squarely facing the individual. Such a position increases the clinician's degree of contact with the client and is a sign of openness to what the client has to say. Folded arms by either the client or dental professional might bring a meaning of rigidity into focus. A slouched or slumped position generally indicates boredom or lack of interest.

When the client and clinician meet, the clinician should observe the client's facial expression. The client's facial expression sets the stage for the clinician's mind to collect preconceived notions about the client's thoughts and feelings. Hopefully, the dental professional will be focusing in the eye area. Eye contact provides the clinician with the most information about the expression of the client. The length of time of the eye contact can give information to the dental hygienist about the client's willingness to interact. A short glance implies shyness or disinterest, while extended but relaxed eye contact shows friendliness and interest. Although a message from the client is being delivered to the dental hygienist through the length of eye contact or the lack thereof, it is impossible to interpret the complete message the client is communicating without further interaction.

The client's gestures also convey a message. In dentistry the most noticeable or talked about gesture is the vivid picture of the client's white knuckles clenching the dental chair indicating an uncomfortable experience is expected. A clinician's finger pointing in the direction of the client usually implies a lecture or reprimand is on its way. An example of a positive gesture is to extend an arm while leading the client to the treatment room. Again, further interaction is necessary to fully understand the true meaning of the nonverbal message.

In the dental office, touching in the head and neck area is common practice. The amount of touching that is necessary depends on the procedure being performed. An extraoral examination will more than likely need to be explained to new clients so they will not be uncomfortable with this touching. This type of examination might be a new experience. The pressure and duration of the touch might also be explained. The clinician's moving the client's head closer or farther away is another means of touching that is common in the dental office. Touching on the arm or shoulder is at times used to show concern on the clinician's part. Should nonverbal discomfort or uneasiness be expressed as a result of any touch, the clinician will realize that this nonverbal behavior is not within the client's realm of comfort; therefore, it is inappropriate.

Treating the whole person versus the oral cavity needs to be fully understood by the dental professional before successfully facilitating change in the client's oral self-care. Dental hygiene clinicians and clients are placed in a very unusual situation when compared to other health care providers due to the close nature of the treatment environment. Clinicians need to be acutely aware, and occasionally reminded of, the close working environment in which they practice. Very early in the development of the clinician/client relationship, the comfort zone of the client is invaded. Dental clinicians find themselves practicing in the intimate distance or space which is from contact to 18 inches (Chambers and Abrams, 1986). Personal distance is defined as 18 inches to 4 feet and social distance is 4 to 12 feet (Chambers & Abrams, 1986).

While reviewing the medical history the clinician is probably seated within the average personal distance, and then quickly moves into the client's intimate space to perform the assessment phase of care. Clinicians do this on a day-to-day basis sometimes neglecting to consider the client's comfort with this close encounter. Consideration of the dental hygienist's invasion into the private space of the client needs to be realized and at times respected. A simple statement acknowledging this intimate space is all that is necessary, particularly if the individual seems to be uncomfortable with the process of care.

*Example of clinician's statement acknowledging client's intimate space:*

*RDH:* I appreciate your cooperation in allowing me to reposition close to you in order to see your back teeth.

*Client:* That's all right.

Encouraging and acknowledging clients' acceptance of the dental professional's closeness during treatment lets clients know that the clinician is aware and involved in making them feel comfortable. Particularly with the new or anxious clients, acknowledging the closeness would be recommended. With returning clients perhaps nothing needs to be said because they are acquainted with the closeness of the treatment in the dental office. Whenever the clinician observes client discomfort with proximity, a comment to assure client comfort is in order.

The voice tone and hesitation in the speech or other audible sound are considered to be nonverbal behaviors. The dental hygienist's ears play an important role in deciphering the message implied by voice tone. Although voice tone obviously requires the use of sound, the main focus is the loudness, intonation, or inflection of the word or "noise" that is heard. The clinician can hear the feelings of the person by listening to the tone of the message. Anger, fear, excitement, and cooperation can be heard in the client's message. Hesitations in the speech pattern and audible sounds during a message causes the listener to think about the speaker's uncertainty in the message being expressed. It can also mean the client does not understand the topic in question. When a client responds to the use of a periodontal aid with "uh-huh" along with hesitation, the dental hygienist will want to question the client's willingness to accept the aid.

Just as nonverbal communication can help clinicians more effectively understand what a client is feeling, it is important not to become consumed with those behaviors. Some clinicians might have a tendency to "read into" what a person is thinking or feeling and incorrectly interpret the client's mannerisms. For example, if the client exhibits a grimace during the fluoride treatment, the clinician could misinterpret the expression as a reaction to a mouthful of tray and fluoride when actually the client finds the pina colada-flavored fluoride distasteful. Through practice, the skilled clinician learns to validate nonverbal behaviors.

**Verbal Behaviors.** This form of communication is the actual spoken message. Verbal behaviors include language, active listening, and paraphrasing (Carr 1979; Geboy 1985). **Language** used in communication needs to be straightforward and delivered in a nonthreatening manner. The words spoken to convey the dental hygienist's or dentist's message are selected carefully for the particular client. The language a dental hygienist or dentist would use with a child would be much different from the language used with an adolescent. Likewise, the language used with an adolescent would be very different from words spoken to an adult. At times clinicians get into a mode in which presenting self-care education includes the same memorized rationale. Individualizing the message presented is important for the client to accept the message. The ability of the clinician to enter the client's frame of reference is reflected by the clinician's capacity to chose words that capture his thoughts and feelings.

*Example of selected language for various client age groups:*

*RDH:* (statement with child) Your teeth are sure pretty when you smile.

*RDH:* (statement to adolescent) You sure have a great smile. I'm excited all your brushing and flossing has really paid off.

*RDH:* (statement to an adult) The brightness of your teeth and the healthy appearance of your gum tissue has really improved. You should be proud of the effort you have put forth to improve your self-care.

At times the clinician makes an error in assuming the comprehension level of the client, and variations need to be made in the presentation. Hopefully, the clinician has not misjudged the level of understanding and insulted the client. In order to make an assumption as to the level of comprehension, the clinician must exhibit exceptional **active listening skills**. There are inherent problems associated with listening. Concentration and focusing are two examples. While the client is explaining his self-care regime, the dental hygienist finds herself concentrating on the response rather than being attentive to what the client is saying and the nonverbals being portrayed. Remember the client is viewing the clinician's interest in what is being said and listening for encouraging responses. Dead silence on the part of the dental hygienist along with a far away look does not encourage the client to continue speaking. A nod, some praise, or a restatement of the client's response would be encouraging and illustrate attentiveness.

Think of the last time you were encouraged by the client's interaction during your self-care instructions. What type of client verbal and nonverbal behaviors demonstrate motivation and focus toward the education? If the person was motivated, she would face toward the clinician, use eye contact, and respond with some form of verbal behavior. These verbal behaviors might include "uh-huh" and/or nonverbal positive behavior such as nodding the head, or a question might be asked seeking additional information. Eye contact is important in both listening and speaking and denotes interest in what is being said. A dead stare is not considered good eye contact and would probably imply daydreaming is in motion. Eye contact involves facing toward the other person and looking generally in the facial area focusing at the other person's eye level.

Improvement in listening requires much concentration and elimination of distraction. Often the message leaves some extra "air time" where the listener's mind has a tendency to wander because some people process language faster (500 to 600 words per minute) than the average speaker can articulate (125 words per minute) (Chambers & Abrams, 1986). Daydreaming enters when the clinician uses the extra "air time" to think about the next appointment or what needs to be picked up at the grocery store after work. Getting caught up in the client's mannerisms and gestures sometimes takes the clinician away from the message. Therefore, focusing actively not only on the spoken message, but also on the nonverbal behaviors keeps the listener's mind in the conversation.

**Paraphrasing** can also be referred to as reflecting, a perception check, or feedback. These similar terms act as an avenue for the listener to repeat what was seen or heard. Paraphrasing corrects any misconceptions and allows for a free flowing interaction including feelings and thoughts. Paraphrasing will give the client a chance to validate or correct the dental hygienist's perception of his verbal and nonverbal behavior. This process helps both parties remain on the same track and be more involved in the conversation.

Paraphrasing also allows the clinician to evaluate the total communication picture, including the spoken message and the nonverbal communication of the client. However, a message three sentences or longer without allowing a response turns the dental hygienist's or dentist's comment into a "lecture" (Patterson & Eisenberg, 1983). The "lecture" style is not appropriate in cooperative communication because the client needs to be included in the discussion. However, the dental hygienist's role in educating the client about the causes and prevention of periodontitis is very limited by this principle. The clinician, therefore, needs to self-evaluate her communication to ensure the client is included in the discussion after three to five sentences at a time have been spoken. Paraphrasing the speaker's message, including both the spoken message and the nonverbal behavior, will increase the accuracy of the message and provide another avenue for the client to interact with language.

Below is an example of interpersonal communication that incorporates many of the concepts of nonverbal and verbal communication.

*Example of interpersonal communication:*

*RDH:* Linda, I notice that behind your last molar you have an area that is red and inflamed. Can you think of any reason why just this area is swollen?

*Client:* No, not really. I brush every day about three times and I floss most days.

*RDH:* Well, it's great you brush three times everyday and floss regularly. Let's take a look at your technique.

*Client:* (client rolls her eyes and sighs)

*RDH:* I notice you rolled your eyes and gave a frustrated sigh. When I ask you to demonstrate your brushing in the molar area how did that make you feel?

*Client:* Like a little kid who after all these years still cannot brush correctly.

*RDH:* My comment on you showing me your brushing and flossing technique made you feel dumb or like a failure with your brushing method.

*Client:* (thinking and responds) No that's not it. I guess I am just embarrassed at my age to still not have my technique perfected.

*RDH:* I appreciate your honesty with me and I can assure you that age has nothing to do with your ability to get your back teeth clean. You are doing a great job on all other areas and this area is very difficult to reach. Perhaps a toothbrush with a smaller head would be helpful.

The clinician allows the individual to speak, ask questions; and at the same time focuses on the client's nonverbal behavior. Note how the dental hygienist discusses the client's feelings, repeats what the client has said, and puts the response in feeling terms. The clinician's perceptions were not correct and the client had a chance to clarify what she actually meant. Dental appointments run smoothly when both parties are on the same wavelength. The dental hygienist should use paraphrasing to understand and evaluate the message from the client, rather than to judge its content.

Unfortunately, when the verbal and nonverbal messages are not congruent, the nonverbal interpretation will win out as being the true message. In the previous example, if the client had said that she knew she was not doing as well as she could in that area while rolling her eyes and sighing, the clinician would receive two different messages. Paying more attention to the nonverbal cues than the spoken words would be the most accurate interpretation of the client's message. Communication through nonverbal and verbal behaviors is much like putting a puzzle together. The clinician must collect all the information both behaviors are displaying and develop the correct message. This interaction between two people includes discussion of both feelings and spoken words to effectively communicate the total message.

## Building Confidence and Trust

Think about the last time you, as a clinician, were successful in providing effective NSPT. The client became motivated and took responsibility for his/her dental disease and for the recommended maintenance therapy after initial treatment. In order for this to happen, you, as the dental hygienist or dentist exhibited characteristics that enabled you to facilitate effective communication where confidence and trust were established. Garza (1982) uses the term **facilitative communication** in describing the interaction that exists between the health care provider and the helpee. In other words, the term facilitative communication is the ease with which the clinician and the client receiving NSPT cooperatively communicate. The dental hygienist acts as the facilitator in the NSPT and works in harmony with the client to successfully achieve common goals set by both parties.

In order for the client/dental hygienist relationship to be harmonious, the clinician needs to approach the client with empathy, respect, warmth, concreteness, genuineness, and self-disclosure. Garza, Childers, and Walters, (1982) define these six characteristics which are necessary for effective communication (see Table 7-2). The first three characteristics of empathy, respect, and warmth are important for the oral health care provider because they are vital to the client's **self-exploration** of her NSPT needs. Clients would discuss with the dental hygienist what dental needs are important to them, what self-care aids they are willing to use, how many times a day they are willing to use these aids, and their commitment to the total treatment plan. During this exploration the dental hygienist would facilitate the process by being nonjudgmental, accepting the client's ideas and thoughts, and placing himself in the client's frame of reference. An example of how to explore a client's needs follows.

*Example of exploring client's needs:*

*RDH:* Brushing and using the interdental brush will be an important part of your self-care during and after initial NSPT. I would suggest increasing your brushing to three times a day and using the interdental brush once a day. Does that seem realistic for you?

*Client:* That much! I can only fit brushing in two times a day. I will be able to brush once in the morning and once at night.

*RDH:* That sounds like a good starting point for you. So you will try to brush twice a day and can you use the interdental brush one of those times, possibly in the evening?

When the client chooses an alternative regime rather than the suggested one, the dental hygienist needs to express encouragement without judging the altered plan. The clinician invites clients to share their feelings about self-care without fear of consequence. Many times clients are afraid of being embarrassed or ridiculed by the lack

**Table 7-2  Six Characteristics of the Helping Professional during Self-Exploration and Action***

| Patient Stages | Characteristics of Clinician | Definition of the Characteristic |
|---|---|---|
| Self-Exploration | • Empathy | • Listening and understanding the emotions and feelings of another; understanding the other person's world |
| | • Respect | • To convey honor or esteem for another |
| | • Warmth | • Display your personal feelings and empathy |
| Action | • Concreteness | • Communicate clearly |
| | • Genuineness | • Communicate openly and honestly |
| | • Self-disclosure | • Share your personal experiences with others |

*These same six characteristics are necessary for the clinician to use in order to understand patient needs and implement "change."

of compliance with the recommendations. The dental hygienist must instill in the client a feeling that something of purpose will come out of the sharing, whether or not the altered plan is the appropriate method for obtaining optimum oral health as the clinician sees it.

If the client's suggested self-care plan is unacceptable to the clinician and would not promote improved oral health, additional education or alteration of that plan is indicated. Remember, if the client is actively involved in the design of the self-care practices, the success rate will likely be more favorable for both the clinician and client (Greenstein, 1992). An example of a response to a person who refuses to comply with the total self-care program that you have recommended is illustrated below.

*Example of noncompliant client treatment:*

Client response to recommendation by dental hygienist for use of periodontal aid.

*Client:* I know I would not use it. Brushing and flossing will have to do.

*RDH:* I'm sure you have a good reason for not using it.

*Client:* Yeah.

*RDH:* Could you tell me why?

*Client:* It has to do with time and patience.

*RDH:* We never seem to have enough time or patience with some things. I know we have discussed the need for the toothpick in the problem areas and the lack of use may result in tooth loss. If you understand this, then there is not any need for me to try and force you to use it.

*Client:* I do understand and I still know I will not use it. Brushing and flossing is enough for now.

*RDH:* OK. I will make a note of this conversation in your chart so that the office is aware of what we have decided for your self care program.

*Client:* Okay.

The next three characteristics of concreteness, genuineness, and self-disclosure are vital characteristics for

the dental hygienist and dentist to possess in order to promote client cooperation and compliance with the NSPT care plan. Professionals who possess these qualities provide the client with a sincere, caring, and earnest outlook that incorporates self-experiences into the treatment of clients. Further, the clinician must be able to incorporate the client's comments concerning daily routines, responsibilities, and limitations, into an individualized NSPT treatment plan. Remember, the empathy, respect, and warmth characteristics of a dental hygienist allow the client to feel comfortable in the practice setting. The client's comments are accepted and encouraged. The clinician does not discourage the client from expressing his wants, needs, and experiences. Then, the next step is to tackle the development of the individualized NSPT client education program utilizing the information disclosed by the client. The important part of this self-exploration stage is to remember that the clinician should listen to what the client says, paraphrase back to the client what is heard, and have the client confirm those comments as illustrated below.

*Example of confirming what the client has said:*

*Client:* I get up each morning at 5:00 and exercise for 20 minutes. It's really the only time I have to myself. Then I shower and get ready for work. My children and I have to leave the house by 6:45 A.M. I get the kids up at 6:00 and they have their breakfast by 6:30. It's a mad house in the morning!

*RDH:* Sounds like your mornings are busy and very tightly scheduled. It doesn't seem like there is any room for more than brushing your teeth in the morning.

*Client:* You're right. I am really busy.

*RDH:* I'm happy to see you are as concerned about your physical health as you are about your dental health. Perhaps evenings would be best for more extensive oral hygiene measures like using the interdental brush.

*Client:* I'll try.

The clinician in this example was being realistic and not trying to push the client into performing additional self-care in the morning. The dental hygienist or dentist could try to suggest more extensive self-care in the morning, but more than likely this would only reinforce to the client that the clinician was not listening. If the clinician keeps pushing, chances are the client might consent to the morning routine just so she does not have to repeat her busy schedule again while thinking that the clinician did not hear the message the first time. This "trying" by the dental hygienist stops communication between the client and clinician and creates a breakdown in the morning self-care plan. Both the clinician and the client would lose in this case, and more importantly the NSPT would be compromised because of lack of full cooperation.

The more effective the dental hygienist or dentist is at implementing the principles of communication, the more likely the chance of a behavior change within the client. Methods that facilitate client compliance with oral hygiene and professional maintenance, increase the likelihood for success in periodontal therapy (Greenstein, 1992).

The NSPT self-care education plan is designed to incorporate all of the needs of the client. It is essential that the client feels ownership in this plan and it is the dental professional's responsibility to involve the client as a cotherapist in treatment. Success of NSPT relies on honesty and openness on both the client's and clinician's parts. Providing an open, honest, and safe arena for the individual to tell the dental hygienist that flossing is not becoming a regular daily occurrence is a sign of workable facilitative communication. When a client does not feel embarrassed or afraid to confess his limitations at completing the NSPT home care plan, an open, friendly, and nonjudgmental arena is created.

### Six Behavior Types and Suggestions for Coping with These Behaviors

There are times in dental hygiene practice when a client seated in your chair exhibits a behavior that makes treatment difficult. During these times the clinician must grasp for her best communication skills to make it through the appointment. The first step in coping is to realize what type of behavior this client is exhibiting. Next, the clinician must put into action the possible ways of interacting with the client to achieve success. Labeling clients according to their behavior is not the point; however, being able to understand the characteristics of the person, note the reasons for the behavior, and deal with the particular behavior are important elements for communicating with clients who exhibit challenging behaviors.

Table 7-3 depicts six different behavior types, the possible behavior characteristics, and suggested ways of handling each behavior (Bramson, 1981). Also included is a dialogue associated with each behavior illustrating the communication techniques suggested for each client

type. The example for all six behavior types will be centered around the same "time issue" scenario because the number of appointments and/or time involved in NSPT is a typical client concern. It is hoped that the use of the same scenario will assist the reader in seeing the different approaches for each behavior type. In this scenario, the clinician has completed the treatment plan and is communicating the case presentation. It is time to discuss the number of appointments needed and the time commitment necessary for success in NSPT.

## DOCUMENTING COMMUNICATION

As reiterated throughout this chapter, the more effective the implementation of principles of communication, the more likely the success of the clinician in affecting behavior change. In turn, behavior change by the client will increase the chance for successful NSPT. Increased communication necessitates increased documentation in the dental records. Many clinicians write notations in the client's chart as if they will be the only persons that will read the notes, or as if they will be around to interpret the message to the next person. This is, of course, not always the case. The written record is the basis for future therapy and is essential for continuity of treatment. In today's age of consumer advocacy, there is an increasing number of malpractice suits, particularly as they relate to some area of personal health or lack thereof (Mitchell, 1991).

A deficiency of clear documentation in client records can contribute to a loss of credibility, even for the best clinician, in the courtroom (D'Eramo, 1979). Written communication, as with verbal and nonverbal communication, can leave the receiver with an entirely wrong impression if incorrectly stated. Whenever a word is used that has more than one meaning, that word must be clarified or replaced with another word. For example, it is likely that a reader does not read the same message that you are attempting to connote. Because juries are sympathetic to clients, it would behoove all clinicians to attend to thorough and understandable documentation.

More and more frequently, courts seem to be saying that clients have a right to know what is written in their records. If the client is involved in writing their record, it helps to "demystify" the record (Mitchell, 1991). Just as the clinician works with the client to set goals that the client will accept, they should work together to document the goals and objectives. Working together does not actually mean that the client writes the record; however, the practitioner might make statements as follows.

*Example:*

RDH: I will just record in your record that we have agreed to a three-month recall interval for periodontal maintenance therapy.

RDH: In our discussion about the recall interval I discovered, we have a difference of opinion. You are thinking six months is early enough to return to the

# Table 7-3 Six Different Behavior Types and Possible Suggestions for Coping with These Behaviors

The table below summarizes 6 difficult behavior types and possible suggestions for the clinician to effectively facilitate NSPT. Responses are based on the following sample statement by the clinician: *"Sarah, as we discussed in the treatment plan for you, we will need to scale and root plane all four quadrants in your mouth. Each quadrant will take approximately 1 hour to thoroughly treat. Therefore, we will need to schedule four 1-hour appointments and another 1/2-hour visit for reevaluation. How do you feel about this appointment schedule?"*

| Behavior | Behavior Characteristics | Possible Explanation for Behavior | Suggestions for Coping with Behavior | Typical or Possible Response to above Sample Dialogue |
|---|---|---|---|---|
| Silent/ Unresponsive | • Reacts to questions or conversation with silence, "yep," "nope," or a noncommittal yes or no. <br> • Offers little information. | • To avoid painful interpersonal situations, express hostility, avoid taking a position on an issue. <br> • Masks fear, sullen anger, or a spiteful refusal to cooperate. | • Get patient to open up and begin to discuss what it is that is on her mind or what is bothering her. | *Sarah* (gripping the arms of chair): humm <br> *RDH:* By the sounds of your "humm" it seems as though you still have a question in your mind. Is that correct? <br> *Sarah:* uh-huh <br> *RDH:* What's on your mind right now? |
| Indecisive Staller | • Habitually indecisive. Will accept a responsibility and then not follow through on it. <br> • Usually agreeable and easy to work with until you need to depend on them. <br> • Typical response is no response. | • The desire to avoid making someone mad or to disappoint someone is the prime force behind the staller's indecisiveness. | • Attempt to engage patient in problem solving by not taking their problems on yourself. <br> • Be open to listening to conflicts and difficulties. <br> • Listen for indirect clues for the underlying issues. | *Sarah:* I don't know how I feel. I know I need this but I'm not sure how I'll fit the time in. <br> *RDH:* What do you suppose we ought to do? <br> *Sarah:* I guess maybe I could come in during my lunch hours . . . are you open during the lunch hour? <br> *RDH:* We try to take our lunch hour from 12-1. Is it possible for you to reschedule your lunch hour? Or have you thought about the possibility of an early morning appointment? or late afternoon? <br> *Sarah:* I hadn't thought of that. Let me think about it. |
| Complainer | • Finds fault with everything. <br> • Feels someone else should be resolving the problem. <br> • Unable to engage in productive problem-solving dialogue; will result in additional complaints. | • They feel powerless to change the situations about which they complain. <br> • They feel they are free from responsibility—take no ownership for the problem. | • Interrupt their cycle of consistent blaming. <br> • Insist that their problems be managed in a problem-solving manner. <br> • Do not agree with or apologize for their complaints. <br> • If all else fails, ask the Complainer "how do you want this discussion to end?" | *Sarah:* Four 1-hour appointments? That's 4 hours!! And I brush my teeth all the time and have them cleaned every year! Now I have to get off work and then . . . <br> *RDH:* Wait a minute. Let me see if I understand what you're saying. The four hours of appointments seems excessive to you because you brush your teeth regularly and have them cleaned once a year, and you're concerned about getting the time off work for these appointments. Right now you seem pretty frustrated about the whole thing. <br> *Sarah:* Well, yes. I still think four more appointments is ridiculous! <br> *RDH:* Sarah, how do you suggest we proceed? |
| Negativist | • Responds to question or proposal with a quick and negative response. <br> • Unable to move from "fault-finding" position to action mode of problem solving—continue in negative and critical mode. | • They feel as if everything is out of their control. <br> • Do not recognize their feelings of powerlessness and pessimism yourself. <br> • Basically bitter about themselves, others, and life in general. | • Engage them in rational problem solving without getting drawn into the negativism and pessimism yourself. <br> • Make optimistic but realistic statements about past successes with similar problems. <br> • Be prepared to take action on your own and announce your plans to do so. | *Sarah:* It won't work. I can't come in here four more times. Can't you do it in less time? <br> *RDH:* I have found with other patients in your similar situation that four appointments are necessary. I want to have enough time to do a thorough job. |
| "The Know-It-All" | • Expert on all matters. <br> • Often react to others' facts or knowledge with irritation, anger, or withdrawal. | • Driven by the need to simplify their own world and make it as understandable and controllable as possible. <br> • Operate on the assumption that the only sure thing is to know it all and to do it all oneself. | • Get them to consider alternatives without directly challenging their alleged expertise. | *Sarah:* That schedule seems to satisfy your needs! I know I have pockets . . . you've told me that before. I've been taking care of them. <br> *RDH:* I realize you're aware of your pocket depths and as you know in order to thoroughly treat those areas, I need additional time. Although I do not think it's in your best interest, we could combine the appointments and schedule two 1-1/2-hour appointments to cut back on the number of visits. |
| Hostile-Aggressive | • Behave in abusive, abrupt, intimidating, and contemptuous manner—victims are left feeling overwhelmed and powerless. | • A strong and driving need to prove to themselves and others that they are always right. <br> • Lack a sense of caring and respect for others—may consider these qualities as weaknesses in others. | • Give them time to run down. <br> • Stand up to them without being drawn into a fight of argument. <br> • Maintain eye contact. <br> • State your own opinion and thoughts forcefully and without apology. <br> • Be friendly and receptive to negotiation. | *Sarah:* There is absolutely no way that I am going to come in here for four more hours to have my teeth cleaned! <br> *RDH:* Sarah, to thoroughly treat each quadrant this time frame is necessary. I do not see any other way of doing this without compromising your care. |

191

office and after my assessment of your periodontal needs, I feel a three-month recall is essential. I will record this discussion and the decision for a six-month recall so there is no question about your decision.

The record does not need to be lengthy, but it requires specificity. There is no room for vagueness in medical documents. The client's chart must say a lot in a little space. The language used must be precise and leave no room for misinterpretation. Clichés should be avoided. The use of adjectives should be limited and verbs should be used to replace adjectives that describe a client behavior. For example, rather than stating in the record "client was a complainer throughout entire appointment, particularly during self-care", the clinician could record in the client's own words the exact complaint(s) and the behavior that accompanied the complaint. A statement by the client such as, "I hate to floss because it shreds between my fillings" can be quoted in the dental record.

To further clarify this problem, an additional follow-up comment should be included, such as, the dentist diagnosed that #4-DO and #5-MOD need to be replaced. The relationship of the shedding floss to the interproximal bulk would be explained to the client. Additional examples of how to document communication encountered during self-care education follow.

*Example record of services entry 1:* Client did not listen to self-care education.

*Corrected entry:* Client stated "I already know about what causes periodontal disease."

*Example record of services entry 2:* Client is not brushing or flossing as recommended.

*Corrected entry:* Client stated "I will brush 1X/day but will not floss at all."

*Example record of services entry 3:* Client is not interested in surgery.

Patient name _____                    Date _____

| Questions to Ask Yourself | Yes | No |
|---|---|---|
| 1. Did I actively listen to what the patient is saying?<br>   a. Attend carefully to messages being presented by patient? | | |
|    b. Listen for basic messages? | | |
|    c. Respond frequently and briefly to the message to show understanding? | | |
|    d. Respond to both the feeling and content of the message? | | |
|    e. Move gradually toward the exploration of sensitive topics or feelings? | | |
|    f. After I responded, did I attend carefully to cues that either confirm or deny the accuracy of my response? | | |
| 2. Did I avoid making judgmental responses about the patient's statements or the patient in general? | | |
| 3. Did I use eye contact while speaking and listening to the patient? | | |
| 4. Was I able to accurately paraphrase the patient's message? | | |
| 5. Are my values and attitudes being expressed in my nonverbal behavior? | | |
| 6. Are my values and attitudes being expressed in my verbal behavior? | | |
| 7. Did I appropriately respond to the patient's nonverbal and verbal behaviors? | | |
| 8. Did I select words that mirrored that of the patient? | | |
| 9. Did I show empathy, respect, and warmth while discussing the patient's needs and expectations? | | |
| 10. Did I speak concretely, genuinely, and incorporate appropriate self-disclosure while discussing the NSPT treatment plan? | | |
| Based upon your answers to the above questions, how would you more effectively communicate with this patient?<br><br>_____<br><br>_____<br><br>_____ | | |

**Figure 7-1** Communication skills: A Self-Assessment.

*Corrected entry:* Discussed periodontal surgery. Client stated "Tooth loss is acceptable and money was not available to do surgery." Client did not consent to care.

The medico-legal record must accurately reflect why the client was seen, what services were performed, and the recommendations for care. Also specific progress or lack of progress must be clearly documented at subsequent appointments. Refer to Chapter 19 for general guidelines on documenting NSPT.

## IMPROVING COMMUNICATION SKILLS

A goal of NSPT is to initiate a behavioral change in the client's self-care practices through higher level learning. As with any skill to be learned, whether it is communication or the use of a periodontal aid, there are guidelines that can be followed to ensure success. Figure 7-1 lists a number of questions that can be answered by the clinician to self-evaluate communication skills. This format could also be used to help clinicians within the office or educational setting to evaluate one another and, therefore, help heighten the level of communication with clients.

When performing a communication assessment, whether on yourself or another team member, pay close attention to what the client is saying and particularly what the client seems to be feeling. The interpretation of nonverbal behavior requires practice and experience. It is important to remember that nonverbals are open to a number of interpretations and that you must be sensitive to the particular situation. The key to effective interpretation is to listen to the entire context without becoming distracted on the specific behavior.

The clinician should always show empathy and genuine interest in the person's concerns. The clinician should not be concerned about agreeing with what the client is saying. Acknowledgment of their feelings is of utmost importance. Showing respect for each client's feelings is often more beneficial to the dental hygienist/client relationship than the actual "being right." If the client is upset, allow them to be. There is probably a reason for their behavior. Acknowledge the problem, "Gee, that is a problem, I don't have an answer to solve it yet, but I'm sure we can figure something out." Try not to become defensive. Use active listening skills to collect all the information given by the client. Asking questions, paraphrasing, and clarifying what the individual has said will assist the skilled clinician in effectively implementing NSPT or any type of dental care. The clinician needs to focus on the problem at hand.

Continuing education courses are another route for clinicians to enhance their skills. Perhaps looking outside the field of dentistry for courses in communication would be beneficial to all team members in the office or clinic. Demonstrating good problem-solving skills will win the client's respect and trust in the clinician, and will allow the dental professional to more truly help the client.

## Summary

The application of communication principles is an often overlooked and underutilized aspect of dental care. Applying proper communication techniques can be just as important to successful NSPT as other "technical" skills. This chapter is intended to heighten the clinician's awareness of the importance of both verbal and nonverbal behaviors in the dental operatory.

Critical to the success of NSPT is the client's involvement in treatment. If the client feels the clinician is competent, the client is more likely to become involved and to cooperate with all aspects of the therapy. In order for cooperation to occur, the clinician must secure the confidence of the client. Lack of, or ineffective, communication can barricade the process of therapy before it really begins.

Whether or not words are being spoken, communication is occurring on several levels throughout the entire appointment period. It is important for clinicians to remain cognizant of client behaviors and not become complacent in the treatment of the client's needs.

## Case Studies

**Case Study One:** Lowell Chilis, a local stockbroker, was appointed for an emergency toothache. When Lowell checked in with the receptionist he was notified that he would have about a thirty-minute wait. Lowell sat in a straightback chair in the reception room, which gave a full view of the receptionist's desk and of the office staff members. As the auxiliaries and dentist approached the receptionist's desk, Lowell observed their nonverbal behaviors. While waiting to be seated he selected a magazine, not from the magazine rack but one that was tossed on one of the couches. The magazine was curled up on the edges and had a date from the previous year. Dr. Colby came in Lowell's view, looked towards Lowell and the reception room, questioned the receptionist, took a deep breath while rolling his eyes, looked at his watch, and walked out of view. Which form of communication was Mr. Chilis experiencing? What impression do you think Mr. Chilis has regarding this practice?

**Case Study Two:** Blake Cole, a 35-year-old amateur golfer, is discussing his treatment plan with his dentist, Dr. Dennis Edwin. Dr. Edwin was discussing Blake's restorative, preventive, and prosthetic needs. The case presentation is being presented in the dental operatory with the restorative tray on the bracket table. Blake is seated in the supine position and is ready for treatment once he agrees to the treatment plan. How would you improve Dr. Edwin's case presentation?

**Case Study Three:** Doug Alan, a 50-year-old pool supply salesman presents for his six-month recall appointment. During NSPT, Lucille Price, the dental hygienist has the following dialogue with Doug:

*Lucille:* Doug, I notice the gingiva around your anterior teeth, these in front with the crowns, is bleeding when I use the probe .

*Doug:* Any of my gums would bleed if you poke them with that sharp pick!

*Lucille:* (Lucille stops probing and puts the probe and mirror in a relaxed position in one hand) Doug, it sounds like you think this probe is causing your tissue to bleed.

*Doug:* Doesn't it?

*Lucille:* No. Can I show you the end of the instrument? (Doug nods yes)

*Lucille:* As you can see the end is blunted. If my technique in using the instrument was incorrect causing you discomfort then bleeding might occur. Is the probing causing you any discomfort?

*Doug:* No. It doesn't hurt. The bleeding must be something else. Right?

*Lucille:* Yes. If you should feel any discomfort at all during your appointment(s), please raise your hand and I will stop.

*Doug:* OK. What were you saying about the bleeding?

*Lucille:* Your gums are bleeding because there is inflammation present in this area. Let me explain it thoroughly.

How did Lucille handle Doug's initial response and rationale for bleeding gums?

**Case Study Four:** Breanne Nicole, a 35-year-old veterinarian, first visited the dental office with an emergency toothache. At that appointment a temporary restoration was placed in tooth #30 and an appointment was scheduled with the dental hygienist for the following week. One week later, Breanne enters the dental hygiene operatory and is seated in the dental chair. Her seated position has the appearance of discomfort. Her shoulders are raised and her eyes are looking in a downward stare at the dental equipment surrounding her and at the hoses from the handpieces that are dangling in her lap. The dental hygienist, Jeff Raudabaugh, flips through Breanne's med-ical history and asks Breanne about her chief complaint of "bleeding gums." While Breanne struggles to describe her dislike for bleeding gums she offers very little information in her one-word sentence responses. During this time she gets little attention from Jeff because he continues to review the medical history. What behavior type fits Breanne? What changes could Jeff make to improve his overall communication focusing on the behavior type of Breanne?

**Case Study Five:** Judi Samuelson, a 40-year-old psychic, is in the middle of a discussion about her self-care needs with the dental hygienist, Jeffrey Dean. During their discussion, Jeffrey suggested that Judi use an additional self-care aid. Judi responded quite negatively toward the use of the aid by stating "No, I will not use that aid." Jeffrey then discusses the result of not being able to effectively remove plaque from pocket areas and furcations. "Judi, the pockets are quite deep adjacent to these teeth (demonstrates the depth in the area with a probe); this tooth has 6 mm pocket depths and this tooth has 5 mm pockets. Additionally, there are furcations on each of these teeth. This wooden toothpick will assist you in removing plaque from the pocket and within the furcation area. If the plaque is not removed the result will be loss of supporting tissues in the problem areas." What is the appropriate chart entry in the above case study?

## Case Study Discussions

**Discussion—Case Study One:** Lowell experienced intrapersonal communication. He spent the half-hour wait, pondering the nonverbal he had observed in the office. The curled up magazines, the disorder of their placement, and the out-of-date magazine might exhibit an unorganized office. The out-of-date magazine might also lead Lowell to question the current dental practices of the professionals. Dr. Colby's nonverbal communication—rolling his eyes, discussion with receptionist, looking at his watch, and walking out of sight all might suggest to Lowell that his reception from the staff might not be a pleasant one.

**Discussion—Case Study Two:** Dr. Edwin's case presentation can be conducted in the operatory. However, the fact that the unit is set up for treatment and Blake is in the full supine position indicates that the treatment decisions have already been made by Dr. Edwin. Open and relaxed communication is lacking. Blake should be seated in the upright position, on an equal seating level with the dentist with the instruments out of his view. Dr. Edwin should face toward Blake, maintain eye contact, explain the treatment, and allow Blake to ask questions and respond to treatment.

**Discussion—Case Study Three:** Doug's questions concerning the reason for his bleeding gums could have been addressed previously in the appointment if Lucille had educated Doug about the probing procedure. Because this was not addressed earlier, Lucille had to stop during treatment and respond. If Lucille had discussed the procedure earlier and Doug still had questions, then stopping is necessary. If the hygienist continued to probe while trying to discuss the bleeding gums she would not be focusing directly on the client's concerns. Stopping the probing procedure lets the client know that the clinician is not in a hurry and is willing to take the time listen. She also made sure Doug understood the characteristics and use of the instrument as well as the reason for the inflammation. Note that the explanation and responses Lucille expressed were limited and gave Doug a chance to ask questions and fully understand what she was saying. Lucille also used paraphrasing in her second response to Doug, "It sounds like you think this probe is causing your tissue to bleed." If this statement was just taken as a joke by the hygienist and dismissed, Doug would not have understood the probing procedure or the cause of bleeding gums.

**Discussion—Case Study Four:** Because Breanne offered little information and answered in one-word phrases, her behavior could be classified as silent/unresponsive. Changes in both Jeff's verbal and nonverbal interaction with Breanne can be improved as follows:

1. Verbal: Silent/unresponsive types need to be encouraged to open up and provide more information. A client such as Breanne will not open up to explain her chief complaint without further questioning and a show of interest from the dental hygienist. Active listening is important to all clients not only the silent/unresponsive type. Facing the client and connecting with eye contact

would encourage her and demonstrate interest in her response.

2. Nonverbal: Jeff's nonverbals, such as looking down and flipping through the medical history are not effective communication. He should, as stated above, face Breanne, engage in eye contact, and nod, when appropriate, to reassure Breanne that he is listening. Breanne's "tense" seated position should have alerted Jeff that something might be bothering her. Questions directly related to Breanne's appearance of being uncomfortable should be addressed immediately. For example, Jeff could ask, "Breanne, is this equipment crowding you?" If Breanne's response to being uncomfortable is not due to the closeness of the equipment, further questioning is needed such as, "Breanne you seem tense, especially in your shoulder area. Am I right?" If the answer is "yes" continue the questioning to find out if the tenseness is dentally-related.

**Discussion—Case Study Five:** An accurate chart entry is necessary not only for legal purposes, but also for future continuity of care. This entry could read: (date) *Discussed the wooden toothpick with Judi for #15 and #14. She responded "No, I will not use that aid." Explained results of non-compliance: gingival inflammation, bleeding, and further periodontal destruction.*

Even though it takes time to record information appropriately, the document must be complete, thorough, and accurate. If legal problems with this client should arise at a later date, it would be necessary to recall what had transpired at each appointment. Reviewing the client's records prior to care will assist the therapist in remembering the client's complete response to treatment, especially comments relating to noncompliance. Note that direct comments made by the client are put in quotes.

## REFERENCES

Bolton, R. (1979). *People skills.* New York City: Simon & Schuster.

Bramson, R. M. (1981). *Coping with difficult people.* New York City: Dell Publishing.

Carr, J. B. (1979). *Communicating and relating.* Dubuque, IA: Wm. C. Brown Publishers.

Cherry, C. (1974). *Human communication: Theoretical explorations.* Hillsdale, NJ: Lawrence Erlbaum Associates.

Chambers, D. W. & Abrams, R. G. (1986). *Dental communication.* Norwalk, CT: Appleton-Century-Crofts.

Covey, S. (1989). *The 7 habits of highly effective people.* New York: Simon & Schuster.

D'Eramo, E. (1979). The office anesthesia record. *Journal of American Dental Association, 98,* 407–409.

David, J. (1987). *People factor training manual & guide.* St. Petersburg, FL: INNERSEE.

Davies, P. (1994). Non-verbal communication with patients. *British Journal of Nursing, 3*(5), 220–223.

Drafke, M. (1994). *Working in health care: What you need to know to succeed.* Philadelphia: F. A. Davis.

Egan, G. (1982). *The skilled helper.* Monterey, CA: Brooks/Cole Publishing.

Geboy, M. (1985). *Communication and behavior management in dentistry.* Baltimore: Williams & Wilkins.

Garza, G. M., Childers, W. C., & Walters, R. P. (1982). *Interpersonal communication.* Gaithersburg, MD: Aspen Publishers.

Greenstein, G. (1992). Periodontal response to mechanical non-surgical therapy: A review. *Journal of Periodontology, 63,* 118–130.

Guralnik, D. K. (Ed.). (1976). *Webster's new world dictionary.* USA: Williams Collins and World Publishing Co., Inc.

Klinzing, D. & Klinzing, D. (1985). *Communication for allied health professionals.* Dubuque, IA: Wm. C. Brown Publishers.

Mitchell, Robert. (1991). *Documentation in counseling records.* 3 vols. Alexandria, VA: American Association for Counseling and Development, 1991.

Patterson, L. E. & Eisenberg, S. (1983). *The counseling process.* Boston: Houghton Mifflin.

Sisty-LePeau, N. (1995). Emphasis on communication. *Journal of Dental Hygiene, 69*(3), 101.

# CHAPTER 8

# Oral Self-Care Education and Case Presentation

## Key Terms

Dental Hygiene Human Needs Conceptual Model
disease theory
external motivational strategies
external motivation
informed consent
internal motivation
Learning Ladder Continuum

management discrepancy
Maslow's Needs Hierarchy
oral self-care
readiness
skill discrepancy
skill enhancement

## INTRODUCTION

Dental hygienists highly value self-care education and case presentation for many reasons. First, these components of care provide the clinician with the opportunity to personalize dental hygiene care through facilitative communication. The relationship of effective communication to self-care education was highlighted in the previous chapter and the reader is referred to its contents for a review of productive communication strategies. Effective communication is also essential to enhance the chances of client informed consent for the proposed nonsurgical treatment plan.

Second, clinicians realize the relationship of a client's self-care practices and informed consent for professional therapy to successful short-term and long-term NSPT. The *Guidelines for Periodontal Therapy* (American Academy of Periodontology [AAP], 1993) recognizes self-care as being an essential component of treatment planning, implementation of care, reevaluation, periodontal maintenance procedures (PMP), and evaluation of therapy. Self-care education and training in personal oral hygiene should be included in all treatment plans. Reevaluation, or posttreatment, should review and reinforce personal daily oral hygiene. Upon completion of active therapy, follow-up PMP should include assessment of the client's bacterial plaque control effectiveness and reinstruction where needed. Upon completion of planned periodontal therapy, the records and a clinical assessment of the client should reveal that counseling regarding why and how to perform an effective daily personal oral hygiene program occurred. Informed consent, the expected result of case presentation, is also

addressed in these *Guidelines* (AAP, 1993). The client is entitled to know the diagnosis, etiology, proposed therapy, alternative treatment, and prognosis with or without the proposed therapy or a limited therapeutic approach. Informed consent also should contain, where appropriate, the recommendations for treatment to be performed by other professionals, inherent risks, potential complications, and the need for PMP.

Third, dental hygienists view self-care education and case presentation as fundamental yet challenging components of their professional care. Frequent challenges include creating the time to provide quality client-centered interactions, creating the atmosphere to foster learning, focusing on the individual's needs and values, and making these aspects of care financially rewarding. This chapter addresses the theory related to self-care education and case presentation, while providing practical suggestions for incorporating these services into NSPT. Self-care education addresses adherence issues, motivation and needs, readiness to learn, and the process of education. Case presentation is discussed by addressing its purpose, components, and implications in providing periodontal care.

## ORAL SELF-CARE

Self-care education is a dynamic and continuous process that occurs throughout each appointment in initial therapy and PMP. **Oral self-care** can be defined as the client removal or reduction of bacterial plaque both supragingivally and subgingivally (1 to 3 mm) to help resolve periodontal inflammation. Many terms are used to describe oral self-care such as oral hygiene measures, plaque control (programs), and mechanical plaque removal. No matter which term is used, the main focus of any oral health education session is to teach the client how to control plaque accumulation. Because education is individualized for each client, the use of the term "program" refers to the general program established in an office or clinical setting. A self-care program does not imply that a single, "canned" approach is effective for all clients.

Other terms incorporated into this chapter include **disease theory** and **skill enhancement.** Disease theory is defined as knowledge shared with the client about periodontal diseases. Theory is related to the cognitive domain and includes, but is not limited to, the causes, classification, and stage of bone loss. Skill enhancement refers to the teaching of brushing, interdental aids, and other self-care devices or practices (i.e., oral rinsing, irrigation) to enhance plaque removal. It is involved with analysis of the client's psychomotor domain. The objectives of client education are to improve the outcome of NSPT in clinical practice and to elicit the client as a cotherapist responsible for daily self-care practices. Empowering clients with this responsibility permits them to realize that they have some degree of control over periodontal disease. The ultimate goal of oral self-care education is to promote client behavior change which will, in turn, enhance long-term results of NSPT.

## Bacterial Plaque and Self-Care

The inflammatory components of gingivitis and periodontitis can be managed effectively for the majority of clients with a combination of a plaque control program and root debridement (American Academy of Periodontology, 1993). Even though research has shown that client removal of supragingival plaque can help decrease the signs of gingival inflammation in relation to gingival bleeding and erythema, self-care alone has a limited effect on clinical conditions associated with periodontitis such as probing depth or attachment level (Bakdash, 1994). In a study designed to analyze the effects of scaling and root planing in subjects who exercised meticulous plaque control, Sato and others (1993) found that in nonscaled quadrants, self-performed plaque control resulted in continued improvement of periodontal sites less than 5 mm deep. Supragingival plaque control does not predictably alter the microbial composition in pockets greater than 5 mm, and therefore, professional subgingival mechanical instrumentation should always be utilized in conjunction with personal self-care (Bakdash, 1994; Corbet & Davies, 1993; Greenstein, 1992).

The relationship that exists between supragingival and subgingival plaque formation must be emphasized to the client. When supragingival plaque is ineffectively removed, microorganisms will quickly recolonize subgingivally after subgingival debridement (Magnusson, Lindhe, Yoneyama, & Liljenberg, 1984). The longer the gingival plaque is allowed to mature in the gingival sulcus and periodontal pocket, the greater the potential for mineralization in the apical areas (Axelsson, 1993). The mineralized deposit or calculus itself, however, is not the primary etiological factor that contributes significantly to the destruction of the periodontium. Instead, when calculus mineralizes it is always overlaid with microbial plaque; thus, calculus is a retentive factor requiring professional removal to facilitate effective oral self-care. In fact, mature plaque that never calcifies is probably more detrimental to the periodontium than calcified plaque. Self-care education requires that clients be given adequate information regarding the cause and effect relationship between the bacterial plaque, host, and periodontal diseases. A thorough explanation of microbial causes is one essential component of fostering effective personal plaque control (Low & Ciancio, 1990). Another component of daily self-care is the client's skill level in actual removal of bacterial plaque with self-care aids that are appropriate for the client's oral conditions. Although host factors play a major role in disease susceptibility, the client has more control over bacterial plaque removal than systemic health problems or genetic predisposition. Therefore, it must be established in the client's mind that his effort in daily oral self-care is the single most important factor in determining a long-term prognosis (Palmer & Floyd, 1995).

## Client Compliance

*Compliance* can be described as the degree to which a client's actions conforms with professional advice about self-care practices and recall interval recommendations (Kühner & Raetzke, 1989; Wilson, 1987). This description can be misleading because it suggests that the client is a passive listener or observer and not an active participant (Wilson, 1987). Currently the term *adherence* is gaining popularity because of the connotation that the client willingly heeds professional advice. Actually, compliance or adherence should be thought of as self-care behavior changes that result from collaboration between the practitioner and client. This "cotherapist" relationship or "therapeutic alliance" is essential to facilitate because client needs, choices, and internal motivation are critical elements to consider when teaching another self-care behaviors. Compliance with self-care practices and periodic maintenance procedures (PMP) are both essential components of successful periodontal care. Researchers, however, have noted that motivation and compliance are usually short-lived resulting in only short-term changes in behavior (Greenstein, 1992; Stewart et al., 1991; Weinstein, 1982). In general, compliance decreases as treatment time or the complexity of the required behavioral changes increase (Wilson, 1987).

Results of a 1993 survey (Proctor & Gamble Educational Series) about dental care and brushing behavior reveal that 85 percent of Americans rate their overall dental health as excellent or pretty good. Fifty percent like to visit the dentist and 64 percent claim they faithfully follow their dental professional's instructions. In relation to brushing behavior, survey results reveal that 80 percent of Americans brush their teeth several times a day; however, only 16 percent rate their current toothbrush as excellent in being able to clean in between the teeth. It is notable that 55 percent of those surveyed wished they could find an easier way to clean in between their teeth. In 1989, 662 dentate adults living in the Detroit metropolitan area were interviewed and asked how frequently they brushed, flossed, and had checkups. Ninety-seven percent reported brushing once a day, 32 percent reported flossing once a day, while 13 percent indicated they did not brush all teeth and about 10 percent of those who flossed daily said they did not floss all teeth (Ronis, Lang, Farghaly, & Ekdahl, 1994). A Swedish national dental survey showed that approximately 46 percent of adults use toothpicks sporadically and 12 percent use them daily. On the other hand, dental floss was used occasionally by 12 percent of the adults and daily by 2 percent; therefore, adults used toothpicks 4 to 6 times more frequently than dental floss (Håkansson, 1978). It was concluded that the toothpick is not only the more common aid, but the more appropriate aid for the majority of adults. Refer to Chapter 6 for further information about appropriate selection of self-care methods and aids.

It seems that self-reported adherence rates are high, and that these rates do not correlate to the estimated prevalence of gingivitis in the American population. If brushing behavior occurs daily, and gingivitis and periodontitis affect the majority of the population, then effectiveness of self-care techniques must be contributing to the prevalence of periodontal diseases. The *effectiveness* of toothbrushing for plaque removal and gingivitis prevention has been established (Walsh, et al. 1989); however, research does not link increased *frequency* of brushing with improved oral health (Gift, 1985; Ronis, Lang, Farghaly, & Ekdahl, 1994). Practicing dental hygienists recognize that the majority of clients do brush, however, the technique usually needs to be modified and refined to enhance effectiveness. Additionally, low adherence with interproximal aids is a common finding that significantly contributes to the prevalence of periodontal diseases and increased need for frequent maintenance procedures.

Often practitioners find it difficult to foster long-term compliance. Noncompliance is recognized in clients with health problems that are both nonsignificant and that are life-threatening (Wilson, 1987). The less threatening the client perceives the problem to be, however, the lower the compliance rate with professional recommendations for behavior change. An example of noncompliance is illustrated by people who continue to use smokeless tobacco or cigarettes, despite the fact that they understand the potential for the development of a life-threatening disease (Wilson, 1987).

A long-term study to evaluate compliance with interproximal aids was conducted in Sweden. A group of 44 subjects with moderate periodontitis was treated with NSPT by student dental hygienists. Results showed that after oral hygiene instruction, less than half of the subjects still used interproximal cleaning aids at the end of three years (Johansson, Oster, & Hamp 1984). Wilson and others (1984) studied 961 patients over an eight-year period to assess compliance with maintenance schedules in a private periodontal practice. Results showed that only 16 percent of the clients had been in complete compliance over the eight-year time span. Also, results indicated that those who previously had periodontal surgery were more likely to have a higher compliance level than clients who had NSPT. Refer to Chapter 17 for information concerning the relationship of compliance and periodontal maintenance procedures.

Because periodontal disease is usually painless and slowly progressive, many clients do not perceive that a problem exists, or have difficulty sustaining required behavioral changes. Therefore, adherence can be a problem in NSPT. Several studies have focused on factors that might improve long-term compliance with self-care recommendations. Positive feedback, successful communication, demonstration of skills, reinforcement of efficacy, and thorough instruction when used concurrently in education, serve to enhance compliance and motivation. These factors will be discussed in the section devoted to the process of self-care education as each factor is related to effective teaching strategies.

## Motivation and Needs

The primary reason for people not to seek dental care or to reject treatment when they do, is that they do not perceive that a need exists (Manji, 1992). Clients will only become motivated to take action when they realize the importance of doing so. The satisfaction gained from a fulfilled need is the goal of any given behavior. Motivation and needs are, therefore, interrelated because the motivation necessary to change behavior often results when a need is unmet or not satisfied. Motivation is defined as the readiness to act, or the driving forces behind our actions (Axelsson, 1993). For example, a client concerned about halitosis might be more motivated to seek regular dental care and to have effective oral self-care practices because of the desire to eliminate breath odor. The desire to prevent halitosis is this client's driving force. Each clinician needs to develop mechanisms for discovering each client's driving forces which may be derived internally or externally.

A client's **internal motivation** refers to an individual's existing desire or willingness to alter behavior, and the ability to attempt behavior change (Weinstein, Getz, & Milgrom, 1991). Those clients who are internally motivated believe they can influence their own lives, that they are responsible for success and failure, and that they can influence life events. This type of motivation will usually result in long-term protective health behaviors. An example follows:

*Client:* My teeth are extremely important to me; therefore, I will do anything to keep my mouth disease free. I understand the importance of good oral hygiene and regular professional care and will perform it on a daily basis.

An individual who is **externally motivated** relies on others' opinions or belief systems to guide them (Weinstein, Getz, & Milgrom, 1991). This is the individual who believes in fate and/or feels he has little control of life events. An example of an externally motivated client is a teenager who is not brushing daily. His peers mention his bad breath, because peer appreciation is important at this age. He brushes daily for two weeks hoping his girl friend will really appreciate him if he has fresher breath. He then realizes that his girlfriend has not noticed his breath and he ceases to brush routinely, resulting in short-term motivation. It is important to try to discover how the client views motivation because it affects the person's ability to change behavior. Dental hygienists will have more success with clients who are internally motivated. Those who are externally motivated require more supervision and direction.

Another way of looking at motivation is in relation to how the professional encourages or instills a behavior change in another regardless of the type of motivation (internal or external) inherent in an individual. Unfortunately, it is recognized that motivation cannot be bestowed upon or taught to the client. The best a clinician can hope to accomplish is to instill in a client some degree of desire to attempt self-care recommendations. Instilling this drive is actually the **external motivational strategies** used by clinicians to encourage behavioral changes. Individual clinicians have different approaches designed to encourage oral self-care depending on each practitioner's style, her skill and experience with facilitative communication, and commitment to this aspect of therapy. Motivational factors for one client certainly differ from those elements that motivate others.

A common way to identify the client's motivational force is to focus on the chief concern (complaint). Clinicians who seek this concern discover that the appointment cannot really proceed until the client's primary need is met. It is surprising how many clients can easily verbalize single or multiple concerns when questioned appropriately. In fact, these goal-directed behaviors are often the reason why clients schedule appointments at the dental office and thus enter into initial NSPT. An example of a chief concern follows:

*Dental Hygienist:* Do you have any concerns about your mouth?

*Client:* Yes, my gums are tender and ache, and they also bleed when I brush.

*Dental Hygienist:* Are you concerned with the uncomfortable feeling?

*Client:* Yes, I want it to go away.

Dental hygienists would typically focus on the primary need, which is inflammation and bleeding, but instead attention should be directed to what is motivating the client. The tender, aching gums are the client's motivational force. Motivational forces or concerns should be assessed at each appointment because once a primary concern is met, another may surface.

The art of motivating a client involves generating interest by displaying enthusiasm, showing concern by personalizing the message, and providing information (Weinstein, Getz, & Milgrom, 1991). Offers of praise, incentives, rewards, or punishment are used to externally motivate others even though this type of motivation usually results in short-term behavior change. To enhance external motivation use verbal phrases such as:

"I would like to see you use the interdental brush with some type of regularity during the next two weeks. What do you think?"

or

"I believe it will be beneficial for you to use the dental floss because, although you are effective with the toothbrush, its use is not enough to reduce the plaque to a level where you do not get gingivitis."

The point of these statements is that the clinician is using "I" statements instead of "you" statements. These verbal messages provide incentive and/or possibility of a reward or verbal praise if incorporated into self-care practices. Helping a client set short-term goals from appointment to appointment is another example of a concrete way to externally motivate another. Verbal praise can then be given when goals are accomplished. Certainly, punishment in the form of scolding or nonconstructive comments is not a motivational tactic that encourages compliance. Positive feedback and reinforcement are used to externally motivate clients and will be addressed in the section devoted to effective teaching.

Some practitioners are not aware of the way in which they identify needs and encourage motivation, while others might have an approach or theory that they use in daily practice. While motivating another to take action is an abstract phenomenon, the needs assessment necessary to initiate the motivational process is more concrete. **Maslow's Needs Hierarchy** is a familiar model dental hygienists learn early in their education to determine a client's needs. This needs theory utilizes human nature to explain the motivational process. Five needs are arranged to show that as one need is satisfied, an individual is then motivated to satisfy the next need, or level, in the hierarchy (see Figure 8-1). According to Maslow, these needs define a person's growth from infancy to adulthood; however, depending on factors within the internal and external environment at any given time, one need may dominate and influence behavior. This means that the client's status will change over time in relation to these levels. Questioning the client at each

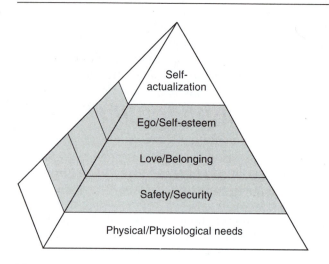

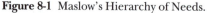

**Figure 8-1** Maslow's Hierarchy of Needs.

**Table 8-1 Dental Hygiene Human Needs Conceptual Model: Four Major Concepts of the Paradigm**

| Term | Definition |
|------|------------|
| Client | A biological, psychological, spiritual, social, cultural, and intellectual person who is an integrated, organized whole, and whose behavior is motivated by fulfillment of his human needs. |
| Environment | The milieu in which the client and dental hygienist find themselves. It affects the client and the dental hygienist; and the client and dental hygienist are capable of influencing the environment. |
| Health/ Oral Health | Health—A relative condition; a state of well-being with both objective and subjective aspects that exists on a continuum from maximal wellness to maximal illness. Oral Health—Oral condition that results from the interaction of individuals with their environment under varying levels of human needs fulfillment. |
| Dental Hygiene Actions | Interventions aimed at assisting clients in meeting their human needs through the performance of those oral health behaviors and practices that lead to optimal oral wellness and quality of life throughout the cycle. |

appointment is critical to assess if life changes have occurred that might affect motivational strategies.

The basic needs such as physiological (food, water, and sleep) and safety (shelter, freedom from anxiety) must be satisfied before any higher level needs are recognized and given priority. If clients have met both their physiological and safety needs, then they are ready to address the next level, which is love or belongingness. Everyone needs to feel a part of a group, family, and culture; and have significant relationships. The fourth level of the hierarchy is self-esteem or ego, which can be defined as an overall belief in oneself. Terms that are synonymous with self-esteem include confidence, self-worth, usefulness, and capability. Lack of achievement of this need creates feelings of inadequacy, helplessness, lack of control, and loss of hope. The highest level of achievement is self-actualization, which is full development of one's ambitions and/or potential. This level enables one to realistically cope with society. Clinicians will find that the three needs most often involved in client education are safety, love, and ego (Scranton-Gluch, 1989).

Recently, dental hygiene theorists have developed a **Dental Hygiene Human Needs Conceptual Model** to be used during dental hygiene care (Darby & Walsh, 1994). The primary purpose of implementing this model during therapy is to assist clinicians in providing care that is scientific, humanistic, and holistic, thereby guaranteeing that treatment is more client-oriented rather then task-oriented. In this model, basic human needs theory is utilized to explain four major concepts of the dental hygiene paradigm: client, environment, health and oral health, and dental hygiene actions (see Table 8-1). Darby and Walsh (1994) further identify eleven human needs as being particularly relevant to dental hygiene care (see Table 8-2) and suggest that a baseline assessment form

be incorporated into clinical practice (see Table 8-3). Avenues for assessment depend on the specific need and include evaluation of the client's verbal and nonverbal behaviors, careful observation of the client, and/or findings of the intraoral and extraoral examination. Dental hygiene diagnoses are made based on deficits in these eleven human needs, and then the planning, implementation, and evaluation of care is designed to meet the unmet needs.

The eleven needs are continually evaluated and applied throughout the dental hygiene process of care and each has specific implications in the process of self-care education. For example, safety can relate to how the client uses an interdental aid or the daily use of an oral rinse. If the aid is used inappropriately creating trauma or the daily oral rinse is hydrogen peroxide, then the safety need is unmet. Freedom from pain or stress can relate to the intraoral pain experienced by inflamed gingiva or the stress a client expresses about progressive recession, root exposure, and sensitivity. Self-determination and responsibility relate to the client's perception of his role

## Table 8-2 Human Needs Related to Dental Hygiene Care

| Human Need | Definition |
| --- | --- |
| 1. Safety | The need to experience freedom from harm or danger involving the integrity of the body structure and environment around the person. |
| 2. Freedom | The need for freedom from pain and stress is the human need for exemption from physical and emotional discomforts. |
| 3. Wholesome Body Image | The need for a wholesome body image is the need for a positive mental representation of one's own body boundary and how it looks to others. |
| 4. Skin and Mucous Membrane Integrity of Head and Neck | The need to have an intact and functioning covering of the person's head and neck area, including the oral mucous membrane and gingivae, which defend against harmful microbes, provide sensory information, and resist injurious substances and trauma. |
| 5. Nutrition | The need to ingest and assimilate sufficient amounts of carbohydrates, proteins, fats, vitamins, minerals, trace elements, and fiber required for growth, repair, and maintenance of structurally and functionally competent body parts. |
| 6. A Biologically Sound Dentition | The need for intact teeth and restorations that defend against harmful microbes and provide for adequate function and esthetics. |
| 7. Conceptualization and Problem Solving | The need to grasp ideas and abstractions, to make sound judgments about one's life and circumstances. |
| 8. Appreciation and Respect | The need to be acknowledged for achievement, worth, service, or merit and to be regarded favorably with admiration and approval by others. |
| 9. Self-Determination and Responsibility | The need to exercise firmness of purpose about one's self and accountability for one's behavior. |
| 10. Territoriality | The need to possess a prescribed area of space or knowledge that a person denotes as one's own, maintains control over, and defends if necessary and is acknowledged by others as owning. |
| 11. Value System | The need to have the freedom to develop one's own sense of the importance of people, institutions, things, activities, and experiences in one's life. |

(Adapted from Darby, M. C. & Walsh, M. *Dental hygiene theory and practice*, W.B. Saunders Co., Philadelphia, 1994, pgs. 32 and 33)

in self-care and his monitoring of active periodontal disease. This need is unmet if the client is not aware that bleeding exists after being taught how to monitor it. For a comprehensive review of this conceptual model, the reader is referred to Chapter 2 of the text, *Dental Hygiene Theory and Practice* (Darby & Walsh, 1994).

Another advantage of using a needs theory in clinical practice is that it can be documented in the client's record. Documentation provides valuable information for initial therapy as well as PMP. Practitioners in an office use this written documentation to assure team members are aware of the client's needs in hopes of enhancing effective communication and client-centered care. In conclusion, motivation is essential to study and keep in mind when teaching clients about self-care. Frequently just being willing to listen and apply effective communication principles allows the clinician to discover the individual's key motivational factors and needs.

## Barriers to Compliance

It is essential to recognize that there are client barriers as well as clinician-induced barriers to compliance. To initiate positive changes in client self-care behavior, both types of barriers must be recognized and used to modify recommendations to an individual. Barrier identification is indeed another important aspect of individualiz-

ing NSPT. Various authors have identified client barriers to positive oral health care practices such as negative health beliefs, low knowledge level, lack of motivation, and differing personal values (Chambers & Abrams, 1992; DeBiase, 1991; Kühner & Raetzke, 1989). These four barrier categories can be specifically described as social economic class, fear and anxiety, ethnic and cultural beliefs, skill level, time restrictions, lack of information, value judgments, cost of care, and laziness. These specific client barriers might be easier for the therapist to identify than the broader concepts of motivation and health beliefs. The following client statements provide examples of such barriers.

*Example of time restriction:*

*Client:* I am incredibly swamped at work, I hardly have time to eat, let alone floss.

*Example of lack of information:*

*Client:* My brother never brushes his teeth and he has never had a cavity. Why are you so concerned about my brushing habits?

The clinician might also create barriers to compliance. A positive relationship between the dental professional and the client serves to encourage compliance. Therefore, it is necessary to identify barriers that the therapist may inadvertently create. These clinician-

**Table 8-3  Baseline Assessment of Eleven Human Needs Related to Dental Hygiene Care**

Below are eleven human needs related to dental hygiene care. Please indicate whether the need is unmet by circling "yes" or "no" in the space provided. If the need is unmet, circle in red the specific deficit listed under each need, and note salient comments.

| Human Needs/Deficits | Unmet? | Comments |
|---|---|---|
| ***Safety*** | Yes/No | |
| • BP outside of normal limits | | |
| • Current serious illness | | |
| • Need for prophylactic antibiotics | | |
| • Concern about: | | |
|   1. Infection control | | |
|   2. Radiography | | |
|   3. Fluoride therapy | | |
|   4. Fluoridation | | |
|   5. Mercury toxicity | | |
|   6. Dental hygiene care planned | | |
|   7. Previous dental experience | | |
| • Potential for injury | | |
| • Other | | |
| ***Freedom from Pain/Stress*** | Yes/No | |
| • Reports or displays: | | |
|   1. Fear/anxiety | | |
|   2. Extra-/intraoral pain or sensitivity | | |
|   3. Discomfort during dental hygiene care | | |
|   4. Oral habits | | |
|   5. Substance abuse | | |
| • Other | | |
| ***Wholesome Body Image*** | Yes/No | |
| • Dissatisfaction with appearance of: | | |
|   1. Teeth | | |
|   2. Gingiva | | |
|   3. Facial profile | | |
| • Other | | |
| ***Skin and Mucous Membrane Integrity of Head and Neck*** | Yes/No | |
| • Presence of: | | |
|   1. Extra-/intraoral lesion | | |
|   2. Tenderness, swelling | | |
|   3. Gingival inflammation | | |
|   4. Bleeding on probing | | |
|   5. Pockets greater than 4 mm | | |
|   6. Attachment loss greater than 4 mm | | |
|   7. Xerostomia | | |
| • Other | | |
| ***Nutrition*** | Yes/No | |
| • Extra-/intraoral manifestations of malnutrition | | |
| • Rampant caries | | |
| • Unbalanced diet | | |
| • High sugar intake on a daily basis | | |
| • Other | | |
| ***Biologically Sound Dentition*** | Yes/No | |
| • Difficulty in chewing | | |
| • Presents with: | | |
|   1. Defective restorations | | |
|   2. Teeth with signs of disease | | |
|   3. Missing teeth | | |
|   4. Ill-fitting dentures, appliances | | |
|   5. Calculus, plaque, or stain | | |
|   6. Abrasion, erosion | | |
|   7. No dental examination within the last two years | | |
| • Other | | |

**Table 8-3 (continued)**

| Human Needs/Deficits | Unmet? | Comments |
|---|---|---|
| ***Conceptualization and Problem Solving***<br>• Has questions or misconceptions associated with dental hygiene care<br>• Does not understand:<br>  1. What plaque is, its relationship to oral disease, and/or the importance of daily plaque control<br>• Other | Yes/No | |
| ***Appreciation and Respect***<br>• Expresses dissatisfaction with clinician and/or dental hygiene care<br>• Reports disapproval from others about oral hygiene status<br>• Other | Yes/No | |
| ***Self-Determination and Responsibility***<br>• Does not verbalize awareness of own role in oral hygiene care<br>• Inadequate oral health behaviors<br>• Does not participate in setting goals for dental hygiene care<br>• Inadequate parental supervision<br>• Other | Yes/No | |
| ***Territoriality***<br>• Verbally or nonverbally expresses discomfort with the proximity of the operator during conversation or dental hygiene care<br>• Expresses a need for confidentiality<br>• Other | Yes/No | |
| ***Value System***<br>• Indicates oral health and hygiene is a low priority<br>• Has history of failing appointments<br>• Other | Yes/No | |

(Courtesy of Darby, M. C. & Walsh, M. *Dental hygiene theory and practice*, W.B. Saunders Co., Philadelphia, 1994 pgs. 30 and 31)

induced barriers can also be the same barriers experienced by the client. Examples of barrier-inducing internal statements made by the clinician and possible resolutions follow:

*Example of time restriction:*

*Clinician:* Because I don't have time to scale/root plane, irrigate, and discuss self-care education, I will show the client how to use the interdental aid at the next appointment if she has any problems with it.

*Example of time restriction barrier resolution:*

*Clinician:* Because I don't have time to scale/root plane, irrigate, and discuss self-care education, I will need to scale/root plane only one quadrant versus the entire mouth. I will then have time to explain periodontal disease and to help her practice the appropriate interdental aid in her mouth.

*Example of lack of knowledge:*

*Clinician:* This client really should floss.

*Example of lack of knowledge barrier resolution:*

*Clinician:* Because you are having difficulty with daily flossing, I will review the research about self-care devices to help find another aid that might be beneficial.

In addition, the communication skills used by the dental hygienist can create barriers.

*Example of poor communication:*

*Clinician:* Mr. Hep, your oral self-care is not good. Have you been doing what I told you to do?

*Example of poor communication resolution:*

*Clinician:* Mr. Hep, as you can see, these areas are free from bleeding, representing healthy gum tissue. Unfortunately, many other areas are still bleeding. Is this a concern of yours?

*Client:* Yes, I am aware that bleeding means infection or disease is present. I have been trying to use that new brush.

*Clinician:* Are you interested in having some help with the interdental brush?

*Client:* Okay.

*Clinician:* Perhaps if I review how you are using the brush I could offer some tips on how to use it more effectively and easily.

A common error made by dental professionals is to judge clients by their different beliefs and values. Dental professionals must be patient, never impose their values on clients, and respect the fact that people will have many different points of view. When first coming into contact with a client, the clinician needs to be aware of the tendency to impose value judgments on statements made by the client. Dental professionals can easily judge the clients' values by their own standards. Because of the knowledge level we have gained through professional education, it is sometimes easy to forget that everyone does not have equal oral health knowledge. Naturally, value judgments will inhibit learning and compliance.

*Example of value judgment from dental hygienist to other team member:*

I can't believe anyone would let their mouth get like that. Don't they know how important it is to have regular dental care?

*Example of value judgment from dental hygienist to client:*

Mr. Trench, I don't understand why you won't use this wooden toothpick to clean the furcations. It is such a simple task and I know you want to keep your teeth from falling out.

In the previous example, the first sentence to Mr. Trench might seem harsh and could be stated less abrasively. The actual value judgment is that the dental hygienist thinks that using the wooden toothpick is a "simple task." It is probably best for the practitioner to openly listen to how Mr. Trench feels about using the wooden toothpick. The clinician can use questioning and paraphrasing to assure that the client's message is being understood. This exercise will help the practitioner to concentrate on the individual and keep from formulating a negative judgment or creating a potential barrier.

The only barrier that can be directly removed through self-care education is lack of knowledge (Kühner & Raetzke, 1989). Clinician lack of knowledge is prevented by continual reading of scientific journals and continuing education. Involvement in lifelong learning gives the professional impetus to continually update knowledge in self-care education theories and practice. Lack of knowledge portrayed by the client is overcome by providing the client with disease theory education about periodontal disease on a need-to-know basis. The clinician can only work with the other barriers and hope that as the client gains knowledge and experience, these other barriers will also diminish.

## Learning

Dental hygienists are accustomed to assessing the client's main problem with self-care performance at home. The gap between the desired performance and the actual performance of self-care has been termed a "performance discrepancy" (Mager & Pipe, 1970; Weinstein, Getz, & Milgrom, 1991). If the client does not have the knowledge and psychomotor ability to perform self-care, then it is most likely that a **skill discrepancy** exists that is rectified by designing an individualized plan to teach the needed skill. If the knowledge and psychomotor ability is present, however, and the skill is not being performed, then a **management discrepancy** exists meaning that the client possesses the know how but does not perform the self-care regularly or adequately. In the latter case the "why" of nonperformance is important. This is the point where the clinician can look into the client's readiness to learn.

**Readiness** is a term used to describe the client's position or attitude toward changing behavior (Weinstein, Getz, & Milgrom, 1991). Factors used to assess "readiness" include willingness to attempt a change, and ability to change at this given time. Willingness refers to the individual's perceived needs and knowledge about periodontal disease and his ownership of the problem. Lack of knowledge and need can be affected by providing disease theory information and skill instruction, but dealing with ownership is more complex. Clearly, it is the client who is ultimately responsible for daily care, but delivering this message and shifting the responsibility to the client is challenging. Nevertheless, the client who does not own the problem will probably not change until he recognizes it is his responsibility to perform daily oral self-care. The ability to change at a given point in someone's life depends on self-care orientation, internal or external motivation, the social support system, and absence of conflict and stress (Weinstein, Getz, & Milgrom, 1991). If the client is not willing or able to change, self-care education still occurs knowing that the potential for success is limited. At a later point in initial therapy or PMP, willingness and ability may occur.

One familiar approach to assessing a client's readiness to learn is based on the concept that learning occurs in a progressive series of steps or intervals referred to as the **Learning Ladder Continuum** (DeBiase, 1991; Harris & Christen, 1995; Wilkins, 1994) (see Figure 8-2). The dental hygienist who uses this approach determines which stage of the ladder the client has reached and then uses the level to plan appropriate individualized education. The ultimate objective, of course, is to assist the client in reaching the top of the ladder.

The first or lowest stage of the learning ladder is unawareness. At this level an individual has incomplete or inaccurate information, such as believing that teeth fall out because of aging and silver fillings cause cancer. The second step, awareness is encountered when the client is given correct information, but it lacks personal meaning.

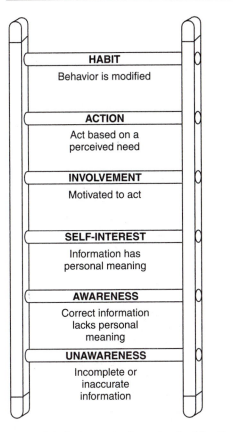

**Figure 8-2** Steps on the Learning Ladder Continuum.

For example, the client knows the relationship of bacterial plaque to periodontal disease, and yet recognizes plaque deposits and inflammation in his own mouth. To help the client's knowledge gain personal importance, the clinician can utilize the conditions in the client's mouth by pointing out areas of inflammation, and comparing them to areas that are healthy or an illustration of healthy gingiva. A discussion about causative factors of inflammation can then follow.

If or when this knowledge becomes personally meaningful to the client, he has then reached the next level, the self-interest stage. During this stage, the client may begin to see the purpose of what you are trying to teach. To assist the client in achieving the next stage, values clarification exercises may be used to help determine what aspects of health care are important to him (DeBiase, 1991). For example, the person could rank-order several different items that range from owning a sports car to keeping teeth to overall body health. Clients may discover that oral health care is much more important than previously thought. Therefore, when this new change in attitude has occurred and the client is motivated to act, then the next stage of the ladder, involvement, has been reached. When the client is at the involvement stage, it is necessary for the dental hygienist to continue to use all communication and motivational resources. During this stage the client may want more information than previously shared because his knowledge level has increased.

This client is now taking ownership for self-care, beginning to problem solve, and can progress up the next rung of the ladder, to the action level. At this level, the professional's external motivation is useful. Clients are stimulated to act when they perceive a need exists, and this can be most easily communicated when the professional points out undesirable consequences of the client's behavior.

*Example of undesirable consequences of client behavior:*

*Hygienist:* Mrs. March, you should be pleased with the overall health of your tissues. I am concerned, however, about the pocket areas that have become deeper. As you can see, these deep pockets are harder to clean at home and deposits have accumulated here. Eventually we may need to discuss periodontal surgery to reduce the pocket depth and help you clean these areas.

During the action stage, the client will abandon old ideas for new concepts and behaviors that focus toward problem solving. An example of the action level would be when the client realizes the consequences of not using a wooden toothpick to remove plaque from open embrasures and furcation areas. After continued daily use of the aid, the client notices a decrease in bleeding and gingival sensitivity. The dental hygienist records decreased pocket measurements and then reinforces this positive behavior. The client begins experiencing self-satisfaction with this accomplishment and is greatly motivated to continue this enhanced oral self-care, and therefore, reaches the habit stage. This stage is the highest level of the learning ladder. Once a habit is formed by this change in cognitive (knowledge) and behavior modifications, the probability of this new self-care regime becoming a long-term behavior is greater.

Several studies have been conducted to determine the effect of behavior intervention (changing behavior) on oral hygiene (Stewart et al., 1991; Wolfe, Stewart, & Jacobs-Schoen, 1989; Tedesco, Keffer, & Fleck-Kandath, 1991). Wolfe, Stewart, and Jacobs-Schoen (1989) suggested that dental hygienists need to make an effort to assess clients' commitment to better oral hygiene prior to teaching self-care skills. Weinstein, Getz, and Milgrom (1991) also feel that self-care often starts too early in the process of care; before the professional gets to know the client and can individualize the message. Using the learning ladder is one way of assessing the client's level of commitment. If the commitment is lacking or the individual does not understand that a need exists, instruction in self-care practices might become pointless. The concepts of the learning ladder could be considered when educating clients in initial NSPT or PMP. By determining which level of the ladder the client has attained, the clinician will better know the extent of disease theory that needs to be discussed or clarified and what type of self-care practices can be recommended. Again, incorporation of this concept into care provides the professional with a means to document stages of learning.

## The Process of Education

The self-care education process is a continuous one because it occurs at each appointment and throughout each appointment. An advantage of NSPT is that initial therapy occurs in a series of appointments and PMP are typically recommended at three-month intervals; therefore, frequent contact with the client is fostered. This frequent contact permits the clinician to deliver the education in intervals while incorporating the fundamental principles of teaching and learning. When developing the initial treatment plan or making recommendations for PMP, adequate time for plaque removal and self-care education must be considered. Keep in mind that thirty-to forty-five-minute appointments for PMP are obsolete. When short appointment blocks for the initial appointment or PMP are scheduled, self-care education is sacrificed. One strategy for ensuring that education is a financially rewarding process is to arrange the client fee based on the number of appointments and the time involved with each appointment. Some insurance companies do pay on the code identified for patient education, and if this is the case, a separate and distinct fee can be charged for education.

The more often the client is seen, the less new information needs to be presented; however, remotivation, assessing oral hygiene, and reinforcement of techniques is always necessary (Rateitschak, 1994). Prior to presenting new information, a review of previously given instruction and an assessment of the client's understanding is always needed. Even though the process of education is similar for each client at each appointment it in no way implies that the discussion and approach are standardized. The individual's needs, motivational forces, and level of commitment to care make each educational session a unique challenge for the clinician.

Four phases are included in self-care education: initiation of education, presentation of disease theory, teaching of skill enhancement, and closure of the educational session. Table 8-4 is a self-evaluation form clinicians can use to assess their thoroughness and effectiveness. Peer evaluation can also be accomplished by having faculty and/or peers observe interactions with clients in the educational setting or in clinical practice.

**Initiation.** It is suggested that initiation of the educational process begins the moment the client enters the operatory and treatment commences. During the review of the health history, the practitioner has the opportunity to educate the client about existing health conditions and their relationship to general dental care and, specifically, to NSPT. Customarily, the chief concern of the client is discovered by the clinician prior to proceeding through the assessment phase of care. Frequently, it is necessary to address this chief complaint in some manner during the assessment. For example, a sensitive tooth might indicate a periapical radiograph, or concerns about chlorhexidene staining can be addressed and discussed

as early in the treatment as possible. If bleeding is a concern, the clinician might choose to check gingival inflammation and probing at the beginning of the assessment and include a discussion of findings with the client. Even if the client's chief concern is not directly related to periodontal disease, it is addressed immediately, and then assessment proceeds.

While the assessment is being completed, the client may be given a hand mirror to watch the process more precisely (Bader, 1989; Scranton-Gluch, 1989). The dental hygienist can explain each procedure such as the extraoral and intraoral examination, the restorative and periodontal charting, deposit identification, indices evaluation, and radiographs. This phase of care provides an opportunity for the clinical hygienist to not only explain the data collection procedures, but to discuss significant findings as well. Client involvement in assessment personalizes the procedure, enhances informed consent, helps reduce apprehension about new or time-intensive procedures, and begins the education that the consumer has the right to receive. For example, explaining the probing procedure as it is conducted permits clients to begin thinking about their gingival tissue and supporting structures and provides an opportunity for clients to develop questions about their conditions. If periodontal charting is not explained during the assessment, the opportunity for client involvement early in treatment is lost and it means the clinician must collectively review all the assessment findings later in the appointment when periodontal disease theory and self-care aids are discussed. Explaining procedures and findings as care progresses facilitates communication and decreases the chances of education being provided as a "lecture-type" presentation.

Also during the assessment, the clinician can be mentally organizing which oral health needs must be addressed, the motivating forces, readiness to learn, and the individual treatment plan. Asking several open-ended questions during the assessment phase to determine current self-care practices, knowledge level, and long-term health goals of the client will promote facilitative communication while helping the clinician to individualize oral self-care instruction. Example questions are represented in Table 8-5. Some practices might have clients address their current self care practices by completing a questionnaire prior to treatment. If this is the case, questions can be employed during the assessment to help clarify the recorded information. Customarily, after the assessment phase is completed, planning client oral self-care education in written form, occurs as part of a treatment plan. Self-care recommendations are interwoven with other therapeutic interactions provided for the client. See Chapter 6 to review care planning recommendations and guidelines for selection of appropriate self-care aids.

**Disease Theory.** The next component of education involves teaching disease theory. This phase of education

**Table 8-4 Self-Care Education Assessment**

DIRECTIONS: Assess each criteria by using a (Y) for Yes, an (A) for Attempted, or an (N) for No. A (Y) indicates the criteria was adequately incorporated during the education session. An (A) indicates the clinician attempted to incorporate the criteria; however, it can be enhanced. An (N) means the topic was not included/addressed.

| Component | Criteria | Self | Peer |
|---|---|---|---|
| Implements Effective Communication Skills | Client and clinician are at eye level (client upright). | | |
| | Maintains eye contact. | | |
| | Listens attentively. | | |
| | Paraphrases and uses reflective responding. | | |
| | Questioning and clarifying are incorporated. | | |
| | A discussion format is employed. | | |
| Applies Assessment Information | Establishes chief concern(s). | | |
| | Identifies client's human needs. | | |
| | Identifies long-term goal for oral health. | | |
| | Determines oral health self-care practices and knowledge level. | | |
| | Identifies current oral self-care practices. | | |
| | Identifies learning ladder level. | | |
| Teaches Disease Theory | Shows client oral conditions present (bleeding). | | |
| | Discusses new or reviews previously given theories. | | |
| | Presents relative, accurate, and sufficient theory. | | |
| | Uses disclosing solution to help client see plaque. | | |
| | Leads client to identify deposits. | | |
| Provides Skill Enhancement | Offers rationale for teaching new techniques or aids. | | |
| | Shows technique on model and/or in mouth. | | |
| | Has client demonstrate technique in their mouth. | | |
| | Modifies technique as indicated. | | |
| | Leads client to set short-term goals for self-care. | | |
| Incorporates Characteristics of Effective Teaching | Presents information in small steps. | | |
| | Employs self-pacing. | | |
| | Encourages active client participation and discussion. | | |
| | Provides specific immediate feedback. | | |
| | Provides positive reinforcement. | | |
| | Teaches client self-evaluation of the skills. | | |
| | Uses indirect approach (open-ended questions). | | |
| | Incorporates effective visual aids. | | |
| | Organizes the session systematically and logically. | | |
| Includes Thorough Documentation | Records session thoroughly in record of services. | | |

(Courtesy of Idaho State University, Department of Dental Hygiene, Pocatello, ID, 1996)

**Table 8-5  Examples of Open-Ended Questions to Assess Client Self-Care, Knowledge, and Long-Term Goals**

| Assessment of: | Open-Ended Questions |
| --- | --- |
| Current Self-Care Practices | • Can you tell me about your daily routine of taking care of your teeth?<br>• Would you share with me how you clean your teeth?<br>• Do you use other aids or rinses besides the toothbrush? |
| Knowledge Level | • Have you heard of gingivitis?<br>• Have you heard of periodontitis?<br>• Do you know what bleeding of the gums means?<br>• What education do you remember receiving at your previous dental visits?<br>• Are you aware of self-care aids other than dental floss that can be used to clean in between your teeth ? |
| Long-Term Goals | • Is there anything you hope to accomplish with your teeth or gums over your lifetime?<br>• Do you have any future goals for improving the health of your mouth?<br>• Have you thought about anything that you would like to improve about the way you clean your teeth? |

usually occurs after the assessment and treatment plan formulation; and prior to case presentation and professional deposit removal. Providing this education prior to the treatment plan discussion facilitates understanding of the recommended therapy and this enhances the chances of receiving informed consent. Another reason for discussing theory prior to initiating any debridement or adjunctive therapy is because once treatment has begun, the etiologic factors have been disorganized and will not seem as significant to the client. When the majority of education is given at the end of the appointment, it might be rushed or eliminated. During a series of initial appointments or maintenance appointments, self-care education should always be initiated prior to any treatment (Bader, 1989).

This time period in the appointment is referred to as the educational session because it is when the dental hygienist teaches preventive oral health behaviors and externally motivates the client. When the educational session begins, typically a pause in professionally rendered care is taken, the client is seated upright, and eye contact is maintained to enhance communication and learning. To assist clients in understanding the importance of adequate plaque removal, it has been suggested that during the education session disease theory be taught prior to teaching skills (Rateitschak, 1994).

Because the client's needs and knowledge level were determined during the assessment phase, the dental hygienist has planned how much or which theory to present (plaque and calculus, gingivitis including inflammation and bleeding, periodontitis including pocket depth, clinical attachment level, recession, furcations, bone loss, scanty or loss of attached gingiva, etc.). For example, if a client does not understand what plaque is, then it would be pointless to begin discussing the role of microorganisms in alveolar bone destruction. A more effective sequence would be to discuss the composition of plaque and how it relates to gingival inflammation and periodontal destruction; and then address other clinical findings such as furcation involvement. Continual questioning to assess the client's understanding is important. If the client is not understanding the message, clarification needs to be attempted prior to presenting new theory. This is also the point where the clinician shares the preliminary periodontal diagnosis with the client. The clinician will have determined if health, gingivitis, or periodontitis exists; while recognizing that this diagnosis could change as therapy progresses, especially if an uncommon form of gingivitis or periodontitis is suspected. The following dialogue represents client and clinician interaction at the initial appointment of active therapy:

*Dental Hygienist:* Are you interested in knowing more about what I found in your mouth?

*Client:* Yes, go ahead.

*Dental Hygienist:* I would like to address the inflammation of the gum, the pockets, and the bleeding we discussed during the assessment I just completed. These findings are all signs of a disease which has many causes, however, the major cause is bacterial plaque. Have you ever heard of periodontitis or periodontal disease?

*Client:* Yes, kind of. Is that what I have?

*Dental Hygienist:* Yes, Dr. Bybee confirmed the findings and we feel the conditions in your mouth indicate that periodontitis is present. Can you tell me what you know about this disease?

*Client:* Not much; just that it can lead to tooth loss and other problems.

*Dental Hygienist:* You are on the right track. It can lead to tooth loss because periodontitis involves more than the gum inflammation, pockets, and bleeding we noticed during the examination of your mouth. Actually, periodontitis is bone loss that occurs from the interaction of the bacterial plaque and your immune system. Are you interested in knowing even more about the causes of this infection?

*Clinician:* Yes, how did the bone loss occur and can it heal?

*Dental Hygienist:* The plaque itself is made up of bacteria that produce by-products called toxins. These substances destroy the bone that supports your teeth.

After the bone is lost it does not replace itself. Unfortunately, the loss is permanent; however, research has shown that the majority of people with periodontitis can control or manage this disease with a combination of professional treatment that I can provide and your self-care of your teeth and gums on a daily basis. What else would you like to know about periodontitis?

*Client:* How to prevent it or stop it, I guess.

*Dental Hygienist:* Well, this infection is chronic in nature meaning that it will always be present. Because bacterial plaque is the main cause, the control of periodontitis involves controlling the plaque. Bacterial plaque is located above your gums and below your gum tissue. Everyone has plaque in their mouth, but different people's plaque contains different types of bacteria. Dentistry does not have an efficient way to routinely evaluate the type of plaque you have, but because I know that bone loss is present, I also know that your mouth contains periodontitis-causing bacteria. There are ways for you to consistently remove or disturb this bacterial plaque. Are you interested in discussing some of these methods?

*Client:* Yes. I know flossing is important.

*Dental Hygienist:* Right, flossing is important for some people. It will probably amaze you to know that although flossing cleans between the teeth well, it is not the best aid for you to use to clean between your teeth. If it is okay with you, I would like to show you another aid in just a few minutes. (Pause for response.) I am concerned that plaque is not being removed from between your teeth because this area is usually where bone loss occurs the quickest and easiest. Would you like to see the bone supporting your teeth by looking at your radiographs? (Explanation of the structures visible on the films includes a review of where the height of the bone would be located in health, and a comparison to the existing bone level. Illustrations of the stages of bone loss in the disease process can be incorporated.) Your bone loss appears to be in only the early stages of the disease. I am glad you came into the office for dental care before it advanced any further, aren't you?

*Client:* Yes, how fast does it progress?

*Dental Hygienist:* It progresses at different rates with different people and dental professionals do not have an exact way to determine how fast it will progress, but again remember that the majority of people can control the disease if they practice effective daily plaque removal and visit their dental hygienist as often as recommended. The advancing of the infection depends on the reaction of your immune system to the bacterial plaque and is related to your general health. [Question client to see if they are interested in discussing pertinent risk factors (smoking, diabetes, cardiovascular disease, etc.)] and if so, proceed to explain their relationship to periodontitis).

In the preceding dialogue, the clinician is trying to let the client lead the discussion. The information presented about periodontitis will depend on the client's questions indicating readiness to learn. In the earlier dialogue, the clinician could choose to stop and teach the interdental aid before discussing the radiographs. Because the clinician should take cues from the client about what she is interested in, the clinician should not have a pat speech or approach in a specific sequential order ready to deliver. The clinician can, however, make mental notes about what information is covered through facilitative communication and can then fill in the gaps to ensure the client leaves the appointment knowing the diagnosis, etiology, relationship to the host, recommended professional therapy, and recommended self-care. How long this discussion takes should be gauged by the client's interest, number of questions, level of knowledge, and needs.

When an unusual and aggressive form of gingivitis or periodontitis is suspected/diagnosed, the clinician is faced with a special challenge in presenting the etiology, diagnosis, therapy, and prognosis. When early-onset periodontitis or juvenile periodontitis is evident, self-care education (and case presentation) should be presented to the parent or guardian as well as to the client. Likewise, when an unusual form of gingivitis is recognized in a child or adolescent the parent should be brought into the self-care education and case presentation. Information to include in the disease theory portion of education includes the following:

1. Why a type of aggressive periodontal disease is suspected. Age (puberty, under 35 years, or over 35 years), generalized or localized radiographic bone loss, and relationship of plaque and inflammation to the destruction are discussed.
2. How this type of periodontitis compares with the more common form of adult periodontitis. Again, age of onset, the rapid loss of bone, and lack of deposits and corresponding inflammation, if appropriate, are compared.
3. The etiology. An explanation of the etiology should include that certain types of bacteria are probably present and that a systemic host defense defect is often suspected or a compromised immune system is involved.
4. Therapy. In addition to the conventional therapy (professional deposit removal and self-care) treatment might include microbial analysis and host modification. Initial therapy is likely to include antibiotics and/or antimicrobials. The goal of therapy is to establish a balance between the bacteria and host so that conventional therapy is effective. In most forms of aggressive periodontitis, surgery is not immediately indicated or is only suggested once the active infectious process is controlled. Surgery may or may not be indicated in the case of aggressive gingivitis.

5. Response to therapy. Unfortunately, the response to conventional therapy is not predictable in the majority of aggressive forms of periodontitis. The response to therapy may be more predictable with gingivitis.

6. Prognosis. The outcome depends on the response to initial therapy and compliance with PMP.

The outline presented is just a framework for clinicians to use to develop an appropriate dialogue for discussions with clients when unusual forms of periodontal diseases are recognized. The etiology, age of onset, specific therapy, and prognosis vary depending on which disease classification is apparent. Refer to Chapter 1 for an overview of the disease classification and to Chapter 6 for further information about care planning for these unique situations.

During the disease theory explanation, plaque accumulation and location should also be identified. The use of disclosing solution is an effective means of assisting the client in visualizing supragingival areas in need of improved plaque removal (Bader, 1989; Palmer & Floyd, 1995; Scranton-Gluch, 1989), especially when key areas are targeted such as the gingival one-third and interproximal surfaces. To encourage active participation, have the client identify the areas that have been stained with the solution and relate these areas to bleeding and/or attachment loss. Subgingival plaque can sometimes be recognized by the client by placing the probe just under the gingival margin or further subgingivally to disturb the plaque and have it adhere to the probe. Encourage the client to suggest methods to improve bacterial plaque removal.

In the past, oral health education focused on the premise that clients would comply with plaque removal instruction if they had a through understanding of the cause and effect of periodontal disease (Wolfe, Stewart, & Jacobs-Schoen, 1989). Current research suggests that the cause and effect relationship is not enough to motivate clients to change. Because an increase in knowledge does not necessarily lead to an improvement in self-care practices, the professional educator needs to identify if the client has a skill discrepancy, management discrepancy, or a combination of both.

**Skill Enhancement.** Teaching the client how to use self-care aids immediately follows or is interwoven with theory presentation. The dental hygienist has the individual demonstrate techniques currently being used at home, and if indicated, suggestions are offered for improving plaque removal. For instance, if moderate plaque was located along the gingival margins, perhaps changing the angle of the toothbrush to 45° towards the gingival margin is indicated or if progressive generalized recession is present, recommending the Stillman's brushing technique is indicated. Another example would be if a client is using dental floss but has Type II embrasure spaces and beginning furcation involvement, then perhaps a wood-

en toothpick is a better interdental cleaning device. Researchers have suggested that the effectiveness of the technique is more important than the frequency or correctness of the technique (Lang, Farghaly, & Ronis, 1994; Ronis, Lang, Farghaly, & Ekdahl, 1994; Stewart et al., 1991; Weinstein, Getz, & Milgrom, 1982). If the client's plaque removal is effective, but the technique is incorrect with nonexistent tissue damage, it is acceptable for the client to continue to use the technique that is most effective.

When teaching self-care skills, both clinician and client demonstrations are essential. The demonstration can be on a model or in the individual's mouth. After the demonstration, have the client verbalize the technique as well as demonstrate the technique in the mouth. Even if a client can accurately verbalize the technique, it does not guarantee that he will be able to perform the task. A statement often made by clients is "I was told about floss, but no one ever showed me how to use it." During the demonstration, provide positive reinforcement which will help encourage and motivate the client.

**Closure.** The closure of the educational session involves asking the client open-ended questions about the information presented. Also, the clinician can answer any additional questions the client may have. It is the responsibility of the practitioner to seek client questions and to establish an environment where the client feels comfortable requesting information. To finalize the session and provide external motivation, the dental hygienist prompts the client to set achievable, specific, and realistic short-term goals for daily oral self-care. For example, a client who has never used dental floss, sets a short-term goal to floss twice a day. This might not be realistic. A more appropriate goal would be to floss every other day at bedtime. After the short-term goal has been identified, relate all this new information to the client's original long-term goal, chief concern and/or motivating force, which was identified during the assessment. At this point, because the client has gained new knowledge and may be moving up the learning ladder, he may want to identify a new long-term goal. Goal setting provides client direction and motivation.

## Effective Teaching

Just as facilitative communication occurs throughout the self-care educational process, so does the incorporation of effective teaching strategies. The original five principles of instruction include presenting small amounts of information at one time (small step size), letting the client set his own pace (self-pacing), supervising the client's practice, providing immediate feedback, and using positive reinforcement (John, 1972; Stanford & Roark, 1974). Over the last two decades, each of these principles has been shown to enhance the effectiveness of teaching. Other teaching strategies that help the client learn disease theory and skills include use of an indirect approach, incorporating visual aids, and organizing the session systematically and logically.

Small step size refers to the increments used in presenting disease theory and in teaching skill enhancement. As a student clinician do you remember the difficulty experienced with the instrument grasp, fulcrum, and adaptation? Learning instrumentation in small steps helped you learn the technical skill as a whole process. Likewise, it is essential to determine your client's present knowledge and skill level to decrease the chance of providing too much information at one time. Concepts to remember are that information needs to be simple and direct, precise yet not overwhelming, and repeated in different fashions to enhance understanding. While sharing knowledge about periodontal disease, periodically ask if the client understands or has questions, and strive to restate the periodontal disease theory in a few different ways. At the first appointment of initial therapy it is probably enough for the average client to leave knowing that he has gingivitis or periodontitis; that this infection is caused by bacterial plaque; that the response to this plaque depends on his immune system; and that the infection has occurred over time. Additionally, understanding the stage of disease progression, recommended therapy, and need for compliance with self-care is essential.

Small step size is also critical with the mastery of psychomotor self-care skills. Not only should the clinician consider the increments used in teaching each aid, but the number of aids necessary to achieve optimal self-care. For example, someone who has never practiced the Bass technique of toothbrushing might need to combine it with the current toothbrushing methods by performing the Bass technique on the buccal surfaces only for a few weeks. Eventually the Bass method could be applied to the entire dentition. Another approach would be to recommend that the client concentrate on using the Bass technique in the quadrant or area that was professionally treated, and to brush nontreated areas with the current method. After each professional care appointment, the Bass method would then be applied to the recently treated area as well as previously treated areas. For most clients, however, brushing the entire mouth with a new technique is achievable over time.

A six-month study evaluated whether client compliance with plaque control recommendations after active therapy varies with the number of self-care aids recommended (Heasman, Jacobs, & Chapple, 1989). Six dental hygienists treated ninety-three subjects with moderately advanced chronic adult periodontitis who were enrolled in a nonsurgical periodontal program. Self-care instructions include the Modified Stillman's method of toothbrushing and additional aids were incorporated as indicated. Aids included single-tufted brushes, interproximal brushes, unwaxed dental floss, triangular woodsticks, and disclosing tablets. Each subject was educated in the use of two, three, or four aids in addition to the toothbrush. These researchers concluded that there is no benefit to the client to increase the number of aids as it was found that plaque scores achieved after therapy and at the six-month recall are comparable regardless of the number of aids used. Compliance with aids decreased as the number of aids increased. It is interesting to note that a higher number of clients abandoned the use of dental floss than other interproximal aids, possibly due to the lack of persistence and the time necessary to achieve results. Subjects also felt disclosing tablets were messy and 57 percent abandoned their use. The authors' final conclusions were that a minimal number of aids should be recommended and their use checked and reemphasized at each treatment visit.

When selecting interdental aids it is best to recommend only one aid in addition to brushing that will achieve the optimal results for diseased sites. Only the extremely motivated client in initial therapy can be expected to achieve optimal results with two or more interdental aids in conjunction with toothbrushing. Success with multiple aids is probably more realistic when the client is in the maintenance phase of care and is compliant with the self-care recommendations and the recall interval. Research demonstrates that employing interdental aids into daily self-care routines is even harder for clients than toothbrushing, as compliance with their use is low. Recommending that the client use the aid in a localized area, meaning the one that was most recently treated by the dental hygienist, is again a good idea. Some clinicians also advocate the use of an interdental aid every other day or a certain number of times per week with the eventual goal of building to daily use. Asking the client which approach is more practical for his daily self-care or lifestyle will enhance compliance and enhance the cotherapist relationship.

Another consideration in gauging small step size is if any additional self-applied supportive treatment such as antimicrobial rinsing or application of an agent for desensitization is being recommended. The more self-care that is requested of a client, the less likely the client will be to optimally perform each skill. The professional has a responsibility to reduce the number of recommendations to those that are essential and also to allow the client to help make decisions about these aids/skills. For example, if the wooden toothpick and interdental brush would be equally effective in cleansing the embrasure spaces, then permitting the client to choose will enhance compliance. If you feel you are recommending too many things, confront the individual with your thoughts and ask her what she feels she will most likely comply with. These examples are further illustrations of a cotherapy approach to self-care education.

The therapist must also be keenly aware of how much and how fast each client can learn (Huntley, 1979). To gauge self-pacing, assess prior knowledge, attentiveness, anxiety, motivation, and trust (Huntley, 1979). Self-pacing is intimately related to small step size because what is a baby step for one individual is an adult step for another regardless of chronological age. Not permitting the client to self-pace your education can lead to a frustrated client who feels failure as early as the first few appointments of initial therapy. To assess self-pacing, observe client verbal and nonverbal messages. A client might directly indicate he has had enough "knowledge" by stating "Wow, this is complicated," or "I lost you when we were discussing the gums." Also, nonverbal communication, such as loss of eye contact or body movement might indicate the client has lost interest.

Supervised practice should occur at each appointment to ensure that the client's application of the psychomotor skills is accurate, that they are not causing ill effects, and that inappropriate habits have not been developed. Practice in the client's oral cavity is the best way to assess these factors. A client may be able to describe exactly how to use a toothpick holder, but during the client's demonstration the aid is used incorrectly; therefore, a skill discrepancy exists. If the clinician had not prompted the client to practice at the appointment, this discrepancy would not have been recognized and corrected. DeBiase (1991) states that skill development is progressive and will improve over time through repetition and reinforcement. In a study conducted to assess client recall of oral health education services delivered in private practice settings, it was found that subjects (N = 199) were able to recall they were given a toothbrush (79 percent) and shown proper toothbrushing technique (71.9 percent) (McConaughy, Toevs, & Lukken, 1995). Less than one-half of these clients (34.8 percent), however, remembered receiving feedback on the technique and remembered being asked to demonstrate brushing in their mouth (30.2 percent).Conclusions included that adult clients have a low recall frequency of oral health education services, which may indicate that providers might not be incorporating effective learning strategies into self-care education. Therapist interaction is critical as the dental hygienist can demonstrate and redemonstrate while eliciting the client's demonstration and redemonstration after instruction.

Immediate feedback includes both positive and constructive criticism. A client needs to know if he is performing a task correctly or if he is communicating disease theory accurately. It is the clinician's responsibility to identify problems and clarify and reteach when necessary by concentrating on the behavior expressed and not the individual. Immediate feedback encompasses more than just reinforcement in a timely manner; it also includes self-evaluation. Huntley (1979) points out that it is important for the professional to teach the client self-evaluation mechanisms because the oral health educator will not be present on a daily basis. Self-evaluation mechanisms can include observation in the mirror, use of disclosing dyes to self-assess plaque removal, peer evaluation (husband/wife, mother/child), and/or written instructions in the form of a task-analysis or checklist format to be used at specified time intervals. See Figure 8-3 for a client evaluation of brushing. Figures 8-4A and B provide the client with a means to evaluate technique with the wood-

en toothpick (A) and bleeding points while using the wooden toothpick (B). Giving the client a copy of the computerized or hand-recorded periodontal charting is another avenue for self-evaluation. The clinician helps the client understand the charting by explaining the tooth numbers, the right and left sides of the mouth, how bleeding is recorded, and how pockets are identified. The charting form could even contain an explanation of the charting symbols and meanings for the client's benefit. The client can then refer to the charting when performing self-care at home.

Client self-evaluation of behavior can be collected as baseline data prior to teaching disease theory or skill enhancement, or it can be collected after self-care education to motivate and reinforce suggested behavior changes. Baseline data, collected for five to fourteen days, is used to plan intervention strategies. Weinstein, Getz, and Milgrom (1991) feel that taking baseline counts gives the professional a way to determine if the new procedure used was effective. It also serves to reinforce the client's positive behavior should it occur. Data can be collected about frequency and/or duration of brushing; frequency of using floss, wooden toothpicks, or interdental brushes; the recognition of plaque and its location; or the frequency or location of bleeding points.

Research has been conducted on the relationship of client self-assessment to periodontal status. Nowjark and others (1995) studied the long-term effectiveness of two self-assessment strategies; one focused on gingival bleeding (Group I), the other focused on plaque (Group II). Fourteen- and fifteen-year-old subjects were examined at baseline and six, twelve, eighteen, and twenty-four months for gingival bleeding on probing, plaque, calculus, and probing depth. Both groups experienced reductions in gingival bleeding (59 percent for Group I; 55 percent for Group II) suggesting that both approaches can be effective in improving long-term periodontal health status. Other researches have also found that bleeding shows promise as a short-term motivational tool and that it can be assessed by clients (Glavind & Attstrom, 1979; Kallio, Ainamo, & Dasadeepan, 1990; Walsh, Heckman, & Oreau-Diettinger, 1985).

Charting of behavior is conducted by the client to make him aware of the behavior and to identify the sequence of events surrounding the behavior. Identifying what precedes and follows the behavior is used to incorporate a self-care change. For instance, a client who watches the news every night at ten o'clock might increase the use of the interdental aid if an agreement is made that she cleans with the interdental brush prior to watching the news. The premise of using sequences of events to incorporate daily self-care practices is based on the assumption that any behavior that has a higher probability of being performed can be used to reinforce any behavior of lower probability by making it depend on the performance of the less frequent behavior (Weinstein, Getz, & Milgrom, 1991). This concept does not involve a "reward" or positive reinforcement per se;

Directions: Observe your toothbrushing in a mirror three times a week on *Monday*, *Wednesday*, and *Friday* at *night*. Evaluate your new toothbrushing method in the *entire mouth* according to the following steps. Place a checkmark by each step that is incorporated into your brushing.

| STEPS | Week #1 | | | | | | Week #2 | | | | | |
|---|---|---|---|---|---|---|---|---|---|---|---|---|
| | M | T | W | F | S | S | M | T | W | F | S | S |
| 1. Set your timer for a minimum of 3 minutes. | | | | | | | | | | | | |
| 2. Use a soft bristle brush. | | | | | | | | | | | | |
| 3. Follow this sequence:<br>• Brush the outsides of the _bottom_ teeth first by starting on the last molar and advancing to the other side.<br>• Brush the insides of the _bottom_ teeth next by starting, again, on the last molar.<br>• Move to the outside of the _top_ teeth starting on the last molar.<br>• Brush the inside of the _top_ in the same manner. | | | | | | | | | | | | |
| 4. Place the toothbrush bristles at a 45° angle to the gumline. (See Figure A) | | | | | | | | | | | | |
| 5. Apply gentle pressure to insert the bristles into the sulcus or pocket (space) just below the gumline. The gums should blanch (whiten) when enough pressure is used. | | | | | | | | | | | | |
| 6. Use gentle vibratory strokes (slight back and forth motion) without removing bristles from the gumline. | | | | | | | | | | | | |
| 7. Use ten strokes in an area before moving to the next area. | | | | | | | | | | | | |
| 8. After 10 strokes, move to the next area, making sure to overlap strokes with the completed area to avoid missing any gum surface and teeth. (See Figure B) | | | | | | | | | | | | |
| 9. When brushing the front teeth on the inside, hold the handle vertically. Use the toe of the brush with short up and down strokes. (See Figure C) | | | | | | | | | | | | |
| 10. After brushing all outside and inside surfaces, brush the tops (biting surfaces) of the teeth by using a back and forth stroke. Press the bristles into the top surfaces of the teeth. | | | | | | | | | | | | |

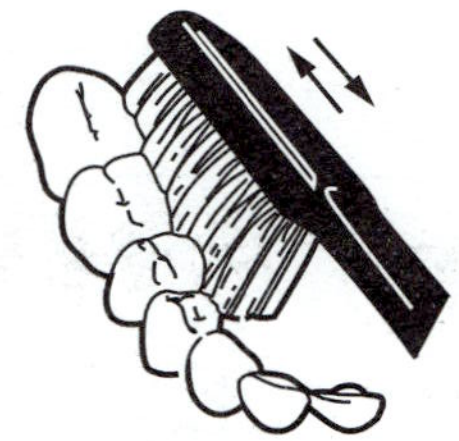

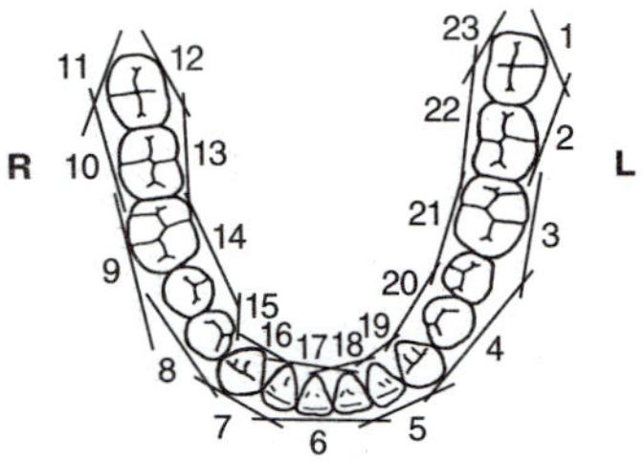

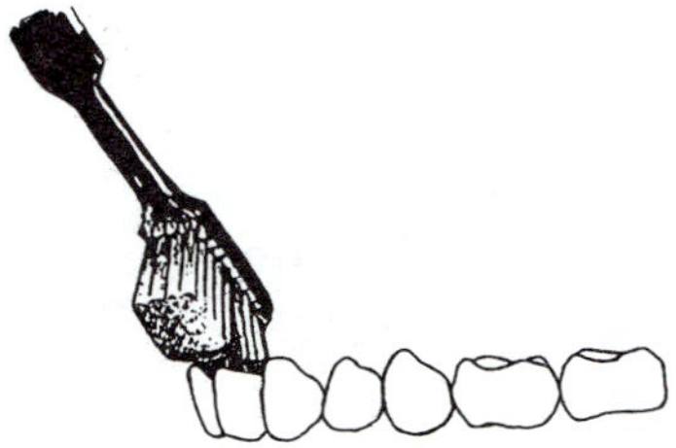

A.

B.

C.

**Figure 8-3** Client self-evaluation of brushing.

CLIENT NAME _____ DATE _____

Directions: Assess your daily use of the round ended wooden toothpick and holder _____*after your morning shower*_____.

| | DAY | | | | | | | | | | | | | | STEPS |
|---|---|---|---|---|---|---|---|---|---|---|---|---|---|---|---|
| | Week #1 | | | | | | | Week #2 | | | | | | | |
| | M | T | W | T | F | S | S | M | T | W | T | F | S | S | |
| | | | | | | | | | | | | | | | 1. Insert toothpick in the holder. Break off the excess. |
| | | | | | | | | | | | | | | | 2. Moisten tip of toothpick with your saliva to soften. |
| | | | | | | | | | | | | | | | 3. Clean the outside of the _____*top six front teeth*_____ first. |
| | | | | | | | | | | | | | | | 4. Start on the left posterior side of the _____*top six front teeth*_____. |
| | | | | | | | | | | | | | | | 5. Move from left to right, tooth by tooth. |
| | | | | | | | | | | | | | | | 6. Place the toothpick tip at a 45° angle to the gumline to remove the plaque just below the gum. (See top figure) |
| | | | | | | | | | | | | | | | 7. Keep the tip at the same angle and follow the gum margin around the tooth and in between the teeth. (See bottom figure) |
| | | | | | | | | | | | | | | | 8. Clean the inside of the _____*top six front teeth*_____ in the same manner. |

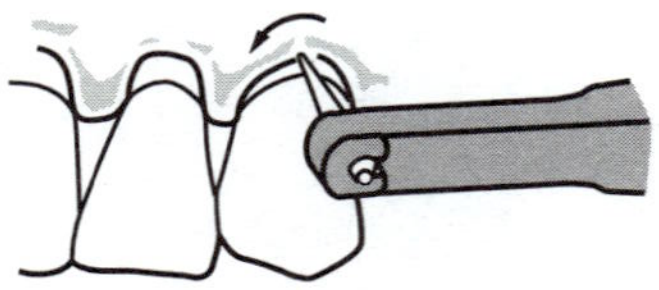

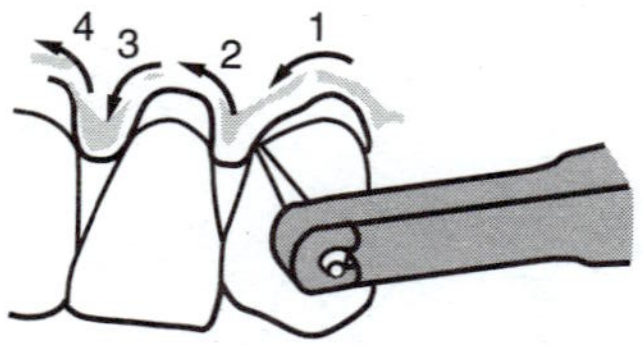

Left side

**Figure 8-4A** Client self-evaluation of the wooden toothpick.

214

To evaluate where your gum tissue bleeds, use a mirror to observe the gum area between each of the ___ *top six front teeth* ___ on the outside front surfaces. Place a red dot on the picture of the gum tissue to indicate where you see bleeding.

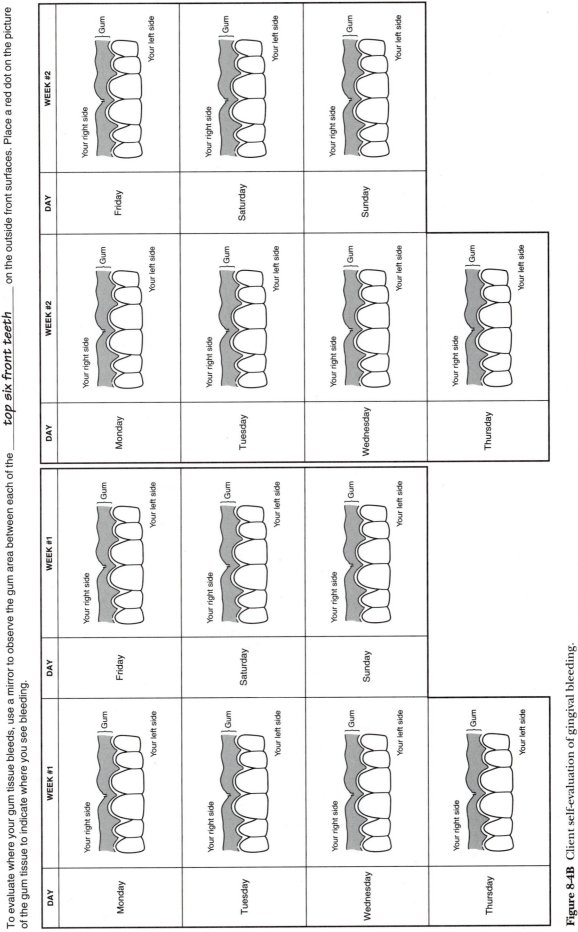

**Figure 8-4B** Client self-evaluation of gingival bleeding.

215

instead, it is a means to link behavior to a consistent habit. The performance of the desired behavior improves the frequency of the event, however, it does not guarantee adequacy of the skill.

Positive reinforcement is probably the most important principle (Huntley, 1979). It includes material rewards, verbal praises, and written comments that are appropriately awarded to the client to enhance external motivation. The goal of this reinforcement is to increase the chances of the behavior being repeated. To select a reinforcer, consider availability in the practice setting and individuality of the client. Any reinforcer should have positive consequences, be strong enough to be of value, be able to be delivered, and be observable by monitoring of some type (Weinstien, Getz, & Milgrom, 1991).

Material reinforcers include toys, clothes, or money. The nature of this type of reinforcer makes it difficult to deliver in dentistry. Some clinical practices might use monetary means to motivate clients. For example, if the client returns for PMP at the recommended interval, then the fee for maintenance care is reduced by a certain percentage. If initial therapy appointments are all attended as planned, and self-care practices are incorporated, then the client is not charged for the reevaluation visit. If a reduction in gingival bleeding is seen as measured by an index at the reevaluation visit and/or for the first maintenance visit, then a fee reduction of 5 percent occurs. Another monetary strategy would be to not charge the client for the fee involved with the consultation visit if the client chooses to comply with the NSPT recommendations including self-care practices. The limitations of these approaches are that the behavior that the cost reduction is based on must be easily measured because the professional must decide if the client deserves the monetary reward or not. Another consideration is that if the cost of care is not a barrier or obstacle, it may not be a useful reinforcer.

Social reinforcers such as verbal praise, acknowledgment, or recognition are the most available and effective type of positive reinforcement. Activity reinforcers are based on activities the client likes to do such as shop, watch television, walk, talk, relax, play games, or read. Dental hygienists can use activity reinforcers to encourage the performance of oral self-care behaviors that are less likely to occur. For example, if a client enjoys watching the late evening news, the clinician could recommend that the Perio-aid™ be used prior to watching television. Watching television will then serve as a reward for using the Perio-aid™. A disadvantage of this type of reinforcer is that the client controls its delivery, which means it can be awarded appropriately or inappropriately. An advantage is that activity reinforcers are often related to social reinforcers because participating in a desired activity frequently involves family or friends.

Positive reinforcement must be incorporated often and whenever possible no matter how small the accomplishment might seem to the clinician. For example, if a client verbally expresses understanding of the role of

bacterial plaque in periodontal disease, but verbally expresses incorrect information about bone loss and furcations, positive reinforcement should be immediately given for the correct verbalization. The clinician can then continue to reteach the concept of bone loss and furcations by an alternate approach and different verbalization. When a client demonstrates difficulty with a psychomotor skill, the clinician understands and acknowledges that most people have difficulty with the task and this will put the client at ease. If a client demonstrates repeated difficulty over time with the recommended aid, the client and clinician will need to work together to choose an alternate self-care aid that can be mastered even though a compromise in potential effectiveness is being made.

Positive reinforcement that is specific and direct is most effective versus one-word acknowledgments such as "yes" and "no." For example, voicing that the client's "correct application of the wooden toothpick in the furcation area on the second try is great as it takes many people more practice," provides specific and detailed positive feedback. Another example would be letting clients know when their theory verbalization of how bone loss occurs is 100 percent accurate. For many people, this process is difficult to understand.

Indirect approach refers to the manner in which the clinician relays the message. A direct approach would involve the clinician telling the client what to do in an authoritarian manner, which prevents the client from taking the responsibility to think about how to initiate change and what changes are necessary. Often people, especially those who are internally motivated, prefer to come to their own conclusion about something versus having someone tell them how and what to do. An indirect approach includes questioning, diplomacy in phrasing verbal messages, and facilitative communication.

Incorporation of visual aids is usually necessary for the client to comprehend the periodontal disease process. Discussion of radiographs, photographs, and illustrations all provide a concrete means of understanding the anatomy of the periodontium and the appearance of different stages of gingivitis and periodontitis. Intraoral photography used prior to, and after, therapy can be a powerful reminder of the benefits of combined professional therapy and self-care. Intraoral cameras used to photograph the client's oral cavity as the clinician performs assessment procedures provide the client with a picture that matches the verbal message being relayed by the clinician. Pamphlets and other literature can also provide visual aids used in education while the client is in the office as well as a reminder at home. Although not a substitute for in-office education, pamphlets from professional associations and commercial companies can supplement self-care education and can be shared with the client's family and friends.

An organized session is inevitably more effective in teaching the client self-care than one that is not systematically or logically planned. Smooth transition from component to component of care, a relaxed atmosphere, and concentration on the client's needs are essential. Logically, clients' needs cannot be incorporated prior to their assessment and self-care practices cannot be modified until current practices are analyzed. As previously mentioned, research does recommend that teaching of disease theory should occur prior to enhancing skills in order to facilitate understanding.

Thinking about these teaching principles aids the clinician in self-evaluation of self-care education and is likely to enhance the chances of initiating a client behavioral change. The more the clinician accommodates the client's needs, the greater the chances of successful self-care education (Wilson, 1987).

## Documentation

Not only is failure to diagnose, treat, or refer clients with periodontal disease common, but also failure to maintain adequate records is frequently discovered (Ray & Staffa, 1993). Documenting oral self-care in the permanent client records involves specific and clear notations about the professional's role in self-care education and the client's role in self-care practices. Teaching of disease theory and skill enhancement should be recorded at each appointment and includes how this information is received by the client. When a human needs model is used, client needs can be summarized in the record of services even when a separate data collection form is employed. It is also important to monitor and document the extent of compliance with self-care recommendations at each appointment. Examples of record of services entries follow:

*Example for initial therapy/first appointment:*

Client informed/educated about adult periodontitis Case Type II. Discussed bacterial plaque, the host response, inflammation, bleeding, and bone loss. Disclosed: generalized moderate plaque at gingival margins. Demonstrated the Modified Bass technique. Patient was able to grasp technique well and set short-term goal to brush for 3 min. before work and at bedtime. Needs deficits identified for safety, stress, and responsibility (see assessment form). Using hydrogen peroxide as a daily rinse. Discussed efficacy, potential side effects, and alteration of rinse to another antimicrobial. Listerine™ was chosen because compliance is expected. Peridex™ was used previously with noncompliance. Client chief concern bleeding; self-evaluation of bleeding discussed. Not able to verbalize how to decrease bleeding; discuss again at next visit.

*Example for initial therapy/second appointment:*

Safety need met—Listerine™ being used daily. Stress reduced as bleeding is only localized. Verbalized relationship of bleeding to reduction of bacterial plaque and Bass brushing. Reevaluated gingival inflammation and clarified the host's role in periodontitis.

Brushing as suggested. Disclosed: moderate plaque at gingival margin on mandibular lingual surfaces. Taught skill enhancement with Bass brushing in this area. Set short-term goal to brush the mandibular lingual surfaces prior to other brushing and to spend 1 minute here. Uses a timer. Client stated "This new brushing technique is easy except for the insides of the teeth; it's easier to use my old method here."

It is difficult to develop record of services examples because notations are dependent on other forms used in the process of care such as needs assessments, treatment plans, current self-care practices, and recommended modifications. Table 8-6 is one example of a form used to record current self-care practices and recommended modifications. It is the clinician's responsibility to write in the record of services' summary notations of information documented elsewhere while focusing on individual client compliance, needs, motivational forces, commitment to learning, and/or relative statements.

Recording actual statements made by clients about self care might prove useful in subsequent education sessions. Examples include "I will never floss" and "I know I need to come in every three months as you recommend." Thorough documentation about self-care not only fulfills a legal obligation, but provides valuable information for any other team members who might be responsible for self-care education. Just as professional therapy is noted in a detailed fashion, it is initially important that self-care education and practices are precisely represented to foster client-centered care. In summary, the AAP (1993) recommends that records and a clinical assessment reveal that the client has been counseled on *why* and *how* to perform effective daily self-care.

## CASE PRESENTATION

After self-care education, it is time to communicate the recommended treatment and various options to the client. The purpose of the case presentation is twofold: to satisfy legal responsibilities for care; and to encourage collaborative treatment efforts between the client and clinician.

### Purpose

Dental hygienists not only have a legal responsibility to provide a case presentation, but an ethical responsibility as well (ADHA Code of Ethics, 1995). One component of the *American Dental Hygienists' Association Code of Ethics, Standards of Responsibility* (ADHA Code of Ethics, 1995) reads: "Provide clients with the information necessary to make informed decisions about their oral health and encourage their full participation in treatment decisions and goals" (p. 161). Presenting the nonsurgical periodontal therapy treatment plan is definitely a challenging communication activity. If the communication has been effective, the prospect of case acceptance is high. Quality case presentations help clients arrive at the best deci-

**Table 8-6  Self-Care Information**

| Current Self-Care Practices: | Recommended Modifications: |
|---|---|
| ☐ Toothbrushing — Type / Frequency / Method | ☐ Toothbrushing — Type / Frequency / Method |
| ☐ Flossing — Type / Frequency / Method | ☐ Flossing — Type / Frequency / Method |
| ☐ Wooden Toothpick — Type / Frequency / Method | ☐ Wooden Toothpick — Type / Frequency / Method |
| ☐ Interdental Brush — Type / Frequency / Method | ☐ Interdental Brush — Type / Frequency / Method |
| ☐ Other Aid — Type / Frequency / Method | ☐ Other Aid — Type / Frequency / Method |
| ☐ Smoking/Tobacco — Type / Frequency / Method | ☐ Smoking/Tobacco — Type / Frequency / Method |
| ☐ Cariogenic Foodstuff — Type / Frequency / Method | ☐ Cariogenic Foodstuff — Type / Frequency / Method |
| ☐ Other — Type / Frequency / Method | ☐ Other — Type / Frequency / Method |

sions; therefore, thorough, clear and concise case presentations are part of our professional responsibility.

Many clinicians are uncomfortable when they must inform a long-term client of the need for periodontal therapy (Dunlap, 1992). Dental hygienists immediately assume the client will feel angry or disappointed in our capabilities as oral health care providers. When the clinician is open and honest with clients regarding their oral conditions and new techniques available for treatment, individuals are usually quite appreciative that the dental professional has taken the time to discuss plans in such detail. One of the best mechanisms for effective case presentation and, thus, case acceptance is through providing adequate self-care education and encouraging client motivation (Manji, 1992; Newman, Kornman, & Holtzman, 1994).

## Recommendations

The case presentation itself should cover at least eight basic components (Darby & Walsh, 1994; Dunlap, 1992; Gommerman, 1994; Woodall, 1993) as follows:

1. Provide a description of existing oral conditions.
2. Provide a brief explanation of the treatment procedures and how therapy differs from previous appointments.
3. Discuss, in a nonthreatening manner, the consequences of rejecting treatment and the outcomes of care.
4. Provide information relative to all treatment options and mention the possible need for future surgical procedures, if appropriate.
5. Identify the client's responsibility as a cotherapist including the necessity for compliance with self-care and recall interval recommendations.
6. Describe fully the benefits and risks of all treatment options involved with the NSPT, if any exist.
7. Allow the client the opportunity to consent initially and to quit or withdraw from treatment at any time.
8. Address the specifics of the time and money requirements of the treatment.

*Example of a brief case presentation with consent :*

Mrs. Baldwin, I would like to share with you what I believe is the best plan for your nonsurgical care. As we discussed during the assessment and educational session, your teeth are in good condition. There are no cavities present and your existing fillings are intact. The main area where there is disease activity present is in the supporting structures that surround the teeth, such as your gums and the bone. Based on your x-rays there are signs of bone loss around your teeth.

As you recall, when I was probing around your teeth I did note several areas where pockets were present. Do you remember when we discussed what normal depths are? (Pause, client statement addressed.)

Currently there are 5 mm pocket probe readings around your back teeth. Also, while I was probing we discussed the significance of the bleeding. Did the relationship of bleeding to disease make sense to you? (Pause and engage in conversation.) I also explored around your teeth for calculus deposits and discovered that there are deposits below your gumline that are harboring bacterial plaque. This build-up is due to plaque not being effectively removed.

It is probable that because you are in the relatively early stages of periodontitis, we should see some healing; however, the results of the disease will never go away. Because of the disease that is present (pockets, plaque, and calculus), we will need to utilize a slightly different approach than simply cleaning your teeth as you have experienced in the past. Instead of cleaning your teeth all at one time, we will need to divide the therapy into four appointments to remove the deposits and one appointment at least four weeks later to assess improvements with your pocket depths and bleeding. Because of the pockets, you have plaque and calculus present on the root surfaces of your teeth and you need periodontal therapy rather than a preventive procedure such as cleaning. I will scale and root plane or remove the calculus from the root surfaces and debride the pockets of plaque to encourage healing. I will only complete a section of your mouth at a time to assure that we are thorough in removing the bacterial irritants that cause disease in your pockets. Can I answer any questions? (Pause, client statement addressed.) At each of these appointments we will discuss this disease process in more detail so you have a thorough understanding of its cause. Also during each appointment, we will work together on your self-care techniques to help you maintain your oral health. You will be responsible at home to work with these recommended techniques on a daily basis because bacteria recolonize every twenty-four hours or so.

Because of the pocket areas, after each scaling appointment you may experience some sensitivity to temperature changes or chewing and your gums may be sore. However, these conditions will last only a day or two and over-the-counter pain relievers are effective. Sometimes root sensitivity can become persistent, and I can then recommend specific agents to reduce the sensitivity. Saline rinses (explain procedure) are also useful if gum sensitivity occurs.

Because your gums are sensitive, I suggest that we use local anesthesia to numb each area for deposit removal. According to your health history, the use of local anesthesia is not contraindicated. There are a few risks associated with anesthesia such as muscle soreness, prolonged numbness, and swelling. I assure you that we will utilize the most efficient method of anesthesia to reduce the chance of those risks and increase your comfort level during treatment. The appointments will be one hour in length. The cost of the treatment includes today's appointment, which includes the x-rays ($95.00) and scaling and root planing each one-fourth or quadrant of your mouth ($145.00/quad). I have checked your insurance policy and it should cover 80 percent of the total cost of the treatment. Your deductible is your responsibility.

You have the right to decline this suggested treatment now or once treatment has begun, however, my concern would be that the disease will only progress and you could lose more of the supporting bone and eventually your teeth. I realize that your teeth are very important to you as you stated when you first came in and we can work together to help you maintain them for a long time. I would be happy to answer any questions you may have. Do you have some questions? Do you consent to this treatment plan?

The example above represents the clinician dialogue without the client interaction or dialogue and only includes information necessary for traditional therapy employing local anesthesia and scaling and root planing/periodontal debridement. When supportive care such as irrigation and overhang removal is indicated, it is also included in the case presentation. When additional therapy such as periodontal fiber placement is recommended at subsequent appointments, a new case presentation is indicated and the process repeats itself.

Student clinicians and private practitioners presenting NSPT might be concerned about the customary length of time it takes to present the case. Ten minutes is the average time necessary for a client receiving initial therapy, and variances occur depending on the number of questions the client has and the scope of indicated care (supportive, restorative, and/or endodontic therapy). The case presentation for PMP or recall visits will take approximately five minutes (Rateitschak, 1994). Again, this time interval will be altered based on client needs, especially if maintenance involves retreatment or surgical intervention.

Clinician challenges with case presentation are to ensure that explanations are not hurried or that the client is not being pushed into a treatment decision. It is equally true, however, that presenters need to be concise in their discussions with clients. When clients are given the opportunity to understand their diseases and the remedies that dentistry has available today, acceptance of periodontal therapy recommendations is nearly a certainty (Dunlap, 1992). In order to achieve a concise presentation, practitioners need to have their thoughts organized in advance of the presentation. The clinician needs to determine what to communicate and how to deliver the message to assure client understanding. Actually, mental planning of the presentation occurs as the assessment data is being examined and recorded. Visual aids such as the periodontal assessment, radiographs,

---

Patient Name _____   Date _____

---

**Directions:** Assess YES (Y) or NO (N) for performance in each criteria.

_____ 1. Information is presented at the appropriate time during dental hygiene care.

_____ 2. The nature of the client's condition is described in understandable terms.

_____ 3. Discusses the care plan (i.e. number of appointments, length, purpose of each appointment, services to be incorporated, a description of the services).

_____ 4. Outcomes of treatment are explained.

_____ 5. Risks of care are described.

_____ 6. The likely outcome of not proceeding with care is explained.

_____ 7. Alternative treatment approaches are offered, if any exist (i.e. ultrasonic vs. curets; radiographs vs. no radiographs; NSPT vs. surgery).

_____ 8. Cost for care is expressed as an estimate.

_____ 9. The client's right to decline care is explained.

_____ 10. Informed consent is requested and a signature obtained on the written informed consent form.

_____ 11. Information is presented by the clinician in a reasonable amount of time (10 minutes).

_____ 12. The presentation is direct, accurate, and concise.

Comments:

---

**Figure 8-5** Case presentation assessment. (Courtesy of Idaho State University, Department of Dental Hygiene, Pocatello, ID, 1996)

and illustrations would be helpful. When you have made these decisions, it is then time to present your treatment plan utilizing effective communication skills and displaying a high confidence level. Careful attention to your clients' nonverbal communication is helpful at this stage in the treatment presentation. Hidden feelings might emerge in the client's posture, tone of voice, or in seemingly irrelevant remarks. Using the communication approaches addressed in the previous chapter will assist you in gaining the trust of the client. In return, the individual should feel comfortable in making an informed decision. To strengthen confidence in presenting the proposed treatment plan, the clinician can self-evaluate the verbal communication (see Figure 8-5). As with self-care education, case presentation can be peer evaluated by engaging a qualified colleague in observation.

## Client Consent for Care

After thoroughly discussing the suggested course of treatment (case presentation) and answering any questions the client may have, informed consent will need to be obtained. Informed consent is legally considered as such only when the previously discussed eight factors pertinent to the case presentation are offered. **Informed consent** is the process by which a client agrees to proposed treatment following a complete case presentation (Buchheister, 1993; Darby & Walsh, 1994; Gommerman, 1994; Searight & Barbarash, 1994). Informed consent should include both verbal and written consent (American Dental Association Council on Insurance, 1987; Searight & Barbarash, 1994; Zarkowski, 1995). A declaration form signed by the client or guardian stating that all treatment, risks, outcomes of treatment, alternative treatments, and the opportunity to ask questions and receive answers to any questions should be furnished prior to treatment (Searight & Barbarash, 1994; Zarkowski, 1995) (see Figure 8-6). The advantage of a written declaration form is that although it does not prevent a malpractice allegation, it aids the dental practitioner in supplying the burden of proof. It is easier to prove that the client was properly informed when it is substantiated through written documentation (American Dental Association Council on Insurance, 1987). It is important that consent

---

Following a complete examination and diagnosis, I have been informed of the recommended treatment plan, alternative treatment, fees for treatment, and the benefits and risks involved with and without treatment.

I acknowledge that no guarantees have been made to me concerning the results of my periodontal therapy. Regardless of treatment, a risk of failure, relapse, or worsening of periodontal conditions may result. Adjunctive treatment or retreatment may be indicated. I recognize that long-term success depends upon my cooperation, self-care practices, and routine maintenance as well. As treatment progresses, if alternative treatment is indicated, I authorize both the dentist and dental hygienist to provide appropriate care.

I am aware that there are potential risks and consequences involved with any diagnostic, surgical, nonsurgical, anesthetic, or analgesic procedure. Several potential risks include:

☐ allergic reactions          ☐ pain                            ☐ other

☐ excessive bleeding          ☐ sensitivity                     _____

☐ gum recession exposing the root  ☐ spaces between teeth       _____

☐ infection                   ☐ temporary/permanent numbness    _____

I have had all my questions answered. Knowing and understanding these risks, I consent to treatment and authorize Dr. _____ and the dental hygienists to provide nonsurgical periodontal treatment as recommended.

Client Signature: _____

Date of Consent: _____

Treatment Option Chosen: _____

Witness Signature: _____

**Option 1:** Referral to a periodontist for an examination and possible treatment.

**Option 2:** A nonsurgical regime of treatment where I accept the responsibility of acting as a cotherapist for my own care. Referral to periodontist may still be indicated.

**Option 3:** Decline all options for care.

**Figure 8-6** Informed consent for periodontal treatment. (Used with permission from Stepping Stones to Success, Pueblo, CO. Adapted from Informed Consent Sample Forms. 1-800-548-2164)

forms comply with state laws, so consultation with an attorney is advisable.

One aspect of case presentation and informed consent that makes dental professionals anxious is the chance that a client will decline therapy. If this situation occurs, the clinician will need to assess what the next step will be. At this point, ask open-ended questions to determine why treatment was declined. Rationale for declining care includes the cost, lack of understanding, or fears. It might be helpful to rediscuss the recommendations for therapy and the consequences of declining treatment. If the client continues to decline an aspect of care, the client will need to complete an informed refusal form (Zarkowski, 1995) or postpone care until other aspects not reliant on the rejected procedure can be completed (Woodall, 1993). The informed refusal form (see Figure 8-7) should include: the proposed treatment; the risks involved without treatment; the list of procedures being refused; the date; and signatures of the client, dentist, and a witness (Zarkowski, 1995). A negotiated or alternative phase of treatment may be discussed collaboratively between the dental professional and client.

Another aspect of the consent process includes alternative treatment options. For example, a client with adult periodontitis that is advanced, might choose NSPT instead of immediate periodontal surgery. Another example could be if a client with moderate bone loss and adult periodontitis selects an oral prophylaxis instead of NSPT after the explanation of the risks associated with refusal of NSPT. The definition of informed consent clearly states that as long as clients understand all outcomes of each treatment, the choice is theirs to make. Should the client decide not to accept any treatment, the professional should advise the client of the consequences. In the previous example, if the client declines both the NSPT and periodontal surgery, the clinician is obligated to discuss the fact that if left untreated, the disease will continue to progress, pain and discomfort can occur, more degeneration can occur, and eventually the teeth might be lost.

---

I understand the current disease and the etiology of this disease present in my mouth. I acknowledge the proposed treatment recommendations made by Dr. _____. Alternative treatment options and risks associated with and without treatment were discussed. I have had all questions answered. I hereby release from liability Dr. _____ , the dental hygienists, and associates from any injury I may currently, or in the future, suffer as a result of my refusal to proceed with periodontal treatment or periodontal referral.

All my questions have been answered satisfactorily. I understand that inadequate or no treatment may result in the progression of my periodontal disease. Several potential results include:

| | |
|---|---|
| bleeding | recession of gums |
| body health compromised | spaces between teeth |
| bone loss | teeth or gum sensitivity |
| infections | teeth loosening/loss |

I fully understand each of these consequences and will assume all responsibility.

I am declining the following aspects of care (list all):

_____

_____

_____

_____

_____

I have carefully read the above and understand this refusal for treatment.

Client Signature: _____

Witness Signature: _____

Date of Refusal: _____

**Figure 8-7** Informed refusal form. (Used with permission from Stepping Stones to Success, Pueblo, CO. Adapted from Informed Consent Sample Forms. 1-800-548-2164)

## Documentation

Once verbal consent has been obtained, documentation in the client's chart is indicated by recording in the record of services that the oral case presentation and implied consent occurred (American Dental Association Council on Insurance, 1987). Even when separate informed consent forms containing the client's signature are used, it is still recommended to record the status of implied consent in the record of services. When an informed consent form is used, a copy should be given to the client and a copy kept in the client's chart. Examples of record of services entries follow:

*Example of consent for case presentation in the record of services when a written declaration form is not used:*

Discussed current oral conditions, brief explanation of treatment, consequences of no treatment, possibility of additional treatment, client's cotherapist role, benefits and risks, client's right to decline treatment, time and cost of therapy. Informed consent was obtained for attached treatment plan.

*Example of when the client consents to the majority of the treatment plan but declines certain aspects of care, and a written declaration form is not used:*

Discussed current oral conditions, brief explanation of treatment, consequences of no treatment, possibility of additional treatment, client's cotherapist role, benefits and risks, client's right to decline treatment, time and cost of therapy. Informed consent obtained for enclosed treatment plan except local anesthesia was declined.

*Examples of informed consent when a declaration form is employed:*

Case presentation: Informed consent was obtained (see enclosed declaration form).

Case presentation: Informed consent was obtained except client declined local anesthesia and topical fluoride treatment (see enclosed declaration form).

## Summary

Success with self-care education and case presentation is dependent on the dental hygienist's communication and teaching abilities. The best way to develop and enhance these assets is to strive to incorporate them into dental hygiene care and to self-evaluate interactions and client compliance. In addition to participating in continuing education courses within the professions of dentistry and dental hygiene, one could take advantage of courses sponsored by other disciplines such as counseling or education. Classes or courses designed to teach interpersonal communication skills and teaching-learning strategies would be worthwhile and rewarding for the professional dental hygienist.

The majority of the hours of each working day are spent sending messages, either verbal or nonverbal, about self-care and professional therapy. Client compliance is a critical component of NSPT and can be cultivated by using effective communication approaches. Wilson (1987) makes suggestions for improving client compliance as follows.

1. Simplify. Clients remember what you tell them first and the simpler the suggested behavior change, the more likely it is to be incorporated into self-care.
2. Accommodate. The more your suggestions match client needs, the more likely they are to comply.
3. Remind clients of appointments. Failed appointments create problems for both the client and therapist. Strive to use appropriate vehicles for reminders including postcards and telephone calls.
4. Keep records of compliance. Advanced systems such as the computer can track individuals who are noncompliant. Communication with the person should be initiated as soon as possible after the noncompliant behavior is noticed.
5. Inform. Instructions and recommendations should be put in writing and given to the client.
6. Provide positive reinforcement. This will enhance client compliance as opposed to a more negative approach to the compliance problem.
7. Identify potential noncompliers. If there is suspicion that compliance will be erratic or difficult, discuss the problems this may create for the client before therapy begins. Generally, the need for compliance is covered in a case presentation for all clients in need of NSPT.

In order for an individual to be compliant with the dental professional's recommendations, communication during all phases of education and case presentation must be productive. It is the responsibility of the practitioner to present a clear and accurate message and to assess the effectiveness of the interaction with the client.

## Case Studies

**Case Study One:** Tom Ashley, a 40-year-old businessman, comes to the office for the first time. When you escort Tom back into the operatory, he says gruffly, "How long is this going to take? I'm behind at work." His medical history is not significant. The plaque and calculus deposits are generalized, and bleeding is present on probing. When viewing the radiographs, horizontal bone loss is present in the posterior regions. You ask Tom when he last visited a dental hygienist. He states, "I had my teeth cleaned ten years ago. I have never had a problem with my teeth, so I only get them polished occasionally. My parents never go to the dentist and they have all their teeth." What would be an appropriate reflecting response statement to the first statement by Tom? At what level of the Learning Ladder Continuum would you classify Tom?

**Case Study Two:** Maude Allen is a 50-year-old elementary school teacher. Maude is in good health. Examination findings include: generalized periodontal pockets from 4 to 6 mm, radiographic crestal bone loss, localized areas of plaque and calculus deposits, and generalized gingival inflammation and bleeding. Maude was able to discuss plaque and calculus theories. She has stated that she never flosses and she brushes once a day. She is concerned that she has bad habits and seems motivated to improve her self-care routine. What level of the learning ladder is Maude probably on? What patient education would you present to Maude at this initial appointment? Develop a plan for proposed treatment and practice a case presentation to Maude.

**Case Study Three:** Molly Max is a 30-year-old nuclear engineer. She comes to the office for the first time and has not received dental care for three years. Her medical history shows good health and her dental history shows she has been having sensitivity to cold. She feels embarrassed that she has not recently seen a dentist, but she had been in graduate school and funds were lacking. Examination findings include: 4 to 5 mm pocket areas in posterior regions, radiographic evidence of crestal bone loss, generalized recession of 2 to 3 mm, Class I furcations in maxillary molar regions, generalized areas of light plaque and calculus, and generalized gingival inflammation and bleeding. Molly was able to discuss plaque and calculus theories and differentiate between gingivitis and periodontitis. She has stated that she flosses daily and brushes three times a day with a hard-bristled brush. She is concerned about the recession and furcations and is motivated to improve her self-care routine. What level of the learning ladder is Molly probably at? At what level of Maslow's Needs Hierarchy is Molly? What human needs, as identified in the Human Needs Conceptual Model, might be unmet? What disease theory would you discuss at this appointment? What self-care instruction would be given?

**Case Study Four:** Clara Budd presented for her PMP visit one month late. During the self-care educational session you question her about the periodontitis present in her mouth, the stage of destruction, the recession, the furcation involvement, and the periodontal pockets. You are pleasantly surprised because she reflects that she understands these entities and she is also able to relate her clinical findings to the disease theory. During the skill enhancement segment of the session, you discover that Mrs. Budd has not been using the interdental brush and she has not offered any rationale for nonuse. You question her about the noncompliance by discussing if she knows how to use the interdental brush and why it is important to her overall oral health. She responds that she feels she knows how to use it and that she realizes it would be best to incorporate it into her self-care practices on a daily basis. What should you as the clinician do next? What type of performance discrepancy is evident? What type of external motivational strategies would you employ to encourage her to use the interdental brush daily?

**Case Study Five:** Using the information from the case study above, suppose Mrs. Budd's performance discrepancy was both skill and management oriented. What suggestions do you have for self-evaluation of her technique at home?

## Case Study Discussions

**Discussion—Case Study One:** Tom is definitely a businessman in a hurry. An effective reflective responding statement could be, "You are very busy at work, and would like your dental treatment to be completed as quickly as possible." Because Tom associates few problems with his teeth to a healthy mouth, he has misinformation that needs to be clarified. He is therefore at the unawareness phase of the learning ladder.

**Discussion—Case Study Two:** Maude has accurate existing knowledge about plaque and calculus theory, but has never made a direct association with the disease process. After presenting existing oral conditions, Maude clearly sees the relationship between her current home care routine and oral health status. She would then be ready for the involvement phase of the learning ladder. Because of the disease conditions, treatment involves NSPT and self-care education. After treatment, a four week reevaluation appointment is indicated and a three-month recall interval for PMP. When presenting the case presentation, make sure to include the eight components (see page 543). Construct a dialogue and then self-evaluate the verbalization using the evaluation mechanism presented in this chapter (see Table 8-5).

**Discussion—Case Study Three:** Molly is very knowledgeable about periodontal disease and is concerned about the areas of recession. She is motivated to maintain these areas because her teeth are important to her. Therefore she is driven by the need of "safety" as identified by Maslow's Hierarchy of Needs. Human needs deficits using the Dental Hygiene Conceptual Model might include safety, freedom from pain and stress, wholesome body image, and conceptualization and problem solving (hard-bristled toothbrush). Because Molly's chief complaint (driving force) was hypersensitivity and she has adequate knowledge about plaque, calculus and the difference between gingivitis and periodontitis, it would be appropriate to discuss periodontitis related to recession and loss of attachment and to modify her toothbrush to a soft or extrasoft brush. Also a discussion of the relationship of plaque to hypersensitivity would be beneficial. The clinician should have Molly demonstrate her current brushing technique and if indicated, modifications should be offered. A desensitizing toothpaste can be recommended and the clinician can also discuss during self-care education and case presentation the incorporation of professional desensitization into her NSPT.

**Discussion—Case Study Four:** You need to review Mrs. Budd's use of the interdental brush by having her demonstrate her technique in her mouth to ensure that she is performing the skill correctly as she stated. If she is performing the technique appropriately, then it appears that she has a management discrepancy. If she is not performing the technique well, then she has a skill discrepancy as well as a management discrepancy. External motivation could be easily employed by incorporating verbal praise into the communications. Praise could be given for being within one month of complying with the suggested recall interval, for remembering about the process of periodontitis and the conditions in her mouth, and for being able to use the interdental brush as recommended. Displaying enthusiasm is important. The office might have other ways of externally motivating clients to achieve compliance like monetary rewards for receiving professional recare on time, as recommended.

**Discussion—Case Study Five:** A self-evaluation form could be developed to meet her needs. It could include information about the correct technique for using the interdental brush. It could also include frequency information by having her evaluate its use on a daily basis. To address the management component of the discrepancy, you could try to establish some type of link between another activity and this self-care practice. Asking Mrs. Budd questions about when it could best be accomplished at home will enhance the cotherapy approach to self-care as well as compliance. This question might also allow you to discover if there is another routine activity that can be performed after the use of the interdental aid. Designing a self-evaluation mechanism for Mrs. Budd would be a valuable activity. Correct technique, frequency, and timing at home should be incorporated into her self-evaluation to meet her needs related to the skill and management discrepancies.

## REFERENCES

American Dental Association Council on Insurance. (1987). Informed consent: A risk management view. *Journal of the American Dental Association, 115,* 630–635.

American Academy of Periodontology. (1993). *Guidelines for periodontal therapy.* Research, science and therapy committee. Chicago: American Academy of Periodontology.

American Dental Hygienists' Association. (1995). Code of ethics for dental hygienists. *Journal of Dental Hygiene, 69*(4), 159–162.

Axelsson, P. (1993). Mechanical plaque control. In N. P. Land & T. Karring (Eds.), *Proceedings of the 1st European Workshop on Periodontology* (pp. 219–243). London: Quintessence Publishing Co.

Bader, H. (1989). *Inflammatory control: Theory and practice.* Quintessence International, *20,* 803–812.

Bakdash, B. (1994). Oral hygiene and compliance as risk factors in periodontitis. *Journal of Periodontology, 65*(5), 539–544.

Buchheister, J. (1993). Confidentiality, informed consent and loyalty. *Journal of the Michigan Dental Association, 75*(7), 22.

Chambers, D. & Abrams, R. (1992). *Dental communication.* Sonoma, CA: Ohana Group.

Corbet, E. & Davies, W. (1993). The role of supragingival plaque in the control of progressive periodontal disease: A review. *Journal of Clinical Periodontology, 20,* 307–313.

Darby, M. & Walsh, M. (1994). *Dental hygiene theory and practice.* Philadelphia: W.B. Saunders Co.

DeBiase, C. (1991). *Dental health education theory and practice.* Philadelphia: Lea & Febiger.

Dunlap, J. (1992). Case presentation for nonsurgical periodontal therapy. *Dental Economics,* 81–85.

Gift, H. C. (1985). Current utilization patterns of oral hygiene practicers. State-of the science review. *Dental Plaque Control Measures and Oral Hygiene Practices.* Bethesda, MD: IRL Press.

Glavind, L. & Attstrom, R. (1979). Periodontal self-evaluation: A motivational tool in periodontics. *Journal of Clinical Periodontology, 6,* 238–251.

Glavind, L., Zenner, E., & Attstrom, R. (1983). Evaluation of various feedback mechanisms in relation to compliance by adult patients with oral home care instructions. *Journal of Clinical Periodontology, 10,* 57.

Gommerman, J. (1994). Informed consent—The process. *Journal of the Canadian Dental Association, 60*(3), 202–203.

Greenstein, G. (1992). Periodontal response to mechanical non-surgical therapy: A review. *Journal of Periodontology, 63*(2), 118–130.

Håkansson, J. (1978). Dental care habits, attitudes towards dental health and dental status among 20- to 60-year-old individuals in Sweden. Thesis, University of Lund, Lund, Sweden.

Harris, N. & Christen, A. (1995). *Primary preventive dentistry* (4th ed.). Norwalk, CT: Appleton & Lange.

Heasman, P., Jacobs, D., & Chapple, I. (1989). An evaluation of the effectiveness and patient compliance with plaque control methods in the prevention of periodontal disease. *Clinical Preventive Dentistry, 11*, 24–28.

Huntley, D. (1979). Five principles of patient education. *Dental Hygiene, 53*, 420–423.

Johansson, L., Öster, B., & Hamp, S. (1984). Evaluation of cause related periodontal therapy and compliance with maintenance care recommendations. *Journal of Clinical Periodontology, 11*, 689.

John, R. (1972). *Developing a plaque control program.* Berkeley, CA: Praxis Publishing Company.

Jupp, A. (1994). A new era in dentistry: Patient education and case acceptance. *Journal of the Canadian Dental Association, 60*(3), 193–195.

Kallio, P., Ainamo, J., & Dasadeepan, A. (1990). Self-assessment of gingival bleeding. *International Dental Journal, 40*, 231–236.

Kühner, M. K. & Raetzke, P. B. (1989). The effect of health beliefs on the compliance of periodontal patients with oral hygiene instructions. *Journal of Periodontology, 60*(1), 51–56.

Lang, W. P., Farghaly, M. M., & Ronis, D. L. (1994). The relation of preventive dental behaviors to periodontal health status. *Journal of Clinical Periodontology, 21*, 194–198.

Low, S. & Ciancio, S. (1990). Reviewing nonsurgical periodontal therapy. *Journal of the American Dental Association, 121*(10), 467–470.

Mager, R. P. & Pipe, P. (1970). *Analyzing performance.* Belmont, CA: Pearon Publishers, Inc.

Magnusson, I., Lindhe, J., Yoneyama, T., & Liljenberg, B. (1984). Recolonization of a subgingival microbiota following scaling in deep pockets. *Journal of Clinical Periodontology, 11*, 193–207.

Manji, I. (1992). Getting patients to say yes: Effective case presentations. *Canadian Dental Journal, 58*(8), 619–620.

McConaughy, F. L., Toevs, S., & Lukken, K. M. (1995). Adult clients' recall of oral health education services received in private practice. *Journal of Dental Hygiene, 69*, 202–211.

Newman, M. G., Korman, K. S., & Holtzman, S. (1994). Association of clinical risk factors with treatment outcomes. *Journal of Periodontology, 65*(5), 489–497.

Nowjack-Raymer, R., Ainamo, J., Suomi, J., Kingman, A., Driscoll, W., & Brown, L. (1995). Improved periodontal status through self-assessment. A 2 year longitudinal study in teenagers. *Journal of Clinical Periodontology, 22*, 603–608.

Palmer, R. M. & Floyd, P. D. (1995). Periodontology: A clinical approach. 3. Nonsurgical treatment and maintenance. *British Dental Journal*, 263–268.

Proctor & Gamble Educational Series. (1993). Survey of brushing behavior. Cincinnati, OH: Proctor & Gamble Educational Series.

Rateitschak, K. H. (1994). Failure of periodontal treatment. *Quintessence International, 25*(7), 449–457.

Ray, A. E. & Staffa, J. (1993). The importance of maintaining adequate dental records. *New York State Dental Journal*, November, 55–60.

Ronis, D., Lang, P., Farghaly, M., & Ekdahl, S. (1994). Preventive oral health behaviors among Detroit-area residents. *Journal of Dental Hygiene, 68*(3), 123–130.

Sato, K., Yoneyama, T., Okamoto, H., Dahlen, G., & Lindhe, J. (1993). The effect of subgingival debridement on periodontal disease parameters and the subgingival microbiota. *Journal of Clinical Periodontology, 20*, 359–365.

Scranton-Gluch, J. (1989). Oral hygiene instruction in dental hygiene care. *Seminars in Dental Hygiene, I*(3).

Stanford, G., & Roark, A. (1974). *Human interaction in education.* Boston: Allyn and Bacon Inc.

Searight, H. R. & Barbarash R. A. (1994). Informed consent: Clinical and legal issues in family practice. *Family Medicine*, (26), 244–249.

Stewart, J., Schoen, M., Padilla, M., Maeder, L., Wolfe, G., & Hartz, G. (1991). The effect of a cognitive behavioral intervention on oral hygiene. *Journal of Clinical Periodontology, 18*, 219–222.

Tedesco, L., Keffer, M., & Fleck-Kandath, C. (1991). Self-efficacy, reasoned action, and oral health behavior reports. A social cognitive approach to compliance. *Journal of Behavioral Medicine, 14*(4), 341–355.

Walsh, M., Heckman, B., Leggott, P., Armitage, G., & Robertson, P. B. (1989). Comparison of manual and powered toothbrushing with and without adjunctive oral irrigation for controlling plaque and gingivitis. *Journal of Clinical Periodontology, 16*, 419–427.

Walsh, M., Heckman, B., & Oreau-Diettinger, R. (1985). Use of gingival bleeding for reinforcement of oral home care behavior. *Community Dentistry and Oral Epidemiology, 13*, 133–135.

Weinstein, P., Getz, T., & Milgrom, P. (1991). *Oral self care: Strategies for preventive dentistry.* (3rd ed.). Seattle, WA: Continuing Dental Education, University of Washington.

Weinstein, P., Milgrom, P., Melnick, S., Beach, B., & Spadafora, A. (1989). How effective is oral hygiene instruction? *Journal of Public Health Dentistry, 49*(1), 32–38.

Weinstein, P. (1982). Humanistic application of behavioral strategies in oral hygiene instruction. *Clinical Preventive Dentistry, 4*(3), 15–19.

Wilkins, E.M. (1994). *Clinical practice of the dental hygienist.* (7th ed.). Philadelphia: Williams & Wilkins.

Wilson, T. G., Glover M. E., Schoen, J., Baust, C., & Jacobs, T. (1984). Compliance with maintenance therapy in a private periodontal practice. *Journal of Periodontology, 55*(8), 468–473.

Wilson, T. G. (1987). Compliance: A review of the literature with possible applications to periodontics. *Journal of Periodontology, 58*(10), 706–714.

Wolfe, G., Stewart, J., & Jacobs-Schoen, M. (1989). Cognitive-behavioral psychology and oral hygiene? A new perspective on an old problem. *Journal of Dental Hygiene, 63*(3), 130–133.

Woodall, I. (1993). *Comprehensive dental hygiene care.* (4th ed.). St. Louis: Mosby-Year Book, Inc.

Zarkowski, P. (1994). Ethical and legal decision making in dental hygiene. In M. L. Darby & M. Walsh (Eds.), *Dental hygiene theory and practice* (pp. 1073–1096). Philadelphia: W.B. Saunders Co.

# CHAPTER 9

# Use of Pain Control Modalities

## Key Terms

analgesia

ball-type flow meter

conscious sedation

electronic dental anesthesia

fail-safe system

local anesthesia

maximum safe dosage (MSD)

pain and anxiety control

psychosomatic methods

topical anesthetics

trituration techniques

vasoconstrictors

## INTRODUCTION

**Pain and anxiety control** includes the use of various physical, chemical, and psychological modalities to prevent or treat preoperative, operative, or postoperative patient apprehension and pain (American Dental Association, 1972). It is involved in all phases of periodontal and restorative care including nonsurgical periodontal therapy (NSPT).

It is estimated that nearly half the people in the United States fear dentistry to some degree (McCann, 1989). Further, an estimated fourteen to thirty-four million adults in America avoid dental treatment because of fear (Malamed, 1995). Because studies of the natural history of periodontal disease clearly demonstrate that the periodontal lesion will progress at a more rapid rate without interference of professional care (Löe, Ånerud, Boysen, & Smith, 1978), it is important that consumers do not avoid oral health care because of fear. More frequent professional care has been shown to reduce the risk of periodontal disease; sites previously affected by periodontitis are at greatest risk for future attachment loss; and patients previously treated for periodontitis require more frequent supportive periodontal therapy (Axelsson, Lindhe, & Nystrom, 1991; Chrissterson, Grossi, Dunford, Machtel, & Genco, 1991; Grbic, Lamster, Celenti, & Fine, 1991).

Incorporation of adequate pain control modalities into treatment plans for nonsurgical periodontal therapy can encourage patient cooperation and compliance. Periodontal treatment methods that facilitate client cooperation and compliance with oral hygiene and professional maintenance are likely to result in greater success (Greenstein, 1992). The most common cause of dental phobia relates to a previous painful or anxiety-producing experience in the dental office (McCann, 1989). Modern day dentistry offers excellent pain control techniques that can be employed to relax and reassure anxious patients, or to prevent pain and anxiety from occurring during the delivery of nonsurgical periodontal care.

Another advantage of using pain and anxiety control techniques relates to the confidence and comfort level of the clinician. The ability of a clinician to perform thorough scaling, root planing, and/or periodontal debridement can be impacted by a variety of factors, one of which is patient pain or discomfort.

Today, use of general anesthesia in dentistry is limited to only a relatively few specialists in anesthesia and oral surgery (Jastak, 1989). Instead, local anesthesia, nitrous oxide-oxygen analgesia and behavioral techniques for managing fear and anxiety are frequently and effectively employed in both restorative and periodontal care plans. Patients who rely on pain control for restorative dental procedures may also require it for nonsurgical periodontal therapy (Stach & Dafoe, 1993). Its use allows dentists and dental hygienists to provide relatively painless oral health services to clients who might otherwise avoid treatment.

This chapter presents an overview of the use of nitrous oxide-oxygen analgesia, local anesthesia, and other pain control techniques commonly employed for the delivery of nonsurgical periodontal care. A discussion of patient evaluation, indications, and contraindications also is presented for selection of appropriate cases. Overviews of related techniques are presented; however, clinicians who provide treatment in conjunction with various pain control modalities must complete formal education and training on a periodic basis (American Dental Association, 1989).

# USE OF NITROUS OXIDE-OXYGEN ANALGESIA FOR CONSCIOUS SEDATION

Nitrous oxide ($N_2O$) is employed in dentistry for the primary purpose of reducing anxiety in the dental client. **Conscious sedation** is a minimally depressed level of consciousness that can be produced by pharmacological means (such as nitrous oxide), by nonpharmacologic methods, or by a combination of both. The client can independently maintain an airway and can respond appropriately to verbal instructions or physical stimulation (Subcommittee on Anxiety and Pain Control, 1994). Conscious sedation, or relative analgesia, obtained through the administration of nitrous oxide is a safe and effective means of anxiety control in restorative dentistry and periodontal therapy. Its use enables dentists and dental hygienists to provide oral health services to many individuals who might otherwise avoid the dental office. The apprehensive client is calmed without loss of consciousness.

Nitrous oxide is a colorless gas with a sweet taste and odor. It is dispensed as a liquid under pressure in a container that is always marked blue for identification. The gas is stable at normal temperatures; it is nonflammable, but will burn readily if ignited. It is a relatively safe gas; however, all gases should be handled with caution. Nitrous oxide is classified as a mildly potent general anesthetic. It is mixed with oxygen in dental inhalation sedation units and administered to obtain **analgesia**, a decreased ability or inability for the patient to perceive pain. Conscious sedation is not a method of absolute pain control and, therefore, should not be confused with general anesthesia and its inherent risks. Nitrous oxide-oxygen analgesia affects the nervous system including, but not limited to the cerebral cortex, the outer surface of the brain's cerebrum, and the thalamus, a part of the brain stem. All pain sensations are relayed from the thalamus to the cortex and pain reaction is based upon past experiences. When applying these concepts to dental pain and anxiety, one can see why a patient might react to an oral injection by jerking or turning the head when the cortex receives the sensation from the oral cavity. If pain reaction, or the patient's response to pain, is to be slowed or dulled, nitrous oxide must have a physiologic effect on parts of the brain (specifically, the cerebral cortex and thalamus). Because nitrous oxide analgesia is particularly effective in reducing pain sensation in soft tissues, it is considered ideal for use during deep scaling, debridement, and root planing procedures (Jastak, 1989). It also can be used in conjunction with local anesthesia when pulpal anesthesia is necessary. A full discussion of pharmacologic effects of nitrous oxide is beyond the scope of this text.

In some states, dental hygienists who are properly educated can legally administer nitrous oxide; in other states, hygienists can monitor or assist with administration. Even if this procedure is not legal for dental hygienists, they must be familiar with indications and contraindications, patient evaluation, and health history considerations, and procedures for monitoring levels of analgesia during the provision of NSPT. Although the dentist may be the one to administer nitrous oxide, the hygienist will be responsible for preoperative and postoperative client assessment and for monitoring signs and symptoms of analgesia.

## Patient Evaluation, Indications, and Contraindications

Dental hygienists often have the responsibility of selecting appropriate cases for administration of nitrous oxide analgesia. An updated, complete personal and health history must be reviewed for each patient prior to administration. Vital signs must also be evaluated, recorded and monitored. A thorough awareness of primary indications, special considerations, and contraindications is essential (Bowen, 1993; Malamed, 1995).

**Primary Indications.** Patients who exhibit fear and anxiety will present patient management problems. They also are more prone to medical emergencies because stress can initiate an exacerbation of their medical problems. Patients who have a history of upsetting or painful experiences in the dental office may be more anxious. Nitrous oxide-oxygen sedation can serve to safely relax most fearful or anxious dental patients. It has been shown to significantly reduce irritability when compared with controls (Fine, Easton, & Skelly, 1991). Some persons, however, are not comfortable with the effects of $N_2O$, and some, such as those with a high drug tolerance or extremely fearful patients, will not achieve adequate sedation at safe concentrations. When adequate sedation cannot be achieved within safe limits, another form of sedative should be selected for that patient. The patient who refuses or is allergic to local anesthesia might benefit from the use of $N_2O$-$O_2$. Although it is not a true substitute for local anesthesia, it can be used to reduce pain sensation when local anesthesia is contraindicated. A prominent gag reflex is a potential problem during many dental procedures. Administration of $N_2O$-$O_2$ will reduce or eliminate severe gagging without jeopardizing protective cough reflexes. Lastly, some patients get impatient at long appointments due to nervousness or stress. Because nitrous oxide reduces the patient's awareness of the lapse of time, it can be beneficial in these cases.

**Indications with Special Consideration.** In the recent past, $N_2O$-$O_2$ sedation has become increasingly important in management of medically compromised clients. It is particularly indicated when these clients are stressed or anxious because stress can result in an oxygen deficit state or cause an acute exacerbation of an underlying medical problem. Nitrous oxide should only be administered to these clients with special consideration given to each case. A physician consultation might be needed prior to administering $N_2O$-$O_2$ sedation in these cases to determine whether the medical condition is under treatment and control. If not, administration of $N_2O$ is not recommended. As long as the medical conditions are not severe, nitrous oxide is the sedative of choice because of its margin of safety and its adjunctive use of oxygen during administration (Malamed, 1995). There are no known allergies to nitrous oxide, so allergic reactions are not a concern.

Medical conditions to consider include cardiovascular disease, cerebrovascular disease (stroke), respiratory disease (asthma), and epilepsy or other seizure disorders because the stress/anxiety of NSPT might trigger an "attack" situation. In each of these conditions, $N_2O$-$O_2$ is the most appropriate agent for conscious sedation of these clients. Its use does not increase heart rate or blood pressure in the presence of cardiovascular disease (Henry & Quock, 1989). It is not recommended, however, within six to nine months following a heart attack or when there is cardiac dysfunction. In clients with a history of stroke or seizure disorders (epilepsy) levels of $N_2O$ beyond 50 percent are not recommended due to the threat of hypoxia, decreased oxygen in the tissue.

Other health history findings that warrant special consideration include thyroid disease, hepatic disease (hepatitis or cirrhosis), prescribed medications that cause depression of the central nervous system (CNS), or the use of alcohol by the client. Thyroid diseases or hepatic diseases routinely raise questions about the administration of drugs during NSPT. Clients with hyperthyroidism or hypothyroidism, however, will usually have normal thyroid activity because of drug therapy or surgical intervention. A physician consult to determine current status is indicated (Malamed, 1995). Clients with hepatic disease can safely receive $N_2O$-$O_2$ since it is not biotransformed in the liver. All drugs taken by clients who are to receive $N_2O$-$O_2$ should be evaluated for effects on the CNS, or for contraindications with anesthetics. Some examples include tranquilizers (diazepam), analgesics (morphine, percodan, meperidine), and hypnotics (barbiturates). Nitrous oxide should not be administered in conjunction with these drugs unless absolutely necessary. If used, low concentrations are essential. Nitrous oxide also is not recommended for clients who are chronic alcohol abusers or for clients who have had a social drink immediately prior to the dental appointment.

**Contraindications.** In some cases, administration of nitrous oxide is *not* recommended. Again a careful review of the health history should be made to rule out medical contraindications such as nasal obstruction, chronic obstructive pulmonary diseases (COPD), debilitating cardiac or cerebrovascular disease and pregnancy. Clients with nasal blockage from the common cold, upper respiratory infections or bronchitis, allergies or hay fever, and deviated nasal septum cannot sufficiently inhale $N_2O$-$O_2$ gases administered.

COPD will prevent the sedative effect of $N_2O$ and contraindicate its use. Clients with emphysema, tuberculosis, eustachian tube blockage, and other chronic respiratory disorders should not receive nitrous oxide. It can result in immunosuppression, abnormal pulmonary function, secondary bacterial infections, or hypoxia. If debilitating heart disease or valvular damage limits a person's daily activities or if clients report cyanosis, dyspnea, need for increased pillows when sleeping, or artery blockage, all CNS depressants (including $N_2O$) should be avoided.

Nitrous oxide administered to a pregnant client does cross the placenta to the fetus and affect the baby's CNS. Studies in animals show that a single dose of $N_2O$ is usually safe when administered in proper concentrations. Nitrous oxide also has been shown to be the most highly recommended sedation agent when one *must* be employed during pregnancy. In the opinion of these authors, however, administration of all drugs should be avoided whenever possible during pregnancy, and particularly during the first and third trimesters. If a sedative is absolutely essential for dental treatment, a medical consultation should be made prior to administration.

Other cases that contraindicate nitrous oxide administration include clients with psychiatric disorders, compulsive personalities, or claustrophobia or behavioral problems. It is difficult to predict the effects of $N_2O$-$O_2$ in clients with psychiatric disorders or compulsive personalities and negative reactions might result. Drugs given to psychiatric clients, such as mood-altering antidepressants, also should be carefully evaluated. Claustrophobic clients are not able to tolerate the nasal mask without a feeling of suffocation. The nasal cannula can be used in these cases; however, this technique is not routinely recommended because of the risk of exposure of trace elements to dental personnel.

Nitrous oxide can be used to control fear and anxiety in most pedodontic clients. Children with severe behavioral problems, however, cannot give the degree of cooperation needed for administration of $N_2O$-$O_2$ inhalation sedation. Forced administration is never recommended. Clients who do not want nitrous oxide should never be forced or coerced to receive $N_2O$ (or any other drug) against their will. Doing so can result in negative side effects or legal repercussions. Refer to Table 9-1 for a summary of indications and contraindications.

### Armamentarium

Several types of machines are available for use in nitrous oxide-oxygen inhalation sedation. The gases generally are transported to the machine at chairside through a series of copper tubings from the central storage area. Some offices have portable nitrous oxide-oxygen machines that house small tanks of $N_2O$ and $O_2$. The portable units usually are employed when nitrous oxide is administered infrequently.

The most common machine used in dentistry has **ball-type flow meters** that indicate the amount of gas

**Table 9-1  Summary of Indications and Contraindications for Nitrous Oxide**

| Primary Indications | Special Considerations | Contraindications |
|---|---|---|
| *Patients who* | *Patients who* | *Patients who* |
| 1. exhibit fear and anxiety. | 1. have medical conditions which trigger "attack" situations. | 1. have nasal obstruction. |
| 2. refuse or are allergic to local anesthesia. | 2. have thyroid disease. | 2. have COPD. |
| 3. have prominent gag reflexes. | 3. have hepatic disease. | 3. have debilitating cardiac or cerebrovascular disease. |
| 4. are impatient with long appointments. | 4. take prescribed medications | 4. are pregnant. |
| | 5. use alcohol immediately prior to appointment, or who are chronic alcohol abusers. | 5. have psychiatric disorders or compulsive personalities. |
| | | 6. are claustrophobic. |
| | | 7. have severe behavior problems (children). |
| | | 8. do not want $N_2O_2$. |

being administered (see Figure 9-1). The machine has an on-off knob that allows the gases to flow into the tubing and nasal mask. Two additional knobs are used to regulate the amount of nitrous oxide and oxygen flow, which is displayed in two separate glass tubings. As each knob is turned to a more open position, more gas enters the glass tubing in the flow meter and a ball floats to indicate how much gas is being dispensed. The flow tubes have markings that are numbered to show how many liters per minute are being dispensed. These two "ball flow meters" (one for $N_2O$ and one for $O_2$) enable the clinician to regulate the flow up to a maximum of 10 liters per minute (lpm). The nitrous oxide can be turned off to 0 lpm, but the knob regulating the flow of oxygen cannot be used to turn the oxygen flow off to 0 lpm. The oxygen flow can only be reduced to about 2.5–3.0 lpm. This safety feature prevents administration of pure nitrous oxide because a minimum oxygen flow is always ensured.

All inhalation sedation units marketed in the United States contain certain safety features to prevent accidents from occurring. Any mechanical device can fail, however, so visual and verbal monitoring of a client is always critical. Dental analgesic units not only are designed so that a minimum of 21 percent oxygen will always be administered, but the **fail-safe system** provides additional safety measures. It is designed so that the nitrous oxide will automatically turn off when oxygen is depleted before the $N_2O$ tank is empty. An audible alarm also sounds to alert the clinician that the client no longer is receiving $N_2O-O_2$.

The nasal hood fits comfortably, yet snugly, over the client's nose. Two types are available. The traditional nosepiece has one hose on each side that is used for inhalation and exhaled gases are eliminated through an

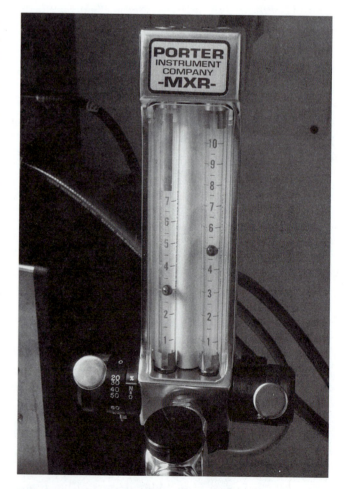

**Figure 9-1** Ball-type flow meters.

exhaling valve located on the top of the nasal hood (Figure 9-2). This exhaling valve creates concerns for occupational exposure; thus, a scavenging nasal hood is recommended. The scavenging nasal hood typically has four tubes (two on each side) connected to it (Figure 9-3). Two of the tubes contain gas(es) flowing from the nitrous oxide machine. The other two tubes carry exhaled gases through a controlled ventilation system (scavenging system) that deposits them outside of the building, or to a safe repository away from the dental operatory. When selecting a nasal hood, the clinician should be sure that it fits the client's nose properly in order to prevent discomfort, but also to ensure minimal or no leakage into the treatment room. Autoclavable nasal hoods, or disposable hoods, are recommended in order to prevent disease transmission. Nasal hoods and tubing also should be checked frequently for cracks, which might allow leakage, and be replaced as needed.

## Technique

After reviewing the client's health history, recording vital signs, and gathering needed armamentarium, the clini-

cian is ready to administer nitrous oxide-oxygen analgesia. An overview of one recommended technique follows (see Table 9-2).

Informed consent must be obtained prior to administration of nitrous oxide. A thorough discussion with the client includes a description of the procedure, an explanation of the effects of $N_2O$, and disclosure of associated risks. Clients can be informed that the technique of inhalation sedation with low to moderate concentrations of nitrous oxide has a remarkable safety record—in over forty-five years of use there has not been any mortality or serious morbidity recorded (Roberts, 1990a). A small proportion of clients feel nausea and an even smaller proportion (less than 0.003 percent) vomit (Roberts, 1990b). These side effects can be minimized or totally prevented with the trituration technique described in this chapter. Clients also can have some control over dosage if effects are unpleasant by breathing room air to dilute the concentration of $N_2O$; however, they should inform the clinician so that the amount being administered can be reduced. The clinician also can show the client the inhalation equipment to be used and describe the positive effects anticipated. A feeling of warmth, perhaps a

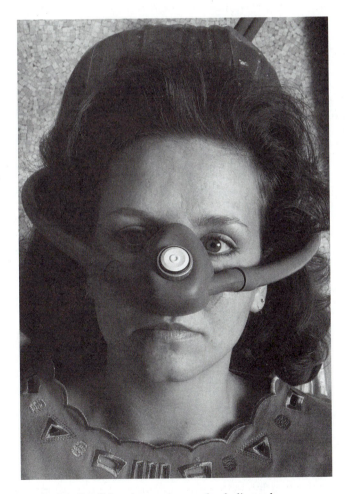

**Figure 9-2** Traditional nosepiece and exhaling valve.

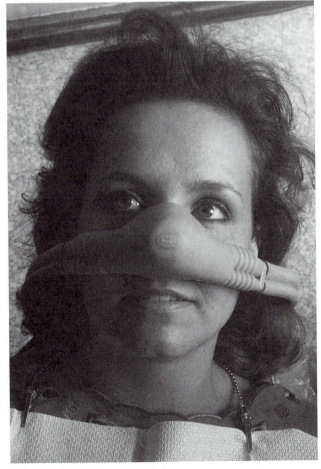

**Figure 9-3** Scavenging nosepiece.

**Table 9-2  Summary of Steps in the Procedure for Administration of Nitrous Oxide-Oxygen Analgesia**

| Procedural Stage | Step Involved |
|---|---|
| Preanesthetic Preparation | 1. Have client visit the restroom.<br>2. Check all equipment.<br>3. Turn on main tanks and analgesic machine.<br>4. Review medical history and take vital signs.<br>5. Explain procedure and effects to client and obtain consent.<br>6. Select appropriate size nosepiece. |
| During Administration | 1. Begin flow of oxygen at 8 liters.<br>2. Place nosepiece over client's nose allowing breathing adjustment time.<br>3. Begin nitrous at 20% concentration (1.5 lpm and oxygen at 80% (6.5 lpm).<br>4. Observe client for one minute prior to changing dosage.<br>5. Increase nitrous by one-half liter and decrease oxygen by one-half liter until desired effect is obtained.<br>6. Monitor clinical manifestations closely, adjusting levels after waiting one minute.<br>7. Oxygenate client until normalcy is regained (minimum 3 to 5 minutes). |

little tingling in the fingers and toes, but most noticeably a very pleasant feeling of relaxation is the goal. Consciousness is fully maintained but altered so that painful sensations are filtered out and an increased sense of well-being remains. After fully explaining risks, benefits, the procedure, and answering any client inquiries, the clinician can request written consent for $N_2O$-$O_2$ analgesia. After consent is obtained, the patient and the inhalation sedation unit can be positioned for use. The preferred patient position is supine; however, partially reclined or upright positioning is acceptable when indicated for a particular procedure or for client comfort.

The flow of oxygen is started at 8.0 lpm and the nasal hood is placed over the patient's nose. Starting the oxygen first will prevent a feeling of suffocation. The patient is asked if breathing is comfortable and volume is adjusted accordingly. Patients also should be reminded to breath through the nose throughout the appointment.

After determining proper flow rate for the client, the clinician can begin administration of nitrous oxide. Various **trituration techniques** allow for gradual increases in the concentration of $N_2O$ delivered to the client. In the trituration technique described herein, the total flow of gases will always remain constant. Thus, if the client is comfortable with breathing oxygen at 8 lpm (liters per

minute), the total flow of gas(es) will always equal 8 lpm. The first adjustment should equal about 20 percent $N_2O$ and 80 percent $O_2$. Since 20 percent of 8 lpm is approximately 1.5 lpm, the nitrous oxide would be started at 1.5 lpm and the oxygen would be reduced (from 8 lpm) to 6.5 lpm. Note that 1.5 lpm and 6.5 lpm equals the eight liters total flow with which the administration was started.

The patient is permitted to breathe this concentration of $N_2O$ for 60 to 90 seconds to allow for the drug to be absorbed into the circulatory system and for the effects to be realized. During this time, the clinician observes the patient for signs and symptoms of sedation (Table 9-3). The typical patient receiving 20 percent $N_2O$ will have little or no effect after 60 to 90 seconds, so trituration of $N_2O$ continues.

Following the initial level of 20 percent, all subsequent increases will be smaller, approximately 10 percent. In this example of 8 lpm total volume, the oxygen would be decreased 0.5 lpm to 6.0 lpm and the nitrous oxide would be increased 0.5 lpm to 2.0 lpm. Wait 60 to 90 seconds and observe the patient's signs and symptoms before making another adjustment. Continue decreasing the oxygen by 0.5 lpm and increasing the nitrous oxide by 0.5 lpm until signs and symptoms of adequate conscious sedation are achieved (see Table 9-3). During this time, the client is asked "What are you feeling?". The patient is then required to give a specific response regarding his/her symptoms. Subjective effects include a feeling of relaxation; happy, euphoric mood changes; changes in body awareness; alterations in time perception; and experiences of a detached, dreamy reverie state, even at 30 percent $N_2O$ (Block, Ghoneim, Kumar, & Pathak, 1990).

The last adjustment of $N_2O$ should be made when the oxygen and the nitrous oxide are each at 4 liters, again totaling 8 liters. At this point, 50 percent $O_2$ and 50 percent $N_2O$ are being administered. This is the highest ratio of nitrous oxide recommended for safe administration without special consideration. The maximum safe dose is considered to be 65 percent $N_2O$; however, chances of side effects such as nausea and headaches are more frequent when concentrations exceed 50 percent (Malamed, 1995). The importance of maintaining an appropriate ratio of oxygen to nitrous oxide cannot be overstressed.

Once the patient is relaxed and conscious sedation is attained, dental or dental hygiene treatment can begin. The only way to accurately determine whether the proper sedation level is achieved is to initiate treatment and observe the patient's response. If adequate sedation has not been achieved, continue the trituration technique until the patient is comfortable and relaxed during treatment.

Observe the patient and the inhalation sedation unit throughout treatment. Patients will appear relaxed and their attention may drift in and out of the environment. They will, however, be responsive to instructions given. Clinical signs and symptoms should continue to be mon-

## Table 9-3 Signs and Symptoms of Adequate Conscious Sedation

| Level of Sedation | Signs and Symptoms |
| --- | --- |
| Light Analgesia | 1. Patient appears normal, relaxed, awake.<br>2. Patient might feel slight tingling in toes, fingers, tongue, and lips.<br>3. Patient might giggle.<br>4. Vital signs remain normal. |
| Conscious Sedation (Relative Analgesia) | 1. Patient may have dreamy look.<br>2. Reactions of patient are slowed.<br>3. Partial amnesia may occur.<br>4. Voice will sound "throaty."<br>5. Patient will feel warm and drowsy.<br>6. Patient may drift in and out of environment.<br>7. Patient may hear pleasant ringing in ears.<br>8. Vital signs remain normal.<br>9. Pain is reduced or eliminated but touch and pressure is still perceived.<br>10. Patient is less aware of surroundings; sounds and smells are dulled.<br>11. Patient remains cooperative and follows instructions. |

(Courtesy of Bowen, D. M., *Journal of Practical Hygiene*, PP&A Publishing, Inc., 1993)

## Table 9-4 Signs and Symptoms of Oversedation

Signs and Symptoms

1. Patient's mouth tends to close frequently.
2. Patient no longer cooperates.
3. Patient becomes angry with hard stare.
4. Patient is totally unaware of surroundings.
5. Patient may hallucinate.
6. Patient's chest may feel heavy.
7. Sensation of flying, falling, or uncontrolled spinning is present.
8. Pupils may dilate.
9. Patient talks incoherently.
10. Patient cries or becomes giddy.

(Courtesy of Bowen, D. M., *Journal of Practical Hygiene*, PP&A Publishing, Inc., 1993)

itored closely for any change so further adjustments can be made when necessary.

If patients become irritated or they can no longer cooperate and their mouth tends to close, oversedation is being approached. This is an indication that the nitrous oxide level is too high. Also, changes in physical symptoms, such as dilation of pupils or nausea, would be an indication of too much nitrous oxide. Table 9-4 outlines signs and symptoms of oversedation (Bennett, 1978; Bowen, 1993; Malamed, 1995). At this point the clinician should take three steps to rectify the situation. First, reduce the level of nitrous oxide or turn it off depending upon severity of the side effect or reaction; second, increase the level of oxygen; and last, reassure the client.

Since emergencies occur without notice and patient analgesia levels fluctuate, it is important to monitor the patient continuously while nitrous oxide is being administered. *Never* leave a patient unattended while under the effects of nitrous oxide. Some references suggest retaking vital signs periodically, at a minimum every 45 minutes, during dental treatment to compare with baseline data (Malamed, 1995; Subcommittee on Anxiety and Pain Control, 1994). Remember, vital signs will remain normal with proper levels of analgesia. The ratio of oxygen to nitrous oxide should be maintained at a comfortable level according to the patient's response.

As dental treatment is terminated, pure oxygen is administered to stabilize the patient before dismissal. Turn the nitrous oxide completely off and increase the oxygen to 8 liters to "oxygenate" or "flush" the client with oxygen. Pure oxygen should be administered for a *minimum* of 3 to 5 minutes following nitrous oxide analgesia. Oxygen should be administered until the client regains "normalcy." It may take longer for some patients to return to normal than others. When oxygenating the patient, inform him/her that you are turning off the nitrous oxide and that, while breathing pure oxygen, the symptoms will disappear. Some of the effects of nitrous oxide are psychological.

Once the client feels normal again, vital signs should be taken and compared to the baseline data. An operator who releases a client who has not regained normalcy can be held legally liable for any harm that results. For this reason, oxygenation is essential. Also, if a client is permitted to breathe room air immediately after inhalation of nitrous oxide-oxygen, "diffusion hypoxia" can result. Diffusion hypoxia can result in headaches or nausea following the administration of nitrous oxide. If the client is adequately flushed with oxygen, this condition can be prevented. Once the client is oxygenated and reports that he/she feels normal, the client can be dismissed. Malamed (1995) suggests administering a connect-the-dots test to clients to test their coordination prior to dismissal.

After completion of treatment, a legal chart entry is recorded. There are two major reasons for being certain to record administration of nitrous oxide completely and accurately. First, in the event of a complaint by the client or a malpractice suit, the dental chart will be considered a primary source of evidence. Second, dosage levels vary from client to client and even with the same client on a day-to-day basis. Factors contributing to the variance include: amount of food or drink consumed

**Table 9-5 Components of a Complete Chart Entry for Nitrous Oxide-Oxygen Analgesia and Local Anesthesia**

| | |
|---|---|
| General | 1. Date. |
| | 2. Preoperative health history evaluation including vital signs. |
| | 3. Name, address, and telephone number of patient's physician. |
| | 4. Discussed advantages and risks of drug administration. |
| | 5. Patient consented to drug without concern (if patient had a concern, record any concern). |
| | 6. Pre- and postoperative instructions given to patient. |
| | 7. Postoperative vital signs. |
| | 8. Any adverse reactions, complications, or side effects (even if telephoned in later). |
| Nitrous Oxide-Oxygen Analgesia | 1. Concentrations of nitrous oxide and oxygen administered. |
| | 2. Length of procedure. |
| | 3. Oxygenation and length of time oxygen administered postoperatively. |
| | 4. Assessment of patient's normalcy prior to discharge. |
| | 5. Name of responsible adult to whom patient is discharged, if applicable. |
| Local Anesthesia | 1. Injection(s) administered. |
| | 2. Type of anesthetic and vasoconstrictor administered. |
| | 3. Amount of anesthetic and vasoconstrictor deposited (number of mg). |

prior to the appointment, mental and/or emotional state of the client at any specific point in time, amount of sleep or physical condition of the client, and increased tolerance with repeated administration. This is one reason that the trituration technique presented in this chapter suggests beginning with pure oxygen and increasing nitrous oxide slowly at each client appointment. It is not safe to assume that the previous analgesic level will be appropriate on sequential visits. A very rapid induction also might cause nausea or other adverse reactions.

Table 9-5 outlines essential information to be included in a complete and accurate chart recording for both nitrous oxide-oxygen analgesia and local anesthesia administration because these pain control modalities are frequently used together. When only one technique is employed, selected components can be recorded. Nitrous oxide concentration is recorded as a percentage of gas volume administered. On some nitrous oxide systems, the percentage can be read on the flow meter; on others the volume is shown in liters per minute (lpm). A formula for calculating percentage of nitrous oxide administered follows (Stach & Dafoe, 1993):

$$\frac{\text{Liters of N}_2\text{O/minute}}{\text{Total flow of N}_2\text{O} + \text{O}_2 \text{ in lpm}} \times 100 = \% \text{ of N}_2\text{O}$$

Example:

$$\frac{3 \text{ Liters of N}_2\text{O}}{3 \text{ L of N}_2\text{O} + 5 \text{ L of O}_2} = 3/8 \times 100 = 37.5\% \text{ N}_2\text{O}$$

By subtracting the liters of $N_2O$ from 100 percent, the percentage of oxygen can also be determined. In the example provided, 62.5 percent $O_2$ was administered (100–37.5 = 62.5). The volume of each gas is recorded in the chart entry following every administration.

Additional considerations necessary for the ethical and legal administration of nitrous oxide should be made. Emergency equipment must be readily available at all times. Be certain to follow all previously discussed precautionary measures including: taking a thorough medical history including vital signs, making sure that the client has regained normalcy prior to dismissal, obtaining informed consent of the client before administration of nitrous oxide, and documenting procedures thoroughly. It is also essential that any clinicians involved in the administration of nitrous oxide complete specific education and clinical training prior to use (American Dental Association, 1989). This education is important for safety of the client as well as legal protection for the operator. The dentist, dental hygienist, and/or assistant can be held liable in any civil or malpractice suits filed by the client. Practitioners should inquire with their malpractice insurance carrier to assure that administration of nitrous oxide (or other drugs such as local anesthetics) are covered by their policy. The administration of nitrous oxide-oxygen analgesia by appropriately educated individuals is a safe and effective means of anxiety control. As stated in the American Academy of Periodontology's Guidelines for the Use of Conscious Sedation in Periodontics, "It is the responsibility of each practitioner who uses conscious sedation to be a continuous student of the art and science of the discipline" (Subcommittee on Anxiety and Pain Control, 1994, pg. 2).

## Occupational Exposure to Nitrous Oxide

Although nitrous oxide is considered to be a safe pharmacologic agent for client administration, there are environmental health concerns for dental personnel chronically exposed to trace amounts of waste nitrous oxide in the operatory (Cohen et al., 1980; Henry, 1992; Mandel, 1993). In 1977, the National Institute of Occupational Safety and Health (1977) established recommendations for nitrous oxide levels absorbed by dental personnel to be limited to a maximum of 25 parts per million during administration of the gas; however, dental offices frequently exceed this level. Refer to Chapter 15 for further information on nitrous oxide as an occupational hazard.

Particularly disturbing is a 1980 report showing increased spontaneous abortion rates for dental assistants and unexposed wives of dentists who used nitrous oxide in their practices (Cohen et al., 1980). This landmark investigation studied health histories of 61,197 dentists and chairside assistants. Results indicated that dentists and dental assistants who worked in offices where $N_2O$ was used more than eight hours per week had higher incidences of liver, kidney and neurological diseases. Dental assistants also had a 2.3 fold increase in number of spontaneous abortions compared to nonusers.

A more recent study of full-time dental assistants has documented a dramatic decrease in their ability to become pregnant if exposed to more than five hours of unscavenged $N_2O$ per week (Rowland et al., 1992). Among over 400 women who participated in this study, those who were exposed over five hours per week were significantly less fertile and only 41 percent as likely to conceive during each menstrual cycle. Most important, no decrease in the ability to become pregnant was found for dental assistants working in offices where $N_2O$ was scavenged regardless of length of exposure, nor in offices where $N_2O$ was unscavenged if exposure was less than five hours per week. These findings highlight the importance of using a scavenging system when regularly using nitrous oxide in dental practice. The study also estimates that there are 175,000 dental assistants, 80,000 dental hygienists, and 15,000 dentists in the United States who are women of reproductive age.

Habitual use of nitrous oxide by dental personnel is also of concern. Professionals should never use nitrous oxide recreationally and self-administration is definitely unsafe. Chronic abuse of $N_2O$ can have pronounced, toxic effects including central nervous system myeloneuropathy (numbness, equilibrium and coordination problems, muscle weakness, headaches, and memory and mood alteration), multiple sclerosis-like symptoms, and hemotologic effects or changes in bone marrow synthesis (Henry, 1992; Jastak, 1991).

To reduce nitrous oxide levels in the dental operatory, the following procedures are recommended:

1. Use an approved scavenging system.
2. Use a proper fitting nasal hood.
3. Be sure $N_2O$ is evacuated outside and away from return air ducts.
4. Use supplemental oral suction to reduce ambient $N_2O$.
5. Minimize patient conversation and thus exhaled gases.
6. Leave the scavenging mask in place until patient oxygenation is completed.
7. Check the $N_2O$ system frequently for leaks and replace hoses, bags, or connectors when leakage is detected.
8. Be sure dental operatory is adequately ventilated.
9. Wear passive dosimeters (badges that measure levels of exposure).

## USE OF LOCAL ANESTHESIA IN NONSURGICAL PERIODONTAL THERAPY

A response to the question "When should local anesthesia be administered during nonsurgical periodontal therapy?" seems obvious: when the client might experience pain. The answer to this question, however, is not as simple as it first appears. Although there are numerous advantages of employing local anesthesia for both the client and the clinician, a number of factors need to be considered when determining whether or not to administer it. Once the decision has been made to use a local anesthetic, additional questions surface. Decisions need to be made for the patient regarding the most appropriate anesthetic to administer and which injections would best benefit the patient's treatment. Also, the clinician must select a suitable way to discuss the need for this "shot" with the patient, who might be very anxious about receiving treatment, let alone the anxiety-ridden injection!

### Background Information

The Subcommittee on Anxiety and Pain Control of the American Academy of Periodontology (1994) defines **local anesthesia** as the elimination of sensations, especially pain, in part of the body by the topical application or regional injection of a drug. Painless and effective local anesthesia is the goal for all injections. Currently, administering local anesthesia is legal for dental hygienists to perform in twenty-two states, and professional associations in many other states are actively working to include this procedure in their respective practice acts (American Dental Association, Department of State Governmental Affairs, 1995). In states not allowing the administration of local anesthesia, hygienists might be hesitant to interrupt the dentist's schedule to provide anesthesia for a patient requiring deep scaling and root planing (Sisty-LePeau, Nielsen-Thompson, & Lutjen, 1992). A busy appointment schedule often does not permit the extra time required for the dentist/employer to suspend treatment in the middle of his/her procedure to anesthetize another patient receiving dental hygiene treatment. The possibility of the need for reinjection during NSPT further complicates the office schedule. Without adequate pain control measures, less-than-ideal therapy could result, particularly while providing services for patients with periodontal disease.

Reports of client reactions to dental hygienists administering injections have been extremely positive. Hygienists' success rate of achieving profound anesthesia is comparable to that of dentists (Lobene, Berman, Chaisson, Karelas, & Nolan, 1974; Sisty-LePeau & Henderson, 1974), and the technique employed by hygienists is often perceived as more comfortable than the technique used by dentists. Possible explanations for this increased comfort are that hygienists often pay closer attention to details of atraumatic technique and display greater empathy for their patients. In summary, both patients and dentists appreciate the skills of dental hygienists administering local anesthesia (Malamed, 1990).

The scope and quality of NSPT can be improved with this procedure. Comfortable treatment helps to decrease client anxiety, which might then be reflected by more frequent maintenance therapy. Colorado dentist/employers reported other positive effects of dental hygienists administering local anesthesia, including a more smoothly running practice, more satisfied patients, and increased productivity of the hygienist (Cross-Poline, Passon, Tillis, & Stach, 1992).

### Factors to Consider When Determining the Need for Local Anesthetic

As reiterated throughout this text, NSPT and effective maintenance therapy are dependent upon thorough removal of bacterial deposits both supra- and subgingivally. Complete elimination of subgingival deposits is difficult, with the effectiveness of deposit removal being proportional to the pocket depth (Greenstein, 1992). The deeper the periodontal pockets, the greater the chance that more deposits will remain, primarily due to decreased accessibility and visibility. The clinician's role is to perfect the exacting instrumentation technique required for thorough scaling and root planing or periodontal debridement, and to facilitate comfortable therapy. In some cases, the quality of these services depends upon effective pain control to ensure patient comfort (Sisty-LePeau, Henderson, & Martin, 1986). It is important to note that many of the studies have documented that NSPT is equally as effective as periodontal surgery in improving periodontal status employed local anesthesia in conjunction with scaling and root planing (American Academy of Periodontology, 1989; Isidor & Karring, 1986; Isidor, Karring, & Attstrom, 1984; Lindhe, Westfeit, Nyman, Socransky, & Haffajee, 1984). Frequently, clinicians feel more comfortable when the patient is anesthetized and, therefore, perform a thorough debridement regardless of the client's degree of sensitivity.

The decision to administer local anesthetic agents should be made prior to the patient experiencing any pain. When deciding whether or not to administer local anesthesia for pain control during clinical treatment, consideration should be given to a variety of factors that are summarized in Table 9-6. These factors are evaluated during the assessment phase of therapy, thus permitting the clinician to consider the use of anesthesia before formulating the treatment plan. Any one, or a combination, of the factors listed might require that local anesthesia be administered in localized or generalized areas of need.

Periodontal assessment factors are related to the comfort level of both the patient and clinician during NSPT. Complete deposit removal is more complex when pocket depth is greater than 4 mm and might be enhanced with the use of local anesthesia. Tight gingival tissue limits accessibility to deeper pockets and corresponding root anatomy. Conversely, when loss of tissue tone results in a "flabby" interdental papillae, the turgor can be enhanced by injecting directly into the papilla. Also, attachment loss that creates areas of cratering or narrow infrabony pockets is difficult to access during NSPT. Local anesthesia should aid in deposit removal adjacent to the attachment. Molar furcation involvement and anatomic variations complicate therapy further by limiting accessibility. For example, instrument adaptation is challenging in furcations occluded by gingiva and in longitudinal depressions found on root surfaces. When the patient is anesthetized, operator confidence is increased while working in more complicated treatment areas.

Patients who experience increased sensitivity from exposed cementum and/or dentin are also likely candidates for local anesthesia. Inflamed tissue that is painful or bleeds upon provocation will require an injection to control discomfort or to provide hemostasis in the area. When hemostasis is a concern, an anesthetic with a vasoconstrictor is employed to help control the bleeding. Patients with low pain thresholds should be identified during the health history review or during the periodontal assessment. For these individuals, the use of local anesthesia will control pain in the area of the injection and assure the clinician that the patient is not experiencing discomfort. It is important for the operator to determine the type of sensitivity (pulpal, soft tissue, or even psychosomatic) the patient experiences in order to choose appropriate pain control modalities. Lastly, the type of instrumentation to be employed (hand versus ultrasonic instruments) might impact the need for pain control procedures. Some patients experience sensitivity with either or both approaches to scaling and root planing.

### Selection of Local Anesthetic Agents

There are a variety of effective agents available on the market and selecting an appropriate anesthetic can be a difficult decision. Unfortunately, some operators are accustomed to selecting whatever agent happens to be available without considering the effects of the drug they are using. This section summarizes the most commonly used local anesthetics today (see Table 9-7) and offers a list of factors to consider when selecting the anesthetic drug most appropriate for a particular client and care plan (see Table 9-8).

Although local anesthetic agents are available as either ester or amide compounds, amides are used almost exclusively in dentistry because they do not exhibit the history of allergic reactions experienced with the esters. Esters are primarily metabolized in the plasma by the enzyme pseudocholinesterase; amides are metabolized primarily in the liver. It is important to know to which chemical group a local anesthetic is classified, because a person allergic to one anesthetic is likely to be allergic to another anesthetic in the same chemical group.

**Table 9-6  Factors to Consider When Determining the Need for Local Anesthetic**

| | Factor | Comment |
|---|---|---|
| Periodontal Assessment Factors | Pocket depth greater than 4 mm | • limited accessibility and visibility decrease chance of complete deposit removal; pain control increases patient comfort and operator confidence |
| | Tissue tone | • tight or nonelastic tissue may limit access to deep pockets or challenging root anatomy<br>• local anesthetic may be used to increase the turgor of the gingiva if injected into an edematous interdental papilla |
| | Pocket topography | • cratering at epithelial attachment or narrow infrabony pockets; pain control enhances deposit removal |
| | Furcations | • limited accessibility and visibility decreases chance of complete deposit removal; pain control increases patient comfort and operator confidence |
| | Root anatomy | Anatomic variations may require pain control for NSPT<br>• limited accessibility<br>  – unusual longitudinal depressions<br>  – deeper pockets with more complex root anatomy<br>• increased sensitivity<br>  – overscaled roots (coke-bottle appearance)<br>  – gingival recession<br>  – abrasion |
| | Inflammation | • inflamed tissue likely to be painful<br>• incidental curettage will occur inadvertently in some areas<br>• hemostasis may be a concern |
| | Hemorrhage | • use vasoconstrictor when hemostasis is a concern such as with bleeding upon probing or spontaneous hemorrhage |
| Patient-Related Factors | Patient pain threshold | • if patient's pain threshold is low, administer local anesthetic to control pain and/or reduce anxiety level |
| | Patient sensitivity | • determine type of sensitivity (pulpal or soft tissue)<br>• determine type of instrumentation (hand vs. ultrasonic instruments) |

As of January, 1996, the only ester-type anesthetic available in dental cartridges in the U.S. (a combination of propoxycaine and procaine) was withdrawn from the U.S. market (Malamed, 1997).Other than giving preference to the amides in all cases, it is difficult to recommend one agent over another. The clinical differences in rate of onset or degree of effectiveness among the amide solutions available are slight. The one significant difference is the presence or absence of a vasoconstricting agent.

Lidocaine was the first amide introduced, is the standard of comparison for other amide anesthetics, and is probably the most popular or frequently used local anesthetic today. Lidocaine is available without vasoconstrictor (plain) or with a vasoconstrictor (epinephrine 1:50,000 or the more commonly employed 1:100,000). Because it has greater vasodilating effects than other amides such as mepivacaine or prilocaine without vasoconstrictors, lidocaine plain exhibits very short-acting (5 to 10 minutes) pulpal anesthesia. Soft tissue anesthesia can be expected to be 1 to 2 hours in duration. It might be used, for example, to infiltrate around a single sensitive tooth on the maxilla because a longer duration anesthetic would not be necessary to scale and root plane

one sensitive tooth. When epinephrine is included, the duration of anesthesia is increased to 60 to 90 minutes for pulpal tissues and soft tissue anesthesia varies from approximately 3 to 5 hours (Astra, 1990; Cook-Waite, 1993; Malamed, 1990).

Prilocaine is the least inherently vasodilating agent and is said to be less toxic than all other local anesthetic agents (Young & MacKenzie, 1992). It is available with a vasoconstrictor (epinephrine, 1:200,000) or without (plain). The duration of action not only varies considerably with the addition of vasoconstrictor, but also with the type of injection employed. When prilocaine plain is administered, infiltration anesthesia produces pulpal anesthesia of 5 to 10 minutes duration and 1 to 2 hours of soft tissue anesthesia, while a nerve block results in longer pulpal and soft tissue anesthesia (40 to 60 minutes and 2 to 4 hours respectively). Regardless of technique used, prilocaine with epinephrine produces anesthesia of much longer duration than plain prilocaine: 60 to 90 minutes pulpal and 3 to 8 hours soft tissue anesthesia. Because the epinephrine (1:200,000) is half of that used with lidocaine 2 percent, 1:100,000, prilocaine with epinephrine is recommended for epinephrine-sensitive

**Table 9-7  Common Local Anesthetic Agents and Vasoconstrictors**

| Generic Name | Lidocaine | Lidocaine | Lidocaine | Prilocaine | Prilocaine | Mepivacaine | Mepivacaine | Bupivacaine | Etidocaine |
|---|---|---|---|---|---|---|---|---|---|
| Trade Name | Xylocaine Lidocaine Alphacaine | Xylocaine Lidocaine Alphacaine | Xylocaine Lidocaine Alphacaine | Citanest | Citanest Forte | Carbocaine Polocaine Isocaine | Carbocaine Polocaine Isocaine | Marcaine | Duranest |
| Classification | amide | amide | amide | amide | amide | amide | amide | amide | amide |
| Concentration of Anesthetic Agent (%) | 2% | 2% | 2% | 4% | 4% | 3% | 2% | 0.5% | 1.5% |
| Amount of Anesthetic Agent (mg/ml) | 20 mg/ml | 20 mg/ml | 20 mg/ml | 40 mg/ml | 40 mg/ml | 30 mg/ml | 20 mg/ml | 5 mg/ml | 15 mg/ml |
| Amount of Anesthetic Agent per carpule (mg/cartridge) | 36 mg | 36 mg | 36 mg | 72 mg | 72 mg | 54 mg | 36 mg | 9 mg | 27 mg |
| Maximum Dose of Anesthetic Agent (mg/lb of body weight) | 2 mg/lb | 2 mg/lb | 2 mg/lb | 2.7 mg/lb | 2.7 mg/lb | 2 mg/lb | 2 mg/lb | 0.6 mg/lb | 3.6 mg/lb |
| Absolute Maximum Safe Dose Anesthetic (total dose) | 300 mg | 300 mg | 300 mg | 400 mg | 400 mg | 300 mg | 300 mg | 90 mg | 400 mg |
| Vasoconstrictor | — | epinephrine | epinephrine | — | epinephrine | — | levonordefrin Neo-cobefrin® | epinephrine | epinephrine |
| Concentration of Vasoconstrictor | — | 1:50,000 | 1:100,000 | — | 1:200,000 | — | 1:20,000 | 1:200,000 | 1:200,000 |
| Concentration of Vasoconstrictor (mg/ml) | — | .02 mg/ml | .01 mg/ml | — | .005 mg/ml | — | .05 mg/ml | .005 mg/ml | .005 mg/ml |
| Amount of Vasoconstrictor per Cartridge (mg) | — | .036 mg | .018 mg | — | .009 mg | — | .09 mg | .009 mg | .009 mg |
| Maximum Safe Dose of Vasoconstrictor (mg) | — | 0.2 mg | 0.2 mg | — | 0.2 mg | — | 1.0 mg | 0.2 mg | 0.2 mg |
| Agent Limiting Max. Volume Number of Cartridges Needed to Reach MSD of Limiting Agent | Lidocaine 8.3 | epinephrine 5.5 | Lidocaine 8.3 | Prilocaine 5.5 | Prilocaine 5.5 | Mepivacaine 5.5 | Mepivacaine 8.3 | Bupivacaine 10 | Etidocaine 15 |
| Duration | short | intermediate | intermediate | short | intermediate | short | intermediate | long | long |
| • Pulpal tissues | 5 to 10 min. | 60 to 90 min. | 60 to 90 min. | infiltration: 5 to 10 min. block: 40 to 60 min. | 60 to 90 min. | 20 to 40 min. | 50 to 90 min. | 1.5 to 5 hours | 1.5 to 3 hours |
| • Soft tissues | 1 to 2 hours | 3 to 5 hours | 3 to 5 hours | infiltration: 1.5 to 2 hours block: 2 to 4 hours | 3 to 8 hours | 2 to 3 hours | 3 to 5 hours | 4 to 9 hours | 4 to 9 hours |

(Information compiled primarily from Malamed's "Handbook of Local Anesthesia" (1997), Moore (1990), and manufacturer's package inserts (1990, 1993))

**Table 9-8 Factors to Consider When Selecting a Local Anesthetic Agent**

| Factor | Comment |
| --- | --- |
| Physical Status of Patient | The medical history must be thoroughly updated and reviewed each appointment; select an anesthetic and vasoconstrictor based on health history findings. |
| Length of Treatment | Short-, intermediate-, and long-acting anesthetics are available; duration times vary for both pulpal and soft tissue anesthesia. Consider length of treatment time required for pulpal and soft tissue and select an anesthetic accordingly. |
| Need for Hemostasis | If bleeding is a concern, always select an agent with a vasoconstrictor. Epinephrine is the vasoconstrictor of choice for hemostasis. |
| Potential for Discomfort after Treatment | If postoperative discomfort is expected, select a long-acting anesthetic to minimize necessity for postoperative analgesics. |
| Possibility of Self-mutilation Postoperatively | Child patients or others who may bite themselves inadvertently when lip is anesthetized should receive an anesthetic with as short-acting soft tissue anesthesia as possible (particularly a concern with the inferior alveolar injection). |
| Personal Preference of Operator | Some clinicians believe they have higher success rates with a particular anesthetic. Always buy anesthetic from a reliable manufacturer. |

clients such as those with cardiovascular disease or hyperthyroidism.

Mepivacaine, like prilocaine, exhibits mild vasodilating properties and is equivalent to lidocaine in potency (Ciancio, 1991). Mepivacaine 3 percent (no vasoconstrictor) can produce pulpal anesthesia that lasts 20 to 40 minutes and soft tissue anesthesia of 2 to 3 hours. It is recommended for clients for whom a vasoconstrictor or a long-acting anesthetic is contraindicated. Levonordefrine (Neo-Cobefrin®), the vasoconstrictor that is added to mepivacaine 2%, produces less cardiac and central nervous system stimulation than epinephrine (Malamed, 1990). For this reason, mepivacaine 2% in a 1:20,000 concentration is an excellent anesthetic for clients with compromised cardiovascular status or other epinephrine sensitivity. It produces pulpal anesthesia of 50 to 90 minutes and soft tissue anesthesia of 3 to 5 hours.

Two long-acting amide local anesthetic agents are also available in dental cartridges. Bupivacaine (Marcaine® by Cook-Waite) and etidocaine (Duranest® by Astra Pharmaceutical Products) were introduced in the United States in July 1983 and November 1985 respectively (Malamed, 1990). These long-acting anesthetics provide effective anesthesia throughout treatment and prevent discomfort postoperatively (Crout, Koraido, & Moore, 1990). Their use is particularly beneficial following oral surgery, endodontics, and periodontics. These long acting anesthetics minimize the need for oral analgesics, because the anesthesia lasts much longer postoperatively. Reports about the duration vary from 1 to 6 hours for pulpal and from 4 to 9 hours for soft tissue anesthesia (Astra Pharmaceutical Products, 1990; Cook-Waite Anesthetics, 1993; Crout et al., 1990; Malamed, 1990; Moore, 1990; Skoglund & Jorkjend, 1991).

Epinephrine, in a 1:200,000 concentration, is included with each of these long-acting local anesthetics. There is evidence that the lower concentration of vasoconstrictor is not adequate when hemostasis is required and, in fact, increased bleeding has been noted during surgical procedures. Also, duration of anesthesia seems to vary according to type of injection administered. A comparative study of bupivacaine, etidocaine, and lidocaine found that the lidocaine 2% with vasoconstrictor provided longer pulpal anesthesia than the others following maxillary infiltration injections, whereas the long-acting amides have greater duration with mandibular nerve blocks (Moore, 1990).

When moderate to severe pain is anticipated, these long-acting local anesthetic agents can be beneficial by delaying the onset of pain following treatment. They are considered to be an effective pain management strategy; however, careful patient selection and education are required. Children, or patients who are likely to bite themselves while anesthetized, are not good candidates for a long-acting anesthetic because of the possibility of self-mutilation. They may inadvertently bite their cheek or lower lip and inflict damage. A short-acting anesthetic is a more suitable selection in these cases. Additionally, patients must be informed how long the anesthetic will last so they do not unnecessarily worry about prolonged numbness or paresthesia.

When selecting which anesthetic is appropriate for use for a particular patient (refer to Table 9-7), consideration must be given to the physical status of the patient; therefore, the medical history must be thoroughly evaluated and updated at each appointment. The choice of both the anesthetic agent and the vasoconstrictor must be based on the health history findings. A thorough knowledge of the properties of all of the local anesthetics is important to be able to relate medical/dental history and periodontal assessment findings with anesthetic selection. It is not enough to know, for example, that a client is sensitive to lidocaine 2%, 1:100,000. The clinician must be able to ascertain if the sensitivity is related to the anesthetic drug itself (the lidocaine), the vaso-constrictor (the epinephrine), the sodium bisulfite which is included to prolong the shelf life of the vasoconstrictor, an associated medical condition, a drug interaction, or a "psychosomatic" consideration. Chapter 2 discusses medical history considerations for selecting an appropriate agent.

As previously discussed, local anesthetics are available in a variety of preparations: short, intermediate, or long-acting. Duration times for each of the agents vary for both pulpal and soft tissue anesthesia; therefore, consideration must be given to the length of treatment time required for both pulpal and soft tissue anesthesia when selecting the appropriate anesthetic. If soft tissue anesthesia is needed but pulpal anesthesia is not a concern, a shorter-acting anesthetic, such as lidocaine plain or prilocaine plain, might be adequate. Examples of therapy that might require soft tissue anesthesia include root planing in shallow pockets where only the tissue is sensitive and not the root, or localized soft tissue curettage. If short acting pulpal anesthesia is required (less than 20 minutes) and hemostasis is not a consideration, Carbocaine 3%, without vasoconstrictor is a good alternative. To obtain profound anesthesia for longer appointments, a vaso-constrictor is necessary or a long-acting anesthetic can also be employed. Half-mouth scaling/root planing with desensitization is an example of therapy that might require profound anesthesia for a long appointment.

Another factor to consider when choosing an anesthetic is the need for hemostasis. Local anesthetics have, to varying degrees, vasodilating properties. Therefore, because hemostasis is usually a concern during deposit removal, select an agent with a vasoconstrictor. Epinephrine is the vasoconstrictor of choice to control bleeding. If the medical history indicates a physical complication with epinephrine, choose levonordefrin (Neo-Cobefrin®) and/or limit the amount of drug administered.

Besides increasing the duration of local anesthesia and providing hemostasis, **vasoconstrictors** also help prevent toxicity related to high levels of the local anesthetic agent. By slowing absorption of the drug into the bloodstream, anesthetic blood levels are lower and the potential for overdose is decreased. For all of these reasons, vasoconstrictors should be employed whenever possible (Malamed, 1990).

Of course, the personal preference of each operator is also a consideration when choosing which anesthetic to administer. Some clinicians believe they have a higher success rate with a particular anesthetic. It is important that the clinician not become complacent in the selection of anesthetic and choose one simply because it is readily available or convenient. Consideration must be given to the other factors discussed. Additionally, quality anesthetic should be purchased from a reliable manufacturer. Note the expiration date and dispose of anesthetic that is outdated, or contaminated or cloudy.

For obvious professional, ethical, safety and legal reasons, clinicians must determine the **maximum safe dosage (MSD)** for each client that receives local anesthesia and use the smallest amount of anesthetic necessary to provide profound anesthesia. Dosage of the anesthetic agents are established according to milligrams of drug per pound of body weight. The absolute maximum safe doses (MSD) listed in Table 9-7 are based on 150-pound healthy adult clients who respond to anesthetic in "an average" manner or within the middle of the normal distribution curve. Drug dosages should always be decreased for children, elderly or debilitated patients, or medically compromised patients (Malamed, 1990).

The MSD is commonly dictated by the anesthetic agent itself. To determine the MSD of anesthetic drug for a particular patient, simply multiply the patient's weight by the maximum dose of anesthetic agent (refer to Table 9-7) allowed for that drug. For example, the maximum safe dose of anesthetic agent for lidocaine 2% is 2 milligrams per pound (mg/lb) of body weight; the amount for mepivacaine 2% or 3% is also 2 mg/lb; however, 2.7 mg/lb is allowed for prilocaine 4%. For a 120-pound healthy patient, the MSD for both lidocaine and mepivacine is 240 mg (2 mg × 120 lb); for prilocaine 4% the MSD is 324 mg (2.7 mg × 120 lb). To determine how many cartridges that 120 pound patient can safely receive, the amount of anesthetic agent in one cartridge must be calculated and that number is then divided into the MSD for the patient. To calculate the number of milligrams of the anesthetic in one cartridge:

1. Determine the concentration of the anesthetic drug. The concentration of the anesthetic (2%, 3%, 4%, etc.) determines the number of milligrams per milliliter (mg/ml). A 2% solution of anesthetic contains 20 mg/ml; a 3% solution converts to 30 mg/ml; a 4% solution converts to 40 mg/ml, etc.
2. Multiply the concentration (mg/ml) by the total ml in one standard dental cartridge (1.8 ml) as follows:
   a. 2% = 20 mg × 1.8 ml = 36 mg/cartridge
   b. 3% = 30 mg × 1.8 ml = 54 mg/cartridge
   c. 4% = 40 mg × 1.8 ml = 72 mg/cartridge

To continue with the above example of a 120-pound patient, the maximum number of cartridges that could be administered before reaching a toxic dose would be as follows:

1. Lidocaine 2%: 6.6 cartridges (the MSD of 240 mg is divided by 36 mg—the number of mg in one cartridge of a 2% solution)
2. Mepivacaine 2%: 6.6 cartridges (the MSD of 240 mg is divided by 36 mg—the number of mg in one cartridge of a 2% solution)
3. Mepivacaine 3%: 4.4 cartridges (the MSD of 240 mg is divided by 54 mg—the number of mg in one cartridge of a 3% solution)
4. Prilocaine 4%: 4.5 cartridges (the MSD of 324 mg

is divided by 72 mg—the number of mg in one cartridge of a 4% solution)

For purposes of legal documentation, the amount of vasoconstrictor administered must also be calculated. How many mg of *vasoconstrictor* are in one cartridge of anesthetic solution? The answer depends upon the concentration (1:50,000, 1:100,000, 1:200,000, etc.) of the vasoconstrictor being considered. A concentration of 1:50,000 means that there are 1,000 mg (1 gram) of vasoconstrictor in 50,000 ml of solution. To calculate how many milligrams in one milliliter (mg/ml): divide 1,000 by 50,000 (or 1/50) = .02 mg/ml. Now, to determine the amount in one cartridge, multiply the number of mg/ml (in this case .02) by 1.8 ml (the size of a standard dental cartridge) to arrive at the answer of .036 mg of vasoconstrictor in one cartridge of 1:50,000 solution. The amount of vasoconstrictor per carpule for other concentrations is listed in Table 9-7; those values are calculated as follows:

1. 1:20,000 = 20/1 × 1.8 = .09 mg/cartridge
2. 1:100,000 = 100/1 × 1.8 = .018 mg/cartridge
3. 1:200,000 = 200/1 × 1.8 = .009 mg/cartridge

Continuing with the above example of the MSDs for a 120-pound client, how many mg of vasoconstrictor have been administered for each of the anesthetics listed:

1. Lidocaine 2%: 6.6 cartridges
   a. plain: does not contain a vasoconstrictor
   b. 1:50,000 (used very infrequently): .036 × 6.6 = .24 mg epinephrine (this amount would exceed the MSD of epinephrine which is .2 mg!)
   c. 1:100,000: .018 × 6.6 = .12 mg epinephrine
2. Mepivacaine 2%: 6.6 cartridges
   1:20,000: .09 × 6.6 = .6 mg levonordefrin
3. Mepivacaine 3%: does not contain a vasoconstrictor
4. Prilocaine 4%: 4.5 cartridges
   a. plain: does not contain a vasoconstrictor
   b. 1:200,000: .009 × 4.5 = .04 mg epinephrine

## Selection of Injections

The NSPT appointment plan will vary according to the classification of periodontal disease (case difficulty), amount and type of deposit, operator efficiency, method of instrumentation, and scheduling needs. When selecting the injection to be administered for a particular appointment, consideration should be given to several factors.

Probably the most obvious factor a clinician needs to consider when selecting the most appropriate injection to administer is the exact area to be anesthetized. The cancellous bone of the maxilla is conducive to infiltrations, while the thicker cortical plate of the mandible requires that a nerve block be administered for maximum effectiveness. A nerve block might not be necessary to anesthetize a single tooth; however, nerve and field

blocks anesthetize broader areas than infiltrations and thus reduce the number of injections/needle penetrations in large areas. Determine the necessity for pulpal versus soft tissue anesthesia. Soft tissue in a localized area can be very easily anesthetized. Pulpal tissue requires more profound anesthesia. A thorough knowledge of the trigeminal nerve and its branches are mandatory to obtain profound anesthesia.

The presence of infection will also have a direct influence on the choice of injection to administer. Local anesthetic agents are less effective in the immediate area of infection, for example an abscess, due to the decreased tissue pH. It is preferable to administer the local anesthetic away from the area of infection rather than directly in that area. Conversely, if hemostasis is required, infiltrate directly in the area requiring hemostasis with an anesthetic containing vasoconstrictor rather than giving a nerve block away from the site of concern.

The age of the client might also be a consideration. Juvenile bone is thinner and more porous than adult bone so juvenile bone is more permeable to anesthetic. It is likely that an infiltration will be effective on the mandible of a child, but would not be effective on an adult.

To some extent, the personal preference of the clinician is also a factor in choosing which injection(s) to administer. Some operators believe they have higher success rates with certain injections. For example, a clinician might chose a Gow-Gates rather than an inferior alveolar nerve block, or an infiltration above individual teeth on the maxilla (requiring multiple needle penetrations) rather than a nerve block (requiring fewer needle penetrations). Once again, legal implications are a factor, because some states allow dental hygienists to administer only infiltration anesthesia, which eliminates the option of a nerve block for NSPT.

Following a thorough patient assessment and classification of periodontal disease, an appointment plan can be developed for each case. Injections can be selected based upon the desired approach to scaling/root planing or periodontal debridement: half-mouth, quadrant, and/or sextant. For maximum patient comfort, anesthesia should be limited to no more than one-half of the mouth per appointment. With a half-mouth approach, the clinician should anesthetize the maxillary and mandibular quadrant on the same side of the mouth. Anesthesia of the entire mandible in one appointment is discouraged and full mouth anesthesia is never a good option.

Table 9-9 illustrates examples of injections that could be administered for different appointment planning options for scaling/root planing/periodontal debridement. The examples listed are provided as guidelines and do not represent the only injections that could be administered. These injections are not individualized according to the specific needs of a patient. Instead, the injections were selected to allow the fewest number of needle penetrations possible while anesthetizing *all* teeth and soft

**Table 9-9  Incorporating Local Anesthesia into NSPT: Appointment Planning Examples**

| # Appts. Planned* | Appt. # | Area to Be Treated | Area by Tooth # | Suggested Injections |
|---|---|---|---|---|
| **1.** Case Type I | 1 | entire mouth | #1 to 32 | Do not anesthetize the entire mouth in one appointment. Full-mouth anesthesia is necessary for this patient, but inappropriate. Reappoint for at least one more session (see example below). |
| **2.** Case Type I or II | 1 | max. right quadrant & mand. right quadrant | #1 to 8 #25 to 32 | PSA, MSA, ASA, GP, NP, IA, L, B |
| | 2 | max. left quadrant & mand. left quadrant | #9 to 16 #17 to 24 | PSA, MSA, ASA, GP, NP, IA, L, B |
| **3.** Case Type II or III (option A) | 1 | max. right sextant & mand. right sextant | #1 to 5 #28 to 32 | PSA, MSA, GP, IA, L, B |
| | 2 | max. left sextant & mand. left sextant | #12 to 16 #17 to 21 | PSA, MSA, GP, IA, L, B |
| | 3 | max. anterior sextant & mand. anterior sextant | #6 to 11 #22 to 27 | NP, right and left: ASA, right and left: Inc. and Li infils. |
| (option B) | 1 | mand. right quad; max. right molars | #25 to 32 #1 to 3 | IA, L, B, PSA, GP (possible MSA) |
| | 2 | mand. left quad; max. left molars | #17 to 24 #14 to 16 | IA, L, B, PSA, GP (possible MSA) |
| | 3 | max. right and left: premolars and anteriors | #4 to 13 | NP, right and left: ASA, MSA, GP |
| **4.** Case Type III or IV | 1 | max. right quad. | #1 to 8 | PSA, MSA, ASA, GP, NP |
| | 2 | max. left quad. | #9 to 16 | PSA, MSA, ASA, GP, NP |
| | 3 | mand. right quad. | #25 to 32 | IA, L, B |
| | 4 | mand. left quad. | #17 to 24 | IA, L, B |
| **5.** Case Type IV or V | 1 | max. right sextant | #1 to 5 | PSA, MSA, GP |
| | 2 | max. ant. sextant | #6 to 11 | NP, right and left: ASA |
| | 3 | max. left sextant | #12 to 16 | PSA, MSA, GP |
| | 4 | mand. right quad. | #25 to 32 | IA, L, B |
| | 5 | mand. left quad. | #17 to 24 | IA, L, B |
| **6.** Case Type V | 1 | max. right sextant | #1 to 5 | PSA, MSA, GP |
| | 2 | max. ant. sextant | #6 to 11 | NP, right and left: ASA |
| | 3 | max. left sextant | #12 to 16 | PSA, MSA, GP |
| | 4 | mand. right sextant | #28 to 32 | IA, L, B |
| | 5 | mand. ant. sextant | #22 to 27 | right and left: Inc. & Li Infils. OR right IA, L, and left Inc., & Li infils. |
| | 6 | mand. left sextant | #17 to 21 | IA, L, B |

*Key to abbreviations used above:*

| | | | | |
|---|---|---|---|---|
| PSA | Posterior Superior Alveolar | IA | Inferior Alveolar | |
| MSA | Middle Superior Alveolar | L | Lingual block | |
| ASA | Anterior Superior Alveolar | B | Buccal | |
| NP | Nasopalatine | Inc. | Incisive | |
| GP | Greater Palatine | Li Infil. | Lingual infiltration | |

*The number of appointments planned correlates with case difficulty. The examples listed assume that the patients require both pulpal and soft tissue anesthesia in all areas of the mouth. Consideration has not been given to prioritizing areas to be treated. In these examples, treatment always begins in the maxillary right area and the goal is to minimize the number of needle penetrations.

tissue treated in each appointment. The number of appointments listed in Table 9-9 correlates with the current insurance classifications of periodontal disease, [i.e., Gingivitis (AAP Case Type I), Early Periodontitis (AAP Case Type II), Moderate Periodontitis (AAP Case Type III), Advanced Periodontitis (AAP Case Type IV), and Refractory Periodontitis (AAP Case Type V)]. The examples have been limited to a maximum of six appointments because private practitioners would usually be limited to no more than six appointments per client.

Length of appointment could vary from 40 to 90 minutes depending on the size of the area and the nature of the deposit.

If the patient requires localized anesthesia, the most conservative injections should be selected. For example, a dental hygienist has determined that only one long appointment is required to complete scaling and root planing, and that he/she would like to anesthetize #3 because of furcation involvement, #29 because of sensitivity, and #30 because of furcation involvement, and a 6 mm pocket on the mesial. Due to the periodontal conditions, pulpal anesthesia is required in these areas. An infiltration over tooth #3 would be more appropriate to administer than a PSA and MSA, because only one needle penetration would be required and a minimum amount of anesthetic would be deposited. A greater palatine injection is not required because only pulpal anesthesia is necessary and the pulpal tissue receives no innervation from the greater palatine nerve. An inferior alveolar nerve block should be administered in the lower right quadrant and buccal or lingual nerve blocks are not necessary because soft tissue anesthesia is not required. Usually, the lingual nerve is incidentally anesthetized during the administration of the inferior alveolar injection because both injections are given during the same needle penetration. As a course of habit, many clinicians will anesthetize the lingual tissue as the needle travels through the tissue to reach the inferior alveolar nerve and only a small amount of anesthetic, less than one-fourth cartridge, is needed to anesthetize the lingual nerve.

## Technique

As mentioned in the introduction, information provided in this chapter is an *overview* of techniques and assumes that the reader has received formal education in the administration of local anesthesia. The goal of the information provided herein is to supplement that knowledge by relating local anesthesia specifically to NSPT. Because of these assumptions, an extensive discussion of technique is not included in this chapter.

The administration of local anesthesia is a procedure that is not to be taken lightly by any clinician who is licensed to administer these drugs. Clinicians have a moral and ethical responsibility to stay abreast of new agents, current research on drug interactions, and medical emergency protocol. The two most common causes of failure to achieve profound anesthesia are anatomic variation and faulty technique (Malamed, 1990). Periodic review of associated nerves, musculature, bony structures and technique, either through continuing education courses or reviewing relevant literature, is necessary. The clinician must maintain the degree of skill and knowledge required to assure a high success rate of obtaining profound anesthesia.

There are fundamental principles that are necessary to apply when administering any injection. Employing each of these principles increases the likelihood of a successful injection for both the clinician and patient. First, the clinician must locate and palpate landmarks. Due to individual anatomic variation is it critical to palpate the proper landmarks prior to inserting the needle. Adjustments in technique are made according to size and shape of skull, location of foramen, and height of vestibule. Next, the injection site must be dried with a sterile gauze square before applying the topical anesthetic. By drying the injection site, the effectiveness of topical anesthetic is increased, and the improved visibility makes it easier to orient the bevel of the needle. Topical anesthetics, like local anesthetics, have maximum safe dosages; therefore, apply only a small amount for the appropriate length of time. Some clinicians also advocate the use of a topical antiseptic either before or after placing the topical anesthetic to ensure a sterile environment prior to inserting the needle.

Always obtain good retraction and keep the tissue taut. A sterile gauze helps to keep the lip from slipping away during retraction and to hold the tissue tense or taut. By extending the tissue until it is taut, the needle slides through the tissue easily, contributing to an atraumatic injection. The clinician should always attempt to obtain a stable fulcrum. Keeping the elbow down and as close as possible to the body offers more stabilization than an arm that is elevated and in a "still frame" position for the entire minute it takes to deposit a cartridge. Next, orient the syringe. The large window of the syringe should always be turned toward the operator during an injection. This orientation allows the operator to easily observe the speed at which the solution is being deposited as well as a positive or negative aspiration.

Many clinicians believe the bevel of the needle should be facing the bone prior to needle penetration so that the anesthetic solution automatically flows toward the nerve. For better control of the syringe during aspiration and deposition, the pad of the thumb should be placed on the thumb ring and the ring should not slide below the knuckle. With the syringe securely placed in the hand, the palm and wrist should be facing upwards toward the ceiling. Again, this allows the operator better control and comfort throughout the injection. Keep the syringe out of view of the patient throughout the appointment period. It is much easier to keep the syringe out of view of the patient by placing the anesthetic tray setup behind the patient's head. For clinicians with across-the-chest delivery systems, it might be necessary to use a "mobile cart" to achieve this arrangement.

The clinician is now prepared to penetrate the tissue with the needle just until the bevel of the needle is embedded in tissue. Drop a few of drops of solution and wait approximately 5 seconds, to anesthetize the area of insertion. Next, advance the needle slowly. This step is critical for administering atraumatic injections. The clinician that advances the needle very quickly can be certain to cause discomfort for the patient. Depositing a drop or two of solution in advance of the needle to anesthetize the area on the way to the deposition site is an acceptable procedure for increasing patient comfort. The operator must be careful to use only a slight amount of anesthetic, however, because the bulk of the solution must be reserved for the nerve(s) to be anesthetized.

Aspirate at the deposition site by pulling back gently on the thumb ring. Aspiration is performed to determine the location of the needle tip prior to depositing the anesthetic. If the aspiration is "positive" blood will enter the cartridge. A "positive" aspiration indicates that the needle is in a vessel and, therefore, anesthetic should not be deposited. In deeper injections, such as the posterior superior alveolar or the inferior alveolar, multiple aspirations should be performed because slight hand movement will relocate the needle tip. Relocation of the tip increases the chance of depositing in a vessel and creating a toxic reaction. Following a negative aspiration, deposit the solution slowly. To increase comfort and decrease the chance of toxicity, the anesthetic ideally should be deposited at a rate of 1 ml per minute (Malamed, 1990). In the clinical setting, a more realistic time frame is no faster than one minute per cartridge. Finally, withdraw the needle slowly from the tissue and replace the protective cap. A variety of commercial needle guards are now available for health care professionals. Needles *must not* be recapped without using one of the many protective barrier devices. It is permissible to use a one-handed "scoop" technique to replace the needle sheath. The needle is immediately discarded in a clearly identified, puncture-resistant, and leakproof sharps container.

The clinician must remember to communicate with the patient throughout the entire procedure. Besides verbal communication (see next section), it is important to observe the patient's face and body for signs of discomfort during the procedure. Speak to the patient in a positive, reassuring manner remembering that the patient cannot answer questions. Do not leave the client unattended after administering local anesthesia. If an adverse reaction occurs, it will usually happen within 10 minutes after the injection is administered.

Table 9-10 presents a detailed summary of the technique for administering common injections. Each of these injections can be given painlessly if clinicians adhere to proper technique. Patients are pleasantly surprised when they receive injections that have been administered with careful attention to atraumatic technique!

## Case Presentation and Documentation

Presenting the need for local anesthesia can be a challenging part of the NSPT, particularly for those who are less experienced with the administration of pain controlling agents. Anxious patients often "overestimate the likely discomfort" of treatment when the procedure is invasive and requires a local anesthetic (Kent, 1990). It is helpful to inform the patient that care is being provided by an "expert." Many patients have never received an injection from a hygienist and need to be made aware of

acquired education and expertise. Patients appreciate an overall description of the treatment and an explanation of what is going to happen during each appointment, prior to beginning therapy. This is an excellent time to obtain the obligatory informed consent (DeBiase, 1991) from the patient. Also an explanation during treatment serves to reinforce the initial case presentation. Such information allows the patient to "ready" himself/herself throughout the treatment and gives the patient a sense of safety by knowing "what comes next."

In preparing for this discussion, it is important for the clinician to review the medical history and consider the chief complaint. If a "bad experience" is listed on the dental history, discuss the specific incident and determine the cause. If it was a bad experience with local anesthesia, openly discuss the actual problem associated with the injection. Was the problem a fear of the needle, a shaking of the lip (used by some clinicians as a distracter technique during the injection), the way the operator talked during the injection, the needle moving too fast, the anesthetic being deposited too fast, or even an unpleasant memory reminding the patient that it "might hurt?" *Listen* to what patients say about their poor experience without any preconceived ideas of what his/her response will be.

The clinician should attempt to determine the *specific* problem prior to formulating thoughts about how to address it. Explain what you can do to eliminate this problem. For example, if your patient states that the injection "always hurts" you can reply with a variation of the following:

*Example dialogue, anxious client:*

There are some techniques I can use to make the injection more comfortable for you. I will apply topical anesthetic with a cotton-tip to "numb" the area first and proceed with the injection very slowly. It may seem like it is taking a little longer than it should, but I assure you that it will make the injection much more comfortable.

If, on the other hand, the patient has a high pain threshold, is not anxious about receiving injections, or has developed coping mechanisms for dealing with local anesthesia, the discussion can simply focus on the need for pain control procedures and obtaining informed consent.

*Example dialogue, need for local anesthesia for NSPT:*

The NSPT we need to complete today is in the lower right quadrant which consists of eight teeth. I realize from your medical history and our discussion thus far that you usually do not experience sensitivity; however, I feel that local anesthesia is indicated for this procedure to assure your comfort. Knowing you will be comfortable throughout the procedure will make it easier for me to thoroughly debride the deep pockets and furcations we discussed.

**Table 9-10  Technique Summary Sheet**

| Injection | Branch of Trigeminal Nerve | Teeth | Gingiva | Volume of Solution (Anesthetic) |
|---|---|---|---|---|
| PSA Block | Posterior Superior Alveolar Max. Division (V2) | Max. molars except mesiobuccal root of 1st perm. molar. | Facial of max. molar region except area of MB of 1st molar. | 1.2 to 1.8 ml 2/3 to full cartridge |
| MSA Field Block | Middle Superior Alveolar branch of infraorbital nerve (V2) | Max. premolars and MB root of 1st perm. molar. | Facial of max. premolar region and MB of 1st molar. | .9 to 1.2 ml 1/2 to 2/3 cartridge |
| ASA Field Block | Anterior Superior Alveolar branch of infraorbital nerve (V2) | Max. centrals, laterals, and cuspids. Often central innervation overlap. | Facial of max. canine and incisors (to midline). | .9 to 1.2 ml 1/2 to 2/3 cartridge |
| Nasopalatine Block | Nasopalatine nerve, branch of pterygo-palatine nerve (V2) | None | Lingual max. canine to canine. | .2 to .45 ml 1/8 to 1/4 cartridge |
| Anterior/ Greater Palatine Block | Anterior (or greater) Palatine nerve, branch of pterygopalatine nerve (V2) | None | Lingual max. molar to canine to midline of palate. | .2 to .45 ml 1/8 to 1/4 cartridge blanch tissue |
| Inferior Alveolar Block | Inferior Alveolar nerve, branch of posterior root of Mandibular (V3) | Mand. molars, pre-molars, canines, and central and lateral incisors. | Facial mand. central incisor to 2nd premolar. | 1.4 to 1.8 ml 3/4 to full cartridge |
| Lingual Block | Lingual nerve, branch of posterior root of Mandibular (V3) | None | Lingual mand. central to 3rd molar, anterior 2/3 of tongue, floor of mouth. | .2 ml 1/8 cartridge |
| Long Buccal Block | Long buccal nerve, branch of anterior root of Mandibular (V3) | None | Facial mand. molars to mental foramen. | .2 ml 1/8 cartridge |
| Mental Nerve Block | Terminal branch of the inferior alveolar nerve | None | Buccal soft tissues from mental foramen to midline and the soft tissues of the lower lip and chin. | .6 ml 1/3 cartridge |
| Incisive Nerve Block | Terminal branch of the inferior alveolar nerve | Teeth anterior to the mental foramen. | Incisive nerve blocks teeth only; however, mental nerve will be anesthetized incidentally when this injection is administered. | .6 to .9 ml 1/3 to 1/2 cartridge |
| Lingual Infiltration | Terminal branch of the lingual nerve | None | Lingual from area of infiltration to midline. | .2 ml 1/8 cartridge |
| Gow-Gates Nerve Block | Mandibular Division (V3) block | Mand. molars, pre-molars, canines, central and lateral incisors. | All facial and lingual gingiva, buccal soft tissues of lower lip and chin, anterior 2/3 of tongue, floor of mouth, auriculotemporal area. | 1.8 ml 1 cartridge |
| Intraligamentary (PDL) | Terminal nerve endings in the area of the injection site | Pulpal tissue localized in the area of the injection (single tooth). | Soft tissues localized in the immediate area of the injection. | .2 ml per root |

**Table 9-10  (continued)**

| Adverse Effect | Landmarks | Injection/Penetration Site | Anesthetic Deposition Location |
|---|---|---|---|
| Penetration of venus plexus. Cutting branch of maxillary artery (hematoma). Scrape periosteum. Mandibular anesthesia if too far lateral. | MB fold in concavity distal to malar process/zygomatic struct. Max. tuberosity. 2nd max. molar. | Over facial roots of 2nd max. molar at height of MB fold. | Paraperiosteal through the mucous membrane and muscle behind the apex of 3rd molar. Posterior, superior, and medial to max. tuberosity. 2/3 to 3/4″; 16 mm deep. |
| Scrape periosteum. Pain. Ballooning of tissue. | MB fold. Malar process (zygomatic strut). Max. premolars. | Height of MB fold. Long axis of 2nd premolar. | Paraperiosteal through the mucous membrane over apex of 2nd premolar. 1/4 to 1/2″; 6 to 12 mm deep. |
| Scrape periosteum. Pain. Ballooning of tissue. | MB fold max. lateral and canine. Canine fossae between lateral and canine. | Height of MB fold mesial to root of canine in canine fossa. | Paraperiosteal through the mucous membrane mesial to the apex of max. canine. 1/4 to 1/2″; 6 to 12 mm deep. |
| Pain. Necrosis of soft tissue from vasoconstrictor is possible. | Max. centrals. Incisive papilla. | To either side of incisive papilla. | Paraperiosteal through the mucous membrane next to incisive papilla. 1/8 to 1/4″; 3 to 6 mm deep. |
| Pain. Necrosis of soft tissue from vasoconstrictor is possible. | Junction of vertical and horizontal surfaces of palate lingual to 2nd max. molar. | Junction of horizontal and vertical planes of hard palate. Midway between midline suture and crown of 2nd molar. | Paraperiosteal through mucous membrane at junction of vertical and horizontal planes of hard palate. 1/8 to 1/4″; 3 to 6 mm deep. |
| Too far medially: medial pterygoid muscle; trismus. Too deep: facial nerve paralysis if anesthetic is deposited in parotid gland. | Medial to internal and external oblique ridges. Height of coronoid notch. Lateral to pterygomandibular raphe. | Center of pterygomandibular triangle. Deepest part of the sulcus. Palpating finger should remain on internal oblique ridge. | Paraperiosteal through mucous membrane and buccinator muscle near post. wall of mand. sulcus. 1 to 1-1/8″; 20 to 25 mm deep. |
| Pain. Shocking pain if lingual nerve touched. | Same as above | Same as above; withdraw needle halfway, aspirate, deposit. | Through mucous membrane and buccinator muscle. 1/4 to 1/2″; 6 to 12 mm deep. |
| Too lateral: masseter muscle. Trismus. Pain. May get hematoma. | External oblique ridge and 2nd molar; retromolar fossa. | Lateral to the internal oblique at height of DB cusp of 2nd molar. Medial to external oblique. | Paraperiosteal through mucous membrane 1/8″; 2 to 4 mm deep. |
| Few complications. May get hematoma. Deposit ahead of needle to avoid discomfort when periosteum is touched. | Mental foramen: usually located between the two premolars. However, it may be either anterior or posterior to this site. | MB fold directly over or slightly anterior to the mental foramen. | Paraperiosteal through mucous membrane. 1/4″; 5 to 6 mm deep. |
| Few complications. May get hematoma. Deposit ahead of needle to avoid discomfort when periosteum is touched. | Same as above. Palpate foramen by placing finger in MB fold in 1st molar area. Move it anteriorly until you feel the bone become irregular. Radiographs are helpful. | Directly over the mental foramen. Sit behind patient to be able to direct the needle toward the foramen, which opens toward the posterior. | Advance the needle 1/4″; 5 to 6 mm. |
| Hematoma | Mucolingual fold next to area of insertion. Tissue will be anesthetized from that point to midline. | Lingual mucosa adjacent to the alveolar bone. | Advance needle 1/8″; 3 mm. |
| Hematoma, trismus, temporary paralysis of cranial nerve III, IV, VI. | Extraoral: intertragic notch, corner of mouth. Intraoral: mesiolingual cusp of max. 2nd molar. | Slightly distal to the max. 2nd molar at height of mesiolingual cusp, coming from opposite side of the mouth. Keep syringe parallel with the line visually drawn from corner of mouth to intertragic notch. | Advance needle approx. 1″; 25 mm until neck of the condyle is encountered. Onset of anesth. is delayed (3 to 5 min.) because of size of nerve and location of deposition. |
| Do not use with periodontally (severe) involved teeth or primary teeth; postop. discomfort, sloughing of tissue. | Periodontal tissues surrounding tooth to be anesthetized. | Mesial root (or mesial and distal of multirooted teeth); depth of gingival sulcus. | Base of the gingival sulcus, next to the tooth structure. Deposit when resistance is encountered. |

*Example dialogue, informed consent:*

The anesthesia will numb your teeth in that area, your tongue and your lower lip for approximately 2 to 3 hours (depending on the drug used). It is important to me that you understand any associated risks and that you have a voice in your treatment. Let me remind you that risks associated with local anesthesia are minimal and extremely rare. They could include a slight temporary stiffness in the jaw or prolonged numbness in the area, some bruising in the area (hematoma), an allergic or toxic response, or some tissue sloughing at the site. Also, you will need to be careful not to bite your lip or cheek while it is numb. If we do not use anesthesia, the chance of deposits remaining is greater. If deposits remain in an area, the inflammation we discussed might continue.

Do you have any questions about anything I have discussed or have not discussed? (*discussion with patient*) Is this treatment acceptable to you? (*patient responds affirmatively*) If at any time you feel any discomfort, please let me know by raising your left hand. I will also ask after treatment how you felt about today's appointment for future reference.

Allowing the patient to raise his/her hand in response to discomfort offers a feeling of maintaining some control in the situation.

When a patient has been treated for fifteen years in the same office by the same clinician and then asks why local anesthesia is needed and/or why is he/she being informed of associated risks, the clinician might respond:

*Example dialogue, change in office procedure:*

I am glad you feel comfortable asking me that. I can see this is quite a change from your appointments fifteen years ago. Our office staff has been keeping informed of the latest techniques through recent continuing education courses. An important aspect of treatment is having you become involved with your own treatment. I will be interested in hearing your response to this new technique after we are finished today.

As with all dental procedures, a thorough, accurate, distinctly written medicolegal chart entry must be documented subsequent to the administration of local anesthesia. Components of a complete chart entry relevant to local anesthesia and nitrous oxide analgesia are listed in Table 9-5. Further discussion of a complete medicolegal document is presented in Chapter 19.

## USE OF ALTERNATIVE METHODS

Alternative methods of pain control might be used in lieu of, or in conjunction with, nitrous oxide analgesia and/or local anesthesia. These modalities may be preferred for particular clients' conditions or preferences, or when administration of local and nitrous are not legal procedures for dental hygienists to perform.

**Psychosomatic methods** of pain control are non-pharmacologic methods used to alleviate the client's dental fear or anxiety. They include behavior management techniques as well as strategies for helping to build a better relationship between the client and the health care provider. These techniques are used routinely during every client visit with or without conjunctive pharmacologic pain control methods. They should be informally interwoven throughout the appointment or, in cases of more extreme dental fear, formal behavioral therapy sessions are required prior to rendering treatment. Pain can be psychologically induced by the client even in the absence of performing dental procedures that can commonly elicit pain (Milgrom, Weinstein, Kleinknecht, & Getz, 1985).

Informal approaches to psychosomatic pain control include simple methods for treating the client as an individual in a caring manner (Bay & Cannon, 1990). Verbal and nonverbal communication skills are essential to ameliorate treatment of the fearful patient. Nonverbal techniques might include caring gestures, a warm smile, calm mannerisms, or reassuring physical contact (for example, placing a hand on the client's shoulder). Verbal techniques might include a thorough explanation of all procedures to be performed, expressions of understanding and empathy, the use of humor, or the use of a soothing voice to help relax the patient.

Creative imagery can be used to help the patient mentally imagine themselves in a more favorable environment (Gawain, 1978). For example, the hygienist could suggest that patients imagine they are at the beach or soaking in a hot bath. Clinicians can use their familiarity with each individual's hobbies and interests to formulate an appropriate suggestion. Dental hygienists are encouraged to expand their knowledge in the areas of communication and management of apprehensive patients.

Technological advances have led to the availability of distraction techniques that can be used to refocus a patient's attention during the delivery of care. Many dental offices and clinics have headphones or television monitors that allow the patient to select from a variety of musical or entertainment programs. White noise, which is a wide range of variable sound frequencies, can be transmitted to patients through earphones to muffle sounds associated with dental procedures.

Other psychosomatic methods that require further training include counseling, hypnosis, biofeedback, or progressive relaxation. Specialists in behavioral management of dental fear or dental professionals with specific advanced training can provide these services for patients with extreme fear and anxiety.

**Topical anesthetics** are used to decrease discomfort associated with the initial penetration of the needle. They also can be used to reduce discomfort during scaling and root planing by applying the topical directly on the adjacent gingival tissue. Topical anesthetics do not penetrate intact skin. They are only effective on abraded skin or mucous membranes. Because the oral mucosa and gingival lining consist of mucous membrane, topical anesthetics can be effective in reducing pain sensation. The topical anesthetic must be applied to the mucous membrane for an adequate length of time. Manufacturer's instructions will specify the ideal time frame for application with varying recommendations. In general, a one-minute application is considered to be the minimum but some types require two or three minutes.

Topical anesthetics are available in gel, liquid, ointment, or spray forms. Like local anesthetics, they are classified into two chemical groups: esters and amides. Unlike local anesthetics, esters are used more frequently and the most common agents are benzocaine and tetracaine. Examples of products available in this group include: Hurricaine, Orident, Benzodent, and Cetacaine. As mentioned previously, allergic reactions are a concern with the use of esters and tissue sloughing is a potential side effect. For these reasons, some clinicians prefer topical anesthetics from the amide chemical group. Lidocaine is available in either a gel or ointment form.

Topical anesthetics do not contain vasoconstrictors and, as with injectable anesthetics, are vasodilators. Blood levels reach a high level quickly, thus increasing their potential for toxicity. For topical anesthetics to achieve maximum effectiveness, they typically are prepared in higher concentrations than their injectable counterpart in order to facilitate diffusion through the tissue. For example, Lidocaine in the injectable form is a 2 percent concentration, but a 5 percent or 10 percent concentration is required to be effective as a topical. MSDs must be adhered to, but because random amounts are applied, it is difficult to control dosage with ointments, liquids, or gels. Most topicals that spray have premetered control devices to assist with controlling the dosage. It is difficult to calculate an MSD; therefore, techniques to minimize dosage should be employed. The operator should limit the amount applied to the cotton tipped applicator, confine the topical to the necessary area (do not spread over a large area), and rinse the area so that the excess is not swallowed.

Technique for application of topical anesthetic will depend upon its form and purpose. If the intended purpose is to control pain in the area of needle insertion, a cotton-tipped applicator is placed (not rubbed) directly at the injection site for the specified time of application. Rubbing can cause tissue sloughing and sensitivity. When using a topical anesthetic for scaling and root planing or debridement, the topical must be placed directly onto the area to be treated. For example, a cotton-tipped applicator may be used to apply a gel or ointment to the gingival margin or papilla in an area of sensitivity or inflammation. Also, a curet or periodontal probe can be used to carry the topical subgingivally in a localized pocket or furcation area and when removing overhanging dental restorations. Application should be limited to no more than three or four teeth at a time. While this technique will help reduce sensitivity, the clinician and patient must realize that topical anesthesia does not provide profound anesthesia.

**Electronic dental anesthesia (EDA)** has been proven to be an effective method of achieving oral anesthesia for pain control in dentistry (Bishop, 1986; Clark et al., 1987; Hockman, 1988; Katch, 1986; Malamed & Joseph, 1987; Quarnstrom, 1988; Quarnstrom, 1989). Studies have shown that fear of the dental environment, specifically fear of the injection using a hypodermic needle ("shot"), is a major reason why almost 50 percent of populations in the western world do not seek dental care on a regular basis. Similar statistics are reported in countries where dentistry is virtually free, indicating that cost is not as large a factor in avoiding dental treatment as is the fear of the treatment itself (Silverstone, 1989).

A needle is not required to achieve anesthesia with EDA. Electrode pads are placed bilaterally in the vestibule next to the teeth being treated. The client is in control of the amount of anesthesia used by increasing the intensity of electrical stimulation from a hand-held control unit. Anytime pain is felt by clients, they can turn the dial placed in their hand to increase the current of electricity. Clients are pleased to be able to leave the office without the feeling of numbness that generally follows the administration of a local anesthetic agent. Another advantage to the use of this noninvasive means of pain control is the fact that no drugs, with their associated risks, need to be administered. Thus, use of EDA to produce pain-free dentistry, without needles, has been a significant contribution to the field of dentistry.

Although the safe use of transcutaneous electrical nerve stimulation (TENS) is not new to medicine, its use has been adapted to dentistry (EDA) since the mid-1960s. Within the past ten years, techniques and equipment have been advanced to the point of now being able to produce adequate anesthesia in the oral cavity for most dental procedures. In fact, research studies reveal a greater than 80 percent success rate in the elimination of pain while performing a variety of dental procedures normally requiring anesthetic (Clark et al., 1987; Hockman, 1988; Quarnstrom, 1988). The highest success rate of EDA has been documented during scaling and root planing with success rates varying from 83 percent (Hockman, 1988) to 100 percent (Clark et al., 1987). The use of EDA during NSPT might be particularly useful in those states where it is not legal for dental hygienists to administer nitrous oxide analgesia or local anesthesia.

An anesthetic state is achieved through electrical stimulation to the nervous system using an electronic anesthesia machine. Although the exact mechanism of action is unclear, several theories exist and are currently being investigated. The most commonly accepted theories involve central nervous system activity and specify a variety of ways in which naturally occurring, pain-inhibiting neurochemicals are released into the bloodstream (Bishop, 1986; Hockman, 1988).

This relatively new modality for controlling pain has wide applications in dentistry, particularly when considering the number of patients who neglect treatment because of their fear of receiving "shots." Contraindications to the use of electronic anesthesia include patients with cardiac arrhythmic disorders, cardiac pacemakers, a history of cerebrovascular attack or stroke, cochlear implants, pregnancy, and communication barriers such as mental handicaps or language problems.

The use of EDA as a pain control modality should include a thorough training program for all personnel who will administer or assist with the administration of electronic anesthesia. The clinical component of the training program should include not only the administration of the EDA but also the experience of receiving electronic anesthesia. There are a variety of machines available on the market and the clinician must become familiar with the operation of the particular machine being used. It is important to remember the psychological factors influencing pain control and to communicate with the patient throughout the procedure.

## Summary

This chapter is not intended to replace any of the excellent textbooks (Bennett, 1984; Evers, Haegerstam & Hankansson, 1981; Jastak & Yagiela, 1981; Malamed, 1990) that are dedicated to the administration of nitrous oxide analgesia or local anesthesia, but rather to supplement those texts by reviewing selected information for clinicians to consider when rendering NSPT. It is essential that clinicians involved in the administration of these drugs complete specific education and clinical training prior to their use. The information provided herein serves only as a supplement to that formal education.

Use of pain control modalities for delivery of non-surgical periodontal therapy provides benefits to both the patient and the clinician. A thorough patient assessment can be used to determine the need for pharmacologic agents such as nitrous oxide or local anesthesia, electronic dental anesthesia, psychosomatic methods, or a combination thereof. Many treatment plans will call for a combination of pain control methods and nearly every patient will benefit from behavioral management techniques. Also, chances of increasing client cooperation and compliance are likely to be improved when nonsurgical periodontal therapy is delivered painlessly. Provision of treatment without patient discomfort and anxiety, or at least with significant reductions in these responses, is positive for all involved.

## Case Studies

**Case Study One:** Mike Peters, a 44-year-old physical therapist, is a new patient in your office. The health history interview reveals that he is nervous about injections and restorations because these procedures always caused pain in the past. Mike has moderate periodontitis with generalized gingival bleeding and sensitivity. Your treatment plan includes a half-mouth approach to nonsurgical periodontal therapy including use of local anesthesia and nitrous oxide oxygen analgesia. Mike is in good general health and there are no contraindications to these pharmacologic agents. You obtain his consent and administer $N_2O$-$O_2$. Mike appears to be responding well and adequate conscious sedation is achieved prior to beginning NSPT. After 30 minutes, however, signs of oversedation become apparent. What signs and symptoms indicate adequate sedation? How would you know that oversedation was approached?

**Case Study Two:** Richard Mince, a 49-year-old golf course groundskeeper, recently has consented to NSPT following an eight-year lapse in dental visits. He has moderate adult periodontitis, with generalized 6 to 7 mm probing depths and furcation involvement on all four first molars. The treatment is planned to be completed in four appointments (quadrant approach) applying ultrasonic instrumentation. Full-mouth anesthesia is indicated for Richard. Hemostasis is not a concern and Richard has no significant health history findings. What injections would be appropriate to administer to anesthetize all pulpal and soft tissue at each fifty-minute appointment? What is an appropriate anesthetic to administer?

**Case Study Three:** Suzanne Clements, a 33-year-old high school counselor, has chronic marginal gingivitis and a periodontal abscess on #15. A local anesthetic is required only for debridement of the abscess and for hemostasis in the area of #25 to #27. What injections are appropriate to administer, and what is the anesthetic of choice for Suzanne's treatment?

**Case Study Four:** Don Door, a 37-year-old corporate lawyer, is "difficult to anesthetize." After depositing two cartridges of lidocaine 2%, 1:100,000 in the mandibular left quadrant, he still complains of sensitivity. Two additional cartridges of mepivacaine 2%, 1:20,000 are administered. How many more milligrams of anesthetic can be administered before reaching Don's maximum safe dose? Don is a healthy 180-pound adult with no medical history complications.

**Case Study Five:** You have completed scaling/root planing/debridement in the maxillary right quadrant for an adult patient. During this appointment you administered nitrous oxide-oxygen analgesia (2 liters $N_2O$ and 5 liters $O_2$) for 45 minutes and you also administered two carpules of lidocaine 2% of 1:100,000 for PSA, MSA, and ASA injections. Complete a legal chart entry for these services.

# Case Study Discussions

**Discussion—Case Study One:** The effects of nitrous oxide would be presented positively to Mike emphasizing a feeling of relaxation and the ability of $N_2O$ to reduce anxiety. Signs of adequate conscious sedation include being relaxed and awake, having slowed reactions, having a throaty voice, and feeling reduced pain or no pain. Most importantly Mike will remain cooperative and be able to follow instructions with adequate conscious sedation. The earliest sign that sedation is approaching oversedation is the client's inability to maintain an open mouth (tends to close). You will know that Mike has approached oversedation when he is no longer cooperative, if he becomes angry, if his chest feels heavy, if he experiences uncontrolled falling or spinning and/or when he talks incoherently. At this point you should reduce the level of $N_2O$ or turn it off, increase the level of $O_2$, and reassure the client.

**Discussion—Case Study Two:** Because there are no areas requiring priority treatment, the following appointment plan is offered:

> Appointment 1: PSA, MSA, ASA, GP, NP (right side)
>
> Appointment 2: IA, Li, B (right side)
>
> Appointment 3: PSA, MSA, ASA, GP, NP (left side)
>
> Appointment 4: IA, Li, B (left side)

Either lidocaine 2%, 1:100,000 or mepivacaine 2% (with Neocobefrin) would be suitable for fifty-minute appointments to obtain profound pulpal and soft tissue anesthesia. An anesthetic without a vasoconstrictor would not be appropriate as it would not offer the duration required for 50 minutes of pulpal anesthesia.

**Discussion—Case Study Three:** PSA nerve block is indicated for the periodontal abscess on #15. An infiltration over #15 is not as effective as a nerve block in this instance. The nerve should be blocked away from the site of infection, if possible, to obtain more profound anesthesia. *Rationale: in an area of infection, the pH of the tissue is decreased so that the acidic anesthetic cannot dissociate as effectively as in an area of normal tissue pH. Less free base of the anesthetic is available to act on the nerve.*

Depositing a small amount of anesthetic into the papillary tissue surrounding #25, 26, and 27 is an acceptable means of providing hemostasis on the mandible. Papillary injections offer a conservative method for providing hemostasis, requiring that only a minimal amount of anesthetic, approximately one-eighth cartridge per papilla, be deposited. An anesthetic with a vasoconstrictor is employed when hemostasis is required. Epinephrine is the vasoconstrictor of choice for hemostasis. Therefore, lidocaine 2%, 1:100,000 would be an appropriate anesthetic to administer. Lidocaine 2%, 1:50,000 is rarely indicated.

**Discussion—Case Study Four:** Don's maximum safe dose (MSD) for either lidocaine 2% or Mepivacaine 2% is 300 mg (refer to Table 9-7). Two carpules of lidocaine 2% (20 mg/ml × 1.8 ml = 36 mg per 2% cartridge) were administered (72 mg) and two cartridges of mepivacaine 2% were administered (72 mg) for a total of 144 mg. Therefore, another 156 mg, which converts to 4 and 1/3 cartridges, of either anesthetic could be administered because they are both 2% solutions.

The amount of vasoconstrictor also should be computed and recorded in Don's chart as follows:

1. Epinephrine 1:100,000: 1/100 = .01 mg/ml × 1.8 ml = .018 mg per cartridge.
   .018 mg per cartridge | 2 cartridges = .036 mg of epinephrine.
2. Neocobefrin 1:20,000: 1/20 = .05 mg/ml × 1.8 ml = .09 mg per cartridge.
   .09 mg per cartridge × 2 cartridges = .18 mg of neocobefrin.

**Discussion—Case Study Five:** A complete chart entry would include the following information: HH review, pre- and postoperative vitals within normal limits, patient consent obtained for nitrous oxide and local anesthesia, 37.5 percent $N_2O$ and 62.5 percent $O_2$ administered for 45 minutes and Xylocaine 2% 1:100,000 2 carpules (72 mg anesthetic and .036 mg epinephrine) administered for PSA, MSA, and ASA in maxillary right quadrant. No complications. Scaling/root planing/debridement maxillary right quadrant. Vitals retaken after 5 minutes of oxygenation; patient reported normalcy prior to dismissal.

## REFERENCES

American Academy of Periodontology. (1989). *Proceedings of the world workshop in clinical periodontics;* Section II. Nonsurgical Periodontal Treatment (pp. II-17–II-23). Chicago: The American Academy of Periodontology.

American Dental Association Council on Dental Education. (1972). Guidelines for teaching the comprehensive control of pain and anxiety in dentistry. *Journal of Dental Education, 36,* 62–67.

American Dental Association Council on Dental Education. (1989). Appendix A: Guidelines for teaching the comprehensive control of pain and anxiety in dentistry. *Journal of Dental Education, 53,* 305–310.

American Dental Association Department of State Governmental Affairs. (1995). *Administration of local anesthesia/nitrous oxide by dental hygienists.* Chart #1. Chicago: American Dental Association.

Astra Pharmaceutical Products. (1990). *Prescribing Information. Dental.* Westborough, MA, Astra Pharmaceutical Products, Inc. 1–22.

Axelsson, P., Lindhe, J., & Nystrom, B. (1991). On the prevention of caries and periodontal disease. Results of a 15-year longitudinal study in adults. *Journal of Clinical Periodontology, 18,* 182–189.

Bay, N. & Cannon, T. M. (1990). Management of the fearful patient. *Journal of Dental Hygiene, 64*(5), 188–191.

Bennett, C. R. (1978). *Conscious sedation in dental practice* (2nd ed.). St. Louis: Mosby-Year Book, Inc.

Bennett, C. R. (1984). *Monheim's local anesthesia and pain control in dental practice* (7th ed.). St. Louis: Mosby-Year Book, Inc..

Bishop, T. S. (1986). High frequency neural modulation in dentistry. *Journal of the American Dental Association, 112*(2), 176–177.

Block, R. I., Ghoneim, M. M., Kumar, V., & Pathak, D. (1990). Psychedelic effects of a subanesthetic concentration of nitrous oxide. *Anesthesia Progress, 37*(6), 271–276.

Bowen, D. M. (1993). Aiding in the administration of nitrous oxide-oxygen analgesia. *Journal of Practical Hygiene, 2*(2), 9–14.

Chrissterson, L. A., Grossi, S. G., Dunford, R. G., Machtel, E. E., & Genco, R. J. (1991). Dental plaque and calculus: Risk-indicators for their formation. *Journal of Dental Research, 71*(7), 1425–1430.

Ciancio, S. (1991). Drugs in dentistry. *Dental Management, 5,* 16–18.

Clark, M. S., Silverstone, L. M., Lindemuth, J. E., Hicks, M. J., Averback, R. E., Kleier, D. J., & Stoller, N. H. (1987). An evaluation of the clinical analgesia/anesthesia efficacy on acute pain using the high frequency neural modulator in various dental settings. *Oral Surgery, Oral Medicine, and Oral Pathology, 63,* 501–505.

Cohen, E. N., Brown, B. W., Wu, M. L., Whitcher, C. E., Brodsky, J. B., Gift, H. C., Greenfield, W., Jones, J. W., & Driscoll, E. J. (1980). Occupational disease in dentistry and chronic exposure to trace anesthetic gases. *Journal of the American Dental Association, 101,* 21–31.

Cook-Waite Anesthetics from Kodak Dental Products. (1993). *Prescribing Information.* New York, Eastman Kodak Co. 1–9.

Cross-Poline, G. N., Passon, J. C., Tillis, T. S. I., & Stach, D. J. (1992). The effectiveness of a continuing education course in local anesthesia for dental hygienists. *Journal of Dental Hygiene, 66*(3), 130–136.

Crout, R. J., Koraido, G., & Moore, P. A. (1990). A clinical trial of long-acting local anesthetics for periodontal surgery. *Anesthesia Progress, 37*(7), 194–198.

DeBiase, C. B. (1991). *Dental health education, theory and practice.* Philadelphia: Lea & Febiger.

Evers, H., Haegerstam, G., & Hakansson, L. (Eds.), (1981). *Handbook of dental local anesthesia.* Copenhagen: Schultz Medical Information.

Fine, S. E., Easton, P., & Skelly, A. M. (1991). Amnesia for dental procedures and mood change following treatment with nitrous oxide or midazolam. *International Clinical Psychopharmacology, 6*(3), 169–178.

Gawain, S. (1978). *Creative visualization.* San Rafael, CA: New World Library.

Grbic, J. T., Lamster, T. B., Celenti, R. S., & Fine, J. B. (1991). Risk indicators of future clinical attachment loss in adult periodontitis. Patient variables. *Journal of Periodontology, 62,* 322–329.

Greenstein, G. (1992). Periodontal response to mechanical non-surgical therapy: A review. *Journal of Periodontology, 63,* 118–130.

Henry, R. J. (1992). Assessing environmental health concerns associated with nitrous oxide. *Journal of the American Dental Association, 123*(12), 41–47.

Henry, R. J. & Quock, R. M. (1989). Cardiovascular influences of nitrous oxide in spontaneously hypertensive rats. *Anesthesia Progress, 36*(3), 88–92.

Hockman, R. (1988). Neurotransmitter modulator (TENS) for control of dental operative pain. *Journal of the American Dental Association, 116,* 208–211.

Isidor, F. & Karring, T. (1986). Long-term effect of surgical and non-surgical periodontal treatment. A 5-year clinical study. *Journal of Periodontal Research, 21,* 462–472.

Isidor, F., Karring, T., & Attstrom R. (1984). The effect of root planing as compared to that of surgical treatment. *Journal of Clinical Periodontology, 11,* 669–681.

Jastak, J. T. (1989). Issues of pain and anxiety control training and continuing education. *Journal of Dental Education, 53,* 293–296.

Jastak, J. T. (1991). Nitrous oxide and its abuse. *Journal of the American Dental Association, 122*(2), 48–52.

Jastak, J. T. & Yagiela, J. A. (1981). *Regional anesthesia of the oral cavity.* St. Louis: Mosby-Year Book, Inc.

Katch, E. M. (1986). Application of transcutaneous electrical nerve stimulation in dentistry. *Anesthesia Progress, 33*(3), 156–160.

Kent, G. G. (1990). Thinking about anxiety. *British Dental Journal, 163*(9), 133–135.

Lindhe J., Westfelt, E., Nyman, S., Socransky, S. S., & Haffajee, A. D. (1984). Long-term effect of surgical/nonsurgical treatment of periodontal disease. *Journal of Clinical Periodontology, 11,* 448–458.

Lobene, R. R., Berman, K., Chaisson, L. B., Karelas, H. A., & Nolan, L. F. (1974). The Forsyth experiment in training of advanced skills hygienists. *Journal of Dental Education, 38*(7), 369–379.

Löe H., Ånerud, A., Boysen, H., & Smith, M. R. (1978). Natural history of periodontal disease in man. The rate of periodontal destruction after 40 years of age. *Journal of Periodontology, 49,* 607–620.

Malamed, S. F. (1995). *Sedation: A guide to patient management* (3rd ed.). St. Louis: Mosby-Year Book, Inc.

Malamed, S. F. (1997). *Handbook of local anesthesia* (4th ed.). St. Louis: Mosby-Year Book, Inc.

Malamed, S. F. & Joseph, C. E. (1987). Electronic anesthesia. Electricity in dentistry. *Journal of the California Dental Association, 15*(6), 12–14.

Mandel, I. D. (1993). Occupational risks in dentistry: comforts and concerns. *Journal of the American Dental Association, 124*(10), 41–49.

McCann, D. (1989). Dental phobia: Conquering fear with trust. *Journal of the American Dental Association, 119,* 593–598.

Milgrom, P., Weinstein, P., Kleinknecht, R., & Getz, T. (1985). *Treating fearful dental patients. A patient management handbook.* Reston, VA: Reston Publishing Company.

Moore, P. A. (1990). Long-acting local anesthetics: A review of clinical efficacy in dentistry. *Compendium of Continuing Education in Dentistry, 11*(1), 22–30.

National Institute of Occupational Safety and Health. (1977). *Criteria for a recommended standard, occupational exposure to waste anesthetic gases and vapors.* Cincinnati, OH: DHEW publication no. 77-140.

Quarnstrom, F. C. (1988). Electrical anesthesia. *Journal of the California Dental Association, 16,* 35–40.

Quarnstrom, F. C. (1989). Clinical experience with TENS and TENS combined with nitrous oxide-oxygen. *Anesthesia Progress, 16,* 66–69.

Roberts, G. J. (1990a). Inhalation sedation (relative analgesia) with oxygen/nitrous oxide gas mixtures: 1. Principles. *Dental Update, 17*(4), 139–142, 145–146.

Roberts, G. J. (1990b). Inhalation sedation (relative analgesia) with oxygen/nitrous oxide gas mixtures: 2. Practical techniques. *Dental Update, 17*(5), 190–196.

Rowland, A. S., Baird, D. D., Weihberg, C. R., Shore, D. L., Shy, C. M., & Wilcox, A. J. (1992). Reduced fertility among women employed as dental assistants exposed to high levels of nitrous oxide. *New England Journal of Medicine, 327*(4), 993–997.

Silverstone, L. M. (1989). Electronic dental anesthesia. *Dental Practice, 27,* 33–34.

Sisty-LePeau, N. L. & Henderson, W. G. (1974). A comparative study of patient evaluations of dental treatment performed by dental and expanded-function dental hygiene students. *Journal of the American Dental Association, 88*(5), 985–996.

Sisty-LePeau, N., Henderson, W. G., & Martin, J. F. (1986). The administration of local anesthesia by dental hygiene students. *Dental Hygiene, 60*(1), 28–32.

Sisty-LePeau, N., Nielsen-Thompson, N., & Lutjen, D. (1992). Use, need and desire for pain control procedures by Iowa hygienists. *Journal of Dental Hygiene, 66*(3), 137–146.

Skoglund, L. A. & Jorkjend, L. (1991). Postoperative pain experience after gingivectomies using different combinations of local anesthetic agents and periodontal dressings. *Journal of Clinical Periodontology, 18,* 204–209.

Stach, D. & Dafoe, B. (1993). Nitrous oxide and oxygen conscious sedation. In I. Woodall (Ed.), *Comprehensive dental hygiene care* (4th ed.), (pp. 699–715). St. Louis: Mosby-Year Book, Inc.

Subcommittee on Anxiety and Pain Control. (1994). *Guidelines for use of conscious sedation in periodontics.* Chicago: American Academy of Periodontology.

Young, E. R. & MacKenzie, T. A. (1992). The pharmacology of local anesthetic agents: A review of the literature. *Journal of the Canadian Dental Association, 58*(1), 34–42.

# CHAPTER 10

# Instrument Selection: Philosophy and Strategies

---

## Key Terms

area-specific curets
cervix
debridement
developmental depressions
developmental grooves
endotoxin

extended shank curets
functional shank
minibladed curets
terminal shank
universal curets
working end

---

## INTRODUCTION

This chapter and the next two chapters address periodontal instrumentation to promote healing of the gingiva, to decrease pocket depth, to create a gain in attachment level, and ultimately to arrest the progression of periodontal disease. Removal of bacterial plaque, calculus deposits and other plaque-retentive risk factors is a critical treatment modality during the implementation phase of nonsurgical periodontal therapy (NSPT). The intent of this chapter is to present an underlying philosophy, recommend an approach to nonsurgical periodontal instrumentation, and highlight recommendations for instrument selection. Instrument selection depends on intraoral conditions discovered in the assessment phase of care as well as clinician preference. The client's periodontal conditions, however, dictate instrument selection more than operator preference because instruments are designed to accommodate specific intraoral conditions. In other words, a single instrument design cannot achieve optimal results in a variety of intraoral situations. For example, deep periodontal pockets, furcation involvements, and root concavities all require careful analysis to determine which instruments are best suited for assessment and therapy. In addition to these anatomical considerations, deposit size, configuration, mode of attachment, and location influence instrument selection.

The underlying philosophy of this chapter is that instrument selection must be directed at removal of subgingival deposits including calculus, bacterial plaque, its endotoxin, and other by-products. However, instrument selection aimed at removal of *only* bacterial plaque and endotoxins will not necessarily result in adequate removal of plaque-retentive calculus because those noncalcified substances are more easily removed. Thus, primary consideration must be given to the removal of calculus and other plaque-retentive factors without disregarding the importance of removal of plaque and its by-products. To attain the treatment goals of NSPT the clinician must be equipped with a variety of instruments to accommodate individual client's preferences and intraoral conditions discovered through a comprehensive assessment. Both hand-activated and ultrasonic instruments are addressed.

First, literature related to efficacy of scaling and root planing and outcomes of nonsurgical and surgical periodontal care is reviewed. Next, the philosophy of periodontal instrumentation is discussed including comparisons of traditional scaling and root planing with periodontal debridement. Thirdly, anatomical considerations and deposit characteristics are reviewed. Lastly, instrument selection strategies are discussed which consider root anatomy, pocket topography, and deposit characteristics.

## EFFICACY OF SCALING AND ROOT PLANING

Drisko and Killoy (1991) reviewed six studies evaluating the effectiveness of scaling and root planing performed with hand-activated and/or ultrasonic instruments, with and without surgical access. The number of surfaces with calculus remaining after closed scaling and root planing by experienced operators ranged from 17 to 64 percent. Calculus remaining after surgical intervention and open instrumentation ranged from 7 to 24 percent. These authors concluded that although complete calculus removal is never 100 percent successful, it is possible on some surfaces. Despite incomplete calculus removal, numerous investigations have reported that nonsurgical instrumentation arrests periodontitis (Greenstein, 1992). Other conclusions from studies evaluating the efficacy of NSPT follow:

1. Effectiveness of removal of plaque and calculus decreases as pocket depth increases no matter if hand-activated and/or mechanized devices are used for nonsurgical therapy (Brayer, Mellonig, Dunlap, Marinak, & Carson, 1989; Caffesse, Sweeney, & Smith, 1986; Fleischer, Mellonig, Brayer, Gray, & Barnett, 1989; Sherman et al., 1990).

2. After subgingival instrumentation, the deepest sites (7 mm or greater) experienced the greatest reduction in pocket depth and gain in attachment levels when compared to shallow pockets (4 to 6 mm). Instrumentation in shallow sites (1 to 3 mm) causes small amounts of attachment loss (see Table 10-1) (Greenstein, 1992).

3. After nonsurgical therapy, probing depth decreases from 1 to 3 mm (see Table 10-1). Only a 1 mm pocket reduction, however, has been reported adjacent to furcation invasions (Nordland et al., 1987).

4. Efficacy is reduced in pockets adjacent to molar furcation defects when compared to nonmolar teeth (Fleischer et al., 1989; Kaldahl, Kalkwarf, Patil, & Molvar, 1990; Kalkwarf, Kaldahl, & Kashinath, 1988; Ramfjord et al., 1987).

5. Inflammation and bleeding both decrease following scaling and root planing (Kaldahl, Kalkwarf, Patil, & Molvar, 1990).

6. Shifts in the composition of subgingival microflora occur after scaling and root planing. Gram-negative flora decrease while gram positive rods and coccal forms increase, representing a shift to health. Spirochetes, motile rods and *Bacteriodes* species are reduced but not eliminated from periodontal pockets. Predictable elimination of *Actinobacillus actinomycetemcomitans*, associated with juvenile periodontitis, does not occur. Because of the latter, scaling and root planing therapy has been questioned for treatment of localized juvenile periodontitis (Greenstein, 1992).

7. There is minimal, if any, osseous repair after scaling and root planing (Dubrez, Graf, Vuagnat, & Cimasoni, 1990; Isidor & Karring, 1986).

Research evaluating the effects of scaling and root planing must be interpreted, however, considering the following factors. The studies were conducted in controlled environments, often with unlimited time; therefore, results are not directly applicable to the average general practice environment. It is also difficult to isolate factors which contribute to the outcomes of these studies such as hand-activated versus mechanized instrumentation, the type of instruments used to scale and root plane (single curet versus multiple instruments and methods), the methods used to evaluated efficacy (microscopic or clinical detection), the instruments used to evaluate the root surface (type of explorer or periodontal probe), the inherent error in repeated probing measurements, and treatment performed by skilled therapists versus less experienced professionals. Additionally, the role of client oral self-care, the length of the study, the interval for professional maintenance during the study, and the evaluation of multirooted or single-rooted teeth affect infer-

**Table 10-1  Probing Depth, Attachment Level, and Recession (mm) after Nonsurgical Therapy Associated with Initial Probing Depths***

| | *Initial Probing Depth* | | | | | | | | | |
| | 1 to 3 mm | | | 4 to 6 mm | | | ≥ 7 mm | | | |
| Reference | Pocket Reduction | Attachment Change | Recession[†] | Pocket Reduction | Attachment Change | Recession | Pocket Reduction | Attachment Change | Recession | Length of Study |
|---|---|---|---|---|---|---|---|---|---|---|
| Morrison et al. | .17 | −.04 | .17 to .21 | .96 | .23 | .73 | 2.22 | .91 | 1.31 | 1 month |
| Hammerle et al. | .03 | −.03 | 0 | 1.03 | .69 | .34 | 2.28 | 1.52 | .76 | 3 to 5 months |
| Becker et al. | .04 | −.27 | .24 | .86 | .49 | .37 | 1.54 | .61 | .93 | 1 year |
| Hill et al. | .04 | −.50 | .04 to .54 | 1.16 | −.10 | 1.16 to 1.26 | 2.76 | .47 | 2.29 | 2 years |
| Kaldahl et al. | .23 | −.03 | .26 | 1.26 | .82 | .44 | 2.31 | 1.59 | .72 | 2 years |
| Pihlstrom et al. | +.15[§] | −.24 | —[|] | .71 | .41 | .30 | 1.21 | 1.07 | .24 | 4 years |
| Ramfjord et al. | +.14 | −.89 | — | 1.08 | −.32 | 1.08 to 1.4 | 2.92 | .59 | 2.33 | 5 years |

(Courtesy of Greenstein, G. Periodontal response to mechanical nonsurgical therapy: A review. *Journal of Periodontology*, p. 120, 1992)

*Data listed as recorded at end of the study. These studies were selected because they provided frequency distributions regarding clinical efficacy of root planing in shallow, moderate, and deeply pocketed sites.

[†]If recession not reported, it was calculated from provided data; if loss of attachment was recorded, the range of recession was calculated.

[‡]Data from Kaldahl et al. precisely reflects changes for initial probing depths 1 to 4 mm, 5 to 6 mm, ≥ 7 mm.

[§]There was increased probing depth.

[|]It was not possible to calculate recession from provided data.

ences made from study results. Lastly, current theory suggests that only certain sites in an individual may actively break down while other sites may be quiescent. If only active sites or only arrested sites were evaluated, research results would yield different interpretations. For example, current research results might reflect sites where periodontitis was already in remission, not necessarily due to therapy. As clinicians realize, there is a multitude of factors influencing the results of periodontal instrumentation. This chapter and the next two chapters address a few of these issues by discussing thorough and careful client-targeted instrument selection and instrumentation technique, two factors that can be controlled by the nonsurgical periodontal therapist.

## NONSURGICAL AND SURGICAL INTERVENTIONS

Many longitudinal investigations conclude that closed instrumentation is as successful as surgical therapy in long-term maintenance of periodontal attachment levels even for those with moderate to severe periodontitis (Badersten, Nilvéus, & Edelberg, 1981 & 1984; Hill et al., 1981; Lindhe, Westfelt, Nyman, Socransky, & Haffajee, 1984; Pihlstrom, Ortiz-Campos, & McHugh, 1981; Pihlstrom, McHugh, Oliphant, & Ortiz-Campos, 1983; Ramfjord et al., 1982). Generalizations about periodontal surgery include:

1. Loss of attachment in shallow sites (1 to 3 mm) occurs following surgery (Greenstein, 1992).
2. Some studies show that gain in attachment after surgery is greater than after root planing; however, other studies reveal that scaling, root planing, and curettage achieve greater attachment gains than surgery (Greenstein, 1992).
3. Reduction in probing depth is greater with surgery than scaling and root planing (Becker et al. 1988; Isidor & Karring, 1986; Pihlstrom, Oliphant, & McHugh, 1984; Ramfjord et al. 1987).
4. At three to five years postsurgery, the probing depth differences noted in #3 are not sustained (Isidor & Karring, 1986; Lindhe et al. 1984).

Greenstein (1992) and Ciancio (1989) agree that if scaling and root planing/debridement eliminates subgingival infection, then surgery is not necessary. If inflammation persists, however, surgery might be indicated (see Chapter 17). In either regime, effective instrumentation defines the outcome of periodontal therapy.

## PHILOSOPHY

Recently there has been a shift in philosophy regarding periodontal instrumentation in the dental hygiene profession from scaling and root planing toward debridement. Reasons for this movement are as follows:

1. Calculus is recognized as a plaque-retentive factor and not a mechanical irritant in the process of inflammation as previously thought. The focus, therefore, of periodontal instrumentation has shifted from removal of calculus and necrotic cementum to the removal of root surface contaminants and plaque-retentive factors.
2. Removal of cementum during the root planing process has been questioned due to the possible sequelae of root sensitivity. Also, it is thought that cementum removal is not necessary to remove endotoxin because it is only weakly adherent to cementum (Cheetham, Wilson, & Kieser; 1988; Hughes & Smales, 1986; Moore, Wilson, & Kieser, 1986; Smart, Wilson, Davies, & Kieser, 1990).
3. It is not realistic to believe that all subgingival calculus deposits are removed as a result of closed instrumentation, although striving to remove all *clinically detectable* deposits is still the goal of nonsurgical therapy. As previously discussed, even though complete calculus removal is not accomplished, adequate healing of the periodontal tissues occurs in the majority of cases.
4. The healing response to NSPT reflects the host's ability to cope with the level of root preparation that was performed. The outcome of periodontal therapy relies on the client's immune response coupled with the level of root surface preparation.

The approach to subgingival periodontal instrumentation described in Chapter 1 suggested a philosophy lying somewhere between traditional scaling and root planing and generalized debridement of every root surface. This approach is suggested for numerous reasons. First, the objective of subgingival instrumentation is to reduce the "critical mass" of subgingival flora and their by-products and plaque-retentive deposits to a level that fosters periodontal health for each individual. The degree of subgingival instrumentation depends on the host immune system and presence or absence of risk factors associated with periodontal diseases; therefore, the degree of subgingival instrumentation necessary to promote oral health is likely to differ between clients. There is universal agreement among professionals that scaling or debridement to remove subgingival plaque-retentive factors is an essential element in NSPT. On the other hand, many researchers and clinicians have concluded that extensive root planing to achieve a glassy smooth root surface in all areas is not necessary or justifiable (Ciancio, 1989; Greenstein, 1992; Kieser, 1993; Nield-Gehrig & Houseman, 1996; Nyman, Sarhed, Ericsson, Gottlow, & Karring, 1986; Smart et al., 1990; Young, O'Hehir, & Woodall, 1993). While current thought reveals that generalized root planing for all clients with periodontitis is not indicated; a need still exists to remove calculus-embedded cementum in order to create the biologically acceptable root surface. This need is probably the greatest during initial or active NSPT. As a client's dental hygiene care progresses over time to the maintenance phase, the need for continual removal of calculus and calculus-embedded cementum should decline. Inevitably, some cementum might be removed in order to achieve the biologically acceptable root. Clearly, deliberate complete cemental removal should not be the goal of subgingival periodontal instrumentation.

Second, the term debridement has different meanings to various dental and dental hygiene professionals. Some think of it as "gross scaling" that precedes scaling and root planing; some use the term debridement synonomously with scaling and root planing; others think of it as defined by Young, O'Hehir, & Woodall (1993) or Nield-Gehrig & Houseman (1996) (see Chapter 1); and still others believe it infers that incomplete removal of detectable plaque-retentive calculus is acceptable because some individuals' immune systems tolerate this option. Debridement can also be thought of as the first step in a sequential instrumentation process in NSPT (Kieser, 1993). Initially, debridement occurs for removal or disruption of the structure of subgingival plaque, which is comparable to supragingival polishing. Next, scaling is performed to remove calcified accretions and, last, root planing removes diseased root cementum. Debridement is also sometimes thought of as being performed via ultrasonic instrumentation while scaling and root planing is accomplished with hand-activated curets. This philosophy was probably initiated when Smart and others (1990) reported that conservative root surface debridement with an ultrasonic instrument was all that was needed to remove endotoxin. Earlier, Cheetham and coworkers (1988) had come to the same conclusion; however, hand instruments were also employed using overlapping instrumentation. There seems to be a need to clarify the definition of debridement.

Third, some authors imply that debridement requires that every portion of root surface is treated with a debridement stroke performed by either hand-activated or mechanized instrumentation (sonic or ultrasonic) (Nield-Gehrig & Houseman, 1996), while others recommend debridement for the treatment of gingival and periodontal inflammation (Young, O'Hehir, & Woodall, 1993). The discussion of how to determine appropriate conditions and sequencing for debridement will continue as the "debridement theory" develops. Questions that remain unanswered include: 1) does debridement create attachment loss if performed in healthy sites, as does scaling and root planing? and 2) is debridement necessary where gingival inflammation is not clinically visible and/or where bleeding on probing does not occur?

Also, sufficient research has not been conducted or reported to test some of the premises of the movement toward debridement. For instance, *deplaquing* (Young, O'Hehir, & Woodall, 1993) as a concept and outcomes of this therapeutic modality have not been clinically tested and/or published to date. The ease of endotoxin removal in vivo is not possible to test because measurement techniques can only be performed in vitro. If the technology should become available, it will be interesting to either confirm present in vitro findings about ease of endotoxin removal or shed new light on its relationship to periodontal disease.

Last, subjective evaluation of this "in between" philosophy applied in clinical practice yields successful outcomes determined by clinical data and client satisfaction. **Debridement** performed to remove detectable plaque-retentive risk factors (including explorer detectable calculus and calculus-embedded cementum, overhanging restorations, etc.) and plaque along with its by-products, without removing undue cementum, is the focus hereafter. Debridement is necessary where clinical data reveals gingival inflammation and/or bleeding, and may create attachment loss in healthy shallow sulcii; therefore, sites that are clinically healthy need not be treated, unless pockets and/or attachment loss are present. It will be interesting to read the results of debridement therapy performed in ongoing clinical trials and relate the findings to clinical practice observations. Professionals with different philosophies about debridement and/or scaling and root planing hopefully will glean some benefits from the following discussion of instrument selection strategies.

## ANATOMICAL CONSIDERATIONS

A review of pertinent anatomical features might aid the clinician in selecting appropriate instruments for specific client conditions. Treating all indicated portions of root surfaces with debridement requires the clinician to mentally visualize root surface anatomy. Five topic areas are discussed: root anatomy, root surface irregularities, furcation involvement, pocket topography, and gingival contour and tone. These factors, although not mutually exclusive, are considered when selecting probes, explorers, files, curets, and ultrasonic inserts. Each factor is related to effective deposit removal, healing, and prognosis.

### Root Anatomy

The anatomical features related to instrument selection include root shape, root width, root length, the cementoenamel junction, contact areas, and root form deviations. Root shapes vary depending on the number of roots (single rooted or multirooted) and on the location of the tooth in the mouth. When viewed in cross section the root can be convex or concave depending on the tooth and surface (see Figure 10-1). Some teeth appear to have a ribbon effect when they have concave areas on both the distal and mesial surfaces (Wong, 1994). On convex surfaces the clinician must roll and pivot the terminal portion of the working end of an instrument effectively to adapt around this curved anatomy. When approaching a concave surface area, continual rolling and pivoting of the tip must occur to ensure continuity of the stroke from the convex surface into the concave area. Concavities and **developmental depressions** are synony-

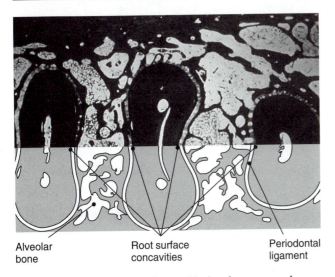

**Figure 10-1** Cross section of roots. Notice the topography adjacent to root surface concavities (ribbon effect). (Courtesy of National Audiovisual Center)

Alveolar bone     Root surface concavities     Periodontal ligament

mous terms defined as cratered, valleylike shapes in the root. Depressions are beneficial because they provide more attachment area increasing periodontal support. The concavity also allows for multidirectional fiber orientation, which makes the tooth more resistant to occlusal forces (Woelfel, 1990). On the other hand, concavities are detrimental because they provide a niche for bacterial plaque accumulation making professional deposit removal challenging and client interproximal cleaning difficult. Researchers frequently find residual deposits in concavities after definitive and controlled scaling and root planing with curets (Jones, Lozdan, & Boyde, 1972; Jones & O'Leary, 1978; Zander, 1953; Zander, 1955). Concavities are more pronounced in the following areas:

1. maxillary first premolars on the mesial surface,
2. the mesiobuccal root of the maxillary first molar,
3. both roots of the mandibular first molars,
4. the mandibular incisors and canines, when compared to the maxillary anterior teeth, and
5. distal proximal surfaces of maxillary first and second molars.

When depressions are 0.5 to 1 mm deep they hinder effective deposit removal. Also, concavities are present coronal to all furcations on all molars. Any tooth can have a concave proximal depression which varies in depth, however, the usual morphology is presented in Figure 10-2.

**Developmental grooves**, which are narrow and deep, usually appear within depressions. They are the result of the union of portions of the crown or root. A notable location for grooves other than proximally, is the maxillary incisors along the palatogingival groove. Palatal grooves are found in 5.6 percent of maxillary lateral incisors and 3.4 percent of maxillary central incisors, and approximately one-half of these have some degree of

associated root defect (Kogon, 1986). Fifty-eight percent of the grooves that extended onto the root traveled more than 5 mm from the cementoenamel junction (Kogon, 1986). The palatogingival groove is a contributing factor in the initiation or progression of periodontitis. Its presence attracts deposit accumulation and decreases the chance of effective instrumentation because of the difficult access, which in turn affects the prognosis of the tooth (Kogon, 1986). The treatment for palatoradicular grooves depends on the extent, depth, and direction of the groove. Virtually none of the grooves are positioned in the midpalatal region of the affected tooth; some are placed mesially or distally. Surgery is a consideration and when a crown is recommended, care must be taken to assess the relationship of the crown margin to the groove. When selecting instruments for concave areas of any depth or width, it is essential that the design matches the need and that adaptation of the instrument considers this anatomical feature.

The width of the root in the bucco/faciolingual dimension is related to the length of the working end of an instrument. Roots are widest at the **cervix** near the cementoenamel junction (CEJ) and gradually taper and become narrower as they ascend to the apex. Table 10-2 identifies the width of specific teeth as well as other dimensional characteristics. The widest teeth in a buccolingual dimension at the junction of the root and crown, or cervix, are the maxillary molars (10 mm). This width reflects the need for an instrument that extends at least 5 mm to reach the midline. The cervix is typically constricted or concave in relationship to the crown. The root surface just below the cervix broadens slightly before the root continues to taper in the apical direction. Deposits are frequently located at the midline of the root surface and, therefore, the clinician must ensure the explorer, ultrasonic insert, or curet can extend to, or cross, the midpoint of the proximal surface. Results of controlled studies evaluating scaling and root planing efficacy reveal that deposits frequently remain on proximal surfaces (Kepic, O'Leary, & Kafrawy, 1990; Sherman et al., 1990). Results also indicate that after instrumentation, deposits remain on proximal surfaces more often than on facial and lingual surfaces, and equally as often in furcations. As the root extends apically, and tapers and narrows, the need for a long working end is reduced; but, conversely, a shorter working end and longer shank are necessary to extend subgingivally.

Root length is significant when assessing the depth of the pocket and the adjacent root topography (see Table 10-2). The length of the root and location of the epithelial attachment bear a relationship to the location of developmental depressions and grooves. The root of a single tooth will feel different depending on the level of attachment. For example, on the mesial surface of the mandibular central incisor, the developmental depression deepens as it advances apically. If the probing depth is 6 mm, the depression at the apical extent of the pocket would be deeper than the depression near the CEJ.

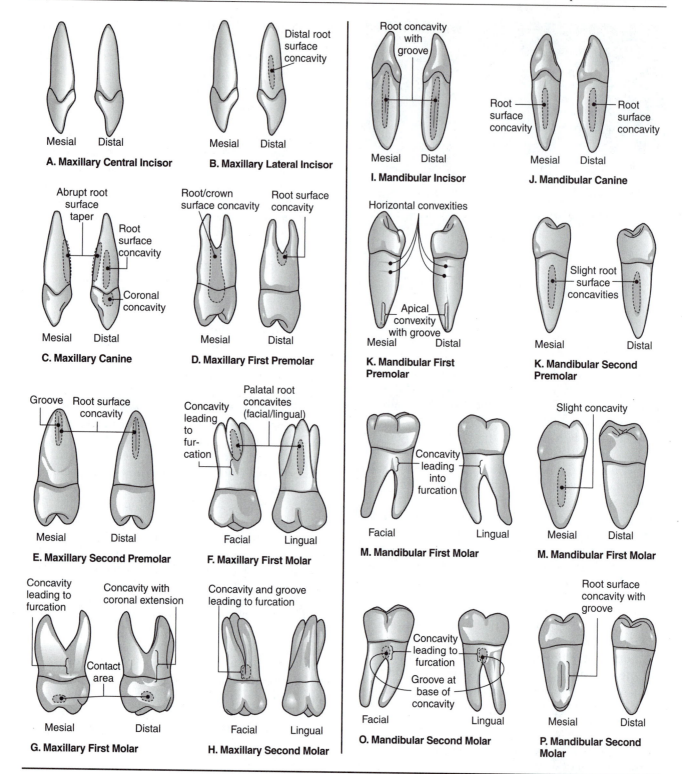

**A. Maxillary Central Incisor**

**B. Maxillary Lateral Incisor**
Distal root surface concavity

**C. Maxillary Canine**
Abrupt root surface taper
Root surface concavity
Coronal concavity

**D. Maxillary First Premolar**
Root/crown surface concavity
Root surface concavity

**E. Maxillary Second Premolar**
Groove
Root surface concavity

**F. Maxillary First Molar**
Palatal root concavites (facial/lingual)
Concavity leading to fur-cation

**G. Maxillary First Molar**
Concavity leading to furcation
Concavity with coronal extension
Contact area

**H. Maxillary Second Molar**
Concavity and groove leading to furcation

**I. Mandibular Incisor**
Root concavity with groove
Root surface concavity

**J. Mandibular Canine**
Root surface concavity
Root surface concavity

**K. Mandibular First Premolar**
Horizontal convexities
Apical convexity with groove

**K. Mandibular Second Premolar**
Slight root surface concavities

**M. Mandibular First Molar**
Concavity leading into furcation

**M. Mandibular First Molar**
Slight concavity

**O. Mandibular Second Molar**
Concavity leading to furcation
Groove at base of concavity

**P. Mandibular Second Molar**
Root surface concavity with groove

**Figure 10-2** Morphology of roots. **A.** Maxillary central incisor. Broad, flat, and convex root surfaces that taper gradually to the lingual. **B.** Maxillary lateral incisor. A convex root surface that tapers to the lingual. The distal may have a root surface concavity. This tooth is prone to abnormal formation and defects. **C.** Maxillary canine. The mesial root surface is flat to slightly convex and tapers to the lingual. The distal root surface is flat, tapers to the lingual, and has a root surface concavity that usually approximates the crown concavity below the distal height of contour. The lingual taper can result in an abrupt contour change in the lingual one-fourth of the root. **D.** Maxillary first premolar. The mesial root surface usually displays a significant concavity contiguous with the coronal concavity. The distal root surface is flat with minimal to no root surface concavity except coronal to the furcation. **E.** Maxillary second premolar. Flat to slightly convex surface with concavity, possible groove, and occasional furcation usually in the apical one-half of the root. The concavity is deeper on the distal root. **F.** Maxillary first molar: facial and lingual views. The root trunk is flat with a concavity leading into the furcation on the facial surface. The palatal root usually is convex but may display shallow facial and lingual

**Table 10-2  Measurements of Teeth. Specifications for Drawing and Carving Teeth of Average Size***

| | Length of Crown | Length of Root | Mesiodistal Diameter of Crown† | Mesiodistal Diameter at Cervix | Labio- or Bucco-lingual Diameter | Labio- or Bucco-lingual Diameter at Cervix | Curvature of Cervical Line—Mesial | Curvature of Cervical Line—Distal |
|---|---|---|---|---|---|---|---|---|
| **Maxillary Teeth** | | | | | | | | |
| Central Incisor | 10.5 | 13 | 8.5 | 7 | 7 | 6 | 3.5 | 2.5 |
| Lateral Incisor | 9 | 13 | 6.5 | 5 | 6 | 5 | 3 | 2 |
| Canine | 10 | 17 | 7.5 | 5.5 | 8 | 7 | 2.5 | 1.5 |
| First Premolar | 8.5 | 14 | 7 | 5 | 9 | 8 | 1 | 0 |
| Second Premolar | 8.5 | 14 | 7 | 5 | 9 | 8 | 1 | 0 |
| First Molar | 7.5 | b   1 12  13 | 10 | 8 | 11 | 10 | 1 | 0 |
| Second Molar | 7 | b   1 11  12 | 9 | 7 | 11 | 10 | 1 | 0 |
| Third Molar | 6.5 | 11 | 8.5 | 6.5 | 10 | 9.5 | 1 | 0 |
| **Mandibular Teeth** | | | | | | | | |
| Central Incisor | 9 | 12.5 | 5 | 3.5 | 6 | 5.3 | 3 | 2 |
| Lateral Incisor | 9.5 | 14 | 5.5 | 4 | 6.5 | 5.8 | 3 | 2 |
| Canine | 11 | 16 | 7 | 5.5 | 7.5 | 7 | 2.5 | 1 |
| First Premolar | 8.5 | 14 | 7 | 5 | 7.5 | 6.5 | 1 | 0 |
| Second Premolar | 8 | 14.5 | 7 | 5 | 8 | 7 | 1 | 0 |
| First Molar | 7.5 | 14 | 11 | 9 | 10.5 | 9 | 1 | 0 |
| Second Molar | 7 | 13 | 10.5 | 8 | 10 | 9 | 1 | 0 |
| Third Molar | 7 | 11 | 10 | 7.5 | 9.5 | 9 | 1 | 0 |

(Courtesy of Ash, M. M. *Wheeler's dental anatomy, physiology, and occlusion,* 7th Ed. Philadelphia: W.B. Saunders Co., 1993.)
*In millimeters. This table has been "proved" by carvings.

The ability of an instrument to extend to the epithelial attachment is a significant factor in selection. Additionally, the size and shape of the working blade selected for instrumentation at this depth should match the potential anatomical features. The length of the root also relates to prognosis. How much bone support has been lost or how much bone support is left is considered when deciding on nonsurgical therapy, surgical therapy, or need for extraction and reconstruction. A 5 mm clinical attachment loss on a maxillary canine with a root length of 17 mm is not as significant as a 5 mm clinical attachment loss on a mandibular central incisor measuring 12.5 mm long. Degree of root taper also influences support. A conical root may have lost more than 60 percent of the periodontal ligament, when only 50 percent of the bone height is lost. This is because 60 percent of the root area exists in the coronal one-half of the root. The apical one-half of the root involves only 40 percent of the root

concavities. **G.** Maxillary first molar: mesial and distal views. Mesial root surface has concavity leading into the furcation. Note the lingual location of the concavity and furcation relative to the contact area. The distal root surface displays a broad shallow surface depression that can extend coronal to the cementoenamel junction affecting crown contour. **H.** Maxillary second molar. The root trunk is flat with the concavity and a possible groove leading to the facial furcation. The palatal root is convex with occasional shallow depressions. **I.** Mandibular incisor. The root surface is flat with nearly universal concavities (distal is deeper) which may run the entire root length. The concavity might contain a groove at the base and occasionally a bifurcation exists in the apical one-sixth. **J.** Mandibular canine. The root surface is broad and flat with well-defined depressions. The mesial depression is more pronounced and deeper than the distal. **K.** Mandibular first premolar. The root surface is convex with slight lingual taper. The coronal one-half might demonstrate horizontal convexities. The apical one-third might demon-strate a concavity with a groove and bifurcation. **L.** Mandibular second premolar. Flat to slightly convex root surfaces with slight concavities on the distal and mesial in the middle one-half of root. **M.** Mandibular first molar: facial and lingual. The root trunk is slightly convex and has a concavity extending greater than one-half the length of the root trunk leading into the furcation area. A groove is sometimes present in the concavity. (See second molar.) The midfacial cementoenamel junction and concavity might have enamel pearls or enamel projections (not pictured). **N.** Mandibular first molar: mesial and distal. The mesial is flat to slightly concave. The distal is flat to slightly convex. **O.** Mandibular second molar: facial and lingual. The root trunk is convex with a concavity leading into the furcation area which may extend the length of the root trunk. (See lingual view.) A groove might be present in the concavity. **P.** Mandibular second molar: mesial and distal. The distal surface is convex. The mesial surface is convex with a midroot concavity and potential groove. (Courtesy of Steven W. Friedrichsen, DDS)

(Woelfel, 1990) (see Figure 10-3). Assessing the potential for furcation involvement also relates to the length of the root and the level of attachment. Quality periapical radiographs are useful in assessing root length (see Chapter 5).

In the posterior teeth the curvature of the CEJ is 1 mm on the mesial surfaces and nonexistent on the distal surfaces; however in the anterior the curvature is much greater ranging from 2.5 mm to 3.5 mm on the mesial surfaces and 1 mm to 2.5 mm on the distal surfaces (see Table 10-2). The most curvature in the anterior occurs on the mesial surfaces of the maxillary central incisors and the least on the distal surfaces of the canine teeth, especially the mandibular canine (1 mm). This information is significant during tactile exploration of the proximal surface and is used to decipher calculus deposits from anatomy. Another factor to consider about the CEJ is the relationship of the cementum and the enamel. The cementum overlaps the enamel in 60 to 65 percent of the teeth, the enamel meets the cementum 30 percent of the time, and the dentin is exposed 5 to 10 percent of the time (Carranza & Ubios, 1996; Wilkins, 1994). It follows that only 30 percent of the time the CEJ will feel smooth, flat, or even from the enamel to the cementum. In the majority of cases, the CEJ will be slightly raised due to the overlapping of tooth tissues and, at times, this overlapping can be quite prominent. If this is the case, the prominence is usually generalized and not localized to a few teeth indicating it is a characteristic of the individual's teeth.

Instrumentation below contact areas is challenging for practitioners and students alike due to the frequent bacterial plaque and calculus accumulation, the anatomy, and the width of curet blades (approximately 1 mm) and sickles. Visualizing the anatomy in this area benefits the instrumentation process because the clinician can relate tactile sensations to the expected location of contacts. If the contact area is usually in the incisal one-third of the crown and the clinician is feeling tactile vibrations near the middle one-third, then the sensation could be calculus. Of course, this reference is only relative if the tooth alignment and contact area locations are normal, and a general appraisal of both would be conducted during the assessment phase of care. A client with contacts broader than normal might readily form calculus in this area, especially if interproximal cleansing is not a daily practice. With age, contact areas become larger and flattened (Woelfel, 1990).

Generally, in the facio/buccolingual dimension contact areas of anterior teeth are centered, whereas in the posterior they are located slightly buccal to the center. Therefore, the lingual embrasure is larger than the buccal embrasure in posterior teeth. During instrumentation, access to the proximal surfaces from the lingual is usually better than from the buccal; therefore, instrumentation initiated from the lingual surfaces removes more deposit and covers more proximal surface than debridement performed from the buccal aspect. When looking at contact areas from the facial (mesiodistal) view, the contacts of anterior teeth are in the incisal third except the maxillary lateral and canine teeth contact at the junction of the incisal and middle one-thirds. Contacts in posterior teeth are near the middle one-third of the crown. The more posterior the tooth, the more cervical the contact area reducing the space in which to activate an instrumentation stroke.

For purposes of teeth carvings, the oval-shaped contact areas of anterior teeth measure 1.5 mm in length and 1 mm in width. Measurements in the posterior teeth are also 1.5 mm long, but are broader in width (2 to 2.5 mm). Below the contact area lies the triangular interproximal space that is filled with interdental papilla in health and early periodontitis. As periodontitis advances, recession and loss of attachment occur, creating open embrasures and exposing the roots supragingivally. The form of the teeth, position and wear of the contact areas, the type of teeth, and the level of eruption all relate to the shape of the interproximal spaces. These factors also determine the shape of the crestal alveolar bone (Ash, 1993).

Infrequently the clinician will be faced with deviations in the root(s) such as dilaceration or flexion, concrescence, fusion, dwarfed roots, accessory roots, or hypercementosis (Wong, 1994). These deviations typically appear near the apical one-third of the root. Dilaceration is the distortion of the root and crown from their normal vertical positions and flexion is a sharp bend or curve in the root affecting only the root portion and not the crown. Concrescence is the fusion of two teeth at the cementum only and is most commonly seen in the maxillary molars and mandibular incisors. Fusion is the formation of a single tooth from the union of two adjacent tooth buds united through the enamel, dentin, and rarely the pulp. Dwarfed roots are those that are smaller in size even though the crown is normal in size. They are most

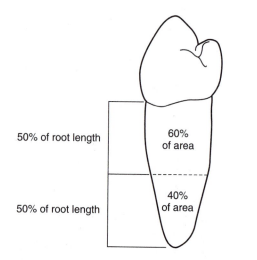

**Figure 10-3** Relationship of root taper, attachment loss, and bone loss. Sixty percent of the root area is present in the coronal one half, while 40 percent of the root area is present in the apical one half.

commonly found in the maxillary teeth or when orthodontic treatment has occurred with rapid tooth movement. Accessory roots are additional roots not normally present and are caused by trauma, pressure, or metabolic dysfunction.

Hypercementosis (cementum hyperplasia) is the excessive formation of cementum around the root of a tooth after eruption. It can be generalized or localized but is found most often on permanent molars at the apical one-third. Hypercementosis is caused from trauma, metabolic disturbances, or from chronic inflammation of the pulp. The cemental thickening is irregular and obliterates the periodontal ligament causing loss of the bony lamina dura. These abnormalities can be viewed radiographically and relate to instrument selection, adaptation, and activation when advanced bone loss occurs. Their presence should be charted for current and future use in NSPT and PMP. Root deviations negatively affect the prognosis of the tooth when periodontitis is present.

## Root Surface Irregularities

Altered cementum, which creates tactile roughness, is not normal anatomy, yet it occurs frequently. Root caries, abrasion, erosion, abfractions, and minute grooves are common occurrences. Root caries could feel concave, rough, or soft with an explorer and are detected by correlating the radiographic appearance, tactile evaluation, and sensitivity expressed by the client. They often do not cavitate like enamel carious lesions. Treatment recommendations are covered in Chapter 4.

Abrasion (mechanical wearing) and erosion (chemical wearing) often exist due to self-care techniques or oral habits. These areas are also concave, but can be distinguished from other concave areas because they are usually smooth, not rough like decay or cemental resorption, and occur adjacent to the CEJ on facial and lingual root surfaces. Due to the etiology, they are not located in the middle or apical one-third of roots. Smooth areas of abrasion or erosion generally do not attract bacterial plaque and plaque-retentive calculus. Abrasion and erosion can be distinguished from one another by the etiology as well as the characteristics of the concave area. Abrasion is usually deep and V-shaped or wedge-shaped whereas erosion is shallow and more trough-shaped.

Abfractions, hypothesized by many researchers, are physical fractures at the cervical region created by interocclusal force (Grippo & Simring, 1995). The horizontal loading forces caused by chewing or bruxing cause a microscopic bending of the anatomical crown with resulting tensile stress in the cervical region on the side of the tooth from which the force is directed. This bending of the tooth from side to side results in the fracturing of the enamel, cementum, or dentin cervical surface layer. Abfractions may represent an initial or continual etiology in the development of all cervical concavities. When a client manifests signs of bruxism or clenching, the role of occlusal stress must be considered. Further study is ongoing to determine if erosion, abrasion, and abfractions are each isolated entities or if cervical concavities are a result of a combination of these etiologies (mechanical, chemical, and/or interocclusal force). The relationship of restoring these surface irregularities to the progression of periodontal disease is discussed in Chapter 4.

Lastly, microscopic grooves or indentations in the root surface are caused by disease, by incorrect and incomplete instrumentation, or developmentally. As discussed in a subsequent section, calculus locks into these irregularities. Resorption lacunae and cemental tears are examples of disease-induced striations. Using the point of a sickle, the toe of a curet, or a file could create grooves in the cementum. Surfaces that have been instrumented and not "finished" or overinstrumented might exhibit indentations that feel rough. The clinician is not always able to distinguish developmental root roughness or disease-induced roughness from clinician-induced roughness. When cementum needs to be "smoothed" because of adjacent gingival inflammation and pocket depth, a curet with a fine flexible shank is preferred over a curet with an inflexible shank because the latter might enhance root irregularities. A precision-thin ultrasonic or sonic insert is also an option.

## Furcation Involvement

Access is gained to the furcation of various multirooted teeth by approaching the tooth based on its anatomical features. A review of furcation anatomy is important when assessing the periodontium, selecting instruments, and removing deposits (see Figure 10-2D, F, G, H, M, O; and Table 10-3). The presence of furcation involvement seriously compromises the future prognosis of the tooth and, therefore, detection at the earliest possible point in NSPT is imperative. Therapists generally encounter difficulty in evaluating the extent of the invasion because of the anatomical variations in the tooth, bone, and gingiva. The morphology of a furcation is usually described in relation to its entrance, called the furcation roof, and its distance from the CEJ, termed the root trunk. Factors affecting the assessment and treatment of furcations include location in relation to the cementoenamel junction, presence of enamel projections, width of the separation of the roots, vertical and horizontal dimensions, and the relationship of the gingiva.

The location of the furcation in relation to the CEJ affects the potential for disease. The further away the furcation entrance is from the CEJ the less likely it is to become diseased, however, once disease is present, the more difficult the area will be to reach. When a 4 mm periodontal probe reading is recorded on a multirooted tooth, and the gingiva approximates the normal contour, a furcation invasion should be suspected. In some cases, especially in mandibular molars where the bifurcation is located only 3 mm from the cervical line, invasion can occur in the early stages of periodontitis with attachment loss of only 2 to 4 mm (Rosling & McGuire,

**Table 10-3  Furcation Anatomy**

| Arch | Tooth | Number of Roots | Location of Furcation | | | Proximity of Roots |
|---|---|---|---|---|---|---|
| | | | Surface | Distance from CEJ | Furcation Entrance Diameter | |
| Maxillary | First premolar | 2 | Mesial Distal | 7 mm 7 mm | unknown | separated |
| | First molar | 3 | Buccal Mesial Distal | 4 mm 3 mm 5 mm | 0.5 mm .75 mm 0.5 to 0.75 mm | all well separated |
| | Second molar | 3 (sometimes fused) | Buccal Mesial Distal | 4+ mm 3+ mm 5+ mm | * | closer together than first molar |
| Mandibular** | First molar | 2 | Buccal Lingual | 3 mm 4 mm | .75 mm 1 mm | widely separated |
| | Second molar | 2 | Buccal Lingual | 3+ mm*** 5+ mm*** | * | close together |

*Diameter is less than reported for first molars due to the close relationship of the roots.

**Root trunk is shorter on mandibular teeth than maxillary teeth.

***Root trunk is longer on mandibular second molars than mandibular first molars.

1992). Refer to Table 10-3 to determine the usual location of furcations in relation to the cervical line.

The presence of enamel projections can confuse clinicians when exploring, probing, or removing deposit from the area. This convex and rounded area could initially be mistaken for calculus deposit. After repetitive instrumentation with no change in configuration, the clinician might conclude that this projection is present. It is likely that a periodontal pocket will exist adjacent to the enamel pearl due to bacterial plaque retention. Also the interface of the epithelial attachment to the enamel tooth surface (instead of the normal connective tissue to cementum attachment) increases the potential for a periodontal pocket. Ninety percent of mandibular molars with isolated involvement of the furcation demonstrate enamel projections (Masters & Hoskins, 1964). The prevalence of these projections is 28.6 percent in mandibular molars and 17 percent in maxillary molars (Masters & Hoskins, 1964). When surgical procedures are attempted to establish a new connective tissue attachment, enamel projections must be removed and exposure of underlying dentin created (Gher & Vernino, 1980).

The width of the separation of the roots in the furcation area is another anatomical factor (see Table 10-3). Widely separated roots permit easier access for instruments. Roots that are close together impede the accurate detection of the degree of periodontal destruction. The roots of the mandibular second molars are not well separated making interpretation of the classification of the furcation difficult. There only exists a 0.75 to 1 mm furcation entrance diameter on first molar teeth, consequently, access with a probe or curet is limited (Bower, 1979a). It is likely that the smaller the furcation diameter the poorer the prognosis due to difficulty in instrumen-

tation when all other factors are held constant (Bower, 1979a). The blade face width of universal and area-specific curets is from 0.75 to 1.1 mm. Area-specific curets (Gracey's) were found to be slightly narrower in blade width than universal designs. When curet blade width is compared to the entrance diameter measurement of furcations, it is easy to see why it is difficult to adequately treat the root with NSPT.

The dimensions of the furcation refer to the width and depth of the periodontal pocket in between the roots. Locating furcations and determining the severity of involvement are essential elements in the active and maintenance phases of NSPT. The extent of periodontal destruction around a tooth determines if nonsurgical or surgical periodontal therapy is indicated. Extent of involvement also impacts the type of interdental aid recommended for client self-care (see Chapter 6). It is well known that maxillary and mandibular molars are lost more often than single-rooted teeth due, in part, to the presence of furcations. Repeated measures of furcation extent must be accurate and standardized with initial measurements in order to make appropriate decisions regarding disease advancement and therapy.

Various clinicians and researchers employ different systems for assessing the extent of involvement of the defect; however, clinicians generally agree that the periodontal probe is best for detecting and classifying furcations. Most classification systems evaluating extent use "degree of horizontal probeability" (Zappa, Grosso, Simona, Graf, & Case, 1993) and 2 mm increments (Ramfjord & Ash, 1979) or 3 mm increments (Hamp, Nyman, & Lindhe, 1975) to describe depth of involvement. Both the Ramfjord Index and Hamp Index use degrees of 0, 1, 2, or 3 to classify the extent of destruction depending on how many millimeters the probe penetrates the defect in a horizontal fashion. These types of indexes are used by researchers and possibly by some practitioners.

Unfortunately, even when access permits, there is a margin of error inherent in probing furcations. Zappa and others (1993) found differences between surgical and clinical measurements to be as much as 9 mm, due to soft tissue interference. Moriarity, Hutchens, and Scheitler (1989) also found probe positioning in grade II and III furcation areas to be invalid when using a pressure-sensitive probe and a Michigan "O" probe with a 0.4 mm tip diameter. Upon histological evaluation it was found that the probe tip did not follow the concave furcation contour. Instead, the tip penetrated into the pocket wall an average depth of 2.1 mm (± 0.6 mm). These authors concluded that measurements should be made adjacent to the roots and not in the interradicular space. Deep concavities, however, in mesial and distal furcation roots complicate probing against the roots. Because attachment level is the most critical clinical means of evaluating periodontal disease, it was recommended that investigations are needed to develop improved means for recording probing attachment levels in furcations.

Bower (1979b) studied the internal concavities of furcations of first molar teeth (see Figure 10-4). The depth of the concavities ranged from 0.1 mm to 0.7 mm depending on the tooth and root configuration. These concavities hinder deposit removal when access permits due to significant furcation invasion. The maxillary first molar also exhibits a root divergence of the buccal roots toward the palatal root. This divergence affects instrumentation because it further limits access to the already narrow furcation entrance (see Figure 10-4A). The internal distance between the mesial and distal roots of mandibular first molars is also limited (Bower, 1979b) (Figure 10-4B). Successful instrumentation within furcations is addressed in Chapter 11.

The relationship of the gingiva refers to the location of the gingival margin to the furcation entrance. A furcation involvement that is occluded by gingiva presents more of a challenge to debride than one that has been exposed by loss of attachment. When the furcation entrance is occluded by gingival tissue, the client is also at a disadvantage in controlling plaque accumulation in the area. Surgical intervention is sometimes recommended in this case to create an environment that can be cleansed by the client and debrided by the professional.

## Pocket Topography

Pocket topography refers to the shape of the pocket that is viewed in cross section (as if looking into the periodontal pocket) or viewed laterally from the buccal, lingual, mesial, or distal surfaces. The topography includes the entire circumference of the periodontal pocket defined by the inner wall, which is the tooth surface, and the outer wall, which is the sulcular or pocket epithe-

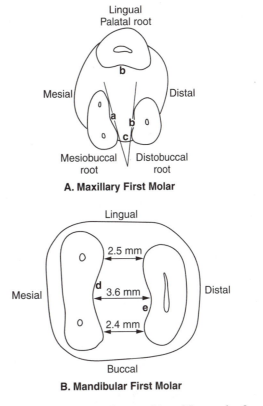

**Figure 10-4** Internal concavities of first molar furcations. *Key:* **a:** Concavity of mesiobuccal root is nearly equal to 0.3 mm deep; **b:** Concavity of distobuccal and palatal roots is nearly equal to 0.1 mm deep; **c:** Divergence or angle toward the palate between the buccal roots is nearly equal to 22°; **d:** Concavity of mesial root is nearly equal to 0.7 mm deep; **e:** Concavity of distal root is nearly equal to 0.5 mm deep. (Adapted from Bower, R. C., "Furcation Morphology Relative to Periodontal Treatment." *Journal of Periodontology, 50,* p. 367, 1979)

lium of the free gingiva. The apical extent of the periodontal pocket is the junctional epithelium. In health, the junctional epithelium is located within 1 mm of the cementoenamel junction (CEJ) and follows the curvature of the CEJ (Itoiz & Carranza, 1996). Refer to Chapter 1 to review the gingiva and supporting structures in health and disease.

Multiple pockets can form on any one tooth, each involving a different area of the root surface (Krayer & Rees, 1993). These pockets terminate independently and are separated from one another by tissue which is either pocket epithelium, junctional epithelium, or connective tissue attachment. Pockets involving different root surfaces on the same tooth can be different depths and types. Pockets in furcation areas are especially challenging to negotiate because they spiral, meaning they originate on one surface of the tooth and twist around to involve another surface (see Figure 10-5) (Carranza, 1996b).

Accurate periodontal probing will reveal differences in the level of the junctional epithelium on the root,

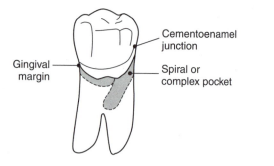

**Figure 10-5** Pockets involving different root surfaces. (Adapted from Carranza, F. A. "The Periodontal Pocket". Carranza & Newman, (Eds.). *Clinical Periodontology*, p. 282, 1996)

however, calculus location, tissue tone, root anatomy, and access hinder the clinician from mentally visualizing the true pocket topography. Nevertheless, combining the periodontal probe measurements and the anatomical features of the root will help the therapist estimate the shape of the pocket. A wide periodontal pocket can be debrided with a variety of instruments whereas a narrow, deep periodontal pocket limits the selection to instruments that have short working ends and long shanks. Even a standard area-specific curet design (Gracey) is not ideal for a deep, narrow pocket. Instead, longer shanked area-specific curets with shorter blades (Mini-Fives™, Hu-Friedy® Manufacturing Incorporated) are an alternative as is an ultrasonic insert that is thin and long (Slimlines, Dentsply Equipment).

### Gingival Contour and Tone

The contour of the gingiva refers to the shape of the gingival margin and interdental papilla. With periodontitis, the contour differs from the normal scalloped appearance seen in health. The interdental papilla often is reduced in height exposing the embrasure space. This exposure permits better access of instruments and self-care devices adjacent to the CEJ and subgingivally.

Tissue tone refers to the resilience or elasticity of the gingiva and is affected by the presence of inflammation. Tight tissue tone hinders subgingival access whereas instrument access is easier when tissue is more "elastic" or when inflammation breaks down gingival fibers or causes edema. Often when calculus deposits are moderate to large in size, or a sufficient quantity or quality of bacterial plaque exists, inflammation is present allowing the clinician to insert instruments subgingivally without tissue resistance. This is not always the case, however, if burnished or smooth calculus deposits exist creating the appearance of healthy tissue due to epithelial adaptation. Thin friable gingiva, usually found in facial surfaces of anterior teeth, is also a consideration when selecting instruments as this tissue is delicate and must not be unduly manipulated. An instrument with a thin shank

diameter, an offset blade (area-specific curets), and a short blade are ideal in this situation.

## DEPOSIT CHARACTERISTICS

Instruments are selected to remove pocket contents including microorganisms and their by-products (enzymes, endotoxins, metabolic products), calculus, crevicular fluid, desquamated epithelial cells, leukocytes, and exudate. The process of instrument selection, however, is aimed at calculus because it is the only entity that can be clinically detected subgingivally with periodontal instruments and it is the most challenging to remove. The principle means of detecting calculus is through tactile sensations created primarily by exploring. Visual inspection with compressed air is useful supragingivally, but this method is limited subgingivally to calculus deposits located just beneath an inflamed gingival margin. The characteristics of calculus that relate to instrument selection include its size, location, and mode of attachment. To understand the origin, composition, and development of calculus it is useful to review bacterial plaque formation as a precursor to calculus formation.

### Bacterial Plaque Formation

Bacterial plaque is the dense, nonmineralized, complex mass of colonies existing in a gel-like intermicrobial matrix (Wilkins, 1994) that is characteristic of a biofilm (binder) (Haake, 1996). Bacterial plaque formation occurs in three stages: pellicle formation, bacterial colonization, and maturation (see Table 10-4) (Wilkins, 1994). These stages represent the average process of bacterial plaque formation; however, slow plaque formers continue to form plaque composed of the cocci species for longer periods of time than fast plaque formers. From days 7 to 14, clinical signs of inflammation are seen and by 14 to 21 days, gingivitis is present. The dense supragingival plaque as it matures forms perpendicular to the tooth surface creating a wall-like appearance. Subgingival plaque then develops by apical growth of microorganisms in the supragingival plaque. The early colonies of bacterial plaque use oxygen which then favors increased colonization, increased density, and the growth of anaerobic microorganisms. Subgingival plaque includes more gram-negative anaerobic and motile organisms. Table 1-1 (in Chapter 1) identifies the microorganisms associated with specific classifications of periodontal disease. The early colonies, the gram-positive variety, use sugar as their energy source and saliva as their carbon source. The mature plaque, composed of anaerobic species, uses amino acids and small peptides as energy sources (Haake, 1996).

Subgingival bacterial plaque is organized in layers of attached plaque, which is adjacent to the tooth surface, unattached plaque within the sulcus/pocket, and

## Table 10-4 Stages of Bacterial Plaque Formation

| Stage | Description | Characteristics |
|-------|-------------|-----------------|
| 1 | Pellicle Formation | • composed of glycoproteins from the saliva<br>• highly insoluble coating over teeth, calculus, restorations, and complete or partial dentures<br>• it is 0.1 to 0.8 µm thick<br>• it is thicker near the gingiva<br>• microorganisms adhere to pellicle<br>• provides a mode of attachment for calculus |
| 2 | Bacterial Colonization | • bacteria multiply and grow within a few hours after pellicle formation<br>• microcolonies form in layers<br>• colonies meet and coalesce<br>• gram-positive microorganisms predominant (*A. viscosus* and *S. sanguis*)<br>• a continuous bacterial mass is formed<br>• transition occurs during this phase from an aerobic to an anaerobic environment |
| 3 | Maturation | • bacteria continue to multiply<br>• bacteria adhere to the plaque surface<br>• bacteria adhere to one another (coaggregation)<br>• the mass increases<br>• the thickness increases<br>• day 1 to 2 cocci exist (*mutans streptococcus* and *Streptococcus sanguis*)<br>• day 2 to 4 filamentous forms and slender rods occur on cocci colonies and gradually replace the cocci<br>• day 4 to 7 rods, filamentous forms, and fusobacteria occurs; spirochetes and vibrios are located in the mature plaque at the gingival margin<br>• day 7 to 14 vibrios, spirochetes, and white blood cells exist<br>• day 14 to 21 vibrios and spirochetes are prevalent; new plaque contains cocci and filamentous forms |

epithelium-associated plaque, which lies next to the inner lining of the sulcus/pocket. Microorganisms have also been shown to invade the connective tissue and reach the bone surface (Carranza, Saglie, Newman, & Valentin, 1983). Microorganisms comprise 70 to 80 percent of the solid components of bacterial plaque. The intermicrobial matrix is derived from saliva for supragingival plaque and from crevicular fluid for subgingival plaque. Embedded bacteria in the matrix exist and proliferate. The gel-like matrix, characteristic of a biofilm or binder, has special characteristics when compared to bacteria that are free-floating. The biofilm is a barrier, meaning that when bacteria produce substances they are retained within the gel-like mass thus increasing the concentration which, in turn, fosters metabolic interactions among the bacteria. Bacteria in the biofilm are also protected from harmful substances such as antimicrobial agents (Haake, 1996). Organic (carbohydrates, proteins, and lipids) and inorganic solids make up 20 to 30 percent of the matrix and the other 80 percent is water. Composition of plaque differs among individuals, differs between the various tooth surfaces of an individual, and changes with age.

The by-products of plaque include cell constituents such as endotoxins, bacterial surface components, and capsular components. Also, bacterial plaque produces enzymes that play a role in the disease process including collagenases, hyaluronidase, gelatinase, aminopeptidases, gelatinase, aminopeptidases, phospholipases, and alkaline and acid phosphates (see Chapter 3). **Endotoxin**, or lipo-oligosaccharide (LOS), is found in the outer cell wall of gram-negative bacteria; therefore, it is found in high concentrations in periodontal pockets. Endotoxin is highly toxic, penetrates gingival epithelium, is released when cells die, and may also be released from viable cells.

Endotoxins do a variety of things such as (Newman, Sanz, Nisengard, & Haake, 1996):

1. produce leukopenia (reduction of the number of leukocytes in the blood),
2. activate factor XII or Hageman's factor (clotting factor) leading to intravascular coagulation,
3. activate the complement (C) system by the alternative pathway versus the classic pathway (see Chapter 1) resulting in an inflammatory response,
4. lead to a localized Scwartzman phenomenon (a localized tissue reaction) creating tissue necrosis after two or more exposures to endotoxin,
5. has cytotoxic effects on cells including fibroblasts, and
6. induces bone resorption in organ culture.

*A. actinomycetemcomitans* produces an endotoxin referred to as leukotoxin. Leukotoxin has a toxic effect on human polymorphoneulear neutropils (PMNs), may enable *A. actinomycetemcomitans* to evade the host defense of phagocytosis, and may be an important property in the virulence of *A. actinomycetemcomitans* (Newman, Sanz, Nisengard, & Haake, 1996).

Bacterial surface components are toxic end products of both gram-positive and gram-negative subgingival bacteria. Fatty and organic acids (butyric and propionic acids), amines, volatile sulfur compounds, indole, ammonia, and glycans are all produced and are capable of tissue destruction. Peptidoglycan, a cell wall component, may affect host responses and is probably capable of stimulating bone resorption and stimulating macrophages to produce prostaglandin and collagenases. Capsular material found on the outermost surface of many bacterial cells may be a factor in tissue destruction and bacterial evasion of host defense mechanisms.

Tactile evaluation of subgingival plaque might feel sticky with an explorer. When calcification is just beginning subgingival plaque can feel slightly rough. Explorers, probes, and curets can retain subgingival plaque although there is no sure way of identifying if it is generalized or localized on a tooth surface. Subgingival bacterial plaque location must be correlated with the presence of calculus, defective or overhanging margins, rough tooth surfaces, and other plaque-retentive factors along with the corresponding gingival inflammation and pocket formation. Bacterial plaque forms a matrix for subgingival calculus formation.

## Calculus Formation

Minerals supplied by the crevicular fluid and inflammatory exudate are deposited in the intermicrobial matrix. Calculus is composed of 75 to 85 percent inorganic matter (calcium, phosphorous, carbonate, sodium, magnesium, and potassium) and the remainder is organic substances and water. About two-thirds of the inorganic matter is crystalline (apatite). Mineralization is actually the crystal formation. Four crystals are involved in this process and each calculus deposit is composed of at least two of these crystals. Hydroxyapatite predominates (58 percent) and is also present in enamel, cementum, and bone. Mature calculus can be more calcified than dentin, cementum, and bone, which points to the challenge encountered in its removal. Other crystal forms include magnesium whitlockite (21 percent), which is more common in posterior regions, octacalcium phosphate (21 percent), and brushite (9 percent), which is common in mandibular anterior regions (Leung & Jensen, 1958). Crystals form not only in the intercellular matrix, but on the surface of bacteria and within bacteria. Mineralization starts in the inner surfaces of the supragingival bacterial plaque and in the attached component of the subgingival plaque. It takes an average of twelve days for undisturbed soft deposit to change to a mineralized form, although the process can start in 24 to 48 hours. Rapid calculus formers mineralize deposits as soon as ten days and slow calculus formers can take up to twenty days. Heavy calculus formers generally have higher salivary levels of calcium and phosphorous than do light calculus formers. Light formers have higher levels of parotid pyrophosphate, which inhibits calcification; therefore,

this substance is used in anticalculus dentifrices. Formation time is influenced by the individual host, roughness of the tooth surface, and client oral self-care practices.

Calculus grows by apposition of new layers. These layers form irregularly on and parallel to the root surface and are separated by lines of pellicle called incremental lines. The pellicle is deposited over the existing calculus, bacterial colonization occurs, mineralization then progresses, and the pellicle becomes imbedded. Thus, calculus is always overlayed by bacterial plaque. The outside surface of the calculus deposit is rough and detectable with explorers, probes, sharp curets, and thin ultrasonic inserts. If the surface was observed microscopically it would appear like peaks, valleys, and pits (Wilkins, 1994). It is this irregular surface that retains the bacterial plaque that is in contact with the inner wall of the diseased pocket.

In conclusion, it is no longer accepted that calculus is a mechanical irritant to the tissue causing periodontal disease (Carranza, 1996a). Instead, it is the bacterial plaque that always covers calculus deposits that is the causative factor in initiating periodontal disease. This bacterial plaque produces endotoxins and other by-products and stimulates the flow of crevicular fluid that contains minerals for subsequent subgingival calculus formation. For these reasons, instrument selection must focus on removal of all plaque-retentive factors including calculus in order to initiate and maintain health. It is rare to find a periodontal pocket in adults without subgingival calculus deposit although it could be only microscopically visible (Carranza, 1996a). Interproximal calculus can be detected, at times, by radiographs however the location does not correlate to the location of the bottom of the periodontal pocket. Plaque exists apical to the deposit that is not radiographically visible (Carranza, 1996a). Regardless of its primary or secondary relationship in pocket formation, calculus is a significant factor in periodontal disease (Carranza, 1996a).

From a clinical standpoint the important characteristics of calculus are size, consistency, configuration (shape), mode of attachment, and location. These five factors are interrelated and when analyzed they help the professional select instruments. Size is described as light, moderate, and heavy and is commonly divided into supragingival and subgingival areas. One interpretation of this subjective classification system is presented in Table 10-5. Defining these terms allows for standardization of classification for practices, clinical situations in educational institutions, or for regional or state testing agencies. Light deposits are characteristically not well attached to the surface and can be removed with flexible shank curets. Moderate or heavy calculus can be either tenacious or not and is often more firmly attached than light deposits. Heavy deposits are usually, but not always, tenacious and attached fairly well to the tooth surface creating a need for ultrasonic instruments, files, sickles, and/or curets. Interproximal calculus is often heavier than facial or lingual deposits, therefore, the mesial and

**Table 10-5 Description of Calculus Size**

| Light | Moderate | Heavy |
|---|---|---|
| • fine, granular, grainy or spicule | • a "bump" with thickness readily discernible | • ledge encircling tooth, thick and dense |
| • located along line angles, marginal areas, and/or under contacts | • a marginal ring or interproximal "click" | • fills interproximal space or is a marginal ledge |
| • slight vibration or roughness detected with explorer | • definite vibration felt with explorer—a "jump," also detected with curet, interproximal deposit sometimes detected from lingual and buccal | • definite vibration, sometimes "binds" explorer, also detected with curet, interproximal deposit detected from lingual and buccal |

distal surfaces are key surfaces on which to focus when selecting instruments. Instrument shank diameter and flexibility relate to deposit size. Increased diameter and less flexibility is needed for heavier tenacious deposits.

Consistency relates to the surface texture. Calculus is either smooth, flat, and dense or irregular and brittle. Smooth deposit indicates it has been present for a long period of time, that it was burnished by a previous clinician, or that it was not removed with previous instrumentation meaning it is residual. Consistency can be determined by comparing it to the root surface. Many times the calculus is smoother than the tooth surface or the tooth surface is flat where a developmental depression should exist. For example, the developmental depression on the mesial of the first maxillary premolar should be prominent and if not, calculus deposit within the depression is a possibility. Frequently with burnished deposit the apical portion is smooth from previous instrumentation, but the lateral borders or coronal portion will have some area of irregularity or roughness. This occurs because the apical portion is where the clinician started scaling and it has been smoothed by instrumentation. To discover burnished deposit, the root surface must be explored from different directions. Tissue response is not a good indicator of burnished calculus because the gingiva can heal over the deposit and appear healthy. When

the area is probed or an instrument is used in the periodontal pocket, bleeding is often seen, indicating infection in the pocket lining. Brittle deposit is easier to remove even if it is moderate or heavy because it is readily detected and fractures piece by piece.

Configuration, or shape, is very useful when determining if the irregularity felt with an explorer is indeed calculus or is anatomic. The shape of calculus is either nodular, crusty or spiny; ledge or ringlike; a thin smooth veneer; finger or fernlike; or like individual islands. Correlating these shapes to anatomy helps the clinician distinguish what is removable and what is not. Calculus usually forms in a horizontal fashion on the root circumference, which is why initial exploratory strokes should be vertical and oblique, not horizontal. Mode of attachment can occur in three ways (see Table 10-6). Calculus that has recently formed and is attached to pellicle is very easily removed as compared to calculus that is mechanically locked into cementum and/or irregularities in the tooth surface. Location relates to the position of the crown or root of the tooth. Calculus located near the margin is easier to reach with any instrument and the farther away it is from the gingival margin the more difficult it is to access requiring an instrument with a long shank. Therefore, calculus of the same size might be removed with different instruments depending on

**Table 10-6 Three Modes of Attachment of Calculus**

| Mode of Attachment | Degree of Attachment | Characteristics |
|---|---|---|
| Acquired Pellicle or Cuticle | Superficial; no interlocking or penetration exists; easily removed | • pellicle is positioned between the calculus and tooth surface<br>• occurs on enamel and recently scaled/root planed/debrided surfaces |
| Mechanical Locking into Minute Irregularities | Challenging to remove because of the locking into the tooth surface | • cemental irregularities include locations of previous Sharpey's fibers, resorption lacunae, instrumentation grooves, cemental tears, or fragmentation |
| Direct Contact between Calcified Intercellular Matrix and the Surface | Hard to distinguish between the cementum and calculus | • inorganic crystals of the tooth interlock with the mineralized bacterial plaque |

the location. This is one reason why multiple instruments are used in one pocket area.

## INSTRUMENT SELECTION CONSIDERATIONS

Instrument identification and description will be reviewed prior to discussing selection of periodontal instruments.

### Instrument Identification

Instruments are identified based on the classification (types); the design name and number; and the manufacturer. The classifications of instruments include probes, explorers, ultrasonic inserts, files, sickles, and curets. Instruments are related to their function in the dental hygiene process of care. Probes and explorers are used during the assessment phase to determine periodontal conditions such as clinical attachment level, width of the attached gingiva, probing depth, presence and extent of furcation involvement, identification of subgingival plaque, scoring of supragingival plaque indexes, calculus location and configuration, and identification of plaque-retentive factors. Ultrasonic inserts, files, and curets are employed in the implementation phase of NSPT to remove deposits and plaque-retentive factors identified during periodontal and restorative assessment. Probes and explorers are again utilized in the evaluation phase of care to assess the effectiveness of the deposit removal and to assess the periodontal status at the reevaluation visit scheduled after the completion of active therapy.

The name printed on the instrument is associated with the individual or school responsible for the design and it usually refers to a type of instrument. Examples include the names "McCall" indicating a universal curet, "Gracey" indicating an area-specific curet, or "ODU" (11/12) referring to a specific explorer. Within each classification, instruments can be further subdivided based on the number which usually relates to the location of use in the mouth. For example, with area-specific Gracey curets a low number such as 1/2 corresponds to an instrument designed for anterior teeth. A high number indicates use in the posterior regions of the mouth such as the Gracey 17/18 designed for the distal surfaces of premolars and molars. Numbers located lengthwise (positioned horizontally) on handles of double-ended instruments appear closest to the working end that corresponds to the number. When the name and number are placed across the handle when the instrument is held vertically, the first number identifies the working end on the top and the second number corresponds to the working end at the bottom of the handle. The manufacturer of an instrument refers to the company that produces the instrument. A variety of companies produce the same instrument; however, these companies design the same instrument in different ways. Two companies might manufacturer universal Columbia 13/14 curets, which look similar when examined side by side; however, upon closer examination differences in the blade width and curvature, shank width and curvature, and other aspects are evident.

### Instrument Description

Various parts of the instrument such as the shank and working end relate to instrument selection because these elements are what makes its design unique (see Figure 10-6). Handle comfort and size also are important factors to consider. Briefly, the shank connects the handle and the working end and can take on many shapes depending on the instrument design. For example, the shank of a curved explorer shaped like a universal curet and of a pocket feeler-type explorer are designed differently to adapt to root surface areas and topography. The curved shank of a universal designed explorer would negotiate convex and concave proximal surfaces better than the straight shank of a pocket feeler, whereas the straighter shank would adapt well in a narrow deep defect. Likewise, the difference in shank designs of universal and area-specific curets is a distinct characteristic affecting their adaptability and activation in the removal of plaque-retentive entities. Shank design can be singular or multiple, meaning that one shank is present (Gracey 1/2 instrument) or up to four shanks might exist (11/12 explorer). Multiple (complex) shanks create more curvature promoting extension into an area that is not easily accessed. The length, angle, and strength of shanks will be highlighted in the selection strategies presented.

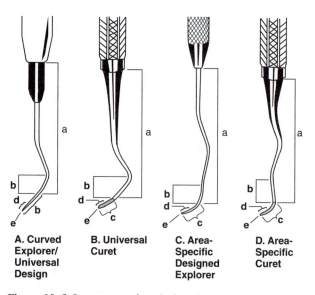

A. Curved Explorer/ Universal Design    B. Universal Curet    C. Area-Specific Designed Explorer    D. Area-Specific Curet

**Figure 10-6** Instrument description.
*Key:* **a:** functional shank: overall distance from working end to handle; **b:** terminal shank: extends between the working end and the first bend in the shank; **c:** working end, distance from terminal shank to point or toe; **d:** tip (explorer) or lower one-third (curet); **e:** point (explorer) or toe (curet).

Shank length refers to the overall distance from the handle to the working end. The shank itself can be divided into two portions: the terminal shank and the functional shank. The **terminal shank** extends between the working end and the first bend in a shank. The **functional shank** is the overall distance from the working end to the handle. A long shank optimizes extension into deep periodontal pockets. Shank angulation is the amount of curvature or bending observed when viewed from the lateral surfaces. Instruments designed for posterior surfaces generally have a more angled or curved shank to facilitate access to the area. Anterior instruments usually have straight shanks because of the ease of access to these teeth.

Shank strength is a function of circumference and the type of metal that is used. Manufacturers differ in amount of shank flexibility. A common system describes three types: rigid, moderately flexible, or flexible (Hu-Friedy® Product Catalog and Reference Guide, 1993). Rigid shanks are designed for removal of heavy calculus and, thus, tactile sense is limited making it difficult to detect light to moderate calculus. Sickles, files, and rigid area-specific curets are examples. The moderately flexible shank is characteristic of universal curet designs. They are designed for removal of moderate to light calculus and provide a sufficient level of tactile sense to detect and remove calculus. Flexible shanks are used to detect and remove light subgingival calculus deposits or plaque. They are characteristic of area-specific curets and explorers and the flexibility provides the best tactile sensation.

The **working end** is the part of the instrument from the terminal shank to the point of an explorer or the toe of a curet. It is the terminal 1 to 2 mm of the working end of explorers and curets that adapts to the tooth to perform the task of detection or removal (Pattison, Pattison, & Takei, 1996). The terminal portion of the working end of an explorer is called the tip and the terminal portion of the curet or sickle is termed the lower, terminal, leading, or toe one-third. Working ends also vary in length and angle as well as width.

When curets or sickles are chosen, blade size becomes a consideration. Size refers to the width of the blade when viewed from the face and thickness or depth of the blade determined by observing the lateral surface. A larger and thicker blade is selected for removal of heavy or tenacious pieces of calculus. Use of a large-sized blade in areas where inflammation is slight and tissue tone is tight will increase trauma and discomfort. Blade angulation is the relationship of the face of the working end to the lower or terminal shank. This angulation is one of the features that differentiates universal curets from area-specific curets. Blade balance occurs when the working ends are centered on an imaginary line that runs through the long axis of the instrument handle. Manufacturers attempt to balance instruments so that when pressure is exerted on the handle of a file or curet it is transmitted to the shank and then to the blade in an effective manner. Manufacturers' product catalogs address blade balance as well as the other characteristics of their instruments.

Although instrument handles do not influence selection of instruments in relation to root or pocket topography, they do relate to a professional's preference for certain instruments and manufacturers. Comfort in handle design is important to the clinician's well-being during NSPT. Handle size refers to its circumference. The larger the handle, the less fatigue the therapist will experience. At the same time, more control is gained with a larger handle than a smaller diameter; however, the larger diameter can restrict movement in posterior areas. Diameter of the handle also affects potential occupational hazards such as musculoskeletal and nerve impairment disorders (see Chapter 15). The weight of handles also differs. A hollow handle will increase tactile sensitivity and decrease muscle fatigue because of the light weight. Conversely, a solid handle reduces tactile sense and increases hand fatigue. The shape of handles varies from company to company. Some are round and others are octagonal. Handles with serrations (scoring or ribbing) enhance control while decreasing hand stress. Conversely, smooth handles decrease instrument control and increase fatigue.

Practitioners are likely to use instruments that they were introduced to in dental hygiene school; therefore, a thorough understanding of instrument design is beneficial to lifelong learning. Being able to evaluate applications for new instruments as they are manufactured is essential when deciding on instruments to purchase for NSPT. The recommendations within this section represent only one philosophical approach to instrumental selection based on root and pocket morphology, and clinical experience. Research evaluating instrument selection is limited, especially in relation to explorers and curets. There is an abundance of literature on periodontal probing, however, to help the practitioner select the best probes for clinical practice.

## Probes

The design of the periodontal probe that is selected for assessment could affect the outcome of the measurements. Use of a periodontal probe for detection of plaque-retentive factors such as calculus and overhanging margins of dental restorations is not addressed in this section because, although calculus can be felt with a probe, its identification, configuration, and location is enhanced when using an appropriately designed explorer. Pocket depth and loss of attachment are perhaps the most important clinical parameters in the assessment of periodontal disease severity. An increase in probing depth has been found to be a valuable indicator in predicting clinical attachment loss (Badersten, Nilvéus, & Egelberg, 1990; Claffey, 1991; Claffey, Nylund, Kiger, Garrett, & Egelberg, 1990). The potential inaccuracy in measuring these parameters has been noted in previous research

(Van der Velden, 1978) and therefore, the value of these diagnostic measures has been scrutinized. Diameter of the probe, probing force, angulation to the tooth, root contour, pocket contour, and errors in reading and recording the measurements affect the outcome of the probing measurements which, in turn, can affect diagnosis of the level of health or disease of a client. The operator can control some of these factors by critical selection of the probe used in daily practice and by self-evaluation of probing technique. The client's inherent intraoral conditions such as root anatomy and tissue tone, can not be controlled per se, but can be addressed by enhancing proper selection and technique.

**Probe Diameter.** Keagle and others (1989) concluded that 0.6 mm was the most discriminatory optimal tip diameter; however, Van der Zee and others (1991) examined a range of probes and concluded that tines themselves vary in accuracy and shape. They also concluded that diameter might affect results of measurements. The measurement error standard deviation for probing attachment loss is between 0.40 mm and 0.54 mm when using probes that measure 0.6 mm at the tip (Kingman, Löe, Ånerud, & Boysen, 1991). Others report that the standard deviation for replicating probing assessments is 0.82 (Kaldahl et al., 1990; Vanooteghem, Hutchens, Garrett, Kiger, & Egelberg, 1987). When using manual probing, two to three millimeters of change of probing attachment level needs to occur for the clinician to feel sure that the change is due to disease and not error (Goodson, Tanner, Haffajee, Sornbager, & Sovansky, 1982; Greenstein, 1994; Jeffcoat, 1994; Lang & Bragger, 1990). This amount of change is not ideal in clinical practice because it encourages the clinician to inform the client of the change *after* significant attachment loss has occurred. An overestimation might be more beneficial because a discussion with the client about enhanced self-care practices and compliance with PMP will occur before significant destruction has occurred, fostering prevention rather than treatment. Fine (1992) points out that the 2 mm change in probing depth set as a standard by Goodson and coworkers assures clinicians that disease detected is indeed progressing; therefore, an underestimation of severity of disease and a delay in disease detection also are assured.

**Force.** If bleeding on probing is to be used as an indicator of disease, correct and standardized force is also an important factor. A wide range of probing force probably exists between clinicians, however, in a study of 58 subjects, different professionals probed with an average of 0.44N force and no significant differences were found in force between students, general practitioners, periodontists, and dental hygienists (Freed, Cooper, & Kalkwarf, 1983). Watts (1987) noted that a force of 0.25N was near the pain tolerance limit for several patients, but Van der Velden and DeVries's (1978) patients tolerated forces up to 0.75N. More recently, it was demonstrated

that probing forces that exceed 0.25N traumatize healthy tissues (Lang, Nyman, Senn, & Joss, 1991). N refers to a newton which is a measurement of force of 1 kilogram at an acceleration of 1 meter per second squared (1 kg · m/s$^2$). N is approximately equal to a gram. Forces from 25 to 50 grams (g) are probably appropriate for clinical practice (Magnusson & Wilson, 1992).

There is a problem with applying research data about force or pressure to clinical use. It is not practical for clinicians using manual probes to estimate force on a constant basis. One means of checking force is to periodically use a metric scale to check the pressure, and then the appropriate force can be reproduced in the mouth (Magnusson & Wilson, 1992). This activity might serve to standardize clinicians in a teaching environment, in a regional or state board examination, or within a practice. Students might be interested in trying this evaluation to make them aware of how probing feels when using force within the range that is acceptable. Clinicians in daily practice can standardize pressure and correlate readings with other clinical data such as sites with inflammation, bacterial plaque accumulation, and radiographic bone loss. The student and practitioner can also self-evaluate pressure by observing clients' reactions to the procedure and questioning them about sensitivity. If generalized bleeding were to occur repeatedly when a client's gingival sulcus was probed and the gingiva otherwise looked healthy, then self-assessment of the technique might indicate that the pressure used was greater than needed. Likewise, if the radiographs show moderate bone loss, the marginal gingiva has normal height and contour, and pockets are not being detected; then the clinician needs to reevaluate probing depths to determine if enough pressure was exerted and/or if deposits were obstructing the accuracy of readings.

**Gingival Condition.** Another factor affecting probing results is the condition of the gingiva. Attachment level measurements are influenced by the density of the connective tissue collar at the margin of the gingiva (Fowler, Garrett, Crigger, & Egelberg, 1982). In healthy tissues and slight inflammation, the probe generally reaches the junctional epithelium, however, in a pocket, the probe tip routinely exceeds the level of the attachment and penetrates into the inflamed tissue. When probing, the tip of the instrument penetrates into the most coronal portion of the connective tissue attachment an average of 0.3 mm (Listgarten, Mao, & Robinson, 1976; Saglie, Johanson, & Flotragh, 1975; Spray, Garnick, Doles, & Klawitter, 1978).

**Force-Controlled Probes.** Force-controlled probes, or automated probes, have been designed to attempt to overcome some of the inherent errors in pressure with manual probing. Because probing for attachment level occurs over time, it is important that force be standardized to reduce error in evaluating loss or gain of attachment. The Florida Probe®, the Toronto Automated

Probe® (TAPP), Peri-Probe® (Dentalair, Netherlands), and the electronic Interprobe® have all been reported to detect small attachment level changes from 0.2 mm to 1 mm depending on the probe and the number of sites evaluated. Rams and Slots (1993) conclude that the Interprobe and Florida Probe systems both tended to produce a more reliable depth measurement when compared to manual probing using a Michigan O-probe. In another study comparing a Brodontic pressure probe with a Williams manual probe (tip diameter = 0.64 mm), it was found that the constant force probe decreased both intra- and interexaminer variation in probe depth readings of sites with chronic adult periodontitis (Walsh & Saxby, 1989).

Automated probes hold promise for future use in detecting and monitoring periodontal disease; however, the clinician should be aware of the inherent weaknesses of these devices. First, researchers conclude that probe readings with the manual probe are deeper than those recorded when using an automated probe (Jendersen et al., 1994; Rams & Slots, 1994). Explanations for the deeper pockets achieved with manual probing are that the deepest portion of the pocket is not always found with automated probes due to the absence of tactile sense and the size, which interferes with optimal interproximal registration (technique), leading to false or less probe readings (Jendersen et al., 1994). Second, the use of the fixed setting for probing force does not allow the clinician to adjust pressure due to the difference in inflammation throughout a single client's mouth. As a result, pain has been associated with automated probing devices. Third, cost is prohibitive for many practices. Chapter 3 reviews some of the most common automated systems.

A workshop sponsored by the National Institute of Dental Research (1979) proposed that periodontal pocket depth-attachment level measurement systems should meet the following criteria (Parakkal, 1979):

1. A precision of 0.1 mm.
2. A range of 10 mm.
3. A constant probing force.
4. Noninvasive, lightweight, and comfortable to use.
5. Able to access any location around the teeth.
6. A guidance system to ensure probe angulation.
7. Complete sterilization of all portions entering the mouth.
8. No biohazard from material or electrical shock.
9. Digital output.

**Manual Probes.** Single- and double-ended probes used for measuring periodontal pocket depth and loss of attachment are manufactured in a variety of designs (see Figure 10-7). Variances occur in the shank angle and length, working end and diameter, the end configuration (blunt rounded, thin tapered, or ball-end), and the measurement indicators (see Table 10-7). Shanks are usually contra-angled, but a newer design has a right angle and reduced shank length to improve access to the posterior

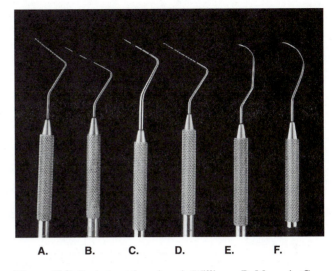

**Figure 10-7** Periodontal probes. **A.** Williams; **B.** Marquis; **C.** Maryland Moffitt; **D.** University of North Carolina; **E.** Nabers, 1N; **F.** Nabers 2N.

regions to enhance accuracy (Novatech™, Hu-Friedy®, see Figure 10-8). The right-angle design can be purchased with a variety of markings such as Williams, Marquis, and screening probe types. Working ends are either an even diameter from the tip to the top of the shank or they can be tapered to a thinner diameter toward the tip and end. Shanks are round, oval, or flat when viewed in cross section. Thinner probes (Marquis type) might provide easier access, however, literature discusses the ease in which the probe tip punctures the epithelium especially in diseased states. For this reason, blunt rounded tip probes are preferred by some clinicians. In fact, the ball-end, initially created for use with the WHO probe (diameter 0.5 mm), was designed to decrease the potential of invading the junctional epithelium to enhance accuracy. Other ball-end probes are now available with plastic or metal handles.

Markings on periodontal probes indicating one millimeter measurement increments are varied in distance and color. For example, the Williams probe, manufactured by a variety of companies, is marked in millimeter measurements of 1, 2, 3, 5, 7, 8, 9, 10, and the Marquis type probe has markings indicating intervals of 3, 6, 9, and 12 mm. Some manufacturers provide black or yellow color coding on the mm markings and/or between the markings to enhance visibility while measuring. A problem with probes that do not have one millimeter intervals marked is the potential for increased error. The clinician must estimate the millimeters to record on the periodontal chart. This is a concern when a variety of professionals are probing numerous clients and making treatment decisions. Repeated measures using periodontal probes with 3 mm gradations are likely to be less consistent or relative to the previous readings. When these considerations are combined with the other errors inherent in the probing process, the likelihood of de-

**Table 10-7  Summary of Manual Periodontal Probes**

| Type | Working Design | Measurement |
|---|---|---|
| • Marquis | round, tapered in diameter | 3-6-9-12 |
| • Goldman Fox | flat | 1-2-3-5-7-8-9-10 |
| • Williams | round, tapered | 1-2-3-5-7-8-9-10 |
| • Michigan-O | round, tapered | 3-6-8 |
| • 15 University of North Carolina | round, tapered | 1-2-3-4-5-6-7-8-9-10-11-12-13-14-15 |
| • Maryland Moffitt | round, tapered, ball-end | 1-2-3-5-7-8-9-10 |
| • Screening Probe | round, tapered, ball-end | • 3.5 to 5.5, 8.5 to 11.5<br>• 3.5 to 5.5 is color coded |
| • Nabers 1N (Mesial and Distal Furcations) | curved shank and working end, round | no markings |
| • Nabers 2N (Facial and Lingual Furcations) | curved shank and working end greater than the 1N, round | • no markings, or<br>• 12-9-6-3 with color coding between 3 and 6 and 9 and 12 |
| • Nabers 3N (Furcation) | straight shank and working end, flat | 10-9-8-7-5-3-2-1 |
| • Novatech™ Right Angle Design | • includes Williams, Marquis, and screening probe (with ball-end) designs | • available with a variety of markings |

creased accuracy in representing the actual clinical state is increased.

A recent development in manual probes is pressure-sensitive probes designed to control the force each time it is used with the same operator or another operator (True Pressure Sensitive (TPS) Probe™, Ivoclar North America Incorporated). The TPS insures a consistent 20-gram force, has a disposable head, and is a plastic screening probe with a ball end. Other companies also manufacture this type of probe.

In conclusion, selection strategies for a manual, straight periodontal probe include evaluation of the diameter (0.6 mm or less), the use of a ball-end to prevent penetration of the probe into the junctional epithelium, and the use of millimeter markings to improve accuracy in measurement. Because of the variances in instrument design and client and therapist factors it is essential for an office or clinical situation to select a single periodontal probe design and evaluate all client's conditions over time with the same instrument. Assessing disease severity and progression by correlating all clinical and radiographic signs of disease is challenging, and introducing different instruments into the process will only increase the inherent errors in using clinical data to assess disease activity. The relationship of initial assessment data to data collected at reevaluation visits and maintenance appointments is subject to increased errors when different probe designs are used for repeated measurements.

The periodontal probe also is used to measure the extent of furcation involvement, in both a horizontal and vertical fashion. A furcation involvement of grade II or greater is extremely significant in periodontal therapy because the interradicular bone is absent, but the facial and lingual orifices are occluded by tissue. In order to detect this type of lesion many clinicians feel the curved Nabers probe is the instrument of choice when compared to a straight periodontal probe because it allows for an accurate horizontal diagnosis (Carranza, 1996b). Others recommend the straight probe for buccal and lingual furcations and the Nabers probe for interproximal furcations on maxillary teeth (Magnusson & Wilson, 1992; Pattison & Pattison, 1992). Considering the small diameter of furcation entrances, a curved explorer is also useful to detect initial involvement.

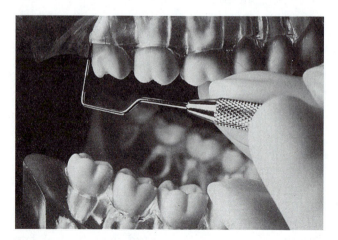

**Figure 10-8** Novatech™ probe on a maxillary tooth. (Courtesy of Hu-Friedy® Manufacturing Company, Inc.)

Nabers probes are designed for specific areas: the 1N is for mesials and distals and the 2N is for facials and linguals (see Figure 10-7). Some Nabers probes have color coded measurements such as the Q-2N (Hu-Friedy® Manufacturing Incorporated). The increments are in 3 mm intervals extending to 12 mm to aid the clinician in determining the millimeters of horizontal penetration within the defect for recording purposes and for decision making for nonsurgical care versus surgery. A 3 mm horizontal depth seems to be a critical point for deciding between osseous resection or guided tissue regeneration (Hall, 1994), along with other factors. Chapter 17 discusses surgical interventions related to furcation involvement. If only the grade of the furcation is recorded, then the use of Nabers probes without markings is sufficient.

## Explorers

Selection of explorers is often related to clinician preference, however, there are anatomical conditions which must be considered such as width of the proximal root surface and the periodontal probing depth. The primary functions of explorers are to detect location and configuration of calculus deposits and other plaque-retentive factors, as well as to assess restorative problems such as contour and marginal integrity. The explorer is a commonly used instrument by dental hygienists and it is the best method to evaluate the subgingival environment during NSPT procedures due to the fine and curved working ends and shanks that other instruments, such as the probe, do not possess. It is used often throughout the debridement process to assess plaque-retentive factors, to evaluate the removal of deposits, and then again at the reevaluation visit to reassess the outcome of care. Because it is the sole primary diagnostic tool in evaluating the quality of deposit removal and removal of overhanging margins its selection is of the utmost importance to success in NSPT.

There are many explorer designs correlating to use and function. Major categories include curved explorers that are paired (#2 and #3 designs), right-angled explorers that are unpaired (#17 and #20—Orban-type), and an area-specific-like design which is paired (#11/12) (see Figure 10-9). Sheperd hooks (#23) and explorers with straight working ends (#6) are unpaired and not used in the debridement process, because they do not effectively adapt to subgingival root topography. The ability to successfully detect and assess results depends on realizing the strengths and limitations of each explorer design.

Curved explorers encompass both the cowhorn and pigtail designs which originally received their name because of their appearance at the working end. Some current literature uses the terms "cowhorn" and "pigtail" interchangeable; however, in the past there were distinct design differences related to the amount of curvature at the working end. For purposes of this text, selection strategies for curved explorers (#2 and #3 designs) will focus on the curvature and length of the working end and shank. Explorers that have extremely curved terminal shanks and working ends (Figure 10-9B & C, #3 designs) are used supragingivally and in normal sulcus depth. They are not well suited to explore periodontal pockets (4 mm or greater) especially as the pocket increases in depth. Tight, nonelastic tissue further decreases the ability of the clinician to adapt this type of explorer due to its curved shank.

Curved explorers with less curvature of the terminal shank and working end are used in healthy sulcus depth and shallow to moderate pockets; they adapt to most surfaces and extend to the midline of proximal surfaces (see Figure 10-9A, E, & F). One such design is the 2R/2L (Suter Dental Manufacturing Company, Inc., see Figure 10-9F). This instrument combines the best features of a curved explorer into one instrument as it has a longer functional shank, terminal shank, and working end than other explorers. The terminal shank and working end measure about 11 mm. The design of the shank and working end combined allow for extension to even the widest proximal surfaces as illustrated in Figure 10-10. The working end curves slightly across planes to adapt to convex and concave surfaces, but the curvature is not so great that extension subgingivally is limited. Table 10-2 on page 259 summarizes the buccal to lingual dimensions of teeth and is useful in selecting explorers that match the root anatomy and deposit conditions.

The Suter 2R/2L also has a unique plastic handle design that is 5/16″ in diameter making it larger than some other explorer handles. The size seems to enhance adaptation in relation to rolling and pivoting of the instrument to keep the tip adapted to the tooth surface. The plastic material enhances tactile sensitivity and insures that the instrument is very light to hold. The cone-socketed shank and working end is available in carbon steel, which also promotes tactile ability.

General limitations of curved explorers include extending to very deep pockets, especially when using a

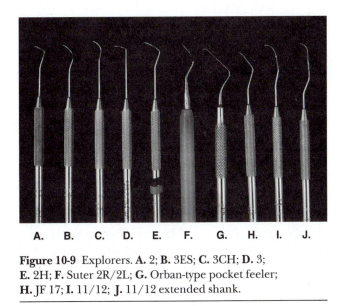

A. B. C. D. E. F. G. H. I. J.

**Figure 10-9** Explorers. **A.** 2; **B.** 3ES; **C.** 3CH; **D.** 3; **E.** 2H; **F.** Suter 2R/2L; **G.** Orban-type pocket feeler; **H.** JF 17; **I.** 11/12; **J.** 11/12 extended shank.

curved explorer with a shorter shank and working end (see Figure 10-9A, #2 design). The 2R/2L is ideal for initial assessment of a client's condition because it adapts to proximal surfaces and root anatomy in any depth of pocket realizing that the deeper the pocket the less effective any instrument will be in NSPT. The explorers discussed in the next section are indicated as adjunct instruments for specific situations such as moderate to deep pockets, furcations, and final evaluation of the root surface. More than one explorer is usually needed to meet the needs of the client in active NSPT.

The #3A design (not pictured) is great for detection in deep pockets on the buccal and lingual surfaces of posterior teeth, anterior teeth, and furcations (Pattison & Pattison, 1992; Perry, Beemsterboer, & Carranza, 1990). Its limitation is the straight shank and working end with no curvature across planes meaning that adaptation on the curved surfaces of teeth (round convex areas and into depressions) is difficult.

Right-angled explorers or pocket feelers (#17 and Orban-type) (see Figure 10-9G & H) are designed to detect fine calculus deposits in deep pockets, to explore amount and configuration of calculus, and to evaluate the product of debridement in relation to removal of calculus embedded in cementum. The long and sometimes thin, fine shank of the Orban-type instrument promotes its extension into deep, narrow periodontal pockets. At the same time, the right-angle design of the working end to the shank and short working end (2 mm) limits its effectiveness in initial calculus assessment where deposits might be large and generalized. Also, it is difficult to adapt the #17 to posterior proximal root surfaces (Huennekens & Daniel, 1992; Perry, Beemsterboer, & Carranza, 1990) because of the straight shank and lack of curvature between the shank and working end. Both types of right-angled instruments are ineffective in negotiating the proximal surfaces because of the straight shank and short tip. Therefore, contraindications for use include normal sulcus depth, gross calculus deposits, and proximal surfaces.

The 11/12 explorer design (see Figure 10-9I & J) is similar to a mesial posterior area-specific curet; therefore, its adaptation would be similar to the Gracey 11/12. Even though it has the shank design of an 11/12 Gracey curet, it has universal surface characteristics (as do other explorers) meaning it adapts to all tooth surfaces by using either side of the working end (Huennekens & Daniel, 1992). Exploration of a quadrant or sextant on the buccal aspects is accomplished with one end of the explorer; likewise, the lingual surfaces are explored with the other end of the explorer. The multi-curved shank and rounded back promote extension subgingivally even when tissue tone is tight.

Strengths of the 11/12 design include adaptation in furcations and moderate to deep pockets, especially those located on the mesial surfaces. The working end is short (about 3 mm), however, and this affects adaptation on proximal surfaces near the cervix in the posterior

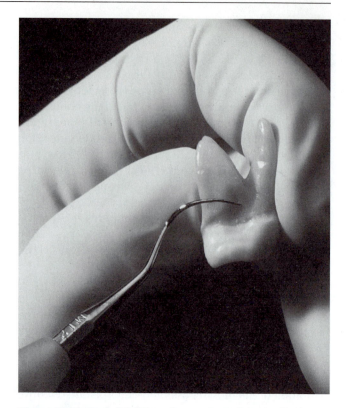

**Figure 10-10** Suter 2R/2L explorer adapted to proximal surface of maxillary right first molar.

regions. The major limitation is the inability of the 11/12 to extend to the midline, especially on distal surfaces of posterior teeth (Pattison & Pattison, 1992). This limitation is represented in Figure 10-11 where it is evident that the tip does not reach the midline affecting adequate coverage of the proximal surface. To reach the midline, the instrument handle would be tilted away from the contact area, the terminal shank would no longer be parallel to the proximal surface, and the point would be directed upward into the contact area. This explorer is available in an extending terminal shank length of 3 mm (11/12 After-Five™, Hu-Friedy® Manufacturing Incorporated) (see Figure 10-9J), which may further enhance its effectiveness in both deep pockets and furcation areas occluded by gingival tissue. When combined with a curved explorer with a long shank and working end, both explorers have the potential for improving the quality of NSPT.

## Ultrasonic Inserts

Standard, traditional ultrasonic inserts used primarily for supragingival deposit removal were introduced into dentistry in the early 1950s. With the advent of thinner tips for ultrasonic instrumentation, referred to as precision-thin inserts, the therapist now has a choice in selecting ultrasonic inserts for either supragingival or subgingival instrumentation. Even when slimmer, precision-thin inserts are used, traditional (larger) inserts are

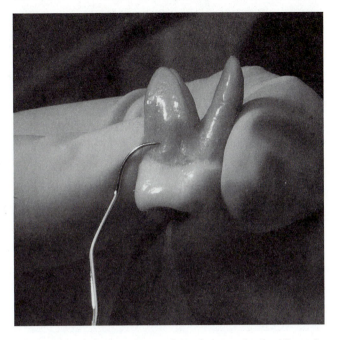

**Figure 10-11** 11/12 explorer adapted to proximal surface of maxillary right first molar.

still necessary for removal of heavy, tenacious calculus deposit and stain. The most common of the designs are shown in Figure 10-12. Many of these designs are available from a variety of manufacturers, and as is the case with hand-activated instruments, companies produce similar inserts that vary in working end length, diameter, and curvature.

The traditional universal design (P10, Cavitron®, Dentsply Equipment) (see Figure 10-12C) is selected by clinicians for removal of heavy and/or tenacious supra-

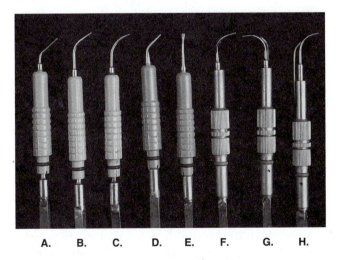

**Figure 10-12** Ultrasonic inserts (Dentsply Cavitron).
**A.** TFI®-EWPP Perio Probe; **B.** Focused Spray Insert (FSI® 10), universal design; **C.** TFI®-10, universal design; **D.** TFI®-3; **E.** TFI®-1; **F.** Precision-thin insert, SLI-10L left; **G.** Precision-thin insert, SLI-10R right; **H.** Precision-thin insert, SLI-10S straight.

gingival calculus deposits and accessible subgingival deposits prior to removal of finer deposits with curets or precision-thin inserts. Another design parallels the shape and size of a periodontal probe (EWPP, Cavitron®, Dentsply Equipment) (see Figure 10-12A). It is indicated for use subgingivally from 1 to 3 mm (or greater) depending on tissue tone, access, and gingival sensitivity. Both the universal design and periodontal probelike design can be used in conjunction with precision-thin inserts because the thinner tip and ultrasonic energy is not always capable of fracturing tenacious deposits.

Use of precision-thin inserts for periodontal debridement is covered thoroughly in Chapter 12. Selection of the precision-tip insert for ultrasonic procedures seems to be, at present, based on therapist preference, client conditions and preference, and the availability of equipment. There are few clinical studies evaluating the effectiveness of precision thin inserts (see Chapter 12); however, research results support the premise that ultrasonic instrumentation and hand instrumentation produce a similar clinical response even though the effect on root surface smoothness remains controversial (AAP, Consensus Report, Discussion Section II, 1989). Once the availability of equipment is overcome, client preference can be a valuable factor in the selection process. Discussing both options with the client including a review of the advantages and disadvantages of each (see Chapter 12) will facilitate collaborative nonsurgical periodontal care. Clients are extremely receptive to ultrasonic instrumentation for subgingival deposit removal and, in fact, may prefer it over hand-activated instruments. Documentation of the client preference in the record of services is useful for the next PMP visit.

A question related to instrument selection frequently asked by clinicians is if hand-activated instruments are needed in conjunction with precision-thin inserts for completion of calculus removal. This question can be answered by considering the following:

1. *Location of deposit.* Deposits found in furcations, deep pockets, and directly under the contact area are detected and removed with the ultrasonic. Because of the length and thin diameter of the precision-thin insert (approximately 0.3 to 0.6 mm), it is potentially more effective than curets in deep pockets and furcations (Dragoo, 1992). Calculus located directly under the contact area is sometimes challenging to remove with these inserts. If the clinician attempts removal in these challenging areas and is not successful, hand-activated curets, files, or sickles are employed.
2. *Variety of insert designs.* If plaque-retentive calculus is located at the proximal midline, then the curved right and left precision-thin inserts are used to reach this area. If a deep pocket exists that needs to be debrided, the straight, universal-type tip is available. Figure 10-12F, G & H shows the right, left, and straight designs.

3. *Therapist experience.* With increased experience, proficiency with these inserts is gained.

The most important consideration in treating the root surface is that it is necessary to employ whatever armamentarium is needed and appropriate to remove the detectable calculus and subgingival plaque. If this goal is accomplished with only ultrasonic instrumentation then hand instruments are not necessary. If, on the other hand, the thin insert is not achieving the desirable results, then hand instruments are employed to complete the debridement process.

Ultrasonic inserts are produced in three basic models depending on how the water spray is channeled to the working tip of the insert (Cavitron®, Dentsply Equipment). First, traditional and precision-thin inserts with a separate water conduit (trombone) (indicated by a "P" prior to the instrument number) are available that are usually less expensive than the other two types (see Figure 10-12F–H). Some therapists feel the water adjustment with this insert is better than with an insert with an internal water flow. The disadvantage is the possibility of bending the water conduit with use and autoclaving, thus, decreasing its longevity and effectiveness. Second, a flow-through model (TFI placed before the insert number) is available that has a casing that encloses the flow of water to the tip (see Figure 10-12A–E). The elimination of the separate water conduit eliminates the problems it creates; however, the casing enclosing the water is susceptible to fractures or cracks. This fracturing produces leakage, dripping, and a decreased water flow to the tip ebbing its effectiveness.

The newest model, the Focused Spray Insert™ (FSI), decreases the surface area of the spray enhancing comfort for the client and visibility for the clinician (see Figure 10-12B). The FSI™ has a narrower tip diameter than the other two models, potentially enhancing its ability to extend subgingivally. At the same time, however, the clinician is cautioned to adapt the side of the tip to the root surface to avoid creating undesirable root roughness or sensitivity. Currently, focused spray precision-thin inserts are also available. A variety of manufacturers produce these different models.

## Files

Files are selected when ultrasonic instrumentation with traditional inserts or precision-thin inserts does not fracture tenacious deposits adequately or efficiently. Files are particularly effective with burnished or smooth calculus. Each file is composed of a head (body), shank, and handle. The round, oval, oblong or rectangular head contains multiple cutting edges that, when adapted parallel to the calculus deposit and engaged, result in the fracturing of the calculus. The portion of the cutting edge of the file that faces the shank and handle, called the lip, is manufactured at either a 90° or 105° angle with the shank (see Figure 10-13). Rank angle refers to the dis-

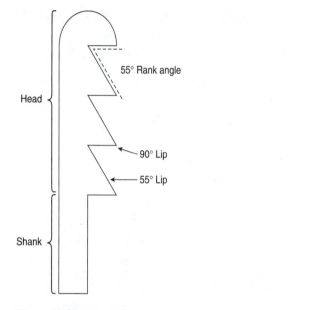

**Figure 10-13** File design.

tance in-between each lip, which approximates 55° depending on the design. The shank of a file is either straight or contra-angled, and varies in length and width to facilitate adaptation.

Three common file designs include the Hirschfeld series (#3/7, 5/11, 9/10) with three cutting edges, the Orban design (#6/7, 8/9, 10/11, 12/13) with approximately six cutting edges, and the Bedbug file (UW B/46) with ten to eleven cutting edges (see Figure 10-14). Each of the cutting edges is sharpened when dullness is recognized (see Chapter 11). The less number of cutting edges the file has, the more likely it is to fracture tenacious calculus deposits efficiently; therefore, the Hirschfeld and Orban designs are superior for fracturing heavy tenacious calculus. The UW B/46 Bedbug file, originally designed as a finishing file for smoothing roots and CEJs (Hoople, 1985), can be used to roughen the outside surface of the calculus deposit to promote removal with a curet or precision-thin insert. The Bedbug design might also be useful for removal of a moderate-sized deposit located on the CEJ on buccal/facial and lingual surfaces. Adaptation of the Bedbug design to proximal surfaces is limited due to the straight shank.

Periodontal instrumentation with files has received considerable criticism because of the potential for creating root surface roughness and gouging. This outcome can be diminished if the file is used *directly on* tenacious calculus deposits. Again it is noted that the file is only adapted to the heavy or moderate deposit, as other instruments (curets or precision-thin inserts) would be used to remove the remainder of the calculus adjacent to the cementum. File use is not indicated in the removal of bacterial plaque or endotoxins because the endotoxin derived from cell walls of gram-negative bacteria is only weakly adherent to periodontally involved root surfaces

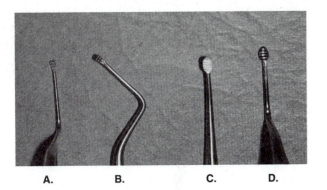

**Figure 10-14** Files. **A.** Hirschfeld 5/11; **B.** Hirschfeld 3/7; **C.** Bedbug design UW B/46; **D.** Orban 12/13.

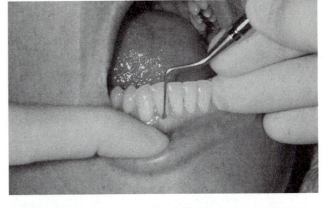

**Figure 10-15** Insertion of a Hirschfeld file subgingivally. Note the tight tissue tone.

(Kieser, 1993); therefore, it is readily removed with other instruments.

Another criticism of files has been their inability to adapt subgingivally to root anatomy due to the bulky design of the head; however, the Hirschfeld files have very small heads permitting easy insertion and adaptation subgingivally. In fact, access with files with very narrow heads is better than curets in some situations. The Hirschfeld designs have a narrower depth diameter (face to back) than the curet, which promotes easy insertion into the periodontal pocket, especially with tight tissue tone (Hoople, 1985) (see Figure 10-15). For this reason, Hirshfeld files are very effective near the junctional epithelium where it is not feasible to insert a curet under the calculus due to lack of space, which ranges from 0.2 to 1 mm (Schmid, 1996). The Hirschfeld designs are also useful for narrow deformities, in furcations with limited access, and between teeth within close proximity of one another (Hoople, 1985). Furthermore, files are useful for removing tenacious deposits from developmental depressions.

Although the use of files in periodontal instrumentation may be limited, when tenacious deposits exist, they are useful in preparing the biologically acceptable root surface. Other indications for files include removal of amalgam overhangs (see Chapters 3 and 14). Files with less cutting edges (Hirschfeld/Orban) are used to remove the bulk of the amalgam and files with many cutting edges (Bedbug) refine the restorative margin.

## Sickles

The single-ended or double-ended sickle is not used for deep subgingival debridement because of the straight design of the cutting edge limiting adaptation to the curvature of the root surface, the bulky working end limiting comfortable subgingival placement, and the pointed tip increasing the chance of producing rough roots. Sickles are useful, however, for removal of supragingival deposits, especially those located directly below contact areas in anterior regions of the mouth. When the inter-

dental papilla is healthy and fills the embrasure space, a sickle can be successfully adapted 1 to 2 mm subgingivally to remove deposit adjacent to contact areas. Anterior sickles have a straight shank and posterior designs have contra-angled shanks. The blades can be parallel to one another creating a triangular-shaped face as with the #30/33 designed for the anterior, or #31/32 for the posterior. The H6/H7 is an area-specific sickle with a straight shank designed for the anterior. The cutting blade (one on each end of the instrument) is slightly curved enhancing adaptation to contact areas. The sickle design is popular for implant maintenance instruments.

## Curets

Practitioners and students are familiar with both universal and area-specific curets due to their ability to adapt to all tooth surfaces, and the fact that for many decades they have been the instrument of choice for treating root surfaces. **Universal curets** were so named due to their ability to adapt to mesial and distal surfaces by alternating the dual cutting edges, adjusting fulcrum placement and positioning, and changing operator and client positioning. Popular designs are the Columbia series including the 4R/4L(posterior), 2R/2L(anterior), and the 13/14; as well as the Barnhardt 1/2 (posterior) and 5/6 (anterior). The Columbia 4R/4L and 2R/2L are chosen when calculus is moderate to heavy and tenacious because the shank is longer, wider (stronger), and less flexible than the 13/14 design. Barnhardt designs tend to have a narrower, straighter, and longer terminal shank than the Columbia design facilitating extension across the proximal surfaces and subgingivally. As with other instruments, universal designs differ slightly from manufacturer to manufacturer. The universal configuration is also commonly manufactured in unfilled plastic for implant maintenance.

**Area-specific curets** were introduced in dentistry over fifty years ago when Dr. Clayton Gracey recognized the need for a curet that would adapt to deep and nonaccessible periodontal pockets without traumatic distention of the gingiva (Hu-Friedy®, Product Catalog and Reference Guide, 1993). Gracey curets are available in an array of blade and shank designs numbered from 1 through 18; the lower the number, the more anterior in the mouth it is used (see Table 10-8). In review, the area-specific design refers to instruments made to adapt to specific areas or surfaces of the dentition. These instruments and their modifications have been said to be the best instruments for subgingival scaling and root planing because they adapt well to complex root anatomy (Pattison, Pattison, & Takei, 1996). The single cutting blade on each end of the double-ended instrument is "offset" indicating that the face of the blade is beveled at a 60° angle to the shank, unlike the universal design that has a face to shank angle of 90°. The blade curves in two planes meaning it curves upward and to the side. Rigid shanks are appropriate for removing moderate or heavy deposit while flexible shanks are indicated for light deposit and finishing of the root surface. In fact, an extra rigid shank is now available for the Gracey 5/6, 7/8, 11/12, and

13/14. The extra rigid shank, achieved by increased shank diameter, is marketed as having a unique shank angulation for enhanced "biting" action for powerful calculus removal (Hu-Friedy® Manufacturing Incorporated). The blade size is the same as standard Graceys.

Other area-specific designs are also available such as the Turgeon Modified Gracey Curets and Furcation Curets. The Turgeon series has a working end that is somewhat pie-shaped in cross section which is reported to improve blade sharpness and insertion (Hu-Friedy® Manufacturing Incorporated Product Catalog, 1993). The Furcation Curets are available in either buccal-lingual or mesial-distal designs. They were developed for scaling root concavities and furcations and have two blade widths: either 0.9 mm or 1.3 mm wide. Based on the figures previously presented about furcation entrance diameters, the 0.9 mm would be the best option.

A limitation of area-specific curets that is worth investigating is the extension of the working end on proximal surfaces of molar teeth where they are the widest, at the cervix. When adapted appropriately to the proximal sur-

**Table 10-8  Area-Specific Gracey Curets***

| Design | Number | Purpose | Shank Length and Angulation |
|---|---|---|---|
| Standard | 1/2 | Anterior teeth | Slight contra-angle |
| | 3/4 | Anterior teeth | Short contra-angle |
| | 5/6 | Anterior and premolars | Medium contra-angle |
| | 7/8 | Premolars and molars, facial and lingual surfaces | Medium contra-angle |
| | 9/10 | Molars | Long contra-angle |
| | 11/12 | Mesial surfaces of posterior teeth | Angulated |
| | 13/14 | Distal surfaces of posterior teeth | Angulated |
| | 11/14** | Mesial and distal surfaces of posterior teeth | Angulated |
| | 12/13** | Mesial and distal surfaces of posterior teeth | Angulated |
| | 15/.16 | Mesial surfaces of posterior teeth | Angulated |
| | 17/18 | Distal surfaces of posterior teeth | Angulated |
| Extended Shank | available in all patterns except 9/10 and 17/18 | Pocket depth 5 mm or greater | • Shank length is 3 mm longer than standard design<br>• Working end is not as wide as standard design |
| Mini-bladed | available in all patterns except 9/10 and 17/18 | • Normal pocket depth (5 mm or greater)<br>• Facial and lingual surfaces<br>• Furcations | • Shank length is 3 mm longer than standard design<br>• Working end is not as wide as standard design<br>• Blade length is 50% less than extended shank or standard design |

(Adapted from the Hu-Friedy® Manufacturing, Inc. Product Catalog and Reference Guide, 1993)

  *Instruments can be adapted in other areas than they were originally designed for.

**Designed to complete an entire facial or lingual sextant without changing instruments to increase efficiency.

face, the working end extends about 4 mm toward the midline potentially preventing overlapping of strokes in this area and extension into depressions and grooves. To reach the midline, the clinician would have to adapt the entire blade and activate the instrument with the shank near or touching the contact area. This is the same limitation recognized with the 11/12 explorer due to similarities in their designs. A universal curet design enhances removal in this area because the handle and shank of the instrument can be directed away from the contact area, which extends the terminal portion of the blade toward the midline to effectively engage deposit. This principle is similar to the adaptation of the Suter 2R/2L explorer to the proximal surface illustrated in Figure 10-10. Figure 10-16 compares the extension of the universal and area-specific curet on a proximal surface. Results of research studies comparing deposit detection and removal with various instruments at the midline of proximal surfaces would be valuable for application to NSPT.

The design features of universal and area-specific curets are compared in Table 10-9. In most cases where considerable debridement is necessary, both types of curets are needed. Universal curets are especially helpful in removing calculus and plaque located at the midline of the interproximal surface, on line angles, just beneath the gingival or crown margin, and for furcation involvement when access permits. Their limitation is that the shank is not as long as the area-specific design nor is the blade honed at an offset angle which limits effectiveness in deeper pockets. Typically, universals can be used in 4 to 5 mm probing depths depending on tissue tone. Area-specific designs are useful for negotiating irregular

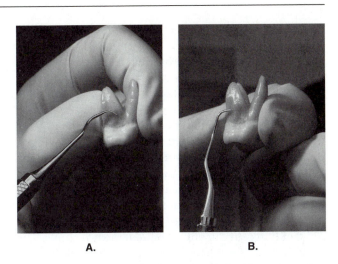

**A.**                                          **B.**

**Figure 10-16** Comparison of the extension of the universal and area-specific curet on a proximal surface. **A.** Universal curet adapted to proximal surface of maxillary first molar. **B.** Area-specific curet adapted to proximal surface of maxillary first molar.

pocket topography, reaching deposits located in deeper periodontal pockets, and for furcations. The recent development of area-specific designs with extended shanks (After-Five™, Hu-Friedy® Manufacturing Incorporated; Gracey +3 Access Curets, American Eagle Instruments, Incorporated) and mini-blades (Mini-Five™, Hu-Friedy® Manufacturing Incorporated; Gracey +3™ Access Curets, American Eagle Instruments, Incorporat-

**Table 10-9 Comparison of Universal and Area-Specific Curet Designs**

| Feature | Universal Design | Area-Specific Design |
|---|---|---|
| Blade Angle to Shank | When viewed in cross section from the toe, the face of the blade is perpendicular (90°) to the terminal shank | When viewed in cross section from the toe, the face of the blade is not perpendicular to the terminal shank; it is angled 60 to 70° from the lower shank |
| Number of Cutting Edges | Two | One; the lower (inferior) blade when viewed perpendicular to the floor or the blade with the largest outer curve |
| Curvature of the Blade When Viewed from the Lateral Surface | Curves slightly upward from the shank to the toe | Curves slightly upward from the shank to the toe |
| Curvature of the Blade When Viewed from the Face | Blades are parallel to one another | Blades are not parallel to one another and the toe is curved to the side |
| Shank Strength | Moderate | Flexible, moderate, rigid, or extra rigid |
| Deposit Recommendations | Light, moderate, or heavy | Flexible shank for light calculus deposit and debridement, increasing shank strength is needed for moderate to heavy calculus |

ed ) have further refined the access and effectiveness of these curets.

**Extended shank curets** have a terminal shank that is 3 mm longer than the standard area-specific design to negotiate periodontal pockets of 5 mm or greater. The blade is also thinner than the standard design allowing for easier insertion and reduced tissue distention. Nagy and others (1992) evaluated the effectiveness of subgingival scaling and root planing with rigid longer shank Gracey curets and rigid standard Gracey curets. One hundred forty maxillary and mandibular incisors, canines, and premolars were evaluated. With stereomicroscopic evaluation of the root surface there was no statistically significant difference in effect between the two curets. The mesial root surfaces had less calculus remaining (27 percent) than the other root surfaces (44 percent); and the distal surfaces had the most calculus remaining. The majority of remaining calculus was located in root flutes, below CEJs, and on root surface line angles which concurs with the findings of other researchers (Brayer et at., 1989; Fleisher et al., 1989). Mean curet efficiency subgingivally ranged from 1 mm to 3.46 mm depending on the root surface and not on the curet used. A limitation of this study noted by the authors was that the presence of tenacious calculus was present requiring more time for instrumentation than was permitted (15 minutes per tooth was used). The authors also noted that results might differ if different operators participated, if ultrasonics were employed, if fiberoptic illumination was utilized, and if multiple appointments were employed (versus one appointment).

The **mini-bladed curet** combines the features of the extended shank designs with a 50 percent reduction in blade length as compared to the extended shank or standard designs. Minibladed curets offer better adaptation to narrow facial and lingual surfaces of anterior teeth, furcations, and root surfaces in narrow and deep periodontal pockets. A limitation of miniblades is the extension to the midline of the interproximal surface. Both the extended shank and mini-bladed versions are available in any pattern except the 9/10 and 17/18 (Hu-Friedy® Manufacturing Incorporated). The 9/10 and the 17/18 designs both have accentuated shank bends and long terminal shanks enhancing their use in deeper pockets and difficult to reach areas even without the extended shank feature.

The Vision™ Curvettes represent another variation of an area-specific design (Hu-Friedy® Manufacturing Incorporated). The blade is 50 percent shorter than the traditional Gracey curets, thus the blade length is similar to minibladed curets. The blade, however, turns upward at the terminal portion unlike other area-specific designs. Curvettes were designed to enhance adaptation on incisor teeth with deep periodontal pockets (Long & Singer, 1992). There are four configurations: the Sub-Zero, the 1/2, 11/12, and 13/14. The Sub-Zero has a long shank for instrumentation on the facial and lingual surfaces and around line angles on premolars and ante-

rior teeth. The 1/2 is for anterior and premolar surfaces. The 11/12 is for mesial surfaces on molars and it is marketed for furcations. The 13/14 is for distal surfaces of molars and furcations. Both the 11/12 and 13/14 come in extended shank designs. Other features of the Vision™ Curvettes are that the tip of the blade and shank are centered over the handle and 5 and 10 mm shank markings are added to aid in visual assessment of pocket depth while instrumenting. Due to the short working end, their limitation is extension towards the midline of proximal surfaces especially of premolar and molar teeth. Another limitation might be the upward curvature of the blade that requires the clinician to carefully adapt the tip to the tooth surface to prevent gouging or striations. Singer and coworkers (1992) compared subgingival deposit removal with the Sub-Zero curvette and the Gracey 1/2 curet. Incisor teeth were tested in an in vitro model (a dentiform). Results indicated that the Sub-Zero curvette removed significantly ($p$ less than 0.0001) more of the surface material (black enamel paint) than the curet (60.7 percent and 46.3 percent respectively). Additional studies with in vivo comparison are needed.

Other curets for periodontal instrumentation include the Langer curets that feature area-specific shank designs coupled with universal curet blades. The Langer 1/2 has a shank resembling the 11/12 Gracey, but it is for both mesial and distal mandibular posterior surfaces. The Langer 3/4 has a shank similar to the Gracey 13/14 and is suitable for mesial and distal maxillary posterior surfaces. The Langer 5/6 has a shank similar to the Gracey 5/6 and it is designed for mesial and distal anterior surfaces as well as premolars. The new Langer 17/18 combines the accentuated features of the Gracey 17/18 and the blade with two cutting edges to treat both the mesial and distal surfaces of posterior teeth. The Langer set of instruments is recommended for debriding the entire dentition and they can be ordered in extended shanks, miniblades, or rigid shanks.

## SELECTION STRATEGIES

Selecting instruments for NSPT for clients who are returning for multiple appointments and for those new to the practice requires different decision making. Once the assessment data are collected, the clinician has the information available to make decisions about the best instrument options for that individual. When organizing tray setups at the beginning of the work day or clinical session, the clinician correlates the therapy planned for the appointment with the client's conditions. A review of the periodontal assessment; care plan; personal, dental, and medical history; and record of services are in order. A client who experienced sensitivity with hand-activated instruments during a previous appointment or who commented on the noise produced with a sharp curet might be interested in trying the precision thin ultrasonic inserts. If standard tray setups are arranged for the therapist by team members, then the hygienist has the option to package unique instruments such as the mini-bladed curets to add to the basic setup. A variety of prearranged trays is an option that provides both convenience and individuality in instrument selection.

If the client is new to the clinic or practice, screening over the telephone when making the appointment could aid in instrument selection. Frequently office coordinators will ask questions about length of time between dental hygiene visits, discomfort experienced at past visits, bleeding, or past dental records that can be forwarded prior to the appointment. This information can be somewhat useful in selecting instruments. Generally, however, with the new client the dental hygienist needs to anticipate a variety of conditions and select instruments that meet the needs of most clients. For example, the explorer that provides the best initial assessment of anatomical features and deposits such as the Suter 2R/2L is chosen for the new client. The most ideal and practical manual probe is selected. If furcation involvement is discovered accompanied by deep pockets filled with tenacious calculus, the extended shank 11/12 explorer, Nabers probe, working files, precision-thin ultrasonic inserts, and extended shank curets with miniblades might be chosen.

Another selection strategy involves the need to remove different calculus deposits within the same periodontal pocket requiring the use of multiple instruments. For example, a 5 to 6 mm pocket is present with heavy tenacious calculus located near the gingival margin and light calculus located apically near the epithelial attachment. In this case, different instruments are indicated for the coronal portion of the pocket as compared to the apical portion. Ultrasonic inserts and files are first used for removal of the tenacious deposit and then universal and area-specific curets with moderate to flexible shanks, or precision-thin inserts, are used to remove the light calculus and debride the subgingival plaque. Figure 10-17 is a self-evaluation mechanism to aid the student or practitioner in the instrument selection process.

---

1. Is therapy for a new client, reappointment, or maintenance?  _____ new   _____ reappointment   _____ maintenance

2. Are there any contraindications for ultrasonic instrumentation (see Chapter 12)?  _____ no   _____ yes   explain:

3. Does the previous record of services contain notes about instrument selection for reappointment or maintenance clients?  _____ no   _____ yes   explain:

4. Did I consider the size of the calculus deposit?  _____ light   _____ moderate   _____ heavy

5. Did I consider the location of the calculus deposit?

_____ near the epithelial attachment   _____ adjacent to contact areas   _____ proximal surfaces

_____ less than 5 mm subgingivally   _____ 5 mm or greater subgingivally

_____ generalized anteriors   _____ localized anteriors

_____ generalized posteriors   _____ localized posteriors

6. Did I consider the mode of attachment of the calculus deposit?  _____ tenacious   _____ not tenacious

7. Are instruments also selected for removal of bacterial plaque and its by-products?  _____ no   _____ yes   explain:

8. Does the tissue tone allow for insertion of the instrument(s) selected?  _____ no   _____ yes   explain:

9. Did I include different shank designs, diameters, and flexibility as needed?  _____ no   _____ yes   explain:

10. Are furcations and/or mobility present requiring specific instrument selection?  _____ no   _____ yes   explain:

SUMMARY:

Instruments selected include: _____

_____

Additional considerations include: _____

_____

_____

**Figure 10-17** Instrument selection self-assessment.

## DOCUMENTATION

It is extremely helpful to document instruments selected for NSPT in the client's permanent record of services. At subsequent appointments, efficiency and comfort are enhanced if references are available about client selec-tion preferences (ultrasonic versus hand-activated), or clinician strategies. Examples of clinician strategies include files for tenacious deposits and amalgam over-hangs, miniblades for the mandibular anterior segment, and generalized use of precision thin inserts.

# Summary

The clinician's ability to reach a therapeutic goal in NSPT is determined by professional knowledge, skill, experience, availability of biotechnical equipment/sup-plies, and the host response (AAP, Consensus Report, Discussion Section II, 1989). The therapeutic goal of ini-tial or active NSPT is healing, which is dependent on the thoroughness of microflora-toxin removal (AAP, Con-sensus Report, Discussion Section II, 1989). Proper judg-ment in instrument selection is one factor that can enhance operator skill and improve the chances for optimal healing. Another factor is the application of a sound theoretical knowledge base in periodontal therapy in relation to root anatomy, gingival contour, pocket topography, furcation architecture, and the heal-ing process (see Chapter 1). The characteristics of cal-culus and other plaque-retentive factors is a third consideration.

It is challenging to keep abreast of all the new devel-opments in dental hygiene instrument design and func-tion. A practitioner should feel confident, however, in trying new instruments because an analysis of the design characteristics will reveal the purpose and use of the instrument. It is recognized that instrument selection is a subjective and somewhat personal issue and, therefore, dental hygienists have different philosophies about how they select instruments for their clients. It is hoped that the content of this chapter brings forth new ideas for the professional and a desire to match anatomy, deposit characteristics, and instrument design for the welfare of the client in NSPT.

# Case Studies

**Case Study One:** Compare and contrast scaling, root planing, and debridement. Address purposes, indica-tions, sequelae, endpoint, and related instrument selec-tion for each using a chart similar to Table 10-10.

**Case Study Two:** Briefly identify and discuss the anatom-ical characteristics of root surfaces that affect instrument selection. Address root anatomy, root surface irregulari-ties, furcations, pocket topography, and gingival con-tour and tone.

**Case Study Three:** Berk Higgins presents for care as a new client. He was referred to your office by another client of record and reported the following to the receptionist who scheduled his first ninety-minute appointment:

- "bleeding gums"
- "deep pockets on the top back teeth"
- "loosening of the bottom front teeth"

Client records from another practice are not extremely relevant because his last appointment was seven years ago. Perhaps radiographs and periodontal assessment from this last dental hygiene visit would be useful for comparing periodontal conditions. What instruments would you select for initial assessment of the periodontal conditions?

**Case Study Four:** During the assessment of Berk Higgins, you discover the following:

- 6 and 7 mm pocket depth on the maxillary molars and mandibular anteriors,
- only 1 mm of recession in some of the above areas indicating 7 to 8 mm of clinical attachment loss,
- generalized 4 to 5 mm periodontal pocket depth in other areas,
- Class II furcations on the facial surfaces of the max-illary molars,
- generalized bleeding,
- no health history contraindications for an ultrason-ic instrument,
- supragingival and subgingival calculus deposit is only light and generalized throughout the mouth,
- subgingival bacterial plaque is noticed when probing and exploring.

Would you use hand-activated instruments if you initial-ly used precision-thin inserts? If you only had hand-activated instruments, would instrument selection change?

**Case Study Five:** Consider case study four. What if all the periodontal conditions remain the same, but, the calcu-lus size changes as follows:

- heavy tenacious calculus deposits in maxillary molars located near the attachment, adjacent to the cementoenamel junction, adjacent to the contact areas, and at the midline of proximal surfaces,
- all other root surfaces have light to moderate calculus deposits located subgingivally on proximal surfaces, at the cementoenamel junction, and near the epithelial attachment.

What instruments would you select for periodontal instrumentation? Consider assessment, removal of calculus deposit, and removal of bacterial plaque and its by-products.

## Case Study Discussions

### Discussion—Case Study One:

**Table 10-10  Comparison of Scaling, Root Planing, and Debridement**

| | Purpose | Indications | Sequelae | Endpoint | Instrumentation |
|---|---|---|---|---|---|
| Scaling | To remove bacterial plaque and calculus from tooth crowns and root surfaces | Usually performed only where calculus deposits exist | Possible gingival sensitivity and hemorrhage, root sensitivity would not result because intentional removal of cementum does not occur | After oral prophylaxis where supra- and subgingival scaling is performed with polishing | Mechanical and hand-activated instrumentation; mechanical is used primarily for supragingival and gross, heavy deposit; subgingival calculus removal is performed with hand-activated instruments |
| Root Planing | To remove cementum and dentin that is rough, permeated with calculus, or contaminated with microorganisms or toxins | Treatment of established periodontal disease; rough root surfaces | Possible gingival sensitivity and hemorrhage, root sensitivity occurs in selected cases or sites | Glassy, smooth and calculus-free root surface as judged by clinical detection with an explorer; 4 to 6 week reevaluation is recommended for assessment of root surface smoothness and healing | Hand-activated instrumentation; area-specific curets are used most often with a finishing/root planing stroke |
| Debridement | Suggested as an alternative to scaling and root planing; removal of tooth and root surface irregularities to the extent that adjacent soft tissues maintain or return to health | Used where clinically detectable calculus, calculus-embedded cementum, and other plaque-retentive factors are present; also subgingival plaque and endotoxin removal occurs where clinical data reveals gingival inflammation, bleeding, pocket depth and/or attachment loss | Possible gingival sensitivity and hemorrhage | Health as defined by no bleeding, no gingival inflammation, reduced or eliminated pocket depth, and maintenance or gain in attachment level; assessed at a 4 to 6 week reevaluation visit | Mechanical and/or hand-activated instrumentation; with mechanical (ultrasonic) instruments) both traditional inserts and precision-thin inserts are used; with hand-activated instruments moderate to light pressure is indicated depending on the purpose of the stroke |

**Discussion—Case Study Two:**

Root anatomy:

1. *Root shape:* convex and concave surfaces (the ribbon effect) (see Figure 10-1); developmental depressions and grooves exist that must be considered; locations of concern are depressions located approximately at the midline of proximal surfaces and coronal to furcation entrances.
2. *Root width:* related to length of working end of the instrument on the proximal surfaces; roots are widest at the cervix and taper as they extend apically (see Table 10-2); research results indicate that deposits frequently remain on proximal surfaces after instrumentation.
3. *Root length:* bears a relationship to location of depressions and grooves and to prognosis as illustrated in Figure 10-3.
4. *Curvature of the CEJ:* expected location (see Table 10-2) must be considered during instrumentation to decipher calculus deposits from anatomy; the relationship of the cementum and enamel also affect assessment and removal of deposits.
5. *Contact areas:* expected anatomy is considered; appraisal of the contact areas of each individual client occurs during the assessment phase of care; instrumentation started on the lingual surfaces is more efficient because the lingual embrasure space is larger.
6. *Deviations in the root:* usually occur in the apical third; therefore, they are considerations when advanced bone loss is present; are viewed radiographically and related to instrumentation; they negatively affect the prognosis.

Root surface irregularities:

1. *Root caries:* creates tactile roughness; indents are concave; can be sensitive; detected by correlating radiographic findings, tactile evaluation, and client sensitivity; advanced lesions might be concave.
2. *Abrasion, erosion, and abfractions:* occur in the cervical one-third; they are smooth and concave; therefore, surface texture is not granular like calculus.
3. *Grooves or indentations:* are usually microscopic yet some are detectable with an explorer; they feel narrow and long and are not completely eliminated with calculus removal or debridement strokes, reevaluation of these areas is imperative to assess if healing occurred or if further instrumentation is indicated.

Furcation involvement: (see Table 10-3)

1. *Location in relation to the CEJ:* The further away the furcation entrance is from the CEJ the less likely it is to be diseased, but when disease occurs, access to the area is difficult.
2. *Enamel projections:* Confuse clinicians; the projections are convex and rounded; they are not

removed with repeated instrumentation; increased potential for pocket depth exists.

3. *Width of the separation of the roots:* The wider the root, the easier the access and, therefore, the more effective the instrumentation; roots of mandibular second molars are not well separated; first molar teeth have an average furcation entrance diameter of 0.75 to 1 mm; the blade width of curets is around 1 mm, therefore, adaptation in the furcation entrance at the roof is difficult.
4. *Vertical and horizontal dimensions:* The width and depth are measured with a periodontal probe; however, a margin of error exists in probing the dimensions; the depth of furcations should be considered when exposure indicates the need to debride the areas (see Figure 10-4).
5. *Relationship of the gingiva:* Exposed furcation involvement is easier to debride than when the gingival occludes the defect; an exposed furcation involvement is also easier for the client to cleanse.

Pocket topography:

1. *Shape of the pocket:* involves the entire circumference of each pocket; shape can vary; pockets in furcation areas may spiral, increasing the difficulty for thorough debridement.
2. *Multiple pockets:* can form on any one tooth each involving a different area; accurate periodontal probing is a must.

Gingival contour and tone:

1. *Shape of the gingival margin and interdental papilla:* is usually not normal with periodontitis; as recession and loss of attachment occur, loss of interdental papilla is likely creating a supragingival environment more accessible than when interdental papilla is at normal height creating a subgingival environment.
2. *Tissue tone:* refers to the elasticity of the gingiva; tight tone hinders subgingival access; burnished or smooth calculus might be present even when tight tissue tone exists, indicating a healthy state when visually inspected and a diseased state when probed; moderate to heavy calculus deposits usually relate to elastic inflamed tissue where access is possible without tissue distention.

**Discussion—Case Study Three:** For assessment, a periodontal probe and explorer is indicated. The ideal periodontal probe would have a round working end with a diameter of 0.6 mm or less, a ball-end configuration, and a straight or right-angled shank. Millimeter measurement indications would be ideal such as those on the Williams or UNC. A periodontal probe that meets all the specified qualifications is the Maryland Moffitt design. Because of the deep pockets in the maxillary posterior areas, 1N and 2N Nabers furcation probes are indicated.

If a screening system is used, a specific probe will be incorporated that meets most of the ideal qualifications of a manual probe. If an automated probe is used, a standard manual probe is not necessary.

Explorers employed would include the After Five 11/12 design due to the client's description of deep pockets and mobility. Another explorer would be added to the armamentarium to negotiate proximal surfaces. The Suter 2R/2L is an ideal choice or another explorer design that would facilitate reaching the midline of proximal surfaces.

**Discussion—Case Study Four:** It is possible to debride all areas with precision-thin inserts. These thinner inserts are ideal considering the periodontal pocket depth, need to extend to the epithelial attachment, the furcations, the generalized bleeding, and the size and location of calculus. There is a chance that hand-activated instruments are also needed for debridement if precision-thin inserts do not remove detectable calculus in some areas. If this is the case, mini-bladed area-specific curets and universal curets might be indicated.

If precision-thin inserts are not available, mini-bladed area specific curets and universals might be adequate to complete periodontal debridement. The mini-bladed instruments would debride near the epithelial attachment, in the furcations, at the line angles, and adjacent to the cementoenamel junction and contact areas. A sickle might also be incorporated for contact areas. The universal design would be helpful at line angles, near the cementoenamel junction, and at the midline of proximal surfaces.

**Discussion—Case Study Five:**

*Assessment:* Ideal periodontal probe, furcation probes, and multiple explorers are needed as identified in the discussion of case study one.

*Calculus removal:* If ultrasonics are employed, standard inserts and precision-thin inserts are indicated. The precision-thin inserts are not likely to remove the tenacious deposits in the maxillary molars and mandible anterior regions. A file will be necessary to fragment the tenacious deposits. Precision-thin inserts are ideal; however, for the periodontal pocket depth and furcations, and mobility once the heavy deposit is reduced in size. A sickle is indicated for the contact areas should precision-thin inserts not be adequate in this location. Extended shank minibladed area-specific curets and a universal design might also be needed for calculus removal if precision-thin inserts are not effective.

*Bacterial plaque removal:* The ultrasonic instrument will accomplish removal of bacterial plaque and its by-products. If ultrasonics are not used, debridement can be accomplished with extended shank area-specific designs and universal designs. A universal design with a long working end is recommended to debride midline areas of molar teeth due to their proximal width near the cervix.

## REFERENCES

American Academy of Periodontology. (1989). Consensus Report, Discussion Section II, 1113–1120. In *Proceedings of the world workshop in clinical periodontics*. Chicago: American Academy of Periodontology.

Ash, M. M. (1993). *Wheeler's dental anatomy, physiology, and occlusion* (7th ed.). Philadelphia: W.B. Saunders Co.

Badersten, A., Nilvéus, R., & Egelberg, J. (1981). Effect of nonsurgical periodontal therapy. I. Moderately advanced periodontitis. *Journal of Clinical Periodontology, 8*, 57–72.

Badersten, A., Nilvéus, R., & Egelberg, J. (1984). Effect of nonsurgical periodontal therapy. II. Severely advanced periodontitis. *Journal of Clinical Periodontology, 11*, 63–76.

Badersten, A., Nilvéus, R., & Egelberg, J. (1985). Effect of nonsurgical periodontal therapy. VI. Localization of sites with probing attachment loss. *Journal of Clinical Periodontology, 12*, 351–359.

Badersten, A., Nilvéus, R., & Egelberg, J. (1990). Scores of plaque, bleeding, suppuration and probing depth to predict probing attachment loss. 5 years of observation following nonsurgical periodontal therapy. *Journal of Clinical Periodontology, 17*, 102–107.

Becker, W., Becker, B. E., Ochserbein, C., Kerry, G., Caffesse, R., Morrison, E. C., & Prichard, I. (1988). A longitudinal study comparing scaling, osseous surgery and modified Widman procedures. Results after one year. *Journal of Periodontology, 59*, 351–365.

Birek, P., McCollough, C. A., & Hardy, V. (1987). Gingival attachment level measurements with an automated periodontal probe. *Journal of Clinical Periodontology, 14*, 472–477.

Bower, R. C. (1979a). Furcation morphology relative to periodontal treatment. Furcation entrance architecture. *Journal of Periodontology, 50*, 23–27.

Bower, R. C. (1979b). Furcation morphology relative to periodontal treatment. Furcation root surface anatomy. *Journal of Periodontology, 50*, 366–374.

Brayer, W. K., Mellonig, J. T., Dunlap, R. M., Marinak, K. W., & Carson, R. E. (1989). Scaling and root planing effectiveness: The effect of root surface access and operator experience. *Journal of Periodontology, 60*, 67–72.

Caffesse, R. G., Sweeney, P. L., & Smith, B. A. (1986). Scaling and root planing with and without periodontal flap surgery. *Journal of Periodontology, 60*, 402–409.

Carranza, F. A. (1996a). Dental calculus. In F. A. Carranza & M. G. Newman (Eds.), *Clinical periodontology* (8th ed.). Philadelphia: W.B. Saunders Co.

Carranza, F. A. (1996b). The periodontal pocket. In F. A. Carranza & M. G. Newman (Eds.), *Clinical periodontology* (8th ed.). Philadelphia: W.B. Saunders Co.

Carranza, F. A. & Ubios, A. M. (1996). The tooth supporting structures. In F. A. Carranza & M. G. Newman (Eds), *Clinical periodontology* (8th ed.). Philadelphia: W.B. Saunders Co.

Carranza, F. A., Saglie, R., Newman, M. G., & Valentin, P. L.

(1983). Scanning and transmission electron microscopic study of tissue-invading microorganisms in localized juvenile periodontitis. *Journal of Periodontology, 54,* 598.

Cheetham, A. H., Wilson, M., & Kieser, J. B. (1988). Root surface debridement: An in vitro assessment. *Journal of Clinical Periodontology, 15,* 288–292.

Ciancio, S. G. (1989). Nonsurgical periodontal treatment. In *Proceedings of the world workshop in clinical periodontics.* Chicago: American Academy of Periodontology.

Claffey, N. (1991). Decision making in periodontal therapy. The reevaluation. *Journal of Clinical Periodontology, 18,* 384–389.

Claffey, N., Loos, B., Gantes, B., Martin, M., Heins, P., & Egelberg, J. (1988). The relative effects of therapy and periodontal disease on loss of probing attachment after root debridement. *Journal of Clinical Periodontology, 15,* 163–169.

Claffey, N., Nylund, K., Kiger, R., Garrett, S., & Egelberg, J. (1990). Diagnostic predictability of scores of plaque, bleeding, suppuration and probing depth for probing attachment loss. 31/2 years of observation following initial periodontal therapy. *Journal of Clinical Periodontology, 17,* 108–114.

Dragoo, M. R. (1992). A clinical evaluation of hand and ultrasonic instruments on subgingival debridement. Part I. With unmodified and modified ultrasonic inserts. *International Journal of Periodontics and Restorative Dentistry, 12,* 312–323.

Drisko, C. L. & Killoy, W. J. (1991). Scaling and root planing: Removal of calculus and subgingival organisms. *Current Opinion in Dentistry, 1,* 74–80.

Dubrez, B., Graf, J. M., Vuagnat, P., & Cimasoni, G. (1990). Increase of interproximal bone density after subgingival instrumentation. A quantitative radiographical study. *Journal of Periodontology, 61,* 723–731.

Fine, D. H. (1992). Incorporating new technologies in periodontal diagnosis into training programs and critical care: A critical assessment and plan for the future. *Journal of Periodontology, 63,* 383–393.

Fleischer, H., Mellonig, J., Brayer, W., Gray, J., & Barnett, J. (1989). Scaling and root planing efficacy in multirooted teeth. *Journal of Periodontology, 60,* 402–409.

Fowler, C., Garrett, S., Crigger, M., & Egelberg, J. (1982). Histologic probe position in treated and untreated human periodontal tissues. *Journal of Clinical Periodontology, 9,* 373–385.

Freed, H. K., Copper, R. L., & Kalkwarf, K. L. (1983). Evaluation of periodontal probing forces. *Journal of Periodontology, 54,* 488–492.

Garnick, J. J., Keagle, J. G., Searle, J. R., King, G. E., & Thompson, W. O. (1989). Gingival resistance to probing forces. II. The effect of inflammation and pressure on probe displacement in beagle dog gingivitis. *Journal of Periodontology, 60,* 498–505.

Gher, M. E. & Vernino, A. R. (1980). Root morphology—clinical significance in pathogenesis and treatment of periodontal disease. *Journal of the American Dental Association, 101,* 627–633.

Goodson, J. M., Tanner, A. C. R., Haffajee, A. D., Sornbager, G. C., & Sovansky, S. S. (1982). Patterns of progression and regression of advanced destructive periodontal disease. *Journal of Periodontology, 9,* 472–481.

Greenstein, G. (1992). Periodontal response to mechanical nonsurgical therapy: A review. *Journal of Periodontology, 63,* 118–130.

Greenstein, G. (1994). Diagnosis of periodontal diseases. *Compendium of Continuing Education in Oral Hygiene, 3,* 2–13.

Grippo, J. O. & Simring, M. (1995). Dental erosion revisited. *Journal of the American Dental Association, 126,* 619–630.

Haake, S. K. (1996). Periodontal microbiology: Host bacteria interactions in periodontal diseases. In F. A. Carranza & M. G. Newman (Eds), (8th ed.). *Clinical periodontology.* Philadelphia: W.B. Saunders Co.

Hall, W. B. (1994). Furcation involvements. In W. B. Hall, W. E. Roberts, & E. E. LaBarre (Eds.), *Decision making in dental treatment planning.* St. Louis: Mosby-Year Book, Inc..

Hamp, S. E., Nyman, S., & Lindhe, J. (1975). Periodontal treatment of multirooted teeth. Results after 5 years. *Journal of Clinical Periodontology, 2,* 126–135.

Hill, R. W., Ramfjord, S. P., Morrison, E. C., Appleberry, E. A., Caffesse, R. G., Kerry, G. J., & Nissle, R. R. (1981). Four types of periodontal treatment compared over two years. *Journal of Periodontology, 52,* 655–662.

Hoople, S. (1985). Files provide desirable results in patient treatment procedures. *RDH,* Nov/Dec, 22–24.

*Hu-Friedy®, product catalog and reference guide.* (1993). Chicago: Hu-Friedy® Manufacturing Incorporated.

Huennekens, S. C. & Daniel, S. J. (1992). Task analysis of the ODU 11/12 explorer. *Journal of Dental Hygiene,* January, 24–26.

Hughes, F. J. & Smales, F. C. (1986). Immunohistochemical investigation of the presence and distribution of cementum-associated lippolysaccharides in periodontal disease. *Journal of Periodontology Research, 21,* 660–667.

Isidor, F. & Karring, T. (1986). Long-term effect of surgical and nonsurgical periodontal treatment. A 5-year clinical study. *Journal of Periodontal Research, 21,* 462–472.

Itoiz, M. A. & Carranza, F. A. (1996). The gingiva. In F. A. Carranza & M. G. Newman (Eds.), *Clinical periodontology* (8th ed.). Philadelphia: W.B. Saunders Co.

Jeffcoat, M. K. (1994). Diagnosis of periodontal diseases: Building a bridge from today's methods to tomorrow's technology. *Journal of Dental Education, 58*(8), 613–619.

Jendersen, M. D., Allen, E. P., Bayne, S. C., Donovan, T. E., Hansson, T. L., Klooster, J., & Kois, J. C. (1994). B. R. Lang (Ed.), Annual review of related dental literature: Report of the committee on scientific investigation of the American Academy of Restorative Dentistry. *Journal of Prosthetic Dentistry, 72,* 39–77.

Jones, S. L., Lozdan, I., & Boyde, A. (1972). Tooth surfaces treated in situ with periodontal instruments scanning electron microscopic studies. *British Dental Journal, 132,* 57–64.

Jones, W. A. & O'Leary, T. J. (1978). The effectiveness of in vivo root planing in removing bacterial endotoxin from the roots of periodontally-involved teeth. *Journal of Periodontology,* 337–342.

Kaldahl, W. B., Kalkwarf, K. L., Patil, K. D., & Molvar, M. P. (1990). Relationship of gingival bleeding, gingival suppuration, and supragingival plaque to attachment loss. *Journal of Periodontology, 61,* 347–352.

Kalkwarf, K. L., Kaldahl, W. B., & Kashinath, D. W. (1988). Evaluation of furcation region response to periodontal therapy. *Journal of Periodontology, 59,* 794–804.

Keagle, J. G., Garnick, J. J., Searle, I. A., King, G. F., & Morse, P. K. (1989). Gingival resistance to probing force. Determination of optimal diameter. *Journal of Periodontology, 60,* 167–171.

Kepic, T. J., O'Leary, T. J., & Kafrawy, A. H. (1990). Total calculus removal: An attainable objective? *Journal of Periodontology, 61,* 16–20.

Kieser, J. B. (1993). Nonsurgical periodontal therapy. In N. P. Lang & T. Karring (Eds), *Proceedings of the 1st european workshop on periodontology.* London: Quintessence Publishing Co., Ltd.

Kingman, A., Löe, H., Ånerud, A., & Boysen, H. (1991). Errors in measuring parameters associated with periodontal health and disease. *Journal of Periodontology, 62,* 477–486.

Kogon, S. L. (1986). The prevalence, locations, and confirmation of palato-radicular grooves in maxillary incisors. *Journal of Periodontology, 57,* 231–234.

Krayer, J. W. & Rees, T. D. (1993). Histologic observations on the topography of a human periodontal pocket viewed in transverse step-serial sections. *Journal of Periodontology, 64,* 585–588.

Lang, N. P., Nyman, S., Senn, C., & Joss, A. (1991). Bleeding or probing as it relates to probing force and gingival health. *Journal of Clinical Periodontology, 18,* 257–261.

Lang, N. P. & Bragger, V. (1990). Periodontal diagnosis in the 1990s. *Journal of Clinical Periodontology, 18,* 370–379.

Leung, S. W. & Jensen, A. T. (1958). Factors controlling the deposition of calculus. *International Dental Journal, 8,* 613.

Lindhe, J., Westfelt, E., Nyman, S., Sovansky, S. J., & Haffajee, A. D. (1984). Long term effect of surgical/nonsurgical treatment of periodontal disease. *Journal of Clinical Periodontology, 11,* 448–458.

Listgarten, M. A., Mao, R., & Robinson, P. J. (1976). Periodontal probing: The relationship of the probe tip to periodontal tissues. *Journal of Periodontology, 47,* 511.

Long, B. A. & Singer, D. L. (1992). A new curet series: The Gracey Curvettes. *Journal of Dental Hygiene, 12,* 48–52.

Magnusson, I. & Wilson, T. G. (1992). Examination of patients with periodontal disease. In T. G. Wilson, K. S. Kornman, & M. G. Newman (Eds.), *Advances in periodontics,* pp. 15–38. Chicago: Quintessence Publishing Co., Inc.

Masters, D. H. & Hoskins, S. W. (1964). Projection of cervical enamel into molar furcations. *Journal of Periodontology, 35,* 49–53.

Moore, I., Wilson, M., & Kieser, J. B. (1986). The distribution of bacterial lipopolysaccharide (endotoxin) in relation to periodontally involved root surfaces. *Journal of Clinical Periodontology, 13,* 748–751.

Moriarty, I. D., Hutchens, L. H., and Scheitler, L. E. (1989). Histological evaluation of periodontal probe penetration in untreated facial molar furcations. *Journal of Clinical Periodontology, 16,* 21–26.

Nagy, R. J., Otomo-Corgel, J., & Stambaugh, R. (1992). The effectiveness of scaling and root planing with curets designed for deep pockets. *Journal of Periodontology, 63,* 954–959.

Newman, M. G., Sanz, M., Nisengard, R. C., & Haake, S. K. (1996). Host-bacteria interactions in periodontal diseases. In F. A. Carranza & M. G. Newman (Eds.), *Clinical periodontology* (8th ed.). Philadelphia: W.B. Saunders Co.

Nield-Gehrig, J. S. & Houseman, G. A. (1996). *Fundamentals of periodontal instrumentation* (3rd ed.). Baltimore: Williams & Wilkins.

Nordland, P., Garrett, S., Kiger, R., Vanooteghem, R., Hutchens,

L., & Egelberg, J. (1987). The effect of plaque control and root debridement in molar teeth. *Journal of Clinical Periodontology, 14,* 231–235.

Nyman, S., Sarhed, G., Ericsson, I., Gottlow, J., & Karring, T. (1986). The role of "diseased" root cementum for healing following treatment of periodontal disease: A clinical study. *Journal of Clinical Periodontology, 15,* 464–468.

Parakkal, P. F. (1979). Proceedings of the workshop on quantitative evaluation of periodontal diseases by physical measurement techniques. *Journal of Dental Research, 58,* 547–553.

Pattison, A. M. & Pattison, G. L. (1992). *Periodontal instrumentation* (2nd ed.). Norwalk, Connecticut: Appleton & Lange.

Pattison, A. M. & Pattison, G. L. (1996). Principles of periodontal instrumentation. In F. A. Carranza & M. G. Newman (Eds.), *Clinical periodontology* (8th ed.). Philadelphia: W.B. Saunders Co.

Pattison, A. M., Pattison, G. L., & Takei, H. H. (1996). The periodontal instrumentarium. In F. A. Carranza & M. G. Newman (Eds.), *Clinical periodontology* (8th ed.). Philadelphia: W.B. Saunders Co.

Perry, D. A., Beemsterboer, & Carranza, F. A. (1990). *Techniques and theory of periodontal instrumentation.* Philadelphia: W.B. Saunders Co.

Pihlström, B. L., McHugh, R. B., Oliphant, T. H., & Ortiz-Campos, C. (1983). Comparison of surgical and nonsurgical treatment of periodontal disease. A review of current studies and additional results after 6 1/2 years. *Journal of Clinical Periodontology, 10,* 524–541.

Pihlström, B. L., Oliphant, T. H., & McHugh, R .B. (1984). Molar and nonmolar teeth compared over 6 1/2 years following two methods of periodontal therapy. *Journal of Periodontology, 55,* 499–504.

Pihlström, B. L., Ortiz-Campos, C., & McHugh, R. B. (1981). A randomized four-year study of periodontal therapy. *Journal of Periodontology, 52,* 227–242.

Ramfjord, S. P. & Ash, M. M. (1979). *Periodontology and periodontics.* Philadelphia: W.B. Saunders Co.

Ramfjord, S. P., Caffesse, R .G., Morrison, E. C., Hill, R. W., Kerry, G. I., Appleberry, E. A., Nissle, R. R., & Stults, D. C. (1987). Four modalities of periodontal treatment compared over 5 years. *Journal of Clinical Periodontology, 14,* 445–452.

Ramfjord, S. P., Morrison, E. C., Burgett, F. G., Nissle, R. R., Shick, R. A., Zann, G. J., & Knowles, J. W. (1982). Oral hygiene and maintenance of periodontal support. *Journal of Periodontology, 53,* 26–30.

Rams, T. E. & Slots, J. (1993). Comparison of two pressure-sensitive periodontal probes and a manual periodontal probe in shallow and deep pockets. *International Journal of Periodontal Restorative Dentistry, 13,* 521–529.

Rosling, B. G. & McGuire, M. K. (1992). Mild chronic adult periodontitis. In T. G. Wilson, K. S. Kornman, & M. G. Newman (Eds.), *Advances in periodontics.* Chicago: Quintessence Publishing Co.

Saglie, R., Johanson, J. R., & Flotragh, L. (1975).The zone of completely and partially destructed periodontal fibres in pathological pockets. *Journal of Clinical Periodontology, 12,* 198.

Schmid, M. O. (1996). Preparation of the tooth surface. In F. A. Carranza & M. G. Newman (Eds.), *Clinical periodontology* (8th ed.). Philadelphia: W.B. Saunders Co.

Sherman, P. R., Hutchens, L. H., Jewson, L. G., Moriarity, J. M.,

Genco, G. W., & McFall, W. T. (1990). The effectiveness of subgingival scaling and root planing I. Clinical detection of residual calculus. *Journal of Clinical Periodontology, 61*, 3–8.

Singer, D. L., Long, B. A., Lozanoff, S., & Senthilselvan, A. (1992). Evaluation of a new periodontal curet: An in vitro study. *Journal of Clinical Periodontology, 19*, 549–552.

Smart, G. J., Wilson, M., Davies, E. H., & Kieser, J. B. (1990). The assessment of ultrasonic root surface debridement by determination of residual endotoxin levels. *Journal of Clinical Periodontology, 17*, 174–178.

Spray, J. R., Garnick, J. J., Doles, L. R., & Klawitter, J. J. (1978). Microscopic demonstration of the position of periodontal probes. *Journal of Periodontology, 49*, 148.

Van der Velden, V. (1978). Influence on periodontal health on probing depth and bleeding tendency. *Journal of Clinical Periodontology, 7*, 129–139.

Van der Velden, V. & De Vries, J. H. (1978). Introduction of a new periodontal probe: The pressure probe. *Journal of Clinical Periodontology, 5*, 188–197.

Van der Zee, E., Davies, E. H., & Newman, H. N. (1991). Marking width, calibration from tip and tine diameter of periodontal probes. *Journal of Clinical Periodontology, 18*, 576–580.

Vanooteghem, R., Hutchens, L. H., Garrett, S., Kiger, R., & Egelberg, J. (1987). Bleeding upon probing and probing depth indicators of the response to plaque control and root debridement. *Journal of Clinical Periodontology, 14*, 226–230.

Walsh, T. F. & Saxby, M. S. (1989). Inter- and intra-examiner variability rising standard and constant force periodontal probes. *Journal of Clinical Periodontology, 16*, 140–143.

Watts, T. (1987). Constant force probing with and without stent in untreated periodontal disease: The clinical reproducibility problem and possible sources of error. *Journal of Clinical Periodontology, 14*, 407–411.

Wilkins, E. M. (1994). *Clinical practice of the dental hygienist* (7th ed.). Baltimore: Williams & Wilkins.

Woelfel, J. B. (1990). *Dental anatomy: Its relevance to dentistry* (4th ed.). Philadelphia: Lea & Febiger.

Wong, M. G. (1994). Root morphology. In M. L. Darby & P. M. Walsh (Eds.), *Dental hygiene theory and practice.* Philadelphia: W.B. Saunders Co.

Young, S. N., O'Hehir, T. E., & Woodall, I. R. (1993). Periodontal debridement. In I. R. Woodall (Ed.), (4th ed.). *Comprehensive dental hygiene care,* St. Louis: Mosby-Year Book, Inc.

Zander, H. A. (1953). The attachment of calculus to root surfaces. *International Journal of Periodontology, 24*, 16.

Zander, H. A. (1955). The role of calculus in the etiology and treatment of periodontal disease. *Academy Review, 3*, 14.

Zappa, V., Grosso, L., Simona, C., Graf, H., & Case, D. (1993). Clinical furcation diagnosis and interradicular bone. *Journal of Clinical Periodontology, 64*, 219–227.

# CHAPTER 11

# Hand-Activated Instrumentation

## Key Terms

assessment strokes
calculus removal work strokes
channeling
debridement work strokes
finger activation
lateral pressure

maintenance sharpening
pivoting
retipping
rocking
rolling
universal characteristics

## INTRODUCTION

The previous chapter discussed the philosophy and efficacy of nonsurgical periodontal instrumentation prior to reviewing instrument selection. This chapter is devoted to instrument sharpening and hand-activated instrumentation, two challenging skills. Dental and dental hygiene practitioners agree that subgingival instrumentation is a technically demanding skill (APA, 1989; APA, 1993;Greenstein, 1992; Pattison & Pattison, 1996).

The outcome of periodontal debridement is affected by the fundamental instrumentation principles employed by the clinician in conjunction with the sharpness of hand-activated curets and files used during therapy. Instruments adapted and activated correctly that are not sharp do not deliver the anticipated result in a reasonable amount of time. Conversely, ill-adapted but sharp curets also are not efficacious. The need to sharpen hand-activated instruments is a disadvantage when compared to ultrasonic instrumentation; however, initial periodontal therapy requires use of hand-activated instruments to some degree even when mechanized devices are available.

First, geometric principles related to sharpening and instrumentation will be highlighted. Next, sharpening rationale, objectives, procedures, and armamentarium are discussed. Last, instrumentation is reviewed including fundamental principles, adaptation, and activation of probes, explorers, curets, and files.

## GEOMETRIC TERMS

A review of geometric terms related to sharpening and instrumentation is included as background for readers (see Table 11-1 and Figures 11-1 through 11-4). Application of these terms to clinical practice requires that a relationship between two objects or surfaces be recognized

**Table 11-1  Geometric Terms**

| Term | Definition |
|---|---|
| Angle | A figure formed by two lines extending from the same point such as a 45°, 60°, 70°, or 80° angle. <br>• acute angle—less than 90° <br>• obtuse angle—greater than 90°, such as 100° or 110° <br>• right angle—at 90° (see Figure 11-1) |
| Bisect | Divide into two approximately equal parts; intersect (see Figure 11-1). |
| Vertical | Perpendicular to a plane or surface; upright; a line extending upward (see Figure 11-1). |
| Perpendicular | Being at right angles to a line or a plane (see Figure 11-1). |
| Horizontal | A plane parallel to the horizon or to a baseline (see Figure 11-1). |
| Oblique | Neither perpendicular nor parallel; at a 45° angle to the right; diagonal (see Figure 11-1). |
| Cross Section | A cutting off or segmenting of a piece of an object at right angles to an axis (see Figure 11-2). |
| Plane | A surface that contains every straight line; joining any two points lying in it; a plane can be vertical, horizontal, oblique (diagonal), or circumferential (see Figure 11-3). |
| Arc | A curved line or object; part of a circle (see Figure 11-3). |
| Parallel | Lines or surfaces that extend in the same direction and are equidistant apart (see Figure 11-4). |
| Long Axes | Imaginary lines through the center of a tooth; a single long axis is visualized in a mesiodistal dimension and/or a faciolingual dimension (see Figure 11-4). |

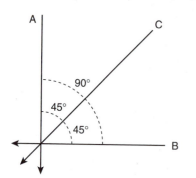

**Figure 11-1** Line A and B extend from the same point forming a 90° angle. Line C *bisects* this angle to form two separate angles, each of which is 45°. Line A is a *vertical* line *perpendicular* to line B. Line B is *horizontal* to the horizon or the bottom of this page. Line C is an *oblique* (diagonal) line.

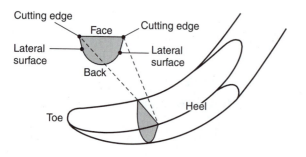

**Figure 11-2** The shaded area is a *cross section* of a universal curet.

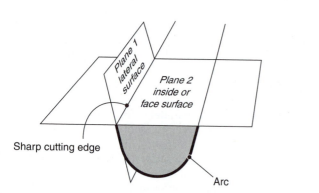

**Figure 11-3** Cross section of a curet and associated *planes.* Plane 1 (lateral surface) and plane 2 (the face) join to create an acute, sharp cutting edge. The bold curved line represents an *arc.*

such as the tooth and curet blade or the terminal shank and the surface being instrumented. To clarify verbal descriptions of instrumentation it is helpful to use these geometric terms and include the relationship between objects being discussed. For example, "The instrument is adapted parallel to the long axes" is not a clear message. Instead, "The handle of an anterior Gracey curet is positioned parallel to the faciolingual long axis of the tooth" is a specific message. Comprehending this message

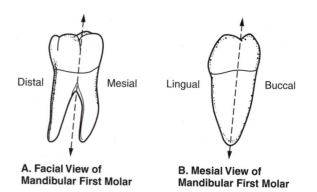

**Figure 11-4 A.** The dashed line represents the long axis in the mesiodistal dimension. The posterior teeth are tilted toward the midline of the dental arch. **B.** The dashed line represents the long axis in the buccolingual dimension.

requires that clinicians understand the geometric meaning of the terms "long axis" and "parallel" as well as the design features of curets (see Chapter 10). The student's and practitioner's continual self-evaluation of instrumentation techniques can also include these geometric terms and relationships.

## INSTRUMENT SHARPENING

When hand-activated instruments are selected for therapy the clinician must consider the quality of the cutting edge. Students and practitioners alike appreciate sharp instruments for deposit removal. Ultimately, a sharp instrument improves the *quality* of periodontal debridement. A sharp edge enhances tactile sensitivity and reduces the amount of lateral pressure needed, resulting in less fatigue and strain for the operator, increased comfort for the client, and efficiency beneficial for both parties. Therapists have experienced how a sharp instrument removes calculus or excess restorative material more effectively than a dull edge. A cutting edge that is acutely sharp enhances detection of calculus and overhanging margins because of the vibrations sent to the operator during the removal process. The sharp edge readily engages the plaque-retentive entity preventing the use of excessive pressure. Use of excessive pressure could negatively affect the short- and long-term health of the operator's hand and forearm as well as the root surface being treated. Excessive pressure is also detrimental for the patient because he feels the extra force compared to the instrument that was initially sharp, or to another clinician who has used a sharp blade.

Efficiency is another concern of both parties in NSPT. Multiple appointments are required at the onset of NSPT; therefore, efforts to streamline deposit removal are beneficial for the client's personal time, the operator's appointed time, and the office's or clinic's scheduling. Both dull and sharp instruments can eventually achieve a satisfactory result (Benfenati, Montesan, Benfenati, &

Nathanson, 1987), but it takes much longer with a dull instrument. There is also a question about whether the dull blade is "smoothing" plaque-retentive calculus into the root surface or removing it. Nonetheless, use of a dull instrument creates frustration on the part of the clinician. Detecting calculus and being ineffective in removal is an unrewarding and time-consuming problem. Therefore, a keen understanding of the principles of effective sharpening and maintenance of acute cutting edges is essential.

The following discussion addresses routine sharpening techniques for curets and files and includes suggestions for maintenance of sharp edges. Recontouring of curets also is discussed. It is important that other instruments such as sickles and explorers are sharpened, however, they will not be reviewed in this text. It is hoped that the principles discussed will be transferred to other hand-activated instruments.

## Objectives of Sharpening

The objective of sharpening is not only to produce an acute, sharp cutting edge but to maintain original contour. Inherent in this definition is the quality of the cutting edge defined by the angle formed between the face and lateral surface, by smoothness of the edge, by its relative sharpness or dullness, and by the presence or absence of metallic projections (Tal, Panno, & Vaidyanathan, 1985). The internal angle of curets and sickles refers to the angle created by the union of the face of the instrument and the lateral surface. Ideally, this internal angle is 70° to 80° because it creates an optimal cutting edge for calculus removal. This internal angle is maintained on curets by placing the stone against the lateral surface so that the angle between the face and the stone is 100° to 110° (see Figure 11-5A). When an internal angle less then 70° is created from wear or sharpen-

ing, the edge is extremely sharp and thin, but the acute cutting edge is rapidly lost during calculus removal. This scenario is suspected when the clinician sharpens, instruments for a minimal number of strokes (5 to 20), and discovers that the blade is dull. To problem solve this situation it is important to recognize what caused the internal angle to be less than 70°. When the stone is placed against the lateral surface creating a stone-to-face angle of greater than 110°, the internal angle of the curet is reduced to less than 70° (see Figure 11-5B).

On the other hand, when the instrument is sharpened with a stone-to-face angle of less than 100°, the cutting edge is not acutely sharp requiring heavy lateral pressure to remove calculus deposits. The use of heavy lateral pressure leads to frustration, discomfort, and inadequate calculus removal. This situation is suspected when the clinician sharpens, uses the instrument, and does not feel or hear the sharp cutting edge against the tooth. Sharpening with the stone against the lateral surface of the curet at an angle less than 100° causes the internal angle of the curet to be 90° or more (see Figure 11-5C).

The smoothness of the blade is visualized by magnification. Smoothness refers to the regularity of the cutting edge which is controlled by the fineness of the abrasive used to sharpen (Paquette & Levin, 1977a). Therefore, fine abrasive stones such as the Arkansas are preferred. Synthetic stones have been reported to remove metal unnecessarily, to create rough root surfaces, and to leave metal projections (Antonini, Brady, Levin, & Garcia, 1977).

The relative sharpness in clinical practice is evaluated by visual and tactile tests. The difference between a dull cutting edge and a sharp one is determined by the visual appearance, performance during instrumentation, and the internal angle of the instrument. When the instrument cutting edge is dull, it is rounded creating a flat surface (facet or bevel) of measurable width that is visible with magnification or the naked eye. Even though it is questionable if this bevel equates to dullness, it is reasonable to assume that there is a relationship. Some researchers have suggested a negative relationship between bevel dimensions and effectiveness of root planing (Tal, Panno, & Vaidyanathan, 1985), although not all researchers agree. Hoffmann and others (1989) question whether bevel width is appropriate to use to indicate sharpness. In conclusion, a sharp cutting edge is more important for effective removal of mineralized calculus than for removal and smoothing of cementum in traditional root planing.

The presence of metal projections relates to wire edges observable on new or sharpened instruments. Research reveals that new instruments directly from the manufacturer have numerous wire edges (Clark & Veno, 1990; DeNucci & Mader, 1983; Hoffmann et al., 1989; Huang & Tseng, 1991; Tal, Panno, & Vaidyanathan, 1985); therefore, new instruments should be sharpened prior to use. Because wire edges are not clinically visible, proper sharpening technique must be used to prevent

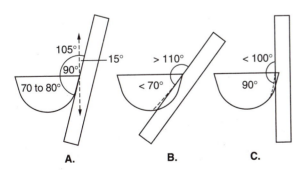

**Figure 11-5** Relationship of the stone to the face of a universal curet. **A.** The stone placed at an angle of 105° to the face of the curet produces an ideal internal curet angle of 70° to 80°. **B.** If the stone-to-face angle is greater than 110°, the internal angle of the curet will be less than ideal (less than 70°). **C.** If the stone-to-face angle is less than 100°, the internal angle of the curet will be greater than ideal (90° or more).

their occurrence. Finishing each segment of the cutting blade with a downward stroke versus an upward stroke prevents wire edges.

Many other factors affect the quality of the edge such as the hardness of the edge-forming surfaces, the design of the cutting edge, and the cutting forces applied to instruments. Stainless steel and high carbon steel curets have been compared prior to and after root planing. It was found that the high carbon steel was more resistant to wear (Tal, Kozlovsky, Green, & Gabbay, 1989). In clinical practice, however, stainless steel instruments are used more routinely resulting in a greater need to

sharpen often to prevent dullness. While these other factors are recognized, they are not all controllable in clinical practice on a day-to-day basis. Factors that are within the clinician's control are the routine sharpening of instruments with each use, use of proper technique, and accurate assessment of sharpness.

## Technique Recommendations for Curets

The sharpening sequence for the movable stone, stationary instrument method is reviewed in Table 11-2. This technique was chosen because clinicians seem to

### Table 11-2  Sharpening Evaluation: Curets

Performance:
S = satisfactory or accurate performance
U = unsatisfactory or improvement needed

Instrument Observed:

| Criteria | Self-Evaluation | Peer/Instructor Evaluation |
|---|---|---|
| 1. Collects complete and proper armamentarium. | | |
| 2. Uses adequate and direct lighting. | | |
| 3. Identifies cutting edge(s) to be sharpened. | | |
| 4. Identifies where the cutting blade is dull. | | |
| 5. Points the blade toe towards the operator and positions the facial surface of the blade parallel to the floor. (see Figure 11-6A). | | |
| 6. Braces the instrument on the mobile cabinet or counter for stabilization throughout the procedure. (see Figure 11-6A). | | |
| 7. Stone is initially placed at a 90° angle to the face of the blade. | | |
| 8. Stone is opened 10° to 20° to achieve the correct 100° to 110° angle for sharpening. | | |
| 9. Begins at the heel and rotates toward the toe, sharpening the cutting edge(s) in segments. (area-specific curet = 6 segments; universal curet = 5 segments; sickle = 3 segments). (see Figures 11-6B and C). | | |
| 10. Continues sharpening to round the toe properly. Back is rounded if necessary. | | |
| 11. Uses short up and down strokes with the most pressure being placed on the downward stroke. | | |
| 12. Uses consistent and light pressure. | | |
| 13. The correct angle of the stone to the instrument is maintained throughout the sharpening sequence. | | |
| 14. Avoids formation of a wire edge by finishing each segment with a downward stroke. | | |
| 15. Sharpens each segment until a sledge of metal shavings and oil appears on the face. | | |
| 16. Tests for sharpness visually and tactilely. | | |
| 17. Asepsis is maintained. | | |
| 18. Stone is cleaned for autoclaving. | | |

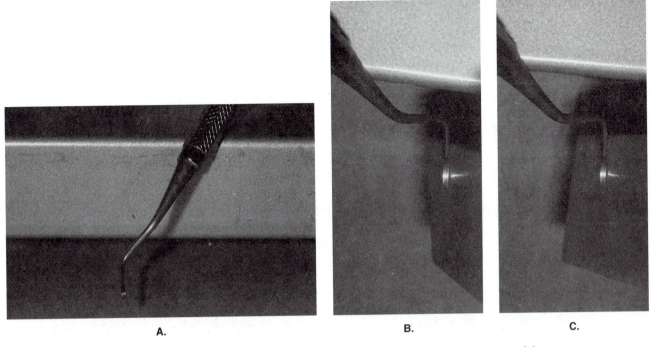

**A.**                          **B.**                          **C.**

**Figure 11-6** Sharpening curets. **A.** Area-specific curet braced against a stable counter. Notice the face of the curet
is parallel to the bottom of the picture (floor). **B.** Stone placed against the cutting edge of a universal curet at approximately
105° to the face. The operator is sharpening the cutting edge segment closest to the shank of the instrument. **C.** The operator is
now sharpening a middle segment of the cutting blade. Notice the stone is not touching the heel portion of the cutting edge.

have the most success when they can observe the contour
of the instrument, keep the instrument stationary, and
move the stone across the instrument's lateral surface.
Biller and Karlsson (1979) compared the two most common methods of sharpening: the movable stone, stationary instrument, and the stationary stone, movable
instrument. Results indicated that 75 percent of the
instruments were sharp when examined with scanning
electron microscopy when the instrument was kept stationary and the stone moved, and only 50 percent of the
curets were classified as sharp when the curet was moved
over the stationary stone. Most likely, increased visualization of the process with the movable stone, stationary
instrument method contributes to this success. It is
important to note that the way an acute, thin, sharp edge
is created is by removing the metal from the lateral surface of the curet and not by actually sharpening the cutting edge.

Some clinicians prefer to remove metal from the
facial surface; however, many authorities do not recommend this technique (American Eagle Instruments, 4th
edition; GC American Hygienists Instruments and Supplies, 1986; Hu-Friedy® Product Catalog and Reference
Guide, 1993; Pattison, Pattison, & Takei, 1996). Sharpening the face requires removal of significant amounts of
metal, which reduces the blade depth (face to back
dimension). This reduction affects the blade's stiffness
and strength that is derived from its depth and not width
(Paquette & Levin, 1977a). An advantage of removing
metal from the lateral surfaces is that the blade width is

reduced allowing for better access and adaptation on
the root surfaces. The disadvantage of sharpening on the
lateral surface, however, is that the clinician must ensure
that the curvature of the blade is maintained by sharpening the cutting edge in segments (see Figures 11-6B
and 11-6C). The convex cutting edge of area-specific
curets, universal curets, and some sickles necessitates
rotating the stone from the shank portion (heel) to toe
in many segments (see Figure 11-7). The advantage of
sharpening one small section of the cutting edge at a time
is that clinicians become very familiar with the original
contour of different curets, enhancing proper sharpening technique and selection of instruments for NSPT.
The number of vertical strokes needed to sharpen each
section varies based on need. Usually the terminal portion of the blade is the dullest due to increased use; however, it is still important to sharpen the blade in segments
to maintain original contour. The number of strokes
needed adjacent to the heel is often less than the number
of strokes needed near the toe.

The steps in the sharpening process build upon one
another and if the first step is incorrect, then all steps that
follow are also incorrect. If the face of the curet is not sit-
uated parallel to the floor (step 5, Table 11-2, see Figure
11-6A) then placing the stone to the lateral surface at an
apparent 90° angle (step 7) and opening the stone 10° to
20° (step 8) to achieve a 100° to 110° stone-to-face angle
is inaccurate. The result is that the ideal internal angle of
the curet is altered as previously described. If step six,
bracing the instrument to maintain stabilization, is not

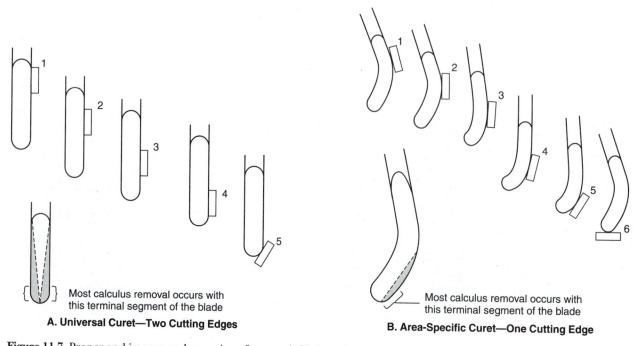

Most calculus removal occurs with
this terminal segment of the blade

**A. Universal Curet—Two Cutting Edges**

Most calculus removal occurs with
this terminal segment of the blade

**B. Area-Specific Curet—One Cutting Edge**

**Figure 11-7** Proper and improper sharpening of curets. **A.** Universal curet, two cutting edges. The stone is rotated in five or more increments to produce a sharp cutting edge on each segment of the blade and to maintain original contour. **B.** Area-specific curet, one cutting edge. The stone is rotated in six increments to produce a sharp cutting edge on each segment of the blade and to maintain original contour. The shaded areas represent the portion of the cutting edge and lateral surface removed if sharpening is performed by dividing the blade into only one or two segments.

achieved, then the pressure exerted on the lateral surface with the stone will cause wobbling of the instrument. This movement produces an uneven edge that will negatively affect efficacy.

Use of a protractor placed behind the face of the blade helps the clinician estimate the stone-to-face angle (see Figure 11-8). Because the relationship of the stone to the instrument is so critical in producing a sharp edge and appropriately contoured instrument, many manufacturers have developed guides (Sharpen-Rite®, Thierman Products, Incorporated) to assess instrument and stone placement. Guides might benefit clinicians striving to perfect their sharpening technique, although an understanding of the original contour of the instrument, goals of sharpening, and tests for sharpening are still necessary. Guides are useful when more than one person is sharpening instruments that are being shared with other professionals (Ellingson, 1993). The guide may help standardize the angulation between the stone and face of the blade at subsequent sharpening times.

Recently, a modification of the traditional technique for the movable stone stationary instrument has been suggested. This teaching strategy is described in a self-instructional videotape and manual called *It's About Time to Get on the Cutting Edge* (Hu-Friedy, 1995). The main difference between the traditional method and the modified-strategy is in the way a clinician assesses correct stone placement. With the traditional method "degrees of angulation" are used. In the new strategy, positions of the

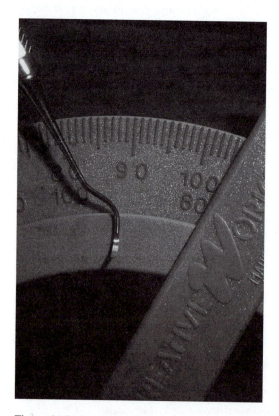

**Figure 11-8** A protractor placed behind a universal curet to approximate angles used for sharpening. The cutting edge is adjacent to the 90° measurement. The stone is then placed near 100°.

hands on a clock are used to judge correct stone placement against the curet's lateral surface. The terminal shank of a sickle or curet is aligned to certain clock positions and the blade to be sharpened is held vertically at six o'clock. The stone is then positioned correlating to the hands of the clock at 4 minutes after 12 for right-handers and 4 minutes before twelve for left-handed clinicians. Stone placement at 4 minutes before or after twelve o'clock corresponds to the recommended 100° to 110° placement of the stone to the curet face (see Figure 11-9). Whichever technique is used, the objectives of sharpening are the same.

**Evaluating Sharpness.** Three tests are used to evaluate sharpness; 1) visual examination, 2) biting into a test stick, and 3) sound created by applying lateral pressure on the tooth surface. Use of these tests occurs prior to seating the client, during therapy, or at maintenance intervals. **Maintenance sharpening** is performed for all instruments at a routine time, not in the presence of a client. For example, students learning sharpening procedures often schedule a time period each week to examine and sharpen instruments in preparation for the next week's clinical experiences. Maintenance sharpening allows the student to concentrate on the technical process of sharpening as well as offering an unlimited time period to practice the procedure. Maintenance sharpening might also occur in an office if certain team members are responsible for sharpening instruments for other team members.

Visual examination is based on the principle that the rounded edge or facet (dull blade), when placed under light, will appear white and shiny (see Figure 11-10). This white line is observable with a magnifying glass at the junction of the face and lateral surface where an acute cutting edge should be. Students initially find this test difficult, but with practice it becomes easier. The key to accurate observation is to rotate the instrument from face to lateral surface until the cutting edge is facing the central beam of the light. Visual examination also includes evaluation of the quality of the edge. A microscope is useful for assessing blade smoothness and wire edges. Although microscopic evaluation is not practical at chairside, it is helpful for maintenance sharpening or in an educational setting when sharpening skills are being mastered.

Placing a cutting edge against a test stick is also feasible and effective when performed correctly. It is critical that the clinician test the blade against the stick by employing the same angle (approximately 70° to 80°) and lateral pressure used when instrumenting. Both appropriate pressure and angulation can be achieved by

## Clock Face Positions
*Sickle Scalers and Universal Curets*
**Terminal shank at 12:00**

Top of stone at 4 minutes after 12:00 for right-handers

Top of stone at 4 minutes before 12:00 for left-handers

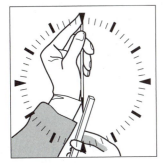
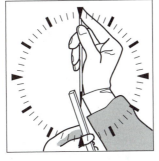

*Gracey Curets*
**Terminal shank toward 11:00**          **Terminal shank toward 1:00**

Top of stone at 4 minutes after 12:00 for right-handers

Top of stone at 4 minutes before 12:00 for left-handers

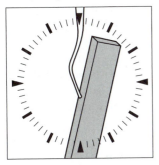
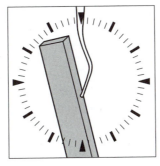

**Figure 11-9** Principles of new sharpening strategy. (Courtesy of Hu-Friedy® Manufacturing Company, Inc.)

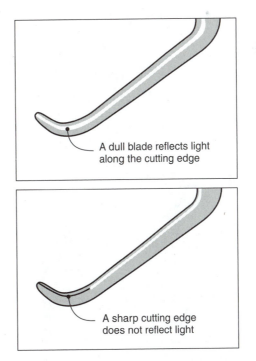

A dull blade reflects light along the cutting edge

A sharp cutting edge does not reflect light

**Figure 11-10** Visual inspection of a dull and sharp cutting edge. (Courtesy of Hu-Friedy® Manufacturing Company, Inc.)

placing a fulcrum on the test stick and initiating a stroke which simulates a calculus removal stroke on the mesial or distal surface of a tooth (see Figure 11-11). If the instrument "bites" into the stick on the first attempt, it is sharp. If, however, the instrument is "dragged" or "pulled" along the stick then additional sharpening is indicated. It is possible to make any instrument appear sharp if improper angles and excessive pressure are applied to the test stick.

The last test is practical to use during therapy. The student or practitioner constantly listens for the *sound* of the instrument during calculus removal and, if absent, the instrument is dull. A sharp instrument during instrumentation will produce an audible metallic sound and when this is no longer present the clinician stops and sharpens. It is wise for students and practitioners to also evaluate the relationship of the blade to the tooth to ensure the proper angle is being used. Improper angulation could account for the lack of sound.

Continual sharpening throughout the debridement process is the key to maintaining sharp curets that do not need recontouring. When a clinician makes the choice to not sharpen during nonsurgical periodontal instrumentation, the detrimental effects previously mentioned occur. In addition, when sharpening is finally initiated the process is difficult because the blade is extremely dull. An extremely dull edge requires removal of excess metal decreasing the instrument's longevity and increasing the financial burden of ordering new instruments.

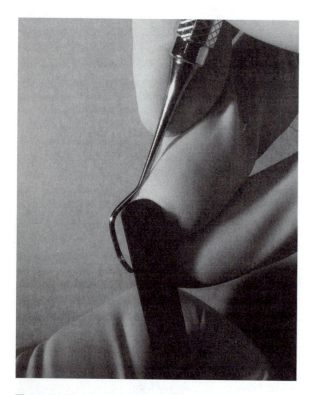

**Figure 11-11** The terminal 1 millimeter of a universal curet being tested against the test stick.

Students learning instrument sharpening usually ask how many strokes or how long they can instrument before sharpening is needed. The answer to this question depends on the initial sharpness of the blade, size of the deposit, tenacity of the deposit, and force exerted by the clinician. Researchers usually implement 45 strokes when studying sharpness in relation to traditional root planing, because it was assumed that this number represented the most strokes realistically employed in one area in a clinical setting (O'Leary & Kafrawy, 1983). After 45 root planing strokes a significant bevel is usually formed (Huang & Tseng, 1991; Tal, Panno, & Vaidyanathan, 1985). These estimations were conducted with the premise that root planing is performed to create a hard, glassy, smooth surface. Even though this philosophy is changing, estimation of stroke numbers might be useful in clinical practice. Removing tenacious calculus and/or heavy deposit creates a dull edge much faster than when debriding subgingival plaque due to the increased lateral pressure needed for calculus removal.

**Armamentarium.** Flat stones are available in three types: Arkansas, India, and ceramic. The stones vary in abrasiveness from fine to medium. The stone most frequently used is the Arkansas, made of natural stone from mined mineral deposits that produces variations in surface texture (Huntley, 1982b). Artificial (India and ceramic) stones are made of nonmetallic substances impregnated with abrasive particles creating a more uniform surface texture (Huntley, 1982b). Other options include rotary-mounted stones and specialized hand-held or mechanized devices. Strengths of the rotary method are that it is fast and can produce a quality edge. Limitations are the difficulty in controlling the handpiece, the frictional heat generated, which is claimed to affect the temper of the instrument (Hu-Friedy® Product Catalog and Reference Guide, 1993), and the coarseness of the stones, which remove a significant amount of metal (Pattison, Pattison, & Takei, 1996). Mechanized devices produce quality cutting edges; however, drawbacks are that they are time-consuming and chairside asepsis is difficult to achieve.

Huang and Tseng (1991) compared the Arkansas, India, synthetic, and ceramic stones by sharpening 21 new Gracey 1/2 curet blades after simulated root planing on extracted teeth. Results indicated that the ceramic stone was the least effective (p < 0.01) and the fine- and medium-abrasive India stones achieved the best results. Clark and Veno (1990) compared the uniformity of the cutting edge on new instruments to those sharpened with a ceramic stone and a portable electronic sharpener (Minisharpener, G-C International Corporation). The most variance in cutting edges was seen on the new curets, which demonstrated wire edges and striations on the lateral and facial surfaces. The edges that were hand sharpened were uniform, met in a clean line, and were without wire edges 75 percent of the time. The curets sharpened with the portable device exhibited quality cutting edges with no wire edges, but the process was cited as being too lengthy and impractical (Clark & Veno, 1990).

## Recontouring Curets

The need for recontouring will diminish as students and practitioners gain experience and proficiency with sharpening technique. Recontouring is needed for two reasons: 1) to remove a significant bevel on the cutting edge, and 2) to restore the original contour of the instrument. The bevel is created by improper sharpening or excessive wear without sharpening. It is eliminated by removing enough metal from the lateral surface to reform the sharp cutting edge. The stone is placed at an angulation of about 110° to the face of the curet or sickle. The larger the bevel, the more time-consuming the procedure because more metal must be removed than if the instrument had a narrow bevel.

If the original shape of the curet has been compromised, it is probably because the cutting edges were not sharpened in segments or the toe was not rounded (see Figure 11-12). These problems are corrected by using proper sharpening skills to remove metal from the needed areas to restore the original contour. For example, if the middle of the cutting edge of an area-specific curet is flattened, then metal must be removed from the toe and heel one-thirds of the blade significantly reducing blade width. If the toe is narrow and pointed, then sharpening to round the toe is indicated, which reduces blade length. A shorter blade decreases the strength of the instrument making calculus removal more challenging. The reduced length is particularly significant with minibladed curets. While recontouring of curets and sickles is possible, it is usually not indicated for files due to their extremely small cutting edges making visual testing for sharpness difficult.

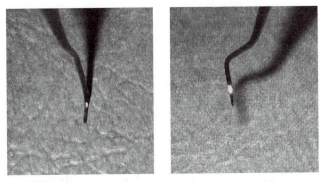

**A. A Gracey 1/2 Curet**     **B. A Universal Curet**

**Figure 11-12** The results of improper sharpening. **A.** A Gracey 1/2 curet. The terminal portion of the blade lost its original curvature because this area was not sharpened in segments. This instrument cannot be recontoured. **B.** A universal curet. The curvature of the blade is lost, the toe is not round but pointed, and the facial dimension is significantly reduced. This instrument cannot be recontoured.

When an instrument is improperly contoured, the clinician must decide if enough metal remains to warrant recontouring or if the instrument should be replaced or retipped. Indications for replacement include loss of one-half the width of the blade or bending occurring when lateral pressure is exerted during scaling (Wilkins, 1994). Comparison of new and used instruments is valuable in making these decisions. Not recognizing the need for new instruments endangers the client, results in considerable risk for the professional, and negatively affects the quality and efficiency of instrumentation. The instruments in Figure 11-12 need to be replaced.

**Retipping** is no longer supported because it compromises the constructional integrity creating a risk for clients and practitioners (Hu-Friedy® Product Hygiene Catalog and Reference Guide, 1993). Reduced quality may lead to tip loss, cracks in the handle, lack of balance, and undue wearing due to inferior steel. Proponents of retipping claim the instruments are strong and can be resharpened repetitively. The cost is certainly less than buying new instruments. The disadvantages are the need for enough instruments to work with during the retipping process, which takes an average of two weeks. Occasionally wrong angulation on some tips was reported by 3 of 23 evaluators (Clinical Research Associates Newsletter, 1994). Retipping services can be located in dental hygiene journals and professional literature. For a student, some instrument manufacturers are willing to replace instruments for a cost less than the original cost of the instrument. This replacement service, however, is not available to practitioners.

CryoEdge™ is a process that treats the cutting edge. According to the manufacturer (EdgeWise Technology Incorporated) these treated instruments stay sharper longer and are easier to sharpen. Instruments are sent to the company for this processing. This manufacturer advocates sharper edges due to the type of metal used and to the special processing.

## File Sharpening

The objectives of sharpening a file are the same as for a curet. It is important to ensure that each of the multiple cutting edges is sharpened to efficiently engage a calculus deposit or amalgam overhang. The rake angle of the file must first be recognized (see Chapter 10, Figure 10-13). The tanged file is then placed within the rake so that the tanged file is positioned towards the handle; thus, the 55° angle portion of the lip is sharpened (see Figure 11-13). Sharpening the 90° angle (lips parallel to the end of the file head) will result in wear in a vertical direction and an increase in the rake and the lip angles. These two effects decrease the file's longevity and increase the time necessary to achieve sharpness (Hoople, 1985). To sharpen the file, the clinician must ensure the tanged file is parallel to the cutting edge on both sides of the file's head. The file head is first positioned parallel to a surface (a counter or the floor). The tanged file is then placed with the rake

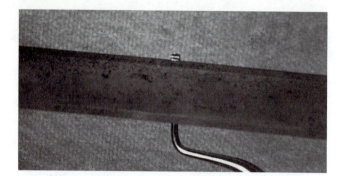

**Figure 11-13** A Hirschfeld file being properly sharpened.

parallel to the file head and surface of the floor. Once positioned, the tanged file is moved back and forth (horizontally) in short strokes across each adjacent cutting edge while maintaining the parallel relationship.

One way to stabilize the sharpening device and instrument is to hold the tanged file in a palm grasp with one hand, grasp the instrument with the head supported on the index finger of the other hand, and tuck arms close to the body for stability. The clinician holds the instrument with no movement and moves only the sharpening device (tanged file) in the back and forth motions that are straight and even (Hoople, 1985). The same positioning is achieved by bracing the file against an object (counter) to keep it stationary, ensuring that the face is parallel with the floor, and moving the tanged file appropriately. The final product is not easily evaluated with a magnifying glass because the "white line" on a beveled cutting edge of a curet is not visible on a file. Therefore, the best tests for evaluating file sharpness are tactile ones: biting on a test stick and evaluation (gripping) on the deposit. In an educational setting, a microscope is useful to examine the cutting edges.

## INSTRUMENTATION PRINCIPLES

Periodontal instrumentation differs from basic instrumentation in relation to extent. *Extent* refers to both the conditions necessary to instrument as well as the time required to perform quality care. With advanced periodontal conditions such as deep periodontal pockets, attachment loss, and furcations, some alterations in fundamental techniques are required; although, basic principles such as grasp, fulcrum, positioning, adaptation, and activation are still essential. For example, to debride a deep periodontal pocket, traditional fulcrum placement might be adjusted to negotiate the apical portion of the periodontal pocket; however, a sound fulcrum is still mandatory to perform efficient and gentle periodontal instrumentation. By virtue of the advanced periodontal conditions, more appointment time is necessary to provide the client with thorough debridement.

Three key areas are discussed in this section: fundamentals, adaptation, and activation. *Fundamentals* refer to the basic principles that students strive to attain in preclinical courses prior to caring for their clients. Once in direct client care, these principles are vitally important for proper and comfortable activation of instruments during NSPT. *Adaptation* is defined as the correct placement of the working end of an instrument against the tooth surface. *Activation* is the movement of the instrument around the convex and concave surfaces of the tooth root and crown. Just as in instrument sharpening, the latter stages of instrumentation (activation) depend on proper adaptation and application of the fundamental principles of instrumentation.

### Fundamentals

Fundamentals include positioning, grasp, fulcrum placement, and mirror use. Each of these principles will be discussed prior to a review of instrumentation with the different classes of instruments.

**Positioning.** There are various recommendations, strategies, and terminology suggested by dental hygiene authors for client and operator positioning. If indicated, a review of the basic principles of positioning can be accomplished by referring to a dental hygiene textbook such as *Fundamentals of Periodontal Instrumentation* (Nield-Gehrig & Houseman, 1996), *Clinical Practice of the Dental Hygienist* (Wilkins, 1994), *Periodontal Instrumentation* (Pattison & Pattison, 1994), *Dental Hygiene Theory and Practice* (Darby & Walsh, 1994); and *Comprehensive Dental Hygiene Care* (Woodall, 1993). Table 11-3 summarizes the key elements for proper client and clinician positioning, and Table 11-4 summarizes one philosophy of clinician positioning. Positioning of the therapist varies depending on the instrument design, pocket depth, positioning of teeth in the dentition, and clinician hand size. Refer to Chapter 15 for recommendations on how to avoid musculoskeletal problems.

**Grasp.** Clinicians are accustomed to using the modified pen grasp for periodontal instrumentation. A proper grasp facilitates tactile sensation, adaptation, activation, and comfort for both the clinician and client's benefit (see Figure 11-14). Typically, the thumb and index finger are placed across from one another on the instrument handle near the junction of the shank and handle. Finger placement might move up the handle (away from the working end) when fulcrums are used other than the conventional built-up position. With a proper grasp, the thumb and index finger should not touch. **Rolling** the instrument in between the thumb and index finger is an essential movement, and if these fingers touch this movement is negatively affected. The instrument can actually roll out or off of the clinician's fingers requiring repositioning and a loss of efficiency. This concept can be tested by placing the thumb and index fingers in proper and improper grasp relationships. When the thumb and index finger touch, rolling should be difficult.

**Table 11-3 Positioning Principles**

| Person | Area | Suggested Position |
|---|---|---|
| Clinician | Back | • against the back of the seat |
| | Thighs | • parallel to the floor or raised slightly upward |
| | Knees | • parallel with thigh or raised slightly higher than thighs<br>• keep apart from one another |
| | Feet | • flat on floor |
| | Arms | • upper arms—aligned with long axis of your body<br>• lower arms—operate with arms at waist level and a 90° angle to your upper arms |
| | Head/Neck | • aligned with long axis of your upper body |
| Patient | Back | • nearly parallel to floor in supine position |
| | Thighs | • slightly raised as compared to the chest and head |
| | Knees | • higher than chest |
| | Feet | • slightly higher than tip of nose |
| | Arms | • relaxed; crossed over stomach area |
| | Head | • nearly parallel with floor<br>• top of head even with top edge of headrest<br>• can move to right or left for clinician access<br>• chin-up position—used for maxillary arch<br>• chin-down position—used for mandibular arch |
| Relationship of Patient to Clinician | Patient Nose | • at or below the clinician's waist |

The thumb and index finger actually hold the instrument and the middle and ring fingers *rest* on the index finger. The side of the fingertip of the middle finger contacts the shank of the instrument. This contact enhances detection because the side of the fingertip is a tactilly sensitive area. The middle finger, however, does not hold the instrument. To test this concept in a laboratory setting or practice session, lift the middle finger off the shank and see if the instrument is dropped (Nield-Gehrig & Houseman, 1996). If so, the middle finger is being incorrectly used in the grasp. The ring finger, or finger rest, is maintained on the tooth for stability during instrumentation. A split grasp is when the middle and index finger are apart. This position is detrimental because it decreases instrument stability. In addition, a split grasp encourages activation with only the fingers versus the wrist and forearm motion.

To self-assess your grasp, evaluate the relationship of the fingers to one another as well as the relationship of the instrument handle to the hand. The handle should rest between the middle joint of the index finger and the joint located where the finger and hand meet (see Figure 11-14). Handle placement within this one and one-half inch area depends on the operator's hand size, the instrument being used, the fulcrum placement, and the area of the mouth being treated. The fingers should always be relaxed and curved away from the instrument handle in an inverted "C" shape ("Ɔ"). When the tip of an instrument is incorrectly adapted to a root surface, the grasp should be reevaluated. An improper grasp can contribute to inappropriate adaptation. Likewise, if an instrument is not activated properly against the tooth, the grasp could be the cause. A proper working stroke is challenging for the clinician when the grasp and fulcrum are not adequate.

**Fulcrum.** Periodontal instrumentation requires the use of alternative fulcrums with different instruments and areas of the mouth (see Table 11-5). As student clinicians advance in the curriculum and understand the concepts of adaptation and activation, a variety of fulcrums are appropriate. Also, development of hand strength is important for correct application of alternate fulcrums. Fulcrums are often recommended for the dental mirror, but they are essential when using probes, explorers, files, and curets. The most important rule for fulcrum selection is the ability to reach all subgingival surfaces with correct adaptation (Pattison & Pattison, 1992). In fact, placement of the working end subgingivally may occur prior to deciding on the exact location for the fulcrum.

It is best to use built-up fulcrums with each type of fulcrum. When the middle and ring fingers are positioned touching one another, the greatest control and power can be exercised. Infrequently, a split fulcrum might occur where the middle and ring finger are apart. Although not ideal, this split might occur when alternate fulcrum positions are employed. An important concept of self-evaluation is to assess if the instrument is stabilized and the tip/blade is adapted. If so, the split fulcrum is satisfactory for a short period of time, but extended use adds extra strain on the operator's fingers and hands.

Fulcrums also vary in placement of the ring finger (finger rest) on the tooth, orientation of the palm to the occlusal or incisal edges of teeth, and intraoral or extraoral positioning. The finger rest need not always be directly on the tip of the finger or in the center of the

**Table 11-4 Operator Positions**

| Arch | Area | Position for Right-Handed Operators |
|------|------|-------------------------------------|
| Maxillary | Right buccal posteriors and left lingual posteriors | • Preferred: 10:00 to 11:00 with palm-up position<br>• Optional: 8:00 to 9:00 with palm-down position where necessary |
| | Left buccal posteriors and right lingual posteriors | • 10:00 to 11:00 |
| | Anterior facial and lingual surfaces | • 12:00 |
| Mandibular | Right buccal posteriors and left lingual posteriors | • Preferred: 8:00 to 9:00<br>• 10:00 to 11:00 useful for mesial surfaces |
| | Left buccal posteriors and right lingual posteriors | • 9:00 to 10:00 (distal surfaces from 9:00; buccal/lingual surfaces and mesials 10:00 to 11:00) |
| | Anterior facial and lingual surfaces | • 8:00 for facial and lingual surfaces towards the operator<br>• 12:00 for surfaces away from the operator |

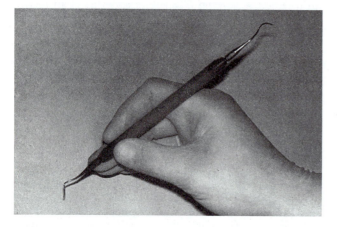

**Figure 11-14** Proper grasp with an explorer. Notice the relationship of the thumb to the index finger and the index finger to the middle and ring fingers. The instrument handle is located between the appropriate joints. The grasp appears relaxed.

occlusal or incisal edge. At times, the side of the fingertip is placed on the buccal or lingual surface near the occlusal or incisal edge. Notice in Figure 11-15 the finger rest involves different portions of the ring finger. Generally, the tip of the finger is used with conventional fulcrum placement and the side of the fingertip is needed with alternate fulcrums. During activation, the clinician pivots and rocks on the finger rest to move the instrument across the convex and concave tooth surfaces. **Pivoting** is the movement of the hand, wrist, and forearm in an arc within the same plane or across planes. If pivoting can be achieved while the hand, wrist, and forearm are in a neutral position, then less strain occurs decreasing predisposure to musculoskeletal disorders (see Chapter 15). The purpose of pivoting is to advance the instrument across tooth surfaces and particularly to ensure that the instrument reaches the midline of the proximal surfaces.

**Rocking** allows the clinician to move the instrument from the epithelial attachment to portions of the root and crown positioned coronally. It is the up and down motion created by moving the wrist from left to right. Both pivoting and rocking require movement on the finger rest to negotiate tooth structure topography.

The palm-up and palm-down positions are so called because of the relationship of the palm to the incisal or occlusal surfaces. These terms are often associated with extraoral fulcrum placement but, for this text, they are used for intraoral fulcrum placement. The palm-down position is the traditional position of the palm facing the occlusal surfaces of the mandibular teeth (see Figure 11-15A). Maxillary teeth can be debrided with the palm-down position, however, it creates a straight and rigid fulcrum finger that does not facilitate pivoting. Therefore, the palm-up position is used on the maxillary posterior buccal surfaces (right-handed operators) (see Figure 11-15C), and the maxillary posterior lingual surfaces when seated at nine o'clock. Figure 11-16 demonstrates the use of a palm-up position with a conventional fulcrum. A palm-up orientation is also used on the facial and lingual surfaces of the maxillary anterior teeth when seated at the twelve o'clock position (versus eight o'clock).

The use of extraoral fulcrums is a matter of preference. An advantage of intraoral fulcrums is the increased comfort for the client. A finger rest and lateral pressure exerted on hard tooth structure is likely to be more comfortable than a fulcrum on soft tissue. Fulcruming on hard tooth structure also affords the clinician more stability than when activating the instrument from a soft tissue fulcrum.

**Mirror Use.** Effective use of the mirror helps the clinician retract and use indirect vision, reflection, and transillumination. Retraction refers to the moving of the client's cheeks and tongue out of the field of vision. It is best to retract with the back of the mirror so that the front

**Table 11-5 Fulcrum Positions and Descriptions**

| Type | Description | Instruments Used With |
|---|---|---|
| Conventional | • Established on tooth surfaces close to the tooth being treated (see Figure 11-15A).<br>• Usually located on an adjacent tooth, however, could be placed as many as 4 teeth away. | Periodontal probes, explorers, sickles, curets, and files. |
| Cross Arch | • Established on tooth surfaces on the other side of the same arch (see Figure 11-15B).<br>• Often used to instrument the mandibular lingual surfaces. | Universal curets, curved explorers, and files. |
| Opposite Arch | • Established on the opposite arch from the area being treated (see Figure 11-15C).<br>• Frequently placed on mandibular tooth surfaces when instrumenting the maxillary posterior sextants. | Area-specific curets and the 11/12 explorer. |
| Finger-on-Finger Rest | • Established on the index finger or thumb of the nonoperating hand.<br>• Employed with missing teeth and mobility. | All instrument designs. |
| Built-up | • Refers to the middle and ring fingers together to provide stability, power, and control.<br>• Used with each of the fulcrums previously identified (see Figure 11-15A, B, and C). | All instrument designs. |

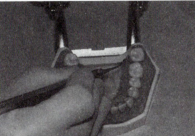

| | | |
|:---:|:---:|:---:|
| **A. Conventional** | **B. Cross Arch** | **C. Opposite Arch** |

**Figure 11-15** Fulcrum placement with a curet.

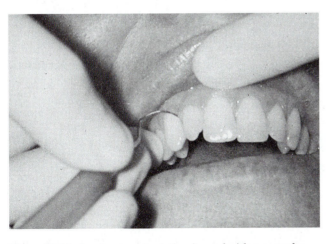

**Figure 11-16** A palm-up orientation is used with a curved explorer on the maxillary right buccal surfaces.

mirrored surface can be used for indirect vision, reflection, or illumination. Reflection is when the dental light directed at the mirror surface bounces light onto the tooth and enhances visibility. Another term for reflected light is "indirect illumination."

Transillumination is used to reflect light through a tooth. Transillumination is frequently used on anterior teeth, but can also be accomplished on posterior teeth if retraction of the cheek and tongue are effective. The therapist uses transillumination to see if any discolored (grayish, yellowish, or white), shadowed, or dull areas appear on the tooth surface. Caries, deposits (hard and soft), fractures, composite restorations, and pit and fissure sealants are detected with the aid of transillumination due to a change in translucency as compared to sound tooth structure. When checking the anterior teeth using transillumination, apply the mirror in a variety of positions in relation to the lingual and buccal tooth surfaces. The mirror is placed parallel to the lingual surface, and then rotated to the right or left in an arc. This rotation reflects light in different positions to help distinguish tooth surface from other entities. Frequently, veneer calculus is visible in one mirror position, but not in another. Movement of the mirror to view the convex and concave surfaces of the tooth facilitates complete deposit and stain removal.

The mirror is also useful for subgingival deposit detection if the gingival tone is elastic due to inflammation. The mirror is positioned above the sulcus and rotated to reflect light in different directions while compressed air is directed into the sulcus or pocket to distend the tissue. Sometimes subgingival calculus is visible. This technique is especially useful in identifying flat and dark calculus adjacent to the cementoenamel junction (CEJ). In conclusion, improper use of the mirror can affect a clinician's instrumentation performance. If indirect vision is needed and the clinician attempts direct vision, the clinician's body positioning, adaptation, and activation are negatively altered.

## Adaptation

Instruments are adapted to tooth surfaces by contacting the appropriate portion of the working end to the calculus, cementum, or enamel depending on the procedure being performed. For assessment, calculus removal, and debridement of bacterial plaque, the principle consideration is that the terminal portion of the working end must be effectively adapted to the tooth topography. Adaptation requires: 1) correct selection of the working end (explorers, curets, sickles, files) and cutting edge (curets and sickles), 2) correct insertion into the sulcus or pocket, 3) use of the terminal 1 to 2 millimeters of the working end, and 4) use of the appropriate cutting edge (blade)-to-tooth angulation.

**Working End Selection.** The correct working end of explorers and curets is determined by multiple concepts. First, the terminal portion of the working end should be directed toward the surface being debrided. For example, to debride the buccal and mesial of the mandibular first molar, the explorer point or curet toe will be directed toward the mesial surface. If the point or toe is directed toward the distal surface when the buccal and mesial surfaces are being treated, then the incorrect side of the explorer tip, curet working end, or curet blade is adapted.

Secondly, the position of the terminal shank serves as a visual cue to the correct working end and tip/blade selection. First, position the handle as parallel as possible with the long axis of the tooth in the buccolingual dimension. If the terminal shank is nearly parallel to the proximal surface, then the correct working end and tip/blade have been chosen. On the other hand, if the terminal shank crosses the proximal and buccal or lingual surfaces diagonally or horizontally, the incorrect working end and tip/blade are being adapted.

For area-specific curets, the correct cutting edge can be selected *prior* to adaptation by viewing the instrument looking down onto the face when it is held so that the terminal shank is perpendicular with the floor. The correct cutting edge is the one that is seen as the larger, convex curve. This cutting edge is also described as the cutting edge farthest away from the handle, the inferior cutting edge, or the leading edge (Pattison & Pattison, 1992). Another way to select the correct cutting edge is to adapt the cutting edge that tilts away from the terminal shank (Nield-Gehrig & Houseman, 1996).

**Insertion.** An instrument is inserted with a blade-to-tooth angulation as close to 0° as possible. This angulation is easy to accomplish with a file that is adapted parallel to the calculus deposit, but with a curet or sickle an angle of zero degrees requires that the face of the curet be completely closed against the tooth surface. To accomplish this 0° blade-to-tooth relationship, the clinician would need to rotate the shank and handle so that it is positioned perpendicular (instead of vertical) to the long axis of the tooth. This position is impossible to achieve in all periodontal pockets, especially on mesial posterior surfaces. Therefore, the goal with a curet is to insert subgingivally with the most closed angle possible to facilitate extending to the epithelial attachment or below the calculus deposit with minimal tissue distention. Typically, the blade-to-tooth angle during insertion ranges from 20° to 40° depending on the instrument and tissue tone. The explorer and probe are also inserted with a tip-to-tooth angle as near to 0° as possible. This angle is maintained when activating a probe, but is increased (opened) when activating an explorer to adapt only the terminal portion of the working end to the tooth surface.

To detect and remove calcified deposit, the tip/blade must be placed approximately 1 mm apical to the calculus. The placement below the piece of calculus permits the clinician to detect the deposit because tooth surface texture can be compared to calculus texture. Also, the placement of the curet blade below the piece of calculus permits the clinician to engage the deposit with adequate lateral pressure and correct angulation at the time the blade contacts the calculus. If the curet blade is positioned on the apical edge of the calculus and not below the deposit, its apical border will remain after the working stroke.

**Terminal Portion of the Working End.** Once inserted, the same portion of the working end of an explorer, curet, and sickle are adapted to tooth surfaces. The terminal 1 to 2 millimeters of the working end of any explorer is adapted to all surfaces, especially the convex surfaces at line angles and the concave surfaces of developmental depressions. The portion of the curet blade that is adapted is also the terminal 1 to 2 mm, which equates to just less than the terminal one-third of the blade near the toe. A frequent error is to use more of the terminal portion than necessary to detect or remove deposits or restorative margins. Another error is to adapt only the middle one-third of an explorer or curet blade instead of the terminal 1 to 2 mm (see Figure 11-17).

As seen in Figure 11-17, proper adaptation requires that the working end approach the deposit in a diagonal manner. If the entire working end of an explorer is parallel to the deposit, the borders and configuration can not be determined. This decreases the opportunity for the clinician to detect calculus or an overhanging margin because only a minor vibration is transmitted to the operator. Instead, the tip actually needs to bisect the deposit to send a significant vibration to the operator. When calculus exists it must be removed in portions and this occurs by fracturing parts of the deposit, piece by piece. This fragmenting requires that the curet blade also approach the deposit in a diagonal direction (see Figure 11-17A). If the entire blade is placed parallel to the deposit, the incorrect portion is adapted and excessive lateral pressure is needed to initiate fracturing (see Figure 11-17B). Furthermore, client discomfort is inevitable when the terminal 1 to 2 mm of the working end is not adapted to the tooth because the tip or blade is inserted into the sulcular or pocket lining.

**Angulation.** Angulation refers to the angle created between the plane of the instrument face and the plane of the cementum, enamel, calculus deposit, or restorative material. The accepted range is *greater* than 45° and *less* than 90° (see Figure 11-18). Angulation less than 45° will result in burnished deposit and angles greater than 90°

remove soft tissue pocket lining (see Chapter 14—soft tissue curettage). Ideally, the curet or sickle blade meets the tooth surface at a 70° to 80° angle for strokes used to detect and remove plaque and plaque-retentive factors. When calculus is only minimally attached to root surfaces, or when debridement is occurring, a blade-to-tooth angle of less than 70° can be used. To adjust blade angulation, the handle is tilted slightly toward or away from the root surface. Tilting the handle toward the root decreases (closes) the angle. Conversely, tilting the handle away from the root surface increases (opens) this angle.

Although explorers do not have a "face" connecting two lateral surfaces like a curet, they must be adapted to the tooth at a correct angle. Adapting only the terminal 1 to 2 millimeters of the working end ensures the working end to tooth angle is approximately 70°.

**Activation.** Activation involves the use of hand, wrist, and forearm motions to maneuver the strokes used to assess and debride a surface. These motions include rolling, pivoting, and rocking. All three motions occur simultaneously when moving the working end around the tooth surfaces. However, depending on the surface being negotiated, one movement will dominate. For instance, if the clinician is advancing across the buccal surface of a molar, rocking will always occur to allow the tip to travel between the epithelial attachment and the gingival margin. Only minor but constant rolling and pivoting are needed to keep the terminal portion adapted because the buccal surface is only slightly convex. When approaching the line angle, however, the clinician continues rocking, rolls the instrument dramatically to stay adapted to the extremely convex surface, and simultaneously pivots with the wrist in neutral position.

Rolling and pivoting also are required to maintain adaptation from the line angle to the midline of the tooth surface. In particular, pivoting is relied upon to negotiate

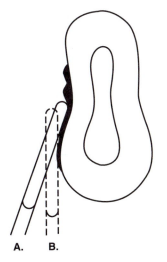

**Figure 11-17** Cross section of a root with calculus in a proximal concavity. To negotiate the midline and deepest portion of the concavity, rolling and pivoting occur. **A.** The terminal 1 to 2 mm of the cutting edge is adapted instead of the middle portion. **B.** An explorer tip is adapted in a similar fashion.

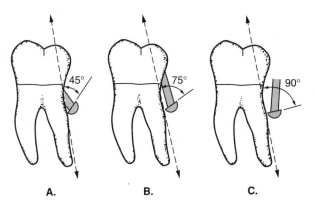

**Figure 11-18** Angulation. **A.** A 45° blade-to-tooth angle is too closed to effectively remove calculus. **B.** A 75° blade-to-tooth angle is ideal for calculus removal and debridement of bacterial plaque. **C.** A 90° blade-to-tooth angle is too open. Notice as the handle is tilted away from the root surface, the blade-to-tooth angle is increased.

the proximal surfaces. If, instead, a clinician relies on only rolling the instrument to stay adapted, eventually the point of an explorer or toe of the curet will meet the tooth surface. In this case, the instrument-to-tooth relationship is inappropriate because of the potential for cemental gouging and ineffective calculus removal. The rock, roll, and pivot are used with probes, explorers, sickles, and curets but not with files. Activation of a file is unique and will be discussed in a subsequent section.

**Three Types of Strokes.** There are three types of strokes associated with activation: assessment (exploratory or placement stroke), calculus removal work stroke, and root surface debridement work stroke (Nield-Gehrig & Houseman, 1996) (see Table 11-6). Supragingival activation is not discussed; however the principles are similar to subgingival activation except that the visualization of the supragingival surfaces enhances the quality and efficiency of removal.

**Assessment strokes** evaluate the root surface for presence of deposits, irregularities, anatomy, or other plaque-retentive factors. This stroke has commonly been called the "exploratory stroke" because it is seeking information about the root surface. Instruments used to assess include probes, explorers, sickles, and curets. Probes assess the pocket depth and topography; and explorers, sickles, and curets detect calculus and other plaque-retentive factors prior to and during nonsurgical instrumentation. The role of assessment in reevaluation cannot be overemphasized. Periodontal probing and exploration always occur during the reevaluation phase of therapy. A periodontal probe can determine if plaque-retentive factors are present, but it can not assess the deposit configuration, texture, or size as well as an explorer. The design characteristics of files limit their use in assessment. Assessment strokes always employ the use of the lightest grasp and lateral pressure possible. In fact, it is best to glide the instrument over the tooth surface during assessment without consciously applying any lateral pressure. Strokes are usually moderate in length and must be overlapping on all surfaces.

**Calculus removal working strokes** are employed with instruments that have cutting edges (curets, sickles, files) to remove calculus and associated bacterial plaque. This stroke is also employed to remove overhanging restorative margins (see Chapter 14). The difference between assessment strokes and calculus removal working strokes is that the latter are activated by **lateral pressure**, which is the force exerted against the deposit with a cutting edge of a sickle, curet, or file. Lateral pressure is achieved by the following:

1. Use the ring finger, the finger rest, to firmly stabilize the stroke. The amount of pressure used depends on the purpose of the stroke and class of the instrument. Probes and explorers require a stable fulcrum, but pressure is not needed on the fulcrum because the stroke does not remove a plaque-retentive factor. Firm, but not heavy, pressure is exerted on the fulcrum when a file, sickle, or curet is activated because their purpose is removal of calculus or overhang.
2. Lightly press the finger rest (ring finger) into the tooth surface. The force will be on hard tissue where the client will only feel pressure and not discomfort. If the pressure is placed on the instrument only, the client will feel discomfort and the stroke will be uncontrolled and ineffective.
3. Slightly flex the index finger and thumb to exert pressure on the instrument. The pressure must be

**Table 11-6  Comparison of Assessment, Calculus Removal, and Root Surface Debridement Strokes**

|  | Assessment | Calculus Removal Work Stroke | Root Surface Debridement Work Stroke |
|---|---|---|---|
| Purpose | to assess root/crown surface topography including plaque-retentive factors | calculus (and overhang removal) | remove or disrupt bacterial plaque and endotoxin |
| Hand-Activated Instruments Used | explorers, probes, curets, sickles | curets, sickles, files | curets with flexible shanks |
| Stroke Direction | vertical, oblique, and/or horizontal | vertical, oblique, and/or horizontal | vertical, oblique, and/or horizontal |
| Insertion | 20° to 40° | 20° to 40° | 20° to 40° |
| Tip/Blade to Tooth Angulation | 70° to 80° with explorers, curets, and sickles; 0° to 10° with probe | 70° to 80° | 70° to 80° or less |
| Stroke Motions | rock, roll, and pivot | rock, roll, and pivot | rock, roll, and pivot |
| Stroke Length | moderate length; longer than working strokes | short, powerful (1 to 3 mm) | moderate length |
| Lateral Pressure | none | light to moderate | light |

evenly distributed between the index finger and thumb. Putting the majority of pressure on the instrument with only the thumb will cause the clinician to push the instrument against the tooth. In this case, the operator will lose control of the instrument. Try this by exerting lateral force on a typodont with only your thumb and then with even pressure distributed between your thumb and index finger. The latter should enhance control.

No matter where the fulcrum is placed, the amount of pressure placed on the finger rest is related to the amount of pressure needed on the instrument blade and deposit. If more pressure is placed on the finger rest, then more pressure is transmitted to the deposit and tooth surface. The amount of pressure needed depends on the purpose of the stroke, the mechanism of attachment of the plaque-retentive factor, and the sharpness of the blade. Assessment with probes and explorers requires a very light approach as does debridement of bacterial plaque. Strokes initiated to remove calculus or an overhanging restoration require more moderate pressure. Heavy pressure on the finger rest is never indicated because of the stress on the operator and effects on the client. Excessive pressure on mandibular teeth can result in temporomandibular joint discomfort. If heavy pressure is recognized, two factors should be evaluated: instrument selection and sharpness. Perhaps another instrument design is needed or sharpening is indicated.

The wrist rock initiates movement of the instrument on the tooth surface, after achieving proper lateral pressure. The movement of the wrist, to the right and left (back and forth), causes the instrument to move vertically (up and down) on the enamel or root surface. It is important that the wrist rock for calculus removal be an extremely minimal movement. If the rock is too great, the deposit will be burnished because the blade-to-tooth angle will be changed with each stroke. Self-evaluation is critical to ensure that the blade-to-tooth angle remains the same with each subsequent stroke. The opposite of the wrist rock is **finger activation** where the finger(s) and thumb move back and forth to push and pull the instrument. Pulling constantly will tire the fingers rapidly even though finger activation results in deposit removal. Strained fingers are the result of not using wrist motion.

The result of correct activation is efficient and effective bacterial plaque and calculus removal. **Channeling**, or removing the mineralized calculus deposit piece by piece, is the result of short, powerful, controlled wrist rocks while rolling and pivoting the instrument to keep the terminal portion adapted. Channeling strokes are approximately 1 mm long. On the proximal surfaces, the goal is to channel calculus by advancing to the contact area in a constant upward movement while maintaining proper adaptation. The approach to channeling mineralized deposit depends on the width and length of the calculus. A deposit that is very wide but only 1 mm in length (apical to coronal dimension) can be channeled by advancing from the distal portion of the deposit to the mesial portion in small (1 to 2 mm) segments. (see Figure 11-19A) On the other hand, calculus that is narrow and wide (apical to coronal dimension) is still channeled from distal to mesial; however, due to the vertical height it also needs to be channeled in 1 to 2 mm segments from the apical border to the coronal border (see Figure 11-19B). Calculus that extends more than a few millimeters from its apical to coronal border can not be effectively removed with one long channel stroke.

Root surface **debridement work strokes** employ only light lateral pressure because their purpose is to remove residual calculus remaining after calculus removal work strokes, and to remove or dislodge bacterial plaque and its endotoxins. Debridement strokes are automatically performed with calculus removal work strokes. On the other hand, debridement strokes might occur independently from calculus removal when gingival inflammation, bleeding on probing, and/or pocket depth are present and calculus is not detected with assessment strokes.

Debridement strokes employ the use of very light lateral pressure, are multidirectional, and cover the entire root surface. In debridement, unnecessary removal of cementum is avoided because of the light lateral pressure used and limited number of strokes employed as compared to traditional root planing technique. Curets with flexible shanks are recommended to further decrease the chance of unwarranted cemental removal. Root planing strokes performed solely to produce smooth, glassy polished surfaces in all locations are not advocated.

**Stroke Directions.** Various stroke directions are advocated to facilitate adequate root surface preparation. Vertical and oblique strokes with a curet or explorer are the most common; however, horizontal strokes are also

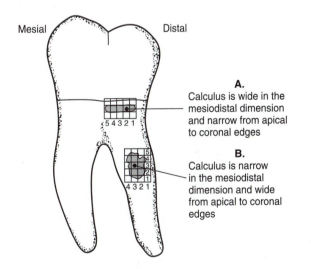

Mesial        Distal

**A.**
Calculus is wide in the mesiodistal dimension and narrow from apical to coronal edges

**B.**
Calculus is narrow in the mesiodistal dimension and wide from apical to coronal edges

**Figure 11-19** Channeling in segments. **A.** Five segments are illustrated. Each calculus removal stroke will extend from the apical to the coronal edge. **B.** Four segments are indicated in the distal to mesial direction, and five segments in the vertical dimension.

important. Use of only one stroke direction is detrimental because it encourages incomplete root coverage and striations in the root surface. Oblique strokes are commonly used on buccal and lingual surfaces, vertical strokes on proximal surfaces, and horizontal strokes at line angles, in deep narrow pockets, near furcation entrances, and on narrow facial and lingual surfaces of anterior teeth. Horizontal strokes are also effective beneath facial/buccal and lingual restorative margins and apical to abrasion, erosion, or abfractions. To perform horizontal strokes with a curet or explorer, a toe-down approach is used, meaning the curet toe or explorer point is directed toward the attachment (see Figure 11-20). The traditional vertical upright handle position is rotated toward the gingiva and, as a result, the shank and handle are diagonal or perpendicular to the buccal or lingual surface of the tooth depending on the instrument design.

All three stroke directions are needed to instrument a surface, although two directions might be adequate depending on the location and width of the periodontal pocket. Using only one stroke results in undetected deposits because of the irregular formations of calculus and the fact that deposits can be minute in size. For example, routine use of horizontal strokes decreases accurate detection of plaque-retentive entities because calculus frequently forms in horizontal directions, and restorative margins extend in a horizontal direction. If only horizontal strokes are used and the clinician is coronal or apical to a deposit, it will go undetected. Likewise, if only horizontal strokes are used below a restorative margin then an improper margin (deficient, open, or overhanging—see Chapter 4) could be missed. Use of vertical and oblique strokes is necessary to evaluate the relationship of the restorative margin to the tooth surface.

## Techniques

The following sections address instrumentation with each class of instruments. It is important that student clinicians

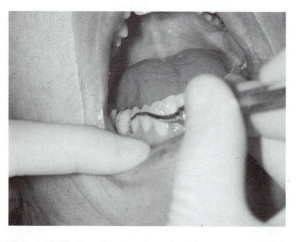

**Figure 11-20** Toe-down approach with an area-specific curet.

and practitioners alike continually self-evaluate instrumentation technique. With any skill, bad habits can develop that are usually harder to correct when repeatedly practiced. In fact, calculus can be removed with ineffective techniques, but these compromises have consequences for both the client and clinician. Client discomfort results and clinician discomfort, predisposition to occupational hazards, inefficiency, and frustration are common.

**Manual Periodontal Probes.** The straight periodontal probe is inserted with a gentle motion to the epithelial attachment where soft resiliency should be felt. If calculus impedes insertion, it will feel hard and resistant to movement of the probe. If calculus is present, probing around the deposit can be attempted to achieve accurate periodontal pocket measurements. If generalized calculus interferes with probing, initial probe readings are recorded immediately after heavy calculus removal and before final completion of the segment(s) planned for the appointment. Thus, these readings become the baseline probe depths.

The working end of the probe is adapted parallel to the root surface being probed. The tip is placed at a zero-degree angle to the root surface and the remainder of the working end is angulated at approximately 10° to the root surface (see Figure 11-21). This angle permits the gentle and smooth walking of the periodontal probe with small vertical motions of about a millimeter in height. Insertion commonly occurs mesial to the distal line angle for the distal surface of posterior teeth and near the midline for anteriors. When the distal line angle is reached, the same probe-to-tooth angulation must be maintained by rolling and pivoting. The probe is then reinserted on posterior teeth distal to the distal line angle and near the midline on anteriors to negotiate buccal/lingual and mesial surfaces. On the distal or mesial surfaces, the clinician must achieve two things: 1) the working end against the contact area, and 2) extension of the tip of the probe to the midline of the proximal surface (see Figure 11-21). Knowing the width of the root surface at the cervix is beneficial for estimating the extension to the midline (see Chapter 10, Table 10-2). If the tooth is 10 mm wide, the probe must be extended approximately 5 mm to reach the midline, depending on the depth of the periodontal pocket. If the width at the cervix is only 6 mm such as in an anterior tooth, then the probe need only be extended 3 mm toward the midline.

Six point probing is conducted by walking the circumference of the sulcus or pocket and recording measurements in a standardized fashion. Significant measurements in between the six points routinely probed are also recorded. This practice facilitates the visualization of the pocket topography. Clinical attachment loss is also critical to measure with the periodontal probe as described in Chapter 3. Standardized techniques for both probing depths and clinical attachment loss are important because they will be repetitively measured at

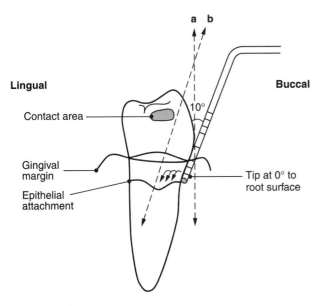

**Figure 11-21** The periodontal probe is inserted to the epithelial attachment with the working end parallel to the root surface. The arrows indicate the 1 mm movement when walking the probe from the buccal to the midline of the proximal surface.
*Key:* The dashed line **a** represents the angle of the probe to the root surface if it was applied parallel to the buccal surface of the crown. This adaptation would result in incorrect measurements and probe tip placement into the sulcular epithelium. The dashed line **b** represents the correct adaptation of the probe to the midline of the proximal surface.

maintenance appointments to determine future therapy needs. Correct technique with the same type of periodontal probe is the best avenue to enhance standardization of measurements for a particular client. Refer to Chapter 3 for the relationship of probing to periodontal assessment including automated probing and screening systems.

Nabers probes, for furcation detection and assessment, are adapted and activated in a different manner than the straight periodontal probe. When gingiva occludes the furcation entrance, the curved Nabers probe must be inserted subgingivally with the tip very closed (as close to 0° as possible) and rolled gently into the furcation entrance. When recession exposes the defect on the buccal or lingual surface, the tip of the Nabers probe can be inserted directly into the defect. It is important that the clinician visualize the suspected root anatomy to accurately adapt the Nabers probe to determine extent and classification of the furcation involvement.

**Explorers.** Explorer technique depends somewhat on the instrument design. For purposes of this text the technique will be divided into that for curved explorers that are designed like universal curets (see Chapter 10) (e.g., 2R/2L, Suter Dental Manufacturing Company; and EXD2 and EXD2H, Hu-Friedy® Manufacturing, Inc.)

and the 11/12 explorer, which is designed like the Gracey 11/12 area-specific curet. Although explorers do not have the cutting edge or blade width and depth of curets, the design of the working end and shank affects adaptation to the root surface.

All explorers, regardless of design, have **universal characteristics** meaning that both sides of the tip can be adapted to all surfaces on the buccal or lingual by alternating the side of the tip. For example, the buccal surfaces of teeth #31 to #28 can be explored with the same end. The distal surfaces are explored with one side of the tip and the buccal and mesial surfaces are explored with the other side of the tip. When the opposing surfaces (linguals) are assessed, the other end is used.

General principles for exploration include:

1. Insertion to the epithelial attachment on all surfaces to ensure complete coverage of the root surface. This can be estimated by placing a probe next to the explorer working end and shank to estimate the needed depth of penetration subgingivally.
2. Visualization of the normal anatomical features of the tooth in combination with the radiographic appearance of the root. The radiograph might indicate alterations in the root structure on proximal surfaces.
3. Use of vertical and oblique strokes that overlap one another to reduce the chance of missing a deposit.
4. Application of horizontal strokes where appropriate (line angles, erosion/abrasion/abfractions, restorative margins, furcations, narrow pockets, and facials/linguals of anterior teeth).
5. Methodical and slow coverage of the root surface.
6. An extremely light grasp and finger rest/fulcrum are always used. The explorer should be held so lightly that a tap on its handle would move the instrument. A moderate or heavy grasp decreases tactile vibrations, accurate interpretation, and comfort for the client and operator.

Principles of correct adaptation and activation with curved explorers follow:

1. *Fundamentals.* Grasp, fulcrum, positioning, mirror use, and adaptation recommendations previously discussed apply. Conventional and cross arch fulcrums are used. Conventional fulcrum placement is possible most everywhere in the normally aligned dentition. Cross arch fulcruming with the curved explorer often occurs on the mandibular lingual when exploring the distal surfaces if the operator is seated at nine o'clock. When exploring the direct lingual surfaces and the mesial lingual the clinician will move the fulcrum closer to the working area. Another modification of a fulcrum and seating position might be the maxillary posterior areas and lingual of the maxillary anteriors

when seated at eleven to twelve o'clock. A palm-up orientation is ideal to negotiate the root surface topography in these areas as seen in the previous Figure 11-16.

2. *Adaptation.* In the posterior, the explorer is placed slightly mesial to the distal line angle and inserted subgingivally with the side of the tip against the epithelial attachment. Assessment of the shank placement with the 2R/2L design shows that the terminal shank is parallel to the distal surface (see Figure 11-22). Remember to only adapt the terminal 1 to 2 mm of the tip. A 70° angle between the tip and root surface will be achieved by tilting the handle slightly away from the tooth. Care must be taken to prevent the point from entering the epithelial attachment causing discomfort and inaccurate assessment.

3. *Activation (Distal Posterior Surfaces).* Rocking occurs to extend from the epithelial attachment to the gingival margin. When at the line angle, the roll motion dominates and the clinician pivots away from the tooth on the fulcrum while *slightly* dropping the handle. This movement is very subtle and the purpose is to achieve a working end orientation to the distal surface that bisects the surface (see Figure 11-23). The handle is tipped slightly away from the tooth in order to direct the tip toward the midline; therefore, the handle is perpendicular to the long axis of the proximal surface. If the pivoting motion was not incorporated and the terminal shank remained parallel to the distal surface, then the midline area might not be thoroughly explored because the tip would not extend to this region. At the same time the tip must still be extended to the epithelial attachment and if not possible due to the pocket depth, the 11/12 explorer would be used. The 11/12 extended shank design (see Chapter 10) would be advantageous in a deep pocket.

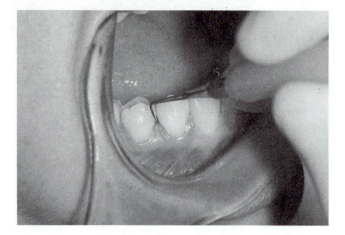

**Figure 11-23** A curved explorer (Suter 2R/2L) adapted to the distal surface. Continual pivoting occurs to keep the tip adapted to the root surface.

a. Once around the line angle, the clinician continues to perform all three motions especially the pivot to explore the distal surface thoroughly. Because the area from the contact to the buccal or lingual surface is broad, it must be divided into sections. Vertically it can be divided into three sections as illustrated in Figure 11-24. Section one is explored first before advancing to sections 2 and 3. As section 1 is completed with the rocking motion, the clinician rolls and pivots to reach section 2. After completion of section 2, rolling and pivoting occur again to advance the explorer to the contact area.

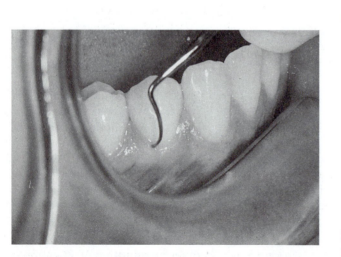

**Figure 11-22** A curved explorer (Suter 2R/2L) inserted at the distal line angle.

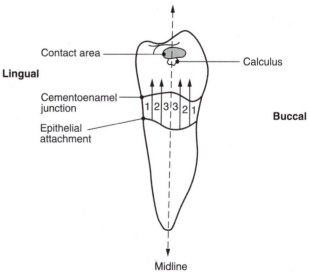

**Figure 11-24** The proximal surface is divided into sections. A piece of calculus wedged beneath the contact area is challenging to detect; exploration from the buccal or lingual must extend to section three.

b. Remember that the contact area has dimension and that calculus accumulation is often present here, especially in anterior teeth (see Chapter 10). Calculus located in the contact area can be deceiving because the explorer sends back a vibration that stops or binds the explorer which simulates what is felt when the contact area is reached. The reason for this is that it is difficult to feel the top of a piece of calculus wedged in the contact area (see Figure 11-24). Only the bottom of the deposit is felt, which makes the clinician think it is tooth structure. To remedy this situation, ensure that exploratory strokes are extended about 1 mm past where you think the teeth contact. In other words, follow through with the assessment stroke into the contact area and slightly occlusal to where the contact seems to be. When this approach is taken, the edge of the top of the piece of calculus is tactily transmitted to the clinician.

4. *Activation (Buccal/Lingual and Mesial Posterior Surfaces).* In the posterior, the tip is reinserted distal to the distal line angle and the buccal or lingual surface and mesial surface are negotiated as previously described. The tip, shank, and handle orientation on the mesial surface (refer to Figure 11-16) simulate the distal surface.

5. *Activation (Anterior Surfaces).* In the anterior, initial insertion is slightly to the side of the midline (buccal or lingual) and the instrument is moved toward either the distal or mesial surface. Because of the narrow distal/mesial dimension of the anterior teeth (5 to 7 mm), rolling and pivoting must occur rapidly. It will only take a few strokes to rock to the line angle located just 2.5 to 3.5 mm from the midline. Then rolling takes place to keep the tip adapted to the convex surface. Once around the line angle, the proximal surface from the line angle to the contact is divided into sections. Even though the faciolingual dimension of anterior teeth is less than posterior teeth, three sections are still advised. After all the proximal surfaces are explored from canine to canine in one direction (toward or away from the clinician), the instrument end is changed and the clinician proceeds with the same process in the other direction. In the anterior region, the clinician stands vertically on the fulcrum to position the tip as seen in Figure 11-25.

The use of the 11/12 explorer is similar to the curved explorers in that the grasp and portion of the tip adapted to the surface are the same. Differences between the techniques occur in fulcrum placement in some areas, and orientation of the shank and handle to the tooth surface. These differences are related to the design features. Conventional fulcrums are used with the 11/12 in most areas with opposite arch placement being indicated

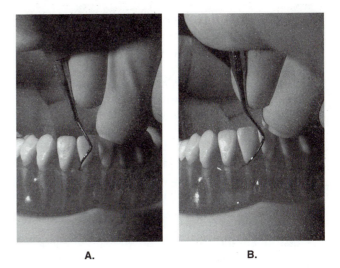

**A.**                              **B.**

**Figure 11-25** Use of a curved explorer (Suter 2R/2L) in the anterior. **A.** A conventional fulcrum is placed on the incisal tooth edge and rolling takes place to keep the tip adapted. **B.** If rolling does not occur, the tip will project into the sulcular tissue causing discomfort.

in maxillary molar regions, especially when deep pockets are present. When approaching the line angle in the posterior, the instrument handle is not dropped. In fact, the clinician must stand vertically on the fulcrum and establish parallelism between the handle, terminal shank, and tooth surface while rolling the instrument around the line angle on all surfaces (see Figure 11-26). If the instrument handle is "dropped," as previously described with curved explorers, the tip will be directed coronally towards the contact area and not the midline.

**Curets.** Universal and area-specific curet designs and selection are reviewed in the previous chapter. Positioning, grasp, fulcrum placement, and adaptation correlate

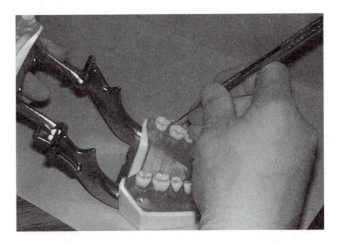

**Figure 11-26** Adaptation of the 11/12 explorer on the distal surface of a posterior tooth.

to the explorer technique recommendations discussed in the previous section. Universal curets are adapted like the curved explorer and area-specific curets are adapted like the area-specific explorer. As previously stated, the difference between explorer technique and curet technique lies within the activation phase. Both universal and area-specific curets are activated with the same principles as follows:

1. Apply the positioning, grasp, fulcrum placement, and adaptation principles discussed previously.
2. With a working stroke, firm pressure is exerted on the finger rest for stability. The thumb and index finger are both flexed applying pressure on the instrument handle. Moderate pressure is needed to remove most calculus, but pressure is dependent on the calculus size and mode of attachment. Heavy lateral pressure is never needed unless an instrument is dull or the calculus is extremely tenacious. To remedy the first case, the instrument is sharpened and maintained routinely, and in the second case another instrument is selected such as an ultrasonic device or file. Light, but firm pressure is exerted on the finger rest for the debridement work stroke.
3. Activate the stroke from the hand, wrist, and forearm as a unit. Once the proper blade to tooth angulation is established and the force placed on the fulcrum finger, the curet is moved coronally to reach the top of the deposit or the contact area. This is accomplished via the rocking motion.
4. During the movement of the instrument, ensure that the blade-to-tooth angle is maintained. If the blade-to-tooth angle is rotated closed (less than 70°) calculus will be burnished. If the stroke is opened, over 90° calculus will also be burnished because the lateral surface of the curet will eventually contact the calculus. Remember the objective is to remove the deposit by placing the sharp cutting edge at the ideal angle to the tooth surface depending on the type and purpose of the stroke. An effective way to think of this motion is to scale into the contact area (coronally) or straight up the tooth. This does not imply that the stroke is one long vertical motion. Instead it is a series of shorter vertical motions (1 to 2 mm).
5. Remove the deposit by channeling or biting into the calculus. Channeling encourages removal of the calculus piece by piece starting at the apical-most portion. A frequent clinician error is trying to remove light, moderate, or heavy calculus layer by layer (outermost surface to innermost surface) with minimal strokes. This creates burnishing and incomplete removal. For beginning clinicians it seems as though channeling takes a fair amount of time; however, in reality, quality results are achieved much faster if slow and methodical channeling occurs.

6. After each stroke, pause momentarily and relax the grasp. Do not move the instrument apically. Instead, reexert the pressure on the grasp and fulcrum and engage another working stroke coronally.
7. Once a series of strokes (channeling) occurs reaching the uppermost portion of the deposit, lighten the pressure and assess its removal with the curet blade. If still present, replace the stroke approximately 1 mm apical to the remaining deposit and repeat the process. If the debridement work stroke is being used in the absence of detectable calculus deposit, a light grasp and light lateral pressure are employed. Channeling with lateral pressure is not used; however, debridement strokes must overlap one another to ensure complete root coverage.

When treating multirooted teeth, the task is complicated if the epithelial attachment is located below the furcation entrance. The location of the furcation involvement, relationship of the gingiva to the furcation entrance, and the pocket depth are also factors to consider when deciding how to treat the area. The best approach is to treat each root as a separate tooth and with a combination of strokes. The distal surfaces of each root are instrumented, and then the buccal/lingual and mesial surfaces of each root are treated, ensuring overlapping strokes on the surface where the roots meet (see Figure 11-27). Next, concentrate on the concavity coronal to the furcation entrance by employing horizontal and oblique strokes with a toe-down approach where the internal portions of each root meet the root trunk. An area-specific curet designed for mesial surfaces (11/12) or one with a straight shank (1/2 or 7/8) can be used in the concavity. When the gingiva occludes the furcation, the periodontal pocket is shallow, or the furcation

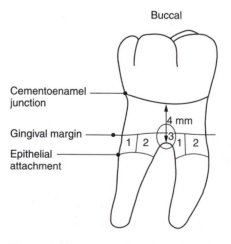

**Figure 11-27** The distal portions of each root (sections 1) are debrided, then the buccal and mesial surfaces are debrided (sections 2). Lastly, the concavity is debrided (section 3). A combination of strokes is used in all areas. Horizontal strokes with a toe-down approach are especially useful in section 3.

entrance is barely detectable, treating each root separately may not be feasible. Instead, the area is treated with a combination of strokes including the horizontal, toe-down approach to treat the concavity coronal to the furcation and the limited furcation opening. A combination of universal and area-specific instruments are effective depending on anatomy, deposit size, and location.

Maxillary molar mesial and distal furcations present a unique instrumentation challenge. Access to the mesial furcations is best from the lingual surface because the furcation entrance is located lingually and not directly in the midline (see Chapter 10, Figure 10-16 to review this anatomy). The portion of the furcation entrance toward the buccal still needs to be debrided however. An area-specific mesial surface design and a universal instrument with a long terminal shank and working end might be needed to access the mesial entrance. The distal furcation entrance is located near the midline of the tooth, therefore, approaching it with a distal area-specific and appropriate universal curet from both the lingual and buccal provide equal access. When furcation involvement is present on maxillary proximal surfaces, extreme rolling and pivoting is needed to adapt explorers and curets into the defect. Chapter 10 includes a review of furcation anatomy. Pattison and Pattison (1992) provide the reader with a comprehensive review of advanced root instrumentation in furcations.

Mobility might also be encountered. The clinician's mirror hand can be used to stabilize the tooth during instrumentation. Stabilization might occur on the incisal or occlusal edge if only slightly mobile. If significant mobility exists, stability might be needed on the surface opposite or adjacent to the one being scaled. For example, if the facial surface of a mobile mandibular anterior tooth is being instrumented, then the index finger on the mirror hand can be placed on the lingual surface near the incisal edge. If the mesial surface of a molar is being treated, the lingual surface might again be stabilized. Mobile teeth sometimes interfere with optimal fulcrum placement. A clinician needs to be creative and use alternative fulcrums when the tooth chosen for the finger rest is not steady.

**Files.** Design features of files (Hirschfeld 317, 5111) used to remove tenacious calculus were reviewed in the previous chapter. Adaptation and activation of files differs from curets in blade-to-tooth relationship and stroke activation. Positioning, grasp, and fulcrum placement are maintained to adapt the file head parallel to the surface being treated. A working file is placed on top of calculus and not on the root surface. Because it is not possible to assess calculus location and configuration with a file, the clinician needs to explore the deposit well and mentally visualize its location and size. The file is then placed to match the visual image and, hopefully, the bulk of a heavy deposit is detectable.

With the working file parallel to the deposit the cutting edges are engaged by applying pressure on the finger rest, thumb, and index fingers. A long pull stroke is not used because eventually the file's cutting edges would reach root surface not covered with calculus causing cemental striations. Instead, the stroke should be directed into the calculus to force the deposit into the rake angle and result in crushing and fragmenting. After each of these strokes, the clinician relaxes the grasp and replaces the file head on the deposit. To effectively fracture deposit, the file head is adapted to the calculus in various ways. The deposit can be approached vertically, obliquely, and horizontally. To do so, a variety of fulcrums is needed. Most frequently, conventional fulcrums are used. Cross arch fulcrums can be employed for mandibular lingual proximal surfaces and opposite arch fulcrums for maxillary posterior areas.

## ENDPOINT OF INSTRUMENTATION

No matter if the terms scaling and root planing or debridement are used to describe the removal of plaque-retentive factors, the endpoint of NSPT is the same. Endpoint is defined as the restoration of gingival health. Gingival health is accomplished through the client's participation in appropriate oral self-care, the clinician's professional instrumentation, and other supportive therapy performed for the client's benefit. Gingival health can only be expected after an appropriate time interval has passed subsequent to the completion of active non-surgical therapy. The four- to six-week reevaluation appointment is, therefore, necessary to evaluate the endpoint of therapy. Without an appropriately timed reevaluation visit, the endpoint of active therapy is never assessed.

Immediately after removal of plaque-retentive factors, the reassessment of the subgingival environment with an explorer is a clinical endpoint that only measures the tooth surfaces preparation for healing to take place. As previously discussed, the clinical endpoint is to remove all detectable plaque-retentive factors knowing that all indicated root surfaces have been treated with the debridement work stroke. In contrast, the endpoint of therapy as measured at the reevaluation visit includes the measurement of clinical criteria such as probing depth, clinical attachment level, and gingival inflammation accompanied by bleeding. Ideally, the goals are a reduction in probing depth, a gain in clinical attachment level, and resolution of gingival inflammation and bleeding. If bleeding and inflammation are present, site-specific therapy is performed including additional instrumentation, consideration of chemotherapeutic agents, and further client education in self-care practices.

The next question asked is, how does one evaluate the clinical endpoint of instrumentation? Because the removal of subgingival plaque and its by-products cannot be measured clinically, the topography of the tooth surface is the best alternative. The clinical endpoint for the majority of clients is a relatively smooth tooth surface devoid of detectable plaque-retentive factors. In NSPT, the explorer examines the subgingival environment, and the explorer accompanied by air and illumination are used to assess the supragingival environment. If a subgingival area remains rough or irregular and calculus is suspected, the clinician should attempt to remove it. To assess when the instrumentation process should halt, the clinician considers many factors: the self-evaluation of proper instrumentation technique, the progress towards removing the irregularity, the probable anatomy in the area, the radiographic appearance of the tooth surface, the extent of gingival inflammation, the extent of periodontitis, and the generalized characteristics of the client's calculus and other plaque-retentive factors.

If instrumentation technique is sound and further instrumentation is not producing results, then the clinician must make a decision to continue or halt instrumentation. This decision is made by evaluating the extent of periodontal disease and the host risk factors identified from the health history. If extensive disease exists and the client is a heavy smoker, the clinician might decide to continue instrumentation for a short period of time. On the other hand, if a medically healthy client has little gingival inflammation, localized sites of chronic periodontitis with early bone loss, and no probing depth or attachment loss in the area, then a decision is made to leave the minute roughness or discrepancy. This area is then reexamined at the reevaluation visit. When clinicians are "in doubt" about certain areas, these sites can be recorded on the record of services to ensure their reevaluation at the next visit during active therapy, or at the reevaluation visit. This practice builds the clinician's NSPT skills because it is a means for self-assessment of the clinician's choice as to when instrumentation should end. If the area demonstrates clinical health upon reevaluation, then the decision was sound. If not, the decision is reevaluated and further therapy is provided. It is noted that the client's role in self-care is also a factor in the healing process and, therefore, homecare must be reevaluated along with the clinical parameters of health.

## INSTRUMENT SEQUENCING

Sequencing of nonsurgical instrumentation is directly related to the care plan. First, the area must be confined to what is reasonable for the time period scheduled. Hopefully, the time period has been adjusted to meet the needs of the client in a particular area. For example, a half-mouth approach might be indicated in a ninety-minute appointment. When in doubt about the extent of the area to treat, restrict the area to a sextant or quadrant to ensure complete instrumentation. Taking on too much of an area will result in ineffective treatment. Within the area defined decide if there are different deposit types and sizes, and different pocket topography. If so, remove the heaviest deposits first, selecting the appropriate instrument design. Treating all areas with heavy tenacious calculus first with a file or ultrasonic device and then changing to other instruments is effective. Use of the

explorer after removal of heavy calculus is indicated before selecting curets. If heavy calculus remains, reinstrumentation with the file or an ultrasonic device is indicated. Also a curet with a rigid shank and large blade might be needed. Not using the explorer to evaluate progress in this situation often results in burnished calculus because an instrument such as an area-specific curet with a flexible shank is used that does not remove heavy tenacious deposit. After removal of heavier deposits, the clinician progresses to other instruments based on deposit size, area being treated, and pocket depth.

Within the area being treated, limit the area first approached. For example, if working on the mandibular right posterior sextant treat all the lingual surfaces first (with the largest embrasure spaces) before proceeding to the buccal surfaces. If treating the entire quadrant, perform removal of tenacious areas in the entire quadrant with a file; next treat the posterior teeth with curets, and move to the anterior and treat them with curets. Dividing the posterior and anterior regions when using curets is recommended because of the differences in instrument selection. Posterior area-specific curets and universal curets are commonly used in posterior regions while area-specific curets are often solely used in the anterior. The procedure, however, would depend on the instruments selected and available. Use of ultrasonic instrumentation affects sequencing because of the limited insert designs. More teeth are treated with one insert reducing operator time in changing inserts when compared to hand-activated instrumentation.

Use of the explorer during the sequence is related to therapist experience and the conditions of the client. The clinician will want to use an explorer prior to instrumentation. Curets should be used whenever possible to assess calculus removal during instrumentation, but the final product (clinical endpoint) is always evaluated with an explorer.

Quality debridement depends on a methodical approach. The clinician must be relaxed, concentrate, and be persistent in achieving the desired results. Perhaps perseverance is a characteristic inherent within the clinician, however, it is enhanced by empathy for the needs of the client; appropriate appointment planning and scheduling; and concentration during the technical removal of deposits. Stress due to time, frustration with removal, lack of concentration, and quitting prior to the clinical endpoint of therapy negatively affect the outcome.

## DOCUMENTATION

The client's record of service is useful for recording information about instrumentation techniques that were effective. For example, if a file was needed for tenacious calculus in the mandibular right quadrant, in addition to ultrasonic instrumentation, then it is anticipated that it will be needed in other areas. If specific instrumentation was effective in a Class II furcation involvement on the mandibular first molar, notes to this effect can expedite the instrumentation process during reevaluation and maintenance.

Notes about areas that were difficult to access and treat are indicated for evaluation and retreatment at subsequent appointments. If the therapist feels calculus or an overhanging margin remains in an area after repeated efforts, notes in the record of services will remind the professional to reexamine the area at the next appoint-ment. The record of services might also reflect the discussion of the purpose of debridement and how it differs from the traditional scaling and root planing. The approach to instrumentation will be discussed during the case presentation but further discussion is likely to occur during the instrumentation phase of therapy. Clients' reactions to instrumentation (gingival or root sensitivity or extreme comfort as compared to previous visits) are also noteworthy.

## Summary

Table 11-7 provides the reader with a summary of instrumentation principles. Just as the steps of instrument sharpening build upon one another, so do the steps in the instrumentation process. Periodontal instrumentation for those with periodontitis varies from basic instrumentation for clients in need of an oral prophylaxis in extent and time necessary to achieve effective results. It is every clinician's responsibility to strive to acquire the appropriate time necessary to thoroughly debride clients in active or maintenance NSPT. Additionally, professionals have the responsibility to educate the client about the need for ample time to instrument and the positive outcome that instrumentation has on the healing process. Even though clinicians use a variety of instrument designs and techniques to accomplish debridement, the instrumentation principles including fundamentals, adaptation, and activation always apply. The approach discussed herein is novel in that periodontal instrumentation with universal curets parallels that of curved explorers and area-specific curet instrumentation parallels exploration with the 11/12 explorer. Table 11-8 provides the reader with a self-assessment for explorer and curet use in NSPT.

## Case Studies

**Case Study One:** You are helping a peer, Ellen Fitsgarald, sharpen instruments and she comments that she understands the principles of sharpening yet her curets only stay sharp for a minimum number of strokes. Ellen asks for your opinion about her sharpening technique and problem with maintaining sharp edges. What would you do to help Ellen solve this problem?

**Case Study Two:** Observe the photograph of a file being sharpened (see Figure 11-28). Identify correct and incorrect technique considerations.

**Case Study Three:** You ask your clinical instructor to observe your instrumentation with area-specific curets. You are using the Gracey 1/2 as illustrated in Figure 11-29. Your instructor asks you to self-evaluate your own technique using the format in Table 11-8 as a guide. What do you evaluate for each of the principles of instrumentation?

**Case Study Four:** Herman Herros is returning for a reevaluation visit. He initially presented for care with 4 to 5 mm pocket depth, attachment loss, generalized diffuse gingival inflammation, generalized bleeding, generalized heavy to moderate subgingival calculus, and subgingival bacterial plaque. Upon reevaluation you notice that your client's gingiva is not as inflamed or bleeding on the buccal/facial surfaces as it was upon initial periodontal assessment. The interdental papilla, how-ever, still bleed upon probing and appear edematous and erythematous. The client reports using the interdental brush daily as you recommended. What do you suspect is the cause of the partial healing and how would you correct this problem?

**Case Study Five:** Based on sound fundamental principles of periodontal instrumentation, develop a trouble-shooting guide for instrumentation with curets. On the left-hand side, identify potential problems that could occur when using a curet. On the right, identify how to correct the problem.

## Case Study Discussions

**Discussion—Case Study One:** Observing Ellen's technique would be the best way to help her. Based on her statement you suspect she is overangulating her stone in relation to the face of the curet blade. Asking her if you can observe her instrumentation technique would be a first step in problem solving. You could also ask her to verbalize the steps in the sharpening process. You might also ask her questions directed at the placement of the stone against the lateral surface. When you observe her technique it is important to evaluate the first steps (positioning of the curet) because they are critical for correct stone placement. It might be that the positioning of the curet face parallel with the floor is not accomplished.

**Table 11-7 Summary of Instrumentation Principles**

| Instrument | Fulcrum | Point of Insertion | Stroke Direction | Tip/Blade-to-Tooth Angulation | Visual Cue |
|---|---|---|---|---|---|
| Gracey 1/2 (Anteriors) and 11/12 Explorer | Conventional | Slightly to the side of the midline to overlap strokes. | Oblique and horizontal on direct facial or lingual, vertical on proximals. | 70° to 80° | Handle and terminal shank are parallel to the long axis in the faciolingual dimension. Terminal shank parallel to the root surface being treated. On proximal surfaces, the handle and shank are tilted slightly toward the midline of the buccal/lingual surface. |
| Gracey 12/13 or Gracey 11/14 (Posteriors) and 11/12 Explorer | Conventional and opposite arch (maxillary positions) | 1 to 2 mm mesial to distal line angles; ensure overlapping of strokes at the line angle. | Oblique and horizontal on buccal and lingual, vertical on mesials and distals. | 70° to 80° | Terminal shank is parallel to the root surface being treated. Toe directed to opposite side of tooth (buccal or lingual). |
| Universal Curets (Posteriors) and Curved Explorer | Conventional and cross arch (mandibular distal lingual surfaces) | 1 to 2 mm mesial to distal line angles; ensure overlapping of strokes at the line angle. | Same as Gracey 1/2, 12/13, and 11/14. | 70° to 80° | Proximal surfaces—Terminal shank bisects the long axis of the distal or mesial surface in the posterior. Toe directed to the opposite side of the tooth (buccal or lingual). Handle is tilted away from the buccal or lingual surface; therefore is not parallel to the buccolingual long axis. Buccal/Lingual surfaces—Terminal shank is oblique to the surface. Handle is parallel to the buccolingual long axis. |
| H6/H7 Sickle (Anteriors) | Conventional | Facial—mesiofacial or distofacial line angle. Lingual—mesiolingual or distolingual line angle. | Vertical. | 70° to 80° | Handle and terminal shank are parallel to the long axis in the faciolingual dimension. Terminal shank is parallel to the root surface being treated. On proximal surfaces the handle and shank are tilted slightly toward the midline of the buccal/lingual surface. |
| Periodontal Probe | Conventional | Anteriors Midline. Posteriors Distal line angles. | Walk or bob on attachment. | Insert parallel to tooth surface and maintain parallelism (0° to 10°). | Must visualize root position and morphology/shape to maintain parallelism of the probe. Ensure midline of proximal is reached; top of working end should touch the contact area. |
| File | Conventional, cross arch, or opposite arch | On top of calculus. | Engage into calculus, only a short pull on top of calculus. | Head is placed parallel to deposit (0°). | Must visualize the relationship of the root anatomy, deposit, and file head. |

**Table 11-8  Self-Assessment: Explorers and Curets**

| Factor | Self-Assessment | Notes |
|---|---|---|
| Sharpness | • when a curet is used, the cutting blade is acutely sharp | |
| Grasp | • index finger and thumb across from one another and not touching<br>• handle rests between the middle joint of index fingers and joint where the finger and hand meet | |
| Fulcrum | • conventional, built-up the majority of the time; placed within 4 teeth adjacent to the tooth being treated<br>• cross arch fulcruming used on distal surfaces of mandibular lingual surfaces with universal designed instruments (curved explorers and universal curets)<br>• opposite arch fulcrum used in maxillary molar regions with area-specific designed instruments (11/12 explorer and area-specific curets)<br>• finger rest is maintained on the tooth surface<br>• palm-up orientation is used on maxillary teeth when appropriate<br>• pressure exerted on the finger rest is appropriate (stable but light with assessment strokes and debridement strokes; firm and moderate with calculus working strokes) | |
| Mirror Use | • grasp and placement are appropriate<br>• retraction is applied where indicated<br>• reflection (indirect illumination) is used<br>• transillumination is incorporated for supragingival assessment<br>• transillumination for subgingival assessment is used when indicated | |
| Adaptation | • the correct working end is selected<br>• inserts in the posterior 1 to 2 mm on either side of the distal line angle depending on surface being treated; inserts in the anterior 1 to 2 mm to the right or left of midline depending on surface being treated<br>• insertion is gentle, as closed as possible, to the epithelial attachment, and prevents tissue distention (20° to 40° blade-to-tooth angle with curet)<br>• calculus removal strokes are placed 1 mm apical to the deposit<br>• the terminal 1 to 2 mm is adapted to the convex or concave root or crown surface | |
| Activation | • assessment strokes are used with an explorer prior to and after curet use; curets are used during instrumentation to assess<br>• calculus removal work strokes are employed, with channeling as needed, applying appropriate *light to moderate lateral pressure* at a 70° to 80° blade-to-tooth angle.<br>• root surface debridement work strokes occur with a curet where indicated with *light lateral pressure* at a 70° to 80° blade-to-tooth angle or less<br>• short (1 to 2 mm) vertical, oblique, and/or horizontal strokes are employed as indicated<br>• the rock, roll, and pivot occur continuously<br>• the epithelial attachment is always reached during assessment and root surface debridement work strokes<br>• the midline of proximal surfaces is always assessed and treated | |

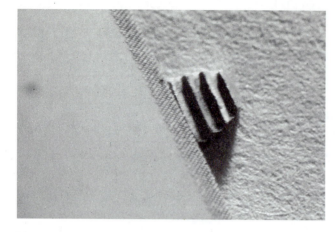

**Figure 11-28** Sharpening a file (Case Study Two).

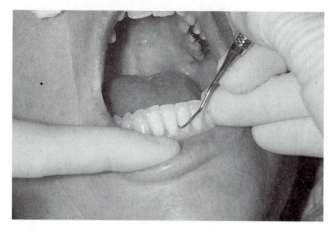

**Figure 11-29** Instrumentation with a Gracey 1/2 (Case Study Three).

This affects stone placement, which will negatively affect the sharpness of the blade. If Ellen positions the curet correctly, the stone placement is then evaluated. It is likely that the stone is placed against the lateral surface at an angle greater than 110°. If this is the case, use of a protractor will help Ellen better estimate the angle. A sharpening guide is another option.

**Discussion—Case Study Two:** Correct technique: The head of the file appears parallel to the surface beneath it. The tanged file is placed on the lip surface facing the shank. Incorrect technique: The tanged file is not placed flatly against the lip. If horizontal strokes are performed with the tanged file in this position, the cutting edge formation will be uneven, not sharp, and ill-contoured. The tanged file should be removed and replaced on the same lip surface so that it is positioned flatly within the rake angle and parallel to the file head.

**Discussion—Case Study Three:** Notes to record on the evaluation form include the following:

*Grasp.* Incorrect: The index finger and thumb are not positioned across the shank from one another. Correct: The thumb, index finger, and middle finger are touching one another for stability.

*Fulcrum.* A conventional built-up fulcrum is being used that is appropriate for the area and instrument design.

*Adaptation.* The terminal shank is not parallel with the tooth surface. In fact, the terminal shank is perpendicular to the mesial surface. Adapting in this manner causes many problems. The depth of the sulcus/pocket is not debrided because the toe of the instrument is directed toward the contact. If calculus is located in this area, it would be effectively removed because the terminal 1 to 2 mm of the blade is not adapted to the surface. To correct this error, the finger rest should occur on the tip of the ring finger resulting in a vertical positioning of the shank and handle. By "standing up" vertically on the finger rest, the handle will also be parallel with the long axis in the faciolingual dimension.

*Activation.* Although activation can not be evaluated from the photograph, the rock would be difficult to perform with the instrument in this position. The instrument would probably be activated with a pull motion out and away from the tooth surface resulting in ineffective calculus removal and root surface debridement.

**Discussion—Case Study Four:** The purpose of the reevaluation visit is to assess healing as it has occurred in the case description. To reevaluate the subgingival environment, the explorer is employed with proper assessment strokes. Because of the location of the bleeding and inflammation, you suspect incomplete debridement in the interproximal areas. The fact that the gingiva healed on the buccal and lingual surfaces leads you to believe that the lack of healing is not due to a compromised immune response. Exploration reveals some calculus deposit in addition to bacterial plaque on the curet blade. To remove the residual deposit, the midline of the proximal areas must be reached. Effective pivoting with the curet is necessary to reach this area. Use of a file (or ultrasonic insert) might be indicated if the deposit is engaged with a curet, and is too tenacious to remove. Other factors that can be self-evaluated with both calculus removal and debridement strokes are adaptation and activation on the proximal surface. Ensuring that the terminal 1 to 2 mm is adapted to the convex line angle and concavity on the proximal surfaces, reassessing the curet blade-to-tooth angle, and observing channeling with calculus removal strokes are indicated. Last, time allotted for care and sequencing might impact the quality of care. It is necessary to spend ample time at this visit to reinstrument interproximal areas. If enough time has not been scheduled, then reappointment is necessary.

**Discussion—Case Study Five:** See Table 11-9.

**Table 11-9 Troubleshooting Guide for Instrumentation with Curets**

| Factor | Common Problems | Solutions |
|---|---|---|
| Sharpness | • Blade is not engaged when activating a calculus removal stroke.<br>• Heavy lateral pressure is being exerted due to ineffective calculus removal. | • Stop and sharpen; always have sterilized stone available.<br>• Sharpen at the first sign of dullness. |
| Grasp | • Split grasp.<br><br>• Placement of the middle finger is on the terminal shank rather than near the junction of the shank and handle; the middle finger then pushes on the instrument to activate. | • Place thumb, index finger, and middle finger together and activate in this position.<br>• Move the grasp to the appropriate point. Use the middle finger to anchor the index finger. Activation can then occur by flexing the thumb and index fingers. |
| Fulcrum | • Fulcrum is too far away from the root surface.<br>• Using palm-down on the maxillary arch.<br><br>• Dropping the fulcrum from the vertical upright position when using area-specific curets. | • Use a conventional built-up fulcrum or alternate fulcrum.<br>• Palm-up is effective even on the maxillary right buccal and maxillary left lingual surfaces (right-handed operators).<br>• Stand up on the tip of the finger rest. |
| Mirror Use | • Reflection (indirect illumination) is not used. | • Use where appropriate. |
| Adaptation | • Select inappropriate cutting edge.<br>• Use of the middle one-third of the blade.<br><br>• Insert and initiate the stroke *on* calculus.<br>• Use of equal pressure for insertion and activation.<br>• Area-specific curets: the terminal shank is perpendicular to the surface being debrided.<br>• Universal curets: the terminal shank is parallel to the proximal surface. | • Assess visual cues prior to placement and once inserted.<br>• Use the terminal 1 to 2 mm. Rolling must be continuous to keep the terminal 1 to 2 mm adapted.<br>• Place the blade 1 mm *below* the calculus to remove the apical border.<br>• Insert gently; increase lateral pressure slightly when activating.<br>• Apply the finger rest to the tooth so that the terminal shank is parallel to the tooth surface.<br>• Pivot to adapt to proximal surfaces by slightly dropping the fulcrum at the line angle to achieve a perpendicular relationship of the terminal shank to the root. |
| Activation | • Activate by moving the handle away from the tooth, which increases the blade-to-tooth angle.<br><br>• Use of finger activation.<br>• Use of inappropriate angle for purpose of stroke.<br>• Trying to remove a moderate to heavy deposit with one stroke. | • Rock the instrument with strokes maintained at the same angle. Advance up the tooth toward the contact. Observe the relationship of the handle to the tooth.<br>• Activate with wrist and forearm.<br>• Open the blade-to-tooth angle to 75°. For debridement the blade can be closed somewhat if desired.<br>• Remove calculus with channeling. Debride with overlapping strokes covering the root surface. |

*(continues)*

**Table 11-9  (continued)**

| Factor | Common Problems | Solutions |
|---|---|---|
| Activation (continued) | • Strokes are too long to effectively remove calculus. | • Keep channel strokes 1 to 2 mm and debridement and assessment strokes can be slightly longer. |
| | • Using inappropriate lateral pressure. | • Grasp, fulcrum, and adaptation must be sound. Use light lateral pressure for debridement; moderate for calculus removal. Do not use moderate lateral pressure for debridement. |
| | • Calculus is still located at the epithelial attachment after instrumentation. | • Reassess probe readings and instrument selection. Evaluate extension to the attachment by measuring the shank length that is inserted subgingivally and comparing it to the probe readings. |
| | • Calculus is located at line angles, beneath cementoenamel junctions, in concavities adjacent to furcation entrances, apical to restorative margins, or apical to abfractions. | • Employ horizontal strokes in these areas. |
| | • Calculus is located at the midline of proximal surfaces. | • Pivot more to extend the instrument to the midline. |

## REFERENCES

American Academy of Periodontology. (1993). *Treatment of gingivitis and periodontitis.* Chicago: American Academy of Periodontology.

American Academy of Periodontology. (1989). *Proceedings of the world workshop in clinical periodontics.* Consensus Report, Discussion Section II (pp. II-13–II-20). Chicago: The American Academy of Periodontology.

American Eagle Instruments, Inc. 4th ed. Manufacturer catalog. Missoula, MT: American Eagle Instruments, Inc.

Antonini, C. J., Brady, J .M., Levin, M. P., & Garcia, W. L. (1977, January). Scanning electron microscope study of scalers. *Journal of Periodontology,* 45–48.

Benfenati, M. P., Montesan, M. T., Benfenati, S. P. Nathanson, D. (1987). Scanning electron microscope: An SEM study of periodontally instrumented root surfaces, comparing sharp, dull, and damaged curettes and ultrasonic instruments. *International Journal of Periodontics and Restorative Dentistry, 2,* 51–67.

Biller, I. R. & Karlsson, V. L. (1979). SEM of curet edges. *Dental Hygiene, 53,* 549 and 554.

Clark, S. M. & Veno, H. (1990). An examination of periodontal curettes: An SEM study. *General Dentistry, 38,* 14–16.

Clinical Research Associates Newsletter. (1994). "Retipping" and resharpening process can extend life of scalers. Provo, UT: Clinical Research Associates.

Darby, M. L. & Walsh, P. M. (Eds.), 1994. *Dental hygiene theory and practice.* Philadelphia: W.B. Saunders Co.

DeNucci, D. I. & Mader, C. J. (1983). (1994). Scanning electron microscopic evaluation of several resharpening techniques. *Journal of Periodontology, 54,* 618–628.

Ellingson, P. (1993, November/December). Instrument sharpening. How to solve your sharpening problems. *Journal of Practical Hygiene,* 23–25.

GC American Hygienists Instruments and Supplies. (1996).

Greenstein, G. (1992). Periodontal response to mechanical nonsurgical therapy: A review. *Journal of Periodontology, 63,* 118–130.

Hoffmann, L. A., Gross, K. B. W., Cobb, C. M., Pippin, D. J., Tira, D. E., & Overman, P. R. (1989, October). Assessment of curet sharpness. *Journal of Dental Hygiene,* 382–387.

Hoople, S. (1985). Files provide desirable results in patient treatment procedures. *RDH,* Nov./Dec., 22–24.

Hu-Friedy® Product Catalog and Reference Guide. (1993). Chicago: Hu-Friedy Manufacturing Company.

Huang, C. & Tseng, C. (1991). Effect of different sharpening stones on periodontal curettes evaluated by scanning electron microscopy. *Journal of the Formosan Medical Association, 90,* 782–787.

Huntley, D. E. (1982a, July/August). A fine edge: Instrument sharpening, Part I. *RDH,* 15–18.

Huntley, D. E. (1982b, September/October). Honing your technique: Instrument sharpening, Part II. *RDH,* 51–54.

Margquam, B. J. (1988). Strategies to improve instrument sharpening. *Dental Hygiene, 62,* 334.

Nield-Gehrig, J. S. & Houseman, G. A. (1996). *Fundamentals of periodontal instrumentation* (3rd ed.). Baltimore: Williams & Wilkins.

O'Leary, T. J. & Kafrawy, A. H. (1983). Total cementum removal: A realistic objective. *Journal of Periodontology, 54,* 221–226.

Paquette, D. E. & Levin, M. P. (1977a). The sharpening of scaling instruments: I. An examination of principles. *Journal of Periodontology*, 163–168.

Paquette, D. E. & Levin, M. P. (1977b). The sharpening of scaling instruments: II. A preferred technique. *Journal of Periodontology*, 169–172.

Pattison, A. M. & Pattison, G. L. (1992). *Periodontal instrumentation* (2nd ed.). Norwalk: Appleton & Lange.

Pattison, A. M. & Pattison, G. L., & Takei, H. H. (1996). In. F. A. Carranza & M. G. Newman (Eds.), *Clinical periodontology* (8th ed.). Philadelphia: W.B. Saunders Co.

Pattison, A. M., Pattison, G. L., & Takei, H. (1996). The periodontal instrumentarium. In F. A. Carranza & M. G. Newman (Eds.), *Clinical periodontology* (8th ed.). Philadelphia: W.B. Saunders Co.

Perry, D. A., Beemsterboer, P., & Carranza, F. A. (1990). *Techniques and theory of periodontal instrumentation*. Philadelphia: W.B. Saunders Co.

Tal, H., Kozlovsky, A., Green, F., & Gabbary, M. (1989, June). Scanning electron microscope evaluation of wear of stainless steel and high carbon steel curettes. *Journal of Periodontology*, 320–234.

Tal, H., Panno, J. M., & Vaidyanathan, T. K. (1985). SEM evaluation of wear of dental curettes during standardized root planing. *Journal of Periodontology, 56*, 532–536.

Wehmeyer, T. E. (1987). Chairside instrument sharpening. *Quintessence International, 18*, 615.

Wilkins, E. M. (1994). *Clinical practice of the dental hygienist* (7th ed.). Baltimore: Williams & Wilkins.

Woodall, I. R. (Ed.). (1993). Comprehensive dental hygiene care (4th ed.).

# CHAPTER 12

# Ultrasonic Periodontal Debridement

## Key Terms

autotuned unit
amplitude (power)
cavitation
frequency (tuning)
insert
magnetostrictive unit
manual tuned unit

piezoelectric unit
precision-thin tips
subgingival ultrasonic periodontal debridement
tip displacement
transducer
ultrasonics

## INTRODUCTION

Ultrasonic periodontal debridement involves removal of bacterial plaque and retentive factors from the crown and root surface to promote health of the gingiva and periodontal tissues. The goal of **subgingival ultrasonic periodontal debridement** is to remove accessible subgingival bacterial plaque, its by-products, and calculus to provide a root surface that is biologically acceptable for tissue healing and regeneration. Additionally, removal of other plaque-retentive factors located subgingivally must be accomplished. Historically, ultrasonic scaling instruments were used for gross debridement followed by hand instrumentation with curets. Recently, new ultrasonic insert designs coupled with specific ultrasonic techniques, have been shown to be as effective as hand instruments in periodontal therapy (Copulos, Low, Walker, Trebilcock, & Hefti, 1993). These newly designed inserts are thinner in diameter than the original, standard inserts and are referred to as **precision-thin inserts**. Their narrow design facilitates adaptation subgingivally and in hard-to-reach areas such as furcations and narrow periodontal pockets. Other terms for the precision-thin insert are modified tips or microultrasonics.

The purpose of this chapter is to familiarize the reader with precision-thin tips and their applications in NSPT. It is assumed that readers will have background knowledge in traditional ultrasonic therapy with standard insert designs. A brief review of the literature is included to enhance background knowledge about ultrasonic devices and their applications in clinical practice. Principles of ultrasonics and recommendations for ultrasonic instrumentation in periodontal therapy will also be discussed.

## HISTORY OF ULTRASONIC SCALING DEVICES

Ultrasonics were initially introduced in dentistry for cavity preparations in the mid 1950s; however, they did not gain popularity with the dental profession until they were introduced into the field of Periodontics for removal of calculus (Zinner, 1955). Early research results concluded that ultrasonic instrumentation should be confined to the removal of supragingival deposits of plaque and calculus. In the 1950s and 1960s, studies produced conflicting reports regarding client safety, efficiency of calculus removal, and its effects on root surfaces. Among the dental community it was believed that ultrasonic instruments inherently damaged root surfaces and created root surface irregularities (Kerry, 1967; Stende & Schaffer, 1961). At this time, a glassy smooth root-planed surface was the endpoint of instrumentation and ultrasonic instruments were thought to create root surface roughness that would contribute to the adherence of bacterial plaque and calculus. Therefore, by default, hand instruments became the instrument of choice for scaling and root planing.

Later, an increasing number of favorable reports about ultrasonic instrumentation began to appear in the literature. Ultrasonic scaling devices were reevaluated and evidence surfaced supporting their safety and effectiveness (Breininger, O'Leary, & Blumenshine, 1987; Garnick & Dent, 1989; Jones, Lozdan, & Boyde, 1972; Leon & Vogel, 1987; Oda & Ishikawa, 1989). In the 1980s it was concluded that hand instrumentation and ultrasonic scaling were equally effective in subgingival plaque removal (Breininger, O'Leary, & Blumenshine, 1987; Leon & Vogel, 1987; Oosterwaal et al., 1987; Thorton &

Garnick, 1982). Checchi and Pelliccione (1988) also concluded that both methods were equally effective in the removal of endotoxins from root surfaces in vitro. Clinically, reduction of pocket depth and maintenance of attachment levels posttherapy have been recognized with both methods (Biagini et al., 1988; Badersten et al., 1981; Badersten et al., 1984; Leon & Vogel, 1987; Oosterwaal, Matee, Mikx, van't Hof, & Renggli, 1987; Torfason et al., 1979). In 1990, Kepic and others found that handheld curets and ultrasonic instruments were equally effective in removing calculus.

When evaluating past research, it should be remembered that these studies were conducted with traditional, bulky ultrasonic inserts used primarily for supragingival and easily accessible subgingival deposit removal. Hence, these results do not reflect the potential efficacy of the recently designed precision-thin inserts.

## PRINCIPLES OF ULTRASONIC INSTRUMENTS

Ultrasonic instrumentation is based upon the conversion of electrical energy into mechanical energy in the form of rapid vibrations. Ultrasonic units generally have four components that perform unique functions. When an ultrasonic unit is plugged into an electrical outlet and the foot pedal is activated, an electrical current is sent through the generator, or base of the unit, to the handpiece, which holds the transducer. The **transducer**, or **insert**, actually converts the electrical energy to mechanical energy which, in turn, causes the working end to vibrate. This mechanical vibration of the working end removes calculus, bacterial plaque, and root surface constituents when they are directly in contact with the tip. The diagram in Figure 12-1 clarifies the components of an ultrasonic unit and insert. For purposes of this text, the working end is divided into the point and tip. Often the terms "insert" and "tip" are used interchangeably; however, the term "tip" will be used in this text when referring to the portion of the insert that is adapted to the tooth surface. Use of these terms will help the student clinician who has fundamental knowledge in basic instrumentation to identify the parts of the working end. These terms are especially useful when discussing adaptation and activation of the ultrasonic insert.

All ultrasonic units are not exactly alike in design and function. There are two types of ultrasonic units: piezoelectric and magnetostrictive. Both types of units consist of the four basic components; however, they differ in that the transducers are made of different materials, the working ends usually operate in different patterns, and the working ends vary in the number of surfaces that are activated. A **piezoelectric unit** houses a crystal transducer. The source of vibration occurs when alternating electrical currents are applied to the crystal transducer creating a dimensional change that is transmitted to the tip in the form of a vibration. The movement of this vibration is in a linear pattern (see Figure 12-2). Only two sides of the working tip are activated, limiting the tip's ability to adapt to the topography of the tooth surface on all sides. The crystal transducer is contained within the handpiece of the piezoelectric instrument. The working end itself

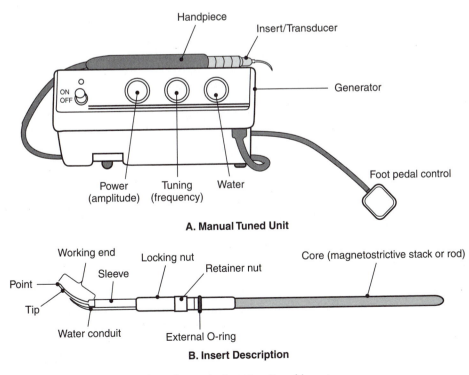

Figure 12-1 Components of an ultrasonic dental unit and insert.

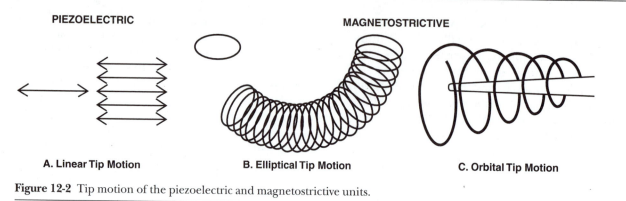

**PIEZOELECTRIC**

**MAGNETOSTRICTIVE**

**A. Linear Tip Motion**

**B. Elliptical Tip Motion**

**C. Orbital Tip Motion**

**Figure 12-2** Tip motion of the piezoelectric and magnetostrictive units.

is threaded into the handpiece and is not connected to the transducer like the insert used with a magnetostrictive unit.

The insert in the **magnetostrictive unit** is a core, which is either a stack of metal (nickel-cobalt) strips or a ferromagnetic rod attached to the working end (see Figure 12-1). Inside the handpiece is a coil of copper wire which, when the current is turned on and the insert is in place, causes the core to become magnetized and demagnetized. When magnetized, the core contracts and when demagnetized, the core returns to its original size. The constant alternating electromagnetic field causes the working end of the insert to vibrate in an elliptical or orbital motion (see Figure 12-2). Unlike the piezoelectric units, the working end can be used on all sides enhancing its adaptability to tooth surfaces.

The amount and direction of change in the magnetostrictive transducer are influenced by the nature and previous treatment of the magnetostrictive material, the degree of magnetization, and temperature (Sweeney, 1957). Heat is a by-product of the dimensional change of the transducer and the oscillating tip when in contact with the tooth surface. Cool water is needed to control the generation of the heat and, thus, to prevent damage to the tooth surface. It is best not to have a heating mechanism in the operatory water lines because cool or unheated water functions to reduce heat production. As

water flows to the end of the insert and contacts the moving tip, a spray results. This phenomenon is called **cavitation**. When water passes over the intense vibration of the oscillating tip, rapid formation and destruction of small air cavities occur at maximum vibrating points along the working end.

The term **ultrasonics** describes a range of acoustical vibrations that cannot be heard by the human ear. In the application of dentistry, ultrasonic frequencies range from approximately 20,000 vibrations per second to 50,000 vibrations per second. These ultrasonic vibrations are a unit of frequency often referred to as cycles per second (cps) or hertz (Hz). When an ultrasonic device is plugged into an electrical outlet, the unit converts ordinary house current (115 volts or 50/60 Hz) to hertz current. If a 25,000 Hz current is produced in the generator, it creates 25,000 cycles per second which, subsequently, creates 25,000 cycles per second in the transducer and causes the rapid, microscopic tip vibration. Unlike their counterparts, sonic scaling devices are air driven and vibrate at lower frequencies of 2,500 to 7,000 cycles per second. These reduced frequencies decrease their ability to remove heavy calculus, although some units have been shown to effectively remove light to moderate calculus (Densonic, Dentsply International; MM 3300, Medidenta International; and Titan SW, Star Dental) (Clinical Research Associates Newsletter, 1993). Figure 12-3 illustrates the cycles per second in the sonic and ultrasonic devices.

## CURRENT TRENDS IN ULTRASONIC EQUIPMENT

Because manufacturers of ultrasonic instruments offer various types of units and inserts, selection of proper equipment can often be confusing and time-consuming. First, a basic knowledge of the types of equipment and their advantages and disadvantages must be gathered. Secondly, an assessment of the needs of clients, clinicians, and the dental practice must be considered. The following information will give the professional a greater understanding of the types of ultrasonic equipment on the market today.

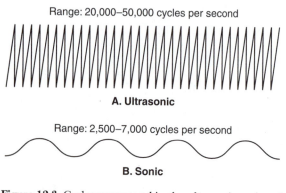

Range: 20,000–50,000 cycles per second

**A. Ultrasonic**

Range: 2,500–7,000 cycles per second

**B. Sonic**

**Figure 12-3** Cycles per second in the ultrasonic and sonic devices.

## Units

At this time, neither of the two basic types of ultrasonic units, piezoelectric or magnetostrictive, have proven therapeutic superiority over the other. Ultrasonic units are either autotuned or manual tuned units. The difference between the two units lies in the clinician's ability to adjust the frequency. **Frequency** refers to the number of cycles per second which affects the speed of movement of the tip. The **autotuned unit** has a preset frequency within the device which automatically tunes the cycles per second to maximum efficiency for each insert within the handpiece. This autotuning feature minimizes the clinician's choice to decrease energy output to reduce the rapid movement of the tip. In comparison, the frequency of a **manual tuned unit** can be adjusted by the professional via a frequency control or tuning knob. The clinician's ability to control the frequency or energy being used is a decisive advantage of manual tuned units. This control permits adjustment of the speed of movement of the tip when needed for certain oral and client conditions. For example, a person with little calculus deposit and gingival inflammation would require use of the lowest frequency possible to ultrasonically debride the subgingival environment. At this time, a limited number of manufacturers produce manual tuning units (examples are J H Maliga Engineering, Ultrasonic Services Incorporated, Tony Riso Company). Advanced ultrasonic instrumentation is equipment specific and technique sensitive. As interest and demand rises for quality ultrasonic equipment, market availability will too. Table 12-1 identifies some of the ultrasonic units being marketed.

Both autotuned and manual tuned instruments have power and water control knobs. The power setting on the unit affects the amplitude of the vibration. **Amplitude** controls the distance the tip travels in one single vibration, referred to as **tip displacement**. For example, one manufacturer reports that its unit has an amplitude from .001 to .008 of an inch (Ultrasonic Services Incorporated, 1993). The greater the amplitude, the further the distance the tip travels in the vibration (see Figure 12-4). Tip displacement creates energy to dislodge calculus and bacterial plaque. Researchers have studied this relationship and concluded that as amplitude increases, the output of power increases enhancing the efficiency of the "chipping" action of the tip (Wamsley, Laird, & Williams, 1986a). These researchers also found that displacement amplitude varied between each insert that was tested indicating different energy transduction efficiencies. There-

**Table 12-1  Ultrasonic Dental Units**

| Type of Unit | Name and Manufacturer | Frequency/Cycle per Second | Insert Availability and Compatibility |
|---|---|---|---|
| Piezoelectric | Amdent 830, Amdent AB | 25,000 Hz | four designs available by Amdent |
| | Piezon Master 400, Biotrol International | 32,000 Hz | five designs available by EMS International Manufacturer |
| | PS Prophy, Young Dental | 40,000 Hz | six designs available by Young |
| | Sensor SG/RP, Professional Dental Technologies | 45,000 to 50,000 Hz | contact the manufacturer |
| Magnetostrictive | Autoscaler, Southeast Instrument Corporation | 25,000 Hz | accommodates Cavitron™ 25K inserts |
| | Cavitron 3000/Cavi-Med 200, Dentsply International Equipment Division | 30,000 Hz and 25,000 Hz | multiple inserts available; 30K design for 30,000 Hz unit and 25K design for 25,000 Hz unit |
| | Turbo 25-30, Parkell | 25,000 Hz | four inserts available from Parkell; accommodates 25K and 30K Cavitron™ designs |
| | *Microson 101, J H Maliga Engineering | 25,000 Hz | contact the manufacturer |
| | Odontoson, PERIOgene | 42,000 Hz | three inserts available by PERIOgene |
| | Sonatron S3X, Simplified System Incorporated | 25,000 Hz | accommodates Cavitron™ 25K designs |
| | *USI, Ultrasonic Services Incorporated | 25,000 Hz | six inserts available; accommodates Cavitron™ 25K inserts |
| | *Model 2530, Tony Riso Company | 25,000 Hz and 30,000 Hz | six inserts available; accommodates Cavitron™ 25K and 30K inserts |

*Manual tuned unit. All other units are autotuned.

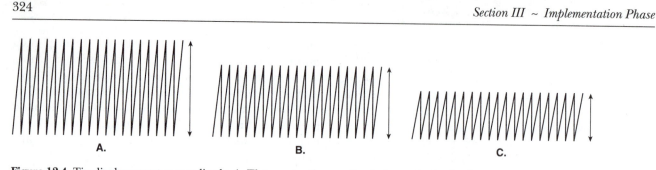

**Figure 12-4** Tip displacement or amplitude. **A.** The greater the amplitude (power), the further the tip travels in the vibration. **B.** and **C.** As the amplitude is decreased, the length of each movement decreases. Amplitude and frequency are interdependent: one cannot exist without the other.

fore, it can be concluded from this study that not only does the amplitude of the unit affect the energy output, but so do the transduction efficiencies of the varying inserts. When energy is needed for the autotuned unit, only the power knob can be adjusted to affect the amplitude and tip displacement. Both frequency and amplitude are measures of ultrasonic energy (see Figure 12-5).

The water control knob adjusts the volume and temperature of the flow from the handpiece to permit the operator to acquire the correct cavitation. Water supplied from the ultrasonic unit has several advantages during instrumentation. Water acts as a coolant for the transducer in the magnetorestrictive handpiece and for the oscillating tip. It also increases visibility, stems bleeding, provides lavage for flushing debris and promoting gingival healing, removes superficial root surface constituents, and serves to irrigate periodontal pockets. A piezoelectric unit does not require a coolant; however, the water produced serves the other identified functions. With a magnetostrictive unit, the proper volume of water spray is critical in decreasing potential damage to the root surface and pulp of the tooth and in enhancing client comfort. The greater the water flow, the lower the water temperature and, conversely, a decreased water flow creates a higher water temperature. Water flow does not relate to the energy generated from the tip. Instead, it is a by-product of the mode of operation of the unit and serves essential functions in providing quality client care.

The clinician must employ critical thinking skills to adequately regulate the water to cool the handpiece and unit. The size of the water spray is adjusted by varying the rate of water flow, the frequency output of the generator (if possible), and the amplitude or power. Cavitation is also used as a guide in tuning an ultrasonic unit. The largest spray of water not accompanied by large water droplets, coupled with a high pitched hissing noise indicates the correct adjustment is achieved. This ideal adjustment has been called "in phase."

### Inserts

The availability of inserts for a unit is an important factor in selecting equipment. As with hand instrumentation, a variety of insert designs improves the quality of periodontal debridement. The following information reviews the relationship of energy to the insert, designs available, and current research on modified inserts.

**Relationship to Energy.** In addition to energy generated by the power and frequency settings, other factors influence the energy emitted from the working end (Clark, 1969; Holbrook & Low, 1989) as follows:

1. *Time of exposure.* The longer the time spent on crown or root structure, the greater amount of energy delivered to the tooth.
2. *Applied pressure.* Increased pressure will increase the effects of the vibrating tip, up to a point of dampening or stopping the vibrating tip.
3. *Relative sharpness of the tip.* The sharper the tip, the greater the energy output of the tip. Consequently, blunt or round inserts with no sharp edges are preferred for periodontal debridement.
4. *Angle of application.* The greater the angle of application (up to 90°), the greater the energy output. The ideal angle of tip application should be 15° or less to the tooth surface being treated.
5. *Surface of the working end in contact with the tooth surface.* Piezoelectric inserts emit the greatest energy from the back and front surfaces of the tip.

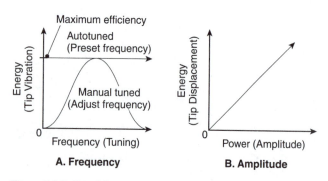

**Figure 12-5** Graphic representation of frequency and amplitude. **A.** The frequency on the manual tuned unit can be adjusted to control the energy and tip vibration. The frequency on the autotuned unit is preset and cannot be adjusted. **B.** As the amplitude or power knob is increased, the energy and tip displacement are also increased.

The side surfaces generate the least amount of energy. In comparison, magnetostrictive inserts deliver energy from all surfaces of the working end: the point, the front or concave surface, the back or convex surface, and the side or lateral surface. The point generates the greatest amount of energy while the lateral surfaces generate the least (see Figure 12-6). This information is highly significant in various situations such as areas of root hypersensitivity, or light versus heavy calculus. Understanding the subtle differences in energy output of the tip when in contact with the root cementum or enamel will enhance patient comfort and instrument efficiency.

**Design.** Ultrasonic inserts are available in various sizes and designs. They contain either an internal water aperture or an external water conduit for cooling and irrigating. Most precision-thin inserts have an external water conduit because the internal water aperture can not be achieved with their small diameter. Depending on the design of the unit, inserts can screw on or snap into the handpiece. As in hand instrumentation, instrument selection requires that the clinician select the best design based upon access, type of deposit, and other client conditions. A bulky insert can not adapt subgingivally in tight or narrow pockets nor small proximal embrasures or furcations; therefore, large inserts are still reserved for gross debridement of supragingival and easily accessible subgingival deposits.

Hou, Chen, Wu, and Tsai (1994) found that the mean buccal furcation entrance dimension (FED) of maxillary and mandibular first and second molars measured from .63 to 1.04 millimeters depending on the anatomy of the molar (first or second) and on the location of the furcation (buccal, mesial, or distal). Mandibular molars FEDs measured from 0.71 to 0.88 mm, again depending on anatomy and location. The considerably large, unused P-10 Cavitron® insert measured an average of 0.56 mm in diameter while the width of a new Gracey

curet blade measured from 0.76 mm to 1.0 mm. The majority of mean FEDs in second molars were less than the blade width of unused Gracey curets and the majority of mean FEDs of first molars were similar to the Gracey curet blade width. These authors concluded that the combined use of cavitron inserts and curets is necessary, versus the use of curets alone, because the cavitron insert tip was narrower than the mean FEDs of maxillary and mandibular molars. Certainly, the reduced width of precision-thin inserts would enhance effective debridement in furcations.

Pocket topography illustrations tend to indicate that all periodontal pockets are bathtub shaped. In reality, the progression of the attachment levels vary from tooth surface to tooth surface according to the pathway of periodontal destruction (see Chapter 10, Figure 10-5). This factor and many others make thorough root debridement challenging. Factors limiting the effectiveness of the curet include the need to adapt the cutting edge to the tooth surface at the proper angle, the need to activate the curet in a precise manner, and maintenance of a sharp cutting edge. With handheld curets, the clinician must place the cutting edge apical to the deposit to engage it for removal. Unlike hand instruments, the tip of the insert can remove a deposit starting at the most coronal aspect of the deposit and moving toward the apical extent (decreasing distention of the epithelial wall). Ultrasonic instruments do not require that a specific blade-to-tooth angle be maintained. Also, ultrasonic instruments do not have a toe-to-shank difference (3 mm to 4 mm for an average curet) nor do they share a blade width of 0.75 mm to 1.0 mm. In fact, the average diameter of a precision-thin tip is 0.3 mm to 0.6 mm (see Figure 12-7). This small diameter is significant when debriding close proximal surfaces, deep periodontal pockets, root concavities, narrow root surfaces, and furcations (see Figure 12-8). Unlike hand instruments, an

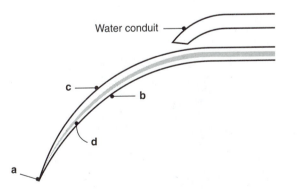

**Figure 12-6** Surfaces of the working end and the order of energy generated.
*Key:* **a**: point—generates the greatest amount of energy; **b**: concave—generates the second greatest amount of energy; **c**: convex—generates less energy than the point or concave surfaces; **d**: lateral—generates the least amount of energy.

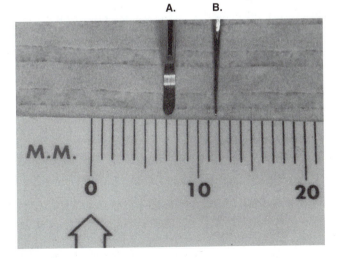

**Figure 12-7** Comparison of the width of (**A**) an anterior Gracey curet blade and (**B**) the tip of a precision-thin insert. (Courtesy of Dr. Thomas E. Holbrook)

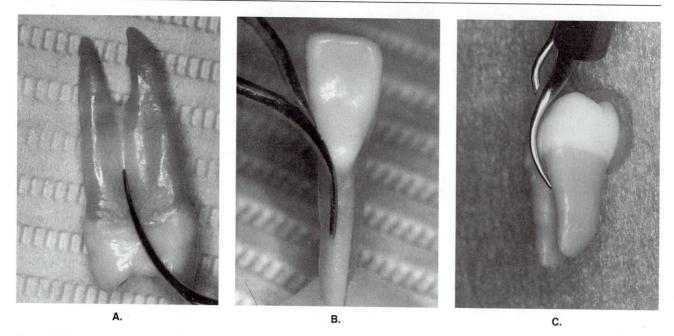

A.                                                    B.                                                    C.

**Figure 12-8** A precision-thin insert in a: (**A**) a root concavity on the maxillary first premolar; (**B**) a narrow root surface on a mandibular lateral; (**C**) a furcation on the mandibular second molar. (Courtesy of Dr. Thomas E. Holbrook)

ultrasonic tip is effective in a static position. Ultrasonic instruments do not need bulk for strength nor a cutting edge for calculus removal; thus, they can be precisioned to the dimension of a periodontal probe and do not need to be sharpened.

Thomas E. Holbrook, D.D.S., realized the limitations of hand-activated instruments thirty years ago and began modifying the size and shape of Cavitron® P-10 inserts (Dentsply International) to resemble a periodontal probe. Recently, manufacturers followed his lead by designing precision-thin inserts (Slimlines, Dentsply International; P-100s, Tony Riso Company; Ultrathins, Ultrasonic Services Incorporated; and Thinlines, Odontoson Unit by PERIOgene) (see Figure 12-9). Slimline inserts are advertised as being 40 percent thinner than standard inserts allowing instrumentation to depths of up to 7 mm (Slimline Ultrasonic Inserts, 1994). They are available in three shapes; straight, right, and left. Other manufacturers also produce their inserts in these three shapes. Currently, a furcation design insert is being marketed with a small ball-end (Hu-Friedy®).

Some companies design units with inserts that are not interchangeable with other units (Odontoson Unit and Thinline Inserts, PERIOgene). On the other hand, some manufacturers sell inserts that are compatible with a variety of units (Slimlines, Dentsply International; P-100s, Tony Riso Company; Ultrathins, Ultrasonic Services Incorporated). It is important to ensure that inserts are compatible with the unit(s) the office already is using, or with a new unit being purchased. The insert must frequently match the hertz of the unit. For example, Dentsply International manufactures 25K and 30K inserts to be used with 25,000 Hz and 30,000 Hz units

respectively (see Table 12-1). Checking directly with the manufacturer, dental supply salespeople, or dental hygiene educators can be valuable when shopping for equipment.

**Research with Modified Inserts.** Recent studies conducted by Herremans (1989), Dragoo (1992), and Copulos and coworkers (1993) utilized modified P-10 Cavitron® inserts reduced in circumference to a thinner, slightly curved probe shape for greater access into periodontal pockets as recommended by Holbrook and Low (1989). These studies not only used similar inserts but fol-

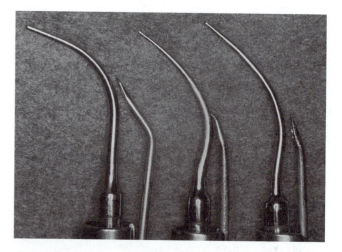

**Figure 12-9** Precision-thin inserts—three different manufacturer's straight insert designs. (Courtesy of Dr. Thomas E. Holbrook)

lowed similar ultrasonic techniques. Herremans (1989) conducted an in-vitro investigation to examine the effects of the modified ultrasonic insert on root surface topography as compared to hand instruments. Twenty periodontally involved extracted teeth were carved into a three split root design, each sample specimen acting as its own control. Specimens were randomly assigned to receive either hand or modified ultrasonic treatment. Scanning electron photomicrographs were taken at 3000X of the experimental surfaces following instrumentation to examine root surface topography (see Figure 12-10). Categories of root smoothness were scored for each photomicrograph by an examiner blind to the treatment assigned. Surface measurements from the modified ultrasonic insert were compared to surfaces scaled with curets. Results indicated that debridement with the modified ultrasonic instrument resulted in a significantly smoother root surface than debridement with curets; however, both hand and ultrasonic instruments produced a significantly smoother root surface than the control (no treatment) group. Dragoo (1992) reported that the ultrasonic insert had greater efficiency in reaching the epithelial attachment, produced less damage to the root surface, and was more efficient in removing subgingival irritants than hand instruments.

Copulos and others (1993) conducted an analysis to compare the effects of a modified ultrasonic insert tip and a Gracey curet on the clinical parameters of periodontal disease. A split mouth design was utilized to treat nine subjects in maintenance therapy with ten sites (N = 90) at the zero-, three-, and six-month intervals. A plaque index, a gingival index, bleeding upon probing, probing depths, attachment levels, microscopic evaluation of supragingival plaque samples, and presence of elastase were assessed at each interval. The investigators reported that both the modified ultrasonic insert and Gracey curets were equally effective in periodontal therapy based upon the clinical parameters examined. They found that significantly less time was needed for debridement with the modified ultrasonic insert as compared to hand instruments. Dragoo (1992) also evaluated time and reported that it took less time to remove calculus using a modified insert then when hand instruments were used. These findings do not

imply that less time is needed for the periodontal maintenance appointment, but that less time is needed to physically remove calculus. Therefore, additional appointment time can be used to provide instructions in self-care and other supportive therapy.

The single most important factor in selecting proper ultrasonic inserts for negotiation of deep, periodontal pockets is access to the pocket. Thin, probe-shaped tips are especially suited for subgingival debridement. The smaller diameter decreases the relative resistance of the gingival tissues and increases access into close proximal embrasures and deep periodontal pockets. Other features to consider when selecting ultrasonic equipment may include finding a unit with various tip shapes and sizes, elliptical or orbital tip movement, wide range of energy levels (provides ability to control energy as needed), power level foot control pedal (provides instantaneous energy to the tip as needed), manual control of frequency, autoclavable handpiece and inserts, fiber optic handpiece option, swivel handpiece connection, light flexible handpiece hose, instantaneous medicinal irrigation, and minimal aerosol. At this writing, no ultrasonic contains all these features.

## BACKGROUND INFORMATION

To accurately assess the conclusions drawn from the literature about ultrasonic instrumentation, one must first review the variables that can be controlled by the clinician. Factors previously mentioned include the amplitude and frequency settings on the unit, length of time allowed for instrumentation, the pattern of the stroke, the surface of the working end contacting the tooth, the angle of application, insert design (dull or sharp, thick or thin), and the amount of pressure applied during instrumentation. Each of these entities will determine the efficiency and/or effectiveness of ultrasonics in periodontal therapy (Holbrook & Low, 1989).

Two important variables are insert design and power setting. Most researchers investigating the effects of ultrasonic instruments on root surfaces used the standard, commercially available P-10 Cavitron® inserts (D'Silva, Nayak, Cherian, & Mulky, 1979; Garnick & Dent, 1989;

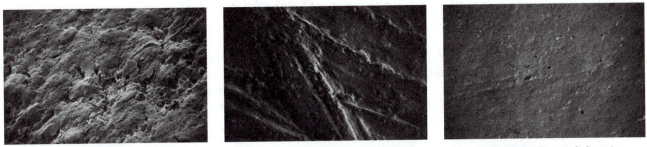

**A. Control**  **B. Curet**  **C. Modified Ultrasonic Insert**

**Figure 12-10** Scanning electron photomicrographs taken at 3000X to evaluate root surface topography.

Green & Ramfjord, 1966; Hunter, O'Leary, & Kafrawy, 1984; Jones, Lozdan, & Boyde, 1972; Stende & Schaffer, 1961). Therefore, research results are affected by the large size and contour. Also, the manufacturer's recommendations for power (amplitude) were often followed, which invariably resulted in settings on medium or high. Hence, a medium to high amplitude would generate the greatest energy output from the ultrasonic insert during instrumentation possibly resulting in undesirable root surface characteristics. Most importantly, it should be understood that either a hand or ultrasonic instrument can destroy the root surface if instrumentation is performed in a careless manner.

These varying results apparent in the literature may be partly due to the lack of standardization of research methods among investigators and the lack of controlling variables. The following brief review of the literature is subdivided by the focus of the study.

## Calculus Removal

The effectiveness of calculus removal with traditional ultrasonic instruments has been reported by various investigators (D'Silva, Nayak, Cherian, & Mulky, 1979; Jones, Lozdan, & Boyde, 1972; Moskow & Bressman, 1964). In some instances it has been documented that calculus removal with traditional ultrasonic instruments and curets is equally effective (Jones, Lozdan, & Boyde, 1972; Moskow & Bressman, 1964; Nishimine & O'Leary, 1979; Stendhe & Schaffer, 1961). Hunter, O'Leary and Kafrawy (1984) reported that neither method, even in open flap root planing, was capable of removing all the calculus at the stereomicroscopic and light microscopic levels.

Thorough subgingival calculus removal is a difficult task. A variety of obstacles must be overcome when providing professional and thorough periodontal debridement. As offered by O'Leary (1986), many factors limit the effectiveness of root planing such as anatomy of roots, depth of pockets, position of teeth, area of mouth being treated, size of mouth, elasticity of cheeks, range of opening, dexterity of operator, and inadequate instruments for diagnosis and treatment. Rateitschak-Pluss, Schwarz, Guggenheim, Duggelin, and Rateitschak (1992) also identified tortuous pocket morphology as a limitation when root planing deep pockets in cases of advanced periodontitis. Instrumentation with curets to the base of the pockets was not achieved completely on 75 percent of the scaled and root-planed surfaces. These researchers concluded, however, that during nonsurgical therapy the surfaces that can be reached with curets are usually free of plaque and calculus.

Dragoo (1992) evaluated instrument efficiency and instrument limitations of various hand instruments, standard ultrasonic instruments (P-10 Cavitron insert), and modified ultrasonic instruments (EW P-10R and EW P-10L). The generators used had a range of 25,000 Hz

and medium power was used. Ten clinicians each with a minimum of ten years of clinical experience were randomly assigned to scale and root plane designated paired teeth with either hand or ultrasonic methods. Instrument efficiency was calculated by measuring the subgingival area free of plaque, calculus, gouges, and scratches after instrumentation. The mean values for instrument efficiency were 3.45 mm for hand instruments, 4.65 mm for modified ultrasonic instruments, and 3.13 mm for standard ultrasonic instruments. Instrument limitations were described as areas where instruments had come in contact with the root surface but were ineffective in removing the remaining plaque and calculus. The mean distance between instrument efficiency and instrument limitation (the distance where the instrument was no longer effective) was 1.65 mm for hand instruments, 0.82 mm for the modified ultrasonic inserts, and 3.05 mm for the standard ultrasonic insert. When compared to hand instruments, the modified ultrasonic insert increased efficiency by 26.9 percent on the mesial, 38 percent on the buccal, 16.6 percent on the lingual, and 18.6 percent on the distal surfaces. Instrument efficiency decreased on all surfaces using a standard ultrasonic insert. Conclusions included that the modified insert removed the most calculus and reached the closest to the epithelial attachment.

Clinical detection of calculus is another factor affecting thorough calculus removal. Sherman and others (1990) found high false negative responses in the clinical detection of residual calculus with the periodontal probe and explorer. In other words, 77.4 percent of the surfaces with microscopic calculus were clinically scored as being free of calculus following subgingival instrumentation, while 11.8 percent of the surfaces microscopically free of calculus were clinically determined to have calculus. It has been reported that operators feel the use of the modified inserts increases their tactile sensitivity when compared to standard inserts, and at times, modified inserts enhance the ability to feel the epithelial attachment and root aberrations when compared to hand instruments (Dragoo, 1992). Even though calculus detection is challenging, it is still essential to evaluate its removal with an explorer to the best of one's ability when using ultrasonic and/or hand instrumentation.

## Root Planing

The longheld belief that cementum was embedded with contaminants promoted overvigorous root planing to decontaminate surfaces. Cheechi, Wilson, and Kieser (1988) reported that lipopolysaccharide (LPS) was present on the periodontally involved root surface; however, Moore, Wilson, and Kieser (1986) found LPS had no significant cemental penetration. They found that simple rinsing and brushing alone removed LPS. Studies conducted by Cheetham and Pellicionne (1988) and Smart, Wilson, Davies, and Kieser (1990) found that light, overlapping strokes with hand or ultrasonic instruments removed LPS found on periodontally involved root surfaces. Therefore, the practice of intentional removal of root structure to remove LPS is no longer recommended.

The smoothness of the root surface with hand-activated curets and ultrasonic instrumentation has also been studied. Results of these studies are varied. Some studies have reported no significant difference in root roughness with ultrasonic instruments as compared to hand instruments (Breininger, O'Leary, & Blumenshine, 1987; D'Silva, Nayak, Cherian, & Mulky, 1979; Garnick & Dent, 1989; Moskow & Bressman, 1964; Pameijer, Stallard, & Hiep, 1972). Others have reported ultrasonic instruments were the least likely to create root surface roughness as compared to curets (Dragoo, 1992; Herremans, 1989; Jones, Lozdan, & Boyde, 1972). On the contrary, Kerry (1967), Hunter, O'Leary, and Kafrawy (1984) and Wilkenson and Maybury (1973) reported that ultrasonic instruments produced a significantly rougher root surface than hand instruments. Pameijer, Stallard, and Hiep (1972) concluded that excessive force applied with hand instruments will produce irregular strokes and gouged root surfaces, and incorrect ultrasonic technique will also result in irregular root surfaces.

It should be noted that a major problem with studying this parameter is the lack of objective criteria to evaluate surface smoothness (O'Leary, 1986). During open flap root planing the smoothness of surfaces treated with hand curets and ultrasonic instrumentation were compared (Hunter, O'Leary, & Kafrawy, 1984). These researchers reported that among the hand-scaled teeth, of the 244 surfaces evaluated, 138 or 56.6 percent were considered smooth, and 106 or 43.4 percent were considered rough. Among the 256 surfaces treated with ultrasonics, 48 or 18.8 percent were smooth and 208 or 81.2 percent were rough. This investigation used the criterion that surfaces exhibiting gouges or ripples of less than 50 µm were smooth. It would be interesting to conduct a similar study incorporating precision-thin inserts using this smoothness criteria.

Current trends in periodontal therapy suggest that the clinician use clinical parameters to judge the endpoint or result of instrumentation therapy because the definition of smooth is unclear. The biological relationship between a smooth root surface, pocket reduction, and gain of attachment is still under debate. Nevertheless, a rough root surface would appear to encourage bacterial plaque and calculus reaccumulation. At the four- to six-week reevaluation visit, the clinical signs of restoration of gingival inflammation will indicate if the clinical endpoint of instrumentation for that particular person was satisfactory. If bleeding on probing, pocket depth, or attachment loss continues, then further instrumentation is needed. The debate as to whether hand instruments are superior to ultrasonic instruments in smoothing a root surface is still underway.

## Clinical Parameters

Oosterwaal and others (1987) concluded that hand and ultrasonic treatments were equally effective in reducing pocket depths and bleeding scores. Badersten, Nilvéus, and Egelberg (1981 &1984) studied clinical attachment levels in those with moderately and severely advanced periodontitis. They concluded that the two instrumentation methods are equally effective in maintaining clinical attachment levels. Further research comparing the long-term effects of hand and ultrasonic instrumentation on the clinical parameters of periodontal diseases is warranted.

## Effects on the Microflora

Oosterwaal and others (1987) conducted microscopic and cultural analysis following hand and ultrasonic instrumentation and concluded that no statistically significant differences existed between treatments. Both hand and ultrasonic treatments resulted in a reduction of spirochetes and motile rods and an increase in cocci cells. These reductions were found up to forty-nine days following treatment with either instrument.

An in-vivo and in-vitro investigation was conducted on the effects of ultrasonic and sonic scalers on subgingival microflora (Baehni, Thilo, Chapuis, & Pernet, 1992). Results indicated a significant reduction in proportions of motile rods and spirochetes and an increase in the percentage of coccoid and rods following both sonic and ultrasonic instrumentation. A significant difference was found between the in-vitro specimens treated by ultrasonic and sonic scalers. Results demonstrated a sharp decline in spirochetes after 10 seconds of ultrasonic treatment and spirochetes were practically undetectable after 60 seconds. Only a slight decrease in spirochetes was observed with the sonic scaler. It is the opinion of these researchers that the changes in bacterial plaque composition observed in vitro after sonic instrumentation are due to the effect of the oscillating tip whereas after ultrasonic instrumentation, the effects are due to the physical action of the vibrating tip as well as the cavitational activity. This action causes the bacterial cell wall to lyse, destroying the bacteria.

A study conducted by Leon and Vogel (1987) compared the efficacy of hand scaling and ultrasonic debridement in furcations. They found that both modes of instrumentation were equally effective in changing the gingival crevicular fluid flow and the subgingival flora in Class I furcations. Ultrasonic debridement, however, was significantly more effective in reducing the counts of spirochetes and motile rods in Class II and Class III furcations than hand scaling. These findings could be a result of the cavitational "cleansing effect" from the vibrating tip and the ability of ultrasonic tips to generate energy from all surfaces,, unlike a curet which must be adapted at a precise angle for the cutting edge to remove deposit. Also, the tip of the ultrasonic insert is reported to have a dimensional advantage over the curet, which would aid in negotiating furcations (Hou, Chen, Wu, & Tsai, 1994.)

## Cavitational Activity

In addition to the ability of ultrasonic instruments to mechanically debride a tooth or root surface, the cavitational activity was found to assist in the removal of plaque (Walmsley, Walsh, Laird, & Williams, 1990). These researchers conducted a scanning electron microscopy (SEM) study to examine the effects of cavitation and acoustic microstreaming found in the water supply at the tip of an ultrasonic insert. An in-vitro system of polished gold was utilized to demonstrate the cleansing action of the cavitation around the tip. The water supply from the ultrasonic tip produced areas of erosion (0.66 ± 0.3 mm mean) beyond the oscillating tip on polished gold surfaces. The scanning electron photomicrographs of root surfaces exposed to the water supply demonstrated the erosive or "cleansing" effects of the water (0.7 + 0.3 mm) beyond the oscillating tip. Such evidence has not been reported in prior dental literature. However, the cavitational activity may have been present but masked by the more pronounced mechanical movement of the oscillating tip.

Concern has been expressed that the water supply may not reach the apical extent of some periodontal pockets resulting in inadvertent endodontic problems (Thompson, 1993). Penetration depth of the water coolant of an ultrasonic instrument was evaluated and results indicate that the depth of the water was equal to the penetration depth of the ultrasonic probelike insert (EWPP) with minimal lateral dispersion (Nosal, Scheidt, O'Neal, & VanDyke, 1991).

## Antimicrobial Irrigation during Ultrasonic Debridement

Various studies have been conducted to determine if ultrasonic scaling with an antimicrobial is beneficial. Chapple, Walmsley, Saxby, and Moscrop (1992) designed a split-mouth study to compare the effects of irrigation with 0.2 percent chlorhexidine to water during ultrasonic instrumentation. They found no significant differences between the experimental groups in respect to probing attachment levels, bleeding index scores, or plaque index scores at the three- and six-month post-treatment visits. Taggart, Palmer, and Wilson (1990) examined the effects of a single episode of ultrasonic instrumentation with a low concentration of chlorhexidine (0.02 percent) or water. Results indicate that these irrigants were equally effective in reducing bleeding scores and improving probing attachment levels. These conclusions suggest that short periods of irrigation with chlorhexidine during ultrasonic instrumentation do not produce any advantages in healing diseased tissues when compared to water. In contrast, Reynolds and coworkers

(1992) reported that oral irrigation with 0.12 percent chlorhexidine during ultrasonic instrumentation significantly reduced clinical probing depths that were site-dependent as compared to irrigation with water. With initial probing depths of 4 to 6 mm, the pocket depth reduction with chlorhexidine was only 0.5 mm greater than the probing depth reduction with water.

Rosling and others (1986) found that ultrasonic scaling with a 0.05 percent iodine solution (used as the coolant) obtained significant gains of probing attachment levels as compared to the experimental group, which was irrigated with saline, or the control group. This single study suggests that chemotherapeutics during ultrasonic instrumentation may be useful as an adjunct to traditional therapy. Further long-term investigations, however, are needed to establish the safety and benefits of iodine in conjunction with ultrasonic debridement. In particular, irrigation with iodine solutions is contraindicated for iodine-sensitive patients. The use of iodine on exposed bone surfaces should be minimized since it may inhibit healing (Genco, Goldman, & Cohen, 1990).

There is a need for further investigation of the therapeutic effects of ultrasonic instrumentation in conjunction with antimicrobial agents. The expense of using chlorhexidene, or another antimicrobial solution, does not appear cost effective when considering the limited improvement in localized sites. See Chapter 14 for further information on chemotherapy and subgingival irrigation.

## Effects on Restorations

Because ultrasonic instruments generate mechanical energy to the tooth surface, it follows that the effects of ultrasonic instruments on restorative materials are of concern. An in-vitro study was conducted by Gorfil, Nordenberg, Liberman, and Ben-Amar (1989) to determine the effect of ultrasonics and airpolishing on the marginal integrity of radicular amalgams and composite resin restorations. Margins were subjected to ultrasonic scaling and air polishing, then clinically evaluated for microleakage. Visual and tactile evaluation of the experimental surfaces found no harmful effects from ultrasonic scaling and airpolishing on Class V restorations. The authors suggest, however, that the differences between clinicians, types of instruments employed, length of exposure, and power settings may vary the efficiency and iatrogenic effects created by the ultrasonic scaling device and the airpolishing instrument. Pollack and Kronenberg (1981) reported that the action of the ultrasonic instrument tends to cause marginal leakage around composite resins, especially Class IV and V restorations. If a metal ultrasonic insert inadvertently comes in contact with a composite material, gray or black streaks may appear on the surface of the restoration. The discoloration of the composite resin is the result of removal of metal onto the restoration. Hence, to decrease the wearing down of the metal insert and the undesirable appearance, avoid scaling on composite resin materials.

Reports from Blanchard (1984) and Rajstein and Tal (1984) stated that ultrasonic instruments can damage amalgam restorations. Crasson (1969) examined the effects of ultrasonic scaling on the cement within gold castings. Conclusions were that a burnishing effect occurred on the cervical margins, however, no cement was lost from within the gold castings. Similar findings were noted by McQuade (1978). Results indicated that the ultrasonic device would not affect the retention of properly cemented and well-fitting cast restorations and that scratching of gold restorations could occur if the ultrasonic tip inadvertently contacted them. It is prudent for the practitioner to avoid contacting composite, amalgam, porcelain, and gold restorations with ultrasonic inserts. Radiographs and periodontal charting are invaluable in helping the clinician avoid the margins of restorations while accomplishing subgingival debridement.

Implant maintenance with ultrasonic instruments was examined by Kwan, Zablotsky, and Meffert (1990). A pilot study evaluated the ability of an ultrasonic insert modified with a custom plastic tip to remove calculus on implant abutments and prostheses. Clinical observations suggested that the plastic ultrasonic instrument can remove lightly adherent calculus. Scanning electron photomicrographs of the experimental surfaces were examined for scratching and roughness. Results from the SEM concluded that the modified plastic insert produced microscratches or smearing of plastic on the titanium surface which could be removed by polishing with a fine prophylaxis paste. The use of the traditional metal ultrasonic insert against the titanium surface created noticeable scratching and gouging. Shallow scratches from the metal insert were readily polished smooth, but deeper scratches and gouges remained after polishing. Results from this preliminary study indicate that a plastic insert may be an asset in the professional maintenance of implants. Further studies are needed to substantiate the therapeutic effects and safety of this implant maintenance modality. Currently, plastic ultrasonic inserts are available from limited manufacturers (Tony Riso Company).

## CASE SELECTION

Currently, the application of ultrasonic instrumentation in NSPT is related to the clinician's educational background, participation in continuing education, and preference. While the technique of periodontal debridement with ultrasonic precision-thin inserts is not complicated, it does require a thorough knowledge of the basic principles and theory behind deposit removal and periodontal diseases. Effective debridement with ultrasonic instruments also requires experience and, as with any technical skill, the more experience one has the more effective the results.

There is continuing discussion as to if the periodontal therapist should use hand curets in conjunction with ultrasonic instruments or if ultrasonic instrumentation alone is sufficient. The concepts of root planing and periodontal debridement were discussed in Chapters 1 and 10. No matter what a person's philosophy is about deposit removal, it is fair to say that clinicians strive to remove all detectable deposits and plaque retention factors such as overhangs. It is also reasonable to assume that clinicians strive to achieve clinical parameters which indicate health such as lack of bleeding on probing, decreased or maintained pocket depth, and gain in or stable attachment levels. With these goals in mind the professional dental hygienist must decide when to use ultrasonic instrumentation in therapy and how to evaluate its effectiveness.

Use of the ultrasonic can be incorporated in initial therapy as well as maintenance therapy. It is extremely useful in initial therapy with clients who have gingivitis, and for retreating areas during periodontal maintenance appointments. Table 12-2 lists the contraindications and considerations for use. As in hand instrumentation, a thorough review of the medical and dental history, periodontal assessment and radiographic evaluation is advised before implementing any periodontal therapy procedures. The situations which would clearly contraindicate the use of ultrasonic instrumentation would be nonshielded pacemakers, respiratory risk, problems with swallowing or gagging, and lack of consent to this mode of therapy.

A magnetostrictive ultrasonic unit could produce a risk to the client with a pacemaker because external electromagnetic energy may interfere with the sensing mechanism of the pacemaker (Adams, Fulfor, Beechy, MacCarthy, & Stephens, 1982; Simon, Linde, Bonnette, & Schlentz, 1975). Newer models of pacemakers are shielded and have less potential for magnetic interference; however, the degree of pacemaker susceptibility varies from manufacturer to manufacturer and various models from the same manufacturer will react differently (Sowton, Gray, & Preston, 1970). The client's attending physician or cardiologist should always be contacted for specific guidance prior to instrumentation. In one study, interference in the sensory mechanism of a pacemaker was noted within 6 cm from the handle of the scaling device to the endocardial lead (Adams et al., 1982). The pacemaker lead in some clients may pass through the subclavian or external jugular vein on its way to the heart muscle; therefore, the handpiece of the magnetostrictive ultrasonic in some positions may come close to this distance during therapy. It must be noted that piezoelectric scaling units did not demonstrate any interferences in these tests so their use is not contraindicated for patients with pacemakers. Informed consent might not be given for this procedure because of the client's personal preference or discomfort experienced with previous ultrasonic devices. An explanation of the difference between advanced ultrasonics and traditional methods might be useful in gaining consent. Other factors that the clinician needs to evaluate and discuss with the client when gaining informed consent include root or tissue sensitivity, and the water flow.

**Table 12-2  Contraindications, Considerations, Advantages, and Disadvantages for Advanced Ultrasonic Instrumentation**

| Contraindications | Considerations | Advantages | Disadvantages |
|---|---|---|---|
| 1. Nonshielded Pacemaker: Consultation with the attending physician/cardiologist is recommended. | 1. Restorations—use on porcelain, composite, gold, amalgam, and titanium implant abutments is not recommended; use on the adjacent root surface is acceptable. | 1. Decreased chance for sensitivity. | 1. Decreased tactile sensitivity because of the lack of a cutting edge. |
| 2. Respiratory Risk: Septic material and microorganisms can be aspirated; a history of asthma, emphysema, cystic fibrosis, cardiovascular disease with secondary pulmonary disease, or a breathing problem should be considered. | 2. Demineralized areas. | 2. Extension subgingivally near or to the epithelial attachment due to diameter and length of working end. | 2. Decreased visibility due to water spray. |
| 3. Swallowing Problem (Dysphagia) or Prone to Gagging. | 3. Sensitivity—root and gingival tissue should be considered. | 3. No need to sharpen. | 3. Indirect vision with the use of the mouth mirror is compromised. |
| 4. Lack of Consent. | | 4. When activating, no lateral pressure is needed. | 4. Evacuation needed for water spray. |
| | | 5. Asset in preventing cumulative trauma disorders. | |
| | | 6. Efficiency. | |
| | | 7. Minimal gingival tissue manipulation. | |
| | | 8. Lavage. | |

The considerations related to ultrasonic periodontal debridement usually do not contraindicate use of the instrument; however, they might require that the clinician not use the ultrasonic on certain tooth surfaces. For example, the gingival tissue around the abutment teeth of a three-unit bridge exhibits bleeding upon probing, inflammation, and explorer detectable deposit. The clinician can consider using the ultrasonic device for periodontal debridement in these areas as long as access to the root can be achieved without contacting the restorative work.

When changing treatment modalities from hand-activated curets to the ultrasonic, the client will need to be apprised of why the "new" instrument is being recommended. Discussing recent research results, invention of precision-thin inserts, comfort, and efficiency are important aspects to include in this discussion. The advantages and disadvantages of ultrasonic instrumentation as compared to hand instruments are considered when selecting the method for periodontal debridement and educating the client (see Table 12-2).

## INSTRUMENTATION RECOMMENDATIONS

It is important to recognize that ultrasonic instrumentation is as demanding to learn and effectively practice as hand instrumentation. Although the objectives of hand instruments and ultrasonic instruments are alike, the techniques vary. Ultrasonic instruments require using more complicated equipment and controlling more variables. Ultrasonic instrumentation, like hand instrumentation, requires that the therapist know root anatomy, instrument selection, adaptation, and activation; along with expected healing responses. Also clinicians need to be experienced in applying assessment data to therapeutic treatments. As with mastering any skill, practice and time will enhance the level of proficiency.

There are various approaches to properly adapt an ultrasonic insert. No matter which approach is selected, it is important that basic instrumentation principles are followed in order to enhance efficiency, effectiveness, and client comfort. It is not the intent of this chapter to include all types and styles of ultrasonic equipment and their applications. To implement advanced ultrasonic instrumentation, it is the choice of the author to use a manual tuning magnetostrictive ultrasonic unit with precision-thin inserts. This does not imply that an autotuned ultrasonic unit cannot perform subgingival periodontal debridement. It does infer that a manual tuned unit allows the clinician the ability to adjust the frequency to maximum or minimum efficiency as clinically needed during the procedure. Figure 12-11 summarizes the procedure that follows.

Clinician _____     Observer _____     Date _____

> KEY:  S = Adequate to Superior Achievement
>        U = Needs Improvement
>
> Directions: Request that your technique be observed in a quadrant. Further observation is encouraged should time permit.
>
> | *Criteria* | Self-Evaluation | Observer Evaluation |
> |---|---|---|
> | **1. Prepares Unit** | | |
> | • Equipment is set up *prior* to appointment | _____ | _____ |
> | • Unit and handpiece are disinfected | _____ | _____ |
> | • Barriers are used | _____ | _____ |
> | • Line is flushed | _____ | _____ |
> | • Places insert into handpiece filled with water | _____ | _____ |
> | **2. Client Selection is Appropriate** | | |
> | • Informed consent is gained | _____ | _____ |
> | • Rationale for use are recognized | _____ | _____ |
> | **3. Client Preparation** | | |
> | • Procedure is explained including operation of unit, purpose, noise, evacuation, and client expectations | _____ | _____ |
> | • An antiseptic mouthrinse is used for 1 minute | _____ | _____ |
> | • Barrier techniques are used including face shield/glasses and drape | | |
> | **4. Instrumentation** | | |
> | • Client and therapist positioning are adequate | _____ | _____ |
> | • Evacuation is appropriate | _____ | _____ |
> | • Explores to locate deposit | _____ | _____ |
> | • Appropriate insert is used | _____ | _____ |
> | • Tuning is correct | _____ | _____ |
> | • Approach is systematic | _____ | _____ |
> | • A gentle pen grasp is used with a soft tissue extraoral fulcrum | _____ | _____ |
> | • Handpiece is balanced | _____ | _____ |
> | • Tip is inserted using the back surface | _____ | _____ |
> | • Universal insert is adapted parallel with long axis of tooth at a 15° angle with tooth surfaces | _____ | _____ |
> | • R and L inserts are adapted perpendicular to long axis on proximal surfaces | _____ | _____ |
> | • Tip is in motion all the time | _____ | _____ |
> | • Strokes are multidirectional, brushlike | _____ | _____ |
> | • Pressure is not used | _____ | _____ |
> | • Stops periodically to allow complete evacuation | _____ | _____ |
> | • Evaluates progress and product with an explorer | _____ | _____ |
> | • Identifies endpoint | _____ | _____ |
> | **5. Management** | | |
> | • Manages client appropriately | _____ | _____ |
> | • Efficiency is demonstrated | _____ | _____ |
> | **6. Prepares Equipment for Next Use** | | |
> | • Disinfects | _____ | _____ |
> | • Prepares inserts/handpiece for autoclaving | _____ | _____ |
> | • Hoses are neatly stored | _____ | _____ |
> | • Unit is stored | | |
>
> COMMENTS:
>
> Clinician:_____
>
> _____
>
> Observer: _____
>
> _____
>
> Another observation is suggested due to:     _____ instrumentation     _____ management of client

**Figure 12-11** Ultrasonic instrumentation observation. (Courtesy of Idaho State University, Pocatello, ID. 1996)

To prepare clients for the ultrasonic procedure, hold the instrument in their view to demonstrate tip design and explain the mechanism of action in layman's terminology. Avoid words like "chipping" and "hammering," although "fracturing" may be appropriate. Point out the water aperture on the tip and define the significance of the water flow. Explain placement of the suction and its ability to remove water during the procedure. Assure clients that if they are uncomfortable at any time during the procedure you can make adjustments accordingly. Constant observation of the client helps the clinician to anticipate needs during instrumentation.

## Infection Control

To prepare the unit for client care, wipe all surfaces with a disinfectant. Do not spray disinfectant directly on an ultrasonic unit. To avoid cross contamination, place plastic or latex barriers on unit or control knobs that will be handled during the periodontal debridement procedure. Clear the handpiece with water. Studies have found that flushing the line of ultrasonic units decrease the number of microorganisms in the lines(Gross, Devine, & Cutright, 1976). Flushing the unit for up to 2 minutes prior to use on each client will reduce, not eliminate, microorganisms. Another factor to consider is the quality of water supplied to the unit. In various areas, water is not potable nor would it be acceptable as an irrigant/coolant for the ultrasonic. Separate pressurized water containers for sterile water are commercially available to compensate for these problems. Bacterial counts from the water lines can be reduced by using filters and flushing lines with a hypochlorite and water solution. These choices may be costly and time-consuming, but are necessary for decreasing the bacterial exposure to the client from stagnate water lines.

Sterilize or disinfect the handpiece. Follow manufacturers recommendations for this important aspect of instrument care. Plastic (Dispo-Shield, Ash Dentsply) and latex sleeves are now available for ultrasonic handpieces. Magnetostrictive inserts can be autoclaved in steam under pressure and chemical vapor, however, magnetostrictive inserts with rubber "O" rings can not tolerate dry heat sterilization. Insert tips may become thin over a period of time from use so evaluation of the tip thickness should occur periodically. Extremely thin tips may increase the risk of tip breakage.

For infection control purposes, ask the client to rinse with an antimicrobial rinse for one minute prior to instrumentation. Chlorhexidene rinses, because of their substantivity, are the most beneficial when compared to other oral rinses. Studies demonstrate that aerosols produced from ultrasonic instruments contain microorganisms. Preprocedural rinsing with an antiseptic mouthwash significantly reduces the microbial content of aerosols generated during ultrasonic scaling (Fine et al., 1992). Bentley, Burkhart, and Crawford's (1994) preliminary results show that spatter and aerosol dissemina-

tion may be a significant hazard for dental personnel. Significant spatter was found on upper surfaces of the clinician's arms, lower neck, chest, and face shield. These observations support the need for covering these areas and practicing universal precautions in the treatment of all persons. Results from the pilot study concluded that bacterial contaminated aerosols and spatter are extremely variable and may be dependent on various factors including level of bacterial plaque in the mouth, type of procedure, evacuation system utilized (low or high volume), position of the client in the dental chair, and position of the tooth. It is also recommended to reduce supragingival plaque prior to instrumentation by polishing first or instructing the client to perform self-care. Also, well-adapted multilayered face masks with high filtration levels should be worn. The face mask should be frequently replaced when using or assisting in high-speed dental procedures like ultrasonic instrumentation.

## Positioning

When operating an ultrasonic unit, the console should be placed within reaching distance of the clinician seated in the operator's chair. Ideally, the unit should be placed on the opposite side of the operatory chair from the clinician. This positioning allows the clinician to move to the twelve o'clock position without encumbering access to the unit. Healthy body mechanics and ergonomic principles (see Chapter 15) apply to ultrasonic instrumentation, as well as other dental procedures. In general, operator/client positioning for ultrasonic instrumentation parallels fundamental positioning recommendations (see Chapter 11). When using an ultrasonic device however, client positioning is altered from traditional recommendations because of the need for water evacuation. Client positioning requires turning the head toward the suction and slightly downward to avoid water running to the back of the throat. Sometimes a client might feel comfortable positioned more upright than would usually be expected for therapy with hand-activated instruments. Often this is because of the water flow and the lack of control the client feels with its evacuation.

Efficiency of the suction will help enhance comfort and instrumentation. High volume suction is ideal for reducing aerosols generated from the unit (Bentley, Burkhart, & Crawford, 1994). However, when working solo, the Hygoformic® (Pulp Dent) saliva ejector will provide adequate suction when adapted to a high volume or an efficient low volume evacuation system. To insure effective suction placement, bring the suction hose behind the dental chair to place it in the client's mouth. The weight of the suction hose will help stabilize the saliva ejector. Twist the Hygoformic saliva ejector open and place it on the retromolar pad. Request that the client turn his head to the side where the saliva ejector is placed. Placement in this manner ensures that the buccal mucosa is retracted with the side of the ejector for greater visibility (see Figure 12-12).

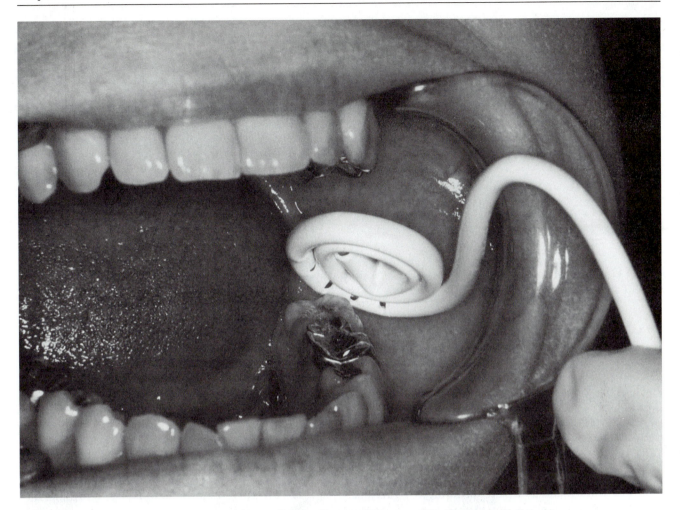

**Figure 12-12** Correct placement of the Hygoformic® Saliva Ejector. (Courtesy of Dr. Thomas E. Holbrook)

Some clinicians request that the client assist in the suction procedure when this type of ejector is not available. The client can place a straight suction piece in either corner of the oral cavity depending on where the clinician is debriding or the client can place the suction into the mouth when the clinician withdraws the insert. Careful attention to the effectiveness of the evacuation is imperative because it relates to the client's acceptance of the ultrasonic procedure.

### Insert Selection

The universal or straight insert, like the periodontal probe, is used for negotiating any sulcus or pocket, especially pockets that are deep and/or narrow (see Figure 12-13A). Right and left (R & L) designs are similar to the Nabers probe and universal curets (Columbia 13/14, Barnhardt 5/6) (see Figure 12-13B). They are used to debride interproximal surfaces of molars and premolars and are ideal to reach deposits located under contacts. Their extension to the depth of a periodontal pocket is limited by the curvature of their design. Other applications for R & Ls include debridement of tipped molars and furcations.

### Tuning the Unit

When using precision-thin inserts, the clinician should begin with the power on the lowest setting and regulate the tip energy by adjusting the frequency (tuning knob). This step minimizes tip displacement and enhances patient comfort and control of the insert. Because tuning a magnetostrictive ultrasonic insert is unique to the manual tuning unit, the following sequence is suggested for preparing the insert.

1. Turn the unit on and set the power control at its lowest setting. Initially adjust the frequency so there are no vibrations emitting from the tip.
2. If tuning an insert with an external water conduit, make sure the conduit is directly centered over the tip and within 1 mm of contacting the tip.
3. Place the insert into the handpiece and adjust the water control. Hold the handpiece in a horizontal position with the tip pointed upward. Adjust the water to gently arch over the upward pointed tip. The water will arch from 1 to 1½ inches over the end of the tip. This step is used to insure adequate water flow to the tip.

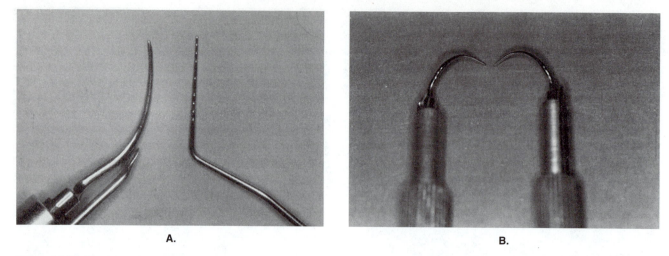

**Figure 12-13** Precision-thin insert designs. **A.** Universal or straight insert compared to a periodontal probe. (Courtesy of Home Study Educators, Inc.) **B.** Right (R) and left (L) inserts. (Courtesy of Dr. Thomas E. Holbrook)

4. With the tip pointed downward, adjust the frequency (tuning) dial so there is a light aerosol emitting from the tip and a fluent stream of water.
5. Repeat this procedure after changing inserts.

### Sequencing

Begin debridement with an intentional sequence of instrumentation. Treat the mouth in an orderly sequence and follow the treatment plan accordingly. To reduce wear and tear on precision-thin inserts and enhance efficiency, utilize standard inserts for gross debridement of supragingival deposits and subgingival deposits located relatively close to the gingival margin (i.e., within 1 to 3 mm). Save precision-thin inserts for other periodontal debridement procedures including moderate to light deposits and subgingival debridement.

To ensure efficiency, complete all areas designated in the treatment plan with the universal precision-thin insert. For example, when treating for half of the mouth, utilize the universal on all indicated surfaces before selecting the appropriate R-insert or L-insert. Needless changing of inserts can be time-consuming because it requires that the clinician retune the insert. The chosen sequence should maximize efficiency by reducing the number of times an insert is changed. Several possible efficient sequences exist when proceeding throughout the entire dentition; however, minimizing repositioning of client and suction also improves time efficiency. Avoid beginning the sequence of ultrasonic instrumentation in the posterior region. Starting in or nearest to the anterior allows time to acclimate the client to the sensation and water spray from the tip.

### Adaptation and Activation

The following are recommendations for advanced ultrasonic instrumentation techniques gathered from the

literature (Holbrook & Low, 1989) and experience of the author.

1. Hold handpiece with a gentle pen grasp (versus a firm modified pen grasp).
2. Balance handpiece to eliminate the torque of the cord. Drape the cord over the inside of the arm to reduce the drag of the cord.
3. Use a soft tissue or extraoral rest for orientation and limitation of movement (versus a fulcrum on hard tissue).
4. Use the lightest possible pressure (allow the instrument to do the work).
5. Activate tip before applying to crown or root surfaces.
6. Adapt the universal (straight) tip parallel (15°) to the long axis of the tooth. If debriding interproximal areas, the tip can be adapted somewhat perpendicular to the long axis of the tooth surface to ensure adequate coverage at the midline of the interproximal space and underneath the contact area. Use of the right and left inserts are discussed in a subsequent section.
7. Insert the tip subgingivally using the back (convex surface) of the tip to avoid tissue trauma (see Figure 12-14A).
8. Use the back surface of the tip to maneuver along the epithelial attachment (See Figure 12-14B–D).
9. Use a brushlike or "vibrato" type stroke with the objective to fully negotiate complete root coverage.
10. After removing the larger deposits, start at the greatest depth of the pocket (or apical extent) and use multiple overlapping strokes moving the tip coronally.
11. Keep the insert moving at all times.

The type or direction of stroke necessary to enhance complete root coverage is an overlapping, brushlike

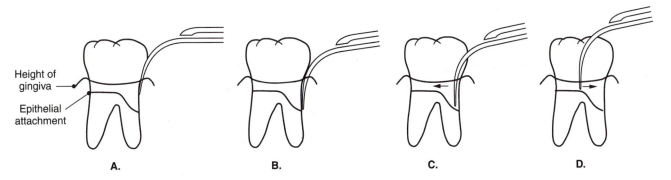

**Figure 12-14** Pocket negotiation. **A.** Enter pocket using the back surface. Keep tip in contact with root and parallel to the long axis of the root. **B.** Negotiate tip to the apical extent of the pocket using minute overlapping strokes. *Note:* The weight of the instrument and the oscillations generated by the tip will guide the tip subgingivally. **C.** To move the tip along the epithelial attachment, use the back of the tip and a pushlike stroke to avoid trauma and patient discomfort. **D.** Avoid using a pull stroke with the front or concave surface when the tip is against the epithelial attachment. Place current periodontal charting and radiographs within view for reference during instrumentation.

stroke. Very little is written about the technique of the stroke; however, thorough complete coverage is recommended. To understand the concept of this stroke, imagine the root surface of a pocket like the canvas of an artist. Begin painting in a bottom corner of the canvas by using minute, overlapping strokes. Move your paintbrush from the corner across the canvas to the opposing, top corner. The objective is to fully negotiate the canvas with a brushlike, overlapping stroke to eliminate evidence of the canvas underneath.

If a tenacious deposit is encountered that cannot be removed with a low-power setting and light overlapping strokes with minimal pressure, first attempt to use a more productive surface of the tip (refer to Figure 12-6). If this alteration does not remove the deposit, increase the frequency of a manual tuning unit to increase the energy output of the tip. If the deposit cannot be removed at maximum frequency, use more pressure and a rapid overlapping stroke. As a last resort, increase the power to medium or high. This step should be minimized whenever possible. Increased power increases tip displacement. Increase power may enhance removal of tenacious deposits; however, it may also increase root roughness or damage. Another alternative may be to switch to a standard insert design.

During ultrasonic instrumentation, visibility may be compromised at times from the cavitational activity of the tip. Use direct vision when possible. If it is not attainable, wipe mirror on the inside of the patient's cheek, spray mirror with water from the tip, and use indirect vision. This step helps reduce mirror distortion from the water spray. Water spray flushes debris from the site of instrumentation and helps maintain a clean field of vision. Magnification lenses also enhance visibility of the root structure, gingival tissue, and deposits.

Endpoint of instrumentation can be assessed by recognizing when no more debris is visibly being flushed out of the pocket; the surface is devoid of deposits and overhangs as evaluated with an explorer; and the entire subgingival root surface (epithelial attachment to the coronal aspect of the pocket) has been contacted with the ultrasonic tip. Further evaluation of the success of debridement therapy occurs when the clinician evaluates therapy at the one-month interval. Lack of bleeding on probing and inflammation; reduced pocket depth; and stable attachment levels all indicate successful therapy. These same clinical parameters are used to evaluate success at the periodontal maintenance appointments (see Chapter 16).

## Special Situations

As stated earlier, R-insert and L-inserts are utilized in specific areas including mesial and distal surfaces, drifted/tipped teeth, furcations, and various curved root anatomy. To debride mesial and distal surfaces, approach adaptation similar to the use of a universal curet, meaning that one working end or insert adapts to both the mesial and distal surface. The therapist can use one side of the R- or L-insert tip on the mesial (and buccal) and the other side of the same insert tip on the distal. Correct insert selection (right or left) occurs when the curvature of tip adapts toward the mesial (see Figure 12-15A). Establish a soft rest for orientation and limitation of movement, close the curvature of the tip by adapting it against the tooth, activate the tip, and direct it under the contact perpendicular to the long axis of the tooth. Roll the handpiece, or turn the insert in the handpiece, to adapt the tip around the line angle (see Figure 12-15B). Extend the tip at least halfway across the interproximal surface toward the opposite side to ensure debridement at the midline (see Figure 12-15C).

To debride curved root anatomy such as the palatal root of a maxillary molar, establish a soft tissue rest and approach the surface from the opposite arch using the back or convex surface of a straight or universal insert design. Correct tip adaptation will follow the curvature of the root (see Figure 12-16). These same principles of tip

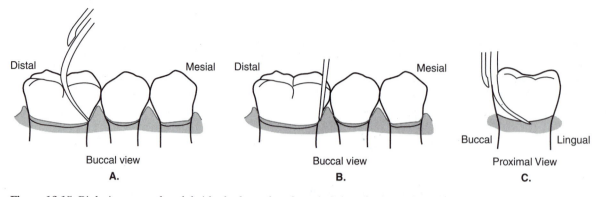

**Figure 12-15** Right insert used to debride the buccal surface. **A.** Select the insert based on its curvature toward the mesial surface. Adapt tip below the contact area. **B.** Roll tip onto the proximal surface. Keep tip against the tooth structure. **C.** Extend tip toward the lingual to negotiate the CEJ and proximal surface.

adaptation will apply in negotiating other curved root anatomy.

To negotiate a furcation, establish a soft tissue rest. Initially place the complete curvature of the right or left insert tip against the crown of the tooth in a closed fashion. As with debriding the mesial surface of a tooth, the correct insert is the one that adapts or curves towards the mesial surface. Activate the insert and place the tip under the gingiva to feel for the furcation entrance. Rotate the tip while pivoting your wrist to access the depth of the bony defect. To reduce tissue distention, keep the tip closed or against the root surface at all times (see Figure 12-17). To negotiate mesial and distal walls of a buccal or lingual bony defect, move the lateral surface of the tip against the mesial of the distal root and use the opposite lateral surface to debride the distal of the mesial root. In other words, the clinician uses the same R-insert or L-insert to debride both walls of the defect. Complete coverage of the roof and lateral walls of a furcation is the objective of debridement in these areas. Depending upon the height of the gingiva and its relationship to the bony defect, selection of inserts and their adaptation may vary.

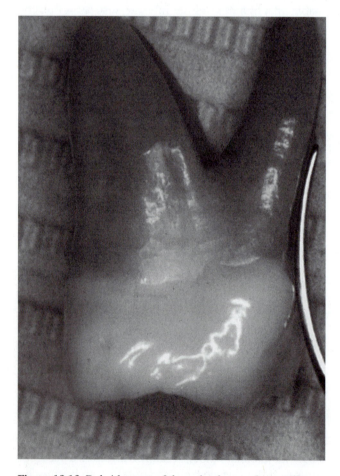

**Figure 12-16** Debridement of the palatal root of a maxillary second molar. Note that the back surface of the working end is adapted to the root. (Courtesy of Dr. Thomas E. Holbrook)

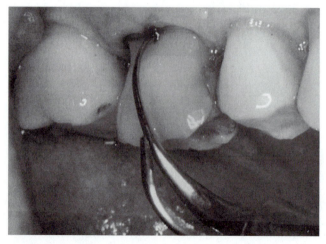

**Figure 12-17** Negotiating a furcation on a maxillary first molar. The tip of the working end is placed within the furcation. All surfaces of the tip are used to debride. (Courtesy of Dr. Thomas E. Holbrook)

## MAINTENANCE OF INSERTS

Follow manufacturer recommendations for sterilization of inserts. Avoid placing magnetostrictive inserts in dry heat sterilization. Steam under pressure or chemical vapor is recommended for magnetostrictive inserts. Over a period of time, rubber "O" rings of magnetostrictive inserts may deteriorate and lose elasticity causing leaking or dripping from the handpiece. If leaking occurs, check to be sure the insert has a complete seal with the handpiece. When an insert is being placed in the handpiece and will not slide in easily, wet the external O-ring. This will facilitate placement in the handpiece while adding to the insert's longevity. Replace external O-rings as necessary.

When autoclaving inserts, avoid placing heavy instruments on top of them. Thin, precision inserts may bend or break if mishandled. If small bends in the tip occur, use orthodontic pliers to gently squeeze out the bends. Some ultrasonic tips are made from metal that is not flexible and they cannot be recontoured or crimped with an orthodontic pliers. Acute or severe bends may indicate need for replacement. Avoid placing magnetostrictive inserts in glutaraldehyde solution for sterilization or as a holding bath.

Metal inserts may be susceptible to corrosion and rust if not properly maintained. To avoid this, dip inserts in antirust and corrosion emulsion prior to sterilization, and properly vent inserts following the sterilization. To remove corrosion, brush sterile inserts with a stiff wire brush. As inserts become too thin from use or break from misuse, do not discard. Some manufacturers will retip or replace inserts (Tony Riso Company, Ultrasonic Services Incorporated). An insert that does not vibrate or cannot be tuned may need repair or replacement. Some factors that may cause lack of vibration include the unit not being plugged into the electrical outlet, insufficient water, the foot pedal or handpiece switch not being activated by the clinician, or a ferromagnetic rod that is fractured from mishandling. These and other factors may limit effectiveness.

## Summary

The focus of this chapter is subgingival periodontal debridement with precision-thin inserts. The mechanism of calculus removal by an ultrasonic device is mechanical in nature. The oscillating tip of an insert produces a rubbing motion at high frequencies to remove deposits. A vibrating ultrasonic tip must be in direct contact with a deposit to remove it from the tooth or root structures. Tip motion is influenced by the size and shape of the insert, power setting, transduction of energy, and the type of ultrasonic unit employed. It is the clinician's responsibility to select the correct power setting, frequency, inserts, coolant/irrigant, and technique best suited to the clinical needs of the client. Proper selection of ultrasonic inserts is dependent on pocket topography, root anatomy, tenacity, amount of calculus, and client comfort during ultrasonic debridement.

The manufacturing of precision-thin inserts has initiated a new approach to periodontal debridement that is particularly applicable to NSPT. Further research comparing the effects of these tip designs and the different types of units is indicated to evaluate the use of advanced ultrasonic therapy in nonsurgical care. No longer should ultrasonics be considered as an adjunct to hand instrumentation, but rather our first choice in the armamentarium for NSPT. The dental hygiene professional is challenged to stay current in this area of therapy by reading peer reviewed literature and attending continuing education courses. Figure 12-18 will aid clinicians when evaluating equipment for advanced ultrasonic instrumentation.

## Case Studies

**Case Study One:** Cindy Donalds identifies that her face is getting wet from the ultrasonic spray. She recently had sinusitis and is having difficulty breathing and swallowing the water spray. What measures can you take to improve her discomfort?

**Case Study Two:** Jimmy Lloyd is experiencing root sensitivity and gingival tenderness when debriding a 6 mm pocket on the distal lingual surface of tooth #30. What steps can you employ to enhance comfort?

**Case Study Three:** Will McNeill has chronic adult periodontitis of moderate severity. Radiographic evaluation and a periodontal assessment reveal a Class II buccal furcation on tooth #30 and a mesial furcation on tooth #14 with a circumferential defect along the palatal root of #14. Mr. McNeill refuses surgical intervention to eliminate the defects; therefore, nonsurgical periodontal debridement is recommended to maintain these areas. Which instrument(s) would you chose for debridement for each of these areas? How would you negotiate (adapt and activate) the root anatomy in each of these situations?

**Case Study Four:** As you are removing deposits during initial therapy, your client, Mrs. Hill, notices the water is getting warmer. Next, she verbalizes that her tooth sur-

Directions: The following evaluation form was created to help you assess the various ultrasonic units and inserts on the market. Please keep in mind your clinical needs when rating the various equipment.

3 = Excellent     2 = Good     1 = Fair     0 = Poor

Design:

_____ 1. Size and shape of tips/inserts compatible with unit
_____ 2. Number of tips/inserts available
_____ 3. Ease of tuning (frequency) inserts
_____ 4. Ease of power (amplitude) adjustments
_____ 5. Ease of foot switch operations
_____ 6. Flexibility of handpiece hose
_____ 7. Handpiece cylindrical and lightweight in design
_____ 8. Ease of disinfecting/sterilizing unit and handpiece
_____ 9. Portability of unit
_____ 10. Ease of changing tips/inserts
_____ 11. Ease of adjusting water/coolant
_____ 12. Provides ability to irrigate with chemotherapeutics

Performance:

_____ 13. Provides access to deep periodontal pockets
_____ 14. Adapts to furcation defects
_____ 15. Removes calculus readily
_____ 16. Amount and direction of water spray
_____ 17. Noise level during use
_____ 18. Tip/insert performance following repeated sterilization and use
_____ 19. Patient comfort during use
_____ 20. Clinician comfort during use

Operation:

_____ 21. User-friendly instructions
_____ 22. Maintenance instructions
_____ 23. Warranty available
_____ 24. Ease of service and repair
_____ 25. Custom tip design services and retipping replacement inserts available
_____ 26. Conveniently positioned handpiece holder

Describe the *best* feature(s) of this unit:

Describe the *least favorable* feature(s) of this unit:

**Figure 12-18** Equipment evaluation.

faces are feeling a little sensitive and you notice your handpiece is feeling very warm to the touch. What steps could you take to remedy the problem?

As you take care of that problem and continue to work, you encounter difficulty in removing tenacious deposits. What can you do to increase the efficiency of the tip?

**Case Study Five:** For the student or practitioner who has not had experience with precision-thin ultrasonic instruments, the following exercises may serve multiple purposes. An objective of this exercise is to allow the clinician to experiment with the ultrasonic unit and accompanying inserts on extracted teeth.

OBJECTIVES:
1. Evaluate the effectiveness of the insert on each side.
2. Practice variable stroke patterns.
3. Demonstrate overlapping, "vibrato" type strokes.
4. Assess the effectiveness of the insert by varying the tuning (frequency), power (amplitude), pressure, and angle of application.
5. Compare energy output from the various ultrasonic units available.

MATERIALS REQUIRED:
A typodont tooth with root anatomy, fingernail polish or model airplane paint, personal protective equipment (gloves, masks, eyewear, and gown), ultrasonic unit, and insert. Note: To stabilize the tooth, mount in plaster or stone with the root surfaces exposed. Cover the exposed root surfaces with polish or paint and let dry.

INSTRUCTIONS:
A. Gradually increase the power while using an insert. How did the tip perform at maximum power when adapted to the root surface?
B. Adapt each surface of the tip to the root (front [concave], back [convex], side [lateral] and point). Did you notice a difference in energy output when using different tip surfaces against the root?
C. Activate the insert and use different hand pressure against the root. How did the tip perform using a heavy hand pressure? What differences did you notice using light pressure versus heavy pressure?
D. Demonstrate a brushlike, overlapping stroke with the tip. Could you obtain complete root coverage with this stroke?
E. Adapt the tip parallel to the long axis of the tooth. Gradually increase the angle of application up to 90°. Did you notice a difference in energy output?
F. (Manual tuning ultrasonic units only.) Gradually adjust the tuning from "in phase" to "out of phase" while using the insert. Did you notice a difference in aerosol and sound? What was the length of the

phase? Could you determine the point of maximum efficiency/vibration for the insert?

# Case Study Discussions

**Discussion—Case Study One:** The clinician should evaluate the evacuation technique using the following criteria:

1. Ensure Cindy's head is tilted far enough to the side corresponding to the side of the mouth in which the water is pooling and the saliva ejector is laced.
2. In addition to making sure Cindy's head is turned to the side, ensure it is also tipped downward to prevent excess flow to the back of the mouth/throat area.
3. When using a Hygoformic saliva ejector, make sure it is twisted open and the holes are placed adjacent to or towards the pooling water.
4. Check the saliva ejector to make sure it is not crimped, which will decrease the efficiency of the evacuation.
5. Check to see if the evacuation hose is arranged effectively. The hose should be positioned behind the chair creating weight on the saliva ejector to keep it stable.
6. Evaluate the supine position to access if Cindy needs to be sitting more upright to be able to tolerate the procedure.
7. Change saliva ejectors to a more effective type if applicable. If a Hygoformic design is available, employ its use. If slow speed is not acceptable, change to high speed. Engage help from an assistant, if available, for this particular situation.
8. If the above steps do not improve the evacuation, discuss the discomfort with Cindy to see if another trouble shooting mechanism can be discovered. If not, discuss whether to continue with the ultrasonic scaling.

**Discussion—Case Study Two:** Gingival sensitivity would lead the clinician to believe that adaptation and activation need to be evaluated. The following steps can be assessed to discover the cause(s) of the discomfort.

1. Check to make sure the lowest power setting is being used.
2. Tune the frequency somewhat "out of phase" to reduce resonance (manual tuning units only).
3. Be sure the tip has no sharp or rough edges.
4. Use the side surface of the tip.
5. Use the lightest pressure possible.
6. Keep the working end moving.
7. Place the insert subgingivally using the back or convex surface.

8. Decrease angulation to the crown/root surface.
9. Check water temperature and evacuation systems to ensure they are not contributing factors.

**Discussion—Case Study Three:** The buccal furcation of #30 should be approached by selecting the curved insert, right or left, which adapts towards the mesial surface. The insert selection is similar to adapting a universal curet to this same buccal surface. Establish a soft tissue rest and place the curvature of the tip against the crown/root surface as close to 0° as possible. This tip angle to the tooth is particularly important if the gingival tissue occludes the furcation. If not, this angle can be opened to greater than 0°. Rotate the tip into the furcation. Because all sides of the working end are activated, the roof, the mesial portion of the distal root, and the distal portion of the mesial root of the furcation should all be debrided. The clinician will need to adapt the lateral surface of the tip to one side of the bony defect, and the opposite lateral surface to the other side of the defect. Depending on the furcation entrance dimension, a straight design might be used exclusively or in combination with the R- and L-inserts. Figure 12-17 is an illustration of correct technique with a curved insert, although it depicts a different tooth.

The mesial furcation on tooth #14 is also approached from the lingual aspect with the appropriate right or left insert. It is debrided with the same procedure as described for #30. The correct insert to use is the one where the curvature of the tip proceeds towards the mesial surface so that when you rotate the tip into the furcation, the curvature adapts into the concave area. It is unlikely that a straight insert design will effectively adapt to this surface.

The correct approach for the palatal root of #14 is illustrated in Figure 12-16 on page 338. A straight or universal insert is employed because of the narrow area limiting access. The back surface is adapted to the root making sure the working end extends the length of the pocket.

**Discussion—Case Study Four:** To remedy the warm sensation felt by you and Mrs. Hill, pay particular attention to the rate of water flow. Increasing water flow will decrease the heat production. Retune and examine the insert to ensure the seal of the external O-ring is adequate and the insert itself is in good shape. If the transducer or stacks of metal are bent, this could contribute to improper tuning. If these procedures do not identify the problem, consider using the insert on a lower power setting and frequency (out of phase) to reduce the sensitivity to the client.

To enhance removal of tenacious deposits, follow this sequence:

1. Use a more productive surface of the working end. Refer to Figure 12-6 on page 325.
2. If this is not successful, increase the frequency (tuning knob), if the unit is manual tuned, to increase the energy and speed of movement.
3. Next, use increased pressure and rapid overlapping strokes.
4. As a last resort, increase the power setting which will increase tip displacement. This is not ideal because it might cause undesirable surface alterations (roughness/striations).
5. If the four steps do not enhance removal, switch the insert to a standard and larger design.

**Discussion—Case Study Five:** Answers to questions A through F should relate to the principles discussed within the content of this chapter. Encouraging the clinician to explain the rationale or reason for each response encourages application of didactic knowledge level information to clinical or psychomotor skills.

## REFERENCES

Adams, D., Fulford, N., Beechy, J., MacCarthy, J., & Stephens, M. (1982). The cardiac pacemaker and ultrasonic scalers. *British Dental Journal, 152,* 171–173.

Badersten, A., Nilvéus, R., & Egelberg, J. (1981). Effect of non-surgical periodontal therapy. I. Moderately advanced periodontitis. *Journal of Clinical Periodontology, 8,* 57–72.

Badersten, A., Nilvéus, R., & Egelberg, J. (1984). Effect of non-surgical periodontal therapy. II. Severely advanced periodontitis. *Journal of Clinical Periodontology, 11,* 63–76.

Baehni, P., Thilo, B., Chapuis, B., & Pernet D. (1992). Effects of ultrasonic and sonic scalers on dental plaque microflora in vitro and in vivo. *Journal of Clinical Periodontology, 19,* 455–459.

Biagini, G., Checchi, L., Miccoli, M.C., Vasi, V., & Castaldini, C. (1988). Root curetage and gingival repair in periodontitis. *Journal of Periodontology, 59,* 124–129.

Bentley, C. D., Burkhart, N. W., & Crawford, J. J. (1994). Evaluating spatter and aerosol contamination during dental procedures. *Journal of the American Dental Association, 125,* 579–584.

Blanchard, J. S. (1984). The periodontal curet and the ultrasonic scaler. Their effectiveness in removing overhangs from amalgam restorations. *Dental Hygiene, 58,* 450–454.

Breininger, D. R., O'Leary, T. J., & Blumenshine, R. V. H. (1987). Comparative effectiveness of ultrasonic and hand scaling for the removal of subgingival plaque and calculus. *Journal of Periodontology, 58,* 9–18.

Chapple, I. L. C., Walmsley, A. D., Saxby, M. S., & Moscrop, H. (1992). Effect of subgingival irrigation with chlorhexidine during ultrasonic scaling. *Journal of Periodontology, 63,* 812–816.

Checchi, W. A., Wilson, M., & Kieser, J. B. (1988). Root surface debridement in vitro. *Journal of Clinical Periodontology, 15,* 288–292.

Cheetham, L. & Pellicionne, G. H. (1988). Hand versus ultrasonic instrumentation in the removal of endotoxins from root surfaces in vitro. *Journal of Periodontology, 59,* 398–402.

Clark, S. M. (1969). The ultrasonic dental unit: A guide for the clinical application of ultrasonics in dentistry and in dental hygiene. *Journal of Periodontology, 40,* 621–629.

Clinical Research Associates Newsletter. (1993). Provo, UT: Clinical Research Associates.

Copulos, T. A., Low, S. B., Walker, C. B., Trebilcock, Y. Y., & Hefti, A. F. (1993). Comparative analysis between a modified ultrasonic tip and hand instruments on clinical parameters of periodontal disease. *Journal of Periodontology, 64,* 694–700.

Crasson, W. (1969). Effects of an ultrasonic instrument on cement with gold castings. *New York State Dental Journal, 35,* 485–487.

D'Silva, I. V., Nayak, R. P., Cherian, K. M., & Mulky, M. J. (1979). An evaluation of the root topography following periodontal instrumentation—a scanning electron microscope study. *Journal of Periodontology, 50,* 283–290.

Dragoo, M. R. (1992). A clinical evaluation of hand and ultrasonic instruments on subgingival debridement. Part I. With unmodified and modified ultrasonic inserts. *International Journal of Periodontics & Restorative Dentistry, 12,* 312–323.

Fine, D. H., Mendieta, C., Barnett, M. L., Furgang, D., Meyers, R., Olshan, A., & Vincent, J. (1992). Efficacy of preprocedural rinsing with an antiseptic in reducing viable bacteria in dental aerosols. *Journal of Periodontology, 63,* 821–824.

Garnick, J. J. & Dent, J. (1989). A scanning electron micrographical study of root surfaces and subgingival bacteria after hand and ultrasonic instrumentation. *Journal of Periodontology, 60,* 441–447.

Genco, R. J., Goldman, H. M., & Cohen, D. W. (1990). Antiinfective and adjunctive management of periodontal diseases. In R. J. Genco, H. M. Goldman, & D. W. Cohen (Eds.), *Contemporary periodontics* (pp. 436–440). St. Louis: Mosby-Year Book, Inc.

Gorfil, C., Nordenberg, D., Liberman, R., & Ben-Amar, A. (1989). The effect of ultrasonic cleaning and air polishing on the marginal integrity of radicular amalgam and composite resin restorations. *Journal of Clinical Periodontology, 16,* 137–139.

Green, E. & Ramfjord, S. P. (1966). Tooth roughness after subgingival root planing. *Journal of Periodontology, 37,* 396–399.

Gross, A., Devine, M. J., & Cutright, D. E. (1976). Microbial contamination of dental units and ultrasonic units. *Journal of Periodontology, 47,* 670.

Herremans, K. L. (1989). *Effects of ultrasonic scaling and hand scaling on root surface topography.* Unpublished thesis, Old Dominion University, School of Dental Hygiene, Norfolk.

Holbrook, T. E. & Low, S. B. (1989). Power-driven scaling and polishing instruments. In J. F. Hardin (Ed.), *Clark's clinical dentistry* (pp. 1–24). Philadelphia: J.P. Lippincott.

Hou, G. L., Chen, S. F., Wu, Y. M.. & Tsai, C. C. (1994). The topography of the furcation entrance in Chinese molars: Furcation entrance dimensions. *Journal of Clinical Periodontology, 21,* 451–456.

Hunter, R. K., O'Leary, T. J., & Kafrawy, A. H. (1984). The effectiveness of hand versus ultrasonic instrumentation in open flap root planing. *Journal of Periodontology, 55,* 697–703.

Jones, S. J., Lozdan, J., & Boyde, A. (1972). Tooth surfaces treated *in situ* with periodontal instruments. *British Dental Journal, 132,* 57–62.

Kepic, T. J., O'Leary, T. J., & Kafrawy, A. H. (1990). Total calculus removal: An attainable objective? *Journal of Periodontology, 61,* 16–20.

Kerry, G. J. (1967). Roughness of root surfaces after use of ultrasonic instruments and hand curettes. *Journal of Periodontology, 38,* 340–346.

Kwan, J., Zablotsky, M. H., & Meffert, R. M. (1990). Implant maintenance using a modified ultrasonic instrument. *Journal of Dental Hygiene, 64,* 422–430.

Leon, L. E. & Vogel, R. I. (1987). A comparison of the effectiveness of hand scaling and ultrasonic debridement in furcations as evaluated by differential dark-field microscopy. *Journal of Periodontology, 58,* 86–94.

McQuade, M. J. (1978). Effects of ultrasonic instrumentation on the retention of simulated cast crowns. *Journal of Prosthetic Dentistry, 39,* 640–642.

Moore, J., Wilson, M., & Kieser, J. B. (1986). The distribution of bacterial lipopolysaccharide (endotoxin) in relation to periodontally involved root surfaces. *Journal of Clinical Periodontology, 13,* 748–751.

Moskow, B. S. & Bressman, E. (1964). Cemental response to ultrasonic and hand instrumentation. *Journal of the American Dental Association, 68,* 698–703.

Nishimine, D. & O'Leary, T. J. (1979). Hand instrumentation in removal of endotoxins from root surfaces. *Journal of Periodontology, 50,* 345–349.

Nosal, G., Scheidt, M. J., O'Neal, R., & VanDyke, T. E. (1991). The penetration of lavage solution into the periodontal pocket during ultrasonic instrumentation. *Journal of Periodontology, 62,* 554–557.

O'Leary, T. J. (1986). The impact of research on scaling and root planing. *Journal of Periodontology, 57,* 69–74.

Oda, S. & Ishikawa, I. (1989). In vitro effectiveness of a newly-designed ultrasonic scaler tip for furcation areas. *Journal of Periodontology, 60,* 634–639.

Oosterwaal, P. J. M., Matee, M. I., Mikx, F. H. M., van't Hof, M. A., & Renggli, H. H. (1987). The effect of subgingival debridement with hand and ultrasonic instruments on the subgingival microflora. *Journal of Clinical Periodontology, 14,* 528–533.

Pameijer, C. H., Stallard, R. E., & Hiep, N. (1972). Surface characteristics of teeth following periodontal instrumentation: A scanning electron microscope study. *Journal of Periodontology, 43,* 628–633.

Pollack, B. F. & Kronenberg, E. B. (1981). A pilot study on the effects of ultrasonic instrumentation in composite resins. *New York Journal of Dentistry, 51,* 151–153.

Rajstein, J. & Tal, M. (1984). The effect of ultrasonic scaling on the surface of class V amalgam restorations—A scanning electron microscopy study. *Journal of Oral Rehabilitation, 11,* 299–305.

Rateitschak-Pluss, E. M., Schwarz, J. P., Guggenheim, R., Duggelin, M., & Rateitschak, K. H. (1992). Non-surgical periodontal treatment: Where are the limits? *Journal of Clinical Periodontology, 19,* 240–244.

Reynolds, M. A., Lavigne, C. K., Minah, G. E., & Suzuki, J. B. (1992). Clinical effects of simultaneous ultrasonic scaling and subgingival irrigation with chlorhexidine. *Journal of Clinical Periodontology, 19,* 595–600.

Rosling, B. G., Slots, J., Christersson, L. A., Grondahl., H. G., &

Genco, G. J. (1986). Topical antimicrobial therapy and diagnosis of subgingival bacteria in the management of inflammatory periodontal disease. *Journal of Clinical Periodontology, 13,* 975–981.

Sherman, P. R., Hutchens, L. H., Jewson, L. G., Moriarty, G. W., Greco, G. W., & McFall, W. T. (1990). The effectiveness of subgingival scaling and root planing. I. Clinical detection of residual calculus. *Journal of Periodontology, 61,* 3–8.

Simon, A. B., Linde, B., Bonnette, G. H., & Schlentz, R. J. (1975). The individual with a pacemaker in the dental environment. *Journal of the American Dental Association, 91,* 1224–1229.

Slimline Ultrasonic Inserts. (1994). Dentsply International, Inc.

Smart, G. J., Wilson, M., Davies, E. H., & Kieser, J. B. (1990). The assessment of ultrasonic root surface debridement by determination of residual endotoxin levels. *Journal of Clinical Periodontology, 17,* 174–178.

Sowton, E., Gray, K., & Preston, T. (1970). Electrical interferences in non-competitive pacemakers. *British Heart Journal, 32,* 626.

Stende, G. W. & Schaffer, E. M. (1961). A comparison of ultrasonic and hand scaling. *Journal of Periodontology, 32,* 312–314.

Sweeney, W. T. (1957). Characteristics of ultrasonic vibrations. *Journal of the American Dental Association, 55,* 819.

Taggart, J. A., Palmer, R. M., & Wilson, R. F. (1990). The individual with a pacemaker in the dental environment. *Journal of the American Dental Association, 91,* 1224–1229.

Thilo, B. E. & Baehni, P. C. (1987). Effect of ultrasonic instrumentation on dental plaque microflora in vitro. *Journal of Periodontal Research, 22,* 518–521.

Thompson, D. (July, 1993). Faster, easier, better root planing with ultrasonics. *Dental Economics,* 80–81.

Thornton, S. & Garnick, J. (1982). Comparison of ultrasonic to hand instruments in the removal of subgingival plaque. *Journal of Periodontology, 53,* 35–37.

Torfason, T., Kiger, R., Selvig, K. A., & Egelberg, J. (1979). Clinical improvement of gingival conditions following ultrasonic versus hand instrumentation of periodontal pockets. *Journal of Clinical Periodontology, 6,* 165–176.

Ultrasonic Services, Inc. (1993). USI-25M periodontal dental scaler. Owner's manual operation. Houston, TX: Ultrasonic Services, Inc.

Walmsley, A. D., Walsh, T. F., Laird, W. R. E., & Williams, A. R. (1990). Effects of cavitational activity on the root surface of teeth during ultrasonic scaling. *Journal of Clinical Periodontology, 17,* 306–312.

Walmsley, A. D., Laird, W. R. E., & Williams, A. R. (1986a). Displacement amplitude as a measure of the acoustic output of ultrasonic scalers. *Dental Materials, 2,* 97–100.

Walmsley, A. D., Laird, W. R. E., & Williams, A. R. (1986b). Inherent variability of the performance of the ultrasonic descaler. *Journal of Dentistry, 14,* 121–125.

Wilkenson, R. F. & Maybury, J. E. (1973). Scanning electron microscopy of the root surface following instrumentation. *Journal of Periodontology, 44,* 559–563.

Zinner, D. D. (1955). Recent ultrasonic dental studies, including periodontia, without the use of an abrasive. *Journal of Dental Research, 34,* 748–749.

# CHAPTER 13

# Clinical Applications for Polishing

## Key Terms

abrasion
cleansing
coronal polishing
extrinsic stain

final polishing
grit or particle size
intrinsic stain

## INTRODUCTION

Authorities in periodontics and clinical dental hygiene agree that "polishing" is a procedure of client care that exists to some degree. Although the polishing procedure is acknowledged, specific recommendations about its technical application to client care are often not presented. Authors in clinical dental hygiene recommend selectively polishing for areas of stain (Daniel, 1993; Nield-Gehrig & Houseman, 1996; Pattison & Pattison, 1992; Tsutsui, 1995; & Wilkins, 1994) versus the traditional generalized polishing of all tooth surfaces. The basic premise for the transition in philosophy is that bacterial plaque reforms within a matter of a few hours; thus, polishing for bacterial plaque removal is a time-consuming procedure with no lasting therapeutic value (Wilkins, 1994). The philosophy of selective polishing places emphasis on the importance of teaching clients effective plaque removal skills (oral self-care) and motivating them to practice these procedures to prevent dental/periodontal disease. Plaque is, therefore, removed by the client and stain is removed by the practitioner. It is also acknowledged that stain removal has no therapeutic or dental disease preventive value (Wilkins, 1994). The only benefit of polishing extrinsic dental stain is to improve esthetics.

Results of current research have prompted a change in professional tooth "polishing" from a routine procedure where the same technique and abrasive agent is applied to all clients to an elective procedure where a decision is made as to whether polishing will or will not be included in the care plan. This chapter recommends polishing strategies for clients who have periodontal diseases. Various philosophies, methods, and concepts of abrasion are included to enhance practitioners' decision making for each client. Recommendations will take into consideration the research, practitioners' views, and the clients' needs and desires to promote practical applications for polishing in NSPT.

## PHILOSOPHIES

Polishing the surfaces of teeth has been a routine procedure practiced by dental professionals since the early 1900s. Philosophies of polishing have been changing from traditional polishing of all teeth to selective polishing to remove only extrinsic stain. Professional mechanical tooth cleaning is yet another philosophy based on oral hygiene training and professional removal of plaque and stain at need-related intervals. Recently, the concept of therapeutic polishing has been introduced as a procedure in periodontal surgery. These four concepts are presented as philosophies because they represent different fundamental beliefs about the manner and purpose of bacterial plaque and stain removal during professional therapy.

### Traditional Polishing

Traditional polishing or **coronal polishing** is the use of an abrasive agent on all accessible tooth surfaces to remove bacterial plaque and stain. Depending on the clinician's interpretation, traditional polishing may include treatment to the exposed root and crown or to the anatomic crown only. Ideally, traditional polishing is a two-step procedure. An abrasive, such as flour of pumice, is applied to all tooth surfaces for the purpose of cleansing the tooth. **Cleansing** is performed to remove acquired pellicle, bacterial plaque, materia alba, and extrinsic stain. **Final polishing** is accomplished by applying a finer abrasive, such as whiting, to the tooth surface to produce a smooth, lustrous surface. With the advent of commercially prepared pastes, clinicians select a single paste to perform both cleansing and polishing functions. Depending on the amount of abrasion created by the commercial paste, final polishing is not always achieved.

In the past, the rationales for traditional polishing included removal of bacterial plaque and stain prior to professional topical fluoride application, creation of a smooth tooth surface, and removal of extrinsic stain. It was thought that complete removal of soft deposit, hard deposit, and stain was necessary for fluoride uptake. Research results identify that removal of acquired pellicle and plaque by professional polishing does not enhance the uptake of professionally applied fluoride (Steele, Waltner, & Bawden, 1982; Tinanoff, Wei, & Parkins, 1974). Steele, Waltner, and Bawden (1982) concluded that cleaning the teeth with a toothbrush and floss prior to application of topical fluoride resulted in greater fluoride uptake than did polishing the teeth with either a fluoridated or nonfluoridated prophylaxis paste prior to applying topical fluoride. Research has also determined that polishing removes some of the fluoride-rich enamel surface, causing a lower concentration of surface fluoride (Tinanoff, Wei, & Parkins, 1974). In children this loss is greater than in adults because a child's enamel is not completely mineralized upon eruption.

The purpose of creating a smooth tooth surface is to retard the rate of bacterial plaque accumulation and to make bacterial plaque removal by the client easier. Opinions differ, however, about the means to create the smooth surface and the degree of smoothness that should be achieved. Dental hygiene authorities emphasize the end product of scaling and root planing is a smooth surface which does not require polishing (Pattison & Pattison, 1992; Wilkins, 1994). Others recommend that polishing be performed in conjunction with scaling and root planing to produce a smooth surface (Carranza & Perry, 1986; Schluger, Yuodelis, Page, & Johnson, 1990; Schmid, 1990). The relationship of debridement to tooth surface smoothness and need for polishing has yet to be studied. Nevertheless, Kenney (1990) points out that the relationship between the degree of surface roughness and bacterial plaque accumulation is undetermined. A study by Rosenberg and Ash (1974) concluded that supragingival plaque accumulation and gingival inflammation are not significantly related to tooth surface roughness. A more recent study, however, identifies a positive correlation between tooth surface roughness and rate of plaque formation (Quirynen et al., 1990). A question arises as to how smooth a tooth needs to be to decrease the rate of bacterial growth and/or improve client plaque removal. Obviously the degree of surface smoothness needed to promote periodontal health depends on multiple factors including client oral self-care practices, client immune response, practitioner expertise in providing professional therapy, and client compliance with periodontal maintenance procedures. Traditional polishing was also performed for extrinsic

stain removal. The removal of extrinsic stain remains a rationale for applying an abrasive agent to the tooth surface. Polishing recommendations began changing in the 1970s because of research invalidating some of the historical rationales and potential effects of the procedure (see Table 13-1).

## Selective Polishing

In 1976, Wilkins presented the concept that routine traditional polishing was no longer recommended. The foundation for this concept was the belief that detrimental side effects occur as a result of traditional polishing, that bacterial plaque should be removed by the client, and that polishing should only be performed to remove extrinsic stain (Wilkins, 1976). These beliefs resulted in a selective polishing philosophy, which refers

**Table 13-1  Detrimental Health and Safety Effects of Polishing**

| Effect | Explanation |
|---|---|
| 1. Removal of fluoride-rich surface layer | • fluoride protection is decreased |
| 2. Increased tooth surface roughness | • due to inappropriate abrasive agent selection, tooth surface can be rougher than it was before polishing |
| 3. Increased scratches and roughness of restorations (gold, composite, and amalgam) | • due to the inappropriate selection of abrasive agents |
| 4. Loss of tooth structure | • the amount removed is dependent on the agent, frequency of abrasive use, method of application, and the type and integrity of tooth structure<br>• may cause increased dentinal hypersensitivity |
| 5. Increased potential for bacteremia | • a result of tissue manipulation, particularly when plaque and inflammation are present |
| 6. Increased risk of disease transmission | • pathogenic microorganisms stay suspended in air<br>• splatter of saliva, prophylaxis paste, or blood contaminated with microbes exists |
| 7. Increased gingival inflammation | • chemicals in commercially-prepared prophylaxis paste have potential to increase gingival inflammatory response |

to the removal of extrinsic stain remaining after professional periodontal instrumentation. Stain removal is accomplished by a rubber cup and paste or by air polishing. The stain removal is for esthetic reasons and is also important when pit and fissure sealants are being placed. Ideally, the selective polishing procedure does not include removal of bacterial plaque. Instead, plaque removal should be accomplished by the patient on a daily basis to prevent disease (Cross & Carr, 1983; Daniel, 1993; Hassel & Kohut, 1981; Rohleder & Slim, 1981; Tsutsui, 1995; Wilkins, 1994). During nonsurgical therapy, teaching effective self-care skills is deemed more valuable than removing bacterial plaque by professional polishing. It is known that pellicle covers the teeth within minutes after completing polishing, that bacterial plaque collects on pellicle within one to two hours, and in twelve to twenty-four hours bacterial plaque is visible with a disclosing agent (Wilkins, 1994).

Literature surrounding the concept of selective polishing has examined the acceptance of this procedure in educational settings. Results of one survey (Hassel & Kohut, 1981), showed that only 38 of 122 responding dental hygiene programs (31 percent) taught selective polishing. Ten years later, results of another survey (Nordstrom, Uldricks, & Beck, 1991) identified selective polishing as an accepted procedure in dental hygiene programs and that educators are utilizing consistent criteria for the implementation of selective polishing. The respondents of the Nordstrom survey included 137 of 176 (76 percent) dental hygiene program directors and 199 of 285 (70 percent) randomly selected dental hygiene faculty members. Cross and Carr (1983) surveyed 424 clients to determine acceptance of selective polishing in dental schools and private practice. Almost two-thirds of the respondents were dental school clients and approximately one-third of the respondents were "recall" clients from private practice. Only 20 percent of dental school clients and 4 percent of private practice clients objected to not having their teeth polished in the traditional fashion. It should be noted that the rationale for selective polishing was provided before the procedure was performed.

To date, there are no published studies that examine the prevalence of selective polishing in the private practice setting. Even though research substantiates the concept of selective polishing, discussions with private practitioners and educators seem to indicate that the concept of selective polishing has not been completely embraced. There appears to be a variety of reasons. First, practitioners view the procedure for selective polishing differently. Some clinicians interpret selective polishing as the removal of both bacterial plaque and extrinsic stain after scaling/root planing or debridement. Others interpret selective polishing as removal of only extrinsic stain after scaling and root planing or debridement because plaque should be removed by the client (Parton, 1994).

Second, dentists and hygienists are reluctant to eliminate "traditional polishing." This reluctance could be due to the perceived client dissatisfaction, a lack of awareness about current research and clinical recommendations, or the practitioner's resistance to change. Most adult clients are accustomed to having their teeth traditionally polished. These individuals could interpret the polishing as the final phase of the dental hygiene care that makes their teeth feel "smooth" and look "white." Walsh, Heckman, and Moreau-Diettinger (1985) surveyed thirty subjects to assess their expectations about procedures that should be included in an oral prophylaxis. One side of the mouth was polished in the traditional fashion and the other side did not receive the polishing treatment. Survey results revealed that 83 percent of the respondents expected polishing, 53 percent stated that they would feel dissatisfied if they paid for care that did not include polishing, and 57 percent noticed some type of desirable difference in the polished side of the mouth. It should be noted that selective polishing was not compared to traditional polishing and that subjects were not educated about the treatment. Another survey of dental school patients identified that 48 percent of the sample objected to the idea of not having their teeth polished as a part of their oral prophylaxis (Schifter, Hangorsky, & Emling, 1981). Again, respondents were not educated about various philosophies of polishing and selective polishing was not a treatment option. In the *Proceedings of the World Workshop in Clinical Periodontics* published by the Academy of Periodontology, it is stated that the psychological benefit and the perception by the patient of a clean mouth warrant continuation of tooth polishing as a part of maintenance appointments (McFall, 1989). It is suggested, however, that a clean mouth can be accomplished by a variety of techniques.

The practitioner's resistance to change is a natural human characteristic. Progress is a result of change, and unless we try something, we cannot evaluate how it works. Hygienists who practice selective polishing have found that many clients, after a brief explanation of rationale, consent to exclude or minimize polishing. In these cases, the client understands that at the completion of the therapy, all visible and detectable plaque, stain and calculus have been removed. The methods of removal have been altered, but not the end product. The client understands that traditional polishing is not necessary because bacterial plaque and stain are removed by oral self-care, ultrasonic or hand scaling, and/or selective polishing. Clinicians who selectively polish also discover that many clients prefer to not have their teeth polished. In this case, clients state they do not like the taste or feel (grittiness, sensitivity) of polishing or are concerned about the purpose of the procedure and the abrasion created.

Last, clinicians are concerned about efficiency. Practitioners are sometimes rushed to complete bacterial plaque removal because the appropriate appointment length was not planned, reappointment to complete therapy is not chosen, and/or the client was not supervised in self-removal of bacterial plaque. In these circumstances, the practitioner might choose traditional polishing instead of selective polishing thinking it will be quicker to polish all teeth versus selecting surfaces. Because a more abrasive agent removes stain and bacterial plaque at a faster rate, an abrasive cleansing agent for rubber cup polishing might be chosen or an air polishing device utilized. In either case, the result is an abraded surface rather than a smooth, polished surface. In summary, selective polishing might not be widely accepted because of differing interpretations of selective polishing, practitioner perceptions, and concern for efficiency.

## Professional Mechanical Tooth-Cleaning

Axelsson (1993a) presents the philosophy of Professional Mechanical Tooth-Cleaning (PMTC) in the *Proceedings of the 1st European Workshop on Periodontics*. PMTC is the selective removal of supragingival plaque and 1 to 3 mm of subgingival plaque from all tooth surfaces, using mechanically driven instruments and fluoride prophy paste (Axelsson, 1993a). This concept stresses a "needs related" approach for client oral hygiene and PMTC. With PMTC, the professional concentrates on "key risk" teeth or surfaces. The key risk teeth are the molars and maxillary premolars, and the key risk surfaces are the proximal surfaces. Axelsson contends that a single thorough scaling and root planing of deep periodontal pockets, followed by meticulous self-care and PMTC at need-related intervals, will prevent further loss of periodontal attachment (Axelsson, 1993b).

Specific equipment and a precise technique are recommended for professional removal of bacterial plaque (Axelsson, 1993b). First, disclosing solution is applied by pressing the cotton pellet or tip into each interproximal space. A syringe is then used to inject fluoride containing prophylaxis paste interproximally. Next, a specially designed prophy contra-angle handpiece (PROFIN© contra-angle) with a reciprocating V-shaped flexible or triangular pointed tip (reciprocating tips such as EVA-123©, EVA-123S©, or EVA-7©) is used to remove proximal surface plaque. These tips are reported to clean 2 to 3 mm subgingivally. The clinician always begins cleaning the proximal surfaces from the lingual aspect of the mandibular molars and then proceeds to the buccal side of the same teeth. Next, the maxillary proximal surfaces are cleaned in the same order. After the proximal surfaces have been cleaned with the reciprocating triangular tip, a standard prophy angle with a rubber cup is used on the lingual and buccal surfaces. The clinician begins on the surfaces most neglected by the client, which frequently are the mandibular linguals. Plaque located at the line angles and 1 to 2 mm subgingivally is removed with the rubber cup and prophy paste. Upon completion of PMTC, disclosing solution is reapplied to ensure all bacterial plaque has been removed. Wilson (1988) presents a similar theory of polishing that includes the use of a rubber cup for lingual and buccal surfaces and definitive polishing of the interproximal area. Prox-

imal surfaces are treated with balsawood sticks, the porte polisher, dental tape, fine linen strips, or a special contra-angle handpiece (EVA© Handpiece [no longer manufactured] or PROFIN©).

Axelsson (1993a) states abrasion of the tooth surface is not a concern with PMTC because pellicle functions as a nonfrictional layer on the tooth surface. Saxton (1975) identified that it takes approximately 5 minutes to completely remove pellicle from the tooth surface. The average PMTC treatment time on each tooth surface is estimated to be 3 to 7 seconds; thus, Axelsson (1993a) concludes that the risk of abrasive damage is not significant. Other considerations in PMTC are that composite restorations are avoided, air polishing is not recommended, and curets may be used to remove partly mineralized plaque in the gingival sulcus or deeper pockets. Air polishing is not recommended because it abrades exposed root surfaces and composite restorations and is ineffective for the proximal surfaces of molars. The rationale for inclusion of PMTC as a component of mechanical plaque control and a procedure that is critical to primary or secondary periodontal disease prevention is summarized in Table 13-2 (Axelsson, 1993a).

Clinical studies reveal that PMTC significantly reduces bacterial plaque and gingivitis based on frequent application of the technique three times per week to one application every second week. In the original "Karlstad studies," plaque and gingivitis in schoolchildren was reduced 60 to 85 percent (Axelsson & Lindhe, 1974, 1977, 1981a; Axelsson, Lindhe, & Wasëby, 1976). Frequent PMTC has also been successfully used in maintenance programs after initial nonsurgical or surgical therapy of moderate periodontitis, as well as for those with advanced periodontal disease (Axelsson, 1993a). This technique was also studied to determine whether the progression of periodontitis could be prevented in adults, and if a high level of oral hygiene could be maintained by repeated instruction and PMTC (Axelsson & Lindhe, 1974, 1978, 1981b, 1981c; Axelsson, Lindhe, & Nystrom, 1991). Three hundred seventy-five subjects were assigned to the test group and one hundred eighty to a control group. Control subjects were seen once per year for six years and provided with traditional care. Test group participants were seen every other month for two years and once every third month for the remaining four years. Reexamination at the end of the third and sixth years revealed, on average, a loss of 1.2 mm of attachment per individual in the control group and the test group subjects did not lose any periodontal attachment. It is noted that the conditions of some subjects in the test group deteriorated (Axelsson & Lindhe, 1978, 1981b). It is clear when reviewing research related to this approach that clinical parameters improve. It should be remembered, however, that these studies are not evaluating the effects of only "polishing"; client self-care, scaling/root planing and debridement, and/or fluoride are part of the intensive dental disease prevention program. PMTC

### Table 13-2 Summary of Preventive Effects of PMTC

| Condition | Effects |
|---|---|
| Bacterial Plaque Removal | • supragingival plaque is removed<br>• 1 to 3 mm subgingival plaque is removed |
| Composition of Subgingival Microflora | • decreases number of microbes associated with etiology of periodontitis |
| Reaccumulation of Complex Plaque | • retarded for several days in the dentogingival region compared to client oral hygiene procedures where plaque reforms in 1 to 2 days |
| Plaque Retention | • plaque retention factors such as dental caries, overhangs, and deficient margins of restorations are prevented |
| Volume of Gingival Exudate | • is decreased continuously during the first 24 to 28 hours and takes one week to return to the pre-experimental level |
| Gingival Tissues | • inflamed gingiva will heal within one week when PMTC is performed three times at two-day intervals |
| Caries | • possible effects on *S. mutans* located on proximal surfaces of molars<br>• fluoride-containing prophy paste increases the potential for enamel remineralization on "key-risk" surfaces |
| Motivation | • feeling of cleanliness increases client motivation |

includes frequent preventive maintenance care that is provided by state supportive health services in various nations. The practicality of PMTC in the United States is questionable as periodontal maintenance procedures are commonly performed at three-, four-, or six-month intervals. Frequently delivered professional care and education of the type provided in PMTC is expensive in relation to manpower and time (Shieham, 1983).

The basic concepts of PMTC and selective polishing are somewhat parallel in that client self-care in both methods is emphasized. PMTC and selective polishing differ, however, in the manner in which bacterial plaque removal is achieved. With selective polishing, greater emphasis is placed on client removal of interproximal and marginal plaque in the home environment and at the dental hygiene appointment. In PMTC, bacterial plaque removal is performed by the professional at the dental appointment.

### Therapeutic Polishing

This concept involves the polishing of root surfaces when they are exposed during periodontal surgery. The purpose of therapeutic polishing is to remove or reduce endotoxin and the microflora on cementum to enhance tissue reattachment and healing (Daniel, 1993). Either a rubber cup with an abrasive agent or an air-powder device is used. The studies evaluating the value of air polishing in surgical periodontal therapy are limited. The results of an SEM study comparing tooth root topography following instrumentation with an air-powder abrasive, a reciprocating contra-angle system, and a hand curet found a smoother root surface was created with the air polishing system than with the other two methods (Toevs, 1985). In another study using an animal model, the effects of an air-powder abrasive system on periodontal tissues for root preparation during surgery were studied. Slightly lower inflammation scores were identified in the surgical sites treated with a Prophy-Jet™ than in the control sites treated with hand instruments alone (Pippin, Crooks, Barker, Walter, & Killoy, 1988). Horning, Cobb, and Killoy (1987) conducted a study to determine the potential for using an air-powder abrasive technique in periodontal surgery to free root surfaces of plaque, calculus, and pathologically exposed cementum. They also compared the root surfaces prepared with the air abrasive to those prepared by conventional root planing. The results of this study indicated that the air-powder abrasive technique produced a root surface comparable to manual root planing with regard to removal of bacterial plaque, calculus, and exposed cementum. The air-abrasive did not remove ledges of calculus but an average of 80 micrometers of cementum was abraded away after 40 seconds of exposure to the air polisher. The advantage of the air polisher was its ability to remove plaque and cementum from areas that are difficult to reach with conventional root planing instruments such as root flutings, furcations, and close root proximities.

An in vitro study by Gilman and Maxey (1986) assessed the root detoxification effects of the Dentsply Cavitron™ and Prophy-Jet™ using calculus-covered root fragments in gingival fibroblast tissue culture. No fibroblast growth took place on the calculus control specimens. Light fibroblast growth and viability was identified on cavitroned specimens. Specimens that were cavitroned and then had the Prophy-Jet™ applied showed superior growth and vitality of fibroblasts. Further discussion of therapeutic polishing will not be included as it is a procedure used during periodontal surgery rather than NSPT.

## METHODS

The most common methods in this country are rubber cup polishing and air-powder abrasive polishing. Each method involves the use of standard techniques and various equipment or materials. In 1916, Fones advocated the use of a porte polisher for the removal of stain, plaque, and films or all soft accretions. Today, the majority of dental practitioners do not use a porte polisher.

## Rubber Cup Polishing

The rubber cup attached to a prophylaxis angle and air-driven handpiece is probably the method most commonly used in clinical practice. Other recommended equipment includes a bristle brush on the occlusals, and dental floss, tape, or linen finishing strips for proximal surfaces. The rubber cup method can be selected when any of the four philosophies of polishing are employed in therapy. With any polishing method, the clinician must first evaluate the client's conditions to identify any contraindications or precautions. An appropriate abrasive agent is then chosen based on intraoral conditions. Selection of a cleansing and/or polishing agent will be discussed in the following section on abrasion. Refer to Table 13-3 for a review of the rubber cup method as it relates to traditional polishing philosophy. When the rubber cup method is used to selectively polish, some professionally accepted steps are not applicable. For example, the cup is not automatically placed in the cervical area and flared subgingivally. Instead, it is placed on the stain in relation to its location on the tooth. Also, flossing, if indicated, occurs with self-care education and not during polishing.

Rubber cups are available in a variety of forms and designs. A screw, snap-on, or latch form is chosen depending on the equipment utilized. The screw-type attaches to a threaded direct insertion prophylaxis angle; the snap-on to a button-end prophylaxis angle; and the latch type to a mandrel attached to a contra-angle handpiece. Standard, flavored, or scented cups are available in a ribbed, webbed, ribbed and webbed, or turbo (Young Dental Manufacturing) design that aid in retaining paste within the cup. Firm and soft varieties are available that represent varying degrees of flexibility. Soft cups are preferred as they are more resilient or flexible than firm ones. Flexibility enhances correct adaptation to the tooth surface contour and reduces the need for excessive pressure. Use of a prophylaxis cup and/or prophylaxis paste containing fluoride is another consideration. The NSPT client may potentially be more caries prone or experience tooth hypersensitivity; thus, maintaining or increasing fluoride levels of the tooth surface is important. The amount of fluoride imparted to the tooth surface via fluoridated prophylaxis paste or fluoride impregnated prophylaxis cups is not as much as the uptake from professional application. Therefore, neither route replaces professionally applied fluoride. However, Stookey and Stahlman (1976) concluded that fluoride-containing prophylaxis cups removed stained pellicle more efficiently with less enamel abrasion than nonfluoride cups.

Bristle brushes are also available in a variety of forms and styles. Their use should be limited to the occlusal

## Table 13-3  Comparison of Traditional and Selective Polishing with the Rubber Cup Method

| Traditional Polishing | Selective Polishing |
| --- | --- |
| 1. Procure the paste in the rubber cup and spread over approximately four to six surfaces prior to activating the rheostat. Start in the most distal portion of a posterior region and proceed systematically. | 1. Procure the paste in the rubber cup and spread over the surfaces where stain exists prior to activating the rheostat. A single cup of paste should cover at least four surfaces. |
| 2. On each surface, begin in the cervical region by flaring the edge of the cup subgingivally. | 2. Place the cup parallel to the stain on the surface being polished. |
| 3. Activate the rheostat and maintain the slowest speed or rotations per minute (rpm) possible. | 3. Activate the rheostat and maintain the slowest speed or rotations per minute (rpm) possible. |
| 4. Apply light to moderate pressure depending on the mode of attachment of the bacterial plaque or stain. | 4. Apply light to moderate pressure depending on the mode of attachment of the stain. |
| 5. Use intermittent brushing or painting strokes directed toward the occlusal/incisal. | 5. Use intermittent brushing or painting strokes directed toward the occlusal/incisal. |
| 6. Pivot the intraoral fulcrum to extend the rubber cup cup as far as possible toward the middle of the proximal surfaces. | 6. If stain is located on proximal surfaces, pivot the intraoral fulcrum to extend the rubber cup far enough to reach the stain. |
| 7. Use dental floss or tape with paste to polish the direct proximal surfaces of all teeth. Finishing strips can be used for stain removal. | 7. If stain is still present in proximal contacts, use dental floss or tape with paste to remove it. A fine, narrow finishing strip can be used. |
| 8. Rinse the client as needed during the procedure and on completion of the procedure. | 8. Rinse the client as needed during the procedure and on completion of the procedure. |
| 9. Use a separate rubber cup for each abrasive if one agent is selected for cleansing and another for final polishing. | 9. Use a separate rubber cup for each abrasive if one agent is selected for cleansing of stain and another for final polishing. |
| 10. A bristle brush is used for bacterial plaque and stain removal in occlusal pits or fissures. | 10. A bristle brush may be used for stain removal in occlusal pits or fissures. |

surfaces. Disposable prophylaxis angles (DPA) are another option available from a variety of manufacturers. An in vivo investigation was conducted to provide practitioners with comparative information about five different brands. The analysis compared reliability, durability, heat production, vibration, and operator preference factors. Eleven dental hygienists completed a questionnaire immediately following routine oral prophylaxis and polishing treatment on 161 subjects. Results indicate the Young Dental disposable prophylaxis angle was more reliable than the other four brands; however, the Teledyne Getz produced significantly less vibration than the other brands (Fleming, Barnes, & Russell, 1991). A large-scale comparison of numerous disposable angles would be advantageous as well as studies comparing disposable and nondisposable brands. Characteristics of a disposable system should parallel those of nondisposable equipment.

Linen or finishing strips are used when the rubber cup and abrasive agent do not remove interproximal stain. Finishing strips are manufactured in extra-fine, fine, medium, and coarse grits. Four widths are available: extra-narrow, narrow, medium, and wide. Only extra-narrow or narrow strips with extra-fine or fine grit are suggested for stain removal (Wilkins, 1994). Use of finishing strips is limited to anterior teeth. They should be applied with caution and used infrequently. Ultrasonic scaling is another alternative for interproximal stain removal.

## Air-Powder Abrasive Polishing

Air-powder abrasive devices were introduced in the early 1980s. The Prophy-Jet™ and other air-powder abrasive devices, such as Prophyflex™, Satelec™, Jet Polisher™, Kavo Prophyflex™ have created interest in alternative polishing methods. These devices use air and water pressure to expel a controlled slurry of water and specially processed sodium bicarbonate to remove bacterial plaque and stain by continuous abrasion. The slurry is propelled through a nozzle at the end of a handpiece when the foot control of the air-powder device is activated (Dentsply International Inc., 1995). Air polishing can be used with traditional, selective, and therapeutic polishing philosophies. It is not recommended for Professional Mechanical Tooth Cleaning (PMTC) because of its contraindications and limitations. Technique recommendations are presented in Figure 13-1.

Several studies have been conducted to determine the effect of air polishing on composite, amalgam, gold, and porcelain restorative materials. The conclusions of these studies indicate that composite is the most affected dental restorative material because significant surface roughness occurs (Barnes, Hayes, & Leinfelder, 1987; Cooley, Lubow, & Patrissi, 1986; Eliades, Tzoutzas, & Vougiouklakis, 1991; Lubow & Cooley, 1986; Reel, Abrams, Gardner, & Mitchell, 1989; The Clinical Research Associates Newsletter, 5:1, 1981). Research

results also indicate that the surface of gold and amalgam metallic restorations are minimally affected by air polishing. The changes identified on amalgam and gold are appreciable dulling of the polished amalgam surface and slight dulling of the gold surface. One research study reported that cement exposed along the margin of cast gold was eroded when air polishing was employed (Barnes, Hayes, & Leinfelder, 1987). Results of another study identify that all the amalgam samples tested presented increased surface roughness and alterations of the amalgam surface composition (Eliades, Tzoutzas, & Vougiouklakis, 1991). The studies evaluating the effects of air polishing on porcelain identified no clinically visible effects. Scanning electron microscopic viewing, however, identified pitting and/or severe glaze cracking (Cooley, Lubow, & Brown, 1988; Eliades, Tzoutzas, & Vougiouklakis, 1991). Cooley and others (1988) recommend that an air polishing device be used cautiously or not at all on porcelain restorations, especially those with stains and/or specific "characterizations." As a result of these studies, prolonged use on composites and restorative margins is not indicated (see Figure 13-1) (Dentsply International, Inc., 1995).

The manufacturers of air polishing devices advocate their use for more effective cleansing of pits and fissures prior to sealant placement. The only published study evaluating the effect of air polishing on the surface of sealants indicates that sealant wear increases with time of exposure to air abrasion. The amount of wear, however, between the increasing time intervals of 10, 30, 60 and 90 seconds was not statistically significant. It was also determined that differences in sealant type, self-curing or light-curing, as well as fissure geometry (medium or wide) are not factors in abrasion rate (Huennekens, Daniel, & Bayne, 1991).

To date, the results of only two studies conducted to identify the effects of using an air-powder polisher with sodium bicarbonate as the abrasive agent on blood pH and electrolyte concentrations have been published. The first study was a pilot study conducted on one participant, a 24-year-old male (Rawson, Nelson, Jewell, & Jewell, 1985). Posttreatment venous blood samples indicated an increase in serum pH and bicarbonate or a disruption of the participant's acid/base balance. The authors conclude that this rise in blood pH could potentially be medically hazardous for individuals who exhibited disease states that compromise their blood buffering systems. The second study was conducted on ten adult mongrel dogs (Snyder et al., 1990). Arterial blood samples drawn after use of an air-powder device using sodium bicarbonate as the abrasive agent revealed no statistically significant differences in blood pH, sodium, or bicarbonate concentrations over time between the experimental and control group.

Studies have also been conducted to evaluate possible systemic effects of other sodium-containing dental therapeutic agents. A study by Herrin and coworkers (1986) measured urinary sodium excretion in partici-

As with all dental procedures, use standard operator preparation (i.e., wear face mask, eyewear or face shield, gloves, and protective gown).

1. Adjust the amount of powder delivery by turning the indicator on the top of the powder chamber. The indicator moves 360°. The twelve o'clock position will deliver the most powder and the six o'clock position will deliver the least amount of powder. Make the adjustment to suit your patient's needs.

2. Position the patient at a 45° angle.

3. Turn the patient's head toward you. Use direct vision and external fulcrums.

4. Place a 2 × 2 gauze on the lip of the working area.

5. A mouthwash-soaked cotton roll or gauze square placed near the tongue will create a pleasant flavor during the procedure.

6. Position saliva ejector or high volume evacuator.

7. Use your thumb and forefinger to grasp the patient's lip or cheek to form a cup.

8. Place the nozzle tip 3 to 4mm away from the tooth on the middle to incisal third of the tooth.

9. Angle the nozzle slightly apically with a 60° angle for anterior teeth, an 80° angle for posterior teeth, and a 90° angle for occlusal surfaces (see diagrams below).

10. Press the foot control to the first position (halfway) to activate the water spray, then to the second position to produce the air/water/powder combination.

11. Use a constant circular sweeping motion going from interproximal surface to interproximal surface.

12. Polish one to two teeth for 1 to 2 seconds (with the foot control on the second position), then rinse the water from the nozzle (with the foot control in the first position).

13. Rinse excess slurry from the patient's mouth often, using the water from the air polishing nozzle.

14. After completing the procedure, clean the nozzle with the wire cleaner and follow the sterilization procedures.

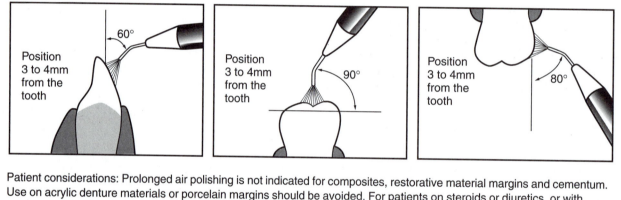

Patient considerations: Prolonged air polishing is not indicated for composites, restorative material margins and cementum. Use on acrylic denture materials or porcelain margins should be avoided. For patients on steroids or diuretics, or with communicable diseases, compromised respiratory conditions or metabolic disorders, consider other polishing methods. Do not direct air polishing spray into the sulcus or onto soft tissue.

**Figure 13-1**  Proper air polishing techniques. (Courtesy of Dentsply International, Inc., 1995)

pants using a baking soda-3% hydrogen peroxide dentifrice and a nearly saturated sodium chloride mouthwash in an oral irrigating device. Findings revealed no increased sodium burden. Kaminsky, Gillette, and O'Leary (1987) measured sodium absorption of a sodium chloride mouthrinse. Participants used a rinse and spit method or a mechanical irrigation device. The results identified a mean absorption of sodium to be 10 percent of the 70 to 90 mg/day recommended for clients on a salt-restrictive diet. Medical literature documents the permeability of mucosal surfaces to electrolytes, yet dental literature has not identified any significant risks attributable to the use of sodium containing therapeutic agents or sodium bicarbonate used with air polishing devices. Snyder and others (1990) recommend that another study

similar to the one on adult mongrel dogs be conducted on healthy human beings. Such a study, as suggested by them, would likely provide a more scientific basis for recommendations for use of sodium bicarbonate with air-powder polishing devices on medically compromised clients who may be affected by alterations in blood pH and electrolyte concentrations.

The production of aerosols and atmospheric contamination is another concern with use of the air-powder devices. Studies to evaluate these problems have been performed using ultrasonic scaling devices and other dental equipment that produce a water spray. A limited number of studies, however, have been conducted using air-powder polishing devices. A study by Glenwright, Knibbs, and Burdon (1985) identified an increase of dust and bacterial levels with the use of an air-powder device verses rubber cup polishing with a prophylaxis paste. The bacterial counts were greatest in the immediate vicinity of the client, but were also significant 2 and 3 meters away. It was found that the movement of the dust particles varied depending on the area of the mouth being treated. The investigators concluded that bacteria in the aerosol produced originated from the client's mouth, but the extent of the potential health hazard is difficult to estimate because the literature does not contain documented cases of dental personnel contracting disease by contaminated aerosol or dust. These researchers, however, recommend that dental personnel use barrier techniques including protective eyewear, face mask, and gloves while using air-powder devices. They also recommended having the client prerinse with 0.2% chlorhexidine for 2 minutes before using the device. Another study, however, indicates that a thirty-second prerinse with 0.12% chlorhexidine or an essential oil mouthrinse had no effect on the quantity or potential respiratory-penetrating ability of microorganisms (Bay, Overman, Krust-Bray, Cobb, & Gross, 1993).

Barnes (1991) published an article that focused on techniques to minimize aerosol production while using an air-powder device. The most common cause of excess aerosol production is incorrect angulation of the handpiece nozzle. High-velocity evacuation, client positioning, and the water-powder ratio are also important factors to minimize aerosols. When working on the client's right side, the head should be positioned as far right as possible and when working on the left side, as far left as possible. Increasing the amount of water in the water-powder spray decreases the number of particles that become aerosolized. Following the manufacturer's recommended handpiece nozzle angulation is not only critical for prevention of excess aerosols, but also for prevention of subcutaneous facial emphysema. Subcutaneous facial emphysema is swelling in the interstices of connective tissue due to the presence of air or gas. Finlayson and Stevens (1988) reported an incidence of subcutaneous facial emphysema caused by inadvertently directing a Cavi-Jet™ nozzle into a periodontal pocket. The client experienced swelling and crepitus on palpation of the area, and was treated with oral penicillin for one week. At the end of one week the condition was no longer present. At the client's next appointment, no adverse conditions remained.

Another aspect of air-powder polishing that has been minimally researched is the potential for bacteremia. Previous studies identified bacteremias following oral irrigation, oral prophylaxis, and periodontal scaling. The results of these studies indicated higher incidence of bacteremia correlated to increased levels of plaque and gingivitis (Connor, Haberman, Collings, & Winford, 1967; Romans & App, 1971; Winslow & Kobernick, 1960). The only study results to date about bacteremia development following air polishing conclude that there is a potential for bacteremia following use of air-powder pol-

ishers and the potential is greater when increased plaque and gingivitis are exhibited (Hunter, Holbrow, Kardos, Lee-Knight, & Ferguson, 1989). Air polishing is also avoided on clients with compromised respiratory conditions (see Figure 3-1) (Dentsply International, Inc., 1995).

From a review of the literature one is likely to conclude that air polishing is not warranted for routine use on all clients and that thorough evaluation of a client's conditions is necessary prior to air polishing. The cases when air-powder polishing would be chosen for those receiving nonsurgical therapy are likely to be limited because it is contraindicated or requires precaution for conditions that are frequently present in those with periodontitis (i.e., exposed cementum or dentin, restorations, implants). Though air-powder polishing devices have been available for over a decade, the results of a recent survey identified that approximately 30 percent or 461 of 1,518 respondents used an air-powder polisher (White & Hoffman, 1991). The majority (83 percent) of respondents were employed in private practice settings, 10 percent were in orthodontic or periodontic practices, and 7 percent practiced in educational or hospital settings. Twenty-two percent of those who used an air-powder device responded that they used it routinely rather than selectively, meaning it was used on all clients as their instrument of choice for polishing. Preference for the air polishing method is most likely due to clinician perceptions about its efficiency and effectiveness.

## Comparing Rubber Cup Polishing and Air Polishing Methods

Results of studies comparing the effectiveness of air polishing to rubber cup polishing for bacterial plaque and stain removal demonstrate that either method is equally effective (DeSpain & Nobis, 1988; Miller & Hodges, 1991; Willmann, Norling, & Johnson, 1980). Some researchers cite air polishers as being more effective for plaque and stain removal in pits and fissures (Garcia-Godoy, & Medlock, 1988; Willmann et al., 1980; Patterson & McLundie, 1984). A few studies have compared bacterial plaque reaccumulation rates after use of air polishing versus rubber cup polishing. DeSpain and Nobis (1987) concluded there was no difference in plaque or stain reaccumulation rates. Baker (1988), however, found the air polisher was not as effective at preventing plaque reaccumulation. Studies evaluating the effect of air polishing and rubber cup methods on the gingiva and soft tissue reveal that both methods cause some gingival trauma; however, it is transient or clinically insignificant (DeSpain & Nobis, 1988; Miller & Hodges, 1991; Mishkin, Engler, Javed, Darby, Cobb, & Coffman, 1986; Munley, Everett, Krupa, Madden, & Suzuki, 1988; Kontturi-Narhi, Markkanen, & Markkanen, 1989; Newman, Silverwood, & Dolby, 1985; Weaks, Lescher, Barnes, & Holroyd, 1984).

There is consensus in the literature that tooth enamel is the tooth structure least affected by air polishing (Galloway & Pashley, 1987; Kee & Allen, 1988). Galloway and Pashley (1987) identified no *clinically* visible effects on enamel after air polishing; however, when viewed under both light and scanning electron microscopes, the air-abrasive system produced a nonuniformly roughened surface. The rubber cup produced shallow curved scratches and the ultrasonic instrument showed linear scratches, running parallel to the path of the tip. The scratches produced by the ultrasonic instrument were deeper and broader than the scratches produced by the rubber cup. Kee and Allen (1988) compared the effects of air and rubber cup polishing on enamel abrasion. Their findings indicated there were no significant differences in coronal enamel thickness or cervical enamel thickness means after using either method.

The only study that actually compared the effects of rubber cup polishing and an air-powder abrasive system (Prophy-Jet™) on various restorative materials was conducted by Patterson and McLundie (1984). This research looked at the effects of these two polishing methods on amalgam, porcelain, extra hard gold and true cast soft gold. Both the Prophy-Jet™ and the rubber cup with pumice caused loss of integrity of the test surfaces. The severity of this loss varied with the hardness and abrasion resistance of the material being tested. The depth of loss appeared to be greater with the air abrasive than the rubber cup. The researchers attribute this difference to the fact that the abrasive slurry was directed at a concentrated spot, whereas, the rubber cup action was over a greater circular area. These authors concluded that widespread use of air polishing as a means of stain removal involves considerable risk of damage to certain restorations and susceptible tooth tissue.

One study has been conducted to assess client preference for either rubber cup polishing with flour of pumice or air polishing (Prophy-Jet™) (Hodges & Miller, 1997). Thirty subjects completed a questionnaire after receiving treatment with both techniques. A split-mouth study design was employed where half of the mouth was traditionally polished with pumice and a rubber cup for 5 minutes and the other half with air polishing for 5 minutes. Survey questions asked subjects about comfort, thoroughness, time, taste, smoothness, gingival sensitivity, tooth sensitivity, sound, and messiness. There was a statistically significant relationship between the rubber cup method and comfort, tooth sensitivity, and messiness. The rubber cup was perceived as more comfortable, less messy, and created less tooth sensitivity than air polishing. There was also a statistically significant relationship between air polishing and time and thoroughness. Air polishing was perceived to be quicker and more thorough than the rubber cup method. Time and thoroughness were both controlled; therefore, it was concluded that these factors were perceived and not true differences between methods. Results about preference for future care revealed that 47 percent would select rubber cup polishing, 40 percent would choose air polishing, and 13 percent had no preference. These researchers recommended that clinicians should consider indications

and precautions for use of the air polisher before offering it as an option. Additionally, client preference should be considered if either method is appropriate for care.

In conclusion, limited studies comparing the two methods have been conducted. Removal of bacterial plaque and stain is at least equally effective with both methods and gingival trauma occurs with both methods although it is transient. Enamel is altered differently by air polishing than by the rubber cup, and is abraded in an equal fashion by either method. Amalgam, porcelain, and gold restorations lose integrity when both methods are applied; however, the depth of loss appears greater with air polishing. It must be noted that studies comparing the abrasion of dentin and cementum with the two methods have not been conducted.

## ABRASION

The amount of tooth structure loss should be considered during NSPT as clients with periodontitis require frequent maintenance. The effects of repetitive scaling and root planing (or debridement) and polishing on the tooth surfaces should be critically analyzed when planning initial therapy or periodontal maintenance procedures (PMP). Minimizing abrasion should be a NSPT treatment goal. For purposes of this chapter, abrasion of tooth surfaces will be approached by considering three factors that interact: the abrasive agent, clinician technique, and the integrity of the tooth surface (see Figure 13-2). These three factors will be discussed in relation to both the rubber cup and air polishing methods. The clinician has some control over the amount of abrasion an agent creates. By selecting an appropriate abrasive agent, self-evaluating operator technique, and evaluating

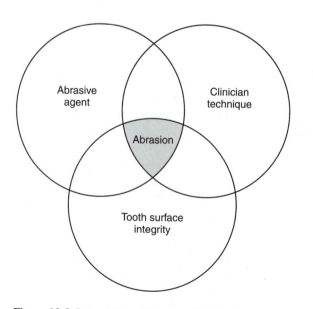

**Figure 13-2** Interaction of factors affecting abrasion.

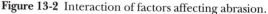

the tooth surface, the clinician can minimize loss of tooth structure. Theoretically, these three considerations can be discussed separately. In clinical practice, however, they are interwoven and interact simultaneously when mechanical polishing occurs.

## Abrasive Agents

The abrasive agent is a substance consisting of particles of sufficient hardness and sharpness to groove or scratch a softer substance when drawn across its surface. It is a substance that causes **abrasion**, or the wearing away of a surface through friction. Generally, the larger the particle size the deeper the scratch produced, and conversely a smaller particle produces a finer scratch. There are a variety of agents categorized as follows: 1) cleansing or abrasive agents, 2) polishing or minimally abrasive agents, and 3) agents that initially have properties of a cleansing agent, then fracture and abrade into a polishing agent. Agent selection based on these categories only is difficult because a single commercial paste can serve both cleaning and polishing functions and some polishing agents create a very smooth and lustrous surface but significantly abrade tooth structure. Clinicians rely on the manufacturer's labeling of commercial pastes, which indicate **grit or particle size** (see Table 13-4). The clinician should apply the smallest particle size or grit that will effectively yet efficiently eliminate the stain while removing minimal or no tooth structure. A medium-sized grit is the largest size applied and a fine or extra fine grit should follow its application to create a final polished tooth surface. If a coarse abrasive is needed, the clinician should reevaluate the method of stain removal. Possibly ultrasonic and/or hand-activated instrumentation are indicated or the stain is intrinsic. Unfortunately, a survey conducted in 1984 (Christensen) indicated that many hygienists use medium (43 percent) or coarse grit size (38 percent) for polishing the tooth surfaces. These abrasives are most likely selected because they remove stain and bacterial plaque in less time than finer abrasives. It is hoped, a decade later, this trend has changed.

The abrasion rate and polishing ability of an agent are not solely linked to particle size. Other characteristics of abrasive particles that influence results are shape, hardness, brittleness, and concentration. Some agents produce a highly polished surface, but remove a significant amount of tooth structure because of the sharpness (shape) and hardness of the particles. The brittleness of the abrasive particles affects how the particle breaks apart. An abrasive particle that maintains its original shape during use will cause abrasion. A particle that is so brittle that it shatters immediately on contacting the tooth surface will be ineffective in abrading that surface. Abrasive particles that are brittle enough to break apart during use might initially produce abrasion, then the sequential fracturing of the particles as they rub against the tooth surface can produce a polished surface. This action explains how some agents (Cleanic and Zircate)

**Table 13-4 Definitions of Grit (Particle Size)**

| Grit | Oral-B Laboratories | Nupro, Ash Dentsply |
|------|---------------------|---------------------|
| Fine | For procedures where cleaning and tooth abrasion are indicated. Mainly used on children and patientson periodontal support therapy. | Ideal for younger patients and prophylaxis procedures requiring minimum tooth abrasion. |
| Medium | Designed for the majority of cleaning needs when a high polish is desired. | Suitable for most cleaning procedures where a high level of polish is desired. |
| Coarse | For heavy stain removal including patients who smoke or consume stain-producing beverages. | For patients with substantial buildup due to smoking or excessive use of stain-producing beverages. |
| Plus | For extremely difficult stain removal needs. | An extra, heavy-duty cleanser for stain buildup difficult to remove with conventional prophylaxis pastes. |

(Courtesy Oral-B Laboratory and Dentsply International, Inc.)

can accomplish cleansing and final polishing with one application. Concentration of the abrasive agent within each paste differs and is reported to be up to 60 percent of the total ingredients (Daniel, 1993; Wilkins, 1994).

Manufacturers consider shape, hardness, brittleness, and/or concentration when testing products. A practitioner must rely on the manufacturer's recommendations when selecting an appropriate agent. When ordering agents, practitioners should inquire about ingredients and functions of the paste. It is increasingly challenging to select agents as more are marketed and standard commercial products are updated. Adding to the problem is the fact that the abrasiveness of prophylaxis pastes is not standardized. The medium grit of one brand might be as abrasive as the coarse or fine grit of other brands (Lutz, Sener, Imfeld, Barbakow, & Schüpbach, 1993). Christensen and Bangerter (1987) even determined variations in the same brand of abrasive agents. Lutz and others (1993) comment that it is unacceptable that most of the market-leading prophylaxis pastes do not polish enamel or dentin; instead, they give restorations a matte finish and aggressively abrade dentin. Currently, two tests are used to evaluate abrasive agents: enamel polishing comparison and enamel abrasion. Refer to Figure 13-3 for information published in 1982 on these two tests (Putt, Kleber, & Muhler, 1982).

Pumice flour is one of the agents tested and is available in a variety of particle sizes (flour or superfine, fine, and coarse). Flour of pumice and superfine can be used to remove stains on enamel only (Wilkins, 1994). The mean abrasive depth of enamel with pumice flour is significant (12.1 micrometers on a scale ranging from 15.6 to 1 micrometer) and it has an average polishing score when compared to the other agents (see Figure 13-3). Calcium carbonate (Chalk or Whiting), not evaluated in the previous study, produces minimal scratches and results in a smooth, polished surface. This would be an appropriate agent to apply when stain is not evident and the client requests traditional polishing.

A limited number of agents are available that initially function as a cleansing agent then are altered in such a manner as to become a polishing agent (Cleanic and Zircate). Cleanic contains perilite, which is natural glass with a sheetlike geometry of particles. This abrasive medium has been compared to conventional prophylaxis pastes containing conventional abrasives. Study results indicate that the three ideal requirements of a prophylaxis paste are met by this agent, whereas conventional prophylaxis pastes only fulfill two of the three requirements (Lutz, Sener, Imfeld, Barbakow, & Schüpbach, 1993). The three ideal characteristics are good cleaning ability, minimal abrasion, and simultaneous polishing. Additionally, the perilite-containing paste functioned as a fine or superfine agent. Further investigation of this product is warranted. The effect of these types of agents on polishing procedure and philosophy will be interesting to observe. A composite polishing agent, Prisma Gloss, is also available. It is recommended when "polishing" is not indicated except by client request and for polishing implant abutments. Toothpastes are also used when "polishing" is not indicated yet traditional polishing is requested by the client. Abrasives in professional polishing pastes are similar to those in toothpastes (Daniel, 1993); however, the major difference between the two is the level of abrasive in the professional pastes is greater. Even so, their degree of abrasiveness is still dependent on clinician technique and tooth surface integrity.

Selecting an appropriate agent can be somewhat controlled when using the rubber cup method, whereas air polishing requires a specific abrasive agent. When the agent and the propelling action of the air polishing of the sodium bicarbonate and water are combined, significant abrasion occurs. Several clinical studies have demonstrated that air-abrasive polishing devices remove significant amounts of root structure, even after short exposure of only 5 to 15 seconds to an air polisher (Galloway & Pashley, 1987; Newman, Silverwood, & Dolby, 1985). Researchers report removal of 10.68 to 25 micrometers of root structure with one exposure of air polishing (Berkstein, Reiff, McKinney, & Killoy, 1987; Petersson, Hellden, Jongebloed, & Arends, 1985). Atkinson, Cobb, and Killoy (1984) found that an average of 636.6 micrometers were removed after a thirty-second application of air polishing which was hypothesized to equal fifteen years of maintenance therapy. Berkstein and others (1987) also estimated fifteen years of maintenance therapy to equal 638.3 micrometers of root structure loss. Cementum is approximately 10 to 50 micrometers thick (Berkowitz, Holland, & Moxham, 1992) therefore, significant removal is caused especially when considering three-month maintenance intervals. Caution should be exercised when the clinician is considering use of an air polishing device on clients with root exposure. Prolonged use on cementum should be avoided (see Figure 13-1, page 352) (Dentsply

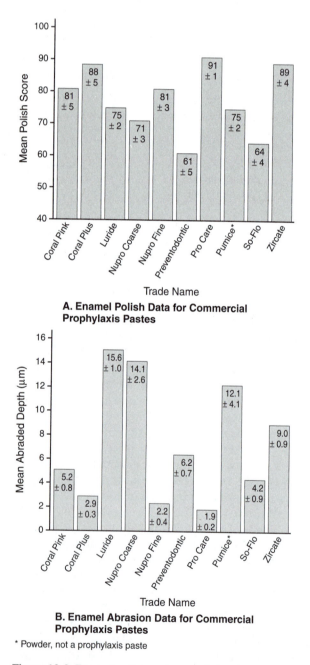

**A. Enamel Polish Data for Commercial Prophylaxis Pastes**

**B. Enamel Abrasion Data for Commercial Prophylaxis Pastes**

\* Powder, not a prophylaxis paste

**Figure 13-3** Enamel polish and enamel abrasion rates of commercial prophylaxis pastes. (Adapted with permission from Putt, M. S., Kleber, C. J., and Muhler, J. C. "Enamel Polish and Abrasion by Prophylaxis Pastes." *Journal of Dental Hygiene, 56,* figures 1 and 2, pp. 42–43, 1982)

International, Inc., 1995). Many clients undergoing NSPT are likely to have root exposure, consequently, use of this device for their therapy is limited.

## Clinician Technique

Self-evaluation of clinician technique is at least, if not more important than selection of an appropriate agent when striving to minimize loss of tooth structure. Technique factors for the rubber cup method include speed, pressure, time, number of particles, and position of the rubber cup. The clinician has some degree of control over each of these entities. Recommendations for speed are discussed in relation to revolutions per minute (rpm) of a rotary instrument used with the rubber cup method. Christensen and Bangerter (1984), in an in vivo clinical study to determine revolutions per minute, time, and pressure, identified the average speed used by twenty-nine dental hygienists to be 2,500 rpms. Because it is difficult to estimate rpm used in the clinical practice, the slow speed handpiece is always rotated at the lowest rpm possible. Applying only the amount of pressure on the foot pedal that is necessary to maintain the rotation of the rubber cup is required. The rpm is too great if "whining" or a high-pitched sound occurs. Most dental units have a gauge that measures air pressure for handpiece connectors in pounds per square inch (psi) and, although this does not indicate speed, operating at 20 psi seems adequate for stain removal (Daniel, 1993). Pressure is the amount of force exerted against the tooth surface. The flaring of the edge of the rubber cup is the clinical characteristic identifying sufficient pressure. Use of a soft, flexible cup permits the clinician to use minimal pressure to achieve the flaring of the edge, as well as ensuring positioning of the rubber cup parallel to the tooth surface. The average pressure has been identified as 150 grams (Christensen & Bangerter, 1984). Grams of pressure are impractical to measure in clinical practice. The use of intermittent strokes with the rubber cup decreases the pressure utilized within any given time period.

Time can be identified in many ways: by surface, tooth, one-half mouth, or full mouth. It is also dependent on the philosophy employed, that is, whether all teeth or selective areas are treated, and whether one or more agents are applied. Regulation of time is achieved by minimizing the interval spent on each surface. Christensen and Bangarter (1984) identified that the rubber cup contacted each tooth surface for an average of 4.5 seconds. Miller and Hodges (1991) estimated it took 10 minutes (3.4 seconds per tooth) to treat the entire mouth when standardizing polishing time in a research study comparing rubber cup and air polishing using traditional philosophy. The number of particles is controlled by applying a full rubber cup of a moist abrasive agent to the lingual or buccal surface of approximately four teeth at a time. The abrasive should always be moist as increased scratching and heat production occur with a dry agent.

Positioning of the rubber cup is the last technique factor which has been shown to have an effect on the tooth surface. Placement of the rubber cup at an acute angle rather than parallel to the tooth surface has been identified as the cause of pronounced scratches and concavities on the root surface just apical to the cementoenamel junction (CEJ). When the rubber cup is positioned correctly, concavities are not produced and the scratches are not prominent. Teeth that exhibit prominent CEJs, malalignment, or less than 2 mm of recession are where improper angulation of the rubber cup most frequently occurs (Christensen & Bangerter, 1987). This study also found increased scratches at the cervical one-third of the enamel surface as compared to the occlusal two-thirds (Christensen & Bangerter, 1987). This result might have occurred because of the relationship of the rubber cup placement as well as the time spent removing plaque in the cervical one-third where the enamel is extremely thin. Refer to Figure 13-4 for a diagram of correct and incorrect adaptation of the rubber cup on enamel. This relationship will vary depending on the constriction of the crown in the cervical area, and the gingival height and contour.

The clinician generally has more control of the technique employed with the rubber cup than with air polishing. To minimize abrasion while air polishing, there are three factors that can be altered: application time, tip angulation, and tip movement. Application time should be minimal, the recommended tip angulation should be maintained, and the tip should be moved in the recommended constant circular motion 3 to 4 mm from the tooth surface. Studies *comparing* the effects of air polishing and rubber cup polishing are limited. The two studies that compared the effects of these two polishing methods on tooth structure both determined that air polishing created deeper grooves or indentations in the

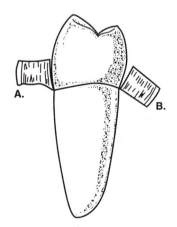

**Figure 13-4** Rubber cup adaptation. **A.** Represents correct adaptation of the rubber cup. The rubber cup is flared at the cervical of the tooth to ensure the cup is parallel to the tooth surface being polished. **B.** Represents the adaptation of a nonflexible rubber cup where an acute angle is created between the edge of the cup and the tooth surface.

tooth surface than rubber cup polishing with pumice (Willmann et al., 1980; Patterson & McLundie, 1984). Therefore, if air polishing is chosen, a final polishing agent should be applied following its use in order to create a tooth surface that is at least as smooth or smoother than the original surface.

## Tooth Surface Integrity

The third factor that affects abrasion is the integrity of the tooth surface in that a less calcified structure will abrade at a faster rate and amount than an area that is more calcified. Tooth surface characteristics to consider include the classification of the tissues being treated (enamel, cementum, dentin), maturation of the enamel, caries, demineralized enamel, erosion or abrasion, and the presence of restorations or implants. Intact enamel is least affected by abrasive agents and dentin is most affected. It is estimated that a thirty-second application of a pumice paste removes approximately 4 micrometers of enamel (Vrbic, Brudevold, & McCann, 1967). Enamel is thickest at the incisal edges and cusps (up to 2.3 mm or 2,300 micrometers) and is not as thick on the lateral surfaces (Berkowitz, Holland, & Moxham, 1992). Removal in either of these areas is not a major concern based on thickness; however, subsurface enamel is not as hard, is more porous, and is less soluble than surface enamel. Therefore, subsurface enamel is likely to abrade at a faster rate and amount than surface enamel. Enamel thins to a knife's edge at the cervical margin and, thus, removal through abrasion is a concern as this is frequently where plaque is located, toothbrushing is aimed, and frequent professional instrumentation occurs. To achieve this treatment goal, polishing exposed root surfaces should be avoided.

Because cementum and dentin are not as calcified as enamel, the same procedures would remove more of these tissues than enamel. Studies have not been conducted to determine the loss of cementum with the rubber cup. Exposed cementum is a concern for those with periodontitis because it is frequently treated with scaling and root planing (or debridement) and polishing. Undue loss of this tissue is damaging to the periodontium and is not necessary to promote healing and enhance postoperative healing (Nield-Gehrig & Houseman, 1996). An in vivo study identified that twenty-six to seventy-one times more dentin than enamel was removed by polishing abrasives.

The effect of rubber cup polishing on newly erupted teeth, caries, demineralized areas, erosion, and abrasion seem self-explanatory. The clinician should, however, be aware of the number and location of restorations and types of materials present. Research indicates that almost all prophylaxis pastes scratch and roughen all types of restorative materials. Roulet and Roulet-Mehrens (1982) evaluated the effect of a variety of commercially prepared prophylaxis pastes on gold, amalgam, conventional composite, microfilled composite, as well as, tooth enamel and dentin. Their research indicated almost all abrasive agents scratch and roughen restorative material and only a few pastes tended to smooth the surfaces of dental hard tissues. Another study evaluated the effects of seven prophylaxis pastes on composite resins. They concluded that the surface of composite resins becomes more roughened with the use of any polishing paste (Serio, Strassler, Litkowski, Moffett, & Kruysa, 1988). Both studies found the degree of roughness varied depending on the prophylaxis paste used. These authors stated that the prophylaxis paste used should be selected very carefully. Serio and others (1988) recommend caution in the selection and use of polishing pastes, especially for clients with composite restorations at or near the gingival margin. Roulet and Roulet-Mehrens (1982), however, recommend avoiding the use of polishing pastes on composites as each polishing increases composite surface roughness. Polishing of implant abutments is covered in Chapter 14. Tooth surface integrity, per se, cannot be controlled by the clinician, therefore, areas of compromised or minimal calcification should not be polished. Eliminating these surfaces from any polishing procedure will ensure undue abrasion is avoided.

It is difficult to determine the exact clinical effect of polishing on the tooth or restorative surface because there are so many variables that affect abrasion. Consequently, studies conducted to evaluate the effect of abrasive agents have differing study designs making the results inconsistent or incomparable. The majority of studies have been in vitro rather than in vivo studies. The validity of the in vitro results to the clinical situation has been questioned (Christensen & Bangerter, 1987; Hunter, Biller-Karlsson, Featherstone, & Silverstone, 1981). Alteration of the grit of an abrasive or even one technique factor can affect abrasion. Altering multiple factors will have a more dramatic effect. For example, the same amount of abrasion can occur if fine grit is applied for more time than a coarse grit agent. In this case, however, the tooth surface treated with the fine grit paste is left smoother than the surface polished with coarse grit. Practitioners must strive to self-evaluate their technique and the integrity of the tooth structure to ensure that the technique and agent applied is providing the desired effect. Table 13-5 summarizes recommendations for reducing abrasion.

## RELATIONSHIP OF POLISHING TO NONSURGICAL PERIODONTAL THERAPY

A final goal of both initial therapy and periodontal maintenance is to produce a relatively smooth and deposit-free tooth and restorative surface, thereby promoting healing. The crown and root should be well prepared to meet this goal after oral self-care education (see Chapter 8) and debridement therapy (see Chapters 10, 11, and 12). Self-care education includes the recurrent theme that bacte-

**Table 13-5  Summary of Recommendations for Reducing Abrasion**

| Factors | Rubber Cup | Air Polishing |
|---|---|---|
| Abrasive Agent | • use the least abrasive agent that will be effective<br>• coarse grit pastes should not be used<br>• medium grit pastes are for stain removal only<br>• toothpaste, extrafine and fine grit pastes combination cleansing and polishing pastes, and composite polishing pastes are recommended<br>• if stain is present after debridement, reevaluate its removal with hand or ultrasonic instruments | • there are no options when selecting an abrasive agent<br>• generally, it is more abrasive than the rubber cup due to its mode of operation |
| Clinician Technique | • correct speed, pressure, time, number of particles, and position of the rubber cup minimize abrasion and can be controlled by the clinician | • correct time, tip angulation, and tip movement decrease abrasion and are the only factors the clinician can control |
| Tooth Surface Integrity | • exposed root surfaces should not be polished<br>• restorations should not be polished<br>• immature enamel, caries, decalcification, and erosion/abrasion should be avoided | • exposed root surfaces should not be polished<br>• restorations should not be polished<br>• immature enamel, caries, decalcification, and erosion/abrasion should be avoided |

rial plaque removal should occur daily by the client. During initial therapy or maintenance appointments, the client is held accountable for bacterial plaque removal with the support and guidance of the clinician. While providing self-care instructions, the dental hygienist encourages the client to practice with the recommended aids to achieve bacterial plaque removal from buccal and lingual tooth surfaces and interdental areas. For instance, if the Bass technique with a soft-bristle toothbrush and a wooden toothpick holder are recommended, then those aids need to be incorporated into the appointment. Small step size with instructions is vital which means, at times, only one aid will be recommended. In this case, the single aid should be practiced until adequate plaque removal is achieved. Ideally, by the last initial therapy appointment, clients should be able to demonstrate adequate use of aids. If this is the case, the client is *capable* of removing bacterial plaque at the final appointment when polishing usually occurs. Debridement removes supra- and subgingival plaque and hard deposits and should leave the enamel and cementum relatively smooth. If root surfaces are cleansed and/or polished after debridement, there is a chance that the amount of abrasion created by the combined procedures is significant and will result in increased sensitivity. It is also possible that polishing will leave the surface rougher than it was after debridement.

It is recognized that there are clinicians who prefer to polish *prior* to periodontal instrumentation to decrease the number of microorganisms and to prevent the introduction of abrasive particles into the "fresh" wounds created during instrumentation. This philosophy differs from author to author (Daniel, 1993; Nield-Gehrig, & Houseman, 1996; Pattison & Pattison, 1992; Tsutsui, 1995; Wilkins, 1994) who recommend polishing be de-

ferred when the client has inflamed gingival tissues that hemorrhage during gentle instrumentation or toothbrushing and immediately after deep subgingival instrumentation. Rationales for these recommendations include:

1. Polishing can cause trauma to the gingival tissues and inflamed tissue is more easily abraded or traumatized.
2. When gingival tissue is abraded, a portal of entry for bacteria is created increasing the possibility of bacteremia.
3. Healing can be prolonged when abrasive particles become embedded in traumatized tissue.
4. Aerosols are created during rubber cup polishing and air polishing.
5. In the presence of gingival inflammation, the risk for disease transmission is increased.

Pre-rinsing or subgingival irrigation with an animicrobial mouthrinse prior to polishing is also an option for decreasing microbial counts.

Ideal care planning for polishing during NSPT requires the clinician to critically analyze philosophy and method, as well as client preference. First, the dental hygienist(s) selects a philosophy and shares it with the employer and coworkers. Selective polishing philosophy is compatible with NSPT because it emphasizes client self-care, considers debridement of the tooth and periodontal pocket by ultrasonic or hand instrumentation, and complements frequent periodontal maintenance appointments. Selective polishing, like NSPT, employs in-office bacterial plaque removal by the client, and professional removal of bacterial plaque and stain via debridement or minimal polishing. Selective polishing is indicated in cases that warrant frequent recall appointments (one to three months), as it will minimize loss of root structure and potential hypersensitivity. This philosophy also supports the recommendations that polishing should not occur on tooth structures that have compromised calcification such as decalcification, caries, or restorations.

Second, methods should be discussed in respect to the NSPT office program. Rubber cup polishing seems to be the method that meets the needs of clients with periodontal diseases. Rationale includes the degree of control the practitioner has over the abrasive agent selected and the technique employed. Other considerations include the recognized precautions and limitations of air polishing. In some practices, the only polishing option is the rubber cup method. In other practices, equipment is available for both rubber cup and air polishing methods. In this case, discussions should focus on the role of each in NSPT.

After philosophy and methods are discussed individualized care planning for clients will occur in a sequence of steps. First, the medical conditions must be considered. Conditions that indicate an increased risk for bacterial infections resulting in a significant medical risk due to bacteremias are important. Circumstances that warrant investigation and possible antibiotic premedication are rheumatic fever with resultant rheumatic heart disease, congenital heart disease, open-heart surgery, organic heart murmur, the presence of cardiac prosthetic devices, some artificial joint replacements, penile implants, cerebrospinal fluid shunts, vascular grafts, pacemakers, or defibrillators (Little, 1994). Persons with respiratory problems such as emphysema, asthma, or allergies also should be evaluated to determine the significance of the problem to decide whether to proceed with polishing. Refer to Chapter 2 for a review of health history precautions and subsequent treatment alterations.

The second step involves examining the characteristics of the enamel and presence of restorations prior to applying an abrasive agent. Reference to the dental and periodontal charting and radiographs are important. Third, through discussion and informed consent, client preference should be determined. Client preference is extremely relevant when deciding which philosophy and method meets individual needs. Because many consumers are accustomed to traditional polishing with either method, it is critical they understand the role of polishing in NSPT. If this is understood, the client will realize that self-care and debridement achieve the goals of NSPT and that polishing is a cosmetic procedure. Remember, Cross and Carr (1983) and other authorities, (Daniel, 1993; Walsh, Heckman, & Moreau-Diettinger, 1985; Pattison, 1992; Tsutsui, 1994; Wilkins, 1994) are in agreement that thorough explanations of the rationale for selective polishing increase client acceptance. Of course, understanding this concept does not ensure informed consent for selective polishing. Some clients might prefer the traditional philosophy.

Polishing philosophies should be discussed with the case presentation during initial therapy and maintenance appointments. An example dialogue for the returning client follows:

*Clinician:* Janice, in the past I have been polishing all your teeth. The latest information indicates polishing does not help prevent inflammation of your gums (gingivitis) or bone loss (periodontitis). As we previously discussed, bacterial plaque is the main reason your gums become infected and bone loss occurs. Therefore, you must remove plaque every day. In fact, it may be detrimental to your teeth to have them polished every time you return for periodontal maintenance care. When I use an abrasive polishing agent on your tooth, a very small amount of tooth surface is removed. This could become a significant amount over many years. For these reasons, I suggest only polishing areas where stain remains after deposit removal. If the stain is removed during debridement (deposit removal), there is no reason to polish. If you prefer, I will still polish all your teeth. Do you have any questions? Are you willing to have me eliminate polishing, polish only the areas with stain, or do you prefer to have me polish all your teeth?

Alterations in the above example can be made to include rubber cup polishing when the client is familiar with air polishing. This discussion should include strengths and weaknesses of each method, why the rubber cup is being recommended, and the fact that air polishing is still an option. The client might be hesitant to make a decision at the first initial therapy appointment. If so, the final decision can be made after the multiple appointments for debridement are completed. Even if informed consent is acquired during case presentation, reiteration of the procedure and method is prudent prior to polishing. The following is an example dialogue to use immediately prior to selective polishing.

*Clinician:* Janice, at your first appointment we discussed the reasons why all your teeth would not be polished. There are six areas where stain remains and so I will polish only these tooth surfaces with a minimally abrasive paste. Do you have any questions or concerns?

Legally, there is not a need to gain informed consent again; however, this discussion provides the client with an opportunity to ask questions and reevaluate the decision.

Last, mechanical polishing occurs, if indicated. The appropriate abrasive agent will be selected and correct clinician technique is self-evaluated. The extent of debridement is considered in reference to when polishing occurs. During initial or active therapy, polishing is performed at the reevaluation visit to allow time for healing to occur. During maintenance appointments, the decision to polish in conjunction with debridement will depend on the extent of polishing needed and the extent of gingival inflammation present.

Realistically, there will be times when selectively polishing stain only cannot be accomplished. When the client is unwilling or not able to perform bacterial plaque removal, polishing therapy will alter accordingly. Unwillingness refers to those who lack the motivation or desire to perform self-care at the dental appointment. Other clients will not be able to perform the tasks due to lack of manual dexterity related to physical or health impairments. In both situations, the clinician has the option to remove bacterial plaque with self-care aids or to mechanically polish. If a mechanical device is chosen, selective polishing can be incorporated by using disclosing solution to identify bacterial plaque. Areas exhibiting bacterial plaque and/or stain are selectively removed and all tooth surfaces need not be treated. When the client prefers traditional polishing, and extrinsic stain is not present, a dentrifice; a polishing agent such as Chalk, Whiting, Cleanic, or Prisma Gloss; or extrafine or fine commercial paste should be selected. Care should be taken to treat only the enamel surfaces and not the exposed root. When coronal stain is present, the least abrasive paste (extrafine, fine, or medium) to effectively remove the stain is applied. A medium grit will often be the abrasiveness chosen for stain removal. Then a fine or extrafine grit or polishing agent is applied to all coronal surfaces.

The clinician must also be aware that there are some tooth stains that cannot be removed. Unlike extrinsic stain, intrinsic stain cannot be removed by ultrasonic or hand instruments or polishing techniques. **Intrinsic stain** is a discoloration incorporated within the tooth structure and **extrinsic stain** is located on the tooth surface or within soft (acquired pellicle, plaque) or hard (calculus) deposit. The dental hygiene clinician develops the ability to differentiate between extrinsic and intrinsic stain to avoid spending unnecessary time and to minimize tooth structure removal. The methods for cosmetic improvement of teeth affected by intrinsic stain include vital and not-vital bleaching, the bonding of composite restorative materials as overlay or laminate veneers, placement of crowns, and enamel microabrasion.

## DOCUMENTATION

Noting the philosophy, method, and abrasive agent used in the record of services aids in documenting informed consent for the procedure. Likewise, the record of services should reflect if polishing is *not* provided. Also, client preference for a philosophy or method should be indicated, especially if it differs from the practitioner's recommendations. An advantage of recording this information in the final record of services rendered is that the clinician can refer to previous notations each time periodontal maintenance care is provided. Because the polishing procedure will be individualized for each client based on needs and preference, it is essential the clinician familiarize herself with former decisions.

## Summary

Research findings indicate that polishing for disease prevention is no longer a valid rationale. Studies have identified loosely adherent bacteria located in the periodontal pocket as the primary etiologic factor in periodontal disease. The individual immune system is also a significant factor in the response of the tissue to bacterial irritation. Current polishing techniques remove adherent bacteria of supragingival plaque but not the loosely adherent plaque bacteria in the periodontal pocket. In fact, adherent plaque bacteria begins to reattach to the tooth surface within hours after removal. Therefore, supragingival and subgingival plaque removal on a daily basis must occur to prevent gingivitis and periodontitis.

There are a variety of polishing philosophies and methods. Authorities in clinical dental hygiene support selective polishing; however, incorporating this philosophy into clinical practice is challenging. The focus of this chapter has been to present background information on each of the polishing philosophies and methods to help the practitioner develop care planning skills for this procedure. A summary of the recommendations for NSPT follows. In cases where the client consents to selective polishing, the following scenarios may be encountered:

1. All tooth surfaces are relatively smooth and free of stain and bacterial plaque. There is no need to selective polish. The case presentation would include this information. This may occur rather frequently in NSPT when periodontal debridement involves the use of ultrasonic instrumentation. The ultrasonic device combined with hand-activated instruments can be used to remove detectable supragingival and subgingival plaque, stain, and calculus.

2. Extrinsic stain remains after debridement is completed. Selective polishing in this case involves the application of an abrasive agent with a rubber cup or bristle brush for stain removal. The least abrasive agent that will remove the stains should be selected. The situations when moderate or heavy extrinsic stains are present after NSPT should be minimal. Moderate to heavy stain is generally more effectively removed by ultrasonic instrumentation or hand scaling than by an abrasive agent. Some practitioners or clients may prefer the air-powder polishing device rather than the rubber cup method. When air polishing is preferred, contraindications and precautions should be

recognized and technique to minimize abrasion applied.

3. Bacterial plaque remains after debridement because the client is not willing or capable to perform self-care at the appointment. Selective polishing, in this case, includes removal of plaque and stain. Bacterial plaque is identified by disclosing solution and/or compressed air. Abrasives are adjusted according to need.

When traditional polishing is preferred, the following situations might occur:

1. All tooth surfaces are smooth and free of stain. A dentifrice, polishing agent, fine or extrafine grit paste may be used. Enamel is polished; exposed root is not. The rubber cup is preferred, especially when root exposure exists. If air polishing is chosen, attempt to limit abrasion by minimizing the time spent and using the correct technique. A polishing agent should be applied following its application.

2. Extrinsic stain and/or bacterial plaque remains after debridement is completed. Apply the least abrasive agent that will remove deposit. If a medium grit paste is needed for cleansing, polish with an appropriate agent afterwards. If air polishing is utilized, incorporate the suggestions in the above example.

Selective polishing using the rubber cup method is the approach recommended for clients with periodontal diseases because it supports client self-care and the goals of professional therapy. Even though this chapter focused on NSPT, the concepts discussed are applicable to those who require only oral prophylaxis.

## Case Studies

**Case Study One:** John Welker, a 45-year-old high school football coach, has been coming to your office for the past eight years for periodontal maintenance procedures at three-month intervals. The assessment identifies several areas with 3 to 4 millimeters of recession, localized abrasion, probing depths no greater than 4 mm, 5 mm of attachment loss in some areas, minimal calculus, minimal plaque, and no stain. All of his restorations are amalgam. Which polishing philosophy and method are indicated? What information would the case presentation include?

**Case Study Two:** Dennis Sparks, a 50-year-old, currently unemployed welder, is a new client in your office. He does not remember when his last dental hygiene appointment was, if ever. He is a heavy smoker (at least a pack a day); consequently, he has moderate to heavy tobacco stains. You determine he has adult periodontitis with moderate bone loss, generalized 4 to 6 mm probing depths, up to 6 mm of attachment loss, furcation involvement, mobility of #3 and #8, and generalized moderate to heavy supragingival and submarginal calculus deposits. He has consented to NSPT. He realizes the cost and has decided it is time to begin taking better care of his mouth. A quadrant approach to debridement is planned using ultrasonic and hand-activated instruments. How would you approach case presentation and care planning for polishing?

**Case Study Three:** Iris Maynard, a 42-year-old housewife and mother of five children, is a client in your office for the first time. She initially scheduled an appointment because of a toothache and bleeding gums. At her initial appointment, it was determined that she has caries in #30, as well as, adult periodontitis with early bone loss. A thorough assessment identified no dental care for the last five years and generalized moderate subgingival calculus deposits. Iris has extensive dental restorative care. All posterior teeth have MOD amalgams, all anterior teeth have mesial and distal composites. She also has significant decalcification at the cervical third on the buccals of all maxillary molars and the buccal and linguals of all mandibular molars. On completion of debridement, she still has light intrinsic stain in a few of the decalcified areas. No extrinsic stain is present. You explain to Iris that polishing is not indicated due to the extensive dental work and the fact that stain is not present. After much discussion, she prefers traditional polishing. How would you approach polishing in this case?

**Case Study Four:** Alfred Rounds, a 63-year-old, returning client in your office had a stroke two years ago. He is right-handed and has not regained complete use of his right arm and hand. He currently uses an automated toothbrush and an interdental brush with a modified handle for bacterial plaque removal. He has generalized recession with hypersensitivity throughout his mouth. Alfred has moderate crowding of his mandibular anteriors. This is the area where he is having the most difficulty removing bacterial plaque. His bacterial plaque removal is effective in all other areas of his mouth. Alfred is on a three-month recall for maintenance. He has limited stain. How would bacterial plaque removal be accomplished at this visit? How would you remove the stain?

**Case Study Five:** Roderick Busby, a 38-year-old banking executive, is a client new to your practice. He moved to the area approximately four months ago. He informs you he has been told he has periodontal disease and that he should seek dental hygiene care every three months. He has been faithfully returning at three-month intervals for two years. He also tells you the last time he was with the hygienist she used a new machine, like a sandblaster, that he really liked. Your assessment identifies a bridge replacing #8 with porcelain fused to metal crowns on #7 and 9. He has 5 mm probing depths on the maxillary molars, recession and abrasion on the buccals of #5, 6, 11, and 12, and up to 7 mm of attachment loss. He has generalized light subgingival calculus and light supragingival calculus on the buccals of #3 and 4. He has some light brown staining on the buccals of #3, 14, 19, and 30. How would you approach care planning and case presentation for polishing?

## Case Study Discussions

**Discussion—Case Study One:** Polishing is not warranted as stain is not present. The case presentation should include the following:

1. Dental/periodontal diseases are prevented by daily bacterial plaque removal.
2. There is currently no research to indicate that professional polishing once every three to twelve months is a factor in preventing dental or periodontal diseases.
3. Studies identify that the tooth surface, particularly the root, is removed or roughened by the abrasive paste. It is best not to apply an abrasive to his teeth because of the exposed root and tooth abrasion.
4. The current approach is to only polish stain. Stain is not present, therefore, polishing can be eliminated.
5. Bacterial plaque was removed during self-care education.

**Discussion—Case Study Two:** Dennis is not sensitized to any type of polishing philosophy or method as he has never had NSPT before. In this case, the clinician does not need to include a *change* in polishing approach in the case presentation. When delivering the case presentation, it should be emphasized that bacterial plaque removal is his responsibility, and that its daily removal, coupled with professional debridement, are necessary to promote healing. Selective polishing philosophy should be reviewed in case this procedure is warranted after debridement. You will have at least four appointments to provide self-care education. If successful, Dennis should be able to demonstrate the use of aids to achieve plaque-free surfaces. Selective polishing is indicated for Dennis because his periodontal status warrants three-month maintenance appointments. When debridement is com-

pleted and tissue healing has occurred, areas of recession may be present. Ultrasonic scaling should effectively remove all the tobacco stain. If some areas of stain remain, an abrasive can be used on the specific areas.

**Discussion—Case Study Three:** The composites and decalcification are areas where an abrasive should not be applied. The least abrasive and indicated method should be employed; therefore, the rubber cup is the best option. Air polishing is not the method of choice due to the composites and cervical decalcification. A dentifrice, extrafine or fine commercial paste, or a polishing agent should be chosen for traditional polishing.

**Discussion—Case Study Four:** Alterations in self-care practices that would help Alfred remove bacterial plaque in the mandibular anteriors should be identified. Appointment time should be utilized to help Alfred practice removing the bacterial plaque in this area. If he is unable to remove all the bacterial plaque or becomes frustrated, you could remove any remaining plaque with whatever oral physiotherapy aid is effective. If selective polishing has previously been included in Alfred's care plan, a discussion of polishing is unnecessary. However, if traditional polishing has been included in previous treatment, the client's consent to selective polishing is necessary. The least abrasive agent that will remove the stain is used.

**Discussion—Case Study Five:** You should question Roderick to determine whether the new machine was an automated scaling device or an air polisher. If it is determined that an air polisher was used, you should explain he has some conditions in his mouth that contraindicate its use. These conditions include the bridge, the teeth with abrasion, and the recommended frequency of his maintenance appointments. You can explain that air polishing scratches/roughens the tooth surface and his bridge, and removes more tooth structure than rubber cup polishing. You should also explain that in his case, the only surfaces where polishing is indicated are the areas where stain remains; the buccals of #3, 14, 19 and 30. Polishing, with any method, is not recommended for his bridge or the areas of abrasion. If the client chooses traditional polishing with the air polisher; however, a discussion and documentation of the effects of doing so every three months is warranted. In this case, the clinician will be very tactful during the discussion to ensure that a negative image of the previous hygienist is not given. The clinician could imply that recent research results on the effects of air polishing have been published that reveal new precautionary measures.

# REFERENCES

Atkinson, D. C., Cobb, C. M., & Killoy, W. J. (1984). The effect of an air-powder abrasive system on in vitro root surfaces. *Journal of Periodontology, 55,* 13–18.

Axelsson, P. (1993a). Mechanical plaque control. In N. P. Lang & T. Karring (Eds.), *Proceedings of the 1st International European Workshop on Periodontology* (pp. 219–242). Chicago: Quintessence Books.

Axelsson, P. (1993b). New ideas and advancing technology in prevention and nonsurgical treatment of periodontal disease. *International Dental Journal, 43,* 223–238.

Axelsson, P. & Lindhe, J. (1974). The effect of a preventive program on dental plaque, gingivitis and caries in schoolchildren. Results after one and two years. *Journal of Clinical Periodontology, 1,* 126–138.

Axelsson, P. & Lindhe, J. (1977). Effect of proper oral hygiene on gingivitis and dental caries in schoolchildren. *Journal of Dental Research Special Issue C, 56,* 142–148.

Axelsson, P. & Lindhe, J. (1978). Effect of oral hygiene instruction procedures on caries and periodontal disease in adults. *Journal of Clinical Periodontology, 5,* 133–151.

Axelsson, P. & Lindhe, J. (1981a). Effect of oral hygiene instruction and professional tooth cleaning on caries and gingivitis in schoolchildren. *Community Dentistry and Oral Epidemiology, 9,* 251–255.

Axelsson, P. & Lindhe, J. (1981b). Effect of controlled oral hygiene procedures on caries and periodontal disease in adults. Results after six years. *Journal of Clinical Periodontology, 8,* 239–248.

Axelsson, P. & Lindhe, J. (1981c). The significance of maintenance care in the treatment of periodontal disease. *Journal of Clinical Periodontology, 8,* 281–294.

Axelsson, P., Lindhe, J., & Nystrom, B. (1991). On the prevention of caries and periodontal disease. Results of a 15-year longitudinal study in adults. *Journal of Clinical Periodontology, 18,* 182–189.

Axelsson, P., Lindhe, J., & Waséby, J. (1976). The effect of various plaque control measures on gingivitis and caries in schoolchildren. *Community Dentistry and Oral Epidemiology, 4,* 232–239.

Baker, D. J. (1988). Effects of rubber cup polishing and an air-abrasive system on plaque accumulation. *Dental Hygiene, 55.* (From Second National Conference on Dental Hygiene Research, Abstract.)

Barnes, C. (1991). The management of aerosols with air polishing delivery systems. *Journal of Dental Hygiene, 65,* 280–282.

Barnes, C., Hayes, E., & Leinfelder, K. (1987). Effects of an air-abrasive polishing system on restored surfaces. *General Dentistry, 35,* 186–189.

Bay, N., Overmon, P., Krust-Bray, K., Cobb, C., & Gross, K. (1993). Effectiveness of anti-microbial mouthrinses on aerosols produced by an air polisher. *Journal of Dental Hygiene, 67,* 312–317.

Berkowitz, K. B., Holland, G. R., & Moxham, B. J. (1992). *Color atlas and textbook of oral anatomy histology and embryology* (2nd ed.). St. Louis: Mosby-Year Book, Inc.

Berkstein, S., Reiff, R., McKinney, J., & Killoy, W. (1987). Supragingival root surface removal during maintenance procedures utilizing an air-powder abrasive system or hand scaling. An in vitro study. *Journal of Periodontology, 58,* 327–330.

Carranza, F. & Perry, D. (1986). *Clinical periodontology for the dental hygienist.* Philadelphia: W.B. Saunders Co.

Christensen, R. (1984). Brand names and characteristics of polishing products used by dental hygienists in the U.S. Results of a survey. *Dental Hygiene, 58,* 222–228.

Christensen, R. & Bangerter, V. (1984). Determination of rpm, time, and load used in oral prophylaxis polishing in vivo. *Journal of Dental Research, 63,* 1376–1382.

Christensen, R. & Bangerter, V. (1987). Immediate and long-term in vivo effects of polishing on enamel and dentin. *The Journal of Prosthetic Dentistry, 57,* 150–160.

Clinical Research Associates. (1981). Oral prophylaxis, Prophy-Jet.™ *Clinical Research Associates Newsletter, 5,* 1–2.

Connor, H. D., Haberman, S., Collings, C. K., & Winford, T. E. (1967). Bacteremias following periodontal scaling in patients with healthy appearing gingiva. *Journal of Periodontology, 38,* 466–471.

Cooley, R., Lubow, R., & Brown, F. (1988). Effect of air-powder abrasive instrument on porcelain. *The Journal of Prosthetic Dentistry, 60,* 440–443.

Cooley, R., Lubow, R., & Patrissi, G. (1986). The effect of an air-powder abrasive instrument on composite resin. *Journal of the American Dental Association, 112,* 362–364.

Cross, G. & Carr, E. (1983). Patients' acceptance of selective polishing. *Dental Hygiene, 57,* 20–23.

Daniel, S. (1993). Cosmetic and therapeutic applications of polishing. In I. R. Woodall (Ed.), *Comprehensive dental hygiene care* (4th ed.), (pp. 648–664). St. Louis: Mosby-Year Book, Inc.

Dentsply International, Inc. (1995). Air polishing, the technology that's taking off. Dentsply/Equipment Division. York: PA.

DeSpain, B. & Nobis, R. (1988). Comparison of rubber cup polishing and air polishing on stain, plaque, calculus, and gingiva. *Dental Hygiene, 62,* 55. (From Second National Conference on Dental Hygiene Research, Abstract.)

Eliades, G., Tzoutzas, J., & Vougiouklakis, G. (1991). Surface alterations on dental restorative materials subjected to an air-powder abrasive instrument. *The Journal of Prosthetic Dentistry, 65,* 27–33.

Finlayson, R. & Stevens, F. (1988). Subcutaneous facial emphysema secondary to use of the cavi-jet. *Journal of Periodontology, 59,* 315–317.

Fleming, L., Barnes, C., & Russell, C. (1991). An in vivo comparison of commercially available disposable prophylaxis angles. *Journal of Dental Hygiene, 65,* 441–444.

Galloway, S. & Pashley, D. (1987). Rate of removal of root structure by the use of the Prophy-Jet™ device. *Journal of Periodontology, 58,* 464–469.

Garcia-Godoy, F. & Medlock, J. (1988). An SEM study of the effects of air polishing on fissure surfaces. *Quintessence International, 19,* 465–467.

Gilman, R. & Maxey, B. (1986). The effect of root detoxification on human gingival fibroblasts. *Journal of Periodontology, 57,* 436–440.

Glenwright, H., Knibbs, P., & Burdon, D. (1985). Atmospheric contamination during use of an air polisher. *British Dental Journal, 159,* 294–297.

Hassel, B. & Kohut, R. (1981). Survey on selective polishing. *Dental Hygiene, 55,* 27–30.

Herrin, J., Rubright, W., Squier, C., Lawton, W., Osborn, M., Stumbo, P., & Grigsby, W. (1986). Local and systemic effects of orally applied sodium salts. *Journal of the American Dental Association, 113*, 607–611.

Hodges, R. & Miller, D. L. (1997). Client preference for rubber cup polishing or air polishing. Unpublished Research, Pocatello, ID: Idaho State University. Grant funded.

Horning, G., Cobb, C., & Killoy, W. (1987). Effect of an air-powder abrasive system on root surfaces in periodontal surgery. *Journal of Clinical Periodontology, 14*, 213–220.

Huennekens, S., Daniel, S., & Bayne, S. (1991). Effects of air polishing on the abrasion of occlusal sealants. *Quintessence International, 22*, 581–585.

Hunter, E., Biller-Karlsson, I., Featherstone, M., & Silverstone, L. (1981). The prophylaxis polish—a review of the literature. *Dental Hygiene, 55*, 36–42.

Hunter, K., Holbrow, D., Kardos, T., Lee-Knight, C., & Ferguson, M. (1989). Bacteremia and tissue damage resulting from air polishing. *British Dental Journal, 167*, 275–278.

Kaminsky, S., Gillette, W., & O'Leary, T. (1987). Sodium absorption associated with oral hygiene procedures. *Journal of the American Dental Association, 114*, 644–646.

Kee, A. & Allen, D. S. (1988). Effects of air and rubber cup polishing on enamel abrasion. *Dental Hygiene, 62*, 55. (From Second National Conference on Dental Hygiene Research, Abstract.)

Kenny, E. B. (1990). Restorative-periodontal inter-relationships. In F. A. Carranza, Jr. (Ed.), *Glickman's clinical periodontology* (pp. 924–955). Philadelphia: W.B. Saunders Co.

Kontturi-Narhi, V., Markkanen, S., & Markkanen, H. (1989). The gingival effects of dental air polishing as evaluated by scanning electron microscope. *Journal of Periodontology, 60*, 19–22.

Little, J. W. (1994). Preventing bacterial infections. Managing the patient with cardiac defects, implants. *Dental Teamwork, 7*, 28–32.

Lubow, R. M. & Cooley, R. L. (1986). Effect of air-powder abrasive instrument on restorative materials. *Journal of Prosthetic Dentistry, 55*, 462–465.

Lutz, F., Sener, B., Imfeld, T., Barbakow, F., & Schüpbach, P. (1993). Self-adjusting abrasiveness: A new technology for prophylaxis pastes. *Quintessence International, 24*, 53–63.

McFall, W. T. (1989). *Supportive treatment. Proceedings of the World Workshop in Clinical Periodontics* (Section IX, pp. 1–23). Princeton, NJ.

Miller, D. L. & Hodges, K. O. (1991). Polishing the surface: A comparison of rubber cup polishing and air polishing. *Canadian Dental Hygiene/PROBE, 25*, 103–109.

Mishkin, D. J., Engler, W. O., Javed, T., Darby, T. D., Cobb, R. L., & Coffman, M. A. (1986). A clinical comparison of the effect on the gingiva of the Prophy-Jet™ and the rubber cup and paste techniques. *Journal of Periodontology, 57*, 151–156.

Munley, M. M., Everett, M. S., Krupa, C. M., Madden, T. E., & Suzuki, J. B. (1988). Air-powder polishing versus rubber cup polishing; efficacy of extrinsic stain removal. *Dental Hygiene, 62*, 49. (From Second National Conference on Dental Hygiene Research, Abstract.)

Newman, P. S., Silverwood, R. A., & Dolby, A. E. (1985). The effects of an air abrasive instrument on dental hard tissues, skin and oral mucosa. *British Dental Journal, 159*, 9-12.

Nield-Gehrig, J. S. & Houseman, G. A. (1996). Extrinsic stain removal from coronal surfaces. In *Fundamentals of periodontal instrumentation* (3rd ed.), (pp. 471–495). Baltimore: Williams & Wilkins.

Nordstrom, N. K., Uldricks, J. M., & Beck, F. M. (1991). Selective polishing, an educational trend in dental hygiene. *Dental Hygiene, 65*, 428–432.

Parton, B. J. (1994). Selective polishing. *Dental Hygienist News, 7*, 16–17.

Patterson, C. J. W. & McLundie, A. C. (1984). A comparison of the effects of two different prophylaxis regimes in vitro on some restorative dental materials. A preliminary SEM study. *British Dental Journal, 157*, 166–170.

Pattison, A. M. & Pattison, G. L. (1992). Polishing. In *Periodontal instrumentation* (2nd ed.), (pp. 313–325). Norwalk, CT/San Mateo, CA: Appleton & Lange.

Petersson, L. G., Hellden, L., Jongebloed, W., & Arends, J. (1985). The effect of a jet abrasive instrument (Prophy-Jet™) on root surfaces. *Swedish Dental Journal, 9*, 193–199.

Pippin, D. J., Crooks, W. E., Barker, B. F., Walters, P. L., & Killoy, W. J. (1988). Effects of an air-powder abrasive device used during periodontal flap surgery in dogs. *Journal of Periodontology, 59*, 584–588.

Putt, M. S., Kleber, C. J., & Muhler, J. C. (1982). Enamel polish and abrasion by prophylaxis pastes. *Dental Hygiene, 56*, 38–43.

Quirynen, M., Marechal, M., Busscher, H. J., Weerkamp, A. H., Darius, P. S., & van Steenberge, D. (1990). The influence of surface free energy and surface roughness on early plaque formation. An in vivo study in man. *Journal of Clinical Periodontology, 17*, 138–144.

Rawson, R. D., Nelson, B. N., Jewell, B. D., & Jewell, C. C. (1985). Alkalosis as a potential complication of air polishing systems. A pilot study. *Dental Hygiene, 59*, 500–503.

Reel, D. C., Abrams, H., Gardner, S. L., & Mitchell, R. J. (1989). Effect of a hydraulic jet prophylaxis system on composites. *Journal of Prosthetic Dentistry, 61*, 441–445.

Rohleder, P. V. & Slim, L. (1981). Alternatives to rubber cup polishing. *Dental Hygiene, 55*, 16–20.

Romans, A. R. & App, G. R. (1971). Bacteremia, a result from oral irrigation in subjects with gingivitis. *Journal of Periodontology, 42*, 757–760.

Rosenberg, R. M. & Ash, M. (1974). The effect of root roughness on plaque accumulation and gingival inflammation. *Journal of Periodontology, 45*, 146–150.

Roulet, J. F. & Roulet-Mehrens, T. K. (1982). The surface roughness of restorative materials and dental tissues after polishing with prophylaxis and polishing pastes. *Journal of Periodontology, 53*, 257–266.

Saxton, C. A. (1975). The formation of human dental plaque: A study by scanning electron microscopy. Unpublished Master's thesis, University of London.

Schluger, S., Yuodelis, R., Page, R. C., & Johnson, R. H. (1990). Debridement of the periodontal tissues: Basic therapy. In *Periodontal diseases—basic phenomena, clinical management, and occlusal and restorative interrelationships* (2nd ed.), (pp. 373–387). Philadelphia: Lea & Febiger.

Schmid, M. O. (1990). Preparation of the tooth surface. In F. A. Carranza (Ed.), *Glickman's clinical periodontology* (7th ed.), (pp. 673–683). Philadelphia: W.B. Saunders Co.

Schifter, C. C., Hangorsky, C. A., & Emling, R. C. (1981). A philosophy of selective polishing. *RDH, 1*, 34.

Serio, F. G., Strassler, H. E., Litkowski, L. J., Moffitt, W. C., & Krupa, C. M. (1988). The effect of polishing pastes on composite resin surfaces. A SEM study. *Journal of Periodontology, 59*, 837–840.

Shieham, A. (1983). Promoting periodontal health effective

programmes of education and promotion. *Journal of International Dentistry, 33*, 182.

Snyder, J. A., McVay, J. T., Brown, F. H., Staffers, K. W., Harvey, R. C., Houston, G. D., & Patrissi, G. A. (1990). The effect of air abrasive polishing on blood pH and electrolyte concentrations in healthy mongrel dogs. *Journal of Periodontology, 64*, 81–86.

Steele, R. C., Waltner, A. W., & Bawden, J. W. (1982). The effect of tooth cleaning procedures on fluoride uptake in enamel. *Pediatric Dentistry, 4*, 228–233.

Stookey, G. K. & Stahlman, D. B. (1976). Enhanced fluoride uptake in enamel with a fluoride-impregnated prophylactic cup. *Journal of Dental Research, 55*, 333–341.

Tinanoff, N., Wei, S. H. Y., & Parkins, F. M. (1974). Effect of a pumice prophylaxis on fluoride uptake in tooth enamel. *Journal of the American Dental Association, 88*, 384–389.

Toevs, S. E. (1985). Root topography following instrumentation. A SEM study. *Dental Hygiene, 59*, 350–354.

Tsutsui, P. T. (1994). Instrumentation theory for professional mechanical oral hygiene care. In M. L. Darby & M. M. Walsh (Eds.), *Dental hygiene theory and practice* (pp. 475–534). Philadelphia: W.B. Saunders Co.

Vrbric, V., Brudevold, F., & McCann, H. G. (1967). Acquisition of fluoride by enamel from fluoride pumice pastes. *Helvetica Odontotogica Acta, 11*, 21–26.

Walsh, M. M., Heckman, B. H., & Moreau-Diettinger, R. (1985).

Polished and unpolished teeth: Patient responses after an oral prophylaxis. *Dental Hygiene, 59*, 306–310.

Walsh, M. M., Heckman, B. H., Moreau-Diettinger, R., & Buchanan, S. A. (1985). Effect of rubber cup polish after scaling. *Dental Hygiene, 59*, 494–498.

Weaks, L. M., Lescher, N. B., Barnes, C. M., & Holroyd, S. V. (1984). Clinical evaluation of the Prophy-Jet™ as an instrument for routine removal of tooth stain and plaque. *Journal of Periodontology, 55*, 486–488.

White, S. L. & Hoffman, L. A. (1991). A practice survey of hygienists using an air-powder abrasive system. An investigation. *Journal of Dental Hygiene, 65*, 433–437.

Wilkins, E. M. (1976). Introduction to polishing. In *Clinical practice of the dental hygienist* (pp. 537–542). Philadelphia: Lea & Febiger.

Wilkins, E. M. (1994). Extrinsic stain removal. In *Clinical practice of the dental hygienist* (pp. 561–565). Baltimore: Williams & Wilkins.

Willmann, D. E., Norling, B. K., & Johnson, W. N. (1980). A new prophylaxis instrument: Effect on enamel alterations. *Journal of the American Dental Association, 101*, 923–925.

Wilson, S. B. (1988). Scaling and root-planing. In D. A. Grant, I. B. Stern, & M. A. Listgarten (Eds.), *Periodontics* (pp. 650–715). St. Louis: Mosby-Year Book, Inc.

Winslow, M. B. & Kobernick, S. D. (1960). Bacteremia after prophylaxis. *Journal of American Dental Association, 61*, 69–72.

# CHAPTER 14

# Supportive Treatment Procedures

## Key Words

antimicrobial therapy
antiseptic
Brannstrom's hydrodynamic theory
dentinal hypersensitivity
endosseous implants
implant system
margination

osseointegration
periimplantitis
peri-implant gingivitis
retrograde implantitis
soft tissue curettage
substantivity
supportive treatment procedures

## INTRODUCTION

Previous chapters have addressed debridement therapy for the control of periodontal disease and maintenance of periodontal health. While these procedures are an integral component of nonsurgical periodontal therapy, periodontal instrumentation is not a sole therapeutic entity. Comprehensive assessment and care planning often include adjunctive therapies that support or enhance the success of nonsurgical periodontal treatment. **Supportive treatment procedures** are those therapeutic interventions that augment debridement for the control of periodontal diseases and maintenance of periodontal health. The procedures include the use of chemical agents and different methods of delivery, desensitization, overhang removal, and special considerations for the care of dental implants. This chapter will discuss the assessment, care planning, implementation, and evaluation of each of these supportive treatment procedures. Integration of supportive therapies in the nonsurgical periodontal treatment plan provides a comprehensive approach to client care.

## OVERVIEW OF CHEMOTHERAPY

Antimicrobial, antibacterial, chemotherapeutic, or chemical agents are all terms used to describe agents employed to control plaque, gingivitis, and periodontitis. These terms are frequently used interchangeably to describe any agent that is used to combat bacterial plaque. **Antimicrobial therapy** is defined by the American Academy of Periodontology (AAP, 1986) as the use of specific agents for the control or destruction of microorganisms, either systemically or at specific sites. Commonly, antimicrobials refer to mouthrinses. Chemotherapy is actually the

prevention or treatment of disease by chemical agents (AAP, 1986). It seems that the term *chemotherapy* is a broader concept. Chemotherapeutics usually refer to administration of antibiotics either locally at a site or systemically. Specifically, chemotherapeutic agents may be used to reduce the quantity of microbial pathogens or to modulate the inflammatory response of the host. Treatment plans for periodontal diseases should indicate, where appropriate, the consideration of adjunctive chemotherapeutic agents (AAP, 1993b). These agents can be added to the basic components of the periodontal plan, which include self-care education, professional removal of plaque-retentive factors and calculus, and posttreatment evaluation. Generally, inclusion of chemotherapeutic regimes is designed to enhance the effects of debridement and is never a substitute for professional and personal mechanical therapy.

To evaluate an antimicrobial agent and its delivery system, the AAP (1991) suggests three criteria. The agent must: 1) be effective in the laboratory against target pathogen(s), 2) reach the site of infection in an effective concentration, and 3) remain at the site long enough to be effective. Because of the intimate relationship between the agent and its delivery system, it is difficult to discuss one entity without the other. Delivery systems have different effects depending on the agent used and the disease treated. Most delivery systems and agents have variable positive effects on gingivitis; however, the same is not true for periodontitis. Because the periodontal pocket presents a unique environment, the delivery mechanism and the agent itself are challenged. Depth of the pocket, gingival crevicular flow, and low fluid volume of the pocket all provide unique situations that are not problematic when treating gingivitis. Further discussion of chemotherapy will be divided into: 1) the agent itself, and 2) the method of delivering the agent.

## Agents

The agents and approaches used for chemical plaque control fall into five categories (AAP, 1994a) as follows:

1. antiseptics that inhibit microorganisms and are broad spectrum,
2. antibiotics that inhibit or kill a specific group of bacteria,
3. single or multiple enzymes that break up or disperse the gel-like matrix that holds bacterial plaque together,
4. nonenzymatic, dispersing, denaturing, or modifying agents that alter the structure or metabolic activity of bacterial plaque; and
5. agents that interfere with attachment of the bacteria to pellicle or to one another.

Most products used by consumers and professionals fall into category one above: antiseptics. An **antiseptic** is any agent that inhibits growth and development of microorganisms (AAP, 1986). Examples include chlorhexidine rinses (Peridex™, Perioguard™) and phenolic compounds (Listerine™). Their purpose is to alter the bacterial composition of plaque, as it is generally accepted that quality rather than the quantity of the bacterial plaque and resultant host resistance interact to create the periodontal infection or disease.

The prevailing philosophy regarding the use of topical or systemic antibiotics is that they are not indicated for the routine control of plaque or gingivitis because their potential for adverse effects outweighs their therapeutic value (Addy, Moran, & Wade, 1994; Ciancio, 1989; Howell, 1991). They are indicated, however, with aggressive gingival disease such as acute necrotizing ulcerative gingivitis and streptococcal gingivostomatitis. Systemic antibiotics are also not recommended for routine treatment of adult periodontitis, again due to potential side effects including resistant bacterial strains and increased growth of opportunistic organisms (AAP, 1993b). Systemic antibiotics are recommended, however, when managing specific types of periodontitis such as prepubertal, localized juvenile, rapidly progressive, and refractory forms of the disease (Ciancio, 1989; Kornman & Wilson, 1992). Topical antibiotics, which are placed subgingivally and slowly released in the periodontal pocket, show promise in the treatment and management of all forms of periodontitis.

Other types of chemical agents identified in categories 3, 4, and 5 above were studied in the 1960s and 1970s and results were inconclusive. Enzymes that have been evaluated include mucinases, pancreatin, protease-amylase, dextranase, mutanase, and glucoseoxidase (Zendium™). Plaque modifiers (ascoxal and urea) have been shown to reduce plaque, but not gingivitis. Agents

that interfere with attachment refer to silicones or polystyrene membranes as a coating on teeth, and, again, this route has not been successful to date. For purposes of this chapter only antiseptics and antibiotics will be discussed.

## Method of Delivery

Methods of delivery include the toothbrush, interdental aids, mouthrinses, irrigation both supragingivally and subgingivally, controlled-release devices and systemic (enteric). The effects of an agent are related to how that agent is delivered. For example, if the same agent were applied in a mouthrinse and in a subgingival controlled-release device, different results would be obtained. The agent applied supragingivally with the mouthrinse would have a potential effect on gingivitis, but not on periodontitis. The same agent applied subgingivally with a controlled-release device would have potential for a positive effect on parameters of periodontitis. The chart presented in Table 14-1 provides the reader with an overview of delivery systems and their potential effects on gingivitis and periodontitis.

The manual toothbrush is the most commonly used method of delivery for dentifrices. Dentifrices appear to have limited value as microbials even though the toothbrush would seem to be a beneficial method of delivery. Incorporation of antimicrobials into dentifrices presents problems of compatibility with the dentifrice components (Bowen, 1995). When an agent is added, it is generally yielded ineffective against plaque and gingivitis as it is inactivated by another chemical or substance. Because the therapeutic effect of this medium has not been documented to date, there is no dentifrice that has received the ADA Seal of Acceptance for its antiplaque and antigingivitis properties. Furthermore, toothbrushing reaches only 1 mm subgingivally, but occasionally it can reach 2 to 3 mm below the gingival margin (AAP, 1991). For this reason, effectiveness is confined to potential improvement of gingival health only; other clinical parameters of periodontitis are not significantly affected. Mechanized or power-assisted toothbrushes are becom-

**Table 14-1 Effects of Delivery Systems on Gingivitis and Periodontitis**

| Delivery Mechanism | Gingivitis | Periodontitis |
|---|---|---|
| Toothbrush/Dentifrice* | Fair/Poor | Poor |
| Mouthrinses* | Fair | Poor |
| Supragingival Irrigation* | Good | Poor |
| Subgingival Irrigation* | Good | Fair/Poor |
| Controlled-Released Delivery | Good | Good |
| Systemic Delivery** | Good | Good |

*Active ingredients with substantivity increase duration and therefore, effectiveness.

**Only recommended for aggressive forms of the disease. Side effects become a risk.

ing increasingly popular. When comparing mechanized methods to manual brushing, improvements in plaque removal, subgingival cleansing, and gingival bleeding are noted (AAP, 1991). Refer to Chapter 6 for more information on toothbrushing alternatives.

Application of antimicrobials with interdental brushes or swab tips is another delivery method recommended by some practitioners for localized periodontal pockets and/or furcation involvement. This method of delivery has not been specifically researched raising questions about effectiveness and penetration. In other words, consideration should be given to the aid's depth of subgingival penetration, if the agent actually reaches the site, and which agent is the best to use. Although the efficacy of this method is not documented, it might motivate clients to perform self-care in the targeted area(s).

A major limitation of rinsing, like dentifrices, is that the agent penetrates subgingivally only a few millimeters. For most forms of gingivitis, the greatest oral hygiene benefit of antimicrobial rinses is to augment the mechanical efforts of clients who are not effective with their self-care (Ciancio, 1989). These antiseptic mouthrinses have a broad spectrum of antibacterial activity and are recommended, when appropriate, despite their high alcohol content. In 1991, researchers (Winn et al.) expressed concern about a possible relationship between high alcohol content of mouthwashes and oral and pharyngeal cancers. The National Cancer Institute did not recommend that clients change mouthwashes as a result of this study. It is incumbent on the clinician, however, to assess the health history to ensure the client is not an alcoholic, recovering alcoholic, or otherwise at risk for these aforementioned types of cancer. People who report xerostomia also should avoid mouthrinses containing alcohol.

Irrigation's role in disease prevention and management is currently inconclusive. Supragingival irrigation can be used as an adjunct to conventional client self-care and it has been reported to improve gingivitis. Supragingival irrigation with a jet irrigator has also been shown to provide secondary subgingival penetration to approximately 3 mm (Ciancio, 1989). This secondary penetration subgingivally might explain why gingival inflammation is frequently diminished despite an unchanged plaque level (Greenstein, 1992). To date, the adjunctive use of supragingival irrigation seems to decrease the gingival inflammatory response in clients with periodontitis; however, there is no evidence to suggest that it changes clinical attachment levels. Further study will continue on the role of supragingival irrigation in the treatment of periodontitis.

The merits of subgingival irrigation in the treatment of periodontitis are controversial. Subgingival irrigation has been reported to penetrate periodontal pockets well; however, the concentration of the chemical used declines rapidly because blood and crevicular fluid levels can deactivate the agent. Controlled-release delivery is thought to produce a more constant and prolonged concentration of the agent compared to systemic and topical delivery systems (oral antibiotics and irrigation). Specifically, these devices use synthetic polymers (fibers) to deliver the chemical agent. Currently, tetracycline hydrochloride fibers are available for use. Studies have reported positive effects on probing depth, bleeding upon probing, significant periodontal disease-causing microorganisms, and attachment levels. Further discussion of chemotherapeutic agents and delivery systems will be divided into subcategories as follows: antimicrobial rinses, irrigation, controlled release devices, and systemic antibiotics. Each of these topics is addressed in a separate section to provide more detail and specific recommendations for clinical practice.

## ANTIMICROBIAL RINSES

It is apparent that, despite professional self-care instructions and recommendations, clients fail to optimally perform daily oral hygiene procedures. Interproximal plaque control is particularly neglected. Surveys indicate that only 2 to 32 percent of patients floss on a daily basis (Murtomaa, Turtola, & Rutomma, 1984; Ronis, Lang, Farghaly, & Ekdahl, 1994). Indeed, floss represents a markedly small percentage of consumer expenditures on oral products. The popularity of mouthrinses, second in sales only to toothpaste, suggests that clients prefer a quick fix to their daily oral hygiene regimen. Consumers frequently select products for home use on the basis of promotional gimmicks and advertised claims. If it tastes pleasant and the manufacturer says it's effective, it must be efficacious.

Dental hygienists, as consumer advocates, strive to educate clients regarding their choice of oral health care products. Today's knowledgeable consumer is keenly aware of the need to fight "plaque" and "gingivitis." Manufacturers are mindful of the consumer's interest in antiplaque and antigingivitis remedies and, desiring to capitalize on current trends, produce a multitude of commercially available products. Dental hygienists will want to base professional recommendations on sound scientific information and therapeutic value rather than perpetuate unfounded marketing claims. In order to accomplish this, students and practitioners must stay apprised of the latest valid information about these products. The American Dental Association (ADA) Council on Dental Therapeutics disseminates information to help professionals make appropriate suggestions for clients. Also, the AAP publishes a position paper entitled, Chemical Agents for Control of Plaque and Gingivitis (April, 1994), which is periodically updated. Current research results are published in peer-reviewed professional journals as well.

### Product Evaluation and Regulation

In 1986, the American Dental Association (ADA) Council on Dental Therapeutics established guidelines that outline the criteria used to evaluate agents for the control of supragingival plaque and gingivitis (American Dental Association, 1986) (see Figure 14-1). These guidelines were developed to encourage properly designed clinical studies that serve as the basis for awarding the ADA Seal of Acceptance. The ADA Seal of Acceptance indicates that a product has met established criteria, that advertised claims are valid, and that the agent is in compliance with instituted standards. The ADA review process for acceptance takes four to six months and must be repeated every three years. It is valuable to recognize that these guidelines do not evaluate the role the agent plays in managing periodontitis. It is also important to note that the American Dental Association is not a regulatory agency. Application for the ADA Seal of Acceptance is strictly a voluntary process for manufacturers of products and does not imply that accepted products are "superior" to nonaccepted products. The concern with products that do not carry the acceptance seal, however, is that they have either not been submitted for review or have been submitted and found to be ineffective in their therapeutic claim (AAP, 1994a). The Food and Drug Administration is the presiding federal regulatory agency and is currently reviewing all over-the-counter products that make therapeutic claims. The results of this review will be forthcoming. Until the FDA completes its review and report on over-the-counter products, the ADA guidelines provide a set of criteria that clinicians can use when professionally evaluating new products. Rinses that carry the ADA Seal of Acceptance due to their therapeutic effect on gingivitis are Peridex, Perioguard, and Listerine. Currently, no mouthwashes or rinses are accepted by the ADA Council on Dental Therapeutics for use in the treatment of periodontitis.

## Substantive and Nonsubstantive Agents

Despite the ability of numerous agents to control plaque in laboratory settings, relatively few demonstrate clinical efficacy. Failure to achieve clinical efficacy may be due to difficulties encountered in product formulation, inadequate exposure time in the oral cavity, and/or lack of bioavailability. The most successful antimicrobial agents to date are those that demonstrate substantivity. **Substantivity** is defined as the ability of an agent to be retained in the oral cavity for extended periods with subsequent slow and sustained release of the active ingredient at effective levels (Scheie, 1989). Substantive agents are effective in both laboratory and clinical testing, when used intraorally due to their retention and release kinetics. To date chlorhexidine gluconate is the only agent commercially available with high substantivity. Because it is antibacterial and is retained and released slowly in the oral cavity, it is classified as a second-generation agent. Comparatively, agents with low to moderate substantivity, or first generation agents, provide short contact times and rapid release providing shorter exposure to obtain a less clinically efficacious result. Phenols and stannous fluoride have moderate substantivity and have been shown to provide some therapeutic benefit in the treatment of gingivitis; however, these agents are less effective than chlorhexidine. While these agents are effective against bacteria in laboratory testing, they are only capable of inhibiting bacteria intraorally for short periods of time. Clinical efficacy of nonsubstantive agents is limited unless used at a frequent rate of four to six times a day. Agents in this group include topical antibiotics, oxygenating compounds, plant root extracts, enzymes, and surfactants.

---

**The following characteristics should be included in clinical studies of plaque/gingivitis control products:**

- Characteristics of the study population should represent typical product users.

- Active product should be used in normal regimen and compared with placebo control, or, where applicable, an active control.

- Crossover or parallel designed studies are acceptable.

- Studies should be a minimum of six months in duration.

- Two studies conducted by independent investigators will be required.

- Microbiological sampling should estimate plaque qualitatively to complement indexes that measure plaque quantitatively.

- Plaque and gingivitis scoring and microbiological sampling should be conducted at baseline, six months, and at an intermediate period.

- Microbiological profile should demonstrate that pathogenic or opportunistic microorganisms do not develop over the course of the study.

- The toxicological profile of products should include carcinogenicity and mutagenicity assays in addition to generally recognized tests for drug safety.

**Figure 14-1** Clinical studies of safety and efficacy.

The graph seen in Figure 14-2 compares the release over time of substantive and nonsubstantive agents (Cummins & Creeth, 1992). Following the first dose of both agents, concentrations of the nonsubstantive agent drop quickly and well below the minimum inhibitory concentration or the concentration needed to be effective. Comparatively, substantive agents retain effective concentrations for a longer period of time requiring less frequent readministration. Recommendations for daily home use of antimicrobial rinses should be based on clinical efficacy related to plaque and gingivitis reduction, safety, and cost effectiveness. Individuals with physical or mental impairments, malpositioned teeth, orthodontics, fixed prosthetics, implants, poor motivation, and/or apthous ulcers might benefit from the use of these rinses. Although chlorhexidine is the most effective agent due to its substantivity, first generation agents will also be reviewed to help the reader gain information to share with clients. Table 14-2 provides the reader with a summary of agents discussed, their use, and effects on gingivitis.

**Chlorhexidine.** Chlorhexidine is the best known and most widely used rinse of the broad spectrum antiseptics (AAP, 1994a). Chlorhexidine is also the most effective antimicrobial agent currently available for the control of supragingival plaque and gingivitis due to its substantivity. Clinical findings suggest plaque reductions of 50 to 55 percent and gingivitis reductions of 45 percent (Banting, Bosma, & Bollmer, 1989; Gjermo, 1989; Grossman et al., 1986). As a compound, chlorhexidine digluconate is a basic lipophilic broad spectrum antimicrobial agent. Chlorhexidine's antimicrobial action results from disruption of the cell's osmotic equilibrium. Positively charged chlorhexidine molecules bind to the negatively charged cell wall, disrupting cellular osmosis and cell wall integrity, ultimately resulting in cell death (Brecx & Theidale, 1984). Chlorhexidine demonstrates pronounced

substantivity resulting from its absorption to oral mucosa, hydroxyapatite and salivary glycoprotein (pellicle) (Rolla, Löe, & Schiott, 1970). Sustained release of chlorhexidine in active form has been demonstrated 8 to 12 hours following application (Bonesvoll, Lokken, Rolla, & Paus, 1974). Approximately 30 percent is retained in the oral cavity after rinsing.

Chlorhexidine was initially used in medicine as a topical disinfectant for burns and ocular infections. It was first used in the United States as an antimicrobial hand soap. Löe and Schiott (1970) conducted the earliest intraoral evaluation of chlorhexidine in an experimental gingivitis study. Varying applications of chlorhexidine have subsequently been evaluated in the form of mouthrinses, dentifrices, gels, and irrigation solutions. Short- and long-term clinical studies show 45 to 60 percent plaque reductions and 27 to 67 percent gingivitis reductions (Addy, Willis, & Morgan, 1983; Flotra, Gjermo, Rolla, & Waerhaug, 1972; Gjermo & Rolla, 1971; Gjermo, Baastad, & Rolla, 1970; Grossman et al., 1986). Chlorhexidine use has demonstrated particular value in reducing plaque and gingivitis during initial periodontal therapy. It is commonly used for the control of gingival inflammation and bleeding prior to and following scaling/root planing and periodontal surgery. It also aids in the control of gingivitis among institutionalized and special patient care groups or orthodontic patients unable to perform adequate mechanical oral hygiene procedures (Brightman, Terezhalmy, Greenwell, Jacobs, & Enlow, 1991; Niessen & Douglass, 1992; Stiefel, Truelove, Chin, & Mandel, 1992). Although FDA approval for its use is limited to the reduction of plaque and gingivitis, it has also been recommended for use with oral candidiasis, apthous stomatitis (Hunter & Addy, 1987), and for the acute symptoms of linear gingival erythema (LGE) and necrotizing ulcerative periodontitis (NUP) in HIV-positive individuals (AAP, 1994b).

Chlorhexidine is currently available for prescription use in the United States as a 0.12 percent mouthrinse (Peridex, Proctor & Gamble; Perioguard, Colgate Palmolive). The mouthrinse contains 11.6 percent alcohol in an aqueous solution with a pH between 5.5 to 6.0. Peridex is approved by the ADA and the Food and Drug Administration. Perioguard is essentially the same composition as Peridex. The recommended and approved use of chlorhexidine mouthrinse is twice daily rinsing with 15 ml for 30 seconds morning and evening. Clients should be advised not to rinse immediately following use as this may reduce the substantivity of the agent. They should also be aware of the potential side effects associated with chlorhexidine use including bitter taste, temporarily altered taste sensation, increased calculus formation, and staining. It is best employed after meals versus prior to eating due to its effects on taste sensations. The yellow-brownish tooth stain associated with use can be removed by scaling, if incorporated in calculus, or polishing procedures. Staining of composite restorations can be removed by applying an appropriate

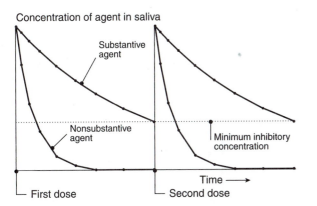

**Figure 14-2** Hypothetical clearance curves for substantive and nonsubstantive agents (Courtesy of Cummins, D. and Creeth, J. E., "Delivery of Antiplaque Agents from Dentifrices, Gels, and Mouthrinses." *Journal of Dental Research, 71,* p. 1440, 1992)

**Table 14-2 Commercially Available Antiplaque and Antigingivitis Agents**

| Product | Active Ingredient(s) | Alcohol | Mechanism of Action | Efficacy | Directions for Use | Adverse Effects |
|---|---|---|---|---|---|---|
| Peridex*, **, ***, and Perioguard*** | chlorhexidine 0.12% | 11.6% | cell wall destruction | 45 to 61% plaque and gingivitis reduction | rinse with 15 ml for 30 seconds, twice a day | tooth staining, altered taste, increase in supra-gingival calculus |
| Gel Kam, Stop | stannous fluoride gels | 0% | interferes with bacterial metabolism | effective in vitro; weak short-term clinical effects | brush twice daily | tooth staining in some patients |
| Gum Care (Crest), Perio-Med™ (Ommi) | stannous fluoride rinses | 0% | interferes with bacterial metabolism | effective in vitro; weak short-term clinical effects | rinse daily | tooth staining in some patients |
| Listerine™ | thymol 0.06%, eucalyptol 0.09%, methyl salicylate 0.06%, menthol 0.04% | 21.6 to 26.9% | inhibits plaque formation and/or adhesion | 19 to 35% plaque reduction 15 to 37% gingivitis reduction | rinse with 2/3 oz. or 4 teaspoonfuls for 30 seconds | sloughing of oral mucosa with prolonged use |
| Cepacol™, Scope™, Clear Choice™ Antiplaque Rinse (Oral-B) | acetylpyridium chloride 0.045 to 0.05% (Scope 0.005% domiphen) | 14% 18% 0% 8% | disrupts cell wall integrity | 14% plaque reduction 24% gingivitis reduction | rinse as directed | tooth staining in some patients, burning, soft tissue irritation |
| Viadent™ | sanquinarine 0.3%, zinc chloride | 10 to 14% | inhibits enzyme activity and bacterial adherence | not significant unless used with the dentifrice | rinse 1 capful for 60 seconds | mucosal irritation |
| Plax™ | sodium benzoate | 7.2% | interferes with bacterial adhesion | 0%, no therapeutic benefit | rinse 1 tablespoon for 30 seconds before brushing | none reported |
| Prevention™ (Regular, Ortho, Perio) | zinc chloride, sodium lauryl sulfate, sodium citrate, hydrogen peroxide (Regular = 0.5%, Ortho = 1.0%, Perio = 1.5%) | 2% | inhibits bacterial adhesion | weak short-term clinical effects, studies in progress | rinse 1/2 capful for 10 seconds | |
| Oxyfresh™ Retar-Dent™ | chlorine dioxide | | inactivates volatile sulfur compounds | 0%, no published randomized controlled clinical trials | | no published safety data |

*Accepted by the Council on Dental Therapeutics of the American Dental Association as an antiplaque/antigingivitis agent.

**Approved by the Food & Drug Administration.

***Demonstrated substantivity.

agent (see Chapter 13); however, the stain might be permanent if the restorative material is pitted. If the level of chlorhexidine is reduced low enough not to stain, it is felt that this antiseptic would lose its effectiveness (Davies, 1992). At least it is recognized that over a two-year period, resistant organisms do not develop when using chlorhexidine (Löe, Schiott, & Karring, 1976) and therefore, it is considered safe for long-term use (AAP, 1994b). It is reported that there might be some advantage in using oxidizing mouthwashes containing peroxyborate or hydrogen peroxide in controlling the stain (Addy, Al-Arrayed, & Moran, 1991; Winer, Chauncey, & Garcia, 1991). Also, foods, beverages, and tobacco use which tend to stain teeth, increase the potential for staining by chlorhexidine.

It also is recommended to allow at least 30 minutes between toothbrushing and chlorhexidine use because of the possible interaction between the sodium lauryl sulfate in the dentifrice and the cationic chlorhexidine that could inactivate the rinse (Barkvoll, Rolla, & Svendsen, 1989). Also, an antagonistic interaction can occur with the fluoride in mouthrinses, toothpastes, and stannous fluoride products so, again, the thirty-minute interval is ideal to ensure the maximum effectiveness of both chemicals.

Chlorhexidine has been studied in other forms including a spray (Francis, Addy, & Hunter, 1987; Francis, Hunter, & Addy, 1987; Kalaga, Addy, & Hunter, 1989) and lozenge (Kaufman, Tal, & Perlmutter, 1989). The spray is advocated for use with those who are physically and/or mentally handicapped. A study evaluating the twice daily use of the 0.2 percent spray as an adjunct to toothbrushing was conducted with physically and mentally handicapped adults attending a day training center (Kalaga, Addy, & Hunter, 1989). Results indicate both clinically and statistically significant lower plaque and bleeding scores, and a reduction in probing depth. These researchers noted that the effects were recognized even with the small dose used, that acceptability and compliance with use was gained, and that tooth staining still occurred.

Building chlorhexidine rinse or any antimicrobials into client care in a practice requires developing an office philosophy. This philosophy would include indications for recommending the rinse, dispensing protocol, follow-up care, and client education. An example of such a protocol exists in Table 14-3. Readers can adapt this model to meet their needs, enhance it by including recommendations for other antimicrobials, and/or provide the client with a modified version of the reappointment and education portions.

**Stannous Fluoride.** Long recognized for their ability to reduce caries, fluorides have also been evaluated as antimicrobial agents. A number of short-term studies indicate that stannous fluoride is a more effective antiplaque agent than sodium fluoride (AAP, 1994a). The proposed mechanism of action of stannous fluo-

ride is associated with the tin component that interferes with bacterial adhesion (Schie, Assev, & Rolla, 1985; Schneider & Muhlemann, 1974; Tinanoff & Weeks, 1979). Laboratory and short-term clinical studies evaluating the effects of stannous fluoride against periodontal pathogens achieved moderate success. Long-term clinical results, however, have been mixed. Contradictory results may be due to the lack of stability in available formulations. Tin is a very reactive element and binds easily to other ions subsequently limiting bioavailability. Stannous fluoride products marketed for client use are available primarily in gels (0.4 percent), mouthrinses (0.64 percent) and dentifrices (0.45 percent). Mouthrinses activated by water and diluted to 0.1 percent, provide weak therapeutic effects against plaque and gingivitis. Recently, improvements in dentifrice stability have improved the availability of stannous fluoride for plaque and gingivitis control. Results from two large six-month clinical trials report 14 to 20 percent reductions in gingivitis and 20 to 33 percent reductions in bleeding (Breiswanger & Perlich, 1995). Side effects associated with use of stannous fluoride include tooth staining, bitter taste, and possible sensitivity resulting from the presence of glycerin in the gels. Stanous fluoride products do carry the ADA Seal of Acceptance for caries protection, but not for the reduction of plaque and gingivitis.

Brecx and others (1993) compared Meridol™, an amine/stannous fluoride solution manufactured in Germany, to chlorhexidine for a three-month period. Plaque and gingival status, as well as tooth staining, were measured. Conclusions include that Meridol was effective in reducing plaque and retarding development of gingivitis, although chlorhexidine was more effective. Both rinses produced staining; however, Meridol stained teeth significantly less than chlorhexidine or the placebo.

Recently, the antimicrobial capacity of mouthrinses containing a combination of chlorhexidine and sodium fluoride at various concentrations has been evaluated in very short-term clinical tests. A two-week period of twice daily use compared to a nonactive placebo control resulted in moderate antiplaque and antigingivitis effects (Jenkins, Addy, & Newcombe, 1993; Joyston-Bechal & Hernaman, 1993). The clinical efficacy of these combined agents must be further investigated in long-term clinical trials and against an active control.

**Phenolic Compounds.** Phenolic compounds, such as Listerine, are also capable of reducing plaque and gingivitis but to a lesser extent than chlorhexidine. A combination of the phenol-related essential oils thymol, eucalyptol menthol and menthyl salicylate has been used as an oral rinse for over one hundred years. Phenolic compounds inhibit plaque formation and bacterial adhesion. Early short-term studies (seven to sixty days) showed favorable reductions of 35 percent in plaque and gingivitis in both the presence and absence of regular oral hygiene (Fornall, Sudin, & Lindhe, 1975; Gomer, Holroyd, Fedi, & Ferrigno, 1972; Lusk, Bowers, Tow, Watson,

**Table 14-3  Recommendations for a Chlorhexidine Rinse**

| Category | Recommendation |
|---|---|
| Indications (for Treatment of Gingivitis) | 1. Healthy gingiva with site specific gingivitis.<br>2. Those with inadequate self-care practices due to lack of motivation or inability to perform skills.<br>3. Special oral or physical situations:<br>  • mentally or physically handicapped,<br>  • crowded teeth,<br>  • poor restorations,<br>  • orthodontics,<br>  • oral candidiasis,<br>  • apthous stomatitis,<br>  • LGE,<br>  • NUP,<br>  • implant management. |
| Prescriptions and Reappointments | 1. Three-month supply equals three bottles. Write Rx for all three at once.<br>2. Reappoint in six weeks to evaluate effectiveness. When possible, combine with the reevaluation visit.<br>3. At the end of three months, reevaluate again. This evaluation might correspond with the recare interval, therefore prophylaxis or nonsurgical therapy might also be indicated.<br>4. If gingivitis is still present, continue with new Rx. If gingivitis reduced or eliminated, discontinue. |
| Education and Instructions for Use | 1. Rinse with 15 ml for 30 seconds morning and evening.<br>2. Do not rinse with water immediately after use.<br>3. Do not brush within 30 minutes of using this rinse.<br>4. Do not use a fluoride mouthrinse, toothpaste, or brush on product within 30 minutes of rinsing.<br>5. Be aware of potential side effects including:<br>  • bitter taste,<br>  • altered tooth sensation,<br>  • increased calculus formation,<br>  • staining of teeth,<br>  • staining of tooth-colored restorations.<br>6. Realize that routine removal of plaque at home can potentially reduce the staining and calculus accumulation. |

& Moffit, 1974). Long-term studies, consisting of six month or greater duration, confirm the antiplaque and antigingivitis properties of this agent. Twice daily supervised rinsing results in a 20 to 34 percent plaque reduction and 28 to 34 percent gingivitis reduction when compared to an alcohol or water control rinse respectively (DePaola, Overholser, Meiller, Minah, & Neihaus, 1986; Gordon, Lamster, & Seiger, 1985; Lamster, Alfano, Seiger, & Gordon, 1983).

Manufacturer's instructions for Listerine mouthwash use include twice daily rinsing, morning and night, with two-thirds ounce for 30 seconds. Reported side effects include burning sensation, objectionable taste and slight tooth staining. Prolonged rinsing exceeding the recommended 30 seconds may lead to chemical irritation and desquamation of oral mucosa. In addition to the active ingredients, the mouthrinse contains 21.6 to 26.9 percent alcohol at a pH of 5.0. Its use is contraindicated for clients with xerostomia, recovering alcoholics, and oral cancer patients. Currently, Listerine is the only over-the-counter product accepted by the ADA for the control of plaque and gingivitis. It is often used in practice when chlorhexidine rinses are not acceptable to clients due to taste, cost, calculus formation, or staining. Listerine toothpaste is also available with some of the same ingredients as the mouthwash. It also contains sodium monofluorophosphate and does not carry the ADA Seal of Acceptance.

**Quaternary Ammonium Compounds.** Quaternary ammonium compounds such as cetylpyridium chloride used at 0.05% (Scope™, Cepacol™, Oral-B Anti-plaque Rinse™), with and without domiphen bromide, have been used in mouthrinses for over fifty years. The mechanism of action of this bactericidal agent is similar to chlorhexidine. Positive ions bind to the negatively charged cell wall effecting permeability and loss of cellular contents. Short-term studies demonstrate a moderate degree of effectiveness; however, the lack of substantivity and rapid clearance of this agent from the oral cavity has resulted in meager long-term clinical results (Carter & Barnes, 1975; Ciancio, Mather, & Bunnell, 1975). Published results from the only six-month study showed a 14 percent reduction in plaque and 24 percent reduction in gingivitis (Lobene & Soparkar, 1977). Side effects associated with use include burning sensation, slight staining, and soft tissue irritation. The lack of subtantivity may be countered by more frequent rinsing to improve efficacy. Client compliance with this regimen is low and may accentuate undesirable side effects. The alcohol content of these products varies from 0 to 18% and the pH is 5.5 to 6.5. None has been accepted by the ADA for the control of plaque and/or gingivitis.

**Sanquinarine.** Sanquinarine is an alkaline extract derived from the bloodroot plant. The proposed mechanism of action inhibits bacterial adherence through alteration of the cell wall. It is commercially available as Viadent™ and has been tested in both dentifrice and mouthrinse formulations containing 0.03 percent sanquinarine and 0.2 percent zinc chloride, a metal salt with antibacterial properties. The pH is 4.5 for both the mouthrinse and dentifrice. The alcohol content of the mouthrinse is 10 to 14 percent. Early short-term studies were conducted with mixed findings (Klewansky & Vernier, 1984; Wennstrom & Lindhe, 1985). Resulting reductions in plaque and gingivitis reported in the literature vary from 0 to 40 percent and appear to be influenced by frequency of use, length of the clinical trial, and procedures for use. Neither the dentifrice nor mouthrinse have demonstrated significant reductions of plaque or gingivitis in long-term clinical trials (Grenby, 1995). The lack of clinical efficacy of this agent may be attributed to the agent's lack of substantivity.

It is important, however, to recognize the favorable results obtained in studies that evaluated the clinical efficacy of the sanguinarine dentifrice and mouthrinse used in combination (Harper, Muellar, Fine, Gordon, & Laster, 1990; Kopczyk, Abrams, Brown, Matheny, & Kaplan, 1991). Plaque and gingivitis were reduced 21 percent and 25 percent respectively following six months of combined dentifrice and mouthrinse use. Professional recommendations for combination use replicate the study regimen, which consisted of brushing, without rinsing afterward and two sixty-second sequential rinses followed by a thirty-minute period of no eating, drinking, or rinsing. Side effects include burning sensation of oral mucosa and objectionable taste. The individual products are not accepted by the ADA. Combined use regimens are not eligible for the ADA Seal of Approval.

**Other Agents.** Various other nonsubstantive agents have been marketed and tested for their ability to reduce plaque and gingivitis. The overall performance of these agents is weak because of the lack of substantivity or efficacy of the active ingredients. Although these agents demonstrate effective antimicrobial ability in laboratory testing, long-term clinical evaluation reveals no therapeutic benefit. Surfactants, oxygenating agents, enzymes, and fluorides other than stannous fluoride are included in this group. Commercially available mouthrinses containing surfactants are marketed as prebrushing rinses (Plax™) claiming to loosen plaque, making toothbrushing easier and more effective. Theoretically, the surfactant lowers the surface tension prior to brushing, which should facilitate plaque removal. Clinical trials have repeatedly failed to substantiate therapeutic effects for gingivitis reduction (Balanyk, 1992; Chung, Smith, & Joyston-Bechal, 1992; Freitas, Collaert, & Attstrom, 1991; Vouros, Sakellari, & Konstantinidis, 1994). No products containing surfactants as the active ingredient are currently accepted by the ADA for therapeutic effects as antigingivitis agents.

Oxygenating agents, such as peroxide and perborates, have also been evaluated for the reduction of plaque and gingivitis. Oxygenating agents produce an effervescent bubbling upon the release of oxygen when in contact with tissue. Anti-inflammatory properties of these agents may be capable of reducing the signs of disease such as bleeding; however, these properties do not reduce the pathogenicity of bacteria (Ciancio, 1992). Additionally, some concern exists regarding safety due to potential delayed wound healing and adverse tissue reaction associated with long-term use of oxygenating agents (Rees & Orth, 1986; Weitzman, Weitberg, Niederman, & Stossel, 1984, Weitzman, Weitberg, Stossel, Schwartz, & Shklar, 1986). Recently, a dual-action mouthwash with baking soda and peroxide has been marketed (Mentadent™). It contains 12 percent alcohol in addition to the other active ingredients. Prevention™ is a low-alcohol, over-the-counter formula, containing zinc chloride, hydrogen peroxide, sodium dodecyl sulfate, and sodium nitrate. In the laboratory setting, this rinse demonstrated a strong antimicrobial activity against a number of microorganisms (Drake, Wefel, Dunkerson, & Hogle, 1993). A six-month clinical trial is underway to test its in vivo effectiveness. It is noted that most long- and short-term studies evaluating baking soda and peroxide paste as an adjunct to self-care have demonstrated no added value over conventional oral hygiene (Bakdash, Wolff, Pihlstrom, Aeppli, & Bandt, 1987; Pihlstrom et al., 1987; Wolff et al., 1987; Wolff et al., 1989). No oxygenating products are currently accepted by the ADA for therapeutic effects as antigingivitis agents.

**Multilevel Marketing.** In addition to the public marketing and availability of over-the-counter and prescription antimicrobial agents, various other oral health care products are available to the public through multilevel marketing programs. These products may be dispensed through dental offices or by nondental representatives. Clinicians should carefully evaluate the claims made by the manufacturers and sales representatives of such products. If these claims are purely cosmetic in nature (i.e., reduce oral malodor, or whiten teeth) they may not be subject to federal regulations governing other therapeutic dental care products. Consumers, however, may be led to believe that these products will improve their dental health. The dental hygienist plays a critical role as an advocate for clients by dispelling such public misconceptions. Dental hygienists must also carefully weigh the ethical dilemma faced by dental practices that choose to market such products for profit. One such agent is chlorine dioxide, marketed as Oxyfresh™ and Retar-Dent™. They are available in dentifrice and mouthrinse formulations only via multilevel marketing representatives. Chlorine dioxide has historically been utilized as an alternative to chlorine for water purification (Lubbers, Chauan, & Bianchine, 1982). This active ingredient reduces volatile sulfur compounds associated with oral malodor and gingivitis (Ng & Tonzetich, 1984; Rizzo, 1967; Schmidt, Missan, Tarbet, & Cooper, 1978). While initial laboratory studies demonstrated reduction of periodontal pathogens, no randomized controlled clinical trials have substantiated the antimicrobial or antigingivitis effects of this agent. The therapeutic value of this agent to date is, therefore, unsubstantiated.

Other multilevel marketing agents include AP-24™ and Melaluca™. AP-24™ is available as a toothpaste, mouthwash, breath spray, and dental floss (AP-24, PharmAssist™, a Summary of Clinical Data, 1994). The manufacturers claim its most significant benefit is client compliance because of the taste and mouth feel. They also state that a reduction in surface-free energy of teeth is the proposed mechanism for the plaque-reducing ingredient defined as an emulsion of polydimenthylsiloxene (dimethicose) in a suitable poloxamer. In other words, it is a surfactant that needs to be applied several times a day. Research comparing its effectiveness to other antimicrobial agents was not reported.

**Future Agents.** Triclosan is a nonionic phenolic-like compound commonly used in antibacterial deodorants and soaps. It has been evaluated for reduction of plaque and gingivitis. Triclosan possesses moderate substantivity evidenced by oral detection up to eight hours after use (Gilbert & Williams, 1987). The mechanism of action is not entirely clear. Clinical studies of six months or longer duration report reductions in plaque of 0 to 30 percent and reductions in gingivitis from 20 to 75 percent (Garcia-Godoy, DeVizio, Volpe, Ferlauto, & Miller, 1990; Svatun, Saxton, & Rolla, 1989; Svaton, Saxton, & Rolla, 1990). Triclosan has recently been approved for oral use in the United States and it is marketed as a dentifrice in Europe and Canada by two leading dentifrice manufacturers.

Delmopinol is another compound under investigation for its effects on plaque and gingivitis. Delmopinol possesses relatively low antimicrobial effects but is thought to reduce plaque through its interaction with oral and bacterial surfaces (Brecx, Theidale, Attstrom, & Glatz, 1987). It is a surface active compound thought to interfere with attachment of bacteria to oral surfaces by lowering the surface-free energy. A dose-related effect has been demonstrated between the concentration of delmopinol used and the reduction of plaque and gingivitis (Collaert, Attstrom, DeBruyn, & Movert, 1992). Initial short-term results over a fourteen-day period indicate an ability to reduce gingivitis comparable to chlorhexidine (Collaert, Attstrom, DeBruyn, & Movert, 1992). The promising results of these short-term investigations has promoted further study of this agent. Elworthy and others (1995) studied the effects of 0.1 percent and 0.2 percent delmopinal mouthwashes on supragingival plaque flora in 141 subjects for a six-month period. Results indicate no effect on bacterial plaque counts or the bacterial population; however, there was a significant decrease in the dextran-producing streptococci when compared to the control group.

## IRRIGATION

In 1966, the first powered irrigation device was introduced in the United States. Since this time, the popularity of oral irrigation subsided; however, recently its potential value in nonsurgical periodontal therapy has been reexamined. The renewed interest in irrigation probably coincided with the discovery of the different types of plaque: supragingival attached plaque, supragingival loosely attached plaque, subgingival unattached or loosely attached plaque, and subgingival attached plaque (see Figure 14-3). The aim of any type of irrigation is to attack the loosely attached plaque both supragingivally and subgingivally.

Irrigation can be divided into three types: supragingival, marginal, and subgingival. Supragingival irrigation involves the use of a pulsating water stream created from a mechanized irrigator, and a tip designed to be placed at a 90° angle to the tooth near the gingival margin. Marginal irrigation (Jolkovsky et al., 1990) is performed with tips that are soft, spongy, and triangular in shape (Pik Pocket™, Teledyne Water Pik), which are attached to a

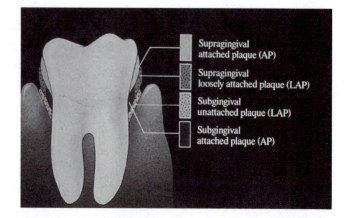

**Figure 14-3** Four types of plaque. (Courtesy of Teledyne Water Pik)

standard irrigating device. The soft tip is actually placed beneath the gingival margin. Marginal irrigation is classified by some authors and researchers as supragingival irrigation, and by others as subgingival delivery. Both supragingival and marginal irrigation methods are used by clients for self-care. Subgingival irrigation involves the use of cannulas placed as far beneath the gingival margin as possible depending on the tissue tone, access, and presence of deposit. Many commercial devices are available for subgingival irrigation including standard irrigating units with a hose and cannula attachment or a handpiece system (Perio Pik™ Handpiece, Teledyne Water Pik). Also, handheld syringes and ultrasonics can be used for this purpose. Generally, subgingival irrigation with cannulas is professionally applied as use of a cannula by clients requires acute dexterity and excellent access to the site. Figure 14-4 is an example of the different tips manufactured by Teledyne Water Pik and their recommended placement. Table 14-4 provides the reader with a summary of the depth of penetration of dye into the periodontal pockets using various tips (Greenstein, 1992). Supragingival, marginal, or submarginal irrigation can be performed with water or a chemotherapeutic agent; again, chlorhexidine is preferred due to its substantivity:

Conclusions about irrigation can be categorized as follows:

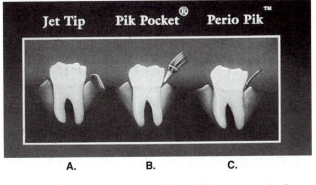

**Figure 14-4** Proper placement of tips. (**A**) supramarginal; (**B**) marginal; (**C**) submarginal (cannula). (Courtesy Teledyne Water Pik)

1. Supragingival irrigation has a positive effect on gingivitis when using water or antimicrobials. Use of antimicrobials, however, improves the clinical and microbial parameters in those with gingivitis when compared to water alone. In general, irrigation with medicaments attains a 30 to 40 percent reduction of the gingival index (Greenstein, 1992). This procedure is valuable for clients with gingivitis who are unable to perform adequate self-care. Because supragingival irrigation

**Table 14-4 Dye Penetration into Periodontal Pockets[a]**

| | | Percentage of Pocket Penetration | | | |
|---|---|---|---|---|---|
| | | Supragingival Irrigation | | | |
| Study | Initial Pocket Depth (mm) | Colgate Via-Jet®,* | Standard Tip[b] | Pik Pocket® | Subgingival Cannula |
| Eakle et al. | 4 to 8 | 42.4 | | | |
| Eakle et al. | 4 to 7 >7 | | 46 56 | | |
| Larner et al. | 4 to 6 7 to 10 | | 9 to 42 29 to 39 | | 67 to 80[c] 41 to 76[c, d] |
| Boyd et al. | 3.5 to 6 >6 | | 29.8 54.3 | | 70.4[e] 74.5[e] |
| Braun et al. | ≤6 >6 | | | 90 64 | |
| Nosal et al. | 3 to 9 | | | | 100[f] |

(Reprinted with permission from *The Compendium of Continuing Education in Dentistry.* Greenstein, G. Supragingival and subgingival irrigation: Practical application in the treatment of periodontal diseases. *Compend Contin Educ Dent 13* (12): 1098–1125, 1992.)

[a] Dyes were delivered with a jet irrigation.

[b] Jet Tip or Water Pik® Tip, which are the same device.

[c] *Max-I-Probe® Side-Window Cannula and *Mono-Ject® Straight-Flow Cannula placed 3 mm subgingivally.

[d] Lower number, 41% reflects presence of calculus.

[e] Perio Pik™—placed to half the pocket depth.

[f] 100% at 86% of the sites evaluated, dye delivered with an ultrasonic tip.

*Vipont Pharmaceuticals, Div of Colgate-Palmolive, Fort Collins, CO 80522.

limits the ability of the agent to penetrate subgingivally, its use in management of periodontitis is questionable.

2. Marginal irrigation clearly results in further penetration of the agent subgingivally; however, comparisons to supragingival irrigation with a standard tip and subgingival irrigation with a cannula are limited. It is, again, effective in managing gingivitis, but its effects on periodontitis need further study.

3. Subgingival irrigation with a cannula and antimicrobial agent decreases plaque indices, gingival indices, and the number of sites that bleed upon probing. Pocket depth has been reduced by less than 1 mm when performed without scaling and root planing and pocket depth has decreased up to 3 mm when performed with root planing (Greenstein, 1992). The role of subgingival irrigation in treating periodontitis is controversial and requires further study. Single episodes of subgingival irrigation, alone or in conjunction with debridement, have a limited effect on gingivitis and periodontitis, but may have some value in reducing periodontal pathogens and encouraging clients to irrigate at home.

The following discussion reviews findings from the literature and clinical applications for supragingival, marginal, and subgingival irrigation.

## Supragingival Irrigation

The primary objective of supragingival irrigation is to flush away bacteria that are located coronal to the gingiva, thereby reducing the potential for gingivitis or decreasing existing inflammation (AAP, 1995a). Client applied mechanized irrigation with a standard supragingival tip results in a range of pocket penetration from 9 to 54 percent. In 1971, Lugassy and coworkers discovered that two zones of hydrokinetic activity were created. The first zone is the direct spray against the tooth and the second zone is created by the deflection of the spray. This second zone results in a flushing action and some penetration into the sulcus as previously mentioned. In order for supragingival irrigation to be successful in managing gingivitis, the client must be educated in self-care through discussion and demonstration. Instructions for use include:

1. Developing a systematic approach to reaching all areas.
2. Placing the tip at a 90° angle to the long axis of the tooth.
3. Focusing on the interproximal space.
4. Starting on a low setting, increasing throughout the procedure if necessary.
5. Spending adequate time to perform the task thoroughly.

Supragingival irrigation does not injure the soft tissue, is particularly beneficial for those who do not perform adequate *interproximal* self-care, and does not increase the number of microbes projected in the tissue (Greenstein, 1992). Recommendations to clients should include the fact that it cannot replace other self-care practices of brushing (AAP, 1995a) and/or interdental cleansing.

Another safety concern studied with client-applied irrigation might be the incidence of bacteremias associated with usage. Irrigation-induced bacteremia is a concern for clients susceptible to bacterial endocarditis. Inconsistent results are reported when the prevalence of bacteremias following irrigation is assessed. The prevalence of irrigation-induced bacteremia ranges from 0 to 50 percent (Berger, 1974; Felix, Rosen, & App, 1971; Lofthus et al., 1991). This range of occurrence, however, is no greater than that associated with bacteremias observed following toothbrushing, flossing or scaling, and root planing. However, as a precautionary measure, the use of self-irrigation in persons susceptible to bacterial endocarditis is contraindicated during periods of active treatment of gingivitis or periodontitis because of the ulcerated epithelium and increased bacteria present (Greenstein, 1992). In other words, self-irrigation therapy for those requiring antibiotic premedication, should only be advised during the maintenance phase of therapy when periodontal health has been established. These clients should further be advised to discontinue irrigation in times of active inflammation (Greenstein, 1992).

Clinicians often wonder about the effects of using water as compared to antimicrobials. Flemmig and others (1990) studied the efficacy of supragingival irrigation with 0.06 percent chlorhexidine when compared to chlorhexidine rinsing, water irrigation, and normal oral hygiene. This study is significant as it had a sample size of 175 and examined the gingival index, bleeding upon probing, the plaque index, pocket depth, the calculus index, and stain at three-month and six-month intervals. Results include that at six months, the greatest effect on gingivitis was seen by chlorhexidine irrigation. Water irrigation and chlorhexidine rinsing were equally effective, although they were less effective than the chlorhexidine irrigation. Other studies comparing chlorhexidine irrigations have been conducted for less than six months and, thus, do not meet the ADA requirements for study duration. Further study is necessary to compare the effects of supragingival irrigation with water and antimicrobials over at least a six-month trial period.

Also, compliance was interesting in the Flemmig (1990) study. At six-months, 91.5 percent were compliant with the chlorhexidine irrigation, 90.6 percent with the water irrigation, 96.8 percent with the chlorhexidine rinsing, and 96.7 percent for the toothbrushing alone. These results initiate questions clinicians frequently have about whether clients will be more likely to use an irrigator or a rinse. The answer probably lies within the client. Through discussion, the clinician must learn which method is most likely to be incorporated into self-care.

When using antimicrobials, oral health professionals should consider the recommended dilutions of the agents. These dilutions are acceptable because oral irrigators deliver medicaments interproximally more effectively than rinsing, these dilutions achieve similar results when compared to higher concentrations or full strength, and the diluted solution might decrease staining (AAP, 1995a). Various companies that produce irrigating equipment and agents provide recommendations about dilutions of a variety of antimicrobials. Some companies even have their own premixed solutions for purchase. Because of the agent's substantivity, only chlorhexidine (Peridex, Perioguard), stannous fluoride (3.28 percent Gel Kam), and a phenolic compound (Listerine) will be addressed. Greenstein (1992) recommends the following:

1. *Chlorhexidine.* To achieve a .02 percent concentration, dilute 5 parts water to 1 part of the product. To acquire a .06 percent solution, the dilution is one to one.
2. *Stannous fluoride.* To achieve a .02 percent solution, the dilution is 164 parts water to 1 part of the product.
3. *Phenolic compound.* Dilute 8 parts water to 1 part product. Ciancio and others (1989) used Listerine at full strength when antigingivitis benefit was documented.

## Marginal Irrigation

This method of delivery is capable of 90 percent penetration of pockets less than or equal to 6 mm and 64 percent penetration of pockets greater than 6 mm (Braun & Ciancio, 1992). While promising in terms of its ability to penetrate subgingivally, the clinical results obtained in terms of reducing gingivitis are similar to those obtained by standard tip designs. This method of irrigation was probably developed to provide the client with a safe, easy, and comfortable means of irrigating subgingivally. Technique recommendations for the use of tips designed for marginal irrigation include:

1. Identification of the specific sites in the mouth.
2. Assessment to see if access to these sites by the client is possible.
3. Use of the lowest pressure setting possible.
4. Demonstration of the insertion of the tip beneath the gingival margin at a 45° angle.
5. Irrigation by the tracing of the margin for 1 to 3 minutes per area.

Because the specialized tip for marginal irrigation has been reported to penetrate periodontal pockets better than the standard tip, it follows that this tip would be recommended for client self-care with those who have gingivitis and pockets associated with Case Type II or early periodontitis, Case Type III or moderate periodontitis, or Case Type IV or advanced periodontitis. Of course, its limitations are recognized since it is probably ineffective in treating periodontitis.

Researchers have studied irrigation with the marginal tip (Fine, Harper, Gordon, Hovliaras, & Charles, 1994; Macaulay & Newman, 1986; Vignarajah, Newman, & Bulman, 1989; Watts & Newman, 1986). Although these studies are valuable contributions to the literature, none were conducted for six months and their designs include different antimicrobials and different in-office and home regimes. Greenstein (1992) comments that client use of these specialized marginal tips may become an integral part of a maintenance program and that this tip plays a role in irrigating deep periodontal pockets that cannot be surgically eliminated.

## Subgingival Irrigation

Subgingival irrigation attempts to reduce the number of microflora in the pocket in an effort to prevent periodontitis or to facilitate its reduction (AAP, 1995a). Professionally applied subgingival irrigation is capable of delivering solutions to the depth of the pocket via handheld syringes, mechanized irrigators, mechanized handpiece, and ultrasonics. Both a disposable, blunt-end needle and/or a cannula attached to a handheld syringe are successful in penetrating deep periodontal pockets. Results of a review of the literature conducted by Greenstein (1992) demonstrate subgingival penetration with cannulas or ultrasonic tips range from 41 to 100 percent depending on the study and equipment used (Boyd, Hollander, & Eakle, 1992; Larner et al., 1989); Nosal, Schiedt, O'Neal, & Van Dyke, 1991). Penetration in these studies is actually a little deeper than expected because of underestimation by the investigators (AAP, 1995, Greenstein, 1992). In general, as pocket depth increases, depth of penetration decreases. The greatest depth of penetration was recognized with ultrasonic instrumentation. Refer to Chapter 12 for further information on ultrasonic instrumentation.

Cannulas can be either side exit or end exit designed. Larner and coworkers (1989) did not recognize a difference in depth penetration of dyes when employing either design. In this same study, however, these researchers demonstrated that calculus on the roots impeded drug delivery in 7 to 10 mm pockets. It is recommended that to maximize drug penetration, calculus needs to be removed prior to irrigation (AAP, 1989a; AAP, 1995a). Subgingival irrigation can suppress microbes; however, they are not eliminated and levels return to baseline in a short time period. This is why most experts do not recommend routine application of subgingival irrigation in the office (AAP, 1989a; Ciancio, 1989; Greenstein, 1992). Although in-office application may not be therapeutic, it does play a role in suppressing microbes prior to scaling and root planing or debridement with either hand instruments or ultrasonics. Other in-office applications include administration prior to an extraction or other surgical procedure, during a surgical procedure, or for implant maintenance. Also, in-office application might be useful when client self-care recommendations include marginal irrigation for targeted areas. Recommended technique suggestions (Teledyne Water Pik, 1992; Rethman, 1992) for use of a cannula and oral irrigating device include:

1. Identification of the purpose: targeted areas or generalized irrigation.
2. Bending the cannula, using its cover, to facilitate access.
3. Use of a fulcrum.
4. Inserting the cannula to the depth of the sulcus, if possible, then retracting about 1 mm.
5. Circumferentially irrigating by walking the cannula around the tooth as if probing.
6. Permitting the solution to flow until it rises over the gingival crest.
7. Irrigating the entire mouth, if applicable, even though deposit removal might have occurred in only one part of the mouth.
8. Disposing of the cannula as you would other "sharps."

Safety issues might be a greater concern with subgingival irrigation than with supragingival irrigation and marginal irrigation. Both side and end-port cannulas are safe as far as pressure used and potential for projecting microbes into the tissues (AAP, 1995; Greenstein, 1992). As with supragingival irrigation, antimicrobials are recommended in certain concentrations as follows (Greenstein, 1992):

1. *Chlorhexidine* (0.12 percent). Use at full strength.
2. *Stannous fluoride* (3.28 percent). Dilute 1 part water to 1 part agent to achieve a 1.64% solution.
3. *Listerine*. Use full strength.

In order to be effective as an adjunct to nonsurgical periodontal therapy, subgingival irrigation must be capable of enhancing the effects achieved by scaling and root planing or debridement alone. These enhanced effects are dependent on the concentrations used, number of applications, and method of delivery. Numerous studies have evaluated various combinations of chemotherapeutic agents and delivery systems in search of a synergistic relationship between scaling and root planing and subgingival irrigation. The majority of studies fails to demonstrate a beneficial effect by the addition of irrigation regardless of the agent utilized (Braatz, Garrett, Claffey, & Egelberg, 1985; Herzog & Hodges, 1988; Krust, Drisko, Gross, Overman, & Tira, 1991; MacAlpine et al., 1985; MacAuley & Newman, 1986; Shiloah & Patter, 1994; Watts & Newman, 1986; Wennstrom, Dahlew, Grandahl, & Heijl, 1987). Antibiotics and high concentrations of chlorhexidine are the only agents shown to enhance the effects of scaling and root planing alone. Four weekly professional subgingival irrigations with 0.5

percent and/or 2.0 percent chlorhexidine improved the clinical response achieved by scaling and root planing alone in short-term studies (Bray, Drisko, & Cobb, 1993; Southard, Killoy, Drisko, & Tira, 1989). These studies utilized four weekly irrigations to simulate the possible results if subgingival chlorhexidine irrigation was applied at each quadrant scaling appointment. Clinical application of these results, however, is limited due to lack of availability and federal approval of chlorhexidine concentrations exceeding 0.12 percent in the United States. Additionally, the samples utilized in these studies were small. The benefits of concentrated subgingival chlorhexidine irrigation need to be validated by studies utilizing a larger sample before this regimen is integrated into clinical use. While routine professional subgingival irrigation with available antimicrobial agents has not been scientifically substantiated, it might be valuable in areas of limited access or sites not responding to other therapy. Clearly, research does not support single episodes of lavage by professionals to increase the impact or duration of root planing (Greenstein, 1992).

Administration of antibiotics via subgingival irrigation generally fails to provide additional benefit. The exception is tetracycline, which is absorbed by root surfaces. Therapeutic levels of tetracycline-HCL are released for up to one week following subgingival irrigation with an 100 mg/ml aqueous solution for 5 minutes. This procedure results in significantly greater gains in attachment levels over a six-month period than achieved by scaling and root planing alone (Christersson, Norderyd, & Puchalsky, 1993). The practicality of irrigating all root surfaces for 5 minutes following scaling and root planing represents a very labor-intensive and costly therapy. Additionally, clients may find the taste objectionable. Again, subgingival irrigation with tetracycline may be valuable in areas of limited access or sites not responding to nonsurgical therapy.

The relatively weak performances of chemotherapeutic agents delivered via subgingival irrigation is due to the inability to sustain adequate concentrations for a sufficient period of time. Continual flow of crevicular fluid from the pocket rapidly clears aqueous agents from the subgingival environment. Even the application of agents in the form of gels only marginally improves subgingival retention. Studies evaluating the clearance of fluorescent gel in periodontal pockets reveals loss of most of the gel in the first 5 minutes after application (Oosterwaal, Mikx, & Renggli, 1990). The need for a delivery system capable of retaining chemotherapeutic agents at high concentrations for extended periods led to the development of controlled-release devices.

## CONTROLLED-RELEASE DEVICES

A sustained release device, or controlled-release delivery, is a system designed to prolong retention of chemotherapeutic agents in periodontal pockets and ensure a regular and steady release of the agent at therapeutic levels. Controlled-release devices theoretically produce more constant and prolonged concentration profiles when compared to systemic and topical applications (AAP, 1994c). This method of delivery is probably beneficial not only because of the chemical effects subgingivally, but because it eliminates the need for self-care requiring client compliance. Many delivery systems have been studied including dialysis tubing, acrylic strips, biodegradable copolymers and drug-filled hollow fibers. These devices have been evaluated with various chemotherapeutic agents including chlorhexidine, metronidazole, ofloxacin, and sanguarine. Most agents and systems reduce gingival bleeding; however, acrylic strips and dialysis tubing with metronidazole showed improved attachment levels and pocket reduction respectively (Addy, Hassan, Moran, Wade, & Newcombe, 1988; Wan Yusof, Newman, Strahan, & Coventry, 1984).

## Tetracycline Fiber Therapy

Although other sustained release devices are expected to be released in the future, to date, only tetracycline fiber therapy is federally approved for clinical use because studies have provided sufficient evidence of efficacy and safety. An advantage of the tetracycline being administered via a fiber as compared to systemic administration is the high concentration of antibiotic that can be placed at the site. Apparently the concentrations in plasma are lower than the systemic route which means controlled delivery minimizes risks of side effects (Rethman, Rethman, & Suzuki, 1995). Tetracycline fiber therapy is capable of reducing pocket depths and bleeding, while increasing attachment. Tetracycline and its derivatives (minocycline and doxycycline) are active, in vitro, against *Actinobacillus actinomycetemcomitans, Porphyromonas gingivalis,* and *Prevotella intermedia.*

**Research Findings.** Research falls into two categories: 1) studies comparing fiber placement to mechanical instrumentation, and 2) studies comparing mechanical instrumentation with and without fiber placement. Goodson and others (1991a & b) conducted a multicenter clinical trial to evaluate the efficacy and safety of tetracycline fibers placed in 113 subjects with adult periodontitis. The subjects were monitored for 3 months with clinical probing and DNA probes were employed to monitor putative pathogens. Diseased sites received one of the three treatments of tetracycline fiber, control fiber, scaling; or no treatment. Results indicate significant improvements in pocket depth reduction, bleeding reduction, and attachment gain with the use of tetracycline fibers. Microbial results indicated that tetracycline fiber and scaling therapies decreased periodontal pathogens except *Actinobacillus actinomycetemcomitans* (Goodson,

Tanner, McArdle, Dix, & Watanabe, 1991). Mandell and others (1986) also reported that fibers did not eliminate *Actinobacillus actinomycetemcomitans* in those with juvenile periodontitis. Possibly these organisms did not respond because they were tissue invasive or because clients had tetracycline-resistant bacteria.

Heijl and others (1991) studied three treatment modalities: tetracycline fibers, scaling, and a combination of fibers and scaling. Sites examined had 6 mm pocket depth or greater and bleeding upon probing. Pocket depth, bleeding upon probing, gingival index measurement, and microbial results were compared at baseline, day 20, and at day 62. The combined therapy of fibers and scaling appeared to be superior over other treatment as evidenced by elimination of *Bacteriodes*, the greatest reduction in viable microbial counts, the complete elimination of bleeding upon probing, and a greater reduction in gingival index. The authors note that these differences, however, were generally not statistically significant. While the results are promising, they call for the initiation of long-term studies.

Newman, Kornman, and Doherty (1994) compared scaling and root planing alone to tetracycline fiber therapy and scaling and root planing in the treatment of localized recurrent periodontitis sites in maintenance clients. Probing depth, bleeding upon probing, and clinical attachment levels were measured on 113 subjects at baseline and one, three, and six months. At one, three, and six months, adjunctive fiber therapy was significantly better ($p < 0.5$) in reducing pocket depth, and reducing bleeding on probing, than scaling and root planing alone. At six months, fiber therapy was significantly better in promoting clinical attachment gain. While all these parameters were statistically significant, it is questionable as to the clinical significance, as differences between treatment groups when comparing probing depth (0.73) and clinical attachment level (0.48) were less than 1 mm in both cases. In contrast, Drisko and others (1994) reported no significant difference in probing depth or clinical attachment when they compared fiber placement, fiber placement and scaling, and scaling over a one-year period.

Only one study with a limited sample size has been conducted evaluating antibiotic resistance of the subgingival microflora when using tetracycline fiber therapy (Goodson & Tanner, 1992). Results indicate no increase in the resistance of gram-negative periodontal organisms to tetracycline, penicillin, or erythromycin after placement of locally-delivered tetracycline. Further study will certainly follow.

**Clinical Application.** Commercially available intrapocket fibers are composed of a 23 cm (9 inch) ethylene vinyl acetate copolymer loaded with 12.7 mg of tetracycline hydrochloride (Actisite™ by Proctor & Gamble). One fiber can treat two or three teeth depending on pocket depth and topography. Typically, t-fibers are indicated as a periodontal maintenance procedure for sites with probing depths of 5 mm or greater accompanied by bleeding upon probing. Use of the periodontal fiber during initial scaling and root planing/debridement represents overtreatment, as deposit removal and self-care are likely to arrest the disease process (Rethman, Rethman, & Suzuki, 1995). Placement of fibers in the distal pockets of terminal molars, pockets less than or equal to 5 mm, and pockets with restricted access or furcations can be difficult. Contraindications for placement include sensitivity to tetracycline, allergy to tetracyclines, acute periodontal abcesses, oral candadiasis (or a history of), and pregnant or lactating women (Rethman, Rethman, & Suzuki, 1995). To date, placement in children is not currently approved.

The manufacturer (Proctor & Gamble) recommends that if multiple sites are indicated, one side of the mouth be treated first to allow for eating on the other side and self-care in all other areas. A gingival retraction cord packing instrument is used to apply fibers in successive layers (see Figure 14-5). The deepest sites are filled first. Once the fiber is moistened in the mouth, it becomes less stiff and more pliable. Floss threaders can be used to pass the fibers between teeth. Any portion of fiber remaining after the pockets have been filled to 1 mm below the gingival margin is trimmed with scissors. After the pockets are filled and excess material trimmed away, a thin layer of cyanoacylate adhesive is placed over the fibers along the gingival margin to hold the delivery system in place. Petroleum jelly should be applied to the client's lips and areas adjacent to fiber placement to avoid contact of the adhesive in these areas.

Time required to place fibers varies from 5 to 20 minutes per site depending on pocket depth, tooth position, need for local anesthesia, and experience of the operator. Assistance with placement is recommended. Fibers are left in position for ten days before removal, and typically, the fiber protrudes from the pocket and is visible at the gingival margin at this time. Care should be taken to remove the fiber in one piece; and if not, residual fiber pieces must be located and removed. Fibers lost prior to day 7 should be replaced. Greenstein (1995) recommends that the client be placed on chlorhexidine rinse during the ten-day period. To date, adverse reactions appear uncommon. The following problems have been noted in fewer than 1 percent of the clients: oral candadiasis, glossitis, allergic response, staining of tongue, pain, severe gingival inflammation, and minor throat irritation (Rethman, Rethman, & Suzuki, 1995). Table 14-5 provides the reader with an overview of the fiber placement procedure. An instructional videotape is also available from the manufacturer. To enhance effectiveness, it might be useful for a client to receive postoperative instructions in writing. It is prudent to telephone the client's insurance provider prior to placement to check on coverage and to request information about proper filing of the claim. Some states do acknowledge that fiber placement by a dental hygienist is within the legal scope of the state Practice Act. Other states are in the process clarifying the hygienist's role in this mode of therapy. The procedure code to use when filing insurance claims is "04381."

## Future Directions

The improvement in attachment levels with controlled-release metronidazole has been previously mentioned. The clinical effects of dialysis tubing with 0.5 percent metronidazole and subgingival irrigation with 0.2 percent chlorhexidine were compared in those with periodontitis (Wan Yusof, Newman, Strahan, & Coventry, 1984). Both treatments reduced the signs of periodontitis, but a greater pocket depth reduction was reported with the metronidazole than with the chlorhexidine. In 1988, a study was conducted in seventy-five subjects over a three-month period. Participants with at least one periodontal pocket received treatment with either chlorhexidine, tetracycline, metronidazole, root planing, or no treatment. Both root planing and controlled-release metronidazole improved attachment levels when compared to chlorhexidine and controlled-release tetracycline.

Chlorhexidine and ofloxacin have also been studied. Chlorhexidine released from an ethyl cellulose matrix was maintained for fourteen days and showed significant reductions in motile bacteria (Soskolne, Golomb, Friedman, & Sela, 1983). Placement of dialysis tubing with 20 percent chlorhexidine reduced gingival bleeding, crevicular fluid flow, and discomfort in nine of eleven subjects treated for only seven days (Coventry & Newman, 1982). Ofloxacin is a synthetic antibiotic which has been shown to alter the subgingival flora when used in a controlled-release device (Higashi et al., 1990). A periodon-

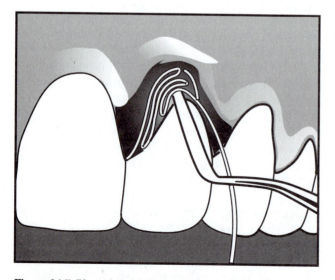

**Figure 14-5** Placement of the periodontal fiber in layers.

**Table 14-5 Periodontal Fiber Placement (Actisite™)**

| Step | Information |
|---|---|
| Armamentarium | Fiber, adhesive and applicator, cotton pliers, petroleum jelly, cotton swabs, scissors, gingival retraction cord packer, probe, mouth mirror, gauze, cotton rolls, floss threaders |
| Placement | 1. Anesthesia is usually not necessary.<br>2. Isolate the area.<br>3. Cut the fiber 3 inches long.<br>4. Place through one interproximal space.<br>5. Guide fiber around the lingual side of tooth.<br>6. Pull through the other interproximal space. Use a floss threader with tight contacts.<br>7. Place one end of the fiber in the deepest portion of the pocket to anchor it.<br>8. Use the gingival retraction cord packer to place the fiber under the gingival margin.<br>9. Layer the fiber within the pocket.<br>10. Use additional segments of fiber when needed.<br>11. Fill the pocket with the fiber to within 1 mm of the gingival margin.<br>12. Trim emerging fiber.<br>13. Avoid overfill, which is indicated by blanching of the gingiva.<br>14. If suppuration is present, fill the pocket loosely with the fiber.<br>15. With a furcation, place a separate fiber in the defect first. Place another fiber in the pocket. |
| Adhesive Placement | 1. Dry tooth; do not overdry.<br>2. Use applicator to apply to the margin.<br>3. Use small drops on the lingual surface first.<br>4. Try not to contact tip with blood or saliva as it will clog the tip.<br>5. With multiple sites, work from the posterior to the anterior. Apply a small amount of adhesive to keep the fiber in place. Then place more adhesive on each site.<br>6. Apply petroleum jelly to site while it is setting. Adhesive sets in 1 minute. |
| Education | Let the client know:<br>1. Not to dislodge the fiber by chewing or self-care.<br>  • Avoid hard, crusty, or sticky foods—peanuts, chips, gum, ice.<br>  • Brush and use interdental aid as recommended except in the fiber sites.<br>2. That gingival shrinkage might make the fiber visible.<br>3. If fiber is lost before seven days, it should be replaced. Telephone the office/clinic.<br>4. Reappointment for removal is needed within ten days.<br>5. Antimicrobial rinse instructions (if professionally recommended). |
| Removal | 1. No anesthetic is necessary.<br>2. Use a curet and/or cotton pliers to remove fiber.<br>3. Flush with water.<br>4. Check distending tissue with air and explorer for any residual calculus.<br>5. Avoid chewing around area for 24 hours. |

tal pocket insert containing 10 percent ofloxacin was compared against a control insert to evaluate its effect on adult periodontitis (Yamagami, Takamori, Sakamoto, & Okada, 1992). Ofloxacin was significantly effective in reducing the plaque index, gingival index, bleeding upon probing, and pocket depth in forty-three subjects. In this study, no mechanical debridement was performed; the only treatment was self-care instruction, and the insert was applied once a week for four weeks.

Nonsteroidal anti-inflammatory drugs (NSAIDs) show promising results for the future. Topically applied, flurbiprofen reduces acute inflammation and alveolar bone loss in beagle dogs (Williams et al., 1988). Others have studied the effects of topical application of meclofenamic acid and ibuprofen in bone loss (Kornman, Blodgett, Brunsvold, & Holt, 1990) and flurbiprofen in a biodegradable subgingival delivery system (Yewey et al., 1991). Rethman and others (1995) point out that it is not unreasonable to expect 2-, 3-, or 4-"tier" controlled-release systems that would deliver agents at selected intervals. For example, the first agent such as tetracycline would be delivered for seven to ten days to control bacteria and the second agent such as NSAID would be released between days 10 to 21 to modulate host responses. The AAP (1994c) states that future research on controlled-release devices will focus on two things:

1. The development of more ideal polymer systems for the local treatment of periodontal disease, and
2. The integration of new bacterial and host modulators into controlled-delivery systems.

## SYSTEMIC ANTIBIOTICS

Use of systemic antibiotics in conjunction with nonsurgical or surgical therapy may be indicated for aggressive forms of periodontitis. Although the dental hygienist will not be responsible for writing prescriptions for systemic antibiotics, a general knowledge of indications and side effects of these drugs will contribute to the success of NSPT for those clients in need of this type of therapy. Antibiotics used in the management of aggressive forms of periodontitis include penicillins, tetracycline-HCl and its derivatives, metronidazole, ciprofloxacin, and clindamycin. Table 14-6 reviews target pathogens, mode of action, resistant strains, side effects, and recommendations for therapy for each antibiotic. To assure optimal concentrations of an antibiotic in the cervicular area, the prescription should be developed considering the highest recommended dose of the antibiotic(s) (Slots & Rams, 1990). When appropriate and feasible, identification of pathogenic organisms along with sensitivity testing should be incorporated into the care plan (APA, 1993a; Morganstein, Blank, & Hasler, 1994).

Success in application of antibiotics to periodontal therapy depends on the following six factors (Morganstein, Blank, & Hasler, 1994):

1. The diagnosis suggests a high probability that impaired host defense mechanisms exist. This application is relevant to all categories of periodontitis except chronic adult periodontitis, which rarely may be managed with antibiotic therapy in conjunction with mechanical therapy.
2. The pathogen must be identified by either culture and sensitivity testing, DNA probing, and/or immunofluorescent testing (see Chapter 3).
3. The pathogen must be susceptible to the antibiotic; potentially more than one pathogen may infect a single periodontal site.
4. The pathogen must not become resistant to the antibiotic. A substantial number of microorganisms in refractory periodontitis are resistant to common antibiotics.
5. The pathogens need to be exposed to effective concentrations of the antibiotic.
6. Minimal side effects; no antibiotic is free of potential side effects.

The use of antibiotics in the treatment of periodontitis should always follow accepted pharmacological principles. If a client has had multiple exposures to tetracycline derivatives or exposure to multiple antibiotics within the past two years, antibiotic resistance may present a problem. Kornman, Newman, and Wilson (1992)

recommend that these individuals should be evaluated for antibiotic susceptibility by means of culture and susceptibility studies.

Combination antibiotic protocols are being considered because of the potential of reaching a broader spectrum of microorganisms. The dosage of each antibiotic when used in combination, is decreased when compared to each antibiotic used separately. Also, the duration of administration may also be less when antibiotics are combined than when each is prescribed alone. Caution must be exercised to ensure the recommended combination does not have negative interactions. For example, tetracycline should not be administered with either penicillin or ciprofloxacin. Table 14-7 provides the reader with example combination regimes and the targeted microorganism(s) (Rams & Slots, 1992).

Clients manifesting systemic diseases that are risk factors to periodontitis should be evaluated carefully prior to recommending systemic antibiotic therapy. Those with LGE and/or NUP in the HIV-positive individual are at risk for potential overgrowth of *candida albicans* and other associated microflora when antibiotics are used. On the other hand, metronidazole has been recommended to prevent overgrowth of *candida* in the management of LGE and NUP lesions (APA, 1994b). Also, sending biohazardous material to laboratories for pathogen identification is not recommended due to the risk it places on those in diagnostic facilities. Chairside diagnosis of pathogens with DNA probes is a consideration. A consultation with the client's physician and identification of pathogens are necessary before therapy is initiated. Persons with diabetes are reported to have *P. intermedia* and *C. rectus* in sites where attachment loss is clinically observed. Also, *P. melaninogenicus, F. nucleatum,* and *E. corrodens* are usually present (Mandell, Dirienzo, Kent, Joshipura, & Haber, 1992). Because of the depressed immune response, myelosuppressed cancer patients need pathogen identification as well as a medical consultation prior to oral health care. Typically, bacteria that are prevalent in the periodontal tissues of the myelosuppressed individual with cancer are *Klebsiella* species, *Pseudomonas* species, enteric rods, *Staphylococcus* species, and *Candida* species (Slots & Rams, 1991).

Currently, studies have not compared the long-term efficacy of locally delivered and systemic administration of antibiotics (Greenstein, 1995). Each route of delivery has advantages and disadvantages. Local delivery of antibiotics are less likely to induce the adverse side effects previously mentioned. Also, higher concentrations of the antibiotic are delivered to the site, and patient compliance with a specific regime is not a factor. On the other hand, the systemic route delivers the antibiotic to the gingival crevicular fluid thereby reaching the base of the periodontal pocket. Many sites can be treated at once versus the need to place periodontal fibers at each site. Also, with the systemic route, bacterial reservoirs on the tongue, tonsils, and saliva are also treated, the antibiotic is delivered *into* the tissues to suppress *A. actinomyceten-*

**Table 14-6 Antibiotics Used in Periodontal Therapy**

| Antibiotic | Active Against | Mode of Action | Duration | Resistant Strains | Side Effects |
|---|---|---|---|---|---|
| Penicillin Derivatives (Amoxycillin, Ampicillin, and Augmentin®) | • Most gram-positive<br>• Many gram-negative anaerobic and anaerobic bacteria | • bactericidal<br>• inhibits bacterial cell wall synthesis | 7 to 14 days | *A. actinomycetemcomitans*<br>*P. micros*<br>*F. nucleatum*<br>*C. rectus*<br>*E. corrodens* | • anaphylactic reaction<br>• drug hypersensitivity<br>• discolored tongue, glossitis, increased thirst, candidiasis, stomatitis<br>• anemia, increased bleeding time<br>• mild to severe gastrointestinal disturbances<br>• headache<br>• vaginal yeast infections<br>• decreased efficacy of oral contraceptives in women<br>• decreased antimicrobial effectiveness of tetracyclines, erythromycins, and lincomycins |
| Tetracycline | • Most periodontal pathogens | • bacteriostatic<br>• binds to the bacterial ribosome<br>• inhibits protein synthesis | 21 days | *Candida* species<br>*Pseudomones* species<br>*Staphylococcus* species<br>*E. corrodens*<br>*P. micros*<br>*P. intermedia* | • teratigenic<br>• bind to forming mineralized tissues (contraindicated for pregnant women and those with developing teeth)<br>• increase impact of anticoagulant therapy<br>• photosensitivity<br>• dermatitis, rash<br>• adsorption inhibited by dairy products, foods, or drugs containing magnesium, calcium, and antacids<br>• decreased efficacy of oral contraceptives in women |
| Metronidazole | • spirochetes and anaerobic bacteria | • targets DNA synthesis at low oxidation-reduction potentials | 7 to 10 days | *A. actinomycetemcomitans*<br>*E. corrodens* | • produces an "antabuse" reaction in those who consume alcoholic beverages<br>• nausea<br>• gastroenteritis<br>• unpleasant metallic taste<br>• dry mouth, glossitis, stomatitis<br>• may increase effect of anticoagulant therapy due to killing of bacteria involved in the synthesis of vitamin K<br>• headache, dizziness, and other CNS effects<br>• carcinogenicity in animals |
| Ciprofloxacin | • gram-positive and gram-negative facilitative bacteria | • bactericidal<br>• does not affect beneficial species consistent with periodontal health (oral streptococci) | 7 to 10 days | *F. nucleatum*<br>*C. rectus*<br>*P. intermedia*<br>*Candida* species | • candidiasis<br>• gastroenteritis<br>• vaginal yeast infection, photosensitivity<br>• unpleasant taste<br>• decreased absorption of sodium bicarbonate<br>• increased action of caffeine |
| Clindamycin (substituted for penicillin in individuals hypersensitive to penicillin*) | • anaerobic bacteria | • bacteriostatic<br>• binds to the bacterial ribosome<br>• inhibits protein synthesis | 7 to 10 days | *E. corrodens*<br>*A. actinomycetemcomitans* | • candidiasis<br>• serious or fatal pseudomembranous ulcerative colitis caused by overgrowth of *clostridium difficile*<br>• decreases action of erythromycin |

*Erythromycin is probably not a viable substitute for penicillin-allergic individuals because most putative periodontal pathogens are resistant to it.

**Table 14-7  Combination Antibiotic Therapy**

| Antibiotics | Dosages and Targets |
|---|---|
| Augmentin® and Metronidazole | 250 mg each t.i.d. 7 days A.a. and P.m. Gram-negative anaerobes |
| Amoxicillin and Metronidazole | 375 mg amoxicillin 250 mg metronidazole t.i.d. for 7 days A.a. |
| Amoxicillin and Metronidazole | 375 mg amoxicillin 250 mg metronidazole t.i.d. for 7 days A.a. and P.g. |
| Ciprofloxacin and Metronidazole | 500 mg each b.i.d. 8 days enterics and pseudomonads facilitative anaerobes |
| Clindamycin and Ciprofloxacin | 300 mg clindamycin 500 mg ciprofloxacin b.i.d. for 8 days P.m. |

Key: *A.a.* = *A. actinomycetemcomitans*, *P.m.* = *P. micros*, *P.g.* = *P. gingivalis*.

(Reprinted with permission from "Antibiotics in Periodontal Therapy: An Update," by T. E. Rams and J. Slots, 1992, *Compendium of Continuing Education in Dentistry, 13*, pp. 1130–1145)

*comitans*, less expense is involved, and combination therapy of antibiotics can be recommended (Greenstein, 1995).

## GINGIVAL CURETTAGE

Gingival curettage, or closed curettage, was widely accepted and utilized in the mid 1900s in an attempt to promote new connective tissue attachment. Gingival curettage is a closed procedure and refers to debriding the soft tissue wall of a periodontal pocket (AAP, 1989b). It may be accomplished manually with sharp curets or by the use of chemicals to facilitate tissue removal. Frequently, the soft tissue lining of the pocket may be unintentionally removed during scaling and root planing with hand or ultrasonic instruments and is referred to as incidental or inadvertent curettage. Incidental curettage can be a normal sequelae to instrumentation and is very different from deliberate curettage. Based on current knowledge of periodontal tissue responses to therapy, the necessity of the procedure is highly questioned. Several studies report no additional benefit by the use of curettage in conjunction with or following scaling and root planing (Echeverra & Caffesse, 1983; Hill et al., 1981; Knowles et al., 1979). It has further been determined that new connective tissue attachment as a result of **soft tissue curet-**

**tage** is precluded by the formation of a long junctional epithelium (Caton & Zander, 1979). Pocket reduction achieved following soft tissue curettage alone is accomplished by tissue shrinkage and reattachment of junctional epithelium rather than by new connective tissue attachment.

Procedurally, mechanical soft tissue curettage is accomplished by anesthetizing the soft tissues and activating a sharp curet at greater than a 90° angle to the tissue wall. Digital pressure is applied to the external gingiva to provide support against scaling pressures. The blade is then moved along the gingival lining, thereby removing the epithelium of the pocket lining. Antiformin, a concentrated alkaline sodium hypochlorite solution, has been investigated as a means of chemically facilitating soft tissue curettage. The solution is delivered to the pocket by means of a medicament loop or curet. The loop or curet is inserted and traced along the pocket wall for 1 minute. Subsequently, citric acid (5 percent) is applied in the same manner for a minimum of 15 seconds to neutralize the antiformin. The area is flushed with water and the resulting gelatinous tissue is easily removed with six to eight strokes of a curet (Kalkwarf, Tussing, & Davis, 1982). Introduced in 1913, antiformin was believed to be an epithelium specific solvent (Hecker, 1913). Later investigations discovered the effects of antiformin were not limited to epithelium and in fact it was found capable of denaturing connective tissue (Kalkwarf, Tussing, & Davis, 1982). Indications and contraindications for chemical curettage are similar to those applied to soft tissue curettage. Chemical curettage is additionally contraindicated in deep pockets (greater than 6 mm), in infrabony pockets and in furcation areas due to an inability to control the solution in these sites. Like mechanical soft tissue curettage, no additional benefit is achieved by the use of chemical curettage as an adjunct or supplement to scaling and root planing (Forgas & Gound, 1986; Lopez & Belvederessi, 1977).

In a survey about teaching gingival curettage in dental hygiene curricula, it was noted that 80 percent taught the procedure (DeVore, Hicks, Whitacre, & Clancy-Schertel, 1993). Reasons cited for inclusion in the curriculum include increased lecture materials, increased utilization leading to a need to achieve clinical competence, an increased emphasis on nonsurgical treatment, a strong belief in bacterial invasion, and a requirement for state licensure. Schools that did not include soft tissue curettage in the curriculum cited the following reasons: conflicting research and questionable benefits, effectiveness of root planing alone, that the procedure is outdated or illegal, that it is not taught to clinical competence, or the increased use of ultrasonics.

In conclusion, the viability of soft tissue curettage was questioned in the 1980s. It is reasonable to assume that quadrant scaling and root planing with curettage as a routine procedure in the treatment of routine adult periodontitis is not warranted. The American Academy of Periodontology (1989c) did call for more evaluation of this procedure to determine its appropriateness in the treatment of compromised clients, maintenance debridement of localized sites of recalcitrated periodontitis, treatment of juvenile periodontitis, and other types of periodontitis when esthetics is of concern. Its usefulness and therapeutic value has been replaced by new, more effective means of promoting pocket reduction and soft tissue attachment. The availability of site-specific drug therapies and guided tissue regeneration offer improved and more predictable results that supersede the use of soft tissue curettage.

## OVERHANG REMOVAL

The effects of dental restorations on periodontal tissues are frequently overlooked (see Chapter 4). Overhanging margins of dental restorations have been implicated as the primary iatrogenic cause of periodontal disease. An overhanging margin is an excess of restorative material extending beyond the margin of a cavity preparation. Overhanging margins may be located supragingivally or subgingivally on any tooth surface. They are associated with a variety of restorative materials including amalgam, composite, gold, or porcelain. Interproximal overhangs are primarily attributed to improper placement of the matrix band and wedge. Other causes include improper manipulation of restorative materials, carving errors, and lack of improper restorative finishing technique. Although ideally identified and corrected immediately after placement, many overhangs are left unnoticed or uncorrected. The prevalence of overhanging margins is quite high. It is estimated that between 16 to 76 percent of all restorations exhibit at least one overhanging margin (Coxhead, 1985; Gilmore & Sheiham, 1971; Hakkarainen & Ainamo, 1980; Leon, 1976). The occurrence of overhangs is greater on interproximal surfaces than on facial and lingual surfaces.

### Relationship to Periodontal Disease

The presence of overhangs has been associated with increased inflammation, bleeding, pocket depths, attachment loss, and bone loss (Gilmore & Sheiham, 1971; Jeffcoat & Howell, 1980; Srivastava, 1979). The deleterious effects on periodontal tissues is attributed to increased plaque retention associated with overhang margins rather than a chemical or physical tissue irritation. Hodges and Bowen (1985) studied the effects of removal of Class II, or moderate size overhangs, on plaque accumulation (Plaque Index), gingival inflammation (Gingival Index), and probing depth prior to removal, at two and four weeks after removal. Results showed that removal did contribute to statistically significant decreases in all three parameters. Overhanging margins as small as 0.2 millimeters have been associated with interproximal bone loss (Bjorn, Bjorn, & Grkovic, 1969). A study examining

the prevalence of overhanging margins in posterior amalgam restorations reports 64.3 percent of pockets adjacent to overhang margins were greater than or equal to 3 mm as compared to 23.1 percent of pockets adjacent to unrestored surfaces and 49.2 percent of pockets adjacent to restorations without overhang margins (Pack, Coxhead, & McDonald, 1990). Overhanging margins may jeopardize the periodontal health of adjacent tissues. Periodontal health can be significantly improved by overhang removal procedures sometimes referred to as **margination** (Hodges & Bowen, 1985; Rogo, 1995).

Successful intervention is dependent on successful recognition or diagnosis. The two most commonly used methods of detecting overhanging margins are clinical exploration with a fine explorer or probe and posterior bitewing radiographs. The radiographic appearance of an overhang is shown in Chapter 5. It is reported that of all interproximal overhangs present, 66 to 74 percent are found radiographically and 62 percent are found clinically (Pack, Coxhead, & McDonald, 1990; Gorzo, Newman, & Strahan, 1979). Radiographic detection can be compromised due to the position of the margin in relation to the beam of radiation (horizontal angulation). Likewise clinical detection may be limited by tight embrasure spaces making instrumentation difficult. Clinicians must recognize that neither method is infallible and both should be employed for the best results.

Due to the potential periodontal destruction associated with overhanging margins, recognition and treatment should be an integral component of initial periodontal diagnosis and treatment. Assessment should include the relation of the overhang to the gingiva (supragingival or subgingival) the tooth surface, its size, and the type of restorative material. Extremely large overhanging margins may require replacement of the entire restoration in order to restore serviceability to the client. A system of quantification of the size of an overhang might be useful in deciding need for removal, method of removal, and armamentarium (see Table 14-8 and Chapter 4, Table 4-2). The presence of overhangs should be charted during comprehensive periodontal assessment. Ideally, overhangs should be removed during the control of plaque retentive factors before or during debridement therapy. Removal of overhanging restorations following debridement may adversely affect postoperative healing.

### Procedure for Removal

The two basic methods of overhang removal are hand instrumentation or motor-driven instrumentation. Hand instruments are useful for removing small to moderate sized overhangs with good accessibility. Hand instruments employed for overhang removal include curets, amalgam files, knives, chisels, and finishing strips. Compared to motor driven methods, hand instrumentation can be time-consuming and operator fatiguing.

**Table 14-8  Classification of Overhang by Size**

| Size | Description | Technique Recommendation |
|------|-------------|--------------------------|
| Type I | • Light catch with explorer | Easily removed with hand instruments |
| Type II | • Moderate definitive overhang<br>• Definite catch with explorer<br>• Restorative material extends beyond the cavosurface proximal area<br>• Generally visible radiographically | A variety can be employed:<br>• directional handpiece system<br>• ultrasonics<br>• handheld instruments |
| Type III | • "Gross" overhang<br>• Usually requires replacement of restoration in order to be functionally serviceable to client<br>• When one-half of the interproximal space is filled, it can be considered "gross" | Restorative treatment is indicated |

Conventional high speed handpieces with flame-shaped finishing burs offer a fast and efficient means of overhang removal. Their usefulness, however, is limited to easily accessible areas due to the potential for significant tissue trauma to adjacent soft tissue. A special flame-tipped scaler insert (Roto-pro™) is available for use in a high speed handpiece with water spray. The tip consists of six flat surfaces for adaptation and is designed to operate in the range of 200,000 rpm. Close examination of the effects of this specially designed tip on amalgam, enamel, and cementum reveals smooth amalgam surfaces with little effect on surrounding dental tissue (Givens, Gwinnett, & Boucher, 1984). This tip appears to remove excess amalgam by a chipping rather than cutting or abrading action. This chipping action favorably removes excess amalgam without adverse effects on adjacent soft tissue. Precision control must be utilized for overhang removal with high speed handpieces to avoid ditching or gouging the surface. Additionally, the oscillating action of ultrasonic devices similarly removes amalgam, producing a smooth even surface without adversely affecting adjacent tissue. The water lavage associated with ultrasonic and high speed handpiece use effectively removes debris, but may also interfere with the field of vision.

Slow speed motor-driven handpieces offer a safe well-controlled alternative means for margination. A reciprocating (back and forth) motion slow speed handpiece (Profin Directional Handpiece™, Dentatus USA, Ltd., New York, NY) with a variety of wedged-shaped abrasive tips is specially designed to recontour porcelain, metal, composite, or amalgam restorations. As described by the manufacturer, it can also be used to refine embrasures and fine finish porcelain or metal margins prior to cementation. This system is similar to the original Eva system developed by Dr. Per Axelsson in 1969. The reciprocating handpiece is designed to operate between 5,000 to 6,000 rpm in two modes. The fixed mode provides directional control of movement in one of six indexing positions and is utilized for improved control

and adaptability for interproximal surfaces. The alternative self-steering mode allows the selected tip to rotate on its free axis for prophylaxis and polishing procedures. The system is equipped with a set of color-coded, autoclavable tips with diamond particles of progressive grain sizes for gross removal to fine polishing. The opposite side of each tip is smooth to prevent damage to adjacent tooth and soft tissues. Plastic polishing tips for interproximal surfaces are also available. Studies comparing the directional handpiece system to curets and ultrasonic scalers report results comparable to that achieved by ultrasonic scalers. While the progressively finer diamond tips produce a fine finished surface, it is a time-consuming process. The pros and cons of each system, as well as the unique circumstances surrounding each overhang, must be considered in order to select the best method of removal. A different system might be necessary for a specific overhang in a single client's oral cavity due to size, access, and operator preferences.

Clients requiring antibiotic premedication for oral health care must be premedicated for this procedure. It is important that the procedure, rationale, time, costs alternative treatments, and consequences of foregoing treatment be explained and consent obtained. The explanation of the procedure will include a description of the removal method selected. Overhanging margins should be thoroughly assessed for contraindications prior to recontouring. Contraindications include overhangs that lack proximal contact, exhibit open margins, or are extensive in size, encompassing greater than one-half of the embrasure space.

The first stage of the process is to remove excessive restorative material. This can best be achieved by ultrasonics or use of coarse tips in the directional handpiece system. The cavosurface margin should repeatedly be evaluated with an explorer during the procedure to determine progress and to determine treatment endpoints. Following gross reduction, the overhanging margin is finished and polished until it is smooth and flush at the margin. A flour of pumice slurry applied by slow speed handpiece or dental tape provides a smooth final surface finish. Upon completion, the area should be thoroughly rinsed and evacuated to remove lingering particles. Refer to Table 14-9 for professional recommendations for margination procedure with hand instruments and a directional handpiece system (Profin™) (Rogo, 1995).

# DENTINAL HYPERSENSITIVITY

Alleviating the pain associated with dentinal hypersensitivity is a concern for both clients and clinicians. A variety of treatment strategies have been developed to resolve this problem. To date, no single therapy has been found to be completely effective in all situations. Successful treatment is often dependent on the knowledge and skill of the clinician in selecting a systematic approach to treatment, which provides relief for the individual. For the dental hygienist, dentinal hypersensitivity is a frequently encountered and sometimes frustrating condition to treat.

**Dentinal hypersensitivity** is defined as pain arising from exposed dentin, typically in response to thermal, mechanical, chemical, or osmotic stimuli that cannot be explained as arising from any other form of dental defect or pathology (Addy & Urquhart, 1992). Although a variety of stimuli may provoke a painful response, studies report approximately 75 percent of patients experience sensitivity to cold and 29 percent to mechanical stimuli (Orchardson, 1987). As the definition suggests, an important aspect in the management of dentinal hypersensitivity is an accurate diagnosis. Dental conditions or pathologies that mimic the symptoms of dentinal hypersensitivity include caries, fractured restorations, and chipped or cracked tooth syndrome.

**Table 14-9  Recommended Margination Procedure with Hand Instruments and a Directional Handpiece System (Profin™)**

| Method | Armamentarium | Suggested Sequence of Removal for Amalgam Restorations |
|---|---|---|
| Hand | 1. Burs<br>  • Diamond or finishing<br>    a. Use for large excess of amalgam<br>    b. Use first where access permits without damage to adjacent tooth or gingival tissue<br>2. Files<br>  • Working files (Hirschfeld files 5/11 and/or 3/7)<br>    a. Use file for removal of bulk<br>    b. Use on the proximal surfaces of posterior and anterior teeth<br>  • Finishing file (Bedbug B46)<br>    a. Use for refinement of cavosurface margin<br>3. Gold Knives<br>  • Use on proximal surfaces of posterior and anterior teeth<br>  • Use on buccal and lingual surfaces<br>  • Use on gingival cavosurface margins<br>  • Use for moderate to slight excess of amalgam<br>4. Curets<br>  • Use to shave or smooth amalgam surface; area specific or universals are used.<br>5. Cuttle Discs<br>  • Use on accessible surfaces on facial and lingual<br>  • Use to refine and smooth amalgam surfaces on proximals<br>6. Abrasive Strips (finishing)<br>  • Use on proximal surfaces of posterior and anterior teeth<br>  • Use to smooth cavosurface margins on the proximal<br>  • Use to smooth amalgam surfaces on the proximal<br>7. Dental Tape and Pumice<br>  • Use on proximal surfaces of teeth to check contact and smoothness<br>  • Use floss in conjunction with pumice to create a smooth, shiny surface<br>8. Explorer and Dental Floss<br>  • Use to check for smoothness of the cavosurface margin | 1. Remove bulk of excess restorative material in proximal area. Use shaving strokes starting at the base and exterior surface of the restorative material. Work from the most apical portion of the overhang toward the contact area.<br>2. Establish smooth and continuous relationship between the tooth surface and the restorative material.<br>3. Maintain and/or create functional anatomy of the proximal areas (embrasures). The angulation of the gold knives, burs, or discs will be critical. |

*(continues)*

**Table 14-9  (continued)**

| Method | Armamentarium | Suggested Sequence of Removal for Amalgam Restorations |
|---|---|---|
| Directional Handpiece Profin™ (Dentatus USA, Ltd., New York, NY) | 1. Supercoarse or coarse tip<br>  • Select depending on the amount of amalgam to be removed<br>  • Color-coding helps identify abrasiveness<br>2. Medium to superfine tips<br>3. Plastic tips<br>4. Handpiece<br>5. Awareness of the modes that can be used for removal and polishing of the surface. Refer to manufacturer's instructions. | 1. Place tip into handpiece in one of the six indexing positions.<br>2. To determine the best position for the tip, hold the handpiece close to the area where amalgam will be removed.<br>3. Move the tip in the handpiece until the abrasive side of the tip is adapted to the amalgam.<br>4. Work from the facial embrasure toward the contact.<br>5. Activate handpiece prior to applying it.<br>6. Use light pressure and continual movement.<br>7. Use for a short time period and evaluate removal.<br>8. Once the facial aspect is completed, repeat on the lingual side.<br>9. Files might be needed should the tip not reach the midline of the interproximal area.<br>10. To smooth the surface, use tips in succession from medium to superfine.<br>11. Polish using a hollow tip filled with a pumice slurry. Place tip in the reciprocating movement by partial insertion. The movement of this tip for polishing is different than the fixed mode used for previous steps.<br>12. Rinse and use another tip filled with a tin oxide slurry. |

## Prevalence and Etiology

Dentinal hypersensitivity occurs in approximately one in seven dentate adults (Orchardson, 1987). Although frequently associated with older populations, virtually one-half of all individuals affected are under age 30. Sensitivity may occur at any site on any tooth, but is commonly associated with the buccal or lingual surface at or below the gingival margin of canine and premolar teeth. Dentinal hypersensitivity is often evidenced in areas of exposed dentin. Exposure to the oral environment occurs as a result of enamel or cementum loss or gingival recession caused by attrition, abrasion, erosion, or a combination of these factors. The common resulting sensitivity in buccal cervical areas illustrates the role of toothbrush abrasion as a contributing factor. Improper or overzealous brushing and/or use of bristles that are not rounded have been shown to cause cervical abrasion. Additionally, dietary acids such as citrus fruits and juices, wine and fruit yogurt may erode enamel or cementum exposing underlying dentin (Addy, Absi, & Adams, 1987).

Of particular interest to the dental hygienist is the dentinal sensitivity experienced by some clients following scaling and root planing therapy. Sensitivity resulting from scaling and root planing typically develops one week after treatment. This iatrogenic sensitivity can be explained by the presence of a smear layer accompanying scaling and root planing. A smear layer is formed when dentin is cut or abraded. Close microscopic examination of the root surfaces after scaling and root planing reveals the resulting smear layer. This smear layer is an organic matrix of hard tissue composed of cementum, dentin, and calculus smeared but not completely removed from the root surface. Over a period of a week, toothbrushing and normal oral function removes the smear layer exposing underlying dentinal tubules. Scaling and root planing associated dentinal hypersensitivity may resolve via natural desensitization mechanisms (secondary dentin formation and tubule obliteration) in a two to four week period or may require professional intervention. It is important to note the effect a new approach to periodontal therapy may have on the incidence of dentinal hypersensitivity. A growing body of evidence suggests vigorous root planing for the removal of "disease altered" cementum may constitute overinstrumentation and, in fact, hinder healing (Drisko, 1993;

Fukazawa & Nishimura 1994; Nyman, Westfelt, Sarhed, & Karring, 1988). A new approach to nonsurgical therapy recommends that removal of cementum be confined to superficial cemental curettage. This approach may theoretically reduce post-therapy hypersensitivity by maintaining the protective cemental layer. Refer to Chapter 10 for more information on scaling and root planing philosophy.

While hypersensitivity is characterized by the presence of exposed dentin, not all exposed dentin is sensitive. Dentin exposure is just one variable in the equation. The presence of cervical abrasion and gingival recession resulting in exposed dentin does not dictate the presence of dentinal hypersensitivity. Why then do some patients with exposed dentin experience painful sensitivity while others do not? The answer lies in an understanding of the etiology of the disease.

The most widely accepted theory describing the mechanism of pain production associated with dentinal hypersensitivity is **Brannstrom's hydrodynamic theory** (Brannstrom, 1986; Gillam, 1995; Hodosh, Hodosh, & Hodosh, 1994). According to this theory, a stimulus, such as cold, applied at the dentinal surface causes fluid within the dentinal tubules to move toward the pulp. This fluid movement displaces or disturbs the pulpal nerve endings causing pain. Differences between sensitive and nonsensitive exposed dentin is associated with differences in the tubules. Scanning electron microscopic examination of exposed dentin reveals eight times more open dentinal tubules in sensitive dentin as compared to nonsensitive dentin. In addition, the diameter of open tubules in sensitive dentin was twice that of nonsensitive dentin (Absi, Addy, & Adams, 1987). These observations may also explain the episodic nature of dentinal sensitivity. Clients experiencing sensitivity fall into two broad categories. Some experience only localized sensitivity of sudden and intense pain. Others experience generalized sensitivity with various degrees of pain over time. Based on our current understanding, dentinal hypersensitivity represents a dynamic equilibrium shifting from periods of sensitivity associated with numerous wide, open tubules and hyperemic pulpal response to periods of remission typified by few, narrow open tubules and weak sensory nerve involvement.

## Current Perspectives on Treatment of Dentinal Hypersensitivity

The primary concern for patients experiencing dentinal hypersensitivity is pain relief. Pain associated with dentinal hypersensitivity is commonly short in duration, sharp in nature, and usually occurs in response to specific stimuli (Addy, 1990). Research regarding the etiology and factors contributing to hypersensitivity has resulted in a variety of treatment options. Patients rely on the knowledge and skill of the practitioner to select the best treatment. This professional decision is further complicated

by the individualized and episodic nature of the disease. A treatment that works for one client may not work for another. In fact, it may be necessary to apply different therapies to different teeth in the same mouth in order to achieve a beneficial response. Clinicians must utilize a systematic approach based on scientifically authenticated information in order to individualize treatment for hypersensitivity.

As previously mentioned in the definition of hypersensitivity, an accurate diagnosis is critical to successful treatment. Caries, cracked tooth syndrome, and fractured or leaking restorations display similar symptoms that mimic the pain associated with dentinal hypersensitivity. Initiating treatment for hypersensitivity in the presence of these conditions is futile. A thorough patient history, radiographic evaluation and clinical exam are all valuable and necessary for making a correct diagnosis. Listening to the client's complaint, however, may provide the best information. Question the client regarding where the pain occurs, how much it hurts, how long the pain lasts, and if sensitivity results from hot or cold beverages, or cold air. In some cases the individual may be able to specify which tooth is the problem. If the sensitive tooth can not be isolated, then clinical application of air, cold, or mechanical exploration of exposed dentinal surfaces may help identify the problem.

Once the diagnosis of hypersensitivity is confirmed, the client should be educated regarding the etiology and contributing factors in order to avoid worsening of the problem. Preventive counseling is helpful in avoiding reoccurrence of the problem. The role of toothbrushing in hypersensitivity is well established. A client's brushing technique should be evaluated and modified if needed to prevent tissue damage. Additionally, dental plaque can invade open dentinal tubules and has been implicated as a pain provoking stimulus. Thus, thorough but safe plaque removal by proper brushing of exposed areas is an important preventive measure. It is also important that clients understand the relationship between dietary factors and sensitivity. Frequent ingestion of dietary acids such as citrus foods may contribute to dentinal hypersensitivity. Individuals should be advised that brushing after intake of dietary acids may accelerate the erosion of tooth surface. Therefore, if necessary, brushing should be completed before meals. Treatment is the next step in achieving relief for hypersensitivity. Figure 14-6 represents the decision making process that occurs once hypersensitivity is identified. A variety of commercial products are available for both professional and client applied therapy as listed in Table 14-10.

**Professional Therapies.** The nature and extent of hypersensitivity is an important consideration in selecting an appropriate and effective therapy. Treatment focuses on occluding dentinal tubules or interrupting neural transmission. Localized sensitivity may be best resolved by professional treatment to seal the open dentinal tubules

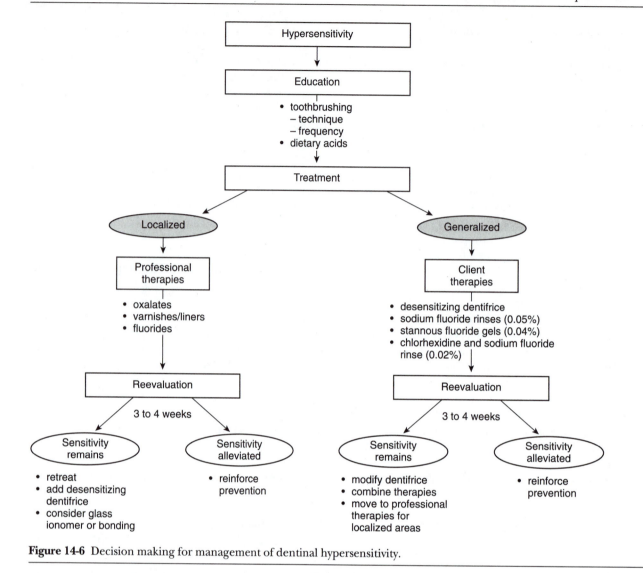

**Figure 14-6** Decision making for management of dentinal hypersensitivity.

of the isolated area. In general, glass ionomers and bonding agents provide longer lasting results than varnishes or liners which are mechanically worn away by brushing and the oral environment. Restorative procedures such as these are warranted when sensitivity persists after use of other therapies. Newly developed oxalates (Protect™ and Sensodyne Sealant Dentin Desensitizing Kit™) are capable of occluding the dentinal tubules because precipitation of crystals block the dentinal tubules and prevent fluid to flow through them (Pashley & Galloway, 1985; Tung & Takagiko, 1990; Yeh et al., 1990); however, longevity is limited due to the vulnerability of the precipitant to mechanical wear. Clinical applications of oxalate salts should include (Muzzin, 1992):

1. Cleansing with a soft toothbrush and a nonabrasive dentifrice if professional therapy has not been performed.
2. Rinsing the area with warm water.

3. Isolation of the area.
4. Drying the teeth with gauze or cotton roll/tip; not air.
5. Application of the agent according to directions.

After application of these agents, use cold water to evaluate the area for reduction of hypersensitivity. The agent can be reapplied immediately, at subsequent visits, or at periodontal maintenance appointments.

Fluorides have been used for many years for the treatment of sensitivity. Precipitation of fluoride ions on the tooth surface can occlude dentinal tubules but is also susceptible to dissolution over time. In general such agents are applied to the tooth surface via a dabbing or burnishing application technique. Recently, lasers have been used to treat dentinal hypersensitivity by creating a smear layer to occlude dentinal tubules. One clinical study reports improved pain tolerance and patient satisfaction after a two-minute treatment exposure with a

**Table 14-10 Commercial Products for Hypersensitivity Therapy**

| Category | Types | Product | Active Ingredient |
|---|---|---|---|
| Professional | Glass Ionomers (Restorative) | Dyract (L.D. Caulk/Dentsply) <br> Fuji II (GC American, Inc.) <br> Geristore (Dent-Mat Corp.) <br> Photac-Fil (ESPE-Premier Sales) <br> Vari-Glass (L.D. Caulk/Dentsply) <br> Vitremer (3M Dental Products) <br> ProBond™ (L.D. Caulk/Dentsply) | polyacrylic acid (approximately 10 to 25%) (mixed with aluminosilicate glass powder) |
| | Bonding Agents (Restorative) | Gluma (Miles) <br> Scotchbond (3M Dental Products) | refer to package insert |
| | Varnishes/Liners | Bibby's <br> Copalite (Bosworth) <br> Zarosen | sodium fluoride <br> solvent mixture and copal resin <br> strontium Chloride (40%) |
| | Oxalates | Protect™ (John O. Butler Co.) <br><br> Sensodyne Sealant Dentin Desensitizing Kit™ (Block Drug) | 3% monohydrogen— monopotassium oxalate <br> ferric oxalate (6%) |
| | Iontophoresis | Various manufacturers | 2% sodium fluoride ion |
| Client | Dentifrices | *Crest Sensitivity Protection <br> *Denquel <br> PreviDent <br> Promise <br> Protect <br> Sensodyne <br> Thermodent | potassium nitrate (5%) <br> potassium nitrate (5%) <br> sodium fluoride (1.1%) <br> potassium nitrate (5%) <br> sodium citrate <br> strontium chloride (10%) <br> strontium chloride (10%) |
| | Stannous Fluoride Gels | Gel Kam <br> Stop | stannous fluoride (0.4%) <br> stannous fluoride (0.4%) |
| | Stannous Fluoride Rinses | PerioMed™ (OMNI) | stannous fluoride (0.63%) |

*ADA Approved

NdYAG laser over a two week period (Renton-Harper & Midda, 1992). The long-term effectiveness and safety of the NdYAG laser was not evaluated in this study and requires additional research before lasers are used for routine treatment of sensitivity.

**Client Therapies.** Comparatively, generalized sensitivity (due to the time and cost effectiveness of professional treatment) often warrants initial therapy utilizing a desensitizing dentifrice. The formulations of available desensitizing dentifrices are designed to occlude dentinal tubules or interfere with neural response (see Table 14-10). The ADA has accepted three categories of dentifrices for desensitizing effectiveness: 1) 10 percent strontium chloride, 2) 5 percent potassium nitrate, and 3) 2 percent dibastic sodium nitrate (AAP, 1989a). Based on the results of clinical investigations, dentifrices containing an abrasive silica capable of occluding dentinal tubules, such as strontium chloride, are the most effective in combating sensitivity (Addy & Urquhart, 1992). The resulting relief achieved by dentifrice use is a slow accumulative process. Therefore, clients should be advised

that beneficial results may not be evident for three to four weeks. If use of the desensitizing dentifrice is successful, clients may return to their regular dentifrice with instructions to return to the desensitizing dentifrice at the first signs of returned sensitivity. Some individuals may require ongoing desensitizing dentifrice use to maintain beneficial effects.

Persons not benefiting from at home use of desensitizing dentifrices may benefit from other client applied therapies. Fluorides have been moderately successful in alleviating dentin sensitivity by stabilizing the dentin surface. Sodium fluoride rinses (0.05 percent) or stannous fluoride gels (0.4 percent) combined with desensitizing dentifrice use may increase efficacy. Fluoride and desensitizing dentifrices should be applied at different times to avoid interaction of the agents. Recently, the combined, sequential use of chlorhexidine (0.12 percent) and sodium fluoride (0.2 percent) rinses used twice daily significantly reduced sensitivity in two to four weeks (Lawson, Gross, Overman, & Anderson, 1991). The prolonged effect of this combined therapy, however, is unknown. Clients not achieving relief from at home therapies should be advised of the professional therapies previously mentioned. Localized or severe sensitivity may require in-office professional therapy combined with at home dentifrice use (Collaert & Fisher, 1991).

## DENTAL IMPLANTS

Modern dental implants are an accepted alternative to conventional techniques for tooth replacement. They are a safe and reliable means of restoring dental function for clients who experience inadequate retention, impaired speech, unpleasant esthetics, pain, soft tissue irritation or psychological problems resulting from partial or complete dentures (Kuebker, 1984 a & b). Although thought of as a product of modern dentistry, various forms of dental implants were used by early Egyptian, Aztec, and Mayan cultures. The emergence of dental implantology as we know it today is delineated by the period from the mid-1930s to the present (Balkin, 1988). The development and use of dental implants has changed rapidly in the past two decades culminating in the most refined and accepted forms currently in use today.

The dental hygienist plays a vital role in education, assessment, and maintenance in implantology. Education includes both the information provided to the client about this option of tooth replacement as well as a general discussion of the surgical procedure. Assessment involves the initial and recurrent evaluations of the implant for health or disease/failure. Maintenance refers to proper professional and self-care needed to prevent failure. Assessment and maintenance contain client education as well. Prior to discussing these responsibilities, background information about the types, structure, and microbiology of implants is addressed.

### Selection Considerations

Implants are recommended for two purposes:

1. To replace teeth for those who are edentulous in one arch or both. This option replaces the need for removable dentures (see Figure 14-7A and B).
2. To replace single or multiple teeth for those who are, thus, partially edentulous. This option replaces the need for a fixed bridge, which involves preparing adjacent, sometimes healthy, teeth (see Figure 14-7C).

Once the client is identified as a potential candidate based on missing teeth, other factors are considered such as systemic health, oral health status, self-care practices, quality and quantity of bone, and the client's needs and desires. It is recognized that these factors are not mutually exclusive.

Systemic health must be scrutinized for any disease(s) that can compromise healing. Uncontrolled dia-

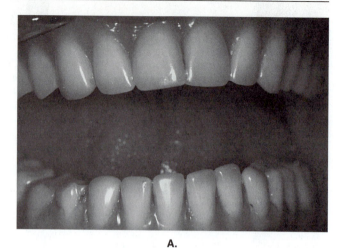

**A.**

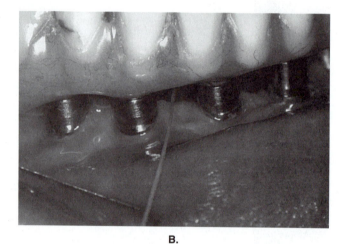

**B.**

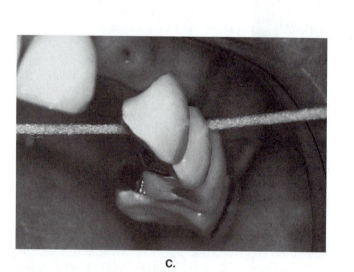

**C.**

**Figure 14-7** Two purposes for implants. (**A**) and (**B**) tooth replacement for edentulous patients, overdentures; (**C**) tooth replacement for partially edentulous patients. The canines and first premolars are implants. A fixture has been placed in the area of the lateral incisor. (Courtesy of Oral-B Laboratories)

betes, blood dyscrasias, or any disease compromising the healing process should be a concern. The oral health of those who are partially edentulous is a consideration in relation to caries activity, gingivitis, and periodontitis. Those who are relatively caries-free and who have stable periodontal health are acceptable candidates, other factors permitting. Self-care habits are important to consider as meticulous control of plaque is mandatory for implant success. Partially edentulous patients should be required to demonstrate effective plaque control around natural teeth before implants are surgically placed. The quality and quantity of bone can be evaluated using periapical, panoramic, and/or computer tomography scans (refer to Chapter 5). When the implant can be placed in cortical bone, there seems to be a greater percentage of implant to mineralized tissue contact than when the implant is placed in cancellous bone (Albrektsson & Sennerby, 1990; Gotfredsen et al., 1991). The client's needs and desires are foremost, as a qualified candidate based on systemic and oral health he might not feel this is the best option for replacing his teeth or current prosthesis. When the client reaches a decision about placement, the surgeon, restorative dentist, and laboratory technician will work as a team to place the implant and construct the prosthesis.

## Types

Implants can be classified according to position, material, and design (Worthington, 1988). Classification according to position delineates three basic implant types (see Figure 14-8A through C). Subperiosteal implants are positioned over the bone. They are used to support removable denture prosthesis. Transosteal implants, sometimes referred to as a staple, are inserted through the bone. Placement of this implant type requires a surgical incision through the anterior mandible to allow passage of the implant from the bottom of the chin up into the mouth. Transosteal implants are generally constructed of gold or vitallium and like subperiosteal implants, are used for denture support. **Endosseous implants** are placed directly in the bone and are the most popular type of implant in use today (Meffert, 1989). Endosseous or endosteal implants are further subclassified into two main forms: blade and root (cylinder) form (see Figure 14-8C). These subclassifications are both utilized as abutments in partially or completely edentulous areas. Root form implants offer a variety of patterns including conical, cylindrical, threaded screw, and perforated or hollow baskets (Worthington, 1988). Root form implants are preferred to blade implants in wide and shallow mandibles (Weiss, 1987).

Materials used to fabricate endosseous implants include polymers, ceramics, and various metals. Titanium is a metal commonly used for implant construction due to its superior biocompatibility. Implant surfaces may be smooth or deliberately roughened to improve the inte-

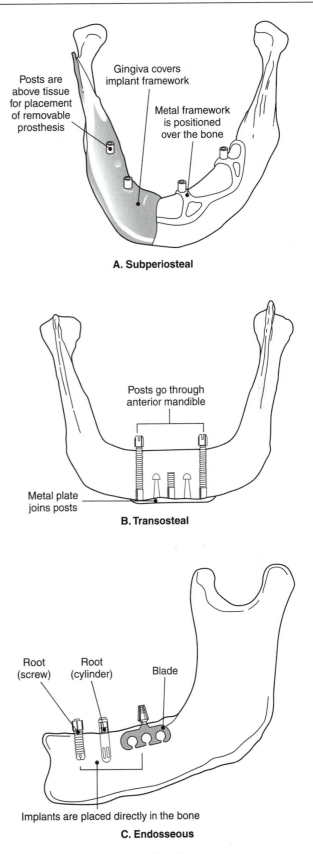

**A. Subperiosteal**

**B. Transosteal**

**C. Endosseous**

**Figure 14-8** Classification of implants.

gration between the implant and bone. Tricalcium phosphate and hydroxyapatite may coat the surface of implants to additionally facilitate bone integration. Selection of implant type should maximize available bone and interface, as well as provide a stable foundation for prosthetic restoration. This is commonly referred to as "loading" the implant.

Implants also differ based on manufacture designs or characteristics. The manufacturer or brand of an implant is referred to as the **implant system**. Implant systems include not only the implant itself, but also the special surgical and restorative equipment necessary for their placement. Selection of one system over another is based on reliability, ease of use, and manufacturer support (Callan, 1991).

## Structure and Function

The two basic patterns of hard tissue integration attained following implant placement and healing are osseointegration and fibro-osteal integration. Fibro-osteal integration results in the presence of a soft tissue zone between the implant and bone. The soft connective tissue attachment surrounding the implant resembles the shock-absorbing feature of the periodontal ligament. For many years this form of integration was considered to be an acceptable means of implant support. The acceptance of this form of integration, however, was challenged in the 1960s by the development of root form implants. Root form implants foster a different type of hard tissue integration referred to as osseointegration. **Osseointegration** can be defined as a direct structural and functional connection between ordered and living bone and the surface of a load carrying implant (Branemark, 1985) (see Figure 14-9). Following an adequate healing period, only a 20 μm space exists between the implant and bone (Albrektsson, Branemark, Hanssen, & Lindstrom, 1981). Longitudinal studies comparing these two contrasting patterns of hard tissue integration conclude osseointegration is essential for the long-term success of dental implants.

The type of hard tissue integration achieved is determined by the physical characteristics of the implant surface and surgical placement. Blade implants are surgically placed and immediately restored or loaded into function. The immediate functional stress resulting from this mode of placement results in the formation of a soft tissue encapsulation or fibrosteal integration. In contrast, root form implants are surgically placed and submerged or buried under the gingiva out of function for a three- to six-month healing period. This extended healing period prior to function allows an intimate contact between bone and the implant to develop. Osseointegration is also favored by the physical characteristics of titanium. Upon exposure to the oral environment, a biocompatible oxide layer is formed on the titanium surface, which enhances the integration to bone. Favorable biocompatibility is

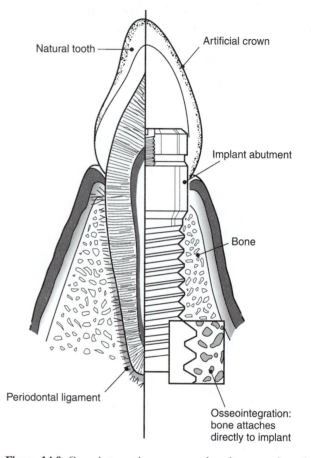

**Figure 14-9** Osseointegration compared to the natural tooth.

also enhanced by utilizing plasma sprayed or hydroxyapatite coated implants. Due to resulting stability, osseointegration is currently accepted as the preferred form of hard tissue integration.

The soft tissue-implant interface in many ways resembles that surrounding natural teeth. Despite efforts to achieve the most beneficial integration of implants, they are not designed or expected to interact in the same manner as natural teeth. An understanding of the distinct structural features of implants is vital for professional care and ultimate success. The gingiva surrounding implants is identical to the gingiva around natural teeth. It consists of a dense lamina propria covered by stratified squamous epithelium. Ideally implants should be positioned within attached gingiva to provide the best support and protection during function. As in the natural dentition, the oral epithelium is continuous with sulcular epithelial lining the pocket wall. The apical extent of the implant sulcus consists of a junctional epithelium attachment histologically similar to natural teeth. A direct adhesion between junctional epithelium and the implant surface is evidenced by the presence of hemidesmosomes (Bower, 1987; James, 1980; McKinney, Steflik, & Koth, 1988). A layer of fibronectin and glycosaminoglycans is thought to serve as the biologic adhesion (Gould, West-bury, & Brunette, 1984; McKinney, Steflik, & Koth, 1988; Meffert, 1989).

Unlike the natural periodontium, implants lack a suprabony fibrous connective tissue attachment. The absence of a cemental layer precludes the development of periodontal ligament or fiber attachments. As a result dentogingival fibers run parallel to the implant surface (Listgarten, 1980). The resulting soft tissue implant interface is referred to as the biological seal (McKinney, Steflik, & Koth, 1988). As opposed to true attachment, the biological seal represents a close association between the surrounding soft tissues and the implant surface. This seal prevents the penetration of plaque bacteria into the internal environment supporting implant. The lack of a true connective tissue attachment and characteristics of the biological seal explain the response of implants in oral health and disease.

## Microbiology

Poor plaque control and subsequent inflammatory disease is a major cause of implant failure. Bacterial invasion of the biologic seal can result in inflammation and eventual implant failure. The inflammatory process resulting from microbial insult to implants closely resembles periodontitis and is referred to as **periimplantitis**. The microflora associated with stable and failing implants closely resembles the microflora associated with healthy and diseased teeth respectively (Mombelli, Van Oosten, Schurch, & Lang, 1987; Mombelli, Buser, & Lang, 1988; Mombelli, Minder, Gusberti, & Lang, 1989; Apse et al., 1989; Newman & Flemmig, 1988). The microbial flora associated with stable implants is characterized by gram-positive cocci and rods with few gram-negative forms (Mombelli, Lang, & Burgin, 1990). Differences, however, have been noted between the floras associated with implants in partially versus fully edentulous mouths (Quirynen & Listgarten, 1990; Lekholm, Ericsson, Adell, & Slots, 1986). These results suggest that implants may be cross infected by the bacterial reservoir from teeth in the same mouth. Patterns of sequential colonization of implants is similar to the natural dentition with gram-positive forms gradually overcome by gram-negative forms. The microbiology of failing implants is homologous to the natural dentition in adult periodontitis. Failing implants are characterized by the presence of gram-negative rods such as black pigmented bacteroides, fusobacterium, and spirochetes (Mombelli, Van Oosten, Schurch, & Lang, 1987; Mombelli, Buser, & Lang, 1988; Apse, 1988).

The response of implants to ongoing or continual microbial insult is comparable to the natural dentition and threatens the success of the implant. Inflammation of the marginal tissues surrounding implants has been referred to as **peri-implant gingivitis** and is histochemically and clinically similar to gingivitis. Plaque-induced implant inflammation results in ulceration of sulcular epithelium and the presence of polymorphonuclear leukocytes in gingival crevicular fluid. As the inflammation progresses into connective tissue and creates peri-implantitis, collagen fibers are destroyed leading to apical migration of the junctional epithelium. Bone loss around dental implants occurs in the same manner as natural teeth. The rate of this resorption, however, is slower when compared to the natural dentition. The absence of any microbial differences to explain the variance in rate of bone loss suggests a potential difference in the susceptibility of peri-implant bone to implant associated pathogens. In other words, osseointegration may afford better defense against inflammatory destruction.

Some disagreement exists regarding the susceptibility of peri-implant soft tissues to disease. The lack of a true connective tissue attachment apparatus suggests increased susceptibility of implants to bacterial insult and subsequent inflammatory disease. Studies examining the association between plaque and disease in clients with implants reveal contradictory results. One study examined the prevalence of gingivitis in ten partially edentulous patients with dental implants (Lekholm, Ericsson, Adell, & Slots, 1986). Gingivitis, in this study, was determined by the presence of bleeding on probing. The prevalence of gingivitis in this study was 80 percent at one or more surfaces and 44 percent at all surfaces. A high correlation was also found between the presence of plaque and gingivitis.

Comparatively, a similar study found little correlation between inflamed gingiva and the presence of plaque. This study also reported a much lower overall prevalence of inflammation of only 8 percent (Adell, Lekholm, Rockler, Branemark, Lindhe, Eriksson, & Sbordone, 1986). The method of assessing gingivitis in this study differed from the previous investigation, utilizing only visual signs of inflammation that did not include bleeding on probing. The resulting level of inflammation in the second study may, therefore, be underestimated. It is also possible that the sites that demonstrated plaque on the day of evaluation may have been plaque-free on other days and, therefore, free of inflammation. The significant role plaque control plays in determining the success and failure of implants suggests an equivalent susceptibility of implants and teeth to inflammatory disease. The failure of visual examination to accurately detect disease emphasizes the need for thorough assessment of implants.

Not all factors that contribute to implant failure have been identified (AAP, 1995b). Some of these factors are related to the procedure itself, such as heat generated during the surgical procedure, improper implant placement or prosthetic design, and functional overloading of the implant. Other factors that occur after successful osseointegration and function and are usually attributed to bacterially induced periimplantitis, as previously discussed, or to functional overloading. Retrograde implant failure, may be due to bone microfractures caused by premature implant loading, overloading, trauma, or occlusal factors, and is called **retrograde implantitis** (Misch, 1990). Retrograde implant failure is suspected when bone loss that does not accompany gingival inflammation is seen radiographically. Rosenberg, Torosian, and Slots (1991) use the terms infectious failure and traumatic failure to describe the differences seen in implant failures. Another difference between those two types of failures lies in the microflora association. While infectious failures is associated with predominately spirochetes and motile rods, retrograde periimplantitis, or traumatic failure is associated with streptococci or microflora that is consistent with periodontal health (AAP, 1995b).

## Assessment

Techniques for implant assessment arise from an understanding of the peri-implant interface. It is important to remember that most implant failures, after primary healing, are due to periimplantitis or occlusal stress. Long-term implant success is dependent on early disease detection and professional intervention. It is sometimes difficult to determine the presence of implants by visual inspection alone. It is critical that clinicians recognize the presence of implants before any type of instrumentation is initiated. Periodontal probing or scaling of an implant in the same manner as natural teeth due to unfamiliarity can inadvertently jeopardize implant integrity.

New client dental histories should include information related to presence of dental implants including implant type, position, date of surgical placement, previous dental professionals responsible for care, and transfer of records. Returning clients with dental implants should be clearly identified by internal and/or external chart notations. Once the implant has been identified special alterations in the assessment and treatment are necessary to avoid undue harm to the implant and surrounding structures. The following techniques and recommendations regarding implant assessment and treatment are derived from extensive research.

Because periimplantitis is one of the leading causes of implant failure following initial healing, thorough peri-implant evaluation is critical. Many traditional assessment methods are applicable to implants because of the clinical and histologic similarities between implants and teeth. It is of the need for subtle, but important, modification of these techniques that the clinician must be aware. The color, contour, and consistency of the peri-implant gingiva should be examined for signs of inflammation. Ideally the implant will be located in attached gingiva; however gingival descriptions will vary if the implant is surrounded by alveolar mucosa. Clinical research has established a positive correlation between elevated plaque scores and increased gingivitis. Increased gingival inflammation is also associated with increased pocket depth (Rams & Link, 1983; Rams, Robert, Tatum, & Keyes, 1984).

Disagreement exists regarding the safety and value of probing dental implant sulci. Because of the lack of a true connective tissue attachment, probing of inflamed gingiva adjacent to the implant may result in penetration of the probe tip through the biologic seal to the crest of alveolar bone. It is accepted by some clinicians and researchers that the likelihood of damage is superseded by the significant relationship between deepened pockets and implant failure. Sulcus depth for stable implants range from 1.3 to 3.8 mm (Apse, 1988; Buser, Warrer, & Karring, 1990; Lekhlom, Ericsson, Adell, & Slots, 1986; Zarb & Symington, 1983). Other clinicians and/or researchers do not recommend probing to assess sulcus depth (Branemark, 1992), except when pathology is observed (Meffert, 1995; Ogren, 1992). Reasons for not probing in a routine manner are that there is no predictable perimucosal seal of the soft tissue to the implant abutment surface and it is difficult to achieve accurate readings due to the superstructure (Meffert, 1995). Unless the superstructure is removed, it is difficult to employ correct probing technique. Meffert (1995) points out that "studies show that probing the dental implant results in the probe proximating bone, thus reaching deeper than in the natural dentition" (p. 13). If probing is performed, special care should be taken to avoid disruption of the biologic seal and plastic probes should be used to avoid scratching the implant surface. The significance of implant surface alteration resulting from professional instrumentation will be further addressed in the section on implant maintenance.

In assessing clinical parameters, there should be no mobility associated with dental implants. The presence of mobility is a good indication of future implant failure. While demonstrating a degree of specificity, traditional mobility assessment, utilizing the blunt end of two instruments, is limited by low sensitivity. In other words, by the time an implant is visibly mobile, failure may be inevitable. The need for a more precise means of determining implant mobility resulted in the development of electronic devices capable of detecting imperceptible changes. The electronic assessment is capable of detecting changes in implant mobility much earlier than traditional clinical evaluation. The same electronic device can also be used to assess the stability of prosthetic attachments.

Radiographic evaluation is an important component of assessing the implant-bone interface. Changes in radiographic density offer a more precise indication of implant status than many other clinical parameters. The integration of more sophisticated techniques such as digitizing radiography will continue to improve the value of radiographic implant assessment. Current recommendations advise periapical radiographic exposure every three months during the first year, and annually thereafter (Young-MacDonald, 1995). These radiographs can then be compared to previous films and the baseline films. Refer to Chapter 5 for additional information on radiographic evaluation of implants.

Because self-care by the client is such an important component of implant success, it should be particularly scrutinized during periodontal assessment. As with natural teeth, notations about plaque and calculus location and amount can be recorded or deposit indices can be used. It is vitally important to focus on control of bacterial plaque in this area as the expense and time the client has invested should be a major concern.

It is evident that traditional periodontal assessment techniques are applicable to implant evaluation with some significant adaptations. Increased gingival inflammation, mobility, radiographic radiolucencies, and evidence of bone loss are indicative of failing implants. Regular clinical and radiographic monitoring are necessary to detect the onset of implant failure and provide an opportunity for successful treatment.

## Maintenance

The long-term success and maintenance of dental implants requires effort by both the client and the dental team. Clients must have a clear understanding of the critical nature daily self-care plays in the stability of their implants. Neither the client's self-care nor professional plaque control measures should alter the integrity of the implant surface or increase plaque retention. It is important to remember that titanium is a relatively soft metal and is susceptible to physical alteration and wear. Self-care education and monitoring should be implemented immediately upon exposure of the implant to the oral environment. Comprehensive self-care instructions are introduced and a baseline assessment of plaque control performance recorded. Self-care should then be monitored for the number of appointments necessary to assure adequate plaque control and absence of inflammation. Following demonstrated plaque control performance, individuals with implants should be placed on a short, regular professional maintenance schedule. It has been suggested that a three-month recall interval is appropriate for the first year with a possible extension to four months if

conditions warrant (Young-MacDonald, 1995). Partially dentulous implant clients may require more frequent maintenance than edentulous implant clients.

Supragingival and subgingival self-care aids and techniques should be modified to accommodate prosthetic design as well as client ability and motivation. For those with multiple implants, it may be necessary to customize instructions for each individual implant. Easily accessible areas may be cleaned with a small, soft-bristled toothbrush. The small head and configuration of an end-tufted brush is particularly suited for use around implants (see Figure 14-10A). Brushes are angled at 45 degrees toward the gingival tissue. Mechanized toothbrushes are also valuable, especially for those with limited or impaired dexterity. Conventional interdental devices such as floss (refer to Figure 14-7B and C), floss with threaders, wooden toothpicks, and brushes (see Figure 14-10B) may be utilized for cleaning less accessible areas around implants and implant-supported prosthesis. The lingual surface and gingival margin are areas frequently missed or neglected. Modification of conventional devices may also be necessary to protect the implant surface from harmful alteration. For example, interdental brushes offer a variety of tip designs for difficult-to-reach areas. The client must be cautioned to use the nylon core tips rather than the metal core tips to avoid potential scratching of the implant surface.

Floss cords (Post Care™, John Butler Co.) or dental tape/ribbon (G-Floss™, 3i Implant Innovations) specially designed for implant use may be more efficient and easier to use than standard floss. Floss can be looped around the lingual side of the implant abutment by threading the floss from the anterior facial interproximal surface around the lingual and back through the posterior interproximal surface. Gauze and yarn can also be used in a similar fashion. The need and cost effectiveness of specialized devices should be carefully considered before they are recommended to clients. Mechanical

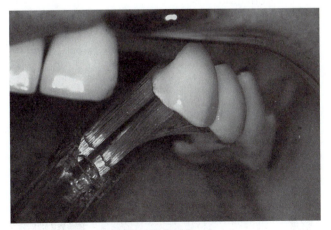

**A. End-Tufted Brush**

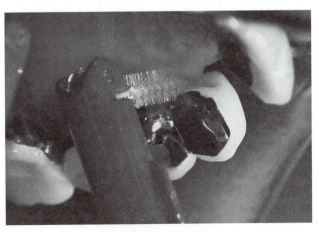

**B. Interdental Brush**

**Figure 14-10** Self-care aids. (Courtesy of Oral-B Laboratories)

self-care may be supported by the use of antimicrobial agents (chlorhexidine) for selected implant clients. These agents may be delivered to the implant surface using a cotton tip applicator, end tufted interdental brush or irrigating device. Pulsating irrigation devices should be used with care around implant sulci to avoid damage to the biologic seal. Clients utilizing these devices should be instructed to use low pressure and direct the stream away from the entry to the sulcus at a 90-degree angle to the long axis of the tooth.

Peri-implant status and self-care should be assessed at each maintenance visit following the evaluation suggestions outlined earlier in this chapter. Each maintenance appointment provides the dental professional an opportunity to review and modify client-performed care based on assessment findings. Soft and hard deposits, if present, should be professionally removed. Calculus formation on implants is generally supragingival and attaches to the supragingival transmucosal cylinder of the implant or to the implant-supported prosthesis. It is similar to the calculus associated with natural teeth. Generally, little calculus forms on the smooth subgingival implant surface due to an inadequate attachment mechanism.

Hand scaling with metallic instruments, ultrasonics or sonic devices is absolutely contraindicated for implants. These instruments can severely scratch the soft titanium implant surface resulting in corrosion and increased plaque retention. The biocompatible titanium oxide layer and hydroxyapatite coating may also be contaminated or dislodged due to the scaling action of metallic instruments. Plastic instruments resembling universal and Gracey curet designs have been developed and marketed for debridement of implant surfaces. Examination of implant surfaces following instrumentation with plastic instruments reveals a relatively unchanged surface (Thompson-Neal, Evans, & Meffert, 1989; Rapley, Swan, & Hallmon, 1990). The calculus removal efficiency of these plastic instruments has, however, been criticized as ineffective due largely in part to plastic's inability to maintain a sharp blade. Single use, disposable plastic instruments are available for deposit removal with a reusable, sterilizable metal handle to improve sharpness. Graphite instruments are also acceptable for implant instrumentation. Additionally, a specially designed plastic tip can be used to cover the metal end of sonic scaler tips to modify the device for use with implants.

Rubber cup polishing of the prosthesis and titanium abutments with a minimally abrasive agent such as tin oxide or superfine commercial pastes is safe. Self-care devices without an abrasive can be applied to the abutment. This is particularly indicated if stain is present on the crown(s). In hard to reach areas, a rubber point and paste can be used. As with polishing of natural teeth, the procedure should be performed on a selected or need basis (refer to Chapter 13). Air-abrasive polishing, however, is contraindicated due to extensive alteration to implant surfaces.

Implant maintenance appointments should allow sufficient time to adequately assess peri-implant status, review and modify client performed plaque control procedures, and debride hard or soft deposits. Some providers recommend the removal of implant-supported prosthesis every eighteen to twenty-four months to provide access for more thorough debridement and evaluation of implant stability (Meffert, 1995). The superstructure can be placed in an ultrasonic cleaning solution. Additional time must be allotted to allow for the removal and replacement of the prosthetic. Table 14-11 provides the reader with a summary of the assessment and maintenance recommendations.

## DOCUMENTATION

Supportive treatment procedures are an integral component of nonsurgical periodontal therapy. By incorporating supportive therapies, the dental hygienist is able to meet clients' comprehensive dental needs. Treatment planning must include evaluation of client factors, technical limitations, and clinician's scope of expertise. Alternative therapies, professional expectations, and the consequences of no treatment (informed consent) must be thoroughly explained and understood by the client before therapy is initiated. Appropriate risk management ensures that all treatment procedures and informed consent be accurately documented in the client's permanent record.

When documenting information about supportive treatment procedures, principles outlined in Chapter 19 will be incorporated. With supportive treatment there are four major points to consider:

1. Documentation of existing conditions on client assessment forms where appropriate (i.e., implants and overhang existence).
2. Notes about a discovered condition in the record of services (i.e., hypersensitivity, localized gingival inflammation).
3. Notations about client self-care education and recommendations in the record of services (i.e., education on causes of hypersensitivity, antimicrobial rinse recommended), and
4. Notations about the actual treatment performed in the record of services (i.e., margination, fiber placement, desensitization, etc.).

The most important factor to remember with supportive therapy is specificity, especially because these procedures are not routine and are based on special needs of the client. Table 14-12 provides examples of Record of Services entries for each supportive therapy discussed. These entries are intended to be a guide and will, of course, vary depending on the client's individualized treatment plan.

**Table 14-11 Summary of Recommendations for Care of the Implant**

| Phase of Care | Recommendations |
| --- | --- |
| Assessment | 1. For a new client, evaluate the health history questionnaire.<br>2. For a returning client, recognize an existing implant by charting notations.<br>3. Evaluate color, contour, and consistency of the gingiva for inflammation.<br>4. Use a periodontal probe to evaluate bleeding. If probing for sulcus depth, do so cautiously.<br>5. Check mobility. None should exist.<br>6. Expose radiographs every three months for the first year, yearly thereafter.<br>7. Assess deposits. |
| Maintenance | 1. Continue the evaluation of deposits and self-care education.<br>2. Recommend appropriate self-care aids including end-tuft brushes, interdental brushes with a nylon core tip, floss cords, and/or an antimicrobial rinse.<br>3. Engage the client in plaque removal with the suggested aid(s).<br>4. Remove supragingival calculus with plastic instruments.<br>5. Polish with rubber cup or point and appropriate agent, if indicated.<br>6. Remove the implant-supported prosthesis yearly to aid in debridement and to check for stability.<br>7. Continue periodic radiographic examination.<br>8. Establish the recare interval. Three-month intervals are suggested for the first year. |

**Table 14-12 Supportive Periodontal Therapy Record of Services Entries**

| Therapy | Sample Treatment Notation |
| --- | --- |
| Antimicrobial Mouthrinse | Rx: Peridex™ mouthrinse. Client instructed to rinse with one capful for 30 seconds after breakfast and before bed after mechanical self-care. Instructed not to rinse after use and told of possible staining and altered taste sensation associated with use. Issued written recommendations for follow-up care. |
| Local Drug Delivery | Tetracycline fiber placed in #14, 18 (Anesthesia use if applicable). Approximately 30 cm of fiber used. Adhesive applied. Patient was instructed not to brush or floss these areas while the fiber is in place, not to eat "hard" foods, and to call the office if the fiber is dislodged. Reappointed in ten days for fiber removal. Issued written recommendations for home care. Previewed education and procedure. |
| Overhang Removal | Marginated Class II amalgam on #3D via Profin™ handpiece and amalgam file. Polished proximal surface. |
| Dentinal Densensitization | Rx: Sensodyne™ Sealant placed on #13, 14, 20, 21, 26, 27. Recommended twice daily brushing with modified Stillman's and to apply the agent liberally to the sensitive areas at bedtime. |
| Implant Maintenance | Endosseous implant in the region of #30 exhibits marginal redness and bleeding on probing. Demonstrated use of an interdental brush in this area. Client instructed to use 3× daily. Area was debrided via plastic curet. Four-week reevaluation visit scheduled. |
| Soft Tissue Curettage | Curettage on #31 to 29 buccal and lingual. Rinsed with saline. Postop instructions given. Informed not to brush vigorously for twenty-four hours. After this time, incorporate routine self-care. No complications. Reappointed in two weeks to check initial healing; four- to- six-week appointment for reevaluation. |

## Summary

The discussion of antimicrobial rinses focused exclusively on their ability to control *supragingival* plaque and gingivitis. The large number of existing and new products marketed and available for client use to control plaque and gingivitis makes it difficult for consumers and professionals alike to evaluate efficacy. Dental hygienists regularly answer client questions and make product recommendations to individuals. Clients frequently select products based on advertised claims, color, and flavor without regard for verified efficacy. It is the dental hygienist's role to provide accurate, reliable and scientifically authenticated information and to counsel clients regarding the use of these products. In order to make accurate and safe recommendations, clinicians must stay abreast of new product releases and independently verify product claims. Criteria and suggestions for the evaluation of antimicrobial agents are presented in Table 14-13 (Cobb, 1993).

In order to be a valuable adjunct to periodontal therapy, antimicrobial agents must also be available and effective against *subgingival* plaque. Although many agents have been evaluated in this capacity, few demonstrate subgingival efficacy. As addressed earlier, the successful application of chemotherapeutic agents for the treatment of periodontal disease is contingent on the ability of the agent to reach the site of action at a concentration greater than or equal to the minimum effective concentration, and to be maintained at the site for a sufficient duration (Goodson, 1985). Failure to meet one of the above criteria might seriously limit efficacy. Numerous studies have demonstrated the success of scaling and root planing for the control and maintenance of periodontal diseases. Favorable clinical response has been observed despite the presence of residual calculus following even the most meticulous scaling and root planing (Fujikawa, O'Leary, & Kafrawy, 1988; Nyman, Sarhed, Ericsson, Gottlow, & Karring, 1986; Sherman, Hutchens, & Jewson, 1990). This implies that while scaling and root planing is not capable of complete calculus removal, it adequately reduces the etiologic irritants below a threshold compatible with health. Despite the general efficacy of scaling and root planing, localized or generalized sites within clients may fail to respond to treatment. Factors such as limited pocket access, operator skill, complex root morphology, and poor host immune response inhibit the success of scaling and root planing. These individualized cases may benefit from the application of antimicrobial agents applied subgingivally via irrigation

**Table 14-13  Suggested Criteria for Evaluation of Antimicrobial Agents/Products**

Question

- Is the agent/product approved by the ADA?
- Are the therapeutic claims substantiated by published research? If so, ask for available studies. Are they published in refereed journals?
- Is the duration of action sufficient to render the desired effect?
- Does the active ingredient exhibit substantivity?
- Are the recommendations for use consistent with the agent/products validated use?
- Is the recommended frequency of use reasonable?
- Was the group (sample) studied appropriate for the intended use of the product/agent?
- Were the methods of measurement valid and reliable?
- Were the examiners blind to treatment group assignment?
- Was the performance of the agent/product compared to an appropriate control group?
- Was the study of appropriate length (at least six months)?
- Despite statistical significance, were the results clinically significant?

or controlled-release devices. Surgical correction may also be warranted.

Other supportive treatment such as systemic antibiotic regimes, margination, desensitization, implant case selection, implant assessment, and maintenance of implants are components of professional care where the dental hygienist has some degree of responsibility. It is imperative that oral health care providers recognize the need for these therapies in the total individualized NSPT care plan.

## Case Studies

**Case Study One:** Jotis Hamilton, a 31-year-old attorney, is a new client in your practice. Health history findings are negative. The dental history reveals routine dental care. He reports his last visit to the dental hygienist was approximately eight months ago. Clinical examination reveals cervical notches and gingival recession on the facial surfaces of #4, 5, 12, 13, 14. Upon questioning, Jotis reports occasional sensitivity to cold. What is your preliminary diagnosis and rationale? What type of treatment is recommended?

**Case Study Two:** You accept a position as a part-time dental hygienist in the growing general practice of Dr. Michael Dean. Another dental hygienist is employed in the office full-time. During the interview, Dr. Dean describes the nonsurgical periodontal care provided for periodontally involved clients. You are excited about the opportunity to utilize your decision-making and clinical skills. Dr. Dean indicates that Pam, the full-time dental hygienist, will discuss the management of those with periodontal diseases with you in greater detail. During your orientation, Pam explains that clients not responding to periodontal debridement/scaling and root planing are treated with chemical curettage. Additionally, all clients are instructed to use a chlorine dioxide dentifrice and mouthrinse sold in the office to reduce plaque and gingivitis. What are your concerns regarding the office nonsurgical management of clients? How would you communicate your concerns?

**Case Study Three:** Sally Jurgens is appointed for her third quadrant of scaling and root planing/debridement. She has been using a 0.12 percent chlorhexidine oral rinse for her generalized gingivitis recognized at the assessment. At the third visit, Sally expressed dissatisfaction with the stain accumulation resulting from chlorhexidine use. What will you tell Sally regarding the importance of chlorhexidine use in conjunction with scaling and root planing? What could you do to satisfy her displeasure regarding tooth staining?

**Case Study Four:** Bill Sanchez has periodontal disease categorized as Case Type III. He presents for initial therapy with generalized marginal gingivitis and generalized 4 to 7 mm pockets. Class II furcations are noted on #2, 3, 14, 15, 18, 19, 31. Self-care instructions are provided and quadrant scaling and root planing/debridement is planned. Would you recommend any chemotherapeutic agent(s) for his nonsurgical care? If so, which ones and why?

**Case Study Five:** The six week reevaluation of Bill Sanchez reveals generalized 1 to 2 mm reduction in pocket depths and resolution of gingival inflammation. The following localized areas, however, show no reduction or an increase in pocket depths, gingival inflammation, or bleeding upon probing: #2ML, 3DL. What supportive therapy would you recommend? How would you document it in the record of services?

## Case Study Discussions

**Discussion—Case Study One:** The preliminary diagnosis is hypersensitivity. The facial cervical regions of the maxillary premolars are a common site for toothbrush abrasion. The enamel and cementum removal has probably resulted from improper toothbrushing contributing to gingival recession and dentin exposure with potential sensitivity. It is important to remember that not all clients with toothbrush abrasion will experience sensitivity; however, individuals exhibiting toothbrush abrasion should receive instructions regarding proper brushing technique and information regarding the harmful effects of this condition. Due to the localized nature of this case, composite restoration and/or dentin bonding could be

offered as the treatment of choice. Other options include desensitizing toothpaste or oxalates. Jotis should be reevaluated in three to four weeks to verify resolution of sensitivity regardless of his treatment choice. If sensitivity persists, the differential diagnosis should be reexamined.

**Discussion—Case Study Two:** Concerns about the management of those with periodontal diseases includes chemical curettage and the dentifrice/mouthwash regime. Although a popular treatment modality in the 1980s, chemical curettage is relatively ineffective for improving the effects obtained by scaling and root planing/debridement. Sites not responding to therapy should first be reassessed to ensure adequate removal of irritants such as plaque and calculus. Occasionally, these areas will benefit from reinstrumentation or subsequent debridement at short maintenance intervals. New sustained release devices, such as tetracycline fibers, are more effective than chemical curettage for treatment of nonresponsive areas. Chlorine dioxide is not accepted by the ADA for the control of plaque and gingivitis. Furthermore, clinical studies show no additional benefit when chlorine dioxide products are compared to a placebo control. The in-office distribution of these products is indicative of a pyramid sales program in which the office stands to gain from the profit of product sales. At the very least, clients need to be informed of its status with the ADA and research results of this agent as compared to other antimicrobials.

It is important that as a well-educated and critically thinking dental hygienist, you try to educate Pam and Dr. Dean regarding the limitations of these treatment modalities. Providing scientific literature from professional journals and/or attending continuing education programs are some examples of how you may elicit change in the office practices. A resistance or unwillingness to change may indicate a need to look for an alternative position.

**Discussion—Case Study Three:** You can reiterate that use of a chlorhexidine oral rinse is a common recommendation during initial periodontal therapy to control plaque and reduce gingivitis with the hope of improving the clinical response to treatment. The benefits of chlorhexidine use should be carefully reviewed with Sally who should make the final decision about continuing oral rinse use. An esthetic polishing and/or scaling to remove stain on a periodic basis may help satisfy her tooth stain concerns. Also, the relationship of diligent self-care practices and reduction of stain can be emphasized. Perhaps rediscussing her self-care recommendations would be beneficial.

**Discussion—Case Study Four:** Because Bill is receiving initial therapy and marginal gingivitis is present, a therapeutic antimicrobial mouthrinse can be included in his treatment plan. Chlorhexidine (Peridex/Perioguard) is recommended knowing it will aid in the healing of gingivitis, but that it will not be effective in combating periodontitis. This concept would be clarified with Bill. Other antimicrobials lack substantivity, so they would not be as useful. Irrigation therapy by Bill is not indicated at this time because it has limited value for routine use in initial therapy. Likewise, t-fiber placement or systemic antibiotics are not indicated. Other chemotherapeutic agents and delivery mechanisms might be recommended if PMP reveal persistent areas of periodontal pocketing and/or bleeding. At the maintenance visit, the classification of periodontal disease can be reevaluated. Reconsideration of other chemotherapeutic agents will be essential if an aggressive form of periodontitis is diagnosed.

**Discussion—Case Study Five:** At this point in therapy, reevaluation of these sites should occur. Self-care practices and professional removal of deposits need to be reassessed. If both are found to be adequate, two alternatives can be offered: retreatment of the area with debridement or tetracycline fiber therapy. If t-fibers are placed, the record of services might read:

Date: Tetracycline fibers were placed without anesthesia in the following pockets not responding to scaling and root planing/debridement procedures: #2ML, 3DL. Fibers were placed circumferentially, overlapped and cyanoacrylate applied. Recommended withholding daily self-care on these teeth for the next ten days. Foods to avoid were discussed and written instructions given. Next appointment: 10 days. Subsequent reevaluation a minimum of 6 weeks post fiber removal for pocket resolution.

## REFERENCES

Absi, E. G., Addy, M., & Adams, D. (1987). Dentine hypersensitivity. A study of the patency of dentinal tubules in sensitive and non-sensitive cervical dentine. *Journal of Clinical Periodontology, 14,* 280–284.

Addy, M. (1990). Etiology and clinical implications of dentine hypersensitivity. *Dental Clinics of North America, 34,* 503–514.

Addy, M., Absi, E. G., & Adams, D. (1987). Dentine hypersensitivity: The effects in vitro of acids and dietary substances on root planed and burred dentine. *Journal of Clinical Periodontology, 14,* 274–279.

Addy, M., Al-Arrayed, F., & Moran, J. (1991). The use of an oxidizing mouthwash to reduce staining associated with chlorhexidine. *Journal of Clinical Periodontology, 18,* 297.

Addy, M., Hassan, H., Moran, J., Wade, W., & Newcombe, R. (1988). Use of antimicrobial containing acrylic strips in the treatment of chronic periodontal disease. A three month follow-up study. *Journal of Periodontology, 59,* 557–564.

Addy, M., Moran, J., & Wade, W. (1994). Chemical plaque control in the prevention of gingivitis and periodontitis. N. P. Lang & T. Karring (Eds.), In *Proceedings of the 1st european workshop on periodontology.* London: Quintessence Publishing Co., Ltd.

Addy, M. & Newcombe, R. G. (1994). Dose response of chlorhexidine against plaque and comparison with Triclosan. *Journal of Clinical Periodontology, 21,* 250–255.

Addy, M. & Urquhart, E. (1992). Dentine hypersensitivity: Its prevalence, aetiology and clinical management. *Dental Update, 19,* 407–412.

Addy, M., Willis, L., & Morgan, J. (1983). Effect of toothpaste rinses compared with chlorhexidine on plaque formation during a 4-day period. *Journal of Clinical Periodontology, 10,* 89–99.

Adell, R., Lekholm, U., Rockler, B., Branemark, P. I., Lindhe, J., Eriksson, B., & Sbordone, L. (1986). Marginal tissue reactions at osseointegrated titanium fixtures. I. A 3-year longitudinal prospective study. *International Journal of Oral Maxillofacial Surgery, 15,* 39–52.

Albrektsson, T., Branemark, P. I., Hanssen, H. A., & Lindstrom, J. (1981). Osseointegrated titanium implants. *Acta Orthopaedica Scandinavia, 52,* 155–170.

Albrektsson, T. & Sennerby, L. (1990). Direct bone anchorage of oral implants: Clinical and experimental considerations of the concept of osseointegration. *International Journal of Prosthodontics, 3,* 30–41.

American Academy of Periodontology. (1986). *Glossary of periodontal terms.* Chicago: American Academy of Periodontology.

American Academy of Periodontology. (1989a). Consensus Report Discussion, Section II. In *Proceedings of the world workshop in clinical periodontitis* (pp. 11-13–11-20). Chicago: American Academy of Periodontology.

American Academy of Periodontology. (1989b). Consensus Report Discussion, Section V (pg. V-20). In *Proceedings of the world workshop in clinical periodontitis.* Chicago: American Academy of Periodontology.

American Academy of Periodontology. (1989c). Tissue Attachment. Consensus Report Discussion, Section V. In *Proceedings of the world workshop in periodontology* (pp. V-20–V-22). Chicago: American Academy of Periodontology.

American Academy of Periodontology. (1991). *Local delivery of antimicrobials: Adjuncts to periodontal therapy?* Research, Science, and Therapy Committee. Chicago: American Academy of Periodontology.

American Academy of Periodontology. (1993a). *Treatment of gingivitis and periodontitis.* Research, Science, and Therapy Committee. Chicago: American Academy of Periodontology.

American Academy of Periodontology. (1993b). *Guidelines for periodontal therapy.* Research, Science, and Therapy Committee. Chicago: American Academy of Periodontology.

American Academy of Periodontology. (1994a). *Chemical agents for control of plaque and gingivitis.* Committee on Research, Science, and Therapy. Chicago: American Academy of Periodontology.

American Academy of Periodontology. (1994b). *Periodontal considerations in the HIV-positive patient.* Committee on Research, Science, and Therapy. Chicago: American Academy of Periodontology.

American Academy of Periodontology. (1994c). *The potential role of controlled-release chemotherapy for periodontitis.* Committee on Research, Science, and Therapy. Chicago: American Academy of Periodontology.

American Academy of Periodontology. (1995a). *The role of supra- and subgingival irrigation in the treatment of periodontal diseases.* Chicago: American Academy of Periodontology.

American Academy of Periodontology. (1995b). *Maintenance and treatment of dental implants.* Chicago: American Academy of Periodontology.

American Dental Association Council on Dental Therapeutics. (1986). Guidelines for the acceptance of chemotherapeutic products for the control of supragingival plaque and gingivitis. *Journal of the American Dental Association, 112,* 529–532.

AP-24, Pharm Assist. (1994). A summary of clinical data.

Apse, P., Ellen, R. P., Overall, C. M., & Zarb, G. A. (1989). Microbiota and crevicular fluid collagenase activity in the osseointegrated dental implant sulcus: A comparison of sites in edentulous and partially edentulous patients. *Journal of Periodontal Research, 24,* 96–105.

Apse, P. (1988). Cross-sectional clinical and microbiological investigation of peri-implant status. *Journal of Dental Research, 67* (Abstract #1398), 287.

Bakdash, M. B., Wolff, L. F., Pihlstrom, B. L., Aeppli, D. M., & Bardt, C. L. (1987). Salt and peroxide compared with conventional oral hygiene—III. Patient compliance and acceptance. *Journal of Periodontology, 58,* 308–313.

Baker, K. (1993). Mouthrinses in the prevention and treatment of periodontal disease. *Current Opinion in Periodontology,* 89–96.

Balanyk, T. E. (1992). Antiplaque efficacy of a prebrushing rinse. *American Journal of Dentistry, 5,* 46–48.

Balkin, B. E. (1988). Implant dentistry: Historical overview with current perspective. *Journal of Dental Education, 52,* 684–685.

Banting, D., Bosma, M., & Bollmer, B. (1989). Clinical effectiveness of a 0.12% chlorhexidine mouthrinse over two years. *Journal of Dental Research, 68,* (Special Issue) 1716.

Barkvoll, P., Rolla, G., & Svendsen, A. K. (1989). Interaction between chlorhexidine digluconate and sodium lauryl sulfate in vivo. *Journal of Clinical Periodontology, 16,* 593.

Bauman, G. R., Mills, M., Rapley, J. W., & Hallmon, W. W (1992). Plaque-induced inflammation around implants. *International Journal of Maxillofacial Implants, 7,* 330–337.

Berger, S. A. (1974). Bacteremia after the use of an oral irrigation device. *Annals of Internal Medicine, 80,* 510–514.

Bjorn, A. L., Bjorn, H., & Grkovic, B. (1969). Marginal fit of restorations and its relation to periodontal bone level. Part I, metal fillings. *Odontologisk Revy, 20,* 311–321.

Bonesvoll, P., Lokken, P., Rolla, G., & Paus, P. N. (1974). Retention of chlorhexidine in the human cavity after mouth rinses. *Archives of Oral Biology, 19,* 209–211.

Bower, R. C (1987). Periodontal considerations of endosseous implants: A philosophy for understanding the tissue implant interface. *Australian Prosthetic Journal,* 25–28.

Bowen, D. M. (1994). Personal mechanical oral hygiene care and chemotherapeutic plaque control. In M. L. Darby & M. M. Walsh (Eds.), *Dental hygiene theory and practice* (pp. 435–460). Philadelphia: W.B. Saunders Co.

Boyd, R. L., Hollander, B. W., & Eakle, W. S. (1992). Comparison of subgingivally placed cannula oral irrigator tip with a supragingivally placed standard irrigator tip. *Journal of Clinical Periodontology, 19,* 340–344.

Braatz, L., Garrett, S., Claffey, N., Egelberg, J. (1985). Antimicrobial irrigation of deep pockets to supplement nonsurgical periodontal therapy. II. Daily irrigation. *Journal of Clinical Periodontology, 12,* 630–638.

Branemark, P. I. (1985). Introduction to osseointegration tissue integrated prostheses. In *Osseointegration in clinical dentistry,* P. I. Branemark, G. A. Zarb, & T. Albrektsson (Eds.), Chicago: Quintessence Publishing Company, Inc., pp. 243, 250, 263, 269, 275–281.

Branemark System. (1992). Clinical Dental Hygiene Slide Services. Nobelpharma USA, Inc.

Brannstrom, M. (1986). The hydrodynamic theory of dentinal pain: Sensation in preparations, caries and the dentinal crack syndrome. *Journal of Endotology, 12,* 453–457.

Braun, R. E. & Ciancio, S. (1992). Subgingival delivery by an oral irrigation device. *Journal of Periodontology, 63,* 469–472.

Bray, K. S., Drisko, C. L., & Cobb, C. M. (1993). Comparison of subgingival irrigation with 0.5% and 2.0% chlorhexidine gel irrigation. *Journal of Dental Research, 72* (Abstract), 360.

Brecx, M., MacDonald, L. L., Legary, K., Cheang, M., & Forgay, M. G. E. (1993). Long-term effects of Meridol™ and chlorhexidine mouthrinses on plaque, gingivitis, staining, and bacterial vitality. *Journal of Dental Research, 72,* 1194–1197.

Brecx, M. & Theidale, J. (1984). Effects of chlorhexidine rinses on the morphology of early dental plaque on plastic film. *Journal of Clinical Periodontology, 11,* 553–563.

Brecx, M., Theidale, J., Attstrom, R., & Glatz, P. O. (1987). The effect of chlorhexidine and Octapinol on early human dental plaque formation. A light and electron microscope study. *Journal of Periodontal Dental Research, 22,* 290–295.

Breiswanger, B. B. et al. (1995). The clinical effect of dentifrices containing stabilized stannous fluoride on plaque formation and gingivitis—a six-month study with ad libitum brushing. *Journal of Clinical Dentistry, 6* (Spec Issue), 46–53.

Brightman, L. J., Terezhalmy, G. T., Greenwell, H., Jacobs, M., & Enlow, D. H. (1991). The effects of 0.12% chlorhexidine gluconate mouthrinse on orthodontic patients aged 11 through 17 with established gingivitis. *American Journal of Orthodontics and Dentofacial Orthopedics, 101,* 408–413.

Buser, D., Warrer, K., & Karring, T. (1990). Formation of a periodontal ligament around titanium implants. *Journal of Periodontology, 61,* 597–601.

Callan, D. P. (1991). Dental hygienist and dental implants. *Practical Periodontics and Aesthetic Dentistry, 3,* 21–25.

Carter, H. G. & Barnes, G. P. (1975). Effects of three mouthwashes on existing dental plaque accumulations. *Journal of Preventive Dentistry, 2,* 6–9.

Caton, J. G. & Zander, H. A. (1979). The attachment between tooth and gingival tissue after periodic root planing and soft tissue curettage. *Journal of Periodontology, 50,* 462.

Christersson, L. A., Norderyd, O. M., & Puchalsky, C. S. (1993). Topical application of tetracycline-HCL in human periodontitis. *Journal of Clinical Periodontology, 20,* 88–95.

Chung, L., Smith, S. R., & Joyston-Bechal, S. (1992). The effect of using a prebrushing rinse (Plax) on oral hygiene in man. *Journal of Clinical Periodontology, 19,* 679–681.

Ciancio, S. G. (1989). Nonsurgical periodontal treatment. In *Proceedings of the world workshop in periodontology.* Chicago: American Academy of Periodontology.

Ciancio, S. G. (1992). Agents for the management of plaque and gingivitis. *Journal of Dental Research, 71,* 1450–1454.

Ciancio, S. G., Mather, M. L., & Bunnell, H. L. (1975). Clinical evaluation of a quaternary ammonium-containing mouth-rinse. *Journal of Periodontology, 46,* 397–401.

Ciancio, S. G., Mather, M. L., Zambon, J. J., & Reynolds, H. S. (1989). Effect of a chemotherapeutic agent delivered by an oral irrigation device on plaque, gingivitis, and sub-gingival microflora. *Journal of Periodontology, 60,* 310–315.

Cobb, C. M. (1993). Evaluation of site-specific chemotherapeutic agents in periodontal treatment. *Current Opinion in Periodontology,* 97–104.

Cobb, C. M., Rodgers, B., & Killoy, W. (1988). Ultrastructural examination of human periodontal pockets following the use of an oral irrigating device in vivo. *Journal of Periodontology, 59,* 155–163.

Collaert, B., Attstrom, R., DeBruyn, H., & Movert, R. (1992). The effect of delmopinol rinsing on dental plaque formation and gingivitis healing. *Journal of Clinical Periodontology, 19,* 274–280.

Collaert, B., Edwardsson, S., Attstrom, R., Hase, J. C., Astrom, M., & Movert, R. (1992). Rinsing with delmopinol 0.2% and chlorhexidine 0.2%: Short-term effect on salivary microbiology, plaque and gingivitis. *Journal of Periodontology, 63,* 618–625.

Collaert, B. & Fisher, C. (1991). Dentine hypersensitivity: A review. *Endod Dent Traunatol, 7,* 145–152.

Coventry, J. & Newman, H. N. (1982). Experimental use of a slow release device employing chlorhexidine gluconate in areas of acute periodontal inflammation. *Journal of Clinical Periodontology, 9,* 129–133.

Coxhead, L. J. (1985). The role of the general dental practitioners in the treatment of periodontal disease. *New Zealand Dental Journal, 81,* 81–85.

Cummins, D. & Creeth, J. E. (1992). Delivery of antiplaque agents from dentifrices, gels, and mouthwashes. *Journal of Dental Research, 71,* 1439–1449.

Davies, R. M. (1992). Rinses to control plaque and gingivitis. *International Dental Journal, 42,* 276.

DePaola, L. G., Overholser, C. D., Meiller, T. F., Minah, G. E., & Neihaus, C. (1989). Chemotherapeutic inhibition of supragingival dental plaque and gingivitis development. *Journal of Clinical Periodontology, 16,* 311–315.

DeVore, C. H., Hicks, M. J., Whitacre, H. L., & Clancy-Schertel, M. (1993). Nonsurgical gingival curettage in dental hygiene curricula. *Journal of Dental Education, 57,* 762–765.

Drake, D. R., Wefel, J. S., Dunkerson, D., & Hogle, K. (1993). The antimicrobial activity of Prevention mouthrinse. *American Journal of Dentistry, 6,* 239–242.

Drisko, C. L. (1993). Scaling and root planing without overin-strumentation: Hand versus power-driven scalers. *Current Opinion in Periodontology,* 78–88.

Drisko, C., Cobb, C., Killoy, W., Lowenguth, R., Pihlstrom, B., Encarnacion, M., & Goodson, M. (1994). Clinical response to tetracycline fiber periodontal therapy. *Journal of Dental Research, 73* (Abstract #1637), 306.

Eakle, W. (1988). Penetration of periodontal pockets with irrigation by a newly designed tip. *Journal of Dental Research, 67* (Abstract), 400.

Eakle, W., Ford, C., & Boyd, R. L. (1986). Depth of penetration in periodontal pockets with oral irrigation. *Journal of Clinical Periodontology, 13,* 39–44.

Echeverra, J. & Caffesse, R. (1983). Effects of gingival curettage when performed 1 month after root instrumentation. *Journal of Clinical Periodontology, 10,* 277–281.

Elworthy, A. J., Edgar, R., Moran, J., Addy, M., Mcovert, R., Kelty, E., & Wade, W. G. (1995). A six-month home-usage trial of 0.1% and 0.2% delmopinol mouthwashes. (11). Effects on plaque microflora. *Journal of Clinical Periodontology, 22,* 527–532.

Felix, J. E., Rosen, S., & App, G. R. (1971). Detection of bacteremia after use of an oral irrigation device in subjects with periodontitis. *Journal of Periodontology, 42,* 785–786.

Fine, J. B., Harper, D. S., Gordon, J. M., Hovliaras, C. A., & Charles, C. H. (1994). Short-term microbiological and clinical effects of subgingival irrigation with an antimicrobial mouthrinse. *Journal of Periodontology, 65,* 30–36.

Flemmig, T. F., Newman, M. G., Doherty, F. M., Grossman, E., Meckel, A. H., & Bakdash, B.M. (1990). Supragingival irrigation with 0.06% chlorhexidine in naturally occurring gingivitis. I. Six-month clinical observations. *Journal of Periodontology, 61,* 112–117.

Flotra, L., Gjermo, P., Rolla, G., & Waerhaug, J. (1972). A 4-month study on the effect of chlorhexidine mouthwashes on 50 soldiers. *Scandinavian Journal of Dental Research, 80,* 10–16.

Forgas, L. B. & Gound, S. (1986). Effects of antiformin on the microbial flora of periodontal pockets. *Journal of Dental Research, 65* (Abstract 349), 208.

Fornall, J., Sundin, Y., & Lindhe, J. (1975). Effect of Listerine™ on dental plaque and gingivitis. *Scandinavian Journal of Dental Research, 73,* 18–25.

Francis, J., Addy, M., & Hunter, B. (1987). A comparison of oral delivery methods of chlorhexidine in handicapped children. II. Parent and houseparent preferences. *Journal of Periodontology, 58,* 456–459.

Francis, J., Hunter, B., & Addy, M. (1987). A comparison of three delivery methods of chlorhexidine in handicapped children. I. Effects on plaque, gingivitis, and tooth staining. *Journal of Periodontology, 58,* 451–455.

Freitas, B. L., Collaert, B., & Attstrom, R. (1991). Effect of a pre-brushing rinse, Plax, on dental plaque formation. *Journal of Clinical Periodontology, 18,* 713–715.

Fujikawa, K., O'Leary, T. J., & Kafrawy, A. (1988). The effects of retained subgingival calculus on healing after flap surgery. *Journal of Periodontology, 59,* 170–175.

Fukazawa, E. & Nishimura, K. (1994). Superficial cemental curettage: Its efficacy in promoting improved cellular attachment on human root surfaces previously damaged by periodontitis. *Journal of Periodontology, 65,* 168–176.

Gage, T. W. & Pickett, F .A. (1996). *Mosby's drug reference.* St. Louis: Mosby-Year Book, Inc.

Garcia-Godoy, F., DeVizio, W., Volpe, A. R., Ferlauto, R. J., & Miller, J. M. (1990). Effect of a triclosan/copolymer/fluoride dentifrice on plaque formation and gingivitis: A 7-month clinical study. *American Journal of Dentistry, 3,* 515–526.

Gilbert, R. J. & Williams, P. E. O. (1987). The oral retention and antiplaque efficacy of triclosan in human volunteers. *British Journal of Clinical Pharmacology, 23,* 579–583.

Gillam, D. G. (1995). Mechanisms of stimulus transmission across dentin—a review. *Journal of the Western Society of Periodontology, 43* (Periodontal abstracts), 53–65.

Gilmore, N. & Sheiham, A. (1971). Overhanging dental restorations and periodontal disease. *Journal of Periodontology, 42*, 8–12.

Givens, E. G., Gwinnett, A. J., & Boucher L. J. (1984). Removal of overhanging amalgam: A comparative study of three instruments. *Journal of Prosthetic Dentistry, 52*, 815–820.

Gjermo, P. (1989). Chlorhexidine and related compounds. *Journal of Dental Research, 68*, 102.

Gjermo, P., Baastad, K. L., & Rolla, G. (1970). The plaque inhibiting capacity of 11 antibacterial compounds. *Journal of Periodontal Dental Research, 5*, 102–109.

Gjermo, P. & Rolla, G. (1971). The plaque-inhibiting effect of chlorhexidine-containing dentifrices. *Scandinavian Journal of Dental Research, 79*, 126–132.

Goldman, H. (1960). A review of current technics in periodontal therapy as practiced in the United States. *International Dental Journal, 10*, 287–309.

Gomer, R. M., Holroyd, S. V., Fedi, P. F., & Ferrigno, P. D. (1972). The effects of oral rinses on the accumulation of dental plaque. *Journal of American Social Preventive Dentistry, 2*, 11–15.

Goodson, J. M., Cugini, M. A., Kent, R. L., Armitage, G. C., Cobb, C. M., Fine, D., Fritz, M. E., Green, E., Imoberdorf, M. J., Killoy, W. J., Mendieta, C., Niederman, R., Offenbacher, S., Taggart, E. J., & Tonetti, M. (1991a). Multicenter evaluation of tetracycline fiber therapy: I. Experimental design, methods, and baseline data. *Journal of Periodontal Research, 26*, 361–370.

Goodson, J. M., Cugini, M. A., Kent, R. L., Armitage, G. C., Cobb, C. M., Fine, D., Fritz, M. E., Green, E., Imoberdorf, M. J., Killoy, W. J., Mendieta, C., Niederman, R., Offenbacher, S., Taggart, E. J., & Tonetti, M. (1991b). Multicenter evaluation of tetracycline fiber therapy: II. Clinical response. *Journal of Periodontal Research, 26*, 371–379.

Goodson, J. M. (1985). Controlled drug delivery: A new means of treatment of dental diseases. *Compendium of Continuing Education in Dentistry, 6*, 27–36.

Goodson, J. M. & Tanner, A. (1992). Antibiotic resistance of the subgingival microbiota following local tetracycline therapy. *Oral Microbiology and Immunology, 7*, 113–117.

Goodson, J. M., Tanner, A., McArdle, S., Dix, K., & Watanabe, S. M. (1991). Multicenter evaluation of tetracycline fiber therapy. III. Microbial response. *Journal of Periodontal Research, 26*, 440–451.

Gordon, J. M., Lamster, I. A., & Seiger, M. C. (1985). Efficacy of Listerine™ antiseptic in inhibiting the development of plaque and gingivitis. *Journal of Clinical Periodontology, 12*, 697–701.

Gorzo, I., Newman, H. N., & Strahan, J. D. (1979). Amalgam restorations, plaque removal, and periodontal health. *Journal of Clinical Periodontology, 6*, 98–105.

Gotfredsen, K., Rostrup, E., Hjorting-Hansen, E., Stoltze, K., & Budtz-Jorgensen, E. (1991). Histological and histomorphometrical evaluation of tissue reaction adjacent to endosteal implants in monkeys. *Clinical Oral Implants Research, 2*, 30–37.

Gould, T. R. L., Westbury, L., & Brunette, D. M. (1984). Ultrastructural study of the attachment of human gingiva to titanium in vivo. *Journal of Prosthetic Dentistry, 52*, 418–420.

Greenstein, G. (1992). Supragingival and subgingival irrigation: Practical application in the treatment of periodontal diseases. *Compendium of Continuing Education in Dentistry, 13*, 1098–1121.

Greenstein, G. (1995). Treating periodontal diseases with tetracycline-impregnated fibers: Data and controversies. *Compendium of Continuing Education in Dentistry, 16*, 448–455.

Grenby, T. H. (1995). The use of Sanguarnine in mouthwashes and toothpaste compared with some other antimicrobial agents. *British Dental Journal, 178*, 254–358.

Grossman, E., Reiter, G., Sturzenberger, O. P., De La Rosa, M., Dickinson, T. D., & Ferretti, G. A. (1986). Six-month study of the effects of a chlorhexidine mouthrinse on gingivitis in adults. *Journal of Periodontal Research, 21* (Suppl. 16), 33–38.

Hakkarainen, K. & Ainamo, J. (1980). Influence of overhanging posterior tooth restorations on alveolar bone heights in adults. *Journal of Clinical Periodontology, 7*, 114–120.

Hardy, J. H., Newman, H. N., & Strahan, J. D. (1992). Direct irrigation and subgingival plaque. *Journal of Periodontal Dental Research, 9*, 57–65.

Harper, D. S., Muellar, L. J., Fine, J. B., Gordon, J., & Laster, L. L. (1990). Clinical efficacy of a dentifrice and oral rinse containing sanguinaria extract and zinc chloride during six-months use. *Journal of Periodontology, 61*, 352–358.

Hecker, R. (1913). *Pyorrhea alveolaris.* St. Louis: Mosby-Year Book, Inc.

Heijl, L., Dahlen, G., Sundin, Y., Wenander, A., & Goodson, M. (1991). A 4-quadrant comparative study of periodontal treatment using tetracycline-containing drug delivery fibers and scaling. *Journal of Clinical Periodontology, 18*, 111–116.

Herzog, A. & Hodges, K. O. (1988). Subgingival irrigation with chloramine-T. *Journal of Dental Hygiene, 62*, 515–519.

Higashi, K., Morisaki, K., Hayashi, S., Kitamura, M., Fujimoto, N., Kimura,. S., Ebisu, S., Sokada, H. (1990). Local ofloxacin delivery using a controlled release insert (PT-01) in the human periodontal pocket. *Journal of Periodontal Research, 25*, 1–5.

Hill, R., Ramjford, S., Morrison, E., Appleberry, E., Caffesse, R., Kerry, G., & Nissle, R. (1981). Four types of periodontal treatment compared over two years. *Journal of Periodontology, 52*, 655–662.

Hodges, K. O. & Bowen, D. M. (1985). Effectiveness of margination procedures in relation to periodontal status. *Journal of Dental Hygiene, 59*, 320–324.

Hodosh, M., Hodosh, S. H., & Hodosh, A. J. (1994). About dentinal hypersensitivity. *Compendium of Continuing Education in Dentistry, 15*, 658–667.

Howell, T. H. (1991). Chemotherapeutic agents as adjuncts in the treatment of periodontal disease. *Current Opinion in Dentistry, 1*, 81.

Hunter, L. & Addy, M. (1987). Chlorhexidine gluconate mouthwash in the management of minor apthous ulceration. *British Dental Journal, 162*, 106–110.

James, R. A. (1980). Peri-implant considerations. *Dental Clinics of North America, 24*, 415–420.

Jeffcoat, M. K. & Howell, T. H. (1980). Alveolar bone destruction due to overhanging amalgam in periodontal disease. *Journal of Periodontology, 51*, 599–602.

Jenkins, S., Addy, M., & Newcombe, R. (1993). Evaluation of a mouthrinse containing chlorhexidine and fluoride as an adjunct to oral hygiene. *Journal of Clinical Periodontology, 20*, 20–25.

Jolkovsky, D. L., Waki, M. Y., Newman, M. G., Otomo-Corgel, J., Madison, M., Flemmig, T. F., Nachnafi, S., & Nowzari, M. (1990). Clinical and microbial effects of subgingival and gingival marginal irrigation with chlorhexidine gluconate. *Journal of Periodontology, 61,* 663–669.

Joyston-Bechal, S. & Hernaman, N. (1993). The effect of a mouthrinse containing chlorhexidine and fluoride on plaque and gingival bleeding. *Journal of Clinical Periodontology, 20,* 49–53.

Kalaga, A., Addy, M., & Hunter, B. (1989). The use of 0.2% chlorhexidine spray as an adjunct to oral hygiene and gingival health in physically and mentally handicapped adults. *Journal of Periodontology, 60,* 381–385.

Kalkwarf, K., Tussing, G., & Davis, M. (1982). Histologic evaluation of gingival curettage facilitated by sodium hypochlorite solution. *Journal of Periodontology, 53,* 63–68.

Kaminske, K., Tung, M., Takagiko, K. (1990). Effects of oxalate and calcium phosphate solutions on dentin tubule obstruction. *Journal of Dental Research, 69,* Abstract 480.

Kaufman, A. Y., Tal, H., Perlmutter, S., & Shwartz, M. M. (1989). Reduction of dental plaque formation by chlorhexidine dihydrochloride lozenges. *Journal of Periodontal Research, 24,* 59–62.

Klewansky, P. & Vernier, D. (1984). Sanquinarine and the control of plaque in dental practice. *Compendium of Continuing Education in Dentistry, 5* (Suppl.), 94–97.

Knight, T. (1969). Erosion-abrasion. *Journal of the Dental Association of South Africa, 24,* 310–316.

Knowles, J., Burgett, F., Nissle, R., Shick, R., Morrison, E., & Ramjford, S. (1979). Results of periodontal treatment related to pocket depth and attachment level. Eight years. *Journal of Periodontology, 50,* 225–233.

Kopczyk, R. A., Abrams, H., Brown, A. T., Matheny, J. L., & Kaplan, A. L. (1991). Clinical and microbiological effects of a sanquinaria-containing mouthrinse and dentifrice with and without fluoride during 6 months of use. *Journal of Periodontology, 62,* 617–622.

Kornman, K. S. (1986). The role of supragingival plaque in the prevention and treatment of periodontal diseases: A review of current concepts. *Journal of Periodontal Dental Research, 21* (Suppl. 16), 5–22.

Kornman, K. S., Blodgett, R. F., Brunsvold, M., & Holt, S. C. (1990). Effects of topical application of meclofenamic and ibuprofen on bone loss, subgingival microbiota and gingival PMN response in the primate: PMN. *Journal of Dental Research, 25,* 300–307.

Kornman, K. S., Newman, M. G., & Wilson, T. G. (1992). The role of microbiology in periodontal therapy. In T. G. Wilson, K. S. Kornman, & M. G. Newman (Eds.), *Advances in periodontics.* Chicago: Quintessence Publishing Co., Inc.

Kornman, K. S. & Wilson, T. G. (1992). Treatment planning for patients with inflammatory periodontal diseases. In T. G. Wilson, K. S. Kornman, & M. S. Newman (Eds.), *Advances in periodontics* (pp. 87–97). Chicago: Quintessence Publishing Co., Inc.

Krust, K. S., Drisko, C. L., Gross, K., Overman, P., & Tira, D. E. (1991). The effects of subgingival irrigation with chlorhexidine and stannous fluoride. *Journal of Dental Hygiene, 65,* 289–295.

Kuebker, W. A. (1984a). Dental problems: Causes, diagnostic procedures, and clinical treatment. I. Retention problems. *Ouintessence International, 10,* 1031–1048.

Kuebker, W. A. (1984b). Dental problems: Causes, diagnostic procedures, and clinical treatment. II. Patient discomfort problems. *Ouintessence International, 11,* 1131–1139.

Lamster, I. B. Alfano, M. C. Seiger, M. C., & Gordon, J. M. (1983). The effect of Listerine™ antiseptic on reduction of existing plaque and gingivitis. *Clinical Preventive Dentistry, 5,* 12–16.

Lang, N. P., Hotz, P., Graf, H., Geering, A. H., Saxer, U. P., Sturzenberg, O. P., & Meckel, A. H. (1982). Effects of supervised chlorhexidine mouthrinses in children. A longitudinal clinical trial. *Journal of Periodontal Dental Research, 17,* 101–111.

Larner, J., et al. (1989). Penetrability of periodontal pockets with various subgingival tip designs. *Journal of Dental Research, 68* (Abstract), 410.

Lawson, K., Gross, K. B. W., Overman, P., & Anderson, D. (1991). Effectiveness of chlorhexidine and sodium fluoride in reducing dentin hypersensitivity. *Journal of Dental Hygiene, 65,* 340–343.

Lekholm, U., Ericsson, I., Adell, R., & Slots, J. (1986). The condition of the soft tissues at tooth and fixture abutments supporting fixed bridges: A microbiological and histological study. *Journal of Clinical Periodontology, 13,* 558–562.

Leon, A. R. (1976). Amalgam restorations and periodontal disease. *British Dental Journal, 140,* 377–382.

Listgarten, M. A. (1980). Periodontal probing: What does it mean? *Journal of Clinical Periodontology, 7,* 165–176.

Lobene, R. R. & Soparkar, P. M. (1977). The effect of acetylpyridium chloride mouthwash on plaque and gingivitis. *Journal of Dental Research, 56*(B) (Abstract), 195.

Löe, H. & Schiott, C. R. (1970). The effect of mouthrinses and topical application of chlorhexidine on the development of dental plaque and gingivitis in man. *Journal of Periodontal Dental Research, 5,* 79–83.

Löe, H., Schiott, C. R., & Karring, T. (1976). Two years use on chlorhexidine in men. (1) General and Clinical Effect. *Journal of Periodontal Dental Research, 11,* 135.

Lofthus, J. E., Waki, M. Y., Jolkovsky, D. L., Otomo-Corgel, J., Newman, M. G., Flemmig, T., & Nachriani, S. (1991). Bacteremia following subgingival irrigation and scaling and root planing. *Journal of Periodontology, 62,* 602–607.

Lopez, N. & Belvedeessi, M. (1977). Subgingival scaling with root planing and curettage: Effects upon inflammation: A comparative study. *Journal of Periodontology, 46,* 354–357.

Lubbers, J. R., Chauan, S., & Bianchine, J. R. (1982). Controlled clinical evaluations of chlorine dioxide, chlorite, and chlorate in man. *Environmental Health Perspectives, 46,* 57–62.

Lugassy, A. A., Lautenschlager, E. P., & Katnana, D. (1971). Waterspray devices. *Journal of Dental Research, 50,* 466–473.

Lusk, S. S., Bowers, G. M., Tow, H. D., Watson, W. J., & Moffit, W. C. (1974). Effect of an oral rinse on experimental gingivitis, plaque formation and formed plaque. *Journal of American Social Preventive Dentistry, 4,* 31–34.

MacAlpine, R., Magnusson, I., Kiger, R., Crigger, M., Garrett, S., & Edelberg, I. (1985). Antimicrobial irrigation of deep pockets to supplement oral hygiene instruction and root debridement. I. Bi-weekly irrigation. *Journal of Clinical Periodontology, 12,* 568–577.

MacAulay, W. J. R. & Newman, H. N. (1986). The effect on the composition of subgingival plaque of a simple oral hygiene system including pulsating jet subgingival irrigation. *Journal of Periodontal Research, 21,* 375–385.

Mandell, R. L., Dirienzo, R., Kent, R., Joshipara, K., & Haber, I. (1992). Microbiology of healthy and diseased periodontal sites in poorly controlled insulin diabetics. *Journal of Periodontology, 63,* 274–279.

Mandell, R. L., Tripodi, L. S., & Savitt, E. (1986). The effect of treatment on *Actinobacillus actinomycetemcomitans* in juvenile periodontitis. *Journal of Periodontology, 57*, 94–99.

McKinney, R.V., Steflik, D. E., & Koth, D. L. (1988). The epithelium dental implant interface. *Journal of Oral Implantology, 13*, 622–641.

McKinney, R. V., Steflik, D. E., & Koth, D. L. (1988). Per, peri or trans? A concept for improved dental implant terminology. *Journal of Prosthetic Dentistry, 52*, 267–269.

Meffert, R. (1989). Implant therapy. In *Proceedings of the world workshop in periodontics.* Chicago: American Academy of Periodontics.

Meffert, R. (1995). Implantology and the dental hygienist's role. *Journal of Practical Hygiene, 4*, 11–13.

Misch, C. E. (1990). Density of bone: Effect on treatment plans, surgical approach, healing, and progressive loading. *International Journal of Oral Implantology, 6*, 123–131.

Mombelli, A., Buser, D., & Lang, D. (1988). Colonization of osseointegrated titanium implants in edentulous patients: Early results. *Oral Microbiology and Immunology, 3*, 113–120.

Mombelli, A., Lang, N. P., Burgin, W. B. (1990). Microbial changes associated with the development of puberty gingivitis. *Journal of Periodontal Research, 25*, 331–338.

Mombelli, A., Minder, C. H. E., Gusberti, F. A., & Lang, D. (1989). Reproducibility of microscopic and cultural data in repeated subgingival plaque samples. *Journal of Clinical Periodontology, 16*, 434–442.

Mombelli, A., Van Oosten, A. C., Schurch, E., & Lang, N. P. (1987). The microbiota associated with successful or failing osseointegrated titanium implants. *Oral Microbiology and Immunology, 2*, 145–151.

Morganstein, W. M., Blank, L. W., & Hasler, J. (1994). *Microbiology of periodontal diseases.* Cincinnati: Target Media, Inc.

Moskow, B. (1964). The response of the gingival sulcus to instrumentation: A histologic investigation. II. Gingival curettage. *Journal of Periodontology, 35*, 112–116.

Murtomaa, H., Turtola, L., & Rutomma, I. (1984). The use of dental floss by Finnish students. *Journal of Clinical Periodontology, 11*, 443–447.

Muzzin, K. B. (1992). Treatment of dentinal hypersensitivity with oxalate salts. *Journal of Practical Hygiene, 1*, 23–25.

National Institute of Health Consensus Development Conference Statement: Dental Implants 1988 7:3.

Newman, M. G. & Flemmig, T. F. (1988). Periodontal considerations of implants and implant associated microbiota. *International Journal of Oral Implantology, 5*, 65–70.

Newman, M. G., Kornman, K. S., & Doherty, F. M. (1994). A 6-month multi-center evaluation of adjunctive tetracycline fiber therapy used in conjunction with scaling and root planing in maintenance patients: Clinical results. *Journal of Periodontology, 65*, 685–691.

Ng, W. & Tonzetich, J. (1984). Effect of hydrogen sulfide and methyl mercaptan on the permeability of oral mucosa. *Journal of Dental Research, 63*, 994–997.

Niessen, L. C. & Douglass, C. W. (1992). Preventive actions for enhancing oral health. *Clinical Geriatric Medicine, 8*, 201–214.

Nosal, G., Scheidt, M. J., O'Neal, R., & Van Dyke, T. E. (1991). The penetration of lavage solution into the periodontal pockets during ultrasonic instrumentation. *Journal of Periodontology, 62*, 554–561.

Nyman, S., Sarhed, G., Ericsson, I., Gottlow, J., & Karring, T. (1986). The role of "diseased" root cementum in healing following treatment of periodontal disease. *Journal of Periodontal Research, 21*, 496–503.

Nyman, S., Westfelt, E., Sarhed, G., & Karring, T. (1988). Role of "diseased" root cementum in healing following treatment of periodontal disease. A clinical study. *Journal of Clinical Periodontology, 15*, 464–468.

Ogren, E. M. (1992). The hygienist's role in successful implant treatment. *Journal of Practical Hygiene*, 29–32.

Oosterwaal, P. J. M., Mikx, F. H. M., & Renggli, H. H. (1990). Clearance of a topically applied fluorescein gel from periodontal pockets. *Journal of Clinical Periodontology, 17*, 613–615.

Orchardson, R. (1987). Clinical measurement of hypersensitive dentine. *International Endodontics Journal, 26*, 5–7.

Pack, A. R. C., Coxhead, L. J., & McDonald, B. W. (1990). The prevalence of overhanging margins in posterior amalgam restorations and periodontal consequences. *Journal of Clinical Periodontology, 17*, 145–152.

Perlich, M. A. et al. (1995). The clinical effect of a stabilized stannous fluoride dentifrice on plaque formation, gingivitis, and gingival bleeding: A six-month study. *Journal of Clinical Dentistry, 6* (Spec. Issue), 54–58.

Pihlstrom, B. L., Wolff, L. F., Bakdash, B., Schaffer, E. M., Jensen, J. R., Aeppli, D. M., & Brandt, C. L. (1987). Salt and peroxide compared with conventional oral hygiene. 1. Clinical Results. *Journal of Periodontology, 58*, 291–305.

Pithcher, G. R., Newman, H. N., & Strahan, J. D. (1980). Access to subgingival plaque by disclosing agents using mouthrinsing and direct irrigation. *Journal of Clinical Periodontology, 7*, 300–308.

Quirynen, M. & Listegarten, M. (1990). The distribution of bacterial morphotypes around natural teeth and titanium implant ad modem branemark. *Clinical Oral Implant Research, 1*, 8–13.

Rams, T. E. & Link, C. (1983). Microbiology of failing implants in humans: Electron microscopic observations. *Journal of Oral Implantology, 11*, 93–100.

Rams, T. E., Robert, T. W., Tatum, H., & Keyes, P. (1984). The subgingival microflora associated with human dental implants. *Journal of Prosthetic Dentistry, 51*, 529–534.

Rams, T. E. & Slots, J. (1992). Antibiotics in periodontal therapy: An update. *Compendium of Continuing Education in Dentistry, 13*, 1130–1145.

Rapley, J. W., Swan, R. H., & Hallmon, W. W. (1990). Surface characteristics produced by various oral hygiene instruments and material on titanium implant abutments. *International Journal of Maxillofacial Implants, 5*, 47–52.

Rees, T. D. & Orth, C. F. (1986). Oral ulcerations with use of hydrogen peroxide. *Journal of Periodontology, 57*, 689.

Renton-Harper, P. & Midda, M. (1992). NdYAG laser treatment of dentinal hypersensitivity. *British Dental Journal, 172*, 13–16.

Rethman, J. (1992). Current concepts in irrigation therapy. *Journal of Practical Hygiene*, March, 11–15.

Rethman, I., Rethman, M., & Suzuki, J. (1995, September/October). Controlled-release periodontal therapy: The evaluation of antimicrobial delivery systems. *Journal of Practical Hygiene* (Suppl.), 1–8.

Rizzo, A. A. (1967). The possible role of hydrogen sulfide in human periodontal disease. Hydrogen sulfide production in periodontal pockets. *Periodontics, 5*, 233–236.

Rogo, E. (1995, May/June). Overhang removal: Improving

periodontal health adjacent to class II amalgam restoratives. *Practical Hygiene*, 15–23.

Rolla, G., Löe, H., & Schiott, C. R. (1970). The affinity of chlorhexidine for hydroxyapatite and salivary mucins. *Journal of Dental Research, 5*, 90–95.

Ronis, D. L., Lang, W. P., Farghaly, M. M., & Ekdahl, S. M. Preventive oral health behaviors among Detroit-area residents. *Journal of Dental Hygiene, 68*, 123–130.

Rosenberg, E. S., Torosian, J. P., & Slots, J. (1991). Microbial differences in two clinically distinct types of failures of osseointegrated implants. *Clinical Oral Implants Research, 2*, 135–144.

Schaeken, M. J. M., Van der Hoeven, J. S., Saxton, C. A., and Cummins, D. (1994). The effect of mouthrinses containing zinc and Triclosan on plaque accumulation and development of gingivitis in a three-week clinical test. *Journal of Clinical Periodontology, 21*, 360–364.

Scheie, A. A. (1989). Modes of action of currently known chemical antiplaque agents other than chlorhexidine. *Journal of Dental Research, 68* (Spec. Issue), 1609–1616.

Scheie, A. A., Assev, S., & Rolla, G. (1985). The effect of SnF$_2$ and NaF on glucose uptake and metabolism in S. mutans OMZ 176. In S. A. Leach (Ed.), *Factors relating to demineralization and remineralization of the teeth*. Oxford: IRL Press Ltd., 99–104.

Schmidt, N. F., Missan, S. R., Tarbet, W. J., & Copper, A. D. (1978). The correlation between organoleptic mouth-odor ratings and levels of volatile sulfur compounds. *Oral Surgery, 45*, 560–565.

Schneider, P. A. & Muhlemann, H. R. (1974). The antiglycolytic action of amine fluorides on dental plaque. *Helv Odontol Acta, 18* (Suppl.), 63–70.

Sherman, P. R., Hutchens, L. H., & Jewson, L. G. (1990). The effectiveness of subgingival scaling and root planing: II. Clinical responses related to residual calculus. *Journal of Clinical Periodontology, 61*, 9–15.

Shiloah, J. & Patters, M. R. (1994). DNA probe analyses of the survival of selected periodontal pathogens following scaling, root planing, and intra-pocket irrigation. *Journal of Periodontology, 65*, 568–575.

Slots, J. & Rams, T. E. (1990). Antibiotics in periodontal therapy: Advantages and disadvantages. *Journal of Clinical Periodontology, 17*, 479–493.

Slots, J. & Rams, T. E. (1991). New views on periodontal microbiota in special patient categories. *Journal of Clinical Periodontology, 18*, 411–420.

Soskolne, A., Golomb, G., Friedman, M., & Sela, M. N. (1983). New sustained release dosage form of chlorhexidine for dental use. II. Use in periodontal therapy. *Journal of Periodontal Research, 18*, 330–336.

Southard, S., Killoy, W. J., Drisko, C. L., & Tira, D. E. (1989). The effects of 2% chlorhexidine digluconate irrigation on the levels of bacteroides gingivalis in periodontal pockets. *Journal of Periodontology, 60*, 302–309.

Srivastava, R. P. (1979). Incidence of periodontal disease in relation to class II silver amalgam restorations. *Journal of Periodontology, 51*, 217–221.

Stiefel, D. J., Truelove, E. L., Chin, M. M., & Mandel, L. S. (1992). Efficacy of chlorhexidine swabbing in oral health care for people with severe disabilities. *Special Care Dentistry, 12*, 57–62.

Svatun, B., Saxton, C. A., & Rolla, G. (1989). A 1-year study of the efficacy of a dentifrice-containing zinc citrate and tri-closan to maintain gingival health. *Scandinavian Journal of Dental Research, 97*, 242–246.

Svatun, B., Saxton, C. A., & Rolla, G. (1990). Six-month study on the effect of a dentifrice-containing zinc citrate and tri-closan on plaque, gingival health and calculus. *Scandinavian Journal of Dental Research, 98*, 301–304.

Teledyne Water Pik. (1992). Learning Resources for Oral Irrigation Therapy (2nd ed.) Ft. Collins, CO: Teledyne Water Pik.

Thompson-Neal, D., Evans, G. H., & Meffert, R. M. (1989). Effects of various prophylactic treatments on titanium, sapphire and hydroxyapatite-coated implants: An SEM study. *International Journal of Periodontology & Restorative Dentistry, 9*, 301–311.

Tinanoff, N. & Weeks, D. B. (1979). Current status of SnF$_2$ as an antiplaque agent. *Pediatric Dentistry, 1*, 199–270.

Vignarajah, S., Newman, H. N., and Balman, J. (1989). Pulsated jet subgingival irrigation with 0.1% chlorhexidine, simplified oral hygiene and chronic periodontitis. *Journal of Clinical Periodontology, 16*, 365–370.

Vouros, I., Sakellari, D., & Konstantinidis, A. (1994). Effect of a new pre-brushing rinse on dental plaque removal. *Journal of Clinical Periodontology, 21*, 701–704.

Wan Yusof, W. Z. A., Newman, H. N., Strahan, J. D., & Coventry, J. F. (1984). Subgingival metromidazole in dialysis tubing and subgingival chlorhexidine irrigation in the control of chronic inflammatory periodontal disease. *Journal of Clinical Periodontology, 11*, 166–175.

Watts, E. A. & Newman, H. N. (1986). Clinical effects on chronic periodontitis of a simplified system of oral hygiene including subgingival pulsated jet irrigation with chlorhexidine. *Journal of Clinical Periodontology, 13*, 666–670.

Weiss, C. M. (1987). A comparative analysis of fibro-osteal and osteal integration and other variables that affect long term bone maintenance around dental implants. *Journal of Oral Implantology, 13*, 3–13.

Weitzman, S. A., Weitberg, A. B., Niederman, R., & Stossel, T. P. (1984). Chronic treatment with hydrogen peroxide—Is it safe? *Journal of Periodontology, 55*, 510–514.

Weitzman, S. A., Weitberg, A. B., Stossel, T. P., Schwartz, J., & Shklar, G. (1986). Effects of hydrogen peroxide on oral carcinogenesis in hamsters. *Journal of Periodontology, 57*, 685–688.

Wennstrom, J., Dahlen, G., Grandahl, K., & Heijl, L. (1987). Periodic subgingival antimicrobial irrigation of pockets. II. Microbiologic and radiological observations. *Journal of Clinical Periodontology, 14*, 573–583.

Wennstrom, J. & Lindhe, J. (1985). Some effects of a sanquinarine-containing mouthwash on developing plaque and gingivitis. *Journal of Clinical Periodontology, 12*, 86–91.

Williams, R. C., Jeffcoat, M. K., Howell, T. H., Reddy, M. S., Johnson, H. G., Hall, C. M., & Goldhaber, D. (1988). Topical flurbiprofen treatment of periodontitis in beagles. *Journal of Periodontal Research, 23*, 166–169.

Winer, R. A., Chauncey, H. H., and Garcia, R. L. (1991). Effect of peroxyl mouthrinses on chlorhexidine staining of the teeth. *Journal of Clinical Dentistry, 3*, 15–18.

Winn, D. M., Blott, W. J., & McLaughlin, J. K. (1991). Mouthwash use and oral conditions in the risk of oral and pharyngeal cancer. *Cancer Research, 51*, 3044.

Wolff, L. F., Bakdash, M. B., Pihlstrom, B. L., Bandt, C. L., & Aeppli, D. M. (1987). The effect of professional and home subgingival irrigation with antimicrobial agents on gingivitis and early periodontitis. *Journal of Dental Hygiene, 63,* 222–227.

Wolff, L. F., Pihlstrom, B. L., Bakdash, M. B., Schaffer, J. R., Aeppli, D. M., & Bandt, C. L. (1989). A four-year investigation of salt and peroxide regimen compared with conventional oral hygiene. *Journal of the American Dental Association, 118,* 67–72.

Wolff, L. F., Pihlstrom, B. L., Bakdash, M. B., Schaffer, E. M., Jensen, J. R., Aeppli, D. M., & Bandt, C. L. (1987). Salt and peroxide compared with conventional oral hygiene. II. Microbial results. *Journal of Periodontology, 58,* 301–307.

Worthington, P. (1988). Current implant usage. *Journal of Dental Education, 52,* 692–695.

Yamagami, H., Takamori, A., Sakamoto, J., & Okada, H. (1992). Intrapocket chemotherapy in adult periodontitis using a new controlled-release insert containing ofloxacin (PT-01). *Journal of Periodontology, 63,* 2–6.

Yeh, K., Dangler, L., Sena, F., Zientek, L., Denooyer, M., & Weddle, L. (1990). Use of ferric oxalate to reduce dentin permeability. *Journal of Dental Research, 69,* (Abstract #479).

Yewey, G., Tipton, A., Dunn, R., Menardi, E. M., McEvoy, R. M., Jensen, J. A., Southard, G. L., & Polson, A. M. (1991). Evaluation of a biodegradable subgingival delivery system for fluorbiprofen treatment of periodontitis in beagles. *Journal of Periodontal Research, 23,* 166–169.

Young-MacDonald, V. L. (1994). Dental hygiene care for the individual with osseointegrated dental implants. In M. L. Darby & M. M. Walsh (Eds.), *Dental hygiene theory and practice* (pp. 823–852). Philadelphia: W.B. Saunders Co.

Zarb, G. A. & Symington, J. M. (1983). Osseointegrated dental implants: Preliminary report on a replication study. *Journal of Prosthetic Dentistry, 50,* 771–776.

# CHAPTER 15

# Prevention and Maintenance of Occupational Hazards

---

## Key Terms

carpal tunnel syndrome (CTS)
cumulative trauma disorders (CTD) or
   repetitive strain injuries (RSI)
ergonomics
job "burnout"
neuromusculoskeletal disorder

neutral wrist position
neutral, balanced body position
occupational exposure
occupational hazard
occupational stress
stressors

---

## INTRODUCTION

All types of workers experience some chance of exposure to occupational hazards; however, some occupations are more hazardous than others. An **occupational hazard** can be defined as exposure or potential for exposure to injury or disease within the workplace environment. Within the dental professions, some of the hazards, such as exposure to infectious diseases, are obvious while others are more subtle. Being able to recognize existing hazards or identify potential hazards is critical to effective prevention and maintenance of occupational hazards for the dental health care worker.

This chapter will provide an overview of some of the more common occupational hazards associated with dental hygiene and dental practice. These hazards will be organized into categories focusing on ergonomic, psychosocial, biological, chemical and physical factors. Within any clinical environment, the practitioner is exposed to a variety of elements in each of these categories. Some exposures might be a one-time event, such as an accidental spill of a toxic chemical. This one-time exposure would be referred to as an *acute dose*. Other exposures might occur over an extended period of time and are termed *chronic exposures*. An example of a chronic exposure would be using an unadjustable operator's chair that results in cumulative damage to your musculoskeletal system (Macdonald, 1987). Additionally, the federal laws that regulate the promotion of safe working environments and the agencies that enforce them will be discussed. Although this content is not unique to nonsurgical periodontal therapy, it is germane. There is a relationship between occupational hazards and the skills performed by oral health care providers who treat those

with periodontal diseases. Traditional dental hygienists spend a great deal of their time scaling and root planing and performing other repetitive skills. The more variance the practitioner can accomplish in a work day, the better the chances of preventing an injury due to repetitive motions or occupational stress and burnout. Also, a general awareness of potential hazards helps the hygienist evaluate the workplace on a daily basis.

## HISTORICAL PERSPECTIVE

Prior to the 1970s, literature regarding occupational hazards for dental hygienists as well as all dental practitioners was limited to studying the effect of long-term exposure to ionizing radiation, musculoskeletal disorders, and communicable diseases. A review of the literature reveals that more research is conducted within the Scandinavian countries than in the United States regarding the identification of occupational hazards, especially in the musculoskeletal area (Rundcrantz, Johnsson,, & Moritz, 1990; Rundcrantz, Johnsson, & Moritz, 1991; Rundcrantz, Johnsson, Moritz, & Roxendal, 1991a; Rundcrantz, Johnsson, Moritz, & Roxendal, 1991b). Since the 1960s reports of dentists and dental hygienists with musculoskeletal problems have been documented in the literature (Bassett, 1982; Boyer, Elton, & Preston, 1986; Fouchard Academy Poll, 1965; Gravois & Stringer, 1980; Kaplan, 1973; Oberg & Oberg, 1993; Osborn, Newell, Rudney, & Stoltenberg, 1990a).

The psychosocial hazards of stress and burnout for dental professionals were initially addressed in the late 1970s and early 1980s; however, recent work in this area concentrates on career and job satisfaction and its relationship to retention within the profession (Bader & Sams, 1992; Boyer, 1994; Dadian, 1993; Deckard & Rountree, 1984; Mellody, 1983; Miller, 1991; Nelson & Newell, 1993a; Nelson & Newell, 1993b; Orner, 1978; O'Shea, Corah, & Ayer, 1984). Chemical and biological hazards have gained attention with the increase in the use of nitrous oxide analgesia; the availability of new products for disinfection and sterilization; the risk of potential exposure to infectious diseases such as hepatitis B, AIDS, and tuberculosis; and the risk of potential exposure to contaminated wastes. Focus was drawn to the physical hazards within the dental environment with the passage of the Consumer Radiation Health and Safety Act, which addresses unnecessary exposure to ionizing radiation. Also, reports of hearing loss due to the use of high speed handpieces and allergies to latex from wearing gloves increased awareness of other physical hazards.

As health care service providers, dental professionals have advocated prevention and maintenance protocols as an integral component of the care provided for their clients. Precautionary procedures have been implemented to reduce or eliminate the risks or the potential risk of harm to our clients. In order to limit harmful exposures to themselves, practitioners must accept the responsibility to recognize existing hazards and identify potential hazards within the work environment. Next, practitioners must take steps to reduce or eliminate such hazards to prevent and maintain their occupational health. For purposes of this text, the hazards will be divided into ergonomic hazards, psychosocial hazards and other occupational hazards such as biological, chemical, and physical.

## ERGONOMIC HAZARDS

**Ergonomics** is a discipline that studies workers and their relationship to their occupational environment. It is an applied science that interfaces the design of work devices, systems, and physical working conditions with the requirements and capacities of the worker (Pollack, 1989). For dental professionals, ergonomics includes concepts such as how we position ourselves and our clients, how we perform our tasks and procedures, how we utilize our equipment and the impact of these actions on our musculoskeletal health. The information on ergonomics will be further divided into musculoskeletal and nerve impairment disorders, risk factors and prevention of such disorders, and a discussion of the ergonomic standard being considered by the Occupational Safety and Health Administration.

### Musculoskeletal and Nerve Impairment Disorders

Musculoskeletal disorders encompass injuries to the tendons, tendon sheaths and the related bones, muscles, and nerves. When there is nerve involvement, it is sometimes referred to more specifically as a **neuromusculoskeletal disorder**. Musculoskeletal pain in dental and dental hygiene practitioners has been most frequently documented in the upper and lower back, neck, shoulders, arms and legs; however, it may occur in any part of the body (Oberg & Oberg, 1993; Osborn et al., 1990; Shugars, Miller, & William, 1987). Shugars et al. (1987) estimated that over 41 million dollars in dentists' annual income was lost due to musculoskeletal pain. He also reported that this type of pain contributed to a reduction in the number of patients treated per day, an increase in time away from the practice, more breaks within the day, and other practice modifications to reduce the pain (Shugars et al., 1987). Osborn and others (1990a), in a study of Minnesota dental hygienists, and Oberg and Oberg (1993), in a study of Swedish dental hygienists, both reported high frequencies of pain in the neck, shoulder, and upper and lower back. Both studies also reported adverse affects on clinical practice such as a reduction in speed and quality of performance, a decrease in endurance, a reduction in days in practice, and a need for practice modifications in positioning and scheduling. In a four-year longitudinal study of nine dental hygienists, eight subjects reported musculoskeletal complaints after four years of practice and four of the nine dental hygienists reported multiple areas of pain (Barry, Woodall, & Mahan, 1992). Barry and others (1992) also reported lower back pain was the most prevalent complaint reported, followed by headaches and neck and upper back pain. The studies reviewed in this section are based on self-reporting of incidence of musculoskeletal pain and do not consider other variables in lifestyle or workplace activities that might contribute to the condition, thereby, limiting a direct cause and effect relationship.

**Cumulative trauma disorders (CTD)** or **repetitive strain injuries (RSI)** as they are sometimes called, are musculoskeletal and nerve impairments caused by repetitive work activities, especially when performed forcefully and/or in awkward postures. Nerves and sometimes blood vessels may become entraped or compressed as they pass through channels in the body formed by muscles, ligaments, and bones. Repetitive action may aggravate the condition by causing inflammation and further compression of the involved nerves or blood vessels (Armstrong, 1986). Common CTDs (see Table 15-1) that involve nerves include carpal tunnel syndrome (CTS), ulnar nerve compression at the elbow, ulnar nerve entrapment at the wrist and thoracic outlet syndrome when the brachial plexus is compressed. CTDs involving vascular compression include illnesses such as thoracic outlet syndrome when the subclavian artery is compressed, and Raynaud's syndrome. CTSs involving compression of connective tissue (muscles, tendons, soft tissue) include conditions such as tenosynovitis (DeQuervain's Disease), tendinitis (rotator cuff tendinitis) and lateral epicondylitis (tennis elbow).

**Table 15-1  Common CTDs, Areas Affected and Symptoms**

| Illness | Area Affected | Symptoms |
|---|---|---|
| Carpal Tunnel Syndrome | Median nerve in the wrist and hand. | Tingling, pain, or numbness in the thumb, pointing finger, the middle finger, and half the ring finger. Symptoms may occur in the back of the hand and in the palm and may be more severe during sleep. Temperature sensitivity and loss of strength may also occur. |
| Ulnar Nerve Compression at the Elbow (Cuptial Tunnel Syndrome) | Ulnar nerve at elbow, forearm, and hands. | Tingling, pain, or numbness in the little finger, half of the ring finger, and the ulnar side of the hand and forearm. Weakness of the hand. |
| Ulnar Nerve Entrapment at the Wrist (Guyon's Canal Syndrome) | Ulnar nerve in the wrist and hand. | Decreased hand strength. |
| Thoracic Outlet Syndrome | Neurovascular compression affecting shoulder, arm, and hands. | Tingling or numbness in the fingers and hands. Atrophying of the hand muscles. Weakness in the hands. Pale or bluish hands. Chronic pain or tired arm sensation. |
| Raynaud's Syndrome | Vascular compression in the hands and fingers. | Tingling or numbness in the hands and fingers that can lead to loss of control. Sensitivity to cold. Pale or bluish hands, especially after exposure to cold. |
| Tensynovitis | Connective tissue or sheath of any tendon overused or injured. | Pain, especially when using hand or arm. Inflammation or swelling may occur. |
| DeQuervain's Disease | Connective tissue at base and side of thumb. | Aching and weakness in thumb. Muscle atrophy. |
| Tendinitis (Tendonitis) | Connective tissue in the shoulder, elbow, or forearm. | Pain or irritation, especially when using the hand or arm. |
| Rotator Cuff Tendinitis | Connective tissue in the shoulder. | Pain, often intense, in the shoulder. |
| Lateral Epicondylitis | Connective tissue at the outside of the elbow. | Pain and tenderness at the outside of the elbow, radiating along the back of the forearm. |

**Nerve Impairments. Carpal tunnel syndrome (CTS)** is the most frequently identified cumulative trauma disorder. The carpal tunnel is a channel within the wrist that is formed by the eight carpal bones and the transverse carpal ligament (see Figure 15-1). Confined within the tunnel are the nine extrinsic flexor tendons of the fingers, the vascular supply, and the median nerve. When the median nerve is compressed in the tunnel, symptoms such as numbness, tingling, pain and a reduced touch sensation may be experienced in the thumb, index, and middle finger and half of the ring finger (Hunter, Schneider, Mackin, & Callahan, 1984; Phalen, 1966). Early symptoms also include an intolerance to cold and sometimes a burning sensation. All of these symptoms might inhibit sleep or awaken an individual from sleep. A weakening or loss of strength, as well as an atrophy of

the thenar muscle at the base of the thumb, may be gradual but progressive over time (Tountas, MacDonald, Meyerhoff, & Bihrle, 1983; Phalen, 1966).

According to a Bureau of Labor Statistics Survey of Occupational Illnesses and Injuries (1992), slightly over 60 percent of approximately 368,000 new cases of occupational illness among workers in the private sector during 1991 were identified as cumulative trauma disorders, and almost 224,000 of the new occupational illness cases were carpal tunnel syndrome. The literature supports the incidence of CTS in the dental hygienist community, however, the prevalence of CTS among dental hygienists is not known (Conrad, Conrad, & Osborn, 1993; Gerwatowski, McFall, & Stach, 1992; Macdonald, Robertson, & Erikson, 1988; Osborn et al., 1990b). All the reported studies except one (Conrad, Conrad, & Oxborn, 1993)

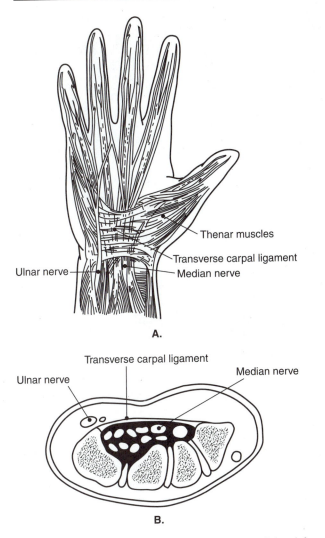

A.

B.

**Figure 15-1** Carpal tunnel area. **A.** Palmar view of the right hand showing median and ulnar nerve distribution. **B.** Cross section of the carpal tunnel area of the right wrist. (Courtesy of "Carpal Tunnel Syndrome: Treatment and Rehabilitation Therapy for the Dental Hygienist," by D. B. McFall, D. J. Stach, and L. J. Gerwatowski, 1993. *Journal of Dental Hygiene,* *67,* p. 127.)

mation and allow for tissue to heal. Aspirin or nonsteroidal anti-inflammatory drugs may be prescribed. Corticosteroids may be injected for relief of pain. Surgical treatment, because of its invasiveness, is usually the last resort. The usual surgical procedure is the complete release of the transverse carpal ligament. An incision of about two inches is made across the wrist and onto the palm to expose the ligament, the ligament is severed, and the incision closed. A dental hygienist can expect to return to work five to eight weeks postsurgery (McFall, Stach, & Gerwatowski, 1993). Microsurgical procedures are also available that require a smaller surgical incision at the base of the hand. Video-endoscopic techniques are used to sever the ligament. The advantages of this type of procedure are smaller scars and a shorter healing time due to less tissue trauma. Exercises to prevent CTS or for posttreatment rehabilitation of CTS are beneficial; however, once CTS symptoms occur and nerve damage exists, only exercises prescribed by the treating health professional should be performed to avoid further nerve damage. The risk factors and prevention strategies for CTS will be discussed later in the text.

The ulnar nerve runs down the arm from the brachial plexus in the shoulder to the hand passing over the humerus bone at the inner side of the elbow. This area of the elbow is often referred to as the "funny bone". When this area is inadvertently bumped a tingling or numbness results in the little finger and part of the ring finger. Repeated trauma to this nerve by repetitive rotations of the lower arm can cause scarring around and within the nerve. Because wrist rotation is anatomically impossible without rotation of the forearm, a practitioner who uses a lot of wrist movement (see Figure 15-2) may be more susceptible to ulnar nerve compression at the elbow or carpal tunnel syndrome. Surgery to have the nerve transposed to the front of the elbow is sometimes recommended when severe symptoms of nerve damage are present. Ulnar nerve entrapment at the wrist or Guyon's canal syndrome is a compression of the ulnar nerve as it passes through the wrist on the little finger side of the carpal tunnel (see Figure 15-1). This illness can result from use of the hand in prolonged or repeated ulnar deviation (see Figure 15-2C) and results in a decrease of hand strength. The sensory branch of the ulnar nerve separates above the wrist and does not pass through the Guyon's canal so that pain, tingling, or numbness is not experienced with this disorder.

The numerous muscles, tendons, and nerves of the shoulder create a multitude of possible injuries. Pain in the shoulder can be caused by many conditions, some not originating in the joint itself. Any practitioner with shoulder pain should seek prompt medical attention. Thoracic outlet syndrome results when the brachial plexus of nerves and often the subclavian artery are compressed by the attached muscles in the channel or space under the clavicle called the thoracic outlet. Practitioners reduce the size of the space and can compress nerves and blood vessels when they elevate their elbows higher then 30°

address medical diagnosis or an analysis of other medical or lifestyle factors that might contribute to the incidence of CTS (Huntley & Shannon, 1986; Macdonald et al., 1988; Osborn et al., 1990b). Although it is clear that additional research is needed to substantiate CTS as an occupational hazard for dental hygienists, the identified risk factors for CTS (repetitiveness, posture, force, mechanical stress, vibration, and temperature) often exist within the dental hygiene work environment (Gerwatowski et al., 1992). A definitive diagnosis must be completed to differentiate CTS from other nerve compression CTDs.

Once the diagnosis is made, the treatment often starts with the most conservative approach such as rest from aggravating activities or immobilization. Medical interventions may be recommended to reduce inflam-

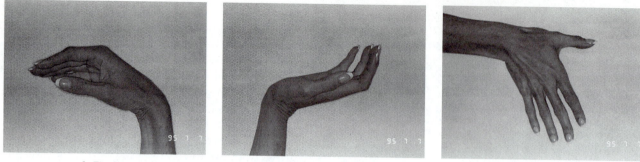

**A. Flexion**          **B. Extension**          **C. Adduction or Ulnar Deviation**

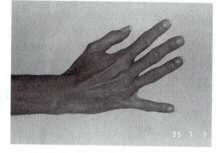

**D. Abduction or Radial Deviation**          **E. Neutral Wrist Position**

**Figure 15-2** Wrist positions.

from the body or work with their shoulders abducted or raised for extended periods of time. When symptoms of ulnar or median nerve compression (tingling, pain or numbness) surface, a differential diagnosis is necessary to determine whether the compression is in the shoulder, elbow, or wrist area. Immobilization of the shoulder using a shoulder sling is traditionally used to open the thoracic outlet space and allow for healing.

**Vascular Compression.** Raynaud's syndrome is a reduction in the flow of blood to the hands by constricted blood vessels. It is often associated with prolonged use of vibrating equipment such as pneumatic tools or jackhammers; however, it has been identified in people with advanced carpal tunnel syndrome or people with connective tissue diseases such as lupus. Individuals with this condition often develop pale or bluish hands, particularly after exposure to the cold and are unusually sensitive to cold. Tingling and numbness of the fingers and hands can also occur.

**Connective Tissue Compression.** Tenosynovitis develops when the sheath (synovium) through which the tendon glides is injured or overused producing excess synovial fluid. As the fluid collects, the synovium swells, reduces its ability to function, an can produce pain in the affected area. DeQuervain's tenosynovitis or disease is a thickening of the sheaths covering the two tendons that pass to the thumb, and is often a result of repetitive motion. Ulnar deviation of the wrist (see Figure 15-2C) during repetitive motion, such as scaling or probing,

may exacerbate this condition (Macdonald, 1987). Symptoms of DeQuervain's tenosynovitis consist of radiating pain at the base of the thumb to the nail and up into the forearm. Immobilization of the wrist can relieve the condition or in severe cases, surgery to release the tendon sheath is necessary.

Tendinitis is an inflammation of the tendon caused by irritation or overuse and can develop in any tendon. When a muscle contracts, strain is put on the tendon that attaches the muscle to the bone. Overuse can cause the tendon to become inflamed, or torn and frayed. Cold packs and immobilization will usually allow the inflammation to subside and the tendon to heal. Rotator cuff tendinitis is an inflammation of the muscles and tendons that form the musculotendinous cuff (rotator cuff) of the shoulder joint. Four major muscles; the subscapularis, the suprasinatus, the infraspinatus and the teres minor, along with their tendons form the capsule of the shoulder joint. These muscles and tendons hold the humerus bone to the glenoid fossa, strengthen the capsule around the joint, and flexibly resist undue movements of the head of the humerus bone in an anterior, superior, or posterior direction. Practitioners who position themselves too far from their clients or supplies and are continually reaching or position themselves too close to their clients could risk this condition. Also, positioning the client too high causing shoulder abduction could contribute to this disorder. Coldpacks and immobilization are effective unless there has been a tendon tear.

Lateral epicondylitis can result from any activity that includes forceful extensions of the wrist with the palm downward or vigorous rotary movement of the forearm against resistance, putting severe stress on the elbow joint. Pain and tenderness at the side of the elbow and radiating pain down the back of the forearm are the common symptoms. If excessive gripping is involved, widespread aching in all the forearm muscles can be present. Such movement is often used with hand instrumentation during debridement procedures when the dental hygienist increases the force and pressure on the instrument in a working stroke to remove tenacious calculus deposits. Coldpacks, massage, and immobilization are the most common treatments, with surgery recommended only in severely disabled clients.

## Contributing Risk Factors and Prevention

The contributing risk factors for CTD fall primarily into two categories: medical and occupational. Pre-existing medical conditions such as arthritis, congenital conditions, traumatic injuries or fractures, and female hormonal changes associated with pregnancy and menopause, and complete hysterectomy with ovary removal have all been related to CTDs, especially CTS (Gerwatoski et al., 1992; Osborn et al., 1990b). Occupational risk factors for CTD have been identified in the literature and include repetitiveness, posture, force, mechanical stresses, vibration, and temperature (Armstrong & Lifshitz, 1987; Cannon, Bernacki, & Walter, 1981; King, 1990; Lukas, 1979). These risk factors are inherent in the daily clinical practice of oral health practitioners. Gerwatowski, McFall, and Stach (1992) modified the earlier work of Armstrong and Lifshitz (1987) to develop a checklist specifically for clinical dental hygiene to analyze these risk factors (see Table 15-2).

**Repetitiveness.** Repetitiveness is defined as the performance of the motion, task, or posture more than 50 percent of the time (Armstrong & Lifshitz, 1987). Dental practitioners, by virtue of the occupation, experience a high degree of repetitive actions. In particular, dental hygienists are involved in repetitive motions especially when performing hand and ultrasonic scaling and rubber cup polishing procedures. Although repetitive motion is used with an ultrasonic instrument, less wrist motion and less force is employed when debridement is accomplished with an ultrasonic instrument.

A California study of 2,400 dental hygienists found statistically significant correlations between CTS symptoms and the numbers of years in practice, number of days worked per week, and the number of clients seen per day (Macdonald et al., 1988). In a study of 440 Minnesota dental hygienists, respondents with lower back pain showed a significant correlation with the number of years in practice and the number of hours a week they were practicing. Significant correlations were also found between the presence of arm pain and full-time practice. Individuals who reported shoulder pain practiced more hours per week than those without shoulder pain (Os-

born et al., 1990a). A study of twenty-eight Swedish dental hygienists who had worked for a mean of 5.2 years and had a 31.5 mean number of working hours per week, exhibited high frequencies of neck and shoulder pain; however, exhibited a lower frequency of lower back pain when compared to secretaries, cleaners, and dentists (Oberg & Oberg, 1993).

The impact of repetitiveness can be greatly decreased with appropriate scheduling. Adequate time to allow for both client and operator needs is recommended. The total number of clients treated as well as the spacing of clients who require intense hand instrumentation should be considered in order to avoid muscle fatigue. The receptionist and other coworkers must be sensitive to this issue to coordinate appropriate scheduling. Clients who require nonsurgical periodontal therapy (NSPT) should not be scheduled consecutively. New client assessments, reevaluation, or child or youth recall appointments can be interspersed between NSPT appointments to avoid muscle fatigue. Scheduling periodontally involved clients for debridement by quadrants and alternating those procedures within the time scheduled provides an opportunity for different muscle groups to rest. A thorough client assessment enables the practitioner to categorize and individualize needs. Treatment can be sequenced to reduce the period of time needed for hand-intense repetitive motions, yet still provide optimum client care. A maintenance client may require the following care: assessment, self-care education, debridement in specific areas, selective polishing, interdental brush education, and radiographs. By interspersing the radiographs, self-care education, and selective polishing into the debridement procedures, repetitive motions will be reduced. For example, after completing debridement and polishing in a quadrant, the practitioner could review the use of the interdental brush and demonstrate its use before continuing with the next quadrant. Shorter recall intervals to reduce the need for heavy scaling and the use of sharp instruments to ease deposit removal also decrease repetitive actions. Selective polishing or using an ultrasonic to remove stain, will also reduce the repetitive motion of polishing procedures. Positioning is often compromised when pressured for time, therefore, allowing adequate time through appropriate scheduling can contribute to maintaining healthy operator/client positioning.

**Posture.** Operators should analyze posture from two perspectives: their own body positioning and the relationship between their position and the client. Posture is one of the most common occupational risk factors (Armstrong, 1986). In evaluating your own body position, you must start with the vertebral column which establishes and maintains the pivotal support for the body. The column is composed of thirty-three vertebrae with a soft disk of cartilage between the first twenty-four vertebrae to separate and cushion the bones (see Figure 15-3). Starting from the top, there are seven cervical, twelve tho-

### Table 15-2 Risk Factors and Prevention Strategies for CTS

| Risk Checklist | Preventive Strategies |
|---|---|
| **Repetitiveness**<br>• Are you scheduling more than two consecutive root planing debridement appointments?<br>• Are you scheduling more than two consecutive difficult clients?<br>• Within an appointment, are you repeating the same hand motion or posture for prolonged periods (scaling for 30 to 45 minutes, then doing other procedures)?<br>• Do you use ultrasonic or sonic scalers infrequently or not at all? | **Repetitiveness**<br>• Allow sufficient time to treat the needs of the client.<br>• Regulate the total number and scheduling of clients requiring hand-intensive motions.<br>• Vary hand-intensive activities by interspersing procedures such as radiographs, self-care instructions, and selective polishing with debridement/root planing.<br>• Use very sharp instruments.<br>• Shorten the client's recare interval.<br>• Maximize the use of ultrasonic scaling devices. |
| **Posture**<br>• Operator Posture<br>  – Are your shoulders elevated and/or one higher than the other?<br>  – Are your wrists flexed or extended during scaling?<br>• Operator/Patient Position<br>  – Are your elbows elevated more than 30°?<br>  – Is your back bent and is your head unsupported by your spine? | **Posture**<br>• Relax shoulders; keep them even and parallel to the floor.<br>• Resist elevating elbows above 30°.<br>• Avoid prolonged ulnar deviation.<br>• Reduce wrist flexion and extension; keep wrist in a neutral position with the hand/arm straight (client height will help control this).<br>• Use full-arm strokes rather than wrist or finger action. |
| **Force**<br>• Are you using a constant, pinching grasp during both exploring and working strokes?<br>• Are your instrument handles smooth? | **Force**<br>• Use minimum pressure in instrument grasp.<br>• Increase pressure with grasp only when deposits are engaged.<br>• Use instruments of adequate weight.<br>• Select instrument handles that are serrated or textured. |
| **Mechanical Stresses**<br>• What are the diameters of your instruments?<br>• Are your instrument handles hexagonal?<br>• Are the cords of your handpieces short or curly?<br>• Are your handpieces unbalanced?<br>• Are your gloves ill-fitting? | **Mechanical Stresses**<br>• Choose larger-diameter, round instruments.<br>• Use contra-angled instruments in anterior regions if they help maintain neutral wrist position.<br>• Avoid heavy and unbalanced handpieces.<br>• Select contra-angled rather than right-angled prophy angles.<br>• Avoid short and curled cords or retractable cords that pull on the wrist.<br>• Wear properly fitted gloves. |
| **Temperature**<br>• Is your operatory cold, or is there a cold air vent directed toward you?<br>• Are your instruments cold when you use them?<br>• Do you wash your hands with cold water? | **Temperature**<br>• Avoid cold drafts and air exhaust, especially on cold hands.<br>• Work in warm rooms or wear warm clothing.<br>• Use warm water to wash hands; maintain 77° finger temperature.<br>• Exercise hand for muscle warm-up and to relax muscles between client appointments. |

(Adapted with permission from "Carpal Tunnel Syndrome: Risk Factors and Prevention Strategies for the Dental Hygienist," by D. B. McFall, D. J. Stach, and L. J. Gerwatowski, 1992, *Journal of Dental Hygiene, 66*, p. 90)

racic, five lumbar, five sacral, and four coccygeal vertebrae. The sacral vertebrae are fused together to make the sacrum, which articulates with the hipbones to form the pelvic girdle. A healthy vertebral column is vertically straight when viewed posteriorly. When viewed from the side, three curves should exist (see Figure 15-3). The cervical segment curves inward (secondary cervical curvature), the thoracic segment curves outward (primary thoracic curvature), and the lumbar segment curves

inward (secondary lumbar curvature). These curvatures along with strong muscles allow us to continually hold our head erect and also to accommodate the internal organs of the thorax and pelvic area. The weight of the head and body is borne primarily by the discs. It has been estimated that the head represents approximately 7 percent of the total body weight (Boyer et al., 1986). Stress to the muscles of the neck and body results when working with the head tilted laterally or bent downward

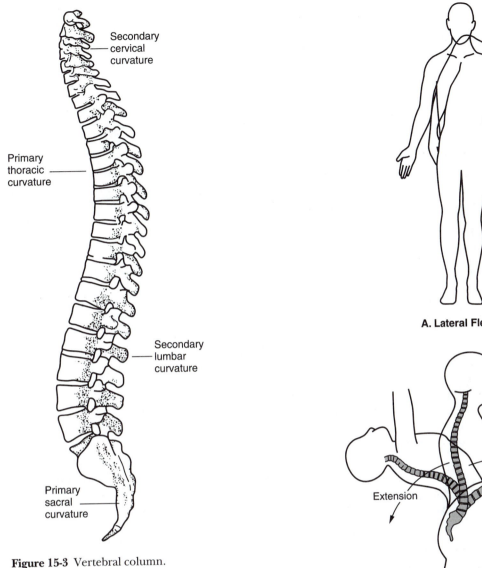

Primary
thoracic
curvature

Primary
sacral
curvature

Secondary
cervical
curvature

Secondary
lumbar
curvature

**Figure 15-3** Vertebral column.

A. Lateral Flexion

Flexion

Extension

**B. Extension end Flexion**

**Figure 15-4** Movements of the vertebral column.

toward the chest at an angle greater than 20°. Twice as much muscle force is needed to counteract the weight of a forward-flexed head as a head held in an upright position (Oberg & Oberg, 1993). When the pressure on the discs is altered, the incidence of joint dysfunctions, disc degeneration, and osteoarthritis may increase.

The movements of the vertebral column are lateral flexion, extension, flexion, and rotation (see Figure 15-4). A **neutral, balanced body position** is that position in which all the muscles are centered and no muscle or muscle group is overworking; the total musculoskeletal structure is in balance. A seated position for performing most dental treatment has been universally accepted. Your weight should be evenly distributed on the operator's chair with your back initially against the back of the chair. The chair should provide complete support for the lumbar segment of the back. The pelvis may tip forward to lean nearer to a client; however, neutral, balanced body position will be maintained. Your thighs should be parallel to the floor. A chair that is too high may cut off

vascular circulation in the back of legs and contribute to leg pain. Separating the knees to form a tripod increases your stability when rotating around the client. Shoulders should be relaxed in a position parallel to the floor. Abduction, or the raising of one or both shoulders and continual lateral flexion of the spine may contribute to nerve entrapment or compression. Shoulder abduction indicates a client being positioned too high. With your shoulders in a relaxed position, the height of your elbows, flexed at 90° to the working plane, indicates the proper client chair height. A supine client at proper height affords your hands, elbows and the client's mouth to all be in the same plane. Efforts should be made to resist elevating elbows more that 30° from the body. The operator should be able to view the working area without bending the neck laterally. The client's mouth should intersect an imaginary line from the operator's eyes to the operator's knees (see Figure 15-5).

Maintaining a **neutral wrist position** (refer to Figure 15-2E), with the arm and wrist in a continuum is critical, especially in the prevention of CTS. It has been reported that the most mechanically efficient position for the wrist is an extension of approximately 30° with fingers that are flexed slightly (Johnson, 1990). Prolonged use of the wrist in ulnar deviation, or cocked medially toward the midline of the arm, has been shown to contribute to both CTS and DeQuervain's tenosynovitis (Johnson, 1990; Macdonald, 1987). Prolonged instrumentation with the wrist flexed may increase rubbing of the median nerve within the carpal tunnel resulting in nerve compression (CTS). A full-arm stroke that employs the muscles of the entire arm, not only reduces wrist strokes and potential for nerve impairment, but also maintains a neutral wrist position and provides more power (Nield-Gehrig & Houseman, 1996; Wilkins, 1994; Woodall et al., 1989). The traditional methods of instrumentation such as pivoting, rocking, and rolling can be accomplished with a full-arm stroke; however, the practitioner might find it necessary to increase the use of extraoral fulcrums. To access different quadrants, the client chair can be adjusted or the client's head may be adjusted to maintain operator body position. A change in position, periodic stretching or even standing, provides necessary muscle relaxation to promote good posture.

**Force.** Undue force is exerted on the fingers, muscles, and tendons when the practitioner applies pressure in grasping or pinching instruments. The force factor increases during a working stroke as opposed to an exploratory stroke. When grasping an instrument, the lightest effective pressure should be utilized (Wilkins, 1994). Increased pressure should only be used in situations such as engaging deposits, or when pressure is necessary in restorative procedures. Force factors may also be affected by the weight and slipperiness of an instrument. When an instrument is too light, there is a tendency to increase pinch pressure to feel the instrument in the hand. A smooth instrument is often perceived as slippery, especially when the practitioner is wearing gloves. Using instruments with serrated or textured handles (see Figure 15-6) will increase retention in the hand so that less pressure or force is used to grasp the instrument and reduce muscle strain (Gerwatowski et al., 1992). Contoured finger grips are available on the handles of some instruments to increase retention and increase the handle diameter. Practitioners should evaluate whether this type of handle is appropriate for them, since hand and finger size vary. These finger grips can inhibit the freedom to move the fingers along the handle for increased access. Intense digital force or pressure on an instrument in combination with postural and mechanical stress factors, may contribute to CTS symptoms (Gerwatowski et al., 1992). Less pressure is used when grasping an ultrasonic instrument because the practitioner is only using pressure to stabilize the instrument. The ultrasonic action of the instrument dislodges the deposits, rather than the force exerted by the practitioner.

**Mechanical Stresses.** Mechanical stresses are evident in the dental environment in numerous situations. Instrument handle size and shape may create both mechanical stress and digital nerve compression. Small-diameter instrument handles can be more difficult to control and lead to muscle strain from increased force. Historically,

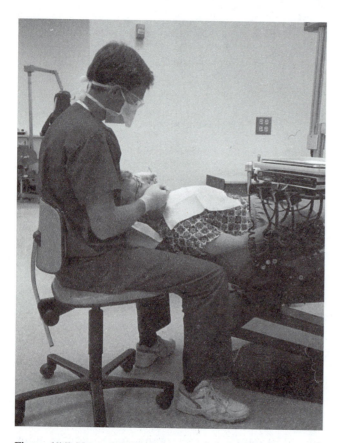

**Figure 15-5** Neutral, balanced operator/client position.

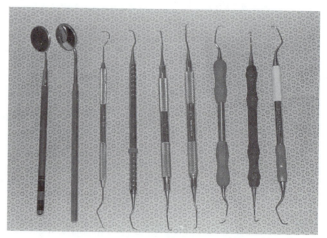

**Figure 15-6** Instrument handle variations.

the #2 handle was the standard handle size. A larger-handled instrument, such as the #4 handle, increases the diameter of the handle, which in turn opens the grasp and decreases the tendency to pinch the instrument. Most instrument manufacturers have the #4 handle available upon request. An instrument handle with hard, sharp edges, such as a hexagonal handle can result in digital nerve compression.

Maintenance of a neutral wrist position is a critical factor in instrument selection and adaptation throughout the mouth. When working on the lingual of the anterior teeth, practitioners may want to consider using a contra-angled instrument such as a Columbia 13/14 universal curet, as opposed to a straight shank instrument such as a Gracey 1/2, which results in more wrist flexion in some situations when properly adapted. This concept should also be considered when using handpieces and prophy angles. A contra-angled prophy angle not only maintains neutral wrist position, but also allows for access to all segments of the mouth. The handpiece should be balanced, lightweight, compact, and easy to handle. A handpiece with the motor weight at one end will require a tighter grasp to offset the weight and resist wrist extension.

Retractable or curled cords on the dental unit are another example of mechanical stresses. These cords retract due to the tension built into them. That tension is transferred to the wrist. To counteract the tension, a tighter grasp and increased muscle strength is used to resist extension of the wrist. This situation is especially harmful when the wrist is in a flexed position (see Figure 15-2A). To reduce this stress, place the cord over the shoulder. For optimal benefits, replace the cord with a straight one of adequate length.

Special attention should be given to choosing gloves that fit properly and are designed to the contour of your hands. Ill-fitting gloves will restrict movement and cause hand fatigue. Examples of gloves that fit improperly include those with short fingers or with a palm width that is smaller than the operator's hands. Tight wristbands may also restrict movement. Gloves that are too large and bunch at the fingers may result in a loss of tactile sensitivity and cause pinch pressure. Another issue to be addressed with ill-fitting gloves is that the thumbs of the hand are not in the same plane as the fingers. The design of many gloves does place the thumb in the same plane as the fingers. This position is an unnatural position for the hand and results in constant muscle action to counteract the stress.

**Vibration.** Numerous studies have been conducted on the use of pneumatic handheld tools, such as drills used in production line assembly, and the effects of vibration on the small blood vessels, nerve injury, and peripheral nerve compressions (Dellon, 1980; Gelberman, Szabo, & Williamson et al., 1983; Lukas, 1979). Vibration has been found to be a contributing factor in the development of nerve neuropathies and CTS in workers who use tools that vibrate in the frequency band of 20 to 80 Hz with an acceleration between 100 and 1,200 m/sec$^2$ (King, 1990; Lukas, 1979). Ultrasonic scaling devices produce vibrations in the range of 25,000 to 42,000 Hz while sonic scalers produce vibration frequencies of less that 16,000 Hz (Gross, Overman, Cobb, & Brockman, 1992). Studies have yet to be conducted and published that examine the relationship of the use of air-driven handpieces, sonic instruments, or ultrasonic devices to the development of CTS or other CTD in practitioners.

**Temperature.** Low temperatures accentuate the symptoms of a nerve-end impairment and reduce manual dexterity (Armstrong, 1986). Exposure to cold air or low room temperatures and manipulation of cold materials or instruments can contribute to cold fingers. Attempting to perform precision work with cold fingers can result in pinching, muscle fatigue, and a loss of tactile sensitivity. It has been recommended that temperatures be kept above 25°C or 77°F to avoid finger dexterity problems (Armstrong, 1986). Cold room temperature or being exposed to cold air drafts directed at the neck and shoulders can also have similar detrimental affects on muscles. A muscle constricts when it is cold, which results in overwork over a period of time. Comfortable room temperatures, redirecting air exhaust fans away from practitioners, warm-water handwashing, and wearing warm garments assist in maintaining appropriate body temperatures to facilitate work.

Exercises can be very beneficial to strengthen muscles to maintain correct posture and to warm up muscles prior to work. Also, exercises (see Table 15-3) are advantageous between client appointments and after work to counteract the muscle action used in work (Gerwatowski et al., 1992; Grossman, 1990; McFall, Stach, & Gerwatowski, 1993).

## Proposed Ergonomic Standard

The Occupational Health and Safety Administration (OSHA) has become increasingly interested in ergonomic issues as a direct result of the tremendous increase of cumulative trauma disorders both in number and as a percent of total illnesses reported. From OSHA's hazard protection perspective, ergonomic issues fall into the areas of repetitive motion, awkward posturing, and vibration and lifting hazards. In 1982, disorders related to repetitive trauma consisted of 21 percent of the total illness cases reported, and by 1991 that percentage had almost tripled (Bureau of Labor Statistics, 1992). OSHA has issued instance-by-instance citations to large corporations since 1988 for alleged repetitive motion-related illnesses in response to this increase, despite the lack of an ergonomic standard. Additionally, these penalties have been issued despite the current controversy between ergonomists and the medical profession as to the scope and validity of the cumulative trauma disorder hypothesis (Vedder, Price, Kaufman, & Kammholz, 1993).

**Table 15-3  Exercise to Reduce Operator Fatigue and Increase Strength**

| Area of the Body | Purpose | Directions |
|---|---|---|
| Back | Stretch and strengthen lower back muscles. | 1. Lie on the floor, pull knees up to chest, and wrap arms around knees.<br>2. Hold for a count of three, release arms, resist arching back and slowly straighten legs.<br>3. Repeat sequence for five repetitions. |
| | Stretch out trunk muscles. | 1. Stand with arms straight down along body.<br>2. Laterally flex back on one side and then the other.<br>3. Perform five repetitions. |
| | Increase natural flexibility of lower spine. | *Extension:*<br>1. Extend back by bending backward with arms held over head for balance.<br>2. Hold in position for a count of two and straighten.<br>3. Perform five repetitions.<br><br>*Flexion:*<br>1. Sit on a chair or stool, lean forward and arch back, with arms hanging toward the floor.<br>2. Hold in position for a count of two and straighten.<br>3. Perform five repetitions. |
| Upper Back and Shoulders | Stretch pectoral muscles. | 1. Stand facing a corner of a room, approximately two feet from the corner.<br>2. Place palms of both hands on side walls in front of shoulders at shoulder height.<br>3. Lean toward corner, supporting your weight with your hands.<br>4. Hold for a count of three, return to original position.<br>5. Perform three repetitions. |
| | Stretch upper back and pectorals. | 1. Clasp hands behind head (not neck).<br>2. Pull elbows back to squeeze shoulder blades together.<br>3. Hold for a count of three, then relax.<br>4. Perform three repetitions. |
| | Encourage stability of upper back and shoulder muscles. | 1. Lift shoulder blades, squeeze shoulder blades together, lower shoulders and then relax.<br>2. Perform three repetitions. |
| | Relax shoulder muscles. | 1. Roll shoulders backward, or in a clockwise direction, in circles for five circles. |
| Neck | Stretch scalenes. | These stretches should be completed on one side and then reversed to stretch the muscles on the other side of the neck.<br><br>1. Sit on a chair or stool with the lower back supported.<br>2. Grasp the edge of the chair with the right hand.<br>3. Place the head toward the left shoulder, then slightly rotate the head to the right.<br>4. Pull the head toward the left shoulder, then slightly rotate the head to the right.<br>5. Hold for a count of six and repeat three times. |
| | Stretch upper tapezius. | 1. Sit on a chair or stool with the lower back supported.<br>2. Grasp the edge of the chair with the right hand.<br>3. Facing forward, turn the head halfway to the left.<br>4. With the left hand on the back of the head, pull the head forward and down in a diagonal direction.<br>5. Hold for a count of six and repeat three times. |

*(continues)*

**Table 15-3** (continued)

| Area of the Body | Purpose | Directions |
|---|---|---|
| Neck (continued) | Stretch levator scapulae (maintains erect head/neck posture). | 1. Sit on a chair or stool with the lower back supported.<br>2. Place right hand on left knee.<br>3. Drop chin to chest.<br>4. Drop left ear to shoulder, and rotate head slightly to the left.<br>5. Hold for a count of six and repeat three times. |
| Wrist | Encourage gliding of radial, median, and ulnar nerves. | Stretches should be completed with one arm and then repeated with the opposite arm.<br><br>1. Extend right arm, elbow straight, palm up, out in front of the body.<br>2. Flex wrist so the palm of the hand is facing the head.<br>3. Extend the wrist by dropping fingers toward the floor.<br>4. Bend and drop the elbow to the side of the body.<br>5. Perform three repetitions.<br><br>1. Extend the arm, elbow straight, palm up, out to the side of the body.<br>2. Rotate the arm backward.<br>3. Stretch the neck by leaning the left ear to the left shoulder.<br>4. Perform three repetitions.<br><br>1. Flex wrist, bend elbow, and raise hand so that fingers are against the forehead.<br>2. Extend wrist so that wrist is against the forehead and slowly straighten elbow until the arm is extended in front of the body.<br>3. Perform three repetitions.<br><br>1. Raise arm to the side, flex wrist, and raise hand to form a 90° angle at the elbow.<br>2. Rotate arm backward.<br>3. Stretch the neck by leaning the left ear to the left shoulder.<br>4. Perform three repetitions. |

(Acknowledgment to Larynne Hashimoto, P.T.)

OSHA issued its Advanced Notice of Proposed Rule-making for Ergonomics Safety and Health Management on August 3, 1992, in order to solicit comments and information as a precursor to standard setting. Numerous responses from the communities of interest, including industry, dentistry, and dental hygiene have been received by the Agency through written submissions and through hearings sponsored by OSHA. Both the American Dental Hygienists' Association (ADHA) and the American Dental Association (ADA) participated in one of the hearings. The ADA testified that there is no scientifically valid evidence of a significant risk for musculoskeletal disorders in the dental office (Jacob, 1994). The Association also indicated that, over time, dentistry has reduced musculoskeletal stress by providing treatment in a sitting position and by using equipment that has been upgraded to avoid ergonomic problems. It was also suggested to OSHA that dental employers would be burdened with ergonomic standards because the majority of dentists are in solo practice and employ an average of 3.9 employees. The ADA pointed out that the ergonomic standards should more appropriately apply to large corporations than to solo or small practices. As an alternative, the Association offered to work with other groups within the dental professions to develop voluntary consensus guidelines that promote the use of the most up-to-date techniques and technology in dental offices. The ADHA presented testimony in support of the development of ergonomic standards based on the published studies highlighted within this chapter. This Association further recommended that the standards address work site analysis to identify ergonomic hazards, ergonomic hazard prevention and control mechanisms, medical management including early recognition and reporting requirements, as well as systematic monitoring, training, and education.

It is uncertain whether the standard will include trigger mechanisms for application of the standard or the traditional exposure limit approach. A trigger mechanism would envoke the protective provisions of the ergonomic standard when "triggered" by the number of musculoskeletal disorders discovered by the employer through worksite analysis. The trigger mechanism might be used because of the lack of scientific data to determine an exposure limit. The traditional exposure limit approach is problematic as there is variability in how many repetitions individuals can be exposed to before they develop early signs or symptoms of cumulative trauma disorders, or how much force individuals can exert before they develop distress. A final standard was anticipated in the spring of 1995; however, in June, 1995, OSHA determined to delay issuing a final standard until further study of the problem. OSHA acknowledged that intense political pressure and opposition from business groups contributed to the decision.

## PSYCHOSOCIAL HAZARDS

Within the work environment we must mentally and physically deal with our own responses to the environment and to employers and coworkers. The way we respond can affect us psychologically and physically in either a positive or a negative manner. Although clinicians might not have control over some conditions or situations within the work environment, each of us needs to be in control of our own responses. Stress is a result of the activities in which we choose to involve ourselves and the way we choose to react to situations. Stress has also been defined as the wear and tear on your mind, body, and emotions (George, Milone, Block, & Hollister, 1986). **Occupational stress** exists when there is disharmony between the individual and the work environment (Mellody, 1983). Sources of stress, or **stressors**, can exist from factors within ourselves, from factors outside of ourselves, and from factors in the environment (George et al., 1986). Factors within ourselves include beliefs, values, responsibilities, and health. Factors outside of ourselves encompass clients, employers, coworkers, family members, and friends. Stressors from the environment include equipment, layout of an office, and scheduling.

How we cope with or manage stress affects the degree of intensity of the negative or positive effects of stress on our well-being. Selye (1974) identified three stages of coping with stress that an individual may experience when confronted with acute stressors. Stage One is the "alarm stage" when you are first faced with the stressor and may experience a strong physical or emotional reaction, especially if you are unprepared or caught off guard. For instance, you arrive at the office to find that during the night a water pipe broke and the office is flooded with water. Stage Two is when you activate yourself both mentally and often physically to solve the problem or counteract the stressor. If one is unable to successfully manage the stress or solve the problem, one might enter the third stage, called "burnout." **Job "burnout"** is the negative psychological reaction to one's work and the workplace environment (Maslach & Jackson, 1981). Successful stress management skills, along with other aspects such as

a healthy work environment, open communication, and fulfillment of career expectations, can contribute to job satisfaction and career retention. Refer to Chapter 18 about career development for further discussion of factors that can contribute to career retention.

### Stress

Stress has evolved within our society to be used in a negative sense, yet stress can actually motivate one to achieve both personal and professional goals. To experience positive effects of stress, we must manage stress effectively to reduce the adverse effects on our physical health and mental well-being. Stress management includes both the management of the sources of stress, stressors, and the management of our responses. Each of us has a different stress tolerance level. The concept of "how much can we take" varies depending on the cumulative effect of the stressors. This concept also is dependent on other factors such as physical health, the body's state of rest, family situations, age, and/or the personal support system. "Stress tolerance" is usually reduced when contributing factors are present such as major life changes including death, divorce, pregnancy and birth, a serious illness or accident in the family, or relocation. Conversely, working with people whom you can trust, who share similar values, and who you know you can depend upon can increase your working environment stress tolerance level (George et al., 1986).

In the dental work environment, sources of stress exist for every member of the office (Cooper, Mallinger, & Kahn, 1978; Mellody, 1983; O'Shea et al., 1984). Anxiety from concern regarding the potential exposure to infectious diseases might be reduced with the application of universal precautions, however, the risk may still be present. Working with clients who demonstrate high levels of fear or anxiety regarding treatment may elevate your stress level. The financial strain of establishing and building a practice, compounded with school loans is a definite source of stress. Being paid by commission in a practice with a high degree of clients who fail to arrive for appointments can cause stress. It seems that all dental professionals have felt scheduling pressures including walk-in emergency clients, a new amalgam restoration fracturing while the occlusion is being evaluated, a crown being displaced during debridement, or inadequate time being scheduled to care for an individual's needs. A lack of understanding in regard to performance expectations by employees, or a continual lack of acknowledgment of knowledge and skills by employers is a two-way street between employees and employers. Stress can be reduced when the dental hygienist knows that thorough assessment, including extraoral and intraoral soft tissue examination, restorative and periodontal assessment, radiographs, dental hygiene diagnosis, treatment planning, and self-care education are expected to be accomplished during an appointment with a "new" client. Also, it is important that the dental hygienist knows that the results of the client assessment will be reviewed and taken into consideration during a consultation with the dentist. At the same time, acknowledgment provided by a dental hygienist to a dentist of a well-completed three-unit bridge, or a thorough, extensive restorative treatment plan can be recognition that the dentist successfully met the challenge of coping with stress in Stage Two. Interpersonal conflicts with coworkers, differences in ethical values, or sexual harassment situations are examples of sources of stress that may necessitate leaving a specific working environment.

A thorough interview process that includes discussion of practice philosophies, personal and professional goals, performance expectations, practice protocols, communication styles, equipment availability, and, compensation can greatly reduce misunderstandings and subsequent stress. Employment contracts (refer to Chapter 18) that delineate specific job responsibilities, compensation packages, and time intervals for performance reviews can assist in mutual employer/employee understanding.

Identifying our personal sources of stress is the first step in being able to effectively manage stress. Compiling a personal stress inventory helps us to focus on all the stressors that affect us. An inventory should include events, conditions, responsibilities, commitments, problems, and disappointments as well as new challenges, projects, or goals that you have accepted or are working toward. Table 15-4 provides an example of this type of inventory.

We have learned how to respond to stress in a variety of methods, depending on our own personal history. Our family behavior patterns, expectations of behavior by our peer groups, and previous history of experiences all impact our current stress reactions. When we encounter stress, our body initiates a stress response, which is a nonspecific physiological response to the event, responsibility, or pressure from our environment. The stress response is considered nonspecific because our body responds the same physiologically to the stress, and the response only varies in degrees of intensity. For instance, our body will have the same physiologic response, although not as intense, from breaking an instrument tip subgingivally in a client's sulcus as it will from having the

**Table 15-4 Stresses Inventory**

| Stresses | Stressors | Degree of Stress: High, Medium, Low | Feasibility of Change: High, Medium, Low | Action Plan |
|---|---|---|---|---|
| Personal | ***Ongoing Stresses*** <br> 1. School loans | H | M | 1. Develop monthly budget and adhere to budget. |
| | 2. Household maintenance | M | H | 2. Delegate chores to family members. |
| | 3. Transportation to children's activities | H | H | 3. Contact other parents to arrange carpool. |
| | 4. Diet control and exercise program | H | M | 4. Reduce sweets, purchase fat-free groceries, walk three to four times per week. |
| | ***Recent Events*** <br> 1. Death of father | H | L | 1. Share with family lessons learned from father and happy experiences you shared. |
| | 2. Dishwasher broke | M | M | 2. Rotate dishwashing to all family members. Obtain repair estimates and schedule repair. |
| Professional | ***Ongoing Stresses*** <br> 1. Staff does not work collaboratively; however, each is highly skilled. | H | H | 1. Develop practice goals and plan to implement staff meeting. Increase staff meeting efficiency by developing and distributing agendas. Select full staff workshops to promote team efforts. |
| | ***Recent Events*** <br> 1. Dental assistant gave two-week notice. | H | H | 1. Schedule exit interview to determine reason(s) for leaving. Place ads. Meet with staff to develop interim plan. |
| | 2. X-ray unit breakdown. | H | H | 2. Schedule repair. Reschedule clients. |

client go into anaphylactic shock. When the central nervous system receives and processes information regarding the stress, it activates the autonomic nervous system and the endocrine system. These two systems together prepare the body to deal with the situation through what is referred to as "fight or flight." The body prepares to either stand firm and "fight" the stress, or run in "flight" from the stress. The autonomic nervous system releases epinephrine and norepinephrine into the bloodstream, which subsequently causes the heartbeat to accelerate, blood pressure to rise, blood to be directed to the skeletal muscles, and our senses to become more acute. Breathing can become more rapid in order to increase oxygenation, and the blood sugar level rises to provide more energy to the cells. Digestion is also inhibited during this process. The endocrine system speeds up the process of synthesis and secretion of hormones, which among other actions, inhibits inflammatory reactions and limits the action of the defense cells within the immune system. All of these responses are necessary to meet the body's challenge of "fight or flight." Once some type of physical action has been taken, the changes begin to subside. If no action is taken and the stress continues, the physiologic changes subside at a much slower rate, or the body may try to adapt to the changes. Adverse reactions such as heart irregularity, hypertension, or gastrointestinal problems may result if the body is exposed to these physiologic changes over a prolonged period of time.

Successfully coping with stress on a psychological level contributes to reducing the intensity of the physiological response. Once we have identified our sources of stress we can begin to analyze the most appropriate course of action. The action may be as simple as replacing a piece of equipment that continually breaks down causing delays in client treatment, to a complex situation of conflict between several coworkers that may necessitate the use of team building interventions. Perhaps a coworker has an addiction problem that is impacting her job performance and professional intervention is necessary. Some of the common interventions that may be helpful within the dental environment are time management, team building, and conflict resolution including negotiation and delegation (George et al., 1986; Paine, 1982) (refer to Chapters 18 and 19). How time is used for work and life activities usually affects values. Your values influence your motivation to work. If your motivation for work is to provide for your family and because you truly enjoy providing oral health care, you may manage your time differently than someone whose motivation is centered around the need to repay school loans and be in a specific income bracket by the time age 40 is reached. Realizing that individuals within the work environment come together with a variety of values that impact their work habits and motivation aids in being able to understand, accept, and cope with differences.

Time pressures can become major causes in stress overload. Time management problems are often a result of failure to plan. Planning should take into considera-

tion priorities and capabilities, as well as provide flexibility to allow for unanticipated situations such as emergency client visits, equipment failures, or staff illness. Participation of all staff members in time management planning enables each member to analyze the span of his or her daily and weekly work responsibilities so that final planning represents realistic work time expectations. Individual participation in planning also increases commitment to the plan.

Teamwork requires a variety of qualities such as communication, creativity, cooperation, and trust. A team is a group of individuals who are striving for a common purpose. Each member brings a unique contribution. Regardless of the differences among team members, they share basic psychological needs, such as the need to contribute, the need to feel competent, the need to achieve results, and the need to have their efforts recognized and rewarded. The boundaries that are set by the manager or leader of a team define the ground rules. These boundaries would include deadlines, measurable goals, clearly stated expectations, limits imposed by authority, limits imposed by responsibilities, and responsibilities assigned to others. The ground rules provide all team members an equal advantage. These might include setting time limits on staff meeting discussions, guidelines for presenting information or an opinion during staff meetings, a process for resolving conflicts, an agreed upon style for critiquing new ideas, or a protocol for how information will be communicated to all team members. Establishing a bond among team members by creating a shared goal, projecting a positive attitude, communicating consistently and clearly in a timely manner, and treating all team members with respect will contribute to successfully creating a cohesive team (Mallory, 1989).

It is inevitable that conflict will periodically surface within the work environment. Conflict exists when the concerns or wants of two or more people appear to be incompatible. Conflict can be considered healthy when it is used constructively to clarify expectations, needs, and roles, and to strengthen relationships. Not having an opportunity to be heard creates one of the most stressful working environments. Basic conflict resolution skills include communication, decision making, problem solving, and negotiation. Keep in mind that the most effective approach to conflict resolution is one that enables both parties to come away with positive feelings about the outcome. This positive approach can be called a "win/win" approach or situation.

The concept of delegation is traditionally thought of in terms of delegation of dental procedures to dental hygienists and dental assistants. Beyond that aspect, delegation of other work responsibilities should be considered that contribute to enhancing self-confidence and abilities. For example, different team members might be ultimately responsible for certain fundamental functions in the practice such as the recall system, public relations, continuing education, or an inventory system. The work should be meaningful, not just busy work to use employee time. All workers want to feel that they are contributing to the common purpose and want to feel a sense of achievement in their work. The purpose of this discussion has been to increase awareness of the sources of stress within the dental work environment and provide basic intervention suggestions to deal with some of the more frequent potential stress situations.

## Burnout

Investigation and studies on the concept of burnout in professionals involved in clinical work associated with providing health care surfaced in the early 1970s and continued to appear through the middle 1980s. Maslach and Jackson (1981) have operationally defined *burnout* as a syndrome consisting of a set of symptoms characterized by emotional exhaustion, lowered feelings of personal accomplishment, and depersonalization. A study of Finnish dentists utilized similar characteristics and analyzed psychological fatigue, loss of enjoyment of work, and "hardening" as factors of burnout. "Hardening" factors included attitudes such as insensitivity toward others and treating patients as impersonal objects. Psychological fatigue was the most common aspect of burnout. A significant predictor of psychological fatigue was poor working posture. Improving work posture, and the physical work environment along with reducing the pace of work was demonstrated to be effective in reducing psychological fatigue (Murtomma, Haavio-Mannila, & Kandolin, 1990).

A 1982 study of dental hygienists employed the Maslach Burnout Inventory (MBI) to measure emotional exhaustion, lowered feelings of personal accomplishment, and depersonalization by measuring the frequency and intensity of responses to a list of twenty-two job attitudes. Segments of the Job Diagnostic Survey (JDS) were also used to measure worker perception of job characteristics and satisfactions and to test the theory that the dental hygiene profession and dental environment have a high burnout potential. This nonrandomly selected group of 111 dental hygienists did not exhibit a high incidence of burnout. The sample presented lower than average scores on the frequency and intensity of feeling emotional exhaustion and depersonalization; moreover, these dental hygienists exhibited lower than average scores on experiencing feelings of personal accomplishment when compared to other health and human service professionals. After analyzing both the MBI and JDS findings, the authors hypothesized that the lack of opportunity to use varied skills and to engage cognitive resources to meet challenges and enrich the job resulted in diminished feelings of personal accomplishment (Deckard & Rountree, 1984).

Burnout is initiated when an employee starts to feel his or her work as a stressful experience; progresses to feelings of both stress and fatigue; and, subsequently responds defensively with changes in behavior and attitudes, especially toward clients (Cherniss, 1980). In the final stage of burnout, mental problems, particularly depression, can develop (Freudenberger, 1980). These phases correspond to the three stages of coping with stress as described by Selye (1974) that were previously discussed in this chapter. Studies conducted from the middle 1980s to date have addressed the prevention aspect of burnout from the perspective of analyzing the attributes of job and career satisfaction and retention within the profession. The demand for dental hygienists in the middle 1980s was low; however, in the past fifteen years the demand for oral health care has increased and, subsequently, the demand for dental hygienists has also increased. The impetus for many of the studies on job and career satisfaction has been to reduce attrition and enhance retention within the profession (Body, 1988; Boyer, 1994; Boyer, 1990; Dadian, 1993; Johnston, O'Shea, & Lewis, 1992; Miller, 1991).

## Job and Career Satisfaction

Body (1988) found in a review of the literature regarding dental hygiene job and career satisfaction that the published studies reflected a high level of satisfaction with dental hygiene, although there were characteristics of dental hygiene and dental practice that contributed to dissatisfaction. The variety of work in dental hygiene practice, education level, opportunity for advancement, and dental hygienists' personal value systems were cited (Body, 1988). Miller (1991) focused on determining dental hygiene attrition rates and reported the five most frequently cited reasons for permanently leaving dental hygiene practice. Boredom, inadequate salary, lack of benefits, concern with infectious disease, and lack of decision-making opportunities were identified. Family responsibilities were found to be a major reason for temporarily leaving practice, although they did not affect leaving the profession permanently (Miller, 1991). Her findings are consistent with other studies. The differences between job satisfaction and career satisfaction were emphasized in a study of dental hygienists by Bader and Sams (1992). Individuals may be satisfied with their choice of dental hygiene as a career and at the same time be dissatisfied with their current job situation. Bader and Sams found that the managerial or supervisory style of the employer has a strong correlation with job satisfaction. Respondents with high job satisfaction characterized employer supervisory style as open, clear, two-way, honest, and displaying a willingness to try new ideas and fully utilize office members' talents and capabilities (Bader & Sams, 1992). The literature reports that unsatisfactory working conditions, lack of career progress, unfulfilled expectations, and significant personal or professional changes can result in job turnover, subsequent career dissatisfaction, and the hygienist eventually leaving the dental hygiene profession (Nelson & Newell, 1993a). Nelson and Newell studied the effects of a career planning workshop on career satisfaction. The workshop included information and activities to guide participants through a career planning process to assess their personal skills, knowledge, values, and work options, and to develop and implement a career plan (Nelson & Newell, 1993b). Dental hygienists and dentists need to develop the intervention skills necessary to promote collaboration in the work environment based on mutual respect, sharing different types of professional expertise, and taking responsibility for the excellence of one's performance.

A collaborative client care approach between dentists and dental hygienists has been proposed as a method to provide optimum client care and increase job satisfaction. This approach includes acknowledgment and mutual respect for scopes of practice, and both clinical and decision-making skills. Nonsurgical periodontal therapy can provide an opportunity within the work environment to implement a collaborative approach to assess client status, identify risk factors and needs, utilize decision-making skills in treatment planning, provide treatment involving a variety of therapies (chemotherapeutics, irrigation, mechanical debridement), and evaluate the client's response to care. Practitioners are challenged to expand their capabilities and skill levels as well as their knowledge base by maintaining a current understanding of new technologies.

## OTHER HAZARDS

Oral healthcare professionals should also have an awareness and understanding of the potential occupational hazards in the biological, chemical, and physical arenas. Biological hazards include the risk of exposure or potential for exposure to microbial aerosols, contaminated wastes, and/or infectious diseases. Chemical hazards exist when we are not only exposed to a chemical, but when the chemical, at a toxic dose, has entered the body through inhalation, ingestion, or through cutaneous absorption (Banting & Robertson, 1991). Physical hazards within the dental workplace include potential exposure to ionizing radiation, auditory deterioration due to exposure to high-frequency noise, and damaged vision due to exposure to light-curing devices.

### Biological Hazards

OSHA has defined an **occupational exposure**, with regard to bloodborne pathogens, as "reasonably anticipated skin, eye, mucous membrane, or parenteral contact with blood or other potentially infectious materials that may result from the performance of an employee's duties" (Occupational Safety and Health Act of 1970). While practitioners have been acutely aware of the risks of exposure to bloodborne pathogens and have made control procedures a part of their daily practice, the reemergence of tuberculosis and the mutant, multidrug-resistant tuberculosis, has increased the awareness and need to control airborne pathogens. Research has shown that the use of sonic and ultrasonic equipment and air

polishing devices do produce aerosols that are contaminated with microorganisms (Gross et al., 1992; Barnes, 1991). Preprocedural rinsing with antimicrobial mouthrinses, appropriate use of barrier techniques and surface disinfection using EPA-registered surface disinfectants can minimize exposure (Gross et al., 1992; Barnes, 1991).

Immunization for specific diseases is also a mechanism for practitioner protection. Although OSHA Standards do require employers to offer hepatitis B vaccinations for dental healthcare workers, other immunizations are not mandated. The Centers for Disease Control and Prevention (CDC) has recommended vaccination for dental healthcare workers for influenza, rubella, measles, mumps, polio, and tetanus as may be appropriate (CDC, 1989). As healthcare providers, oral healthcare workers should accept the responsibility of knowing their immunologic status and pursuing preventive measures such as immunizations. Efforts to reduce or eliminate the risk of exposure to many biological hazards have now been mandated by a combination of federal, state, and local regulations. Practitioners should maintain current information regarding compliance with applicable laws and technological advances.

### Chemical Hazards

The American Conference of Governmental Industrial Hygienists (ACGIH) provides recommendations for safe exposure levels of toxic materials. The levels are expressed as Threshold Limit Values (TLVs), which specify the airborne concentration to which a worker can be exposed for eight hours a day, five days a week over an extended period of time without experiencing adverse health effects. Some of the chemicals commonly used in the dental office environment that present the potential for hazard are nitrous oxide, sterilants/disinfectants, mercury, photographic chemicals, and sensitivity to chemicals used in the manufacturing of latex gloves (ACGIH, 1993).

The results of the American Dental Association 1991 Survey of Dental Practice (1992) found that 58 percent of dentists reported having nitrous oxide anesthetic equipment, and 64 percent of those also indicated having scavenging systems. Since then many states have mandated scavenging systems for such equipment. Studies have concluded that exposure to nitrous oxide causes decreases in mental performance, audiovisual ability, and manual dexterity. Reduced fertility and spontaneous abortion as well as neurological, renal, and liver disease are also results of exposure to nitrous oxide (Cohen et al., 1980; National Institute for Occupational Safety and Health, 1977; Rowland et al., 1992). Although these effects have been demonstrated epidemiologically in humans and studied in laboratory animals, the threshold concentration and length of exposure time necessary to produce these conditions are still unknown. Currently,

OSHA does not have a standard for nitrous oxide. ACGIH has stated that a TLV for nitrous oxide is 50 ppm during an eight-hour time limit (ACGIH, 1993). The National Institute of Occupational Safety and Health (NIOSH) recommended in 1977 an exposure limit for nitrous oxide of 25 ppm during the period of anesthetic administration (NIOSH, 1977). NIOSH has further recommended that an operatory should have a room air exchange rate of ten room air changes per hour and that the nitrous oxide delivery system use scavenging evacuation at a rate of 45 lpm to the nasal mask (McGlothlin, Jensen, Todd, Fischbach, & Fairfield, 1989). Ambient levels of nitrous oxide have been reported in dental operatories that far exceed the NIOSH recommendations (Borganelli, Primosch, & Henry, 1993; Donaldson & Orr, 1989; Henry & Jerrell, 1990; Henry & Primosch, 1991; McGlothlin, Jensen, Todd, & Fischbach, 1988; McGlothlin, Jensen, Todd, & Fischbach, 1990). State health departments, public utility companies, and suppliers of nitrous oxide can assist in determining room air exchange rates and ambient levels of nitrous oxide within the workplace. Refer to Chapter 9 for specific recommendations to reduce nitrous oxide levels in the dental operatory.

The uses and concentrations of chemical sterilants and disinfectants have increased over the past years, especially since the enactment of the bloodborne pathogen standard by OSHA, which mandates sterilization and disinfection protocols. Based upon the risk of transmitting infection and the need to sterilize between uses, dental instruments are classified as critical, semicritical, and noncritical. Critical instruments penetrate soft tissue or bone and should be sterilized after each use. Examples include forceps, scalpels, bone chisels, scalers, and burs. Semicritical instruments are described as those that do not penetrate soft tissues or bone, but do contact oral tissues and should also be sterilized. Examples of semicritical instruments include mirrors and amalgam condensers. Critical and semicritical instruments that are heat stable should be sterilized between uses by steam under pressure (autoclaving), dry heat, or chemical vapor following manufacturer's instructions. Some instruments are damaged by heat sterilization and manufacturers advise the use of chemical sterilization. If a chemical vapor sterilizer is used, practitioners should exert caution to avoid inhalation during opening and venting of the unit. Indications for use of liquid chemical germicides to sterilize instruments are very limited and may require up to ten hours of immersion in the chemical agent to obtain sterilization followed by aseptic rinsing with sterile water, drying, and storage in a sterile container. The agent must be registered by the Environmental Protection Agency (EPA) as a "sterilant/disinfectant" to attain high-level disinfection of heat-sensitive instruments.

Noncritical instruments and devices are those that come in contact only with intact skin and have a low level of risk of transmitting infection. Examples of non-critical instruments include external components of x-ray heads or equipment used for external demonstration of oral hygiene. Intermediate-level or low-level disinfection may be used between clients for noncritical instruments. Chemical germicides that are EPA registered as "hospital disinfectant" and labeled for "tuberculocidal" are recommended by CDC. Intermediate-level disinfectants include compounds such as phenolics, iodophors, and chlorine-containing compounds.

Practitioners must insure that appropriate concentrations and solution preparation guidelines are followed for compliance with OSHA standards. Protective barriers such as masks and gloves should be worn during preparation and use of solutions to avoid exposure by inhalation or cutaneous absorption. Many surface disinfectants are manufactured for ease of use as a spray. Repeated daily exposure through inhalation may result in mucous membrane and upper respiratory irritations. Appropriate labeling is required to avoid exposure and prevent accidental exposure by ingestion.

The use of mercury in dental amalgam restorations has gained increasing media attention in recent years, especially as it relates to toxicity levels for clients. Occupational exposure to dental mercury has been addressed by both OSHA and the ADA Council on Dental Materials, Instruments and Equipment (Council on Dental Materials, Instruments and Equipment, 1984; OSHA, 1989). The OSHA limit for mercury vapor is 50 microgram/cubic meter time weighted average in an eight-hour work shift over a forty hour work week (OSHA, 1989). If interested in guidelines to reduce exposure to mercury vapor, refer to *Dental Mercury Hygiene, Summary of Recommendations in 1990*" (Council on Dental Materials, Instruments and Equipment, 1991).

There has been an increase in the reports of latex-related reactions since glove use has become a mandated infection control protocol (Berkey, Luciano, & James, 1992; Boyer & Bolden, 1993; Gonzales, 1992; Stewart, 1992). Symptoms range from dermatitis, conjunctivitis, and rhinitis to anaphylactic shock (Berkey et al., 1992; Stewart, 1992). The impetus for such reactions needs to be carefully analyzed to determine whether the reaction is due to the chemicals used in the manufacturing of latex, the talc powder that many manufacturers use to facilitate putting the gloves on, or a true allergic reaction to the latex (Berkey et al.; Stewart). The only way to determine if a reaction is an actual allergy to latex proteins is verification by skin testing with the allergens in the glove (Spanner, Dolovich, Tarlo, Sussman, & Butto, 1989). The case studies in the literature support that the incidence of reactions is related to the extent and frequency of exposure to the latex. Early reactions include rash, redness, itching, burning, hives, cracking and bleeding of the skin, eye irritations, shortness of breath, and wheezing. Prompt medical evaluation should be sought to identify the causative factor and implement the recommended therapeutic measures.

## Physical Hazards

Technological advances in radiation equipment and an increased awareness of the physical damage caused by overexposure to ionizing radiation has resulted in efforts to reduce harmful exposure. Radiation safety is included within accredited dental and dental hygiene curriculum. Therefore, practitioners in both disciplines should possess knowledge in this area. Key components of operator safety include positioning the operator behind a shielded barrier or at least six feet from the primary beam of the x-ray. Inspections of all radiology equipment is required in all states to analyze compliance with safety requirements. The length of time between inspections varies from state to state. Most state regulations include equipment, operator, and client safety. Monitoring badges are available and recommended for all personnel who work in environments with risk of exposure to ionizing radiation. Refer to Chapter 5 for further guidelines on radiation safety.

Auditory deterioration because of exposure to noise, such as that generated from high-speed dental handpieces, has been both confirmed and denied in the literature (Park, 1978). Subsequent studies utilizing both low-speed and high-speed handpieces have failed to show conclusive evidence that exposure to handpiece noise alone causes hearing loss. Other variables include age, disease, existing hearing condition, and the exposure to nondental noises. Studies have not been published regarding the effect of sonic and ultrasonic instruments on hearing loss. OSHA standards state a 90-decibel (dBA) maximum for eight hours of permissible continuous exposure per day, while the ACGIH has a more stringent guideline of 85 dBA maximum level. It has been estimated that dental use of high-speed handpieces is about 15 minutes per day on an intermittent basis, far below either standard (Man, Neuman, & Assif, 1982). This estimate could vary widely, depending upon individual handpiece preference, practice specialty, and productivity. The *Dentist's Desk Reference* (DDR), published by the ADA Council on Dental Materials, Instruments, and Equipment reports that most ball-bearing high-speed handpieces elicit sound in the 68 to 97 dBA range and that air-bearing handpieces are usually 10 dBA lower than ball-bearing handpieces. Both improper maintenance of handpieces and wear increase noise levels. Therefore, routine maintenance according to manufacturer's recommendations is essential.

Eye injury, eyestrain, and eye damage from exposure to dental light-curing devices have all been reported in the literature (Goldlist, 1979; Wagner, 1985). The wearing of protective eyewear by practitioners dramatically reduces the incidence of eye injury from flying debris such as dislodged calculus, amalgam, tooth particles, or pumice paste. Eyestrain can result from lack of appropriate lighting and overuse of the eye muscles in focusing. Adequate room illumination as well as illumination of the field of operation will assist in reducing eyestrain. Optic adjustment to the contrast in illumination can contribute to eyestrain. Detailed guidelines have been offered that address the ideal ratio of task to room illumination (Preston et al., 1978). Regular optical evaluations to assess personal visual acuity and maintain visual correction will also contribute to reducing the potential for eyestrain. The use of loupes and glasses with adjustable magnification has been found to be beneficial for visual acuity for both dental hygienists and dentists. Also, the use of fiber optics increases the contrast between the room lighting and the light focused on the oral cavity. When using light-curing devices, care should be taken to avoid staring at the light, and filtered eyewear is recommended to reduce the light's intensity. The light emission spectra of various curing units differs. Practitioners should select protective eyewear that matches the spectrum of the light-curing unit being used.

## FEDERAL REGULATIONS REGARDING OCCUPATIONAL HEALTH

There are several federal laws that regulate aspects of our work environment in an effort to protect workers. These include The Occupational Safety and Health Act and The Consumer Radiation and Safety Act. The Occupational Safety and Health Act was passed in 1970, as a result of public demand to force employers to provide safe working conditions (The Occupational Safety and Health Act of 1970). The Occupational Safety and Health Administration (OSHA) of the United States Department of Labor was established to set workplace health and safety standards and to enforce and insure compliance with the standards. The Act mandates that employers must furnish to each employee a place of employment that is free from recognized hazards that are likely to cause death or serious harm to employees. The Act further requires that employees must comply with all occupational safety and health standards, rules, regulations, and orders specified by the Act that apply to the employees' conduct on the job. When employees believe that conditions exist within their workplace that are unsafe or unhealthy, they have the right to file a complaint with one of the regional OSHA offices. The Act protects employees from discrimination or discharge for filing complaints. When a complaint has been filed, an OSHA inspector from one of the regional offices will conduct an inspection of the workplace to evaluate conditions. OSHA may impose citations or fines for violations. To impose sanctions, the Act requires OSHA to prove that 1) a condition or activity in the workplace presented a hazard to an employee, 2) the hazard was recognized, 3) the hazard was likely to cause death or serious physical harm, and 4) a feasible means existed to eliminate or materially reduce the hazard. OSHA also promotes safe working environments by providing voluntary inspections and assistance by OSHA inspectors to insure compliance with standards.

Several OSHA standards and guidelines directly

affect the dental workplace. The Final Standard for Occupational Exposure to Bloodborne Pathogens that became effective March 6, 1992, sets standards to reduce or eliminate the risk of occupational exposures to bloodborne diseases. This standard addresses eight primary categories:

1. Universal Precautions—Infection control procedures are utilized that treat all human blood and certain human body fluids as if they are infected with bloodborne pathogens.
2. Personal Protective Equipment—Refers to clothing and equipment that is worn by workers to protect them from exposure to potentially infectious hazardous material.
3. Work Practice Controls—Those actions or ways in which a procedure is performed that reduce the potential for exposure.
4. Engineering Controls—Devices or methods that isolate or remove the bloodborne pathogen hazard from the work environment.
5. Housekeeping—Protocols that insure a clean and sanitary workplace.
6. Signs and Labels—Identification of an immediate or recognized hazard using universals symbols or labels.
7. Recordkeeping—Mandates employee records regarding immunization, injury, and exposure incidents.
8. Information and Training—Employers are mandated to provide to employees, at no cost, information and training regarding occupational exposure during working hours.

The OSHA Hazards Communication Standard specifies the information that must be posted and available to workers regarding workplace hazards and the protocols for communicating information. OSHA has also issued mandatory guidelines to protect exposed workers against tuberculosis. These guidelines instruct employers on how to apply OSHA standards for inspections in facilities where increased exposure to TB exists (OSHA, 1993).

The Consumer Radiation Safety Act of 1981 set standards for the Accreditation of Educational Programs and the Credentialing of Radiologic Personnel. The states were encouraged to adopt standards that were consistent with the standards set out in the Act. Dental hygienists and dentists, by virtue of graduation from an accredited program, meet the educational requirements of the Act.

Dental assistants and any other dental health care workers who expose radiographs must meet the requirements as set forth by the state.

Other federal agencies that have an impact on dental practitioners' working environments are the Centers for Disease Control and Prevention (CDC), the National Institutes for Safety and Health (NIOSH), and the Food and Drug Administration (FDA) both within the United States Department of Health and Human Services; and the Environmental Protection Agency (EPA). CDC is not a regulatory agency; therefore it has no enforcement authority. It provides guidelines, consultation, and tracks the epidemiology of disease. The CDC has published two documents that provide guidance for dentistry: 1) *Recommended Infection Control Practices for Dentistry* (CDC, 1993) and the 2) *Guidelines for Preventing the Transmission of Mycobacterium Tuberculosis in Health Care Facilities*, 1994 (CDC, 1994). The latter document provides recommendations to reduce the risk of transmission of TB to "health care workers, patients and others in health care facilities" (CDC, 1994). Dental clinics are considered health care facilities. The recommendation for dental settings is to identify and refer clients with TB and to delay elective dental treatment until the client is no longer infectious. Dental care that cannot be delayed should be provided in facilities that can provide TB isolation. Respiratory protection should be used by practitioners.

NIOSH is a research entity that annually publishes a list of the known toxic substances and at which levels of concentration toxicity occurs. In 1994, NIOSH published a booklet *Controlling Exposures to Nitrous Oxide During Anesthetic Administration*, that alerts workers to hazards and provides prevention strategies. The FDA regulates equipment and products that affect living tissue by exposure, contact, ingestion, or inhalation. In the dental environment, this would include items such as products and equipment for sterilization and disinfection, gloves, and radiologic equipment. The EPA is charged with regulating the use and disposal of products and wastes that impact the environment. The EPA registers all chemical products that are used for disinfection, sterilization, and decontamination. OSHA, FDA, and the EPA are regulatory agencies with enforcement authority. Employers and employees must be aware of and comply with the regulations that these agencies impose. However, these agencies also act in a service capacity by providing resources and guidance for compliance.

## Summary

Occupational hazards are inherent within the oral health professions. The ability to recognize existing and potential hazards is the key to successful prevention and maintenance of practitioners' well-being. Awareness and compliance with applicable regulations will contribute to the prevention of unnecessary exposure and to potentially harmful exposure. A collaborative effort by practitioners can reduce ergonomic, psychosocial, biological, chemical, and physical hazards within the workplace environment.

# Case Studies

**Case Study One:** Diane Baum, a 42-year-old dental hygienist who has been engaged in clinical practice four days per week for the past twenty years, has been awakened at night with numbness and a progressively increasing burning sensation in her right hand for the past three months. During the past two weeks, she has noticed a loss of strength in her hand during intense debridement procedures. This evening as she was finishing a sweater for her father's birthday present, she experienced pain and tingling in her thumb, index, and middle fingers. What CTD is indicated from Diane's symptoms? How should she proceed to alleviate the condition?

**Case Study Two:** Dr. Steven Jacob has been in practice for five years. After two years as an associate, he purchased an existing practice that includes a high percentage of elderly clients, and he also serves as the staff dentist for three nursing care facilities. The practice is secure financially and he and his staff enjoy a good working relationship. Dr. Jacob is the pitcher on a local recreational softball team, enjoys tennis, and lifts weights. In the last several months, he has experienced aching and tenderness in his right arm and a slight weakness in his right hand. He initially contributed the symptoms to softball since his team had made it to the semifinals; however, the season had been over for three weeks and the symptoms were not subsiding. Dr. Jacob now suspects his symptoms may be related to other aspects of his leisure activities, but is not sure what to change or eliminate. What do Dr. Jacob's symptoms indicate? How should he proceed?

**Case Study Three:** Susan Peters and Jane Dieter, two dental hygienists, have worked together in a solo dental practice for twelve years. Each of them works four days a week. Three days a week they are in the office together, however, they each have their own operatory and sets of instruments. This past year, the office merged with another practice. The group consists of three dentists, five dental hygienists, four dental assistants, and one new receptionist. Although Jane is still working four days a week, Susan reduced her time to three days a week (Monday, Wednesday and Friday) due to family responsibilities. Her original employer has reduced his time to two days (Tuesday and Thursday), thus they do not work together. Susan has become frustrated because when she arrives on Wednesday and Friday the operatory she works in is not as organized as she would like, supplies have not been restocked, and the instrument sets are incomplete. All scheduling is now being performed by the new receptionist and regardless of the time Susan is requesting for her clients' appointments, one hour is being routinely scheduled. Susan has complained to Jane over lunch several times, but Jane does not seem responsive to her concerns. What should she do?

**Case Study Four:** Gail Gage, a dental hygienist, has been practicing for twelve years. She has worn gloves while practicing throughout her career and while a student. During that time she has tried four different brands. The practice switched brands two months ago and she has been pleased with the fit of the glove; however, her hands have become red, cracked, and are bleeding. She read that latex allergies often surface years after wearing gloves, and she is considering switching to a vinyl glove. She is aware that vinyl gloves do not provide a comfortable fit. Gail has been using a nonscented lotion at night to heal her hands. A colleague has suggested she wear cotton gloves under her latex gloves. How should Gail deal with this situation?

**Case Study Five:** Using the format in Table 15-4, complete your individual stress inventory for your personal life and your professional life including both ongoing stresses and recent experiences. Rate from low to high the degree of stress and the feasibility of change. Develop an action plan to address the stresses you have identified.

# Case Study Discussions

**Discussion—Case Study One:** Diane's symptoms appear to be consistent with carpal tunnel syndrome. However, a definitive diagnosis is possible only after thorough assessment by another professional. Phalen's test and Tinel's test are the most common initial assessments. Tingling or numbness is experienced in a positive Phalen's test when the wrists are held for one minute in a flexed position. A positive Tinel's sign results in tingling or a shooting sensation when the median nerve area of the wrist is gently tapped. These tests should be followed with electromyography and nerve conduction studies, which assess the transmission of nerve impulses across the segment of the median nerve in the carpal tunnel. A definitive CTS diagnosis is made when it is determined that the nerve compression is in the carpal tunnel as opposed to another area of the arm or shoulder. Hobbies such as knitting contribute to repetitive actions of the wrist. Therapy may include occupational and lifestyle modifications, splinting and immobilization of the wrist to relax the area, local steroid injections, short courses of oral steroids or nonsteroidal anti-inflammatory drugs, diuretics (if the symptoms are perimenstrual), and exercises to encourage gliding of the median nerve. If nonsurgical treatments do not alleviate the symptoms, surgery to release the transverse carpal ligament to relieve compression of the median nerve should be considered.

**Discussion—Case Study Two:** Dr. Jacob's symptoms can be indicative of several CTDs including lateral epicondylitis, tendinitis, and thoracic outlet syndrome. A thorough assessment is again necessary to provide a definitive, differential diagnosis. The assessment should include a work/leisure activity history, medical history, and clinical tests. Because many clinical tests cannot reliably detect CTDs until they have advanced to a moderately severe state of damage, self-reporting of symptoms and activities can be crucial in identification of conditions in early stages. Dr. Jacob can track the frequency and duration of playing tennis and provide his physician with his weightlifting routine. He can ask his chairside assistant to observe his positioning over a three-day period and to share her observations. Perhaps she reports that when Dr. Jacob treated an elderly patient, he did not tilt the chair back far enough to achieve a supine position, thereby causing him to work with his shoulders and elbows raised. She also reports that he does not request clients to turn their heads to increase visibility, because he chooses to compromise his own position. After conducting a series of electrodiagnostic tests and considering the work/leisure history information provided, Dr. Jacob's physician diagnosed thoracic outlet syndrome. The movements involved in pitching, tennis, and weightlifting in combination with the working positions have caused compression of the brachial plexus and subclavian artery in the thoracic outlet space. Dr. Jacob is then advised to eliminate his leisure activities for one month to reduce inflammation in the area, and to slowly resume activities. He is also advised to consult with a trainer to develop an appropriate weightlifting regime. His physician also requests that he pursue neutral, balanced operator/client positioning. Dr. Jacob and his entire staff have attended several workshops, and are working together to develop a more ergonomically safe environment as well as to assist each other in developing good operator/patient positioning.

**Discussion—Case Study Three:** The merger of two offices will inherently bring about change. How the changes are managed will contribute to the level of stress experienced by all members of the practice. Susan made the choice to reduce her time in the office and must accept that she will be sharing the work environment. She is misdirecting her concerns by complaining to Jane. Susan should identify the specifics that are upsetting her and discuss them with the other dental hygienist who works in the operatory on the days she is not there. Perhaps the other dental hygienist is not clear as to the total expectations of the position, such as restocking supplies or insuring that the instrument sets are organized and

sterilized before she departs at the end of the day. Because Susan and the other dental hygienist do not work on the same days, Susan should take the initiative to arrange a time when the two of them can discuss the situation in a nonconfrontational manner. There may be issues that the other dental hygienist is unhappy about when she arrives, after Susan has been working in the operatory. Susan should also meet with the receptionist to discuss why she is requesting specific appointment time allocations for clients. Perhaps the receptionist is unaware of the need for varying times, or she may have been directed by the employers to schedule all appointments for one hour. If the latter is the case, Susan should then request a time to discuss the situation with her employers.

In any practice it is important for all employees and employers to have a clear understanding of job expectations, responsibilities, and the protocols for the practice. When changes are made or are being considered, the individuals who will be affected need to be aware and understand the reasons for the changes. Staff meetings provide a mechanism to communicate and discuss such changes. All differences among staff members do not need to be aired in full staff meetings. A work environment that allows for coworkers to problem-solve differences among themselves promotes collaboration, respect, and trust. When coworkers are able to effectively problem-solve, they reaffirm that they are competent, mature employees, and they relieve employers of the burden of dealing with such situations.

**Discussion—Case Study Four:** The only way to determine whether Gail has an actual allergy to latex proteins is by skin testing. Gail may be reacting to the specific talc powder used in this brand of glove. She may want to switch back to the brand she was previously using or to a glove with a different type of talc powder to see if the condition clears prior to going through skin testing. If the condition continues, Gail should seek medical consultation and skin testing. Although vinyl gloves remove the exposure to latex proteins, they have a higher pinhole failure rate and do not provide the level of barrier protection that latex gloves provide.

**Discussion—Case Study Five:** This is an activity to improve self-awareness. Results can be discussed in small groups or with friends if persons feel comfortable with this process. Problem solving might be enhanced through discussion with others.

## REFERENCES

ACGIH (1993). *1993–94 threshold limit values for chemical substances and physical agents and biological exposure indices.* Cincinnati, OH: American Conference of Government Hygienists.

American Dental Association. (1992). *The 1991 survey of dental practice: General characteristics of dentists.* Chicago, IL: American Dental Association.

Armstrong, T. J. (1986). Ergonomic and cumulative trauma disorders. *Hand Clinics, 2,* 553–565.

Armstrong, T. J. & Lifshitz, Y. (1987). Evaluation and design of jobs for control of cumulative trauma disorders. *Ergonomic interventions to prevent musculoskeletal injuries in industry.* Chesea-Lewis Publishers, Inc.

Bader, J. D. & Sams D. H. (1992). Factors associated with job and career satisfaction among dental hygienists. *Journal of Public Health Dentistry, 52,* 43–51.

Banting, D. W. & Robertson, J. M. (1991). Dealing with risks in the dental office. *Journal of the American Dental Association, 122,* 16–17.

Barnes, C. M. (1991). The management of aerosols with air polishing delivery systems. *Journal of Dental Hygiene, 65,* 280–282.

Barry, R. M., Woodall, I. R., & Mahan J. M. (1992). Postural changes in dental hygienists: Four-year longitudinal study. *Journal of Dental Hygiene, 65,* 147–150.

Bassett, S. (1982). Back problems among dentists. *Journal of the Canadian Dental Association, 49,* 251–256.

Berkey, Z. T., Luciano, W. J., & James, W. D. (1992) Latex glove allergy: A survey of the U.S. Army Dental Corps. *Journal of the American Medical Association, 268,* 2695–2697.

Body, K. L. (1988). Dental hygiene job and career satisfaction: A review of the literature. *Dental Hygiene, 62,* 170–175.

Borganelli, G. N., Primosch, R.E., & Henry, R.J. (1993). Operatory ventilation and scavenging evacuation rate influence on ambient nitrous oxide levels. *Journal of Dental Research, 72,* 1275–1278.

Boyer, E. M. (1990). Job satisfaction among dental hygienists. *Journal of Dental Hygiene, 68,* 235–238.

Boyer, E. M. (1994). Factors related to career retention among dental hygienists. *Journal of Dental Hygiene, 68,* 615–674.

Boyer, E. M. & Bolden, A. J. (1993). Occupational problems associated with glove use. *Journal of Dental Research, 72,* 313.

Boyer, E. M., Elton, J., & Preston, K. (1986). Precautionary procedures: Use in dental hygiene practice. *Dental Hygiene, 60,* 516–523.

Bureau of Labor Statistics. (1992). *Survey of occupational illnesses and injuries.* Washington, DC: U.S. Department of Labor, Bureau of Labor Statistics.

Cannon, L. J., Bernacki, E. J., & Walter, S. D. (1981). Personal and occupational factors associated with carpal tunnel syndrome. *Journal of Occupational Medicine, 23,* 255-258.

Centers for Disease Control. (1989). *Immunization recommendations for health care workers.* Atlanta, GA: CDC, Division of Immunization, Centers for Prevention Services.

Centers for Disease Control. (1993). Recommended infection control practices for dentistry, 1993. *MMWR, 41,* 1–12.

Centers for Disease Control. (1994). Guidelines for preventing the transmission of *mycobacterium tuberculosis* in health care facilities, 1994. *MMWR, 43,* 3.

Cherniss, C. (1980). *Staff burnout.* Beverly Hills, CA: Sage.

Cohen, E. N., Gift, H. C., Brown, B. W., Greenfield, W., Wu, M., & Jones, T. W., et al. (1980). Occupational disease in dentistry and chronic exposure to trace anesthetic gases. *Journal of the American Dental Association, 101,* 21–31.

Conrad, J. C., Conrad, K. J., & Osborn, J. B. (1993). A short-term, three-year epidemiological study of medican nerve sensitivity in practicing dental hygienists. *Journal of Dental Hygiene, 66*(2), 76–80.

Cooper, C. L., Mallinger, M., & Kahn, R. I. (1978). Identifying sources of occupational stress among dentists. *Journal of Occupational Psychology, 51,* 227–234.

Council on Dental Materials, Instruments and Equipment. (1984). Recommendations in dental mercury hygiene. *Journal of the American Dental Association, 109,* 617–619.

Council on Dental Materials, Instruments and Equipment. (1991). Dental merçury hygiene, summary of recommendations in 1990. *Journal of the American Dental Association, 122,* 112.

Dadian, T. (1993). Dental hygienists' career promotional behaviors and attitudes. *Journal of Dental Hygiene, 67,* 318–325.

Deckard, G. & Rountree, B. (1984). Burnout in dental hygiene. *Dental Hygiene, 58,* 307–313.

Dellon, A. J. (1980). Clinical use of vibration stimuli to evaluate peripheral nerve injury and compression neuropathy. *Plastic Reconstructive Surgery, 65,* 466–476.

Donaldson, D. & Orr, J. (1989). A comparison of the effectiveness of nitrous oxide scavenging devices. *Journal of the Canadian Dental Association, 55,* 535–537.

Freudenberger, H. L. (1980). *Burnout: The high cost of high achievement.* New York: Anchor Press.

Fouchard Academy Poll. (1965). One of every three practitioners afflicted with back trouble. *Dental Survey, 41,* 69–70.

Gelberman, R. H., Szabo, R. M., & Williamson, R. V., et al., (1983). Sensibility testing in peripheral-nerve compression syndromes: An experimental study in humans. *Journal of Bone Joint Surgery, 65,* 632–638.

George, J. M., Milone, C. L., Block, M. J., & Hollister, W. G. (1986). *Stress management for the dental team.* Philadelphia: Lea & Febiger.

Gerwatowski, L., McFall, D. B., & Stach, D. S. (1992). Carpal tunnel syndrome. Risk factors and preventive strategies for the dental hygienist. *Journal of Dental Hygiene,* 89–94.

Goldlist, G. I. (1979). Ocular injuries in dentistry. *Canadian Journal of Optometry, 41,* 315–339.

Gonzales, E. (1992). Latex hypersensitivity: A new and unexpected problem. *Hospital Practice,* 137–151.

Gravois, S. & Stringer, R. B. (1980). Survey of occupational health hazards in dental hygiene. *Dental Hygiene, 54,* 518–523.

Gross, K. W., Overman, P. R., Cobb, C., & Brockman, S. (1992). Aerosol generation by two ultrasonic scalers and one sonic scaler: A comparative study. *Journal of Dental Hygiene, 66,* 314–318.

Grossman, R. S. (1990). CTS. *RDH, 10,* 12–13.

Henry, R. J. & Jerrell, R. G. (1990). Ambient nitrous oxide levels during pediatric sedations. *Pediatric Dentistry, 12,* 87–91.

Henry, R. J. & Primosch, R. E. (1991). Influence of operatory size and nitrous oxide concentration upon scavenging effectiveness. *Journal of Dental Research, 70,* 1286–1289.

Hunter, J. M., Schneider, L. H., Mackin, E. J., & Callahan, A. D. (1984). *Rehabilitation of the Hand* (2nd ed.) (pp. 158, 373). St. Louis: Mosby-Year Book, Inc.

Huntley, D. E. & Shannon, S. A. (1986). Carpal tunnel syndrome: A review of the literature. *Dental Hygiene, 62*(7), 316–320.

Jacob, J. (1994). ADA sees no science for ergonomic rule. *ADA News, 25*(15), 23.

Johnston, D. W., O'Shea, R. M., & Lewis, D. W. (1992). Career commitment and satisfaction among American and Canadian dental hygienists. *Journal of Dental Hygiene, 66*, 210–215.

Johnson, S. L. (1990). Ergonomic design of handheld tools to prevent trauma to the hand and upper extremities. *Journal of Hand Therapy, 3*, 86–93.

Kaplan, D. (1973). More on coping with posture-related backache. *Journal of Dental Practice, 49*, 47.

King, J. W. (1990). An integration of medicine and industry. *Journal of Hand Therapy, 3*, 45–50.

Lukas, E. (1979). Lesions of the peripheral nervous system due to vibration. *Work—Environment—Health, 7*, 67–81.

Macdonald, G. (1987). Hazards in the dental workplace. *Dental Hygiene, 61*, 212–218.

Macdonald, G., Robertson, M. M., & Erikson, J. A. (1988). Carpal tunnel syndrome among California dental hygienists. *Dental Hygiene, 62*, 322–328.

Mallory, G. (1989). Uniting your team: Psychological and emotional issues. *Teambuilding*, Shawnee Mission, KS: National Press Publications.

Man, A., Neuman, H., & Assif, D. (1982). Effect of turbine dental drill noise on dentists' hearing. *1st Journal of Medical Science, 18*, 475–477.

Maslach, C. & Jackson, S. (1981). The measurement of experienced burnout. *Journal of Occupational Behavior, 2*, 99.

McFall, D. B., Stach, D. J., & Gerwatowski, L. J. (1993). Carpal tunnel syndrome: Treatment and rehabilitation therapy for the dental hygienist. *Journal of Dental Hygiene, 67*, 126–133.

McGlothlin, J. D., Jensen, P. A., Todd, W. F., Fischbach, T. J., & Fairfield, C. L. (1989). In-depth survey report: Control of anesthetic gases in dental operatories at Children's Hospital Medical Center Dental Facility. Cincinnati, OH: U.S. Department of Health and Human Services, Public Health Service, Centers for Disease Control, National Institute for Occupational Safety and Health, Report No. ECTB 166-11b.

McGlothlin, J. D., Jensen, P. A., Cooper, T. C., Fischbach, T. J., & Fairfield, C. L. (1990). In-depth survey report: Control of anesthetic gases in dental operatories at University of California at San Francisco Oral Surgical Dental Clinic, San Francisco, CA. Cincinnati, OH: U.S. Department of Health and Human Services, Centers for Disease Control, National Institute for Occupational Safety and Health, Report No. ECTB 166-12b.

McGlothlin, J. D., Jensen, P. A., Todd, W. F., & Fischbach, T. J. (1988). Study protocol: Control of anesthetic gases in dental operatories. Cincinnati, OH: U.S. Department of Health and Human Services, Public Health Service, Centers for Disease Control, National Institute for Occupational Safety and Health, Division of Physical Sciences and Engineering.

Mellody, M. (1983). What you should know about stress. *Dental Hygiene, 57*, 28–29, 32–34, 36.

Miller, D. L. (1991). An investigation into attrition of dental hygienists from the work force. *Journal of Dental Hygiene, 65*, 25–31.

Murtomaa, H., Haavio-Mannila, E., & Kandolin, I. (1990). Burnout and its causes in Finnish dentists. *Community Dental Oral Epidemiology, 18*, 208–212.

National Institute for Occupational Safety and Health. (1977). *Control of occupational exposure to nitrous oxide in the dental operatory*. Cincinnati, OH: U.S. Department of Health and Human Services, Centers for Disease Control, National Institute for Occupational Safety and Health, DHEW Publication No. 77-171.

Nelson, M. J. & Newell, K. J. (1993a). The effect of a career planning workshop on graduate dental hygienists. *Journal of Dental Hygiene, 67*, 388–397.

Nelson, M. J. & Newell, K. J. (1993b). A career development program for graduate dental hygienists. *Journal of Dental Hygiene, 67*, 398–402.

Nield-Gehrig, J. S. & Houseman, G. A. (1996). *Fundamentals of periodontal instrumentation* (3rd ed.). Baltimore: Williams & Wilkins.

Oberg, T. & Oberg, U. (1993). Musculoskeletal complaints in dental hygiene: A survey study from a Swedish country. *Journal of Dental Hygiene, 67*, 257–261.

Occupational Safety and Health Act of 1970. (1991). 29 USC. 653, Subpart Z, 1910.1030, 29 CFR.

Occupational Safety and Health Administration. (1989). Air contaminants; final rule. *Federal Register, 54*, 2332–2983.

Occupational Safety and Health Administration. (1993). *Enforcement guidance in the face of increased exposure to tuberculosis*. Washington, DC: U.S. Department of Labor, Occupational Safety and Health Administration.

Orner, G. (1978). The quality of life of the dentists. *International Dental Journal, 28*, 20–26.

Osborn, J. B., Newell, K. J., Rudney, J. D., & Stoltenberg, J. L. (1990a). Musculoskeletal pain among Minnesota dental hygienists. *Journal of Dental Hygiene, 63*, 132–138.

Osborn, J. B., Newell, K. J., Rudney, J. D., & Stoltenberg, J. L. (1990b). Carpal tunnel syndrome among Minnesota dental hygienists. *Journal of Dental Hygiene, 63*, 79–85.

O'Shea, R. M., Corah, N. L., & Ayer, W. A. (1984). Sources of dentists' stress. *Journal of the American Dental Association, 109*, 415–451.

Paine, W. S. (1982). *Job stress and burnout. Research, theory and intervention perspectives*. Beverly Hills, CA: Sage.

Park, P. R. (1978). Effects of noise on dentists. *Dental Clinics of North America, 22*, 415.

Phalen, G. S. (1966). The carpal tunnel syndrome. *Journal of Bone Joint Surgery, 48A*, 211–228.

Pollack, R. D. (1989, September/October). Ergonomics: Comfort by design. *Dental Teamwork*. 163–166.

Preston, J.D., et al. (1978). Light and lighting in the dental office. *Dental Clinics of North America, 22*, 431–451.

Rowland, A. S., Baird, D. D., Weinberg, C. R., Shore, D. L., Shy, C. M., & Wilcox, A. J. (1992). Reduced fertility among women employed as dental assistants exposed to high levels of nitrous oxide. *New England Journal of Medicine, 327*, 993–997.

Rundcrantz, B-L., Johnsson, B., & Moritz, U. (1990). Cervical pain and discomfort among dentists. Epidemiological, clinical and therapeutic aspects: A survey of pain and discomfort. *Swedish Dental Journal, 14*, 71–80.

Rundcrantz, B-L., Johnsson, B., & Moritz, U. (1991). Occupational cervico-brachial disorders among dentists: Analysis of ergonomics and locomotor functions. *Swedish Dental Journal, 15*, 105–115.

Rundcrantz, B-L., Johnsson, B., Moritz, U., & Roxendal, G. (1991a). Occupational cervico-brachial disorders among dentists. Psychological work environment, personal harmony and life satisfaction. *Scandinavian Journal of Social Medicine, 19*, 174–180.

Rundcrantz, B-L., Johnsson, B., Moritz U., & Roxendal, G. (1991b). Pain and discomfort in the musculoskeletal system among dentists: A prospective study. *Swedish Dental Journal, 15*, 219–228.

Selye, H. (1974). *Stress without distress.* Philadelphia & New York: J.B. Lippincott Co.

Shugars, D., Miller, D., & William, D. (1987). Musculoskeletal pain among general dentists. *General Dentistry, 535*, 272–276.

Shugars, D. (1984). Managing dentistry's physical stresses: Chairside exercises for dentists and dental auxiliaries. *NCDR, 2*, 11–14.

Spanner, D., Dolovich, J., Tarlo, S., Sussman, G., & Buttoo, K. (1989). Hypersensitivity to natural latex. *Journal of Allergy and Clinical Immunology, 83*, 1135–1137.

Stewart, L. A. (1992). Occupational contact dermatitis. *Immunology and Allergy Clinics of North America, 12*, 831–845.

Tountas, C. P., MacDonald, C. J., Meyerhoff, J. D., & Bihrle, D. M. (1983). Carpal tunnel syndrome: A review of 507 patients. *Minnesota Medicine, 66*, 479–482.

Vedder, Price, Kaufman, & Kammholz. (1993). OSHA and Ergonomics. *OSHA Observer.*

Wagner, M. (1985). How healthy are today's dentists? *Journal of the American Dental Association, 110*, 17–24.

Wilkins, E. M. (1994). *Clinical practice of the dental hygienist* (7th ed.). Philadelphia: Lea & Febiger.

Woodall, I., et al. (1989). Comprehensive dental hygiene care (3rd ed.) (pp. 615–670). St. Louis: Mosby-Year Book, Inc.

# SECTION IV

# EVALUATION PHASE

# CHAPTER 16

# Periodontal Maintenance Procedures

## Key Terms

continuing care
maintenance
palliative SPC
periodontal maintenance procedures (PMP)
primary prevention

recall
recall system
recare
secondary prevention

## INTRODUCTION

Many terms have been used to define the care that follows active therapy. In 1995, the American Academy of Periodontology (AAP) presented a new term, **periodontal maintenance procedures (PMP)**, as the preferred terminology for the care recommended for those who have completed periodontal treatment including surgical and adjunctive therapies (Current Procedural Terminology, 1995; Insurance Coding Update, 1995). Because the term "Supportive Periodontal Treatment" (SPT) had been recommended by the AAP prior to 1995, it has been used to date in current periodontal literature and texts to describe maintenance therapy. Other terms used to describe PMP include supportive periodontal therapy, periodontal recall, periodontal maintenance, the maintenance phase of periodontal care, preventive maintenance, and supportive periodontal care (SPC). PMP encompasses removal of bacterial flora from crevicular and pocket areas, scaling and selective polishing, and a review of self-care practices. Typically, a three-month interval between appointments is the most effective schedule for PMP. When new or recurring periodontal disease is discovered, additional diagnostic and treatment procedures must be considered. The AAP discusses the fact that maintenance care following periodontal therapy is not synonymous with a prophylaxis (Insurance Coding Update, 1995).

A distinction should be made between the terms *maintenance* and *recall*. **Maintenance** refers to the state of being maintained or a means of upkeep in a desirable condition (Riverside Webster's II Dictionary, 1996). All clients need to be maintained even if they have never had periodontitis. **Recall** is actually the process of requesting that a client return for care at a specified interval and, thus, a **recall system** is a method an office or clinic uses to track intervals and notify clients about continuing care. Recently, the use of the term *recall* has been questioned due to the responsibility it places on oral health care professionals to initiate and track compliance with continuing care. Instead, **recare** or **continuing care** have been suggested to represent appropriately timed maintenance care where the client assumes responsibility. An appropriate recare interval is also applicable to those individuals who do not have periodontitis and require only preventive prophylaxis. Therefore, each client visiting a dental office or clinical situation for dental hygiene care will return for continuing care at an appropriate interval. The terms recare or continuing care should not be interpreted, however, to mean that a practice should not notify clients about their recommended PMP interval because periodontal maintenance care with frequent intervals is considered an essential component for long-term success of periodontal therapy.

This chapter will address the following issues surrounding PMP; its goals, effectiveness, components of the appointment, therapeutic considerations, recommended intervals, and compliance. Prevention of new disease and maintenance of the case stability will be discussed for various categories of clients, including those with gingivitis, adult periodontitis, and aggressive forms of periodontitis. Risk factors associated with the periodontal disease process will be enumerated and discussed.

## OBJECTIVES OF MAINTENANCE

Because maintenance represents both preventive care for those without periodontitis and PMP for those with periodontitis, it has two very general objectives; 1) to continue controlling bacterial plaque, and 2) to preserve the health of the dentition and gingival tissues (McFall, 1989). Specifically, the goals of PMP can be summarized as follows: 1) to prevent the occurrence of new disease, 2) to stabilize or control existing disease, 3) to prevent disease recurrence, and 4) to maintain hopeless or compromised teeth. The dental hygienist plays a key role in the education, motivation, and monitoring of the client's dental needs. It is the hygienist who frequently will detect disease progression and actively participate in the client's therapy. The ultimate objective of a preventive program is to retain the individual's teeth for his or her lifetime; however, this objective may not be attainable for all clients. The prevention of disease is complicated by risk factors such as poor compliance, systemic diseases, smoking, various forms of periodontal disease that do not respond well to therapy, race, and the severity of the preexisting disease.

Baehni and Tessier (1993) in Proceedings of the 1st European Workshop on Periodontology recommended the term *supportive periodontal care (SPC)* to describe the continuing care philosophy. The unique characteristic of this approach is that it is a broad concept not restricted to periodontal maintenance alone. It includes **primary prevention** for those who are healthy or for those who have gingivitis. The focus of treatment is to prevent gingivitis from becoming periodontitis. **Secondary prevention** refers to the phase of care after completion of active therapy for clients with periodontal diseases. A modification of this concept includes a third category called **palliative SPC** (Schallhorn & Snider, 1981). Pallative SPC is designed to prevent, slow down, or arrest disease progression in clients who can not receive appropriate treatment because of medical conditions, poor oral hygiene, or lack of compliance. Pallative SPC becomes the optimal treatment given these circumstances. The extent of therapy and the recare interval may vary in an attempt to control disease. Chemotherapy might be an asset in controlling those cases during pallative SPC that do not respond to conventional therapy. When there is evidence of disease progression, the treatment modalities are revised to meet the individual's needs (Baehni & Tessier, 1993). This approach to maintenance is interesting because it emphasizes the role of continuing assessment and care in preventing periodontal diseases and in situations where secondary prevention or PMP requires modification based on the client's status. The remainder of this chapter addresses maintenance in general; however, the primary focus is on secondary prevention and palliative care.

## EFFECTIVENESS OF MAINTENANCE

It is well-known that the cause of dental disease is the accumulation of microbial plaque. Patients who practice effective plaque control will have less dental disease than those who do not (Axelsson & Lindhe, 1978). Ramfjord (1987) stated that "plaque control is the alpha and omega of prevention, healing and maintenance of periodontal health." The essence of preventing or minimizing dental disease is an effective maintenance therapy program. Axelsson and Lindhe (1978; 1981) found that effective maintenance at frequent intervals reduces the risk for caries and periodontal disease. Other investiga-

tors have found that compliance with the suggested recare interval for PMP after active therapy is essential to halt periodontal disease progression (Badersten, Nilvéus, & Egelberg, 1987; Becker, Becker, & Berg, 1984; Isidor & Karring, 1986; Pihlström, Oliphant, & McHugh, 1984; Ramfjord, 1987).

Maintenance care is most effective when it is designed to eliminate or reduce primary and secondary etiologic agents. It has been well-demonstrated that the primary etiology of dental disease is microbial plaque. The secondary etiologies can include defective margins, overhangs on restorations, and calculus. Client self-care is effective for microbial plaque located supragingivally and in shallow subgingival sulcus or pocket areas. The majority of subgingival plaque within moderate to deep pockets must be removed or disrupted by the clinician. Plaque-retentive factors such as calculus, overhangs, or illfitting restorations must be removed or corrected by the clinician. The professional has the responsibility to explain the relationship of self-care and professional therapy to the client while fostering the cotherapy approach to periodontal care.

## Combined Self-Care and Professional Care

Numerous studies during the past decades indicate when a client participates in an effective maintenance program, both caries and periodontal diseases are arrested or decreased over time. Lindhe and Axelsson (1973; 1974) evaluated the effects of controlled oral hygiene and "professional cleanings" on caries and gingivitis in children seven to fourteen years of age. They found that subjects who were enrolled in a program that practiced intense plaque control every two weeks for two years, developed minimal gingivitis. These results helped to affirm the relationship between the accumulation of supragingival microbial plaque and gingivitis. Although gingivitis does not always progress to periodontitis, it is critical that preventive maintenance or primary prevention be reinforced in clinical practice for all ages of patients. It is not known which site or patient with gingivitis will progress to periodontitis. Interceptive treatment of gingivitis can be classified as a form of preventive maintenance (McFall, 1989).

Lovdahl, Arno, Schei, and Waerhaug (1961) evaluated 1,428 adult Norwegians for the effects of subgingival scaling and controlled oral hygiene on the incidence of gingivitis and periodontitis. Subjects received subgingival debridement and oral hygiene instruction every three to six months for five years depending on their dental needs. Findings indicated that gingival health improved by 60 percent over pretreatment values regardless of the level of self-care, and clients with the best self-care lost the fewest teeth.

The relationship of effective self-care to a decrease in gingivitis and early signs of periodontitis has been supported in many other studies (Lightner, O'Leary, Drake, Crump, & Allen, 1975; Suomi, Greene, Vermillion,

Chang, & Leatherwood, 1969; Suomi, Greene, Vermillion, Chang, & Leatherwood, 1971). These longitudinal clinical investigations have shown that regular scaling and root planing, as well as reenforcement of self-care instructions, result in decreased plaque accumulation, reduced gingivitis, and improved clinical conditions.

Axelsson and Lindhe (1981) evaluated the effects of a carefully controlled PMP program on plaque accumulation, probe depth, and clinical level of attachment. Subjects with advanced periodontal disease were instructed in self-care procedures, then received scaling prior to treatment by modified Widman flap surgery. During the first two months following surgery, the subjects were recalled once every two weeks for professional tooth cleaning. At the end of two months, the seventy-seven subjects were examined and fifty-two clients enrolled in a program (recall group) that stressed carefully controlled maintenance care. This care included self-care instructions, meticulous professional tooth cleaning every two to three months. The remaining twenty-five subjects (nonrecall) were referred to the general dentist for traditional dental care that consisted of treatment to minimize or eliminate symptoms rather than to combat the etiology of the disease. Those in the recall group who had continual reenforcement of self-care procedures as well as frequent maintenance at two- to three-month intervals had reduction of the plaque levels with little or no gingivitis. Refer to Figure 16-1 for a graphic representation of the percentage of tooth surfaces covered by plaque

from the initial visit over the six-year period of the study. The baseline data was collected at the completion of treatment, and then at three- and six-year intervals while the patients were in maintenance therapy. Figure 16-2 represents the probing depth of recall versus nonrecall subjects over the six-year period. In the recall group, 99 percent of the tooth surfaces showed either improvement, no change, or less than 1 mm of clinical attachment loss. The subjects in the non-recall group continued to experience loss of attachment (see Figure 16-3). At the six-year examination, 44 percent of those in the nonrecall group had no change or less than 1 mm of clinical attachment loss, while 55 percent of the sites showed loss of attachment from 2 to 5 mm and 1 percent of the sites lost more than 6 mm of attachment.

Axelsson, Lindhe, and Nystrom (1991) continued the investigation for an additional nine years. After a fifteen-year period, findings demonstrated that the preventive program effectively prevented tooth loss, caries, and periodontal disease. The elements of the program included stimulating the participants to improve their self-performed oral hygiene (the mean plaque scores were found to vary between 10 and 20 percent), meticulous subgingival deposit removal when required, and fluoride application through the daily use of a fluoridated toothpaste.

PMP are particularly critical for the treated client with periodontal disease. Becker, Becker, and Berg (1984) reported on clients who received treatment for periodontal disease and then chose not to participate in a maintenance program. Within the group, there was a high incidence of recurrent disease indicated by an increase in probe depths, furcation involvement, and tooth loss. These findings indicate that treatment without

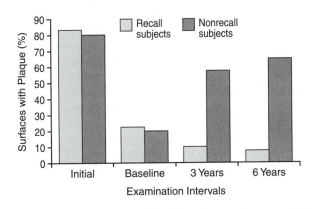

**Figure 16-1** Percentage of tooth surfaces with plaque. This graph represents change in the percentage of tooth surfaces covered by plaque from the initial examination over a six-year period. The baseline is completion of treatment, and the three and six years are the examination periods while the patients were in maintenance. The plaque level remained low in those patients who had constant reenforcement of their oral hygiene (recall). The patients who received traditional dental care (nonrecall) with no emphasis on plaque control had increased plaque accumulation and loss of attachment and probe depths as illustrated in Figures 16-2 and 16-3. (Data from "Effect of controlled oral hygiene procedures in caries and periodontal disease in adults: Results after 6 years," by P. Axelsson, and J. Lindhe, *Journal of Clinical Periodontology*, *8*, pp.239–248, 1981)

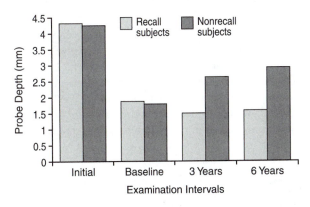

**Figure 16-2** Probe depths. This graph represents changes in probe depth from the initial examination over a six-year period. The reduction and maintenance of shallow depths reflects the low plaque levels in the experimental (recall) group when compared to the traditional (nonrecall) group. (Data from "Effect of controlled oral hygiene procedures in caries and periodontal disease in adults: Results after 6 years," by P. Axelsson, and J. Lindhe, *Journal of Clinical Periodontology*, *8*, pp.239–248, 1981)

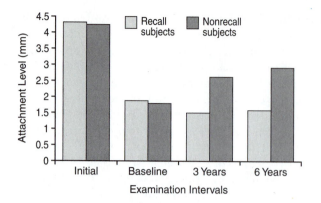

**Figure 16-3** Attachment level. This graph represents change in attachment levels from the initial examination over a six-year period. There was a slight gain of attachment in those with excellent oral hygiene and maintenance. There was loss of attachment over the six-year period in the patients who had no reenforcement of oral hygiene with dental care directed at symptoms rather than etiology (nonrecall). (Data from "Effect of controlled oral hygiene procedures in caries and periodontal disease in adults: Results after 6 years," by P. Axelsson, and J. Lindhe, *Journal of Clinical Periodontology, 8*, pp.239–248, 1981)

PMP is ineffective in preserving periodontal health. Clients who are not effectively maintained have a high incidence of disease recurrence. The aforementioned research represents landmark studies in the field of periodontal maintenance therapy.

There is a significant body of knowledge that indicates the value of PMP in preventing gingivitis and the reoccurrence of periodontitis in children, young adults, and adults after nonsurgical and surgical therapy. Findings reported in the periodontal literature support the fact that persons who are well-maintained and practice effective oral self-care will have fewer sites with new disease, or with disease recurrence. Teeth with advanced disease can be retained for extended periods with PMP. To successfully deal with periodontal disease, the clinician and client must realize that it is a chronic disease and that the concept of a "cure" is transient (Wilson, 1992). PMP which are quality oriented and appropriately timed are the keystone for the maintenance of periodontally involved teeth.

## COMPONENTS OF A PMP APPOINTMENT

During PMP the original dental hygiene process of care is repeated; however, the approach to the five phases of care (assessment, diagnosis, planning, implementation, and evaluation) is modified to meet the individual requirements of the client during the maintenance phase of therapy. The assessment component involves 1) updating of the medical history form, 2) determining the chief complaint, and 3) collecting data pertinent to the oral health care needs from which a diagnosis can be formu-

lated. Data collection allows the dental hygienist to determine whether there is disease stability or progression, to formulate a basic prognosis, to evaluate the self-care, and to determine the location and extent of treatment. It is frequently difficult to determine which sites are progressing; and, consequently, to determine the extent of treatment. Determining the required therapy requires assimilating all the data collected during the assessment of the client and comparing it to the previous data. This comparison assists in aiding the hygienist in formulating the dental hygiene diagnosis and care plan. Once the care plan and dental hygiene diagnosis are determined; case presentation and informed consent are completed. An important component of examination and treatment is documentation and discussion of the findings with the client. Just as facilitative communication was important in initial therapy, it also plays a vital role in PMP. It is essential to inform clients of their dental status, as well as to discuss the restorative and periodontal treatment recommendations presented by the dentist.

The implementation phase consists of self-care reenforcement including skill enhancement based on client needs and interests. The supragingival and subgingival microbial plaque and accumulated deposits are removed by hand and/or automatic instrumentation. The teeth are polished either prior to or following instrumentation. Adjunctive self-care or chemotherapeutic aids may be recommended in an effort to enhance plaque control. A reevaluation appointment may be required if there are sites with disease progression or reappointment might be warranted if the client requires extensive instrumentation.

Prior to initiating PMP, it is incumbent upon the practitioner to review the client's past records for health history implications, previous disease history, and needed alterations in care. A through review also includes examining the restorative and periodontal chartings, the needs assessment information, and prior self care education as well as the therapy performed. The prepared practitioner will appear professional when this review occurs. This routine practice aids in building rapport and enhancing facilitative communication with the client. There are clients who alternate PMP between the periodontist and generalist; therefore, it is also prudent to determine what diagnostic and therapeutic procedures were rendered at the alternating practice. This communication will aid in assessing the effectiveness of the PMP as well as the appropriate recare interval.

### Assessment

The very nature of PMP requires thorough documentation. The information gathered during each appointment will depend on factors such as the type of periodontal disease, disease severity and stability, various risk factors, client compliance with self-care, and with the suggested recare interval. The evaluation criteria to consider are listed in Table 16-1 along with the risk factors

**Table 16-1 PMP Assessment Criteria Procedures and Associated Risk Factors**

| Criteria | Procedure | Risk Factors to Evaluate |
|---|---|---|
| Medical History | Review and update for:<br>• need for prophylactic antibiotics<br>• making sure medications have been taken<br>• new diseases/medications<br>• need for medical consultation<br>• smoking status | • age of client<br>• smoking status<br>• systemic diseases such as diabetes<br>• stress |
| Dental History | Review and determine the chief complaint | • lack of compliance with the PMP recare interval |
| Extraoral and Intraoral Soft Tissue Examination | Examine for significant pathology | • dependent on type of pathology |
| Restorative Examination | Evaluate prothesis (implants), caries activity and risk, and restorations | • overhangs or ill-fitting restorations<br>• the failing implant |
| Periodontal Examination | Examine the following:<br>• gingival conditions for inflammation, position, contour, and mucogingival involvement | • inflammation<br>• progressive recession<br>• minimal or no keratinized gingiva |
| | • probing depth | • 1 to 2 mm increase<br>• moderate to deep probe depths |
| | • attachment loss | • extent and severity of disease; type of disease present; 2 mm loss of attachment in one year |
| | • radiographs | • changes in bone levels<br>• vertical bone loss<br>• presence of caries |
| | • bleeding on probing | • presence indicates risk |
| | • furcation involvement | • presence indicates risk; the more advanced the furcation involvement, the more risk |
| | • mobility | • presence indicates risk; the more advanced the mobility, the more risk |
| | • suppuration | • presence indicates risk |
| Deposit Accumulation | • Evaluate the location and extent of supragingival bacterial plaque | • presence of supragingival bacterial plaque is strongly correlated to gingivitis |
| | • supra- and subgingival deposits | • the type of bacteria present in the subgingival environment (microbiological monitoring)<br>• lack of compliance with oral self-care recommendations<br>• calculus (plaque-retentive factor) |
| Radiographic Assessment | Evaluate the:<br>• risk of advancing disease<br>• clinical findings, especially progressive attachment loss<br>• client radiographic history | • advancing radiographic bone loss |

associated with each parameter. Each evaluation component must be assessed and viewed in a slightly different perspective that relates to the maintenance of periodontal health as well as the *discovery* of new disease during PMP. Points that are germane to reassessment and PMP will be discussed in the following sections.

**Medical History.** Because a client's general health does not remain static, updating of the health history is essential. As a part of the evaluation the therapist should determine if the client requires premedication and whether the appropriate medications have been taken. Medications and/or systemic manifestations that might impact the general well-being of the client as well as his or her periodontal status should be considered. These can include drugs that result in gingival hyperplasia, smoking, and systemic manifestations such as diabetes.

The systemic health of the client might reveal why palliative care is indicated or why routine maintenance has not been followed. For instance, an individual with serious health problems might miss the recommended recare interval because of illness or the general cost of medical care. The client who is a heavy smoker and a poorly controlled diabetic might not be a candidate for periodontal surgery. As a result, the overall prognosis of the dentition may be compromised even with appropriate self-care. A medical consultation might also be indicated when new health conditions are recognized or previous disease history changes significantly. Chapter 2 covers health history assessment and subsequent treatment alterations.

**Dental History.** The dental history is collected at the maintenance visit through verbal questioning and/or by a written format completed prior to entering the operatory. Questioning to determine whether a chief concern or an acute experience has occurred since the last appointment is as significant in meeting client needs at the PMP appointment as it was during active therapy. This questioning sometimes reveals important dental needs the therapist is unaware of, especially if care has been alternating between specialist and generalist offices. Hypersensitivity associated with recession can be a result of initial therapy and is a common example of a client's unmet need or chief concern. The client responses and chief concerns are used to initiate external motivational strategies employed by the professional to encourage further compliance with self-care and recall. Motivation and client needs are discussed in Chapter 8 and the dental history is discussed in Chapter 3.

**Extraoral and Intraoral Examination.** This examination is performed for the purposes of identifying significant pathology as well as other conditions relative to treatment. As a client's health history can change in a short interval of time, so can extraoral and intraoral conditions. If suspicious hard or soft tissue lesions were previously recorded or teeth are periodontally compromised, then close follow-up is imperative. A detailed review of extraoral and intraoral clinical assessment is beyond the scope of this text; consequently, the reader is referred to other references.

**Restorative Examination.** The restorative examination involves assessment of the current charting to detect new areas of decalcification, new carious lesions, defective restorations, or improperly contoured restorations. Of particular interest to NSPT is the evaluation of the root surfaces for caries as the incidence of decay is likely to increase with the occurrence of recession and the age of the patient. Elderly clients may suffer from dry mouth, either as a result of aging or medications. The individual with xerostomia may be at increased risk for dental caries. Overhanging margins and ill-fitting restorations are plaque-retentive factors that enhance the risk of plaque accumulation at a given site. Their role in microbial plaque retention is an excellent point to include in client education and it can also be used as a motivational strategy to gain informed consent for professional removal, repair, or replacement of the inadequate restoration. Occlusion is also evaluated to determine if it has a relationship to fracture of tooth structure, wear facets, or increasing mobility. Chapter 4 highlights the relationship of restorative dentistry to periodontal therapy.

Implant identification and examination is also a part of the restorative and periodontal examination component of PMP. Early identification of periimplantitis is a critical part of the periodic examination. Early interception of progressive periodontal and periimplantitis is a key in exiting the PMP patient from routine maintenance and placing them back into active therapy. Maintenance of implants is discussed in Chapter 14.

**Periodontal Evaluation.** The assessment of periodontal conditions involves reexamination of the following:

1. gingival status
2. probing depth
3. attachment loss
4. bleeding on probing
5. furcation involvement
6. mobility
7. suppuration

The assessment of these clinical parameters should be consistent, beginning from the initial evaluation after active therapy to all subsequent PMP appointments. This practice enhances standardization of clinical findings and permits the clinician to accurately compare previous findings with current findings to determine whether there has been disease progression. When new diagnostic devices such as automated probing or microbial testing are incorporated into the dental practice, it must be determined when and to what extent they are to be used. Options include introducing new procedures into the care of new clients only, or into maintenance care for those who are considered at risk. Procedural changes in the measurement of a clinical parameter require that the clinician recognize the impact the alteration has on care assessment and proposed therapy.

**Gingival Conditions.** Specific attention should be focused on the gingiva for inflammation, changes in position and contour, and for mucogingival involvements (McFall, 1989). The overall health of the gingiva can be evaluated by noting the extent and severity of the inflammation which involves dividing the gingiva into the following zones: 1) papillary (P), 2) marginal (M), and 3) attached (A). The extent and severity of the inflammation can be charted using the abbreviations in conjunction with the location. For example, inflammation that is noted on the lingual of the mandibular anterior teeth and confined to the interdental papilla and marginal gingiva can be described as P/M inflammation on the linguals of 22 to 26. This describes the severity of the gingival inflammation; papillary and marginal, as well as the teeth that are involved: 22 to 26. Because gingival inflammation is a indicator of plaque accumulation, it is an important tool in motivating the client to comply with self-care recommendations and PMP intervals.

The position of the gingival tissues is defined as the location of the most coronal aspect of the gingival margin with respect to the CEJ. Gingival recession is a common clinical finding after initial therapy. Client needs related to recession include desensitization via professional and self-care methods, meticulous self-care to reduce plaque accumulation and thus potential for sensitivity and root caries, and fluoride therapy to decrease the risk of root caries. Gingival recession may require modification in brushing pressure and techniques, as well as an alteration or addition of the interdental aid(s). Most importantly, the client should be educated about the reasons why recession occurred, and the possibility of surgical correction if there is lack of keratinized gingiva or if there are esthetic concerns.

The amount of attached and keratinized gingiva is also determined and sites with minimal or no attached, keratinized gingiva, or mucogingival involvement are recorded. Researchers have evaluated the role of PMP in maintaining areas with minimal attached gingiva (Dorfman, 1985; Lindhe & Nyman, 1980; Wennstrom, 1983). Results indicate that gingival inflammation can be controlled and attachment levels are maintained by regular maintenance care, regardless of the amount of keratinized gingiva (Baehni & Tessier, 1993). Care must be taken not to "overinstrument" sites with little keratinized gingiva. Aggressive instrumentation can increase the severity of gingival recession. Compliance with the suggested maintenance schedule might be a critical factor in determining whether periodontal surgery is indicated to treat sites with minimal keratinized gingiva or mucogingival involvement. An evaluation of the area(s) by the dentist or periodontist may be indicated to determine if

surgical intervention is required (see Chapter 17, Surgical Intervention).

**Probing Depth.** Traditionally, periodontal probing has been the most critical component of the periodontal maintenance evaluation because it remains the most used indicator of periodontal destruction (McFall, 1989). Probe depth is determined by measuring, in millimeters, the distance from the gingival margin to the depth of probe penetration to the epithelial attachment. The depth of probe penetration is frequently dependent on the amount of inflammation present. It is generally accepted that the accuracy and ability to reproduce this measurement depends on the probe diameter or tine, pressure exerted, the presence of inflammation, contour of the teeth, and technique. The more often periodontal probing is performed over time, the more meaningful the measurements become (Ryan, 1985). Shallow sites should not be ignored for 2 to 3 mm probe depths can become 4 to 6 mm pockets.

Because of the inherent limitations to probing , it is suggested that an increase of 2 to 3 mm over time is an indicator of true change (Kornman, 1987; Ramfjord, 1987; Ramfjord et al., 1987; Ryan, 1985). The problem with judging disease progression by a 2 to 3 mm standard is that it appears to be an insensitive measure of early disease progression indicated by attachment loss (Theil & Heaney, 1991). There can be significant disease progression before it can accurately be detected. Clinically, clinicians will want to take a close look at professional therapy; self-care practices and recommendations; and the recall interval when probing depth changes are from 1 to 2 mm.

**Attachment Loss.** Because clinical attachment loss is currently the "gold standard" by which disease progression is determined, it is important to recognize when loss of attachment has occurred and what this means to the clients' future therapy. Clinical attachment loss of 2 mm on any tooth or teeth indicates disease progression and interceptive therapy, which may include referral (AAP, 1989; Ramfjord, 1987). Attachment loss can be from 0.1 mm per year for healthy sites to several millimeters in several months for acute situations. Loss of attachment is calculated by measuring the recession in millimeters (the distance from the CEJ to the gingival margin), and adding this measurement to the sulcus or pocket depth measurement. Another approach to clinical recording of attachment loss is to use negative and positive values indicating the relationship of the gingival margin to the CEJ. When the gingival margin is coronal to the CEJ it is given a negative value, and when it is apical to the CEJ, a positive value.

Measurement and determination of clinical attachment levels is a time-consuming procedure, but at present, it is the only method of accurately detecting disease activity. The advent of automated probes has not made this much easier. At present there is no automated probe on the market that determines the position of the CEJ and calculates attachment loss. The disease status must be evaluated to determine how frequently attachment levels are to be completed. Clients with advanced disease, refractory or progressing periodontitis, or areas of generalized recession with minimal attached and keratinized gingiva should have attachment levels recorded at least yearly.

Risk factors associated with attachment loss that is a manifestation of disease progression include smoking, diabetes, and age. These factors are assessed during the medical history update and review. Grossi and others (1994) conducted a cross-sectional study of 1,426 subjects ranging in age from twenty-five to seventy-four years. They found that an increased incidence of smoking was associated with greater attachment loss. Diabetes was the only systemic disease that had an association with loss of attachment. Loss of attachment increased with the age of the client, and age was found to be the most significant factor associated with loss of attachment.

The importance of microbial transmission cannot be overlooked as a possible etiologic agent in the initiation of new disease or episodes of disease recurrence in the treated periodontal patient. Petit, van Steenbergen, Timmerman, and Van der Velden (1994) evaluated patients with adult periodontitis from twenty-four Dutch families. The prevalence of periodontopathogens in the spouses and children of these subjects was determined. It was concluded, the spouses and children of individuals with periodontitis, have similar pathogens within the subgingival plaque as does the parent with disease. Transmission does not occur easily, but clients whose spouse has periodontitis may be at risk of periodontal breakdown. An interesting statistic was that 26.5 percent of the children examined within the age group of five to fifteen years had loss of attachment. In a separate investigation, Van der Velden and others (1989) evaluated a group of 15- to 16-year-old children from Amsterdam whose parents did not have periodontal disease. They found these children had an incidence of 5 percent of the sites with loss of attachment. These findings may suggest that the children whose parents have periodontal disease are at increased risk for loss of attachment. The treated and maintained periodontal client may be at risk for recurrence if the spouse has untreated periodontitis that can act as a reservoir for periodontopathogens. Microbial transmission may prove to become an important risk factor as further research is undertaken.

**Bleeding on Probing.** The location of bleeding on probing is recorded in the same manner as it was during initial therapy and subsequent PMP appointments. Bleeding on probing is an indicator of inflammation within the gingival connective tissues (Greenstein, Caton, & Polson, 1981). Bleeding while skimming the lateral wall of the gingival crevice is an indicator of early gingivitis (Van der Weijden, Timmerman, Nijbor, Reijerse, & Van der Velden, 1994). Lang, Adler, Joss, and Nyman (1990)

evaluated forty-one subjects in a maintenance program for two and one-half years with recare intervals ranging between two to six months. They found that the absence of bleeding on probing was a better indicator of gingival health than its presence was of disease. The study indicated that nonbleeding sites in subjects returning for PMP did not require further treatment over this time frame. They felt that while instrumentation of sites that bled may result in overtreatment of most areas, from a clinical perspective, this may be acceptable in a client with a history of periodontal disease.

Joss, Adler, and Lang (1994) examined a group of subjects for bleeding on probing, and those patients with a mean bleeding on probing score greater than 30 percent had two-thirds of the sites that suffered loss of attachment. Subjects with bleeding on probing of 20 percent or less, had one-third of sites with loss of attachment. Although bleeding on probing is relatively inaccurate as a method of detecting disease progression, most clinicians feel that these sites should be treated during PMP appointments.

Badersten, Nilvéus, and Egelberg (1990) evaluated nonmolar teeth for five years following nonsurgical periodontal therapy. It was found the diagnostic reliability of plaque and bleeding scores to predict disease activity, reached a predictability of about 30 percent. Results indicated that as many as 30 percent of the sites with plaque at 75 percent or more of the examinations eventually lost attachment. The diagnostic predictability of sites with probe depths of 7 mm or greater that lost attachment increased from 9 percent at six months to 78 percent at five years. Of all the indicators, over time, an increase in probe depth was the most reliable predictor of attachment loss.

Claffey, Nylund, Kiger, Garret, and Egelberg (1990) in a companion study, evaluated the same subjects as did Badersten and coworkers, but over a three and one-half-year period and the sample included molar teeth. When sites with plaque were evaluated, it was found that when plaque was present at more than 75 percent of eight examinations during the 42-month period, 15 percent of the sites had attachment loss. They found an increase in probe depth had an increased predictability for loss of attachment over time, particularly if it was associated with bleeding after probing. They reported that 62 percent of the sites that bleed 75 percent of the time over forty-two months suffered loss of attachment. This finding was particularly true as the probe depth increased. When sites with an increase of 1 mm in probe depth bleed greater than or equal to 75 percent of the time, the diagnostic predictability for loss of attachment was 82 percent. The authors cautioned against placing to much emphasis on bleeding after probing as an indicator of disease activity. It may be more useful as a risk factor, particularly when it occurs with frequency at a specific site. They also suggested that longer monitoring periods increase the accuracy of using traditional clinical indices to predict attachment loss.

**Furcation Involvement.** The location and extent of furcation involvement is recorded. Teeth with furcation involvement are at risk for further attachment loss. Studies have evaluated treated periodontal patients who presented with furcation involvement at the initial examination. McFall (1982) found that 56.9 percent of teeth with furcation involvement at the initial examination were lost over the time subjects were enrolled in a supportive periodontal maintenance program. Hirschfeld and Wasserman (1978) found that 31.4 percent of teeth with furcation involvements were lost. Goldman, Ross, and Goteiner (1986) found that the maxillary and mandibular molars were the most frequently lost teeth.

**Mobility.** The presence and degree of mobility is also determined. Clients with advanced attachment and bone loss might have increased mobility despite frequent professional care and adequate self-care. If areas of mobility are discovered at the recall appointment, then client education must include this discovery. The dentist should determine if the mobility is progressive and requires treatment.

**Suppuration.** The presence of suppuration or exudate indicates an area of concern during the PMP visit. It reflects an inflammatory process within the gingival connective tissue. The presence of exudate does not indicate whether the disease is progressive or arrested. Suppuration is about 30 percent predictive in determining disease progression.

### Deposit Accumulation

Location and extent of microbial plaque, calculus, and stain are recognized. Supragingival bacterial plaque accumulation is commonly recorded by using an index or standardized written notations about extent (light, moderate, or heavy) relative to location. Quantitative assessment does not always correlate to the severity of periodontal disease; however, it serves to evaluate the effectiveness of the client's self-care practices. Plaque accumulation on the day of the appointment does not always indicate the routine status of the client's self-care between visits. It does provide the clinician with a means of initiating self-care education based on plaque accumulation. Disclosing of bacterial plaque also provides an avenue for client self-evaluation of plaque. Qualitative assessment of bacterial plaque is perhaps more meaningful, and as discussed in Chapter 3, routine microbial evaluation in clinical practice is limited at the present time. It might be useful to employ microbiological assessment when progressive disease occurs despite professional therapy. Microbial sampling may be used to monitor the effects of therapy as well as to determine if antibiotics should be prescribed. DNA and RNA sampling can be employed to determine the presence of suspected subgingival pathogens such as *Porphyromonas*

*gingivalis, Prevotella intermedia, Actinobacillus actinomycetemcomitans, Bacteroides forsythus,* and *Eikinella corrodens.*

Supra- and subgingival calculus deposits serve as areas of plaque retention. During the planning of therapy, the clinician must identify the location of calculus deposits to effectively implement scaling and root planing or debridement therapy. The presence of calculus frequently correlates to other significant clinical parameters such as bleeding, pocket depth, and loss of attachment. Stain in itself is not an etiologic factor responsible for the disease process; however, it is an esthetic concern and sometimes relates to a client's needs or chief concerns.

### Radiographic Assessment

Need for bitewing and periapical radiographs should be assessed appropriately realizing that the interval for exposure depends on the risks of advancing disease, the caries index, and other clinical findings that warrant consideration of new films, as well as the client's radiographic history. Clinical attachment loss will precede radiographic appearance of bone loss, so evidence of increased probe depths, loss of attachment or confirmation of clinical findings dictate need for radiographs (McFall, 1989). If caries are not clinically detected or periodontal destruction is not evident, then reexposure of bitewing films should be taken at eighteen- to thirty-six-month intervals. Vertical bitewings are indicated for patients with periodontitis because they reveal more alveolar bone than do regular bitewing radiographs. Chapter 5 reviews recommendations for exposing radiographs as well as interpretation of periodontal disease entities.

## DIAGNOSIS

It is important to establish a tentative or presumptive diagnosis. Diagnosis relates to the classification of periodontal disease and to the determination of which sites are to be treated. The presumptive diagnosis determined at initial therapy or previous PMP visits may, in fact, be altered at subsequent PMP visits due to an increase in severity of disease or nonresponse to therapy. Because there are different forms of periodontal diseases requiring different management, it is important to reevaluate the previous diagnosis in relation to the classification of disease as well as extent. The majority of clients who present for PMP will have adult onset periodontitis. This form of disease appears to be slowly progressing, is treated differently, and responds to therapy in a different manner than does early onset periodontitis or refractory periodontitis. Clients with early onset and refractory periodontitis are at greater risk for severe destruction at an earlier age, and should be treated more carefully and frequently than the client with the adult onset form due to risk for additional periodontal destruction.

Gunsolley, Zambon, Mellott, and Kaugars (1994) evaluated the effects of periodontal therapy on twenty-three patients with severe generalized periodontitis. They found when compared to patients with adult periodontitis, the response to therapy was similar, but the results were less favorable. The reductions in probe depth and gain in attachment following therapy were less than had been reported for the treatment of adult periodontitis with similar involvement.

Gunsolley, Zambon, Mellott, Brooks and Kaugars (1994) evaluated the effects of supportive periodontal therapy on the same group of young adults with severe generalized periodontitis. They found that the frequency of breakdown was higher in this group of subjects when compared to other studies evaluating different forms of periodontitis. It was concluded that more frequent monitoring was indicated and that microbiological monitoring may be an aid in determining the extent and location of therapy.

The therapist must determine which apparent type of disease the client manifests, which sites are stable, which have progressed, and to what extent therapy must be accomplished. There may be areas in the client's mouth that will require retreatment or more aggressive therapy. There are certain factors that may place sites at risk for further disease activity. These may influence the prognosis and treatment needs of the dentition or individual teeth. While these factors in themselves are not predictive in assessing disease activity, the presence of multiple risk factors may increase the risk for disease progression (see Table 16-1).

It is very difficult using traditional clinical indices to detect sites that exhibit disease activity. The loss of 2 mm of clinical attachment continues to be the gold standard for the detection of disease activity. The clinician must evaluate all of the risk factors the client presents with to determine the risk for disease progression, or whether a site is actively breaking down. Sites that have persistent bleeding on probing and an increase in probe depths over time appear to be at relatively increased risk for loss of attachment over extended PMP appointments. Other factors increase the odds of attachment loss. These include furcation involvement, age, and smoking. Treatment decisions and needs for the specific client are influenced by the all risk factors involved.

## PLANNING

A new care plan is developed based on the current clinical findings and diagnosis. It cannot be assumed that the care plan for the last PMP appointment will suffice for the current one. The client must be informed of the PMP treatment needs, especially if there are changes in the disease status. After the case presentation and informed consent, the implementation of care is performed. The data that has been recorded is compared to previous PMP appointments and if there have been indications of increased probe depths and/or loss of attachment, the findings must be discussed with the client.

It may be recommended that the client be exited from PMP and entered into active therapy in an attempt

to control the disease process. The findings and the client's response to the suggested therapy should be documented. When the disease process has been controlled, either by the generalist or specialist, then the client can be reinstated in the PMP program.

## IMPLEMENTATION

The implementation phase of therapy begins with reeducating the client and extending the previous oral self-care education. Treatment during PMP might include periodontal debridement coupled with adjunctive therapy including chemotherapy (antimicrobials and systemic or locally delivered antibiotics) (see Chapter 14).

### Self-Care Education

Educating the client is continued, and past education is reinforced. Inadequate self-care must be addressed and the performance discrepancy identified (see Chapter 8). Additional education is also included on a needs-related basis. Evaluation of client skills with oral hygiene aids is accomplished by questioning and client demonstration in the mouth. Skill enhancement might include reteaching the previously recommended aid(s), changing the aid to another because of client responses, skill levels, motivation, or changes in clinical conditions such as type of embrasure space. The importance of continual reenforcement of supragingival plaque control can not be over emphasized. The patient who performs adequate self-care will have less disease progression and may require less frequent PMP appointments than the individual who does not.

### Instrumentation

The case is selectively instrumented with emphasis on the sites with deeper probe depths and/or progressive attachment loss, as well as those with inflammation and/or bleeding. The sites with bleeding should be carefully inspected for residual calculus. Root planing should be avoided in those areas with probe depths less than 3 to 4 mm. Lindhe, Socransky, Nyman, Haffajee, and Westfeld (1982) coined the phrase "critical probe depth," which is 2.9 mm for root planing and 4.2 mm for surgery. It is defined as that depth below which loss of attachment will occur after instrumentation. Root planing in sites under 2.9 mm will cause irreversible loss of attachment. Care must be exercised during instrumentation, otherwise the therapist, not the disease process, may be the cause of the attachment loss.

The type and extent of instrumentation the patient receives is dependent on what is required to maintain stability. The treatment may range from removing supragingival or subgingival plaque (deplaquing) to definitive periodontal debridement with a local anesthetic. There is evidence the automatic scaling devices are as effective as curets in the removal of subgingival deposits (Badersten, Nilvéus, & Egelberg, 1984) and the method chosen depends on clinician expertise and client preference. Often, instrumentation involves a combination of hand curets and ultrasonic scaling. The flushing action of the ultrasonic instrument may be of benefit in deep pockets, or furcations. Baehni, Thilop, Chapuis, and Pernet (1992) found that ultrasonic scaling resulted in greater reduction of colony forming units in vitro as compared to sonic scaling. When instrumentation is completed, the teeth should be polished to remove stain and residual plaque. Instrumentation is discussed in Chapters 10, 11, and 12.

The clinical findings and therapy performed are reviewed with the dentist during the examination, which can occur at varying times during the PMP appointment. The findings that pertain to the client's treatment needs are documented. The next PMP appointment is scheduled before the client leaves the office. If PMP appointments are alternating between a specialist and generalist, it is important to contact the office that will care for the client at the next recare interval to maintain appointment continuity.

Within the treatment of periodontal patients, there are those who exhibit disease progression, either in localized or generalized sites. The hygienist must be prepared to manage these patients. Sites that are considered at risk have been discussed. The most frequent method to determine disease progression in a practice situation at this time is change in probe depths. When there is a change in probe depths and/or loss of attachment, more aggressive therapy is required. This may include additional debridement or the addition of chemotherapeutics. When there has been a change in the disease, the patient should be appointed for a reevaluation four to six weeks after completion of the PMP appointment. The possibility of referral and more frequent recalls should be discussed at this time. The decision must be made when the client requires additional therapy other than that which can be supplied by the therapist during PMP. The therapist cannot continue to perform PMP on patients who continue to suffer loss of attachment. This is construed as supervised neglect and inadequate treatment. Therapists are professionally and legally responsible for the maintenance of clients' dentition and must decide when they cannot continue to provide adequate therapy within the constraints of a PMP program. The alternatives are more frequent treatment, more aggressive treatment with PMP, and if that fails, reenrollment of the client into the active phase of periodontal therapy.

### Chemotherapy

A decision whether to administer antibiotic therapy is frequently based on clinical judgment and disease progression. Professional mechanical therapy is still the preferred method of altering the composition of the subgingival flora. The routine use of systemic antibiotics for the treatment of adult periodontitis is discouraged.

Antibiotics can be used as an adjunct to mechanical therapy when there is an acute periodontal abscess, or for recurrent and refractory cases that fail to respond to mechanical therapy. Antimicrobial therapy can be delivered by systemic or local routes. Systemic administration may result in complications such as the development of resistant strains of microorganisms, gastric upset, or candidiasis overgrowth. Systemic antibiotics may neutralize the effect of the birth control pill and potentiate the effects of blood thinners.

Local delivery systems are also a viable treatment option. One of the advantages of local delivery is that the drug is available at a much higher concentration at the site as compared to systemic administration. Minimal drug concentrations are found in the serum when the drug is placed into the pocket, so sensitization or the development of resistant bacterial species is minimized. The local delivery systems reduce many of the complications associated with systemic use. Actisite® by Proctor and Gamble is an ethlyene vinyl acetate fiber impregnated with 25 percent tetracycline. The fiber is placed into the pocket and retained for seven to ten days. The drug is released over time at a much higher concentration than when tetracycline is administered systemically. There is evidence that placement of these fibers results in clinical improvement with reduction of probe depths and gain of attachment (Newman, Kornman, & Doherty, 1994). Chapter 14 provides a thorough review of the use of chemotherapy in NSPT.

## SCHEDULING AND FEES

Supportive periodontal therapy appointments are usually 60 minutes in length (McFall, 1989; Killoy, 1995). Longer appointments or reappointment may be required for the necessary documentation and treatment of advanced or progressing cases, or for clients who are noncompliant. Oral health professionals must understand that the person with periodontal disease has examination and treatment needs that are entirely different than one who requires an adult prophylaxis. Time and fee structures must be tailored to fit the specific requirements of the individual being cared for. Cost is a factor relating to compliance with PMP. A large number of clients have dental insurance that may pay a percentage of periodontal posttreatment care. There are several insurance carriers that will only pay for two adult prophylaxis per year (Code 01110), one series of periodontal scaling and root planing (Code 04341) every one to three years, or two PMP services (Code 04910) per year. Unfortunately, the client is led to believe that this coverage is adequate. This individual must be made aware that these intervals are inadequate and may led to disease reoccurrence or initiation of new disease. It may be difficult for the client to understand the importance of more frequent periodontal care, especially when the cost is out-of-pocket. The dental consumer's understanding can be enhanced by involving all office personnel in education toward the value of PMP. The client must be encouraged to pay for the services even though the insurance carrier does not promote the same preventive standard. Education about the periodontal disease process is valuable in helping clients understand why frequent care is the best option for their oral health.

Success has been achieved with some insurance carriers by writing a letter to the company on behalf of the client. This letter documents the need for more care than the existing coverage allows because of systemic disease manifestations, the severity or type of periodontitis, and/or risk factors beyond the control of the individual. It would not be prudent to justify extended coverage for a client when the failure of treatment is related to inadequate self-care, or other factors within their control. Clients are extremely appreciative of the practitioners support of their need for more frequent recare intervals and insurance coverage. This practice usually enhances client compliance with self-care and suggested PMP intervals.

## RECARE INTERVALS

Patients completing nonsurgical or surgical therapy are usually scheduled for three-month intervals for the first year after completion of initial therapy. This is recommended to enhance self-care and evaluate the periodontal status at frequent intervals. It also aids in establishing PMP as a routine component of dental care. Wilson and others (1984) examined 961 maintenance therapy patients in a private practice setting. All subjects were placed on a three-month interval after completion of active therapy. This schedule was later modified as needed. Ninety-two percent of the patients were on a three- to four-month interval. Patients seen at this interval seemed to have less loss of attachment than those on a longer recare interval. Most practitioners find patients have less episodes of disease when seen at three- to four-month intervals. When patients who have been maintained at three- to four-month intervals are compared to those receiving six-month maintenance, or sporadic care, there is less disease progression in the more frequently maintained group. These studies related to tooth loss might form the basis for the three- to four-month interval that is recommended in the literature.

The interval between PMP is determined at the completion of each maintenance appointment or series of appointments. The clinician should consider suggesting a shorter interval for the first year if the case is difficult with complicated prosthesis, furcation involvements, poor crown-to-root ratios, and questionable client cooperation (Merin, 1996). Clients with multiple risk factors, advanced disease, poor oral hygiene, or an aggressive disease will require a more frequent appointment interval ranging from one to three months. When the client's self-performed oral hygiene is assessed, there are a surprising number that lose the motivation to incorporate the recommended practices into daily living. This large group

should be seen at more frequent intervals, especially when they have experienced moderate to advanced loss of attachment. For these clients, a three-month interval over the course of PMP is nearly mandatory.

The PMP interval may also vary over time for individuals, depending on their needs. Clients who exhibit disease stability and practice effective oral self-care may have their recare interval extended. The periodontal status is evaluated at each maintenance appointment, and the interval may be slowly extended or customized to fit the clients needs depending on the case stability. The dental hygienist accumulates the clinical data, evaluates the status of the case, and makes recommendations based on the data to the dentist. From this information and the clinical examination, the PMP interval is established. Refer to Table 16-2 for an overview of suggested recare intervals (Merin, 1996). An important factor in the success of periodontal therapy is patient compliance.

## CLIENT COMPLIANCE

It is accepted that the person who is compliant with self-care recommendations and suggested PMP intervals will have less new disease and disease recurrence. Wilson et al. (1984) evaluated 961 periodontal patients who had been treated within his practice for eight years. Compliance was defined as either complete, erratic, or none. Degree of compliance was calculated by adding the total number of visits during the period of maintenance therapy and dividing by the total number of years in maintenance therapy. It was found that only 16 percent of the patients were considered complete compliers, 50 percent erratic compliers, and 34 percent noncompliers.

His office worked very hard in an effort to improve compliance over a five-year period (Wilson, Hale, & Temple, 1993). They attempted to simplify compliance, maintain records of compliance, inform clients of the effects of noncompliance, and identify noncompliers prior to initiation of therapy. The office staff was educated in the role of compliance in periodontal therapy. The patients were scheduled for the next appointment prior to leaving the office, and then sent a reminder card and notified by telephone before the next appointment. Patients were also notified if they missed an appointment. There was an overall increase in the rate of compliance due to these efforts. After five years the group of complete compliers increased to 32 percent mostly at the expense of the noncompliant group (see Figure 16-4). These investigators suggest that those who comply to recommended periodontal maintenance schedules enjoy better periodontal health and keep their teeth longer than those who do not comply or those whose compliance is erratic. From Wilson's data, it can be seen that initiating and maintaining compliance in treated periodontal patients is difficult, but very necessary for long-term success.

Checchi, Pelleccioni, Gattoi, and Kelescian (1994) evaluated client compliance with maintenance therapy in an Italian periodontal practice. They defined complete

## Table 16-2  Suggested Recall Intervals for PMP

| Characteristics | Recall Interval |
| --- | --- |
| First-year patient—routine therapy and uneventful healing | 3 months |
| *or* | |
| First-year patient—difficult case with complicated prosthesis, furcation involvement, poor crown-to-root ratios, questionable patient cooperation | 1 to 2 months |
| Excellent results well-maintained for 1 year or more | 6 months to 1 year |
| Patient displays good oral hygiene, minimal calculus, no occlusal problems, no complicated prostheses, no remaining pockets, and no teeth with less than 50% of alveolar bone remaining | 6 months to 1 year |
| Generally good results maintained reasonably well for 1 year or more, but patient displays some of the following factors:<br>1. Inconsistent or poor oral hygiene<br>2. Heavy calculus formation<br>3. Systemic disease that predisposes to periodontal breakdown<br>4. Some remaining pockets<br>5. Occlusal problems<br>6. Complicated prostheses<br>7. Ongoing orthodontic therapy<br>8. Recurrent dental caries<br>9. Some teeth with less than 50% of alveolar bone support | 3 to 4 months (decide on recall interval on the basis of the number and severity of negative factors) |
| Generally poor results following periodontal therapy and/or several negative factors from the following list:<br>1. Inconsistent or poor oral hygiene<br>2. Heavy calculus formation<br>3. Systemic disease that predisposes to periodontal breakdown<br>4. Remaining pockets<br>5. Occlusal problems<br>6. Complicated prosthesis<br>7. Recurrent dental caries<br>8. Periodontal surgery indicated but not performed for medical, psychological, or financial reasons<br>9. Many teeth with less than 50% of alveolar bone support<br>10. Condition too far advanced to be improved by periodontal surgery | 1 to 3 months (decide on recall interval on the basis of the number and severity of negative factors; consider retreating some areas or extracting the severely involved teeth) |

(Modified with permission from *Clinical Periodontology*, 8th edition, by F. M. Carranza and M. G. Newman, 1996, Philadelphia: W.B. Saunders Co.)

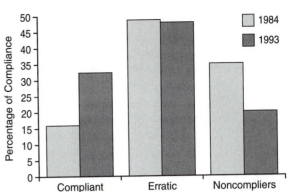

**Figure 16-4** Compliance in PMP. This graph is a representation of the data from the studies by Wilson (and others) published in 1984 and 1993. It depicts the ratio of subjects who were compliant, erratic compliers, and noncompliers. (Data from "Compliance with maintenance therapy on a private periodontal practice," by T. G. Wilson, M. E. Glover, J. Schoen, C. Baris, and T. Jacobs, 1984. *Journal of Periodontology, 55*, pp.468–473; and "The results of efforts to improve compliance with supportive periodontal treatment in private practice," by T. G. Wilson, S. Hale, and R. Temple, 1993. *Journal of Periodontology, 64*, pp. 311–314)

compliance as when the subject completed 100 percent of the scheduled appointments, partial compliance as at least 50 percent completion of the scheduled appointments, and insufficient compliance as less than 50 percent. They found that complete compliance decreased as the number of years after active therapy increased. Complete compliance fell from 38 percent after the first year to 20 percent at the end of four years. They suggest that the first year of PMP is critical in establishing compliance in the treated periodontal patient.

## REFERRAL TO A PERIODONTIST

The decision whether to treat or refer the client to a periodontist is based on 1) the type and severity of disease present and, 2) if you, as a hygienist in a general practitioner's office, possess the required skill and have ample time allotted to maintain periodontally involved clients. Referral to the periodontist depends on the capabilities of the generalist and the staff, as well as the desires of the person undergoing therapy. There are clients who decline referral, either because of cost, geographic constraints, or because they do not want to be exposed to a new office and unfamiliar health care personnel. It must be remembered that the professional maintaining the periodontal patient is responsible for the patient's care. This responsibility includes both professional and legal ramifications.

Most periodontists will alternate visits for PMP with the general practitioner. Clients with advanced periodontal disease, early onset, rapidly progressive, and refractory types of periodontal disease are usually maintained by the periodontist. The individual is referred back to the general dentist for a caries exam at least once a year. Patients with extensive restorative dentistry must be seen periodically by the referring dentist for evaluation. Most general practitioners and their dental hygienists are astute enough to monitor clients for disease progression. The ideal PMP schedule is one that alternates between the general practitioner and the periodontist.

## DOCUMENTATION

Record both the status of the case and the case presentation in the record of services rendered. Make particular reference to the sites at risk or those with disease progression. Record sites with plaque and bleeding as well as areas of inflammation. When there are needs that may include restorative dentistry and periodontal treatment, make note of these. If referral to a specialist was suggested, document this and include the client's response. This documentation will aid in preventing the client from saying, "You never told me I had a problem" at a later date. Documentation of the discussion of the case status is important from a dentolegal perspective, and it serves to inform and protect the clinician. The therapist should note the time of the next PMP appointment and its location, as well as the past compliance. Recommendations, acceptance, or rejection of further therapy such as periodontal surgery should be documented.

# Summary

It has been shown that periodontal therapy that is not followed by adequate plaque control will fail. Nyman, Rosling, and Lindhe (1975) and Axelsson and Lindhe (1981) reported that with regular maintenance that includes professional tooth cleaning, attachment levels can be maintained for years. Stable attachment levels will occur even in those clients with less than perfect oral self-care (Axelsson & Lindhe 1978, 1981; Knowles et al., 1979; Ramfjord et al., 1982). The PMP treatment regimen should be adjusted to fit the needs of the client. Factors that influence the frequency of care include the patient's ability to remove supragingival plaque, plaque-retention factors such as defective restorations, smoking, and systemic diseases that may modify the host response. Other factors that will influence the frequency of PMP are the severity of the loss of attachment, the depth of the residual pockets, and the type of periodontal disease. Three- to four-month intervals for PMP for secondary prevention are customary with more frequent intervals being recommended when the client needs palliative care because of nonresponse to active therapy and/or numerous risk factors for periodontal disease.

During PMP, professionals have the responsibility to recognize sites that are undergoing destruction. Clinical factors strongly correlated to destruction include inflammation, bleeding upon probing, suppuration, increased probe depths of 1 to 2 mm, and/or attachment loss of 2 mm or greater. Conversely, it has been said that two signs of successful periodontal therapy are absence of clinical signs of gingival inflammation and bleeding on probing, as well as stabilization of attachment level (AAP, 1989). Based on the data accumulated during the assessment of the client, the clinician must decide what sites to treat, and what extent to treat them. Clients are always informed of their periodontal status, and continually motivated not only to effectively remove supragingival plaque, but to be compliant with their PMP appointments. Professionals are aware that dentistry is saving more teeth and that as the population ages, there will be more individuals with periodontal diseases and; therefore, more PMP. The therapist faces a difficult challenge and has undertaken a large professional and legal responsibility in assisting the clients who have periodontal disease in retaining their teeth.

# Case Studies

**Case Study One:** A 65-year-old black woman presents to your office. Her chief complaint is "sore gums." Ms. Smith states that it is difficult to eat and, as a result, her physician has directed her to seek dental care in an attempt to improve her ability to eat and to, perhaps, help stabilize or improve her diabetes. She has received sporadic dental care in the past, but now expresses a strong desire to retain her teeth, improve her oral health, and control her diabetes. In the past, she has sought dental care only when there has been a problem usually associated with pain, rather than regular dental examinations.

She is overweight with a resting pulse of 82 and a blood pressure of 180/90. The blood pressure ranges from 180/90 to 160/85 during the course of therapy. She is an insulin-dependent diabetic, and takes 30 units of insulin by injection each day. She is taking Procardia daily (30 mg) for hypertension. A medical consult is obtained prior to therapy. The physician warns against long stressful appointments, and reveals that her glycolated hemoglobin is consistently on the high side. There is no pathology noted, her restorative examination is acceptable, no caries are charted, and her restorations are adequate. Ms.

Smith presents with generalized diffuse inflammation of the gingiva. The papillary, marginal and attached gingiva exhibit acute inflammation. The interdental papilla and marginal gingiva are hyperplastic with varying degrees of fibrosis. The probe depths range from 5 to 6 mm, with 3 to 4 mm of clinical attachment loss. There are Class I and II furcation involvements on most molars. Heavy crown- and root-associated soft and hard deposits are present, and there is evidence of heavy subgingival calculus and generalized horizontal alveolar bone loss.

Ms. Smith states that she brushes once a day, but states this is difficult due to the "sore and bleeding gums." Her diagnosis is Generalized Case Type III adult periodontitis with moderate bone loss. The overall prognosis is fair to guarded. The long term prognosis is complicated by the IDDM. Ms. Smith's compliance is a concern.

Appointment 1: Instruction in self-care with emphasis on brushing is introduced at the first appointment. A chlorhexidine rinse is prescribed for use twice daily in an attempt to reduce the acute inflammatory process.

Appointment 2: At the second appointment, Ms. Smith is taught how to use a wooden toothpick, and a gross supragingival debridement was completed by the use of ultrasonic and hand instrumentation.

Appointments 3 to 6: The removal of subgingival deposits requires several appointments due to the tenacity of the calculus. The self-care is reinforced at each appointment, at which time a plaque index and bleeding upon skimming/probing is recorded in a random quadrant. Each index does decline during the initial therapy, and Ms. Smith now practices excellent self-care.

Midway through her initial therapy, the physician changed her medication from Procardia to Verapamil which has a lower incidence of gingival hyperplasia. As the treatment progresses her glycolated hemoglobin levels decrease. As the nonsurgical therapy progresses, there is a marked decrease in the gingival inflammation. Ms. Smith consistently remarked throughout these appointments about "how much better her gums feel."

**Surgical Therapy.** Surgery is not scheduled at this time. Ms. Smith's care is in early maintenance and her periodontal status is being evaluated.

What are the risk factors to be considered in her case? Will you refer Ms. Smith to a periodontist after initial therapy? Provide rationale for your response.

**Case Study Two:** Using the description provided for the first case study, answer the following questions about Ms. Smith's PMP visits. What recare interval would you suggest for PMP and why? What assessment information will you collect at the PMP visits?

**Case Study Three:** A 28-year-old female, Sue Milder, presents to your office for a dental examination as a new patient. She states she has had routine dental care as well as periodontal therapy by a general practitioner. She tells you, "I have had problems with my gums since I was in my early 20s. I have had bleeding gums for as long as I can remember. My dentist said everyone's gums bleed a little and that's normal. Sometimes my gums swell and I have gum abscesses about every month or so." When questioned about her self-care practices, Sue responds that she flosses once in a while and brushes after every meal. She also uses antitartar toothpaste, because she heard it prevents gum disease.

Sue also shares with you that her general dentist did some "deep cleaning," but never sent her to see a specialist. She was told that she may lose her teeth; however, Sue acknowledges that she wants to keep them for a long time. Her parents had dentures when they were young and their ability to eat was affected.

When you question her as to when she had her last dental appointment, she tells you that it has been a couple of years since she has had a "good deep cleaning." The periodontal examination reveals generalized advanced attachment loss and generalized papillary and marginal inflammation. There is generalized bleeding, and areas of exudate while probing.

What presumptive diagnosis do you suspect and why? Will Sue's care involve PMP? Explain your response. How will you submit Sue's care to her insurance carrier? Is referral to a periodontist indicated?

**Case Study Four:** It is now two years postcompletion of Sue's (case study three) nonsurgical periodontal therapy in your office. She continues to decline referral. There are areas of increased probe depth noted at each appointment. The yearly recording of clinical attachment levels indicate loss of attachment and disease progression. The following teeth exhibit advanced bone loss and a hopeless long-term prognosis: 2, 3, 7 to 10, 14 to 15, 18, 19, 23 to 26, 30, 31. The remainder have a poor long-term prognosis. The probe depths are generally 6 to 10 mm with 4 to 10 mm of clinical attachment loss. There are Class II and III furcation involvements on all of the molars. The molars have Class II mobility and the maxillary and mandibular anterior teeth have Class III mobility.

The gingival health varies at each appointment, with areas of papillary and marginal inflammation. Bleeding on probing is always present. Very little supragingival or subgingival calculus is present. Her self-care is slowly improving; the plaque index is now 35 percent and initially it was 78 percent. Sue still has a history of recurrent periodontal abscesses, even with the use of Doxycycline as an adjunct to therapy.

What recare interval would you recommend for Sue at this point? How much time would you schedule for her PMP? What might the implementation phase of care include?

**Case Study Five:** In Ms. Smith's and Sue Milder's cases, how will you decide when to treat an area and to what extent to treat an area at subsequent PMP visits? How will you decide if the disease process is advancing?

# Case Study Discussions

**Discussion—Case Study One:** Risk factors to be considered in Ms. Smith's case include:

1. Medical risk factors: hypertension, insulin-dependent diabetes, and Procardia-induced gingival hyperplasia.
2. Risk factors: her age, the gingival hyperplasia, the probe depths, clinical loss of attachment, furcation involvement, the severity of the gingival inflammation, and the location of attachment loss. The severe generalized gingivitis may indicate an underlying systemic influence. The poor compliance in the past may be detrimental to long-term success.

Decision Making for the Referral: Treatment of moderate generalized adult periodontitis falls well within the scope of a general practice. Adult periodontitis is usually slowly progressing, and when the tooth associated infection is controlled, the prognosis is generally good. There is a direct correlation between the amount of local factors, the inflammation, and the attachment loss, with generalized horizontal bone loss. These factors should indicate that the response to nonsurgical therapy will be good. In this case, there are several teeth with advanced disease with a complicated medical history and poor compliance in the past. The decision to refer is based on Ms. Smith's desires to go to a specialist, the skills of the general dentist and the dental hygienist, the time needed for NSPT, and the associated fee.

**Discussion—Case Study Two:** Ms. Smith should be seen one month after completion of the initial therapy for evaluation and motivation. She is considered "at risk." Recare intervals of no longer than three months are scheduled for the first year, and depending on the stability of the case, these may be modified to better fit her needs. Throughout her lifetime it is unlikely that her interval for PMP will ever be greater than three months because of the extent of disease and the risk factors associated with her adult periodontitis.

The assessment will include the following:

1. A medical history and dental history update and review.
2. Extraoral and intraoral examination.
3. A restorative examination. A caries examination is completed every six months; however, this interval is dependent on her caries risk. From the previous assessment it appears that Ms. Smith has little caries risk, but this decision is best rendered after completing PMP over time.
4. A periodontal evaluation. The gingiva is examined for signs of inflammation. The location and severity of inflammation will be recorded, and gingival recession and the amount of attached and keratinized gingiva will be assessed. Periodontal probe depths will be recorded at each recare interval and compared to the previous readings. Attachment level measurements are assessed at least yearly, depending on the stability of the case. Bleeding after probing is noted and recorded. The furcations are reexamined and the severity recorded. Teeth, especially those with any further loss of attachment, are checked for mobility. Suppuration is also checked, especially if any areas of acute inflammation are observed.
5. Deposit evaluation. Because tenacious calculus was found initially, residual deposits may be found. Signs of inflammation might indicate that calculus, which is harboring bacterial plaque, is located adjacent to the inflamed area. Ms. Smith can be disclosed in one quadrant or more, and the plaque index recorded. Her oral self-care will be discussed and positive reinforcement given for her progress. Additional education will occur as needed.
6. A radiographic evaluation. Radiographs will not be indicated within the first eighteen months unless risk of further periodontal destruction or caries activity is recognized. An indication for localized radiographs might include an acute episode, which will probably relate to a chief concern.

**Discussion—Case Study Three:** A severe form of periodontitis that may be non-responsive or refractory to therapy is suspected due to her age, dental history information, and advanced loss of attachment. The advanced attachment loss indicates an advanced stage of disease: Case Type IV. Routine PMP are not indicated because of the extent and type of disease and noncompliance with the recare interval or possible unawareness of the need for frequent PMP. Sue needs active therapy again. Although as the treating clinician in the new office, you might consider her care to be initial NSPT, it is probably "retreatment" or maintenance according to the insurance carrier. Her insurance company could look at her care in different ways depending on how the previous dental office submitted the claims for care. Assumably, her "deep cleanings" were previously submitted as scaling and root planing or PMP. In either case, it would be in Sue's best interest to submit a letter with the insurance claim to explain the following:

1. The presumptive diagnosis,
2. The need for frequent PMP that will involve more than routine traditional NSPT, and
3. Why NSPT is indicated at this time versus surgical or continued PMP care.

The ultimate goal of the letter is to request that coverage be extended and or allowed on a more frequent basis than is customary. If the insurance company grants or partially grants the request, it might help Sue adhere to the recommended interval for PMP. Two new resource documents published by the AAP will help with filing the insurance claim:

1. Current Procedural Terminology for Periodontics and Insurance Reporting Manual, 1995
2. Insurance Coding Update, 1995

Referral to a periodontist is indicated due to the type and severity of the periodontal disease. If Sue declines referral it should be documented in the record of services rendered. Continual referral will occur at future PMP visits.

**Discussion—Case Study Four:** Because of her aggressive periodontitis, an interval less than three months is indicated. The recommended interval will most likely depend on Sue's willingness to comply and the response of her insurance carrier to the letter with the special requests. A two-month interval appears to be indicated. A ninety-minute PMP appointment is needed because of Sue's conditions. One hour might not be enough time because of the need for extensive reassessment of the clinical conditions, possible need for radiographs, and adjunctive supportive therapy interventions. There should be adequate time allotted to explain her periodontal conditions to Sue and to remotivate her to comply with self-care recommendations and the recare interval.

The implementation phase will include reeducation about her advancing disease, the recommendation to refer to the periodontist (again), and skill enhancement instruction. Because periodontal abscesses are recurrent and the gingival tissue might be sensitive, the need for local anesthetic and possible nitrous oxide analgesia should be considered. Instrumentation will involve subgingival root surface debridement with hand instruments and/or ultrasonic devices. Subgingival bacterial plaque removal or disruption can be accomplished with ultrasonic instrumentation and its use would be beneficial in the deeper sites and furcation involvements. Localized root planing might be indicated from time to time to enhance disease stability. Coronal polishing for stain could be part of the treatment plan; it also gives the client a feeling of having clean teeth and may motivate her to attain this feeling on a daily basis. Since there is minimal inflammation, chlorhexidene antimicrobial rinse is not indicated. Systemic or local antibiotics may be indicated when there are acute episodes. Microbiological monitoring might be indicated to help chose an appropriate systemic antibiotic or therapy.

The prognosis and treatment needs are discussed and documented. Sue is continually informed of the long-term prognosis of her teeth, including those that are considered hopeless. She is informed that when teeth are lost, replacement will be difficult. Treatment options may be more aggressive therapy by a specialist, partial dentures, or a denture. If Sue was not concerned about keeping her teeth for as long as possible, the implementation phase of care would most likely be altered.

**Discussion—Case Study Five:** The decision to treat an area and to what extent depends on many factors. First the medical and dental histories must be considered to see how they impact care and to assess for any risk factors. The restorative exam might reveal plaque retentive factors such as defective restorations or inadequate restorations that need attention. The periodontal examination will be invaluable in making these decisions. It is imperative that the reexamination of the periodontium be thorough and quality oriented. Inflamed gingiva, increased probe depths, progressive loss of attachment, bleeding on probing, furcation involvement which has advanced in classification or extent, increasing mobility, and/or suppuration are all signs of that which place teeth at risk for further disease. The extent of care relates to the presence of deposits, to the risk factors (refer to Table 16-2 for a review of risk factors), to the type of disease, and to the extent of disease. It was obvious from the previous case study discussions that the extent and type of disease had a extreme effect on the differences in recommendations for therapy for each case and on the recommended interval for PMP.

Disease progression should be considered if periodontal pocket depth or attachment loss has advanced at least 2 mm, and/or if further loss of alveolar bone height is apparent radiographically. Attachment loss will, however, precede alveolar bone loss. Sue is considered a "brittle" periodontal patient who is at continued risk for suffering tooth loss. She represents a classification of periodontal patients that presents a true challenge to the therapist.

---

**REFERENCES**

American Academy of Periodontology. (1989). *Proceedings of the world workshop in clinical periodontics; Section IX.* Supportive Treatment (pp. IX24–IX28). Chicago: The American Academy of Periodontology.

Axelsson, P. & Lindhe, J. (1974). The effect of a preventive programme on dental plaque, gingivitis, and caries in school children. Results after one and two years. *Journal of Clinical Periodontology, 1,* 126–138.

Axelsson, P. & Lindhe, J. (1978). Effect of controlled oral hygiene procedures on caries and periodontal disease in adults. *Journal of Clinical Periodontology, 5,* 134–151.

Axelsson, P. & Lindhe, J. (1981). Effect of controlled oral hygiene procedures on caries and periodontal disease in adults. Results after 6 years. *Journal of Clinical Periodontology, 8,* 239–248.

Axelsson, P. & Lindhe, J. (1981). The significance of maintenance care in the treatment of periodontal disease. *Journal of Clinical Periodontology, 8,* 281–294.

Axelsson, P., Lindhe, J., & Nystrom, B. (1991). On the prevention of caries and periodontal disease. Results of a 15-year longitudinal study in adults. *Journal of Clinical Periodontology, 18*, 182–189.

Badersten, A., Nilvéus, R., & Egelberg, J. (1984). Effect of nonsurgical periodontal therapy. II. Severely advanced periodontitis. *Journal of Clinical Periodontology, 11*, 63–76.

Badersten, A., Nilvéus, R., & Egelberg, J. (1990). Scores of plaque, bleeding, suppuration and probing depth to predict probing attachment loss. 5 years of observations following nonsurgical periodontal treatment. *Journal of Clinical Periodontology, 17*, 102–107.

Badersten, A., Nilvéus, R., & Egelberg, J. (1987). 14-year observations of basic periodontal therapy. *Journal of Clinical Periodontology, 14*, 438–444.

Baehni, P. C. & Tessier, J. F. (1993). Supportive periodontal care. In N. P. Lang and T. Karring (Eds.), *Proceedings of the 1st european workshop on periodontology*. London: Quintessence Publishing Co., Ltd.

Baehni, P., Thilop, B., Chapuis, B., & Pernet, D. (1992). Effects of ultrasonic and sonic scalers on dental plaque microflora in vitro and vivo. *Journal of Clinical Periodontology, 19*, 455–459.

Becker, W., Becker, B. E., & Berg, L. E. (1984). Periodontal treatment without maintenance. A retrospective study in 44 patients. *Journal of Periodontology, 55*, 505–509.

Checchi, L., Pelleccioni, G. A., Gattoi, M. R. A., & Kelescian, L. (1994). Patient compliance with maintenance therapy in an Italian periodontal practice. *Journal of Clinical Periodontology, 21*, 309–312.

Claffey, N., Nylund, K., Kiger, R., Garret, S., & Egelberg, J. (1990). Diagnostic predictability of scores of plaque, bleeding, suppuration and probing depth for probing attachment loss. 3 1/2 year observation following initial periodontal therapy. *Journal of Clinical Periodontology, 17*, 108–114.

Dorfman, H. S., Kennedy, J. E., & Bird, W. C. (1985). Longitudinal evaluation of free autogeneous gingival grafts. A four-year report. *Journal of Periodontology, 55*, 349–352.

Current Procedural Terminology. (1995). *Periodontics and insurance reporting manual* (7th ed.). Chicago: The American Academy of Periodontology.

Goldman, M. J., Ross, I. F., & Goteiner, D. (1986). Effect of periodontal therapy on patients maintained for 15 years or longer. A retrospective study. *Journal of Periodontology, 57*, 347–353.

Greenstein, G., Caton, J., & Polson, A. M. (1981). Histologic characteristics associated with bleeding after probing and visual signs of inflammation. *Journal of Periodontology, 52*, 420–425.

Grossi, S. G., Zambon, J. J., Ho, A. M., Koch, G., Dunford, R. G., Machetei, E. E., Norderyd, O. M., & Genco, R. J. (1994). Assessment of risk factors for periodontal disease. I. Risk indicators for attachment loss. *Journal of Periodontology, 65*, 260–267.

Gunsolley, J. C., Zambon, J. J., Mellott, C. A., Brooks, C. N., Kaugars, C. C. (1994). Maintenance therapy in young adults with severe generalized periodontitis. *Journal of Periodontology, 65*, 274–279.

Gunsolley, J. C., Zambon, J. J., Mellott, C. A., & Kaugars, C. C. (1994). Periodontal therapy in young adults with severe generalized periodontitis. *Journal of Periodontology, 65*, 268–273.

Hirschfeld, L. & Wasserman, B. (1978). A long term survey of tooth loss in 600 treated periodontal patients. *Journal of Periodontology, 49*, 225–237.

Insurance Coding Update. (1995). Chicago: American Academy of Periodontology.

Isidor, F. & Karring, T. (1986). Long term effect of surgical and nonsurgical periodontal treatment. A 5-year clinical study. *Journal of Periodontal Research, 21*, 462–472.

Joss, A., Adler, R., & Lang, N.P. (1994). Bleeding on probing: A parameter for monitoring periodontal conditions in clinical practice. *Journal of Clinical Periodontology, 21*, 402–408.

Killoy, W. J. (1995). Periodontal maintenance therapy. (Recall). In P. F. Fedi & A. R. Vernino (Eds.), *The periodontic syllabus* (3rd ed.). Baltimore: Williams & Wilkins.

Knowles, J. W., Burgett, F. C., Nissle, R. R., Shick, R. A., Morrison, E. C., & Ramfjord, S. P. (1979). Results of periodontal treatment related to pocket depth and attachment levels eight years. *Journal of Periodontology, 50*, 225–233.

Kornman, K. S. (1987). Nature of periodontal diseases: Assessment and diagnosis. *Journal of Periodontal Research, 22*, 192–204.

Lang, N. P., Adler, R., Joss, A., & Nyman, S. (1990). Absence of bleeding on probing: An indicator of periodontal stability. *Journal of Clinical Periodontology, 17*, 714–721.

Lightner, L. M., O'Leary, T. J., Drake, R. B., Crump, P. P., & Allen, M. F. (1971). Preventive periodontic treatment procedures: Results over 46 months. *Journal of Periodontology, 42*, 555–561.

Lindhe, J. & Axelsson, P. (1973). The effect of controlled oral hygiene and topical fluoride application on caries and gingivitis in Swedish school children. *Community Dentistry and Oral Epidemiology, 1*, 9–16.

Lindhe, J. & Nyman, S. (1987). Clinical trials in periodontal therapy. *Journal of Periodontal Research, 22*, 217–221.

Lindhe, J., Socransky, S. S., Nyman, S., Haffajee, A., & Westfelt, E. (1982). Critical probe depths in periodontal therapy. *Journal of Clinical Periodontology, 9*, 323–336.

Lovdahl, A., Arno, A., Schei, O., & Waerhaug, J. (1961). Combined effect of subgingival scaling and controlled oral hygiene on the incidence of gingivitis. *Acta Odontologica Scandinavia, 19*, 537–555.

McFall, W. T. (1982). Tooth loss in 100 treated patients with periodontal disease: A long term study. *Journal of Periodontology, 53*, 539–549.

McFall, W. T. (1989). Supportive treatment. In *Proceedings of the world workshop in clinical periodontics*. Chicago: The American Academy of Periodontology.

Merin (1996). Supportive Periodontal Treatment. In F. A. Carranza and M. G. Newman (Eds.), *Clinical periodontology* (8th ed.). Philadelphia: W.B. Saunders Co.

Newman, M. G., Kornman, K. S., & Doherty, F. M. (1994). A 6-month multicenter evaluation of adjunctive tetracycline fiber therapy used in conjunction with scaling and root planing in maintenance patients. Clinical results. *Journal of Periodontology, 65*, 685–691.

Nyman, S., Rosling, B., & Lindhe, J. (1975). Effect of professional tooth cleaning after periodontal surgery. *Journal of Clinical Periodontology, 2*, 80–86.

Petit, M. D. A., van Steenbergen, T. J. M., Timmerman, M. F. G., & Van der Velden, U. (1994). Prevalence of periodontitis and suspected periodontal pathogens in families of adult periodontitis patients. *Journal of Clinical Periodontology, 21,* 76–85.

Pihlström, B. L., Oliphant, T. H., & McHugh, R. B. (1984). Molar and nonmolar teeth compared over 6 1/2 years following two weeks of periodontal therapy. *Journal of Periodontology, 55,* 499–504.

Ramfjord, S. P. (1987). Maintenance care for treated periodontitis patients. *Journal of Clinical Periodontology, 14,* 433–437.

Ramfjord, S. P., Morrison, E. C., Burgett, F. G., Shick, R. A., Zann, G. J., & Knowles, J. W. (1982). Oral hygiene and maintenance of periodontal support. *Journal of Periodontology, 53,* 26–34.

Ramfjord, S. P., Caffesse, R. G., Morrison, E. C., Hill, R. W., Kerry, G. J., Appleberry, E. A., Nissle, R. R., & Stults, D. L. (1987). Four modalities of periodontal treatment compared over 5 years. *Journal of Periodontal Research, 22,* 222–223.

Ramfjord, S. P. (1987). Maintenance therapy care for treated periodontitis patients. *Journal of Clinical Periodontology, 14,* 433–437.

Riverside Webster's II Dictionary. (1996). New York: Berkley Publishing Group.

Ryan, R. J. (1985). The accuracy of clinical parameters in detecting periodontal disease activity. *Journal of the American Dental Association.*

Schallhorn, R. G. & Snider, L. E. (1981). Periodontal maintenance therapy. *Journal of American Dental Association, 103,* 227–231.

Suomi, J. D., Greene, J. C., Vermillion, J. R., Chang, J. J., & Leatherwood, E. C. (1969). The effect of controlled oral hygiene procedures on the progression of periodontal disease in adults: Results after two years. *Journal of Periodontology, 40,* 416–420.

Suomi, J. D., Greene, J. C., Vermillion, J. R., Chang, J. J., & Leatherwood, E. C. (1971). The effects of controlled oral hygiene procedures on the progression of periodontal disease in adults. Results after the third and final year. *Journal of Periodontology, 42,* 152–160.

Theil, E. M. & Heaney, T. G. (1991). The validity of periodontal probing as a method of measuring loss of attachment. *Journal of Clinical Periodontology, 18,* 648–653.

Van der Velden, U., Abbas, F., van Steenbergen, T. J. M., de Zoete, O. J., Hesse, M., de Ruyter, C., de Laat, V. H. M., & de Graff, J. (1989). Prevalence of periodontal breakdown in adolescents and presence of *Actinobacillus actinomycetemcomitans* in subjects with attachment loss. *Journal of Periodontology, 60,* 604–610.

Van der Weijden, G. A., Timmerman, M. F., Nijbor, A., Reijerse, E., Van der Velden, U. (1994). Comparison of different approaches to assess bleeding on probing as indicators of gingivitis. *Journal of Periodontology, 21,* 589–594.

Wennström, J. L. (1983). Regeneration of gingiva following surgical excision: A clinical study. *Journal of Clinical Periodontology, 10,* 287–297.

Wilson, T. G., Glover, M. E., Schoen, J., Baus, C., & Jacobs, T. (1984). Compliance with maintenance therapy in a private periodontal practice. *Journal of Periodontology, 55,* 468–473.

Wilson, T. G., Hale, S., & Temple, R. (1993). The results of efforts to improve compliance with supportive periodontal treatment in a private practice. *Journal of Periodontology, 64,* 311–314

# CHAPTER 17

# Surgical Intervention

## Key Terms

allografts
autografts
free graft
gingival augmentation
gingivectomy
osteoctomy

osteoplasty
pocket elimination
pocket reduction
resective techniques
regenerative techniques
surgical crown lengthening

## INTRODUCTION

The goal of periodontal therapy has always been the elimination of active disease with the reestablishment of physiologic harmony between the soft and hard tissues of the dental unit (American Academy of Periodontology, 1989). As periodontal therapists, we try to achieve this goal for patients using the most conservative measures possible. Yet, despite our best efforts, there are cases that do not respond to conservative, nonsurgical modalities, and are, therefore, indicated for surgery. In addition, there are various clinical situations, such as lack of attached gingiva, that require surgical intervention to achieve a positive result.

This chapter includes discussion of the following: 1) the indications and rationale for performing periodontal surgery, 2) the surgical evaluative process, 3) surgical case preparation and 4) the scope of specific surgical procedures. Case studies are presented to demonstrate the indications for performing the various procedures.

## PRINCIPLES OF SURGERY

There are numerous reasons for performing periodontal surgery, the most common, and most important, of these being pocket reduction or pocket elimination, resulting from **resective** and/or **regenerative techniques**. Resective osseous surgery involves modification and reshaping of the alveolar bone to create a more physiologic crestal architecture (Ochsenbein & Ross, 1969; Ochsenbein, 1977; Ochsenbein; 1986), thus yielding pocket reduction. While this may result in reduction in the amount of attachment on a tooth, the resultant reduction in pocket depth allows for a better long-range prognosis due to the decrease in probe depths, allowing better access for

oral hygiene care and periodontal maintenance. Fortunately, more recent regenerative surgical methods have been described that offer the surgeon the opportunity to stimulate new periodontal ligament, bundle bone, and root cementum in areas where it was previously lost due to disease (Bowers et al., 1985; Gottlow et al., 1986; Mellonig, 1984; Nabers & O'Leary, 1965; Nyman et al., 1987). The benefit of performing regenerative surgery is that pocket reduction is achieved through regrowth of the lost attachment versus removal of attachment through resection.

While the American Academy of Periodontology states that the ideal goal of periodontal treatment is to restore the tooth and its attachment apparatus to its original form and function, regeneration is not predictably attained in all surgical situations, and is often not indicated. Factors such as defect type (three-walled versus one-walled defects) (see Figure 17-1), bone loss pattern (horizontal versus vertical), root morphology, degree of furcation involvement, and restorative treatment needs all come into play when determining the best way to treat an individual patient.

Previous chapters in the text have discussed different nonsurgical treatment modalities, all with one common endpoint: a reduction in pocket depth with a concomitant elimination of inflammation. However, depending upon the pretreatment probe depth readings, attachment levels, alveolar bone defect types and location of the pockets, this goal is not always attainable by conservative measures (Brayer et al., 1989; Caffesse, Sweeney, & Smith, 1986; Rabbani, Ash, & Caffesse, 1981; Rosenberg, Torosian, & Hammond, 1993). Initial probe depth is a critical factor in predicting the outcome to initial periodontal therapy (Lindhe, 1983; Lindhe et al., 1982). Probing depths greater than 5 mm, particularly in the

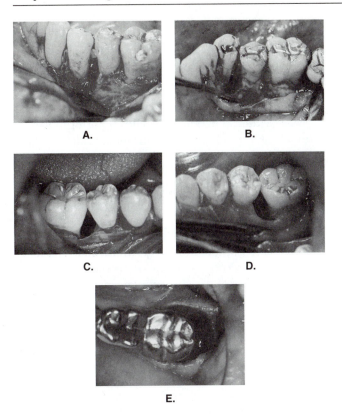

**Figure 17-1** Angular defects. Severe one-walled defect viewed from the buccal and lingual (**A** and **B**). Two-walled defect viewed from the buccal and lingual (**C** and **D**). Circumferential defect on the distal of the second molar (**E**).

ther reduced, due to the irregular nature of the posterior root surface (root concavities are common) as well as the presence of furcations (Fleischer, 1989; Kalkwarf, Kaldahl, & Patil, 1988; Nordland et al., 1987). In these situations, thorough root debridement becomes increasingly difficult to perform (see Figure 17-2). Another important factor contributing to the lack of healing from initial therapy is the alveolar bone loss pattern. Periodontal pockets associated with vertical bone defects are much more difficult to negotiate than similar depth pockets associated with horizontal bone loss.

Where persistent probe depths of greater than 5 millimeters are recognized accompanied by bleeding on probing, surgery is indicated (Becker et al., 1988; Caffesse, Sweeney, & Smith, 1986). Surgical access to these sites enables removal of any residual inflamed granulomatous tissue, thus allowing visual access to the entire root surface. With this improved access, the surgeon is able to visualize and remove any remaining bacterial deposits and thoroughly debride the root surface. The outcome of healing will yield **pocket elimination** (post-treatment sulci of 1 to 3 mm) or **pocket reduction** (a decrease in probe depth with an absence of bleeding), depending upon the presurgical bone loss patterns, degree of furcation involvement, and severity of vertical defects.

Before proceeding to other surgical indications, it is important to make the distinction between a periodontal pocket and a healthy sulcus with increased depth (deep sulcus). A site that demonstrates persistent probe readings coupled with bleeding upon probing after initial therapy is still considered a periodontal pocket. If, on the other hand, a site has persistent probe depth but no longer bleeds after initial therapy, the site is considered a noninflamed sulcus with increased probe depth. Pocket depth associated with bleeding is an extremely useful clinical measure, but it must be evaluated considering the level of attachment. The most important variable for determining whether a pocket (or deep sulcus) is progressive is the level of attachment (Carranza, 1996). Apical displacement of the attachment jeopardizes the health of the tooth, not just the increase in pocket depth.

posterior sextants, typically do not lend themselves to adequate healing after nonsurgical periodontal therapy. In these moderately deep periodontal pockets, persistent probing and inflammation are often seen. The primary reason for this observed phenomenon is that the deeper the pocket, the more difficult it is to adequately debride the root surface of bacterial plaque, calculus, and bacterial toxins (Brayer et al., 1989; Caffesse, Sweeney, & Smith, 1986; Rabbani, Ash, & Caffesse, 1981; Stambaugh et al., 1981). When this increased depth is seen in the posterior sextants, the success of initial therapy is even fur-

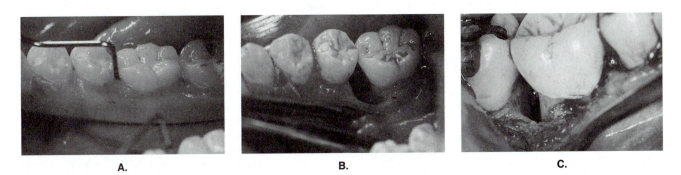

**Figure 17-2** The presence of vertical defects often necessitates surgical intervention. **A.** The mesial lingual aspect of #30 demonstrates a 12 mm probe depth. **B.** The defect visualized at the time of surgery. **C.** This 10 mm vertical defect on the buccal surface was impossible to adequately debride during initial therapy.

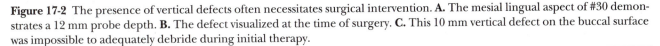

In fact, the increased probe depth can be related to coronal positioning of the gingival margin sometimes seen in inflammation (pseudopocketing). In conclusion, surgery is usually indicated to treat the persistent pocket. In the case of the deep sulcus, however, surgery may or may not be indicated. For example, a 5 millimeter sulcus could be easily maintained on the mesial aspect of a central incisor, but the same situation might not be maintainable adjacent to an exposed furcation on the distal aspect of a maxillary first molar. In this case, the decision of whether or not to perform surgery is made on an individual patient basis, taking into consideration several factors such as ability to perform adequate oral self-care and any restorative needs.

A second reason for performing surgery goes hand-in-hand with the first: creation of a cleanable environment for the patient. Just as the deeper probe depths are more difficult for professionals to treat, they are just as difficult for patients to maintain. By reducing pocket depth, a postsurgical gingival topography is created that is more amenable to oral self-care, thus improving the long-term prognosis.

The treatment or correction of anatomic gingival defects, specifically, inadequate zones of masticatory mucosa/attached gingiva or mucogingival involvement, is another situation requiring surgical solutions. In both situations, mucogingival reconstruction may be indicated via **free graft** or **gingival augmentation** procedures. In the case of narrow zones of attached gingiva or the presence of recession, it needs to be determined if the patient is able to keep the area free of inflammation. The ability to keep the area in question inflammation free or the lack of progression of recession usually obviates the need for gingival augmentation. On the other hand, if a patient is unable to keep their existing zone of gingiva healthy, or if the recession in progressive, gingival grafting is often needed to correct the problem.

Areas demonstrating mucogingival involvement (probing beyond the mucogingival junction) are assessed using the factors previously mentioned. Additionally, response to initial periodontal therapy is considered. A zone of unattached gingiva that is inflamed often reattaches once scaling and root planing has created an environment conducive to reattachment. Mucogingival surgery may be necessary, however, if these areas fail to respond positively to initial therapy.

Other reasons for performing periodontal surgery are in conjunction with restorative dental procedures or for esthetic purposes. Often, surgical crown lengthening is needed when carious lesions have extended so far subgingivally that they impinge upon the connective tissue attachment or crestal alveolar bone violating the biological width (see Chapter 4). A similar situation may exist in subgingivally fractured teeth. In both cases, surgery is necessary to remove crestal bone in order to allow for fabrication of a properly fitted and sealed restoration. Concerning periodontal esthetics, the surgeon is often called upon to create a soft tissue profile that either recreates

normal anatomy or establishes symmetry in an arch. Examples include correction of gingival overgrowth or treatment of altered passive eruption. In these situations, periodontal plastic surgery becomes an invaluable component of treatment.

While it is important for dental professionals to recognize the indications and rationale for performing periodontal surgery, it is just as important to understand the contraindications to surgery. First and foremost, patients must not have systemic disorders that contraindicate surgical treatment. Even though many systemic diseases do not contraindicate surgery, it is incumbent upon the professional to be keenly aware of the patient's medical status, and to investigate *any* potential problems. Cardiovascular (recent history of a myocardial infarction, labile hypertension), hematologic (bleeding disorders, leukopenia), oncologic (history of head and neck radiotherapy), immunologic (HIV, neutropenia) and metabolic disorders (uncontrolled diabetes) are just a few of the potential trouble areas. In all cases, it is imperative to document any changes in a potential surgical candidate's medical history and obtain clearance from the medical team prior to any surgical therapy.

There are some factors that contraindicate surgical treatment. The noncompliant patient (one who presents sporadically for active and maintenance treatment) is not a good surgical candidate. Also, the person who does not fully understand what is involved in performing surgery, despite our best efforts at patient education, is not a good candidate. Finally, patients with poor oral hygiene and inflammatory control are not indicated for surgery. The distinction must be made between the patient who has poor oral hygiene versus the patient who demonstrates improved oral hygiene but cannot remove all deposits due to persistent pocketing. In the case of the former, surgery should not be performed until the level of self-care is acceptable. Surgery would most likely be beneficial in the latter situation, because the result would be pocket elimination and effective oral self-care.

## CASE PREPARATION

Patients need to complete the initial phase of therapy prior to entering the surgical phase of treatment. In the initial phase, or Phase I, care is targeted toward the control of active diseases. From the periodontal standpoint, initial scaling and root planing/debridement and education in proper self-care need to be completed prior to embarking on surgical intervention (Lindhe & Nyman, 1975; Ramfjord et al., 1975). Completion of initial periodontal therapy is important for several reasons. First, it prepares the gingival tissues for the impending surgery by reducing the amount of marginal inflammation and improving tissue tone. This preparation allows for more predictable incisions, flap elevation and suturing, results in decreased surgical bleeding, and imparts an overall improvement in case prognosis.

Second, patient response to initial therapy is assessed, which can relate to the potential for surgical healing. For example, a patient who demonstrates a dramatic reduction in inflammation from scaling and root planing should fare well from surgical treatment. Lack of response to initial therapy may reveal a patient with refractory periodontitis (RFP) or rapidly progressive periodontitis (RPP). Most patients with RFP and certain ones with RPP require systemic antibiotics in conjunction with nonsurgical and surgical therapy to achieve a positive posttreatment result (Rosenberg, Torosian, & Hammond, 1993). Finally, the completion of initial therapy may lead to a reduction in the number of involved teeth in a potential surgical field through pocket elimination on some of the teeth in the quadrant, or even eliminate the need for surgery in a particular quadrant or sextant.

With respect to the other aspects of treatment, all carious lesions should be restored with permanent or temporary restorations, active periapical lesions should be treated endodontically, and all hopeless teeth should be extracted (unless they are to be taken out at the time of surgery). In essence, any active or acute aspect of the patient's diagnosis should be managed prior to surgical intervention.

## SURGICAL EVALUATION

While a tentative surgical evaluation may be completed at the time of initial presentation, the definitive surgical treatment plan is formulated after the completion of Phase I therapy. First, a detailed reexamination of the patient's mouth is performed in order to determine the response to initial therapy. Probe depths, recession, clinical attachment level, mucogingival status, degree of furcation involvement, and mobility are critical clinical factors to document. In addition, bleeding upon probing (bleeding index), the degree of gingival inflammation (gingival index), and the level of oral self-care (plaque index) are recorded. Once this information is obtained, comparisons are made to the pretreatment records, sites are identified that have or have not responded, and a treatment plan is formulated to correct any remaining problems.

Upon determining that surgery is to be performed, the precise procedures need to be identified. The selection of the procedure is made by evaluating the clinical data along with the full series of radiographs. It is simply not enough to know how deep a pocket is; correlating the pocket depth with defect type is essential in determining the exact procedure indicated. For example, the presence of numerous deep pockets associated with vertical defects may warrant regeneration versus aggressive bone contouring, whereas severe bone loss in a furcation site may indicate the necessity to remove a root. In any event, each case's treatment plan is determined on an individual basis, taking into account the clinical and radiographic data as well as the patient's treatment desires

and needs. It cannot be forgotten that there is a human being attached to the mouth we are treating.

## SURGICAL CASE MANAGEMENT

There are numerous surgical procedures available to the periodontist, depending upon the patient's treatment needs and diagnoses. Periodontal flaps are often utilized to treat periodontitis with moderate to advanced bone loss, particularly vertical bone loss, providing the surgeon has access to the teeth and underlying alveolar bone while maintaining the width of gingiva around the teeth (Barrington, 1981; Caffesse, Sweeney, & Smith, 1986; Genco, Goldman, & Cohen, 1990; Goldman & Cohen, 1958; Ramfjord, 1977). In addition, flap surgery allows the surgeon to treat the alveolar bone (Oschenbein, 1977; Oschenbein, 1986; Oschenbein & Ross, 1969) and involved furcations (Lekovic et al., 1989) by resective and/or regenerative methods. When maintenance of the gingiva is not a consideration or its removal is indicated (as with gingival hyperplasia), and where no vertical bone loss exists, a **gingivectomy** (excision of the soft tissue wall of the periodontal pocket by removal of a collar of marginal gingiva) can be utilized to treat persistent pocketing. In the case of mucogingival defects or deficits, there are a host of gingival graft techniques targeted towards augmenting the zones of masticatory mucosa (Carranza & Carraro, 1970; Cohen & Ross, 1968; Grupe & Warren, 1956; Sullivan & Atkins, 1968). It is beyond the scope of this chapter to discuss the full surgical armamentarium; hence, the most commonly performed surgical procedures, periodontal flaps and gingival grafts, will be discussed.

## PERIODONTAL FLAPS AND ALVEOLAR BONE MANAGEMENT

Periodontal flaps are the most common form of surgery used in treating periodontal pocketing. The objective of flap surgery is to reflect the adjacent gingiva from the teeth and alveolar bone, providing total access to debride the root surfaces in order to treat the alveolar bone defects, if necessary. There are two primary flap designs, the modified Widman (Ramfjord, 1977; Ramfjord et al., 1975) and apically positioned flaps (Barrington, 1981; Nabers, 1954), which will be discussed in detail. With respect to alveolar bone management, there are two options available to the surgeon: 1) osseous resection involving removal of bone to modify the defects present (Oschenbein, 1977; Oschenbein, 1986; Oschenbein & Ross, 1969), or 2) osseous regeneration, with the goal being regrowth of lost attachment (Bowers et al., 1985; Froum et al., 1976; Gottlow et al., 1986; Mellonig, 1984; Nabers, 1984; Nabers & O'Leary, 1965; Robinson, 1969; Rosenberg, Garber, & Abrams, 1979).

## Modified Widman Flap

The modified Widman flap (MWF) is a procedure used to gain access to the root surface and alveolar bone defects without apical positioning of the flap margin after suturing (Becker et al., 1988a; Becker et al., 1988b; Ramfjord, 1975; Ramfjord, 1977). The MWF is often used in treating shallow to moderate pockets, for supra-bony or moderately deep infrabony defects, or where esthetics is a major concern.

**Procedure.** Adequate surgical anesthesia is obtained by a block or infiltration technique, with papillary infiltration using 2 percent xylocaine with 1/50,000 epinephrine for hemostasis optional (depending on medical history). A marginal incision is made with the scalpel blade separating the pocket epithelium from the flap. With this technique, the full width of the masticatory mucosa is maintained by the incision design. Full thickness reflection of the soft tissues is then performed using a periosteal elevator: the entire gingival complex, epithelium, connective tissue, and periosteum is reflected from the bone and tooth. The extent of reflection of the flap is usually just beyond the crestal height of bone (just enough to see the roots of the teeth and any alveolar bone defects), but not beyond the mucogingival junction.

Once the flap is elevated, the pocket epithelium and interproximal tissue are removed allowing for direct visualization of the root surfaces and bone defects. At this time, the roots are thoroughly debrided of calculus using hand and ultrasonic instruments, and the bone defects are debrided of granulomatous tissue. Minimal modification of the existing bone profile is performed and regeneration attempted, where indicated. The flaps are then approximated around the teeth at their presurgical heights and secured using simple sutures, resulting in primary closure and minimal postoperative recession.

**Healing.** The resultant healing of the MWF is pocket reduction/elimination by bone repair in the infrabony defects concurrent with a long junctional epithelial attachment of the flap to the debrided root surfaces. While there is not a total regeneration of lost attachment in the bone defects, there is an excellent long-term sustainable gain in clinical attachment and decrease in pocket depth, as compared to pretreatment measurements. Where regeneration was attempted, healing will be by new attachment formation as well.

## Apically Positioned Flap

An apically positioned flap (APF), just as a MWF, is used to gain access to root surfaces and bone defects (Becker et al., 1988a; Becker et al., 1988b; Genco, Goldman, & Cohen, 1990). However, unlike the MWF, the principle of this procedure is quite different. In the case of an APF, the flap is reflected beyond the mucogingival junction, with pocket elimination achieved by repositioning the entire gingival complex apically, approximating the alveolar bone crest after osseous contouring. This results in a free gingival margin apical to its pretreatment height (recession), while maintaining the zone of attached gingiva. The APF is indicated in the treatment of moderate to deep pockets in conjunction with severe vertical bone defects. Also, this flap technique is necessary in treating the involved furcation and for crown lengthening. When performing regeneration, this same flap technique (full MG flap) is used, but the flap margins are then repositioned or positioned coronally, as will be discussed later. Obviously, due to the resultant recession from apical margin placement, an APF is contraindicated when esthetics are a concern.

**Procedure.** Adequate anesthesia is achieved, after which an incision is made in the gingiva down to the crest of bone. Unlike the MWF, the initial incisions can be placed apical to the free gingival margin, depending upon the severity of the disease. For shallower pockets, the incision is made near the free gingival margin, with minimal removal of marginal tissue (similar to the MWF). For deeper pockets, submarginal incisions are used resulting in a collar of gingiva being severed from the flap. The flexibility of incision placement allows for more predictable posttreatment adaptation of the flap, facilitates apical positioning, and allows for more precise control of the marginal tissue thickness and profile.

Once incisions are placed, a periosteal elevator is used to reflect a full thickness flap beyond the mucogingival junction, exposing the tooth, alveolar crest, and buccal and lingual/palatal plates of bone. Thorough root and bone defect debridement is accomplished, after which a decision is made as to how to treat any existing bone defects. In addition, severe furcation involvement can be managed via hemisection or root resection. The flaps are then apically positioned at the alveolar crest of bone, and primary closure achieved with adequate suturing.

**Healing.** Healing following APF surgery will result in pocket elimination by formation of a normal dentogingival complex at a point more apical than the pretreatment level. This healing also results in recession with root exposure, with the exact amount dependent upon the severity of the pocket depths before surgery, and the amount of osseous recontouring performed.

## Osseous Resective Surgery

Surgical debridement alone is frequently inadequate to achieve pocket reduction in the presence of irregular crestal architecture or severe alveolar bone defects. In these instances, treatment of the underlying bony problems, by resective or regenerative techniques, is paramount to achieving the desired goal of therapy. In the case of osseous resection, bone is removed to produce a more physiologic profile/contour of the alveolar crest and process, thus allowing for improved healing and pocket reduction (Goldman & Cohen, 1958; Ochsenbein, 1977; Ochsenbein, 1986; Ochsenbein & Ross, 1986). With regenerative procedures, the goal is to maintain as much of the existing bone around the teeth as possible while attempting regrowth of the previously lost attachment, thus achieving pocket reduction while providing the patient with more attachment than before the procedure.

**Osseous Resection.** It often becomes necessary to remove bone in a surgical site in order to reestablish a more normal physiologic crestal architecture, thus enabling the soft tissues to properly heal. Bone removal may also be indicated for managing vertical defects not amenable to regeneration. In addition, when surgical crown lengthening is the goal (exposure of root structure allowing for a proper restoration to be placed), osseous resection is the only way to achieve the desired result.

After debridement of the surgical field, a close evaluation of the alveolar bone is performed to determine the need for resective therapy. Sites where the marginal crest of bone is thick or where there are marginal exostoses usually require **osteoplasty**, which involves reshaping of the existing bone without exposure of additional tooth structure. Osteoplasty allows the surgeon to modify the existing crestal profile (in the case of irregularities) or remove bony impediments (thickened crestal ledges or tori) that would interfere with the soft tissues healing normally around the teeth, which results in a reduction in pocketing.

If the desired result cannot be achieved by reshaping the bone alone (as is the case with certain vertical and circumferential defects), removal of supporting bundle bone becomes necessary to adequately modify the defects and optimize healing. This procedure is termed **ostectomy**. The other primary indication for performing ostectomy is for **surgical crown lengthening**, which is the exposure of sound root structure apical to deep carious lesions or fractures. In these situations, intentional removal of bone must be completed in order to reestablish the biologic width of the dentogingival complex as well as to allow for fabrication of a properly sealed restoration.

In the case of osteoplasty, no additional root exposure occurs, therefore, there will be no more recession than had the tissues simply been apically positioned. The removal of bone optimizes the long-term healing at the site by creating as ideal a relationship between the bone and soft tissue as possible. Obviously, this is not the case with ostectomy, for there will be additional root exposure. While there are not set guidelines to follow, the surgeon must be keenly aware not only of how much bone needs to be removed, but of how much bone remains. Indiscriminate removal of bone to create the ideal osseous profile can actually worsen a tooth's prognosis and jeopardize its longevity. Taking away too much bone

may result in teeth with insufficient attachment to withstand normal occlusal loading.

## Osseous Regeneration

The ideal goal of periodontal treatment is to restore the periodontium to its predisease levels by regrowth of the periodontal ligament, bone, and cementum (AAP, 1989). While this is not always possible, regeneration can be achieved in certain defect types. Two- and three-walled vertical defects (Gottlow et al., 1986; Nyman et al., 1987), Class II furcation defects (Lekovic et al., 1989; Pontoriero et al., 1988), and circumferential defects offer the best regenerative prognosis, whereas one-walled defects and Class III furcations have a much poorer regenerative potential. As previously stated, after the field is totally debrided, a decision is made whether to close, recontour bone, or attempt regeneration. If the latter is chosen, there are two options available that can achieve this result: 1) guided tissue regeneration, and 2) bone grafts (autografts and allografts).

**Guided Tissue Regeneration.** Guided tissue regeneration involves using a semipermeable membrane as a barrier between the flap epithelium and the underlying bone defect, the purpose of which is to prevent the rapidly proliferating junctional epithelium from populating the defect (which could result in a long junctional epithelium healing) while allowing the slower growing connective tissue cells in the periodontal ligament to reform lost attachment (Gottlow et al., 1986; Isidor, Karring, Nyman, & Lindhe, 1986; Karring, Isidor, Nyman, & Lindhe, 1985; Nyman et al., 1987). Periodontal wound healing is a complex phenomenon, particularly in the ligament space, with the pluripotential connective tissue cells in the ligament space requiring time to differentiate into osteoblasts, cementoblasts, and fibroblasts in order to affect new attachment formation.

After thorough debridement of the defect, the membrane is placed over the affected site, affixed in place, and the flaps positioned *coronally* to cover the membrane. After closure, the membrane allows perfusion of the flap and underlying bone (due to its permeability) while preventing apical migration of the junctional epithelium. When using a nonresorbable membrane (Gore-Tex), it must be removed four to eight weeks after placement. With resorbable membranes (Guidor or Resolute), removal is not necessary. The long-term result of this procedure is pocket reduction by formation of new connective tissue attachment as opposed to a long junctional epithelium (as is the case with the modified Widman flap).

**Bone Grafts.** **Autografts** are bone grafts obtained from the same patient, and are usually harvested from the surgical site (cortical shavings or osseous coagulum) or from another intraoral site (such as cortical or cancellous bone from the tuberosity or an edentulous ridge) (Froum et al., 1976; Nabers, 1984; Nabers & O'Leary, 1965; Robinson, 1969; Rosenberg, Garber, & Abrams, 1979). **Allografts** are processed human cadaver bone (Mellonig, 1984; Quintero, Mellonig, & Gambill, 1982), which are usually freeze-dried and demineralized. Freeze-drying greatly reduces the antigenicity of the graft material (Quattlebaum, Mellonig, & Hansel, 1988), while demineralization results in enhancing the osteogenic potential by exposing the bone-inducing agent bone-morphogenic protein (Urist & Strates, 1971; Urist & Iwata, 1973).

When using bone grafts, the material is placed into the thoroughly debrided defect to the level of the uninvolved crest, if possible, in an attempt to promote bone and attachment to regenerate at the site. With both autografts and allografts, new bone formation is the result of osteoinduction, or the ability of the graft material to modify the course of healing of the bone and ligament cells of the defect. In essence, the graft itself does not become the new bone (osteogenesis), but stimulates the existing tissues to form new attachment. The presence of bone morphogenic protein in the graft material is largely responsible for this process. To a lesser degree, conduction occurs, where the graft acts purely as a scaffolding to allow for new capillary ingrowth with new connective tissue formation.

When attempting regeneration, it is important to understand the limitations and reasonable expectations of the procedures. Regeneration is not 100 percent predictable (the result is not always a new attachment formation), and patients need to know this before proceeding. Also, complete regeneration of the lost attachment, unfortunately, is not always achieved. Postsurgical assessment will often yield partial fill of an involved furcation or incomplete regeneration of an entire vertical defect. Many variables come into play such as the size, shape, and location of the defect, the ability of the surgeon to thoroughly debride the tooth to the base of the defect, as well as individual patient differences in healing. However, it should be noted that even with these "partial successes," some gain is better than none at all.

## Furcation Management

The involved molar furcation is one of the more difficult challenges that faces the surgeon, because this is perhaps the most difficult area for patients to maintain with proper oral self-care. Many times furcation defects can be simply treated with osteoplasty or minimal ostectomy, with the expected results being exposure of the furcation to facilitate oral hygiene efforts. In other instances, regeneration is attempted, with the goal being closure of the furcation. However, in instances where furcation involvement is so severe that osseous surgery will terminally compromise the involved and adjacent teeth, or regeneration has a poor prognosis, then hemisection or root resection is indicated (Newell, 1981).

**Hemisection.** Hemisection is a procedure performed on mandibular molars that involves sectioning the crown and root trunk in half, thus eliminating the furcation and creating two individual, lone-standing roots (Glossary of Periodontic Terms, 1986). In essence, two premolars are created. Once the tooth is sectioned, the stability of each individual root is assessed and a decision made to extract one of the roots or maintain both of them. If both roots are preserved, they can be restored as two premolars. If, on the other hand, one root is removed, the remaining root can be used as an abutment in a bridge (see Figure 17-3).

**Root Resection.** Root resection involves removal of the root from the root trunk without sectioning the crown of the tooth (Glossary of Periodontic Terms, 1986). This is most often executed on maxillary molars due to their having three roots. In this instance, there is usually severe compromise of one of the three roots, with the other two roots having good attachment. When this occurs, removal of the offending root allows for modification of the bone defects while maintaining stability of the tooth itself. Usually the compromised root lends little stability to the tooth with the remaining roots contributing more than enough attachment to stabilize the tooth (see Figure 17-4).

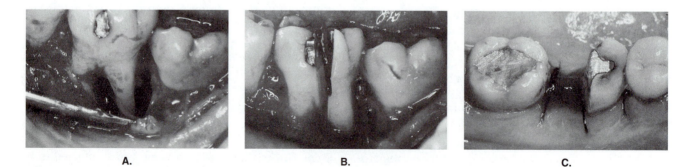

A.                                                                    B.                                                                    C.

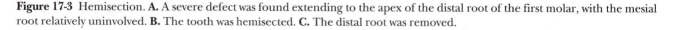

**Figure 17-3** Hemisection. **A.** A severe defect was found extending to the apex of the distal root of the first molar, with the mesial root relatively uninvolved. **B.** The tooth was hemisected. **C.** The distal root was removed.

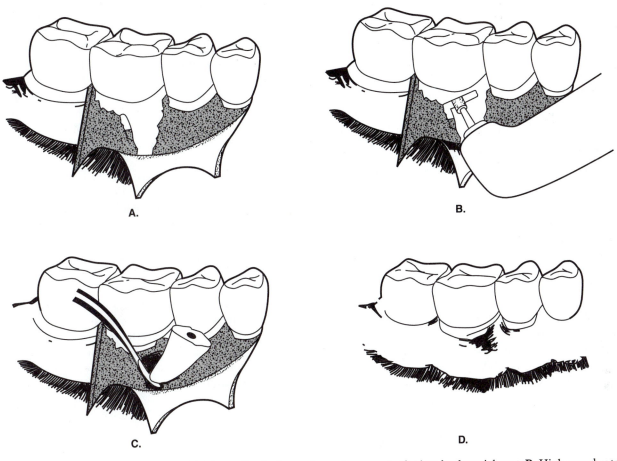

**Figure 17-4** Root resection. **A.** A full thickness flap is elevated to gain access to the involved mesial root. **B.** High-speed rotary instrumentation with irrigation is used to section the root from the remainder of the tooth. **C.** The root is elevated to the facial and the defect debrided. Osteoplasty is performed as necessary. **D.** Final healing. The area is maintained with an interdental brush.

In the case of both hemisection and root resection, the tooth will require endodontic treatment and usually will require crown placement (determined on an individual case basis). And, while the removal of a root creates a larger interproximal space, the soft tissues are allowed to heal, thus reducing pocket depth and creating a local site that is more amenable to cleansing.

## Postoperative Care for Flap Surgery

After the flaps have been sutured and the site determined to be hemostatic, a surgical dressing is placed over the site to maintain primary closure by intimate adaptation of the flap to the teeth and bone. The dressing also provides protection and patient comfort at the surgical site. Postoperative instructions are given to the patient (dietary restrictions, self-care instructions, etc.) as well as any indicated medications (analgesics and antibiotics, if needed).

The surgical patient needs to be seen for several postoperative visits for suture removal, pack changes, tissue assessment, oral hygiene instruction, and evaluation of the healing process. Sutures are usually removed at one week, and the site redressed at the discretion of the surgeon. Once the dressing is removed, patients are instructed in proper home care of the site, taking care that they do not disturb the healing flap. Often, it becomes necessary to supplement mechanical hygiene with a chlorhexidene rinse (Peridex) for two to four weeks after surgery.

In the case of regenerative therapy with nonresorbable membranes (Gore-Tex, W.L. Gore & Associates, Flagstaff, Arizona), the patient is instructed not to perform any mechanical hygiene at the membrane site until after membrane removal, and instructed to simply rely on chemical antiplaque agents (chlorhexidene). If a resorbable membrane has been placed, chlorhexidene rinses are used for approximately six weeks although mechanical plaque removal may be started twenty-one to twenty-eight days postop, depending upon individual healing. Long-term postoperative care involves periodic evaluation of tissue healing, plaque control, and a properly timed maintenance interval (determined on an individual basis).

## MUCOGINGIVAL RECONSTRUCTION

Unlike periodontal flap surgery, where the goal of the procedure is to treat active periodontitis, mucogingival surgery is targeted toward correcting problems associated with attached gingiva or its lack thereof (Barrington, 1981; Carranza & Carraro, 1970; Hall, 1989; Sullivan & Atkins, 1968). While there are numerous surgical options to correct these mucogingival problems, this chapter will only discuss free gingival grafting. For an overview of pedicle grafts (Cohen & Ross, 1968; Grupe & Warren, 1956) and connective tissue grafts (Langer & Langer, 1985), refer to periodontal texts and articles describing these procedures.

### Free Gingival Grafting

Free gingival grafting involves harvesting masticatory mucosa from the palate and placing it at a site with a gingival defect or deficiency. The graft, once placed, will increase the zone of attached gingiva in an area providing long-term stability. The more common indications for performing gingival grafting are areas with lack of attached gingiva (no masticatory mucosa), sites with aberrant frenal attachments, and sites with progressive recession (the presence of recession alone is not enough to warrant gingival augmentation).

**Procedure.** Adequate anesthesia is obtained at the recipient and donor site, using 2 percent xylocaine with 1/100,000 or 1/50,000 epinephrine for hemostasis. The recipient site is prepared first by removal of the surface epithelium over which the graft is to be placed (both over the masticatory and alveolar mucosa), thus exposing a firm connective tissue bed. Once the site is prepared, it is measured (width and height of the graft) and these measurements transferred to the palatal donor site.

At the donor site, the outline of the graft shape is made in the palate with a scalpel blade, and the dimen-sions confirmed. Once it has been determined that the graft is of proper size, an incision is made approximately 2 mm deep into the palatal tissues, and a 1.5 to 2 mm thick graft is harvested from the surface. This results in a free graft of adequate thickness to contain palatal connective tissue, for it is this connective tissue that will allow the graft to succeed. The connective tissue of the donor contains the genetic code for it to form masticatory mucosa at the recipient site. Also, in order for the graft to be accepted, the connective tissue of the donor needs to be placed on the connective tissue of the recipient site.

Palatal hemostasis is achieved by placing a surgical hemostatic agent (Colla-Cote or Colla-Tape) and placing a surgical dressing over the site or inserting a surgical stent (clear acrylic retainer). The donor tissue is then sutured over the recipient site, intimately adapted by proper suturing (using resorbable sutures, when possible), and the area dressed. Patients are seen one week after surgery for a dressing change and evaluation of healing. By the second postoperative week, the dressings can be removed, although the patient must be careful with diet and oral hygiene so as not to disturb the healing graft. As is the case with flap surgery, a chlorhexidene rinse is used for proper plaque control during this critical healing time.

**Healing.** Free gingival grafts are virtually 100 percent predictable when attempting to augment the zone of gingiva. If the graft is properly secured and stabilized, and the patient follows home care instructions, the graft will take with the connective tissues of the donor and recipient, healing as one. When the goal of the procedure is for root coverage (as is the case in progressive recession), the results are not as predictable. The avascular root surface does not provide the same optimal conditions for healing as the highly vascular recipient connective tissue bed. In any event, patients must be informed about effective self-care techniques so as not to recreate the problem for which they were treated.

## Summary

An overview of the most common therapeutic surgical modalities has been presented in an attempt to familiarize the reader with these procedures. This review was not intended to replace any of the quality-oriented publications discussing surgical intervention. For a complete review, the reader is referred to *Clinical Periodontology* (Carranza & Newman, 1996), *Proceedings of the World Workshop in Clinical Periodontics* (American Academy of Periodontology, 1989), *Advances in Periodontics* (Wilson, Kornman, & Newman, 1992), and *Periodontal Regeneration* (American Academy of Periodontology, 1993).

## Case Studies

**Case Study One:** Mr. Jenkins is sixty-two years old and was diagnosed with moderate chronic adult periodontitis. On initial examination, generalized 4 to 7 mm pocketing was found with bleeding upon probing, calculus, and bacterial plaque. Radiographically, there is 20 to 30 percent generalized horizontal bone loss except on the mandibular second molars, isolated, where vertical bone loss is present. Four sessions of quadrant scaling and

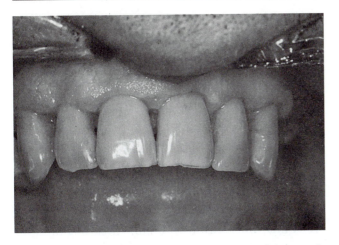

**Figure 17-5** Case Study One: Response after initial therapy; 5 to 6 mm pockets exist interproximally.

root planing were completed, and he was instructed in proper self-care. At the reevaluation examination, there was a dramatic reduction in bacterial deposits with an improvement in marginal tissue tone. However, persistent 5 to 6 mm interproximal pocketing was still seen on teeth #5 to 11 (Figure 17-5) despite his successful response to initial therapy. What procedure would be indicated to achieve pocket reduction in this sextant? Briefly describe this procedure and the expected healing response.

**Case Study Two:** Mr. George Brooks, a 47-year-old male, was initially diagnosed with generalized moderate adult periodontitis with localized advanced periodontitis in the posterior sextants. After completing quadrant scaling and root planing, he had a dramatic reduction in marginal inflammation, although persistent periodontal pocketing remained. In the mandibular right quadrant (see Figure 17-6A and B), apically positioned flap surgery with osseous resection was planned. A crestal incision was placed on the buccal aspect to conserve the attached

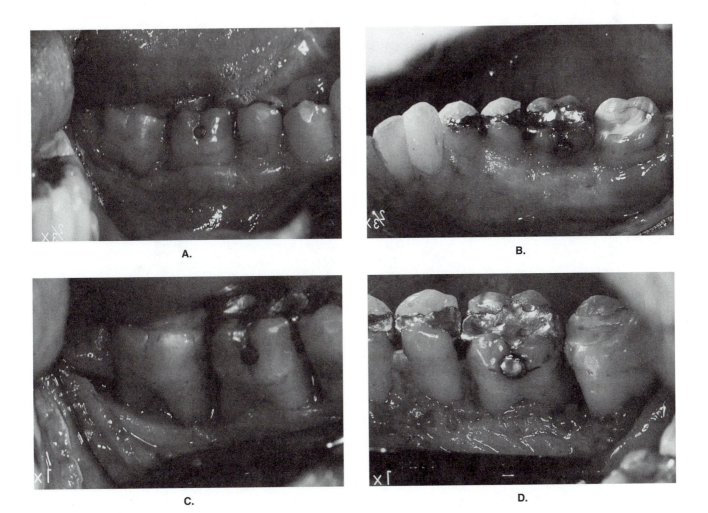

**Figure 17-6** Case Study Two: The buccal (**A**) and lingual (**B**) views prior to surgery. Osseous defects are evident after thorough debridement (**C** and **D**).

gingiva, while submarginal incisions were placed lingually to facilitate apical positioning. After full thickness flap reflection and debridement, it was observed that there were vertical defects on #30D and #31D, a buccal circumferential defect on #31 with furcation involvement, and an irregular alveolar crestal profile (see Figure 17-6C and D). Should any further surgical treatment be performed? If so, what procedure will most likely yield the best results and why? What result(s) is/are expected from this procedure?

**Case Study Three:** Persistent pocketing of 4 to 9 mm was found in the maxillary left quadrant of this 23-year-old female, Susanne Vestal, who was initially diagnosed with rapidly progressive periodontitis despite her positive response to initial therapy (see Figures 17-7A and B). Reflection of a full thickness flap revealed an irregular crestal profile buccally and palatally. A slight vertical defect was noted on the mesiopalatal aspect of #13, with a deep interproximal crater (7 mm) between the molars (see Figures 17-7C and D). Minor osteoplasty and ostectomy adequately managed the problems on #11 to 14.

However, if resective surgery were to be performed to eliminate the crater, severe attachment removal would be necessary, thus jeopardizing the prognosis of both teeth. Can any other surgical procedure be attempted to treat the crater? If so, which one? What is the long-term result of this procedure?

**Case Study Four:** This 31-year-old female, Karen Klinger, presented for evaluation of recession in her maxillary canine. Her initial examination revealed generalized gingival health with an absence of subgingival calculus. Probe depths of 2 to 3 mm were found throughout her mouth except on the direct facial aspect of #11 (see Figure 17-8A), which measured 7 mm. Three millimeters of recession was noted on the facial of #11 (which had increased 1 mm over the past 6 months), though there was an adequate zone of masticatory mucosa present. However, due to the extent of the probe depth, there was no attached gingiva present with mucogingival involvement (see Figure 17-8B). Would a surgical procedure be indicated? If so, which one and why? Would nonsurgical therapy be effective?

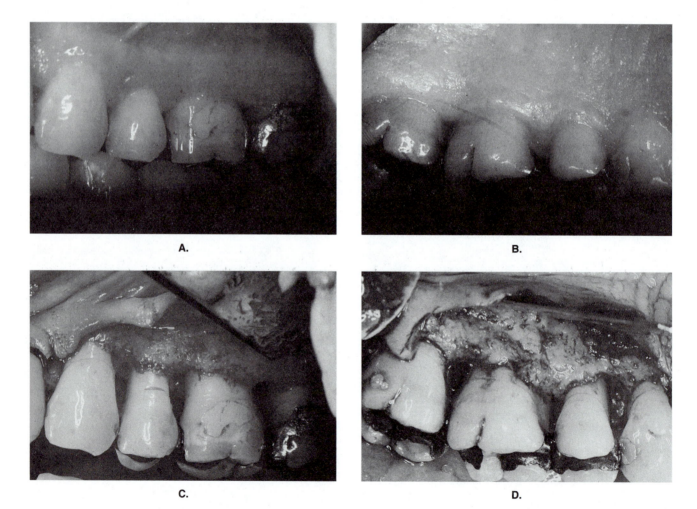

**A.**

**B.**

**C.**

**D.**

**Figure 17-7** Case Study Three: The facial (**A**) and lingual (**B**) views of this 23-year-old patient with rapidly progressive periodontitis prior to surgery. Full thickness flaps were elevated (**C** and **D**) revealing the defects.

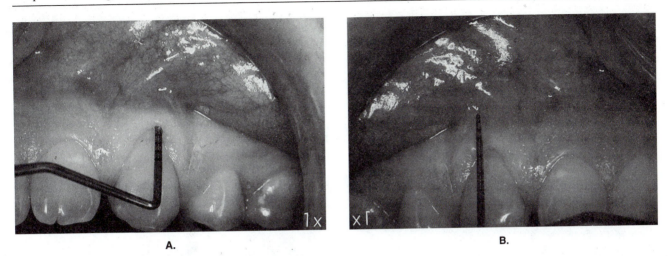

**A.**     **B.**

**Figure 17-8** Case Study Four: The 7 mm probe depth on the facial of #11 (**A**) indicates a lack of attached gingiva and mucogingival involvement (**B**).

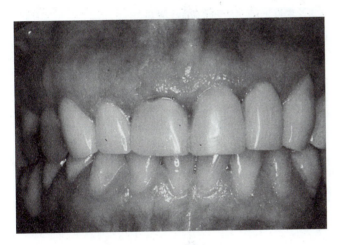

**Figure 17-9** Case Study Five: This patient presented with an unesthetic maxillary splint.

**Case Study Five:** Cheryl Cushman is thirty-eight years old and has recently had a six-unit provisional splint placed from #6 to 11 (see Figure 17-9). The extent of the caries found at the time of the restoration, coupled with the pre-existing localized recession, resulted in a provisional restoration with compromised retention, uneven gingival contours, and unacceptable esthetics. Is surgical intervention indicated? If so, why?

## Case Study Discussions

**Discussion—Case Study One:** A modified Widman flap approach is the procedure of choice to treat this sextant due to the esthetic concerns and the absence of vertical bone loss. After marginal incision placement, minimal reflection of a full thickness mucoperiosteal flap (see Figure 17-10A and B) revealed generalized horizontal

bone loss with sporadic root calculus. After completion of root debridement, it was determined that no contouring of the alveolar bone was necessary; therefore, the flaps were repositioned at their presurgical height (see Figure 17-10 C and D) using continuous vertical mattress sutures. The site was dressed with periodontal pack (see Figure 17-10E) and the Mr. Jenkins was given postoperative instructions.

Figure 17-10F shows the patient at seven days postoperatively (note that the white coating of the flap is simply normal surface epithelial healing). At three weeks (see Figure 17-10G), excellent healing is observed, and the patient resumed normal oral hygiene.

The expected healing response would be pocket reduction from a long junctional epithelial formation. This resulted in a sustained decrease in pocket depth and an elimination of inflammation with generalized 1 to 3 mm probe depths recorded four years posttreatment.

**Discussion—Case Study Two:** Yes. Because of the bony defects and irregular bony profile, osteoplasty and ostectomy are performed on teeth #28 to 31 (see Figure 17-11A and B), which eliminated the vertical and circumferential defects, provided a more physiologic crestal architecture (note the evenness of the alveolar bone), and allowed improved access to the furcation on #31. The flaps were closed primarily using sling sutures, the area packed and postoperative instructions given to the patient. Due to the patient's scheduling constraints, he returned for the suture removal visit fourteen days postoperatively (see Figures 17-11C and D).

This procedure was chosen because it permitted modification of the existing crestal profile to a more physiologic architecture while maintaining the integrity of the teeth. It was determined that actual removal of supporting bundle bone was necessary to adequately modify the defects to promote effective healing. While removal of supporting bundle bone was necessary to promote

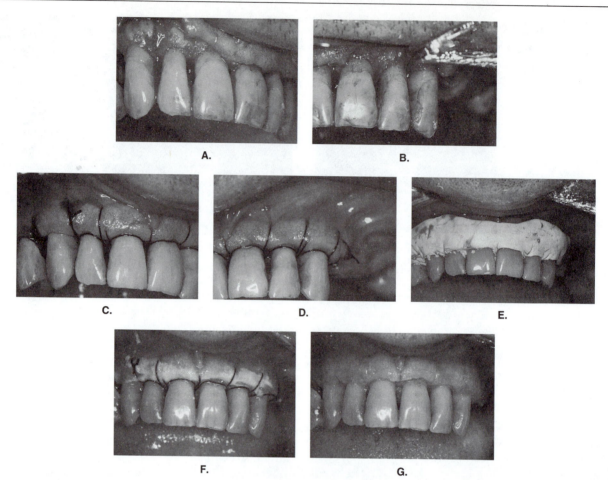

**Figure 17-10** Case Study One Discussion: Modified Widman Flap. A full thickness flap was elevated (**A** and **B**), the area debrided and the flaps repositioned (**C** and **D**), and the area packed (**E**). Postoperative views at one week (**F**) and three weeks (**G**). Notice the minimal recession.

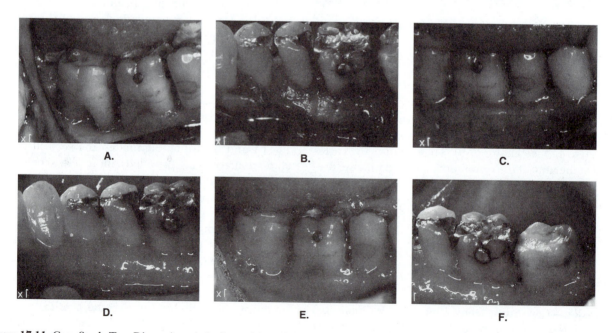

**Figure 17-11** Case Study Two Discussion: Apically positioned flap surgery with osseous resection in the mandibular right quadrant. **A.** The facial alveolar bone after osectomy and osteoplasty to modify defects and provide access to the furcation on #31. **B.** The lingual alveolar bone after resection. **C.** and **D.** The patient at two weeks. **E.** and **F.** The patient at four weeks postsurgically. Notice the improved access for oral hygiene.

effective healing, adequate support remained on the teeth; there was minimal mobility noted after ostectomy. Regeneration, while considered, was not attempted in this case due to the extent and severity of the bone loss pattern (multiple teeth with irregular defects), and the desired result of pocket elimination.

The expected results of this procedure include the formation of a healthy connective tissue and epithelial attachment at the apical crestal margin in conjunction with increased root exposure due to apical positioning of the flap. The long-term result should be an area that is maintainable by Mr. Jenkins, especially in relation to the improved access to the furcation. Excellent tissue healing response was noted, and he was instructed to perform limited mechanical hygiene in conjunction with chlorhexidene rinses. At four weeks (see Figures 17-11E and F), the patient was able to perform normal mechanical hygiene in the quadrant. This resective procedure resulted in an excellent marginal tissue profile and allowed the patient access to reduce or eliminate bacterial plaque accumulation.

**Discussion—Case Study Three:** Yes. It was decided to attempt periodontal regeneration. Autogenous cortical bone chips (harvested from the tuberosity) were mixed with a decalcified, freeze-dried cortical bone allograft (see Figure 17-12A), and the mixture placed into the crater after thorough debridement of the defect with hand and ultrasonic instrumentation (see Figures 17-12B and C). A nonresorbable Gore-Tex periodontal membrane was placed between the teeth covering the defect (see Figure 17-12D) in an attempt to maximize the regenerative potential, and the site was primarily closed with simple suturing. Susanne was placed on postoperative antibiotics and instructed in proper care of the membrane site (no mechanical hygiene at the gingival margin with twice daily Peridex rinsing).

Long-term expected results are pocket reduction by formation of a new connective tissue attachment as opposed to formation of a long junctional epithelium that results from the MWF, although the results are not 100 percent predictable with any regeneration procedure. The outcome depends on the size, location, and

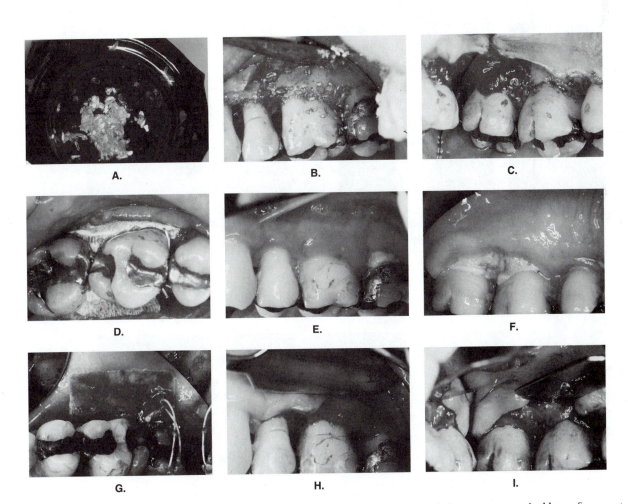

A.   B.   C.

D.   E.   F.

G.   H.   I.

**Figure 17-12** Case Study Three Discussion: Periodontal regeneration is attempted. Autogenous cortical bone fragments are mixed with a cortical bone allograft (**A**) and placed into the molar crater (**B**) and (**C**). They are covered with a Gore-tex membrane (**D**). Membrane removal four weeks later (**E** and **F**) reveals dense, healthy connective tissue in the defect (**G**, **H**, and **I**).

shape of the defect as well as the individual's immune response. After four weeks, the membrane was removed (see Figures 17-12E–G), which revealed a dense, healthy connective tissue fill of the defect (see Figures 17-12H and I). The site was then sutured, and the patient again instructed in proper care of the area. After two years, probe depth in the quadrant has been reduced to 2 to 3 mm with 4 mm interproximal probing (healthy 4 mm sulcus) between two molars.

**Discussion—Case Study Four:** Yes, a surgical procedure is indicated. A free gingival graft was planned, with the primary goal being restoration of the attached gingiva and the secondary goal being root coverage. A connective tissue bed was prepared at the recipient site by removal of the epithelium overlying the masticatory mucosa of #11, extending apically and laterally beyond the root surface (see Figure 17-13A). A surgical template was fabricated

(see Figure 17-13B) to transfer the exact dimensions of the graft to the palatal donor site (see Figure 17-12C), thus minimizing the palatal wound. A 2 mm thick gingival graft was harvested from the palate with a #15 scapel (see Figure 17-13D), and then sutured at the donor site with resorbable gut sutures and one black silk suspensory suture to intimately adapt the graft to the underlying connective tissue bed and root (see Figure 17-12E). The site healed uneventfully, and restored the zone of attached gingiva while decreasing the amount of recession by 50 percent (see Figure 17-13F, six month posttreatment).

Had there been supragingival calculus and pocketing with bleeding, nonsurgical periodontal therapy could have resulted in reattachment of the inflamed masticatory mucosa. Nonsurgical periodontal therapy would not have been effective in this case because, as the area already appeared to be healthy, it cannot restore attached tissue or result in root coverage.

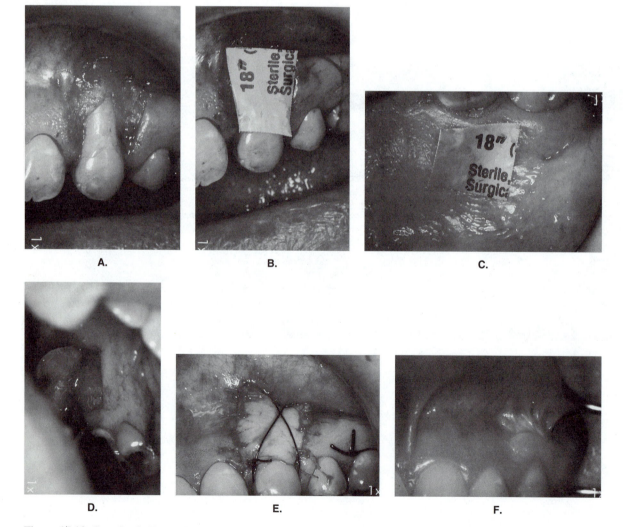

A.   B.   C.

D.   E.   F.

**Figure 17-13** Case Study Four Discussion: A free gingival graft was performed. The recipient bed was prepared (**A**). A template was made of the graft site (**B**) and transferred to the palate (**C**). The graft is harvested (**D**) and sutured at the recipient site (**E**). Six months after surgery, the patient has a wide zone of attached gingiva with no marginal defects (**F**).

**Discussion—Case Study Five:** Yes, correction of these problems can only be solved through surgical intervention. Certainly compromised retention of the provisional restoration, uneven gingival contours, and poor esthetics are not physiologically and cosmetically acceptable. Placement of the initial incisions were performed to address the marginal discrepancy. As can be seen in Figures 17-14A and B, crestal incision placement was executed on teeth #6, 9, 10, and 11, with submarginal placement on #7 and 8, establishing a symmetric gingival profile of the flap. After debridement, it is evident that there is also a discrepancy in the levels of the alveolar crest on #7 and 8 as compared to #9 and 10 (see Figure 17-14C), indicating that the underlying bone is the cause of the mar-

ginal discrepancy. Therefore, intentional ostectomy was performed on #7 and 8 to recreate crestal symmetry around the midline (see Figures 17-14D and E), thus establishing an ideal bony profile for the soft tissues to heal properly, as is evident by the sutured flap (see Figures 17-14F and G).

At the suture removal visit seven days later (see Figure 17-14H), it is evident that the flap is healing in an excellent position. Note the amount of root structure visible on #7 and 8. Had the bone not been removed, the flap margin would have healed at its pretreatment position. Six weeks after healing, a new provisional restoration was fabricated, which demonstrated the improved esthetic results for the procedure (see Figure 17-14I).

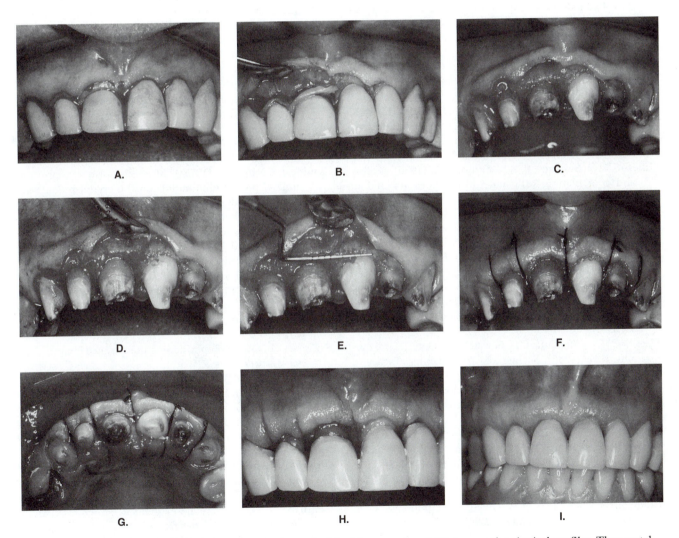

**Figure 17-14** Case Study Five Discussion: A facial submarginal incision was placed (**A**) to even the gingival profiles. The crestal bone discrepancy is seen after debridement (**B** and **C**). Ostectomy is performed (**D**) to even the crestal heights (**E**), and the site is sutured (**F** and **G**). Note the recession created by crown lengthening one week postoperatively (**H**). A new provisional restoration was placed after eight weeks of healing (**I**).

# REFERENCES

American Academy of Periodontology. (1989). *Proceedings of the world workshop in clinical periodontics.* Chicago: American Academy of Periodontology.

American Academy of Periodontology. (1993). *Periodontal regeneration.* Research, Science, and Therapy Committee. Chicago: American Academy of Periodontology.

Barrington, E. P. (1981). An overview of periodontal surgical procedures. *Journal of Periodontology, 52,* 518–528.

Becker, W., Becker, B., Ochsenbein, C., Kerry, G., Caffesse, R. G., Morrison, E. C., & Prichard, J. (1988a). A longitudinal study comparing scaling and osseous surgery and modified Widman procedures—results after 1 year. *Journal of Periodontology, 59,* 351–365.

Becker, B., Kerry, G., Becker, W., Ochsenbein, C., Caffesse, R. G., & Morrison, E. C. (1988b). Changes after three modalities of periodontal therapy. 3-year follow-up. *Journal of Dental Research, 67 (Spec. Issue),* 272, Abstract, No. 1274.

Bowers, G. M., Granet, M., Stevens, M., Emerson, J., Corio, R., Mellonig, J., Lewis, S. B., Peltzman, B., Romberg, E., & Risom, L. (1985). Histologic evaluation of new attachment in humans. A preliminary report. *Journal of Periodontology, 56,* 381–396.

Brayer, W. K., Mellonig, J. T., Dunlop, R. M., Marina, K. W., & Carson, R. E. (1989). Scaling and root planing effectiveness: The effect of root surface access and operator experience. *Journal of Periodontology, 60,* 67–72.

Caffesse, R. G., Sweeney, P. L., & Smith, B. A. (1986). Scaling and root planing with and without periodontal flap surgery. *Journal of Clinical Periodontology, 13,* 205–210.

Carranza, F. A. & Carraro, J. J. (1970). Mucogingival techniques in periodontal surgery. *Journal of Periodontology, 41,* 294–299.

Carranza, F. A. (1996). Clinical diagnosis. In F. A. Carranza & M. G. Newman (Eds.), *Clinical periodontology.* Philadelphia: W.B. Saunders Co.

Cohen, D. W. & Ross, S. E. (1968). The double papilla repositioned flap in periodontal therapy. *Journal of Periodontology, 39,* 65–70.

Fleischer, H. C., Mellonig, J. T., Brayer, W. K., Gray, J. L., & Barnett, J. D. (1989). Scaling and root planing efficacy in multirooted teeth. *Journal of Periodontology, 60,* 402–409.

Froum, S. J., Oritiz, M., Witkin, R. T., Thayer, R., Scopp, I. W., & Stahl, S. S. (1976). Osseous autografts. III. Comparison of osseous coagulum-bone blend implants with open curettage. *Journal of Periodontology, 47,* 287–294.

Genco, R. C., Goldman, H. M., & Cohen, D. W. (1990). *Contemporary periodontics.* St. Louis: Mosby-Year Book, Inc.

Glossary of Periodontic Terms. (1986). *Journal of Periodontology, 57* (Suppl.), 23.

Goldman, H. A. & Cohen, D. W. (1958). The infrabony pocket: Classification and treatment. *Journal of Periodontology, 29,* 272.

Gottlow, J., Nyman, S., Lindhe, J., Karrington, T., & Wennström, J. (1986). New attachment formation in the human periodontium by guided tissue regeneration. Case reports. *Journal of Clinical Periodontology, 13,* 604–616.

Grupe, H. & Warren, R. (1956). Repair of gingival defects by a sliding flap operation. *Journal of Clinical Periodontology, 27,* 92.

Hall, B. (1989). Gingival augmentation/microgingival surgery. In *Proceedings of the world workshop in clinical periodontics.* Chicago: American Academy of Periodontology.

Isidor, F., Karring, T., Nyman, S., & Lindhe, J. (1986). The significance of coronal growth of periodontal ligament tissue for new attachment formation. *Journal of Clinical Periodontology, 13,* 145–150.

Kalkwarf, K. L., Kaldahl, W. B., & Patil, K. D. (1988). Evaluation of furcaton response to periodontal therapy. *Journal of Periodontology, 59,* 794–804.

Karring, T., Isidor, F., Nyman, S., & Lindhe, J. (1985). New attachment formation on teeth with a reduced but healthy periodontal ligament. *Journal of Clinical Periodontology, 12,* 57–60.

Karring, T., Lang, N. P., & Löe, H. (1975). The role of gingival connective tissue in determining epithelial differentiation. *Journal of Periodontal Research, 10,* 1–11.

Langer, B. & Langer, L. (1983). Subepithelial connective tissue graft technique for root coverage. *Journal of Periodontology, 56,* 715–720.

Lekovic, V., Kenney, E. B., Kovacevic, K., & Carranza, F. A. (1989). Evaluation of guided tissue regeneration in class II furcation defects. A clinical study. *Journal of Periodontology, 60,* 694–698.

Lindhe, J. (1983). *Textbook of clinical periodontology.* Philadelphia: W.B. Saunders Co.

Lindhe, J. & Nyman, S. (1975). The effect of plaque control and surgical pocket elimination on the establishment and maintenance of periodontal health. A longitudinal study of periodontal therapy in cases of advanced disease. *Journal of Periodontology, 2,* 67–79.

Lindhe, J., Socransky, S. S., Nyman, S., Haffajee, A., & Westfelt, E. (1982). "Critical probing depths" in periodontal therapy. *Journal of Periodontology, 9,* 323–336.

Mellonig, J. T. (1984). Decalcified freeze-dried bone allograft as an implant material in human periodontal defects. *International Journal of Periodontics and Restorative Dentistry, 4* (6), 40–55.

Nabers, C. L. (1954). Repositioning the attached gingiva. *Journal of Periodontology, 25,* 38.

Nabers, C. L. (1984). Long-term results of autogenous bone grafts. *International Journal of Periodontics and Restorative Dentistry, 4,* 50–67.

Nabers, C. L. & O'Leary, T. (1965). Autogenous bone transplants in the treatment of osseous defect. *Journal of Periodontology, 36,* 5.

Newell, D. (1981). Current status of the management of teeth with furcation involvement. *Journal of Periodontology, 52,* 559.

Nordland, P., Garret, S., Vanooteghem, R., Hutchens, L. H., & Egelberg, J. (1987). The effect of plaque control and root debridement in molar teeth. *Journal of Clinical Periodontology, 14,* 231–236.

Nyman, S., Gottlow, J., Lindhe, J., Karring, T., & Wennstrom, J. (1987). New attachment formation by guided tissue regeneration. *Journal of Periodontal Research, 22,* 252–254.

Ochsenbein, C. (1977). Current status of osseous surgery. *Journal of Periodontology, 48,* 577–586.

Ochsenbein, C. (1986). A primer for osseous surgery. *Interna-*

*tional Journal of Periodontics and Restorative Dentistry, 6*(1), 8–47.

Ochsenbein, C. & Ross, S. (1969). A reevaluation of osseous surgery. *Dental Clinics of North America, 13*, 87–102.

Pontoriero, R., Lindhe, J., Nyman, S., Karring, J., Rosenberg, F., & Sanavi, F. (1988). Guided tissue regeneration in degree II furcation involved mandibular molars. A clinical study. *Journal of Clinical Periodontology, 15*, 247–254.

Quattlebaum, J. B., Mellonig, J. T., & Hansel, N. F. (1988). Antigenicity of freeze-dried cortical bone allograft in human periodontal osseous defects. *Journal of Periodontology, 59*, 394–397.

Quintero, G., Mellonig, J. T., Gambill, V. M., & Pellew, G. B. (1982). A six month clinical evaluation of decalcified freeze-dried bone allograft in human periodontal defects. *Journal of Periodontology, 53*, 726–730.

Rabbani, G. M., Ash, M. M., & Caffesse, R. G. (1981). The effectiveness of scaling and root planing in calculus removal. *Journal of Periodontology, 52*, 119–123.

Ramfjord, S. P. (1977). Present status of the modified Widman flap procedure. *Journal of Periodontology, 51*, 558–565.

Ramfjord, S. P., Knowles, J. W., Nissle, R. R., Burgett, F. G., & Shick, R. A. (1975). Results following three modalities of periodontal therapy. *Journal of Periodontology, 46*, 522–526.

Robinson, E. (1969). Osseous coagulum for bone induction. *Journal of Periodontology, 40*, 503–510.

Rosenberg, E. S., Garber, D. A., & Abrams, B. (1979). Repair of bony defects using an intraoral exostosis as the donor site. A case report. *Journal of Periodontology, 50*, 476–478.

Rosenberg, E. S., Torosian, J. P., Hammond, B.F., & Cutler, S. A. (1993). Routine anaerobic bacterial culture and systemic antibiotic usage in the treatment of adult periodontitis: A 6-year longitudinal study. *International Journal of Periodontics and Restorative Dentistry, 13*(3), 213–243.

Stambaugh, R. V., Dragoo, M., Smith, D. M., & Carasali, L. (1981). The limits of subgingival scaling. *Journal of Periodontics and Restorative Dentistry, 1*, 31–41.

Sullivan, H. C. & Atkins, J. H. (1968). Free autogenous gingival grafts. I. Principles of successful grafting. *Periodontics, 6*, 121–129.

Urist, M. R. & Iwata, H. (1973). Preservation and biogradation of morphogenetic property of bone matrix. *Journal of Theoretical Biology, 38*, 155–167.

Urist, M. R. & Strates, B. S. (1971). Bone morphogenetic protein. *Journal of Dental Research, 50*, 1392–1406.

Wilson, T. G., Kornman, K. S., & Newman, M. G. (Eds.). (1992). *Advances in periodontics.* Chicago: Quintessence Publishing Co., Inc.

# APPLICATION TO PRACTICE

# CHAPTER 18

# Career Development

## Key Terms

base salary plus commission
career
career development
chronological resume
collaboration
combination resume
commission
employee

functional resume
interdependence
independent contractor
networking
proactive
salary
total compensation package

## INTRODUCTION

Do you know how to go about developing your career? Did you ever wonder how you arrived at your present job situation and what your future career will be like? Are you interested in pursuing a career where you can implement NSPT into direct oral care services? A **career** can be defined as "a profession or occupation which one trains for and pursues as a lifework" (Guralnik, 1976). A job, on the other hand, is a position of employment, a situation, or work done by agreement for pay (Guralnik, 1976). Clearly the difference between a career and a job is the emphasis of a career as a lifelong pursuit. **Career development** involves continual growth in both the professional and personal dimensions over time. The result of continued career development should be success in the professional and personal dimensions and thus career satisfaction. Many health professionals tend to let their careers lead them instead of leading their own careers. We have control over our career development by being proactive. **Proactive** means taking the initiative and responsibility to make things happen in one's own life (Covey, 1989). Proactive individuals assume the responsibility and initiative for their career development and do not let circumstances, events, or persons control their future.

Usually students have thought about their careers early in the educational process and, perhaps, have not concretely laid out a plan for its development. The formal process of dental or dental hygiene career development begins when students complete the National Board Examination and prepare for clinical examinations and, licensure. The proactive individual will want to initiate this process by thorough planning. This chapter will guide the reader through a written career plan that will help one achieve a more satisfying career in oral health care. The plan itself is tailored to meet the needs of the dental hygienist who wants to provide nonsurgical periodontal therapy (NSPT) in a practice setting. Professional and personal roles, values, and priorities and decision-making are also discussed to enhance the usability of the career plan. Career retention factors and compensation considerations are reviewed to aid in identifying values and prioritizing their significance to one's career.

## THE CAREER PLAN DESCRIPTION

Career development is facilitated by formulating an individualized plan that reflects one's personal and professional ambitions. This plan serves three purposes: 1) to assess professional and personal roles, values, and priorities, 2) to aid in selecting a practice that is compatible with the plan, and 3) to establish goals for career development. It is designed for the dental hygienist; however, it can be modified to meet the needs of other dental or health professionals. Although it has been developed for the private practice setting, it can be further modified for alternative settings.

To develop and implement this plan, the user follows a series of actions. The reader first recognizes two basic and interrelated self-dimensions: your professional self and your personal self. Next, roles or characteristics of each dimension are identified. Roles are selected based on how individuals view their responsibilities to the profession of dental hygiene or dentistry and how they perceive themselves as persons. The roles are further described by assessing values or standards that have meaning to the individual. Prioritization of the values then occurs because even though each of the selected values has meaning to the dental hygienist, some values might have a higher level of worth than others. Values and priorities are then utilized by the dental hygiene student or practitioner to initiate a job search and develop questions for the inevitable interviews. After several interviewing processes, the plan is finalized by rating each practice using the established values as criteria. To conclude the process, a practice score is calculated that represents how well each environment meets one's needs. Based on the practice score, the recent dental hygiene graduate makes decisions about which practice will be the first place of employment. The practicing dental hygienist can use the career plan to compare multiple new environments to the current setting. The professional who is reentering the field of dental hygiene has the opportunity to compare practices to one another and to previous employment.

This plan can be easily adapted to any phase of career development because roles, values, and priorities are assessed by the user. The senior dental hygiene student or registered dental hygienist who is interested in providing NSPT has the opportunity to develop roles and values that reflect this philosophy of practice. The new graduate's plan will most likely reflect different needs and goals than the practitioner who has experience in private practice. To implement the plan, more information is needed about the roles of a professional and individual; the values that one places within these roles; and the practice rating and scoring.

## Professional and Personal Roles

Dental hygienists are challenged to fulfill many functions, characteristics, or roles in their professional and personal lives. These functions can be interpreted similarly or very differently than others in the same career based on occupational setting, years of experience, educational background, and life values and goals. Because the model career plan being presented has been developed for private practice, the roles selected relate to the dental hygienist who functions as a clinician. At the professional level, the roles include health care provider, team member, employee, and professional. Personal roles include being a family member, a friend, a community member, and an individual. Refer to Table 18-1 for a definition of each role. Each of these characteristics can be viewed separately in the career plan process; however, the roles are not mutually exclusive. In fact, each of the roles should compliment one another and be carried out simultaneously. To personalize the plan, different or additional roles might be selected and defined. These professional and personal roles must be balanced in order to achieve success in one's career.

Career development occurs when professional and personal roles increase in complexity. This complexity is accompanied by increasing relationships and responsibility within the roles (Carney & Wells, 1987). Generally, each role involves a relationship with one or more people. As an employee, your major professional relationship is with a single employer or multiple employers. As a team member in a private practice, you again maintain a relationship with your employer(s) as well as with dental assistants, office managers, receptionists, and other dental hygienists. As a health care provider, your major responsibility is to provide direct oral health care to clients and this responsibility might extend further if you provide oral health education and services in the community. Personal relationships include family, friends, and other members of the community. Increasing the quality of any relationship can lead to professional and personal

**Table 18-1  Role Definitions**

| Dimension | Role | Definition |
| --- | --- | --- |
| Professional | Health Care Provider | Provides quality care to individual or groups of clients as a clinician, educator, change agent, consumer advocate, administrator, or researcher. |
| | Team Member | Collaborates with other members of the oral health care team. |
| | Employee | Provides client care as an employee in a practice environment and is supervised by an employer. |
| | Professional | Performs as a professional within the discipline of dental hygiene by acquiring and sharing expertise in prevention and NSPT. |
| Personal | Family Member | Belongs to a family in the capacity of son/daughter, spouse, parent or extended family member. |
| | Friend | Participates in relationships with friends, other than family members, by enjoying shared activities. |
| | Community Member | Participates in community affairs as a volunteer, politician, or member of a religious or service organization. |
| | Individual | Engages in activities for individual physical, mental, or spiritual well-being. |

growth. The dental hygienist develops relationships with a myriad of other professionals and consumers.

Different levels of relationships exist and in order for them to be quality-oriented, the achievement of the highest level is necessary. **Interdependence** is the highest level where individuals work together by combining their abilities to create something better than could be accomplished alone. The lowest level of relationships is at the dependent level. Dependence occurs when individuals rely on someone else to take responsibility for themselves. Between the interdependent relationship and dependence is independence. Independence occurs when individuals rely on themselves to be responsible (Covey, 1989). Career development is facilitated when professional and personal relationships are managed at the interdependent level. An example of these three levels is illustrated in the following scenario. The private practice dental hygienist is having problems with client scheduling because of frequent cancellations and inappropriate appointment lengths for initial NSPT and periodontal maintenance procedures (PMP). The hygienist in a dependent relationship would rely on the employer or the office manager to rectify the problem. The independent hygienist would try to solve the problem entirely by himself. At the highest level of relationships, the hygienist who is interdependent would enlist the help of the employer, office manager, and other team members to work together to create a solution to the problem.

Practitioners should also strive to develop interdependent relationships with their clients. When interdependence occurs, both parties are considered partners in NSPT because they combine their abilities to repair damage resulting from periodontal disease. The hygienist helps clients develop individual goals and desired results of NSPT by encouraging participation in making decisions about their care. In the interdependent relationship, the client becomes responsible for following the accepted treatment plan, complying with oral self-care recommendations, and returning for continuing care appointments.

Increasing responsibility within a role can also lead to career development. Private practice dental hygiene does not include the traditional career ladder in the same sense as a business where executives climb their way to the top; therefore, dental hygienists must develop *within* their chosen professional environment. For example, a dental hygienist who becomes the manager of the office NSPT program is responsible for supervising other dental hygienists in the practice and coordinating client care, thus leadership is enhanced. In this case, the "Team Member" role is expanded. Other examples of increasing the complexity of the "Health Provider" role include accepting the responsibility for developing a recare system or an OSHA training program for the office. Personal roles can also increase in complexity as a person changes from a "single" to a married relationship, and then to a parental relationship with children. Increased leadership in community activities will again increase

responsibility. This increased complexity in the personal dimension will, in turn, affect the professional role. The next step in developing a career plan is to select values that define each role.

## Professional Values and Priorities

A person's values can be defined as social principles, goals, or standards held by an individual (Guralnik, 1976), who in this case is the dental hygiene or dental student, or practitioner. According to Covey (1989), "Proactive people are driven by values—carefully thought about, selected and internalized" (p. 72). Proactive people are influenced by external stimuli of a physical, social, or psychological nature, but their response is a value-based choice and not a choice driven by feelings, circumstances, or conditions (Covey, 1989). Through self-awareness and reflection, values that are important in one's personal and professional life are identified. The proactive individual assumes the responsibility for making these decisions. In the career plan example in Table 18-2, five values were chosen to represent the "professional dimension": practice is safe; quality care is provided to clients; practice environment is interdependent/collaborative; employer provides support; and professional growth is continued. The five values were derived from a factor analysis presented by Calley, Darby, Bowen, and Miller (1996) based upon research focusing on dental hygiene career retention. The study was conducted on a nationwide sample consisting of 100 hygienists from one randomly chosen state in each of the 12 ADHA districts. Of the 1,200 hygienists surveyed, 755 responses (69.9 percent) were received and 480 (63.6 percent) were employed in a single practice for five or more years.

Below each value, in the sample career plan, statements are placed that define or clarify its meaning. These statements also provide a link between the value and NSPT. The following discussion is centered around each value in hopes of providing readers with ideas for their own career plans. The first definition of a safe practice relates to infection control matters. A factor analysis revealed that for those in practice five years or more, the most important factor in job retention is a work environment that has quality and safety orientation (Calley et al., 1996). These researchers discovered that infection control was a primary concern in retaining dental hygienists in practice. Others have concluded that infection control is a critical factor in the occupation. Boyer (1994) states that the concern for the risk of infectious diseases is a potential and real factor in career retention. Miller (1990) concluded that improving infection control protocol and increasing control in establishing protocol policies are factors that need to be changed to provide incentives for hygienists to reenter the workforce. Other aspects of safe practice could include the application of ergonomic principles (see Chapter 15), employing radiographic equipment that meets state and federal standards (see Chapter 5), and implementation of an

**Table 18-2  The Career Plan: Professional Values**

| Role | Value | Value Priority |
|------|-------|----------------|
| Health Care Provider | ***Practice Is Safe***<br>• Infection control protocol is effective<br>• Ergonomic principles are considered<br>• Radiographic equipment is current<br>• Medical emergency plan and equipment are up-to-date | 2 |
| Health Care Provider | ***Quality Care Is Provided to Clients***<br>• Adequate time for comprehensive NSPT is scheduled<br>• Multiple NSPT appointments are scheduled when indicated<br>• High-quality care is provided by employer<br>• Equipment, instruments, and products are adequate in number, modern, and ordered when necessary<br>• Pain control is incorporated into treatment planning<br>• Recare system considers clients' needs<br>• Pace and stress level are manageable | 2 |
| Team Member | ***Practice Environment Is Interdependent/Collaborative***<br>• Team members perform delegated responsibilities<br>• Employer provides collaboration when necessary<br>• Team members collaborate to provide quality care<br>• Responsibility for NSPT is delegated to the hygienist<br>• Practice philosophy of office is similar to the hygienist's<br>• Office environment is pleasant | 3 |
| Employee | ***Employer Provides Support***<br>• Employer respects and acknowledges education, skills, and expertise of team members<br>• Employer provides positive feedback<br>• Performance evaluations are scheduled every three months<br>• Performance criteria and consequences of evaluation are clearly defined | 1 |
| Professional | ***Professional Growth Is Continued***<br>• Continuing education courses on NSPT are attended and supported<br>• Literature is read to renew information and skills<br>• Relationships are enhanced at the interdependent level<br>• Responsibility in NSPT can be increased<br>• Active participation in local professional societies is encouraged | 2 |

(Score = 10 points)

emergency plan and equipment that is periodically reviewed. These concepts were used to define "safety" in the example career plan; however, the individual designing the plan might define safe practice in other terms.

The ability to provide quality care to clients in a practice is first defined by scheduling adequate time to complete comprehensive NSPT. Having a sufficient, or even maximum, amount of time in which to complete all aspects of NSPT is important for client and practitioner satisfaction. Comprehensive NSPT requires multiple appointments for client instruction in oral self-care, debridement, and supportive treatment. When inadequate time is available, clinicians are forced to make decisions about what aspect of care to withdraw or postpone. The proactive individual will take initiative to evaluate how much time is appropriate for care and schedule accordingly. In return for adequate time for provision of nonsurgical services, the client will be rendered a fee proportional to the quality of care and time spent in pro-

viding therapy. Allowing enough time for procedures and communication with the client is required for effective results in NSPT (Pollack, 1991). NSPT requires a time commitment from the employer, hygienist, and client. The employer commits to providing comprehensive therapy in the practice and establishing appropriate fees for the time involved with therapy. The dental hygienist commits to effectively assessing, planning, implementing, and evaluating comprehensive NSPT. The client commits to receiving the planned NSPT and continuing care in addition to performing oral self-care procedures.

In a study about the perceptions of quality care conducted by Boyer and Gupta (1992), 89.2 percent of the hygienists report that their clients receive the highest quality of care. The major reasons for their ability to provide this type of care is that enough time is allowed for dental hygiene services and the hygienist is responsible for controlling the treatment time. The remainder of the respondents (10.2 percent) indicate that clients do not receive quality care. Inadequate time to treat the client is the major reason and dentist-related issues are the second reason for not providing quality care. These issues include not referring clients to specialists, poor quality of the dentist's work, and lack of positive reinforcement for the hygienist.

Other statements that define quality include adequate equipment, incorporation of pain control, individualized recall system, and a manageable pace and stress level. To provide quality NSPT to clients, sufficient and modern equipment and instruments must be available and working conditions need to be as ideal as possible. In each operatory, the equipment the hygienist uses should be readily accessible and renewed when no longer functioning correctly. Literature and products to distribute to clients for self-care, and use of these during adjunct therapy will enhance the NSPT system. Variety and scope of practice, relating to legalized expanded functions and the variety of services provided on a daily basis contributes to career retention (Calley et al., 1996). Legalized duties and supervision requirements for oral health care team members are described in the Dental Practice Acts in the state where the practice is located. These acts reflect the variety and scope of NSPT services provided to the client. Expanded functions in the area of pain control including local anesthesia and nitrous oxide (see Chapter 9) are essential to NSPT. The variety of services the client receives depends on the comprehensiveness of the NSPT program in the practice and the amount of delegated responsibility to the hygienist.

A system that manages continuing care, or recare, is the "backbone" of every practice. The goal of the system is to involve clients in their own future level of oral health and commitment to continuing care (Lakin, 1988). Continuing care appointments or PMP, as indicated, maintain the periodontal health of clients and the financial viability of the practice. A successful system results from effective management and the oral health care team members' performance of delegated responsibility in that system. Considerable investment by the employer and employees is necessary for client satisfaction and growth of the practice. Clients have difficulty evaluating the quality of their health care; therefore, judgments are made about the practice in relation to the time spent waiting for treatment in the office, time spent to complete treatment, and the comfort level they experience during treatment (Pollack, 1992). The oral health care team needs to provide positive experiences for the clients to ensure their continuing care in a long-term relationship. Clients are the essence of the practice, for without them the healthcare business fails. Approximately 85 percent of the active clients should be involved in preventive and dental continuing care (Pride, 1993) and those patients with periodontitis require PMP.

The pace and stress level of the practice affect the working conditions. The pace is reflected in the number of clients scheduled and the length of the appointment. A high volume and production-oriented practice generally increases the number of clients scheduled and decreases the appointment length, which can increase the stress level of the hygienist. Another stress factor for the hygienist is the time involved with the dentist examining the client after treatment. More than 90 percent of the time, the dentist sees the client at the end of the appointment in the hygiene operatory while the hygienist is present (Boyer, 1990). At the completion of the scheduled treatment, the hygienist notifies the dentist that the client is ready for examination. Once the dentist arrives in the operatory, he spends a mean time of 20 minutes with new adult clients and 13 minutes with recall adult clients. This time is spent gaining rapport, checking the care, confirming the hygienist's examination, and performing his own examination (Boyer & Gupta, 1990). The waiting time and examination time need to be considered when determining appointment length and the overall NSPT care plan to provide the highest quality of oral health care to the client, maintain the office schedule, and reduce stress.

The third professional value identified in the example plan is an environment that is interdependent and collaborative. Interdependence has been previously defined relative to relationships within a role. When the oral health care team, including the employer, work from the interdependent level, they combine their abilities to provide quality NSPT to the client at a higher level than they can accomplish if each works alone. The key to effective management at the interdependent level is appropriate delegation of responsibilities. For delegation to be effective and efficient, the employer and employee must work as partners in providing quality NSPT. The partnership developed between the dental hygienist and the dentist is a "cotherapist" relationship where both partners are offering their professional expertise for the goal of optimum oral health for the client (Darby, 1983). Additionally, **collaboration** means dentists and hygienists working together in an environment of respect and trust, cooperating and being responsible for the care they provide to the client, to achieve the mutual goal of oral health (Darby, 1983). A collaborative management style incorporates the ideas of interdependence with the hygienist responsible for decision making related to assessment, planning, dental hygiene diagnosis, implementation and evaluation of NSPT client care. The lack of decision-making opportunities is one of five reasons that hygienists have permanently left the workforce (Miller, 1991).

Uldricks and others (1993) studied the perceived collaboration between Ohio hygienists and dentists during periodontal assessment. Of the 1,071 dental hygienist respondents, 83 percent agreed or strongly agreed that dentists/employers encourage the concept of cotherapy, 81 percent indicate strong agreement/agreement that dentists acknowledge the dental hygienist's expertise in nonsurgical therapy, and 80 percent strongly agree or agree that there is a collegial relationship between professionals. In an ADHA study, hygienists reported that when providing care to new and recall clients, both independent and collaborative decision making occurred. More collaboration occurred between the hygienist and dentist for care provided to new clients. More independent decisions were made by the hygienist in the treatment of the continuing care clients (Benicewicz & Metzger, 1989). The responsibility for NSPT ultimately belongs to the dental hygienist. As a professional, the dental hygienist provides primary care; is accountable to the client; and is entrusted with assessing disease and health accurately and implementing appropriate care.

The last statements written in the career plan to define the value of interdependent/collaboration are related to the dentists' and dental hygienists' practice philosophies and the office environment. How pleasant the office environment is or needs to be depends on the opinion of the team member. An environment that is extremely pleasant for one practitioner might not be as pleasant for another due to differences in expectations, values, goals, and/or personalities. A pleasant office environment was reported to be significant in retaining dental hygienists in a practice for five years or more (Calley et al., 1996). A common recommendation for those seeking employment is to participate in a working interview, where the dental hygienist observes or works in a practice prior to accepting employment. The working interview (see subsequent interviewing section) permits both parties to compare practice philosophy and the interviewee to assess the office environment.

The fourth value identified in the career plan is employer support. Expectations and needs of the employee define the degree of support that is necessary for career satisfaction. The first statement defining this value relates to the degree of respect and acknowledgment offered to team members. General employer support for the dental hygiene career is evidenced by respect and acknowledgment for the dental hygienist's education, skills, and contribution to the practice. Uldricks and others (1993) report that the hygienists surveyed agreed or strongly agreed with the following statements: 1) the dentist respects the hygienist's education and skills (91 percent), 2) the dentist acknowledges the dental hygienist's role and expertise (85 percent), 3) the dentist acknowledges the dental hygienist's expertise in assessment (80 percent) and NSPT (82 percent), and 4) dental hygiene is an integral part of the practice (91 percent). Respect and acknowledgment through employer support is evidenced by the quality of the interdependent/collaborative relationship and the amount of responsibility and decision making that the hygienist practices.

Employer support is probably also perceived as being related to the style of management employed. Bader and Sams (1992) report a high level of job satisfaction resulting from an interpersonal managerial style of the employer. Personnel management that demonstrates two-way communication, honest feedback, ability to try new ideas and effective use of the oral health care team members' abilities resulted in more job satisfaction. Upgrading the

employer's management and interpersonal skills will enhance job satisfaction for hygienists. The employer's management of the office, including personnel management, was found to be a significant factor in job retention of dental hygienists for five years or more (Calley et al., 1996). Management of the office through policies and procedures that are updated on a regular basis is considered important by dental hygienists. Well-established policies and procedures are an important part of the employer's management. They provide directives and team unity. Policies and procedures need to be reviewed periodically by the entire oral health care team to ensure they remain current and that everyone is familiar with them.

Verbal feedback from the employer on a daily basis is another criteria defining employer support. Verbal comments provide the hygienist with both positive feedback and constructive criticism related to performance. Pritzel and Green (1990) studied the perceptions of working relationships between dentists and hygienists and reported that 55 percent of the dentists perceived that they always provide feedback to the hygienist, while 31 percent of the hygienists perceived that the dentist always provided feedback to them. Daily feedback by the dentist is valued by the hygienist and facilitates communication and collaboration between the two professionals. Another avenue for providing feedback for employees is through oral or written performance evaluations conducted by the employer(s). Performance evaluations are used to evaluate the behavior and expertise of the employees. These evaluations are conducted in many different ways. Chapter 19 discusses their role in evaluating the success of NSPT in a practice. A successful performance evaluation depends on an agreement being made between the employer and employee. The performance agreement includes desired results, guidelines, resources, accountability, and outcomes (Covey, 1989). Positive outcomes include financial, psychological, developmental, and responsibility considerations (Covey). All of these consequences are important to employees; however, the psychological outcomes are more motivating to employees than the others (Covey). Resources that are available to assist the employee in the accomplishment of NSPT are identified in the performance agreement. The employer informs the employee of the practice's resources such as additional employee support, equipment, instruments, products, and other available resources for support. Employees are held accountable for their performance in delegated NSPT responsibilities. In a performance agreement, standards of performance are established and used in the evaluation of the results at specified times. Performance evaluations developed by both the employer and employee create an environment of ownership on the part of both parties.

The last professional value is professional growth is continued. Growth must occur by participating in the learning process throughout one's career. Encouragement by the employer and general support for the career of dental hygiene are cited as factors in career retention (Calley et al., 1996). Often, an employer can offer support for continuing education by addressing travel time, travel expenses, registration fees, and/or accommodations in the employee's benefit package. This benefit is addressed in the section of this chapter about compensation. It is not always possible for dental team members to attend the variety and scope of courses that is desired because of finances and employment responsibilities. An alternative to attendance is the regular reviewing of literature. Subscriptions to professional journals stimulate one to enhance practice modalities and upgrade skills. It is interesting for team members to share articles with one another on any aspect of care that would improve team and client relationships. Other considerations in professional growth include enhancement of relationships, increased responsibility for NSPT, and participation in local professional associations.

It is recommended that a minimum of four to a maximum of six total values be selected for the career plan. After the professional values are written and defined, each should be prioritized by assigning points. Prioritizing the values is accomplished by assessing the significance of each value to the individual. Values that are most significant to the individual should receive the greatest number of points. The total number of points that is assigned to all of the professional values combined is ten. The ten points are divided between the five values as indicated in Table 18-2 on page 482, within the "Value Priority" column. In this example, the value in the "Team Member" role is considered the most important and is assigned three points. The two values listed in the "Health Care Provider" role and the one value in the "Professional" role are considered equally important and are each assigned two points. The value in the "Employee" role is considered the least important and is assigned one point. If the practitioner felt that all the values were of equal importance, each value could have been assigned two points.

## Personal Values and Priorities

These values are often overlooked, but impact career development. Personal values can be dramatically different between hygienists. The lifestyle that one leads determines the complexity of the roles and values. In the example plan, an additional five values were chosen to represent the personal dimension (see Table 18-3). Again, statements are listed under each personal value to clarify its meaning. Values will be briefly discussed using these statements. Spending quality time with the family has a different meaning for each individual. Family values depend on the complexity of the relationships and responsibilities in this role. Values can relate to the amount of quality time spent with the family unit and the responsibilities of contributing to the household man-

**Table 18-3  The Career Plan: Personal Values**

| Role | Value | Value Priority |
|---|---|---|
| Family Member | *Spend Quality Time with the Family*<br>• Foster children to develop their capabilities<br>• Contribute to the household maintenance<br>• Commute within a thirty-mile radius<br>• Limit evening and weekend employment<br>• Flexible working schedule | 3 |
| Family Member | *Contribute to the Financial Support of the Family*<br>• Work three days per week for $25 to $30 per hour<br>• Flexible benefits including family dental care, malpractice insurance, vacation, sick days, and personal days | 3 |
| Friend | *Participate in Activities with Friends*<br>• Go fishing and camping with friends<br>• Meet a friend for lunch once a week | 1 |
| Community Member | *Involvement in Community Activities*<br>• Involvement in children's school, scout, and sports activities<br>• Participate as a member of the Greenway Commission<br>• Provide service to the church | 1 |
| Individual | *Personal Growth Is Continued*<br>• Exercise regularly<br>• Read novels<br>• Complete hobby projects<br>• Read personal growth books | 2 |

(Score = 10 points)

agement. These considerations impact the commuting distance and the amount of travel that one is willing to endure. Other concerns that relate to the work schedule include employment during evening hours and weekends, and having a flexible work schedule.

Contributing to the financial support of the family is a relatively important value to most hygienists. The financial contribution that the hygienist makes to the family unit is a personal consideration. The amount of the contribution whether it be sole, major, or minor determines the number of hours worked per week and compensation that can be accepted for employment. Financial support of the family includes wages and benefits; and both are part of the **total compensation package**. A 1993 survey revealed that part-time hygienists, working an average of 25 hours per week, are paid a higher salary than full-time hygienists who work an average of 35 hours per week (Burt, 1993b). On the other hand, full-time hygienists generally receive more benefits than their part-time counterparts (Willis & Butters, 1993). The national average hourly rate in 1993 for part-time employment was $28.68 and for full-time employment was $22.09. The amount of contribution that the hygienist makes to the family influences the benefits desired. Insurance benefits such as health, life, and disability insurance are more important to hygienists that are sole contributors to the household. When hygienists were given a choice between an increase in salary or benefits, those that are sole and major contributors to their household preferred an increase in benefits (Willis and Butters, 1993). Regardless of the employment status and contribution to the family budget, total compensation is an important consideration. The lack of adequate salary and benefits are two reasons that hygienists have permanently left dental hygiene (Miller, 1991). Increasing compensation is a method of facilitating reentry of hygienists into the workforce (Miller, 1990).

Relationships with others outside the family are usually important to an individual. Values related to participating in activities with friends should be considered in the career plan. Activities usually refer to social and recreational engagements. While involvement in community activities will vary depending on the individual and family unit. Activities can include but are not limited to school, politics, service organizations, recreation, sports, and religious affiliations. The statements in the roles of "Friend" and "Community Member" will vary between individuals , as some will have minimal involvement, while others will have a greater commitment to friends and the community. These two values often overlap as friendships are developed through community involvement.

Continued personal growth of a person as an individual is important; however, it is often ignored due to the complexity of other roles. Development at the physical, mental, and spiritual levels can lead to a well-rounded person. It is recommended that four to six personal values are created for the career plan. Refer to the column "Value Priority" for an example of prioritization of these values (see Table 18-3). The personal values that are most important to the individual are assigned more points. The total number of points assigned to personal values is also ten. In this example, the points are divided between the five values, with three points being awarded to each of the values listed under the "Family Member" role. Two points are awarded to the value in the "Individual" role. The values in the "Friends" and "Community Member" roles are awarded one point each. This process of defining values and determining their priority is a necessary step to complete prior to the job search. The hygienist uses the career plan to develop questions for the interviewing process. Those values that are given the highest priority need to be discussed thoroughly with the potential employer.

## Practice Rating and Scoring

Evaluation of each practice occurs after the interview (see the subsequent section, Interviewing Strategies). To rate each practice, the compatibility of the practice with the career plan is determined by considering how well it meets, or has the potential to meet, the personal and professional values. Within the career plan format, the column "Practice Rating" has been added for this purpose (see Table 18-4). The following scale is used to rate each practice relative to each value:

5—Excellent, the job meets the total value

4—Good, the job meets most of the value

3—Average, the job meets half of the value

2—Fair, the job meets less than half of the value

1—Poor, the job does not meet the value

An additional column has been added to the career plan in Table 18-4 called the "Practice Score." This score is a calculation using the numbers in the "Value Priority" and "Practice Rating" columns. To compute the "Practice Score" for each value, multiply the numbers in the aforementioned columns and place the resulting number in the "Practice Score" column. A "Total Score" for the practice is then calculated by adding the numbers in the "Practice Score" column. The highest score a practice can earn is 100 points. The proactive hygienist then decides an acceptable range of scores that indicates compatibility with the career plan. An example of score evaluation follows: 1) a score above 80 means that the practice is compatible with the practitioner's career plan, 2) scores between 60 to 79 mean that the practice is fairly compatible and that serious consideration of the values that scored low on the career plan is necessary, and 3) a score below 60 means that the values and the practice are not compatible. Several practices can be compared based on the "Total Score" for each practice. The practice that receives the highest score is the one that is the most compatible with the career plan.

**Table 18-4  The Career Plan**

| Dimension | Role | Value | Value Priority | Practice Rating | Practice Score |
|---|---|---|---|---|---|
| Professional | Health Care Provider | Practice is safe | 2 | 5 | 10 |
| | Health Care Provider | Quality care is provided to the client | 2 | 4 | 8 |
| | Team Member | Practice environment is interdependent/collaborative | 3 | 5 | 15 |
| | Employee | Employer provides support | 1 | 3 | 3 |
| | Professional | Continue professional growth | 2 | 4 | 8 |
| Personal | Family Member | Spend quality time with family | 3 | 4 | 12 |
| | Family Member | Contribute to the financial support of the family | 3 | 5 | 15 |
| | Friend | Participate in activities with friends | 1 | 5 | 5 |
| | Community Member | Participate in community activities | 1 | 4 | 4 |
| | Individual | Continue personal growth | 2 | 4 | 8 |

(Score = 88 points)

Ideally, a practitioner would like to select employment in a practice that earns a 100 percent score on the career plan; however, in reality this scenario is unlikely. When a position has been offered by an employer and the employment agreement has been finalized, the dental hygienist must make a decision to accept or reject the offer. Decision making is a difficult process and is best approached by following several steps. These steps include determining a realistic view of the facts related to the decision, listing the alternative decision choices and the consequences of each choice, and then selecting one choice that constitutes the final decision. This process is accomplished by writing each step on paper and enlisting the help of family, friends, or colleagues. To illustrate the decision-making process, consider the following scenario:

A recently graduated hygienist has interviewed at Practice A, B, and C and used the career plan to compute the "Total Score" for each practice; Practice A scored 50, Practice B scored 83, and Practice C scored 71. Practice A has offered employment to the hygienist and Practice B and C have not made employment decisions. Practice A has given the hygienist two days to make the final decision to accept or reject employment.

Refer to Table 18-5 for an example of how to complete the first two decision-making steps. After careful consideration of all the choices and the resulting consequences, the last step in the decision-making process is to make the final decision by selecting one choice. This choice is based on the "best" choice for the individual. Once the final choice is selected, the practitioner should honor the decision. Even if the decision is determined to be inappropriate at a later date, the practitioner will learn from the experience. The next time the process is used, the individual will be better prepared to make a decision.

## THE EMPLOYMENT SEARCH

The employment search is a mutual search for an employer and employee. Employers make a large investment in hiring and retaining oral health care employees in the practice (de St. Georges, 1991). The negative impact of employee turnover is that it decreases productivity and causes stress in the practice, all which impact the provision of quality care to the client (Loiacono, 1989). The hiring process is paramount in recruiting employees who possess the knowledge, skills, experience and personal characteristics that the job description requires. The employer needs to look beyond the technical skills and consider personal characteristics that compliment the practice (Manji, 1991).

The purpose of the job search for the practitioner is to locate employers who need an employee to provide client care. All avenues of job searching are used to produce leads for employment. Newspaper and journal advertisements are accessible; however, they provide a limited amount of information about employment. Networking with personal and professional contacts will broaden the job search and make it more successful. According to Fry (1991), **networking** means establishing an organized system of relationships with contacts from common skills, backgrounds, or interests. The network is

**Table 18-5 Decision-Making Process**

STEP 1: DETERMINE A REALISTIC VIEW OF THE FACTS SURROUNDING THE DECISION

- Compatibility of each practice with the career plan.

  Total Practice Scores—Practice A = 50, Practice B = 83, Practice C = 71.
  Practice B is the most compatible, Practice C is moderately compatible,
  and Practice A is least compatible.

- Employment offers

  Practice A has offered employment and must have a decision in two
  days. Practice B and C may not offer employment in the future.

STEP 2: LIST ALTERNATIVE DECISION CHOICES AND THEIR CONSEQUENCES

| Choices | Consequences |
|---|---|
| • Accept the position at Practice A even though it is not compatible with the career plan. | • The hygienist might be unhappy and short-term employment may result. |
| • Accept the position at Practice A and when an offer is made by Practice B and/or C, accept the offer of the practice that is most compatible. | • Behavior may be seen as unethical and the possibility of a negative reputation within the dental community may result. |
| • Reject the offer from Practice A. | • Unemployment will result if Practice B or C does not offer employment. |
| • Ask Practice A for an extension of time before the decision is made. | • Practice A may agree to an extension and Practice B and C may or may not make their employment decision.<br>• Practice A may answer negatively to the extension and the hygienist has to make a decision. |
| • Stall on the decision by not calling Practice A in two days. | • Practice A may offer employment to someone else.<br>• Practice A may wait a few more days for the decision. |
| • Ask Practice A for another interview to renegotiate employment terms. | • Practice A may agree to renegotiate. After renegotiation, the practice may or may not be more compatible with the career plan.<br>• Practice A might decline to renegotiate and status quo exists. |

built on the idea of a mutual exchange of information between contacts about employment opportunities, practice environment, and ranges of wages and benefits. Networks are not responsible for finding employment, but are responsible for sharing information about employment leads (Drafke, 1994).

## Creating a Resume

Networking will produce employment leads that require a resume to be submitted to the potential employer. The resume is usually the first contact that the hygienist has with the employer. The objective of the resume is to create a good impression that results in securing an interview. Employers spend approximately 30 seconds reviewing a resume (Good & Fitzpatrick, 1993; Kennedy & Laramore, 1990). During that precious time, the prospective employee must highlight his abilities and accomplishments on the resume relative to the personal characteristics that the employer is seeking (Good & Fitzpatrick, 1993). The employer can form a preinterview impression of the hygienist from the resume. This impres-

sion can cause the interviewer to conduct the interview in a manner that confirms the preinterview impression (Linden & Parsons, 1989). This impression can be influenced by the information provided and the appearance of the resume. Considering the impact of the resume on the interview, the construction of the resume is extremely important. There are several guidelines that the dental professional can use to produce a successful resume. Resumes are individually constructed, similar to care plans and client education. The best way to initiate the writing process is to develop a laundry list of accomplishments and credentials and start categorizing the information by topic, such as Professional Activities.

Then the writer will want to select an appropriate resume style. The three types of resumes are chronological, functional, and a combination of the previous two types. The practitioner selects the resume style that will best portray his abilities and accomplishments. A **chronological resume** lists abilities and accomplishments under headings that present information in reverse chronological order, beginning with the most recent experience. Headings are titles (such as Community

Service) given to each section of information presented, and serve to categorize or organize information for the reader. The information presented shows a progression of abilities and achievements over a period of time (see Figure 18-1). It is the resume style that is most popular with job seekers and employers (Beatty, 1991; Good & Fitzpatrick, 1993). A chronological resume is less effective when the practitioner wants to omit information about certain previous employment and large gaps of unemployment for reasons such as family responsibilities or carpal tunnel syndrome. Suggestions for headings used in a chronological resume are reviewed in Table 18-6. Headings are selected based on the experiences that the practitioner wishes to emphasize. Other headings may be created by the resume writer to individualize the resume.

---

## ERIN O'CLEARY

Temporary Address:
427 Westwood Lane
Pocatello, Idaho 83204
(208) 837-2650

Permanent Address:
301 Harriman Avenue
Boise, Idaho 87620
(208) 555-6726

### CAREER GOAL

To secure a part-time position as a dental hygienist in a progressive practice in the Boise area that emphasizes individualized preventive and nonsurgical periodontal therapy as part of total body health.

### EDUCATION

1995 **Bachelor of Science Degree.** Idaho State University.
Curriculum required extensive clinical experience in nonsurgical periodontal therapy, pain control, and restorative expanded functions.

- Clinical Achievement Award
- Sigma Phi Alpha, Honor Society
- Dean's List, three semesters

1991-1993 **Prerequisite Courses.** Boise State University.
Curriculum required extensive coursework in the sciences.

- GPA, 3.2 on a 4.0 scale
- Financed 50% of educational expenses

### WORK EXPERIENCE

Summer 1993, 1994 **Sterilization Assistant.** Sunshine Dental Group, Boise, Idaho.
Modified infection control protocol to meet OSHA standards. Responsible for disinfection of four operatories and sterilization of instruments. Monitored autoclave spore testing, biohazardous trash and sharps disposal. Ordered and inventoried infection control supplies.

1990-1993 **Counterperson.** Blockbuster Video, Boise, Idaho.
Applied interpersonal skills while assisting customers with videotape selection. Recorded purchases on the computer. Collected and accounted for money for videotape rentals.

### LICENSURE AND CERTIFICATION

1995 **Western Regional Board Examination.** Results pending.
Licensure expected in July for Idaho and Utah.

1995 **Expanded Functions Certificate.** Experience in local anesthesia, nitrous oxide-oxygen analgesia, and placing and finishing restorations.

1995 **National Dental Hygiene Board Examination.** May.

1994, 1995 **Cardiopulmonary Resuscitation,** American Red Cross. Updated annually.

*(continues)*

**Figure 18-1** Chronological resume.

## PROFESSIONAL ACTIVITIES

1995    **Table Clinic.** "A Comparison of Polytetrafluoroethylene Floss and Waxed Dental Floss." Idaho State University, Alumni Reception.

1995    **Seminar Attended.** "Update on Nonsurgical Periodontal Therapy," ADHA District XII Annual Meeting.

1993-1995    **Student American Dental Hygienists' Association.**
- Member, Community Service Committee, 1993–1994
- Treasurer, 1994–1995

1994    **Seminar Attended.** "OSHA Standards: What It Means to Practitioners", Idaho Dental Hygienists' Association Annual Session.

## COMMUNITY SERVICE

1995    **Volunteer.** Fort Hall Indian Reservation. Fort Hall, Idaho. Performed preventive and nonsurgical periodontal therapy for Native American patients.

1994, 1995    **Volunteer.** Idaho State University Children's Dental Health Fair. Educated children and parents about plaque and tooth brushing. Over 1,000 people attended.

## REFERENCES

**Clinical Coordinator:** Kathleen O. Hodges, RDH, MS
Associate Professor
Campus Box 8048
Idaho State University
Department of Dental Hygiene
Pocatello, Idaho 83201
(208) 263-2787

**Previous Employer:** Dr. Gregory Smith
Sunshine Dental Group
105 Mulberry Lane
Boise, Idaho 87962
(208) 555-6934

**Previous Supervisor:** Jeffrey Kline
Blockbuster Video
5 Main Street
Boise, Idaho 87960
(208) 555-5234

**Figure 18-1** (*Continued*)

The **functional resume** organizes abilities and accomplishments under headings that describe broad skill or ability areas (see Figure 18-2 on page 492). Dates are not included on a functional resume and this can negatively impact an employer (Coxford, 1995). The functional resume is an acceptable style of listing abilities and accomplishments, especially for people who are reentering the workforce (Kaplan, 1990). This style of resume is useful for the practicing clinician who wants to emphasize a particular skill, such as practical experience in NSPT, for the purpose of a specific position. Functional resumes are also useful for practitioners who have been employed for a long period of time and have varied experiences or increased responsibility within the practice. Headings are organized in a manner that presents the strongest skills or abilities first (Beatty, 1991).

The last style, the **combination resume**, uses both the chronological and functional format combined into one resume. The combination resume follows the traditional chronological style that employers are familiar with and emphasizes functional skills that provide depth to the resume. This resume style is generally used by an expe-

**Table 18-6  Resume Headings**

| Resume Type | Headings |
|---|---|
| Chronological | • Personal Objective, Career Goal or Employment Objective<br>• Summary or Profile<br>• Education<br>• Experience, Work Experience, or Employment History<br>• Licensure and Certification or Licensure/Certification*<br>• Community Service*<br>• Research*<br>• Professional Activities<br>• Professional Membership*<br>• Continuing Education or Seminars<br>• References |
| Functional | • Objective, Employment Objective, Career Goal or Professional Goal<br>• Summary or Profile<br>• Clinical Skills<br>• Health Educator Ability or Health Promotion Capacity<br>• Managerial Capacity<br>• Leadership Ability<br>• Communication Skills<br>• Motivational Skills<br>• Teaching Ability |
| Combination | • Employment Objective, Career Goal, or Professional Goal<br>• Summary or Profile<br>• Education (chronological)<br>• Experience (chronological and functional headings)<br>• Select other chronological and/or functional headings |

*These headings can be combined within the Professional Activities heading.

rienced clinician. The chronological style is used for the "Education" and "Experience" headings; however, within the "Experience" section, skills and abilities may be emphasized using functional headings. Additional functional headings may be selected based on experiences that the practitioner wishes to emphasize.

## Cover Letter Preparation

Each resume is sent to the potential employer with an accompanying cover letter. The letter is the first contact with the employer and entices the reader's interest in the enclosed resume. The key to a successful cover letter is to personalize the contents to the specifics of the position and emphasize contributions that the employer will value. Standard phrases should be replaced with unique thoughts in order to attract the reader's attention. Writing a cover letter will take time; however, the time that is invested will lead to success in getting the employer to read the resume.

The body of the letter contains three paragraphs, each with a specific purpose. The first paragraph states the reason that the letter is being written and names the specific position of interest. Also described is where this position became known to the practitioner (newspaper or journal advertisement). When a networking contact refers a practitioner to a job, identify the person within the first paragraph. If a letter is being sent and no position is available at the present time, discuss how interest in the practice originated.

The second paragraph highlights the abilities (knowledge and skills), accomplishments (experience and professional activities), and personal characteristics of the practitioner. The information in this paragraph presents the applicant's qualifications in an overview style and does not restate everything on the resume. It is intended to stimulate the employer to read the resume for details concerning the highlighted qualifications. Professional skills such as experience in providing NSPT, pain control, expanded functions, and radiology are examples of abilities that can be highlighted. Write this paragraph with the employer's needs in mind, particularly when an advertisement lists requirements for the position. The hygienist can coordinate the advertised requirements with her abilities and accomplishments in this paragraph. When an advertisement does not list requirements for the position, networking contacts are useful for securing information about the employer and designing the contents of this paragraph around that information.

The second paragraph also includes sentences about personal characteristics. These can be difficult to write. To begin, practitioners should think about the personal characteristics they possess. Characteristics might include willingness to take responsibility, initiative, leadership, communication, and interpersonal skills. A close friend or colleague might help the practitioner focus on her positive characteristics. The goal of the second paragraph is to balance sentences around the personal and professional characteristics. In one of the sentences in the second paragraph, refer to the enclosed resume. It is important for the writer to consider the length. If the second paragraph is too short (two sentences or less), the employer might conclude that the dental hygienist has little to offer. On the other hand, if the paragraph is too long and verbose, the employer might deduce that the hygienist is overconfident.

The last paragraph states that the practitioner will telephone to discuss the employment opportunity and arrange an interview. State the amount of time that will lapse before the call to the employer will be made. A specific date or a general date such as "within a week" may be selected. Two weeks is an acceptable interval in which to make the call. The employer is also thanked for his con-

**GLORIA LENSAK, RDH**

30 Lexington Avenue
Seattle, Washington 98750
(206) 327-1287

**PROFESSIONAL OBJECTIVE**

To provide quality nonsurgical periodontal therapy and restorative expanded functions in collaboration with the dentist and other team members. Seeking employment as a dental hygienist in a challenging practice in Seattle that allows personal and professional growth.

**CLINICAL SKILLS**

**Preventive/Nonsurgical Periodontal Therapy Skills.** Twelve years of experience in practice. Assessed medical history and periodontal health/disease. Implemented corresponding therapy including debridement/scaling/root planing, ultrasonic instrumentation using precision-thin inserts, and periodontal fiber placement. Reevaluated clients' therapy. Success rate for decreasing periodontal pockets, bleeding, and/or gain in attachment level from initial therapy to maintenance therapy was 80%.

**Pain Control.** Achieved effective pain control using local anesthesia and nitrous oxide-oxygen analgesia with 40% of the periodontally involved clients.

**Restorative Expanded Functions.** Performed amalgam and composite restorative procedures on a part-time basis for five years.

**MANAGERIAL CAPACITY**

**Dental Hygiene Team Leader.** Five years of experience. Supervised three full-time and two part-time hygienists. Planned and conducted bimonthly team meetings. Identified that 96% of clients needed nonsurgical periodontal therapy.

**Dental Hygiene Treatment Plans.** Formulated treatment plans for new and maintenance clients. Case acceptance rate was 98%.

**Dental Hygiene Fees.** Established fees for preventive and nonsurgical periodontal therapy which increased productivity 30% in a six-month period.

**Dental Hygiene Appointment Schedule.** Reorganized system to 10-minute increments for dental hygiene services thereby increasing client services 25%.

**Recare System.** Redesigned the recare system that increased maintenance visits by 50%.

**Figure 18-2** Functional resume.

*(continues)*

sideration in a uniquely constructed sentence. When this message is personalized it leaves the employer with a positive impression. An example of a quality cover letter focusing on NSPT is provided in Figure 18-3 on page 494.

## Interviewing Strategies

The cover letter and resume have been effective when an interview has been secured. At this time, more preparation is necessary to ensure a successful interview. A thorough interview process requires three separate interviews, each with an intended purpose. This process is lengthy; however, it allows the employer and the practitioner an opportunity to evaluate each other's needs and make an educated decision about employment. Investing time in these interviews will prevent unfulfilled needs for both parties that could ultimately lead to short-term employment.

The first interview is used by the employer and interviewee to screen each other and to provide a mutual exchange of information. The interviewee should anticipate questions that may be asked by the interviewer (see Figure 18-4 on page 494) (Bolles, 1995; Coxford, 1995; & Grappo, 1994). Inevitably, questions will arise that seem to require a negative answer. Responses to these questions should be prepared in advance and in a manner that makes the response positive. Questions such as "What are your weaknesses?" can be answered in a positive manner by stating "Sometimes I'm too enthusiastic about promoting oral health." Likewise, the interview provides an opportunity for the hygienist to ask the employer questions (see Figure 18-5 on page 495). Revis-

**SPECIAL SKILLS**

**Computer Skills.** Efficient data entry during assessment of client's condition, treatment planning, recording services rendered, and posting fees for service.

**HEALTH PROMOTION CAPACITY**

**Client Education.** Provided clients with the knowledge and skills to prevent dental diseases. Used a wide variety of oral health aids and products to enhance client compliance. Designed a dietary counseling program for clients with a high caries rate.

**Elementary School Education.** Provided children in grades 3–5 with information about dental health.

**Nursing Home Education.** Planned and presented an inservice program to nursing home staff about dental healthcare for their clients.

**LEADERSHIP ABILITY**

**President.** Seattle Component, American Dental Hygienists' Association. Membership increased 10%. Planned Annual Session including four continuing education courses and product company exhibitors. Two hundred participants.

**LICENSES/CERTIFICATION**

**Washington State Dental Hygiene License.** #2302.

**Oregon State Dental Hygiene License.** #5789.

**CPR Certification.** American Heart Association.

**REFERENCES**

| | |
|---|---|
| **Colleague** | Mary McCarthy, RDH, MEd<br>30 Rock Place<br>Seattle, WA 98746<br>(206) 782-0113 |
| **Former Employer** | Martin Sims, DDS<br>672 Sterling Avenue<br>Seattle, WA 98752<br>(206) 783-5961 |
| **Former Employer** | Wesley Anderson, DDS<br>32 Fishkill Road<br>Bellevue, WA 95643<br>(206) 224-5516 |

**Figure 18-2** (*Continued*)

iting the professional and personal values on the career plan can be helpful to determine the content of other questions. The practitioner also formulates hypothetical and actual situational questions for the interviewer, as previously described. The interviewing process should be undertaken with the view that employment is mutually beneficial to the employer and interviewee. Cooperation and negotiation between both parties is necessary to establish an agreement that fulfills each party's needs and enhances long term employment.

The second interview is a working interview that allows the employer and interviewee to work together for a period of time to mutually evaluate the professional in the practice environment. When an interviewee has not received her license before the interview, observing in the practice is an alternative to the working interview and can accomplish the same goal for the interviewee. Figure 18-6 on page 496 lists questions to consider during the working interview. It would be most professional to ask one of these questions directly after the interview itself or when not in the presence of a client. The third interview is used to negotiate the final terms of employment that are mutually beneficial to both parties.

Both the employer and the dental hygienist need to take responsibility when securing the terms of the employment agreement. Most practices rely on a verbal agreement that can be subject to misunderstandings due to an unwillingness of the employer or employee to adhere to the agreement terms. The lack of a solid agreement between the two parties is a potential source of dis-

(Spacing varies. Use this space to center the letter on paper)

427 Park Place
Suffern, NY 10901
(914) 357-2650
May 15, 1996

(5 spaces)

Gloria Smith, DMD
209 Custer Avenue
Tuxedo, NY 10987

(2 spaces)

Dear Dr. Smith:

(2 spaces)

As a recent graduate, I am interested in employment as a dental hygienist in the Tuxedo area. While speaking to Linda Morris I learned of an employment opportunity in your office.

The clinical experiences in the dental hygiene program have prepared me to provide preventive, nonsurgical periodontal therapy, pain control, and expanded functions services. In a practice setting, I will continue to emphasize individualized quality care and collaborate with the dentist regarding client care. As the enclosed resume indicates, my experience includes being a sterilization assistant. This experience has taught me that a team approach to client care is important. As a dental hygienist, I will continue the team spirit through effective communication and commitment to the practice.

During the week of May 22, I will be in Tuxedo and would be interested in interviewing for the available position. I will contact the office within two weeks to arrange an interview. I have confidence that this endeavor will be mutually beneficial to both of us. Thank you for your consideration and I look forward to discussing my qualifications with you in person.

(2 spaces)

Sincerely,

(4 spaces)

Suzette Garbly, RDH, BS

(2 spaces)

Enclosure

**Figure 18-3** Cover letter.

- Tell me about yourself.
- Why are you interested in this job?
- What do you like least about your present job?
- What are your strengths and weaknesses?
- Why did you become a dental hygienist?
- What do you think you will be doing in five years?

- What are your long range career objectives?
- What contributions can you make to this job?
- What was your greatest accomplishment in your last job?
- What are the reasons for leaving your present position?
- How do you work under pressure?

**Figure 18-4** Questions asked by interviewers. (Adapted from Bolles, 1995; Coxford, 1995; and Grappo, 1994)

---

**Philosophy of Practice**

- What is the philosophy of practice or mission statement?
- Are there other goals or objectives for the practice?
- How does the dental hygienist's role fit into the philosophy, goals, or objectives?
- Does the practice focus on NSPT?
- What conditions exist when a client is referred to a periodontist?
- Is referral a collaborative decision made between the dental hygienist and the employer?

**Working Conditions**

- How many days per week are available to work?
- What are the specific days?
- What are the hours that the practice is open on each of the days?
- Lunch time is during what hour on each day?
- Are there certain hours that the employer will not be present in the office and the practitioner will provide client care? (If supervision laws permit)
- How much time is usually scheduled for a new adult and new child client?
- How much time is usually scheduled for periodontal maintenance therapy for an adult and child client?
- Are multiple appointments scheduled for periodontally-involved clients?
- Are appointments scheduled for reevaluation of client care?
- How much time is scheduled for a reevaluation appointment?
- Is an assistant provided for the dental hygienist on a part or full-time basis?

**Responsibilities**

- What are the responsibilities related to clients who are new patients or recare patients?
- What is the medical history protocol for antibiotic premedication and high blood pressure?
- What are the radiographic exposure recommendations for new and returning clients?
- What periodontal assessment procedures are completed on each client?
- Who is responsible for planning multiple appointments for the client?
- Who is responsible for scheduling appointments for the dental hygienist?
- Who is responsible for planning the recare interval?
- What are the responsibilities related to the recare system?
- Does the employer perform an examination while the client is in the hygiene operatory?
- When does the examination occur, before, after, or during the dental hygiene treatment?
- How much time is generally needed to complete the dental examination?
- What pain control methods are used in the practice?
- What other responsibilities related to client care or maintenance of the office are required?
- Are the fees for services determined by the employer or the employee?
- Do responsibilities include inventory management and ordering of instruments and products?
- Are staff meetings scheduled and is compensation provided for the meeting time?
- What other team members are in the office and what are their responsibilities?
- Are other dental hygienists employed in the practice?
- What is their philosophy of practice and does it include NSPT?

**Figure 18-5** Questions for the dental hygienist to ask the employer at the first interview.

---

illusionment and short-term employment. To prevent misunderstandings, a written agreement can be mutually beneficial to both parties (see Figure 18-7 on page 497). A written agreement is useful in a practice, whether or not written personnel policies exist in the office manual. When written policies exist, the written agreement is useful for augmenting specifics about the hygienist's employment (responsibilities, working conditions, compensation). Interviewing varies greatly between practices and employers. The interview can range from a well-organized mutual exchange of information between both parties to a disorganized grilling procedure by the interviewer. The quality of the interview can be reflective of the quality of the practice and the employer.

## COMPENSATION

Compensation is a personal need depending on the lifestyle that one leads. It is important for the dental hygienist to explore compensation issues as they are critical in determining the practice rating and score. The method of compensation, the wage received, and the benefits provided affect the compatibility of the practice with one's professional and personal goals. Compensation factors are related to values about employer support, continued professional growth, and the ability to participate in family vacations and activities. Compensation most directly affects the financial support one can offer the family unit. Before deciding on the amount of

**Safety and Quality Orientation of the Practice**

- Who is responsible for sterilizing instruments and how often is sterilization completed?
- What method is used for the preparation and sterilization of instruments?
- What is the procedure followed to disinfect the operatory between clients?
- Are barriers used to protect the unit?
- Where are the biohazardous trash and sharps disposed?
- Does the OSHA manual provide specific information related to occupational exposures, vaccination, and testing?
- Does the employer adhere to OSHA standards in the practice?
- Is quality care provided to the clients?

**Office Management**

- Does the practice have an office manual that describes policies and procedures related to client care and personnel management?
- Is the manual current and are team members following the policies and procedures?
- Is there a collaborative relationship between the employer and team members?
- Does the dental hygienist make independent decisions related to client care?
- Is an adequate amount of verbal feedback provided to team members?

**Employer and Team Members Support**

- Does the employer show respect and acknowledgment for the dental hygienist's and other team members' roles and skills?
- Do team members show respect and acknowledgment for the employer's and dental hygienist's roles and skills?
- Does the employer have good communication and interpersonal skills with team members and clients?
- Do other team members have effective communication and interpersonal skills with the employer, other team members, and clients?

**Work Environment**

- Is there a pleasant office environment considerate of the employer, team members, and clients?
- Is the pace of the office reasonable, rushed, or slow?
- Is an adequate amount of time scheduled for client care?
- Are periodontally-involved clients' treatment-planned for continuing care appointments when necessary?
- What is the procedure used for the employer performing the dental examination?
- If the exam is performed in the hygiene operatory, how long is the waiting time for the employer and how long is the examination time?

**Operatory/Equipment**

- Is therapy provided in one operatory or multiple operatories?
- What equipment (ultrasonic instrumentation device and inserts, nitrous oxide-oxygen analgesia, irrigation, radiographic, etc.) is in each operatory?
- What types of hand-activated instruments are available for use, and is there an adequate number of each type of instrument?
- What products are available for distribution to the client?
- What products (fluoride, desensitization, antimicrobials, anesthetics) are available for client care?
- What system is used to monitor and order needed inventory?
- Who is responsible for inventory management and ordering?
- What method is used to develop and mount radiographs?

**Client Charts**

- Do responsibilities include pulling and refiling client's charts?
- What type of periodontal and dental charting forms are used?
- How is the NSPT treatment plan documented in the client's chart?
- How often are medical histories completed by the client?
- How are significant findings from the intra/extraoral exam noted in the client's chart?
- How are significant findings from the initial dental exam noted in the client's chart?
- What information is listed in the Record of Services?

**Emergency Plan**

- What is/are the emergency procedures for the practice?
- What emergency equipment is available in the office and where is it located?
- What team members have CPR or First Aid certification?

**Figure 18-6** Considerations for the working interview or observation.

**1. DATE OF AGREEMENT, EMPLOYER, AND EMPLOYEE NAME**

**2. POSITION TITLE WITH RESPONSIBILITIES**

Dental hygienist responsible for management of NSPT

*Management*

- Perform as dental hygiene team leader
- Organize and conduct staff meetings with team members
- Standardize client care
- Perform dental hygiene productivity analysis

- Introduce new innovations in NSPT
- Supervise OSHA standards/infection control
- Manage inventory and equipment maintenance for NSPT
- Manage recare system

*Client care*

- Perform thorough medical history assessments by taking vital signs, completing medical consults, and modifying treatment based on findings.
- Complete restorative assessment by charting existing conditions and identifying areas in need of treatment for dentist to confirm.
- Complete periodontal assessment by charting probing pocket depth, bleeding points, furcation involvement, mobility, loss of attachment, and scanty attached gingiva.
- Expose and develop diagnostic radiographs; interpret and chart findings.
- Individualize dental hygiene treatment plan for NSPT based on assessment findings.
- Obtain written informed consent for NSPT.
- Educate client about dental diseases, existing oral conditions, proper oral health methods, and products.
- Implement individualized NSPT to increase the client's periodontal health by providing quality care during debridement/scaling/root planing, and stain and plaque removal, using appropriate equipment and instruments during NSPT, and providing comfortable treatment by using pain control methods.
- Implement other legalized duties such as fluoride treatments, sealants, desensitization, irrigation, amalgam polishing, overhang removal, dietary counseling, tobacco cessation programs, and periodontal fiber placement to promote total patient care.
- Perform reevaluation of NSPT.
- Coordinate care with the dentist.
- Collaborate with the dentist concerning patient referrals.
- Share new ideas, techniques, and equipment with team members.
- Document clients' conditions and care thoroughly in the chart.
- Use proper infection control methods to prevent disease transmission.
- During cancellation time, use time to sharpen instruments, stock operatory with supplies, work on recare system, assist the dentist, or help the receptionist.

*Professional*

- Communicate effectively with clients and other team members.
- Function as an interdependent team member and support others.
- Maintain the clients' confidentiality.
- Maintain current state licensure.
- Perform in accordance with ADHA's Code of Ethics.

**3. WORKING CONDITIONS**

*Work schedule including days and hours*

- Monday, Wednesday: 9:00 to 12:00, 1:00 to 6:00
- Tuesday, Thursday: 10:00 to 1:30, 2:30 to 7:00

*Client scheduling*

- New adult (18 years and older) appointment: 1½ hours.
- New youth (12 to 17 years) appointment: 50 minutes.
- New child (up to 16 years) appointment: 50 minutes.
- PMP appointments for adult, youth and pedo clients individually determined.
- Multiple appointments (length and number) are individually determined.

*Staff meeting attendance*

- Attendance at monthly dental hygiene team meetings is required.
- Attendance at bimonthly team meetings with all team members is required.

*(continues)*

**Figure 18-7** Example employment contract.

## 4. COMPENSATION

### Calculation of wages

- Salary will be paid at a rate of $25/hour to the nearest fifteen minute interval for work beyond the specified working hours. The dental hygienist will receive regular pay when the office is closed by the dentist on a day that the dental hygienist normally works. The dental hygienist will receive regular pay for staff meeting time.
- Each payment period begins on Thursday and ends on the following Wednesday. Weekly checks are received on Thursday.
- In addition, a monthly incentive bonus is computed at a rate of 5 percent of dental hygiene productivity. Checks are received on the first Thursday of the month.

### Record keeping

- At the end of each day of work the hygienist will complete a time card and have it initialed by the dentist. When the dentist is not in the office, the office manager will initial the card. Wages will be computed from the time card.
- At the end of each day the office manager will provide a copy of the dental hygiene productivity to the dental hygienist. The incentive bonus will be computed from the daily productivity sheets.
- Any discrepancies in the time card or productivity sheet must be reported to the dentist within one week of the day of the discrepancy, otherwise the information on the time card or productivity sheet cannot be changed.

### Benefits

- During the first year of employment, the dental hygienist will receive fifteen days in Paid Time Off Bank (PTO). This time can be used for vacation, holidays, sick, and personal days. Vacation and holidays must be scheduled three months in advance. Sick and personal days must be scheduled 12 hours in advance. Unused time in the PTO can be carried over to the next year.
- Dental care will be provided at no cost to the dental hygienist for prevention, amalgam restorations, extractions, orthodontics, and endodontics performed in the office. The dental hygienist will pay for the laboratory work when it is a required part of care. Dental care for the dental hygienist's family will include no cost for prevention and 50 percent of cost for other work performed in the office.
- The dental hygienist will receive 6 hours of paid continuing education registration fees. The dental hygienist will receive salary for scheduled work missed when attending the continuing education course.

## 5. PERFORMANCE EVALUATION

### Evaluation time intervals

- After the initial employment period (3 months), a performance evaluation will be conducted. The results of this evaluation will determine the time interval for the next evaluation, as described in the "Consequences of Performance" section.

### Evaluation criteria

- The criteria used for the performance evaluation are the statements listed in this contract under "Responsibilities."

### Scale of performance

- Each criteria is rated using the following scale (modified from Drafke, 1994):
  - 3– Superior Performance: Performance is consistent and surpasses the expected standard of the performance criteria. Minimal supervision and improvement is required.
  - 2– Quality Performance: Performance is consistent and meets the expected standard of the performance criteria. Normal supervision and minor improvement is required.
  - 1– Improvable Performance: Performance is inconsistent and does not meet the expected standard of the performance criteria. Major supervision is required. Major improvement requiring additional education is necessary.
  - 0– Unacceptable Performance: Performance consistently does not meet the expected standard of the performance criteria. Performance has endangered the well-being of the client and/or other team members. Constant supervision and additional education is required.

### Performance evaluation score

- A performance score is computed by dividing the total number of points earned from each performance criteria by the total number of points possible from the performance criteria.

### Performance evaluation rating

- The performance score is used to determine the performance rating.
  Superior rating: 90 to 100
  Quality rating: 80 to 89
  Improvable rating: 70 to 79
  Unacceptable rating: Less than 70

**Figure 18-7**  (*Continued*)

***Consequences of performance rating***
- Superior rating: Renegotiation of wages and benefits. Next performance evaluation at contract renewal.
- Quality rating: Renegotiation of wages and benefits. Next performance evaluation in six months.
- Improvable rating: No renegotiation of wages and benefits. Next performance evaluation in three months. When three successive Improvable ratings are received, the termination process is initiated.
- Unacceptable ratings: No renegotiation of wages and benefits. Next performance evaluation in three months. When two successive unacceptable ratings are received, the termination process is initiated.

***Performance evaluation process***
- The employer will complete the performance evaluation and will base the evaluation on personal observation and feedback from other team members and clients.
- The results of the performance evaluation will be discussed with the dental hygienist in a time frame no longer than one week after the evaluation has been completed. The dental hygienist will sign the performance evaluation and a copy of the signed evaluation will be given to the dental hygienist.
- When the dental hygienist disagrees with the results of the evaluation, the dental hygienist can submit a written statement which will be attached to the performance evaluation.

**6. EMPLOYMENT PROVISIONS**
- The initial employment period (probationary period) is three months in length, calculated from the first day of work. During that time, the employer or the dental hygienist can initiate the termination process. At the end of the three months, a performance evaluation will occur.
- The termination process is initiated by either the employer or the dental hygienist, by sending a certified letter to the other party notifying them that the termination process has been initiated. A period of fourteen days is established as advance notice. If either party breaks the advance notice period, the other party will be compensated for the remaining time. The employer will be reimbursed for the employment of a temporary dental hygienist and the employee will be reimbursed with regular salary.
- Renegotiation of this contract can occur during the one-year contract period. Renegotiated changes in the contract will be attached as addenda.
- This contract is one year in length and will be automatically renewed unless the other party is notified thirty days or more before the contract expires. Notification must be made by certified mail.

**Figure 18-7**  (*Continued*)

income that one needs, a thorough and realistic determination of an individual's budget should be completed. All expenses should be projected on a yearly basis then divided into twelve segments to represent the amount needed to be earned on a monthly basis. Figure 18-8 lists expenses to be considered in a budget. When an employer pays expenses listed on the individual's budget as a benefit (health and dental insurance, continuing education), the wages earned are worth more.

## Methods

Oral health care providers are compensated for the services that they provide in one of two ways: as an **employee**, or an **independent contractor**. A significant difference exists between these two methods of compensation. Both designations relate to definitions for tax purposes and are separate entities from supervision or practice regulations. States have their own laws concerning these definitions. To standardize their use at a national level, legislation was introduced to the Senate, but never passed (Sack, 1995). As an employee, the employer withholds income, social security, and

1. Home – rent or mortgage
2. Utilities – gas, electric, sewer, water, garbage, telephone, cable television
3. Entertainment – professional and nonprofessional
4. Clothing
5. Car – loan, insurance, registration
6. Insurance – life, disability
7. Medical and Dental Care
8. Professional Expenses – license renewal fee, liability insurance, continuing education courses, dues
8. Loan Payments
10. Credit Card Payments
11. Savings
12. Other – donations, retirement, educational fund

**Figure 18-8** Budget expenses.

Medicare tax from the employee's wages. The employer also pays federal unemployment insurance, and a share of the social security and Medicare tax (U.S. Department of Treasury, 1993). The state may require that the employer carry workmen's compensation and disability insurance for the employee. As an independent contractor, the contracting practitioner is self-employed and the contractor (i.e., dentist, employment agency) pays for services rendered. As an independent contractor, a hygienist is self-employed and responsible for paying all income, social security, and Medicare taxes. The accounting and paperwork associated with self-employment are also the hygienist's responsibility. Definite advantages exist when an employer/contractor designates an individual as an independent contractor. The usual deductions from employee compensation are not taken and the employer/contractor does not have to pay his share of employment taxes, thereby reducing paperwork and money involved with this process. The hygienist also has advantages to this method of compensation in that expenses can be deducted from the gross income. The disadvantages for the practitioner include no liability or workmen's compensation coverage from the contractor. For specific information about this classification, the advantages and disadvantages, consult a certified public accountant (CPA).

Some employers assume that when they compensate an individual on a commission basis, it automatically qualifies the individual for the independent contractor status. The method of compensation is not the only factor that determines this status. The IRS has twenty factors to consider when deciding whether employment is an employer/employee or an independent contractor relationship. Not all these factors are applicable to each situation. Several of these factors are listed in Table 18-7. These factors and specific information for determining the employment relationship are contained in Publica-

tion 937 which can be secured by contacting a local IRS office. It may interest the reader that in an example contained in the Publication, a dental hygienist is employed in a dental practice under general supervision where the employer specifies the work days. Although the hygienists are paid straight commission, they are considered employees.

When an employer wrongfully classifies an employee as an independent contractor, the employer can be held liable for the employment taxes for the employee. When income, social security, and Medicare taxes are not withheld from an employees wages, the employer can be held personally liable for a penalty that equals the amount of taxes that should have been paid. An employer who has questions concerning an independent contracting relationship can file Form SS-8, Determination of Employee Work Status for Purposes of Federal Employment Taxes and Income Tax Withholding, with an IRS District Director (U.S. Department of the Treasury, 1993). Both the employer/contractor and the practitioner should be aware of the advantages and disadvantages of the employee and independent contractor designation. Mutual decisions related to the practitioner's status should be made and collaborated by both parties in consultation with a CPA and the IRS.

## Wages

An employee receives wages on the basis of salary, commission, or a combination of these two mechanisms. Refer to Table 18-8 for a list of compensation considerations for wages. **Salary** is paid on an hourly, daily, weekly, monthly or yearly basis. **Commission** is paid as a percentage of the gross receipts for services that the hygienist provides. The commission rate varies between geographic regions and ranges between 40 percent to 60 percent (Burt, 1993a). **Base salary plus commission** is a

**Table 18-7  Employee/Independent Contractor Factors**

| Factors | Employee | Independent Contractor (IC) |
|---|---|---|
| Working Hours | Employer sets working hours and employee may be required to work full-time. | IC generally controls own working schedule (for whom and when IC chooses to work) and number of hours worked. |
| Place of Work | Usually works on employer's premises. | IC works from own place of business (pays rent) and has a significant investment in the facilities used. |
| Materials and Supplies | An employer usually provides these items. | IC usually provides own items. |
| Control of Work Results | Employer has the right to control how the work results are achieved. | IC controls own work results. |
| Expenses | Business and travel expenses are generally paid by the employer. | IC pays own business and travel expenses. |
| Profit or Loss | Employer can make a profit or suffer a loss, not the employee. | IC can make a profit or suffer a loss. |

**Table 18-8 Compensation Considerations: Wages**

| Considerations | Factors | Options |
|---|---|---|
| Method of Payment | Salary | hourly, daily, weekly, monthly, or yearly |
| | Commission | 45 to 60% of assessments, examinations, radiographs, NSPT, oral prophylaxis, periodontal fiber placement, and/or sealants, etc. |
| | Base salary plus commission | high salary and commission on *limited* services or low salary and commission on *numerous* services |
| Additional Compensation | Overtime | paid by straight salary, compensation time is received or not paid |
| | Staff meetings | full, partial, or no compensation |
| | Office closure | work under general supervision (if legal); or receive full, partial, or no compensation for not working |
| | Benefits | profit sharing, incentives, and/or bonuses |
| Recordkeeping | Tracking time | employer, office manager's, or employee's responsibility via written or mantime clock/card |
| | Payment period | weekly, bimonthly, monthly, on a specific date (15th and 30th) or day (Friday) |
| Renegotiation | Frequency | six months, yearly, or no specified schedule |
| | Basis | productivity, performance, evaluation, cost of living, and/or fixed percent increase |

combination of the two previous forms of compensation. In this case, salary is paid until the gross receipts for dental hygiene services reaches a specified amount, then the hygienist receives commission on the receipts above that amount. To compute the specified amount of receipts before commission, multiply the base salary by three (Burt, 1993a). If a hygienist earns a base salary of $200.00 per day, multiply by three, which equals $600.00. When production reached $600.00, receipts above that amount would be considered for commission.

Benefits for health care positions are computed to be 15 to 20 percent of the total annual wages and for non-health care positions are 30 to 35 percent of the annual wages (Le Bel, 1992). When benefits are not provided, higher wages are necessary for the employee to personally purchase benefits. A hygienist who receives a salary of $20.00 per hour without benefits can consider the actual worth to be 15 to 20 percent less than the hourly rate. Wages and benefits vary based on number of years of experience and geographic region of practice. Interestingly enough, an increase in the number of years in practice does not necessarily mean an increase in salary (Burt, 1993b).

## Benefits

Benefits provided to hygienists vary between practices and employment status, part-time and full-time employment. Table 18-9 lists potential benefits for the compensation package. Full-time and part-time hygienists perceive the same four benefits as important; paid vacation, holidays, dental care, and continuing education (Willis & Butters, 1993). The benefits that hygienists receive as a full or partial benefit are paid vacation, sick days, family dental care, pension/retirement plan, and medical benefits for the employee (Burt, 1993c). Employers should weigh the needs of the hygienist and offer an individual benefit plan based on these needs (Willis & Butters, 1993). Flexible benefit plans offered to employees are increasing in popularity. One type of flexible plan is called a "Paid Time Off" (PTO) Bank. Employers provide an allotment of days off and allow the employee to use them at their own discretion. The allotment of PTO can apply to sick days, vacation days, holidays, and personal days. Some employers combine vacation and sick days into the PTO bank, while others combine holidays and personal days ("Companies Are Offering Flexibility," 1994).

Another flexible benefit plan is called a "cafeteria plan." This is a term used when employees are allowed to select benefits from a variety of choices within an allotted amount designated by the employer. One type of cafeteria plan is a "Section 125 plan." The section refers to an IRS code that allows employees to designate funds before tax dollars to a group health insurance plan. The employee's portion of the insurance premium is deducted from the taxable income and is not subject to social security, federal, and most state taxes. Besides the tax break, this plan allows the employee to select benefits to fit their personal needs (DeCenzo & Holoviak, 1990). Benefits that

**Table 18-9 Compensation Considerations—Benefits**

| Benefit | Options |
| --- | --- |
| Continuing Education (CE) | Employee is compensated for CE registration fee<br>• Full or partial registration fee is paid<br>• Limit on number of CE credits that employer pays each year<br><br>Employee is compensated for travel expenses for CE course<br>• Full or partial payment of travel, accommodations, and meals<br><br>Employee is compensated for work missed while attending CE<br>• Partial or full payment of normal compensation<br>• No compensation, select CE course on a nonworking day |
| Dental Care | Family members covered<br>• Employee, spouse, children<br><br>Care provided at no cost<br>• NSPT, sealants, restorative treatment<br><br>Care provided at employer's lab fee cost<br>• Gold restorations and prosthodontic treatment<br><br>Care provided at a dental specialty office<br>• Orthodontic, endodontic, periodontic, maxillofacial treatment |
| Disability Insurance | Amount of employer's contribution towards the premium<br>• Partial or full payment<br>• Policy can be continued after employment is terminated<br><br>Disabilities covered<br>• Work- or nonwork-related injuries<br>• Coverage of pregnancy and carpal tunnel syndrome<br><br>Insurance specifics<br>• Process used to report the disability<br>• Length of time before disability benefits are received<br>• Method used to compute the dollar amount of disability<br>• Maximum amount or length of time that benefits are paid<br>• Partial payment of benefits when employee returns to work on a limited basis |
| Health Insurance | Type of health insurance<br>• Traditional (Blue Cross/Blue Shield), HMO (Health Maintenance Organization), PPO (Preferred Provider Organization)<br><br>Amount of employer's contribution towards the premium<br>• Partial or full payment for employee and other family members<br><br>Family members covered<br>• Employee, spouse, children<br><br>Medical treatment covered<br>• All prevention including immunizations<br>• Partial or full payment of medications<br>• Coverage of elective or nonelective surgery<br>• Coverage of vision and psychiatry<br><br>Deductible amount before reimbursement (traditional)<br>• Individual or family deductible amount<br>• Dollar amount: $100.00, $250.00, $500.00, $1,000.00<br><br>Reimbursement rate for medical treatment (traditional)<br>• Percent of reimbursement: 50%, 80%, 100%<br>• Dollar limit that insurance pays: yearly or lifetime basis<br><br>HMO<br><br>PPO |
| Holidays | Compensated holidays<br>• Legal holidays: Martin Luther King Day, Memorial Day, Fourth of July, Labor Day, Thanksgiving, Christmas<br>• Other holidays: other religious and recognized holidays |
| Life Insurance | Amount of employer's contribution toward the premium<br>• Partial or full payment<br>• Policy can be continued when employment is terminated<br><br>Type of insurance offered<br>• Whole or term life insurance policy |

**Table 18-9 (continued)**

| Benefit | Options |
| --- | --- |
| Life Insurance (continued) | Worth of life insurance policy<br>• Dollar amount: $20,000, $50,000, $100,000, $200,000<br>• Policy's cash value schedule<br>• Option of borrowing on policy's equity<br><br>Dividends earned from policy<br>• Dividends are paid to employee or used to pay premium<br>• Dollar amount of dividends<br>• Length of time before dividends are paid |
| Malpractice Insurance | Amount of employer's contribution toward the premium<br>• Partial or full payment of premium<br>• Employer pays premium directly to company or employee pays then is reimbursed<br><br>Malpractice liability<br>• Dollar amount: $20,000, $50,000, $100,000, $200,000<br><br>Procedures covered by policy<br>• Traditional treatment, NSPT<br>• Local anesthesia, nitrous oxide<br>• Restorative procedures |
| Professional Dues | Amount of employer's contribution toward dues<br>• Full or partial payment<br><br>Method of payment<br>• Employer pays dues directly to the association<br>• Employee pays and is reimbursed by the employer |
| Retirement Plan | Type of retirement plan<br>• Keogh, annuity, 401K plan, pension fund<br><br>Amount of employer's contribution<br>• Full or partial payment, employer will match employee's contribution<br><br>Dollar investment in the plan<br>• Maximum or minimum dollar amount at initial investment<br>• Maximum or minimum dollar amount invested yearly<br><br>Retirement plan specifics<br>• Plan begins after a specified time of employment<br>• Minimum number of hours worked each year to qualify<br>• Plan can be continued when employment is terminated<br><br>Rules for money withdrawal from plan<br>• Minimum wage<br>• Dollar amount that can be withdrawn<br>• Time frame for withdrawal: yearly, monthly, lump sum distribution, fixed monthly income |
| Sick Days | Method used to compute sick days<br>• Sick days begin to accumulate after six months<br>• Four hours per month are accumulated<br>• Six days per year are allowed for sickness<br><br>Unused sick days<br>• Unused sick days are lost at the end of each year<br>• At the end of the year, employee is compensated for unused sick days<br>• Unused days can be applied to vacation or personal days or maternity leave<br>• Unused sick days accumulate on an ongoing basis |
| Vacation Days | Computation of number of vacation days<br>• One week after one year of employment<br>• Two weeks after three years of employment<br><br>Amount of advance notice before vacation<br>• Two, three, six months<br><br>Restrictions on vacation days<br>• Vacation time must be taken at the same time as the employer<br>• Consecutive or split vacation days |

are offered by the plan include, but are not limited to medical, dental, vision, prescription, disability, and life insurance. Nontraditional benefits are important to explore. In rural geographic areas, benefits associated with transportation include compensation for travel time and gasoline associated with the commute. In large metropolitan areas, tolls and parking expenses are potential benefits. Paid child care during employment is another benefit that employers can provide. For hygienists who had left the workforce but intended to return, family responsibilities are cited as the number one reason for leaving (Miller, 1990). Pregnancy or child care is the most frequently stated reason for considering leaving or leaving dental hygiene (Boyer, 1994). Hygienists are concerned about contracting infectious diseases. As a benefit, employers can provide periodic testing for these diseases, treatment and extended leaves for contracted diseases (Le Bel, 1992).

The dental hygienist should consider purchasing health insurance, malpractice insurance, a retirement plan, disability insurance, and life insurance when the employer does not offer these as benefits. Health insurance coverage is necessary for payment of medical expenses for the individual and family. Malpractice insurance for the individual practitioner helps protect the hygienist in the event that money is awarded from a malpractice litigation. When the practitioner administers local anesthesia, this procedure should be covered by the policy. Although retirement is generally a long-range endeavor, careful financial planning is necessary through the purchase of a retirement plan. In the event that the hygienist becomes disabled for a short or extended period due to a work- or nonwork-related injury, disability insurance can help the hygienist supplement income while being unable to work. The purchase of life insurance is also recommended if no other mechanism is in place to pay for this unforeseeable event. Consultation with a financial planner or insurance agent is recom-

mended when purchasing these insurances and plans. The hygienist should consider participating in continuing education (generally necessary for relicensure) and joining the American Dental Hygienists' Association (ADHA) and other professional associations even when these are not part of the compensation package.

## FUTURE CAREER DEVELOPMENT

When a practice is selected for employment, the hygienist should refer to the career plan to determine the values that received a low "Practice Rating." These values provide the impetus for establishing goals that can lead to career development. Being proactive means taking the initiative for career development by formulating short- and long-term goals. Goals describe concrete achievements to be accomplished relative to the professional and personal values. Short-term goals describe achievements accomplished over a short period of time such as a week or month. Long-term goals can extend to six months and one or more years. Writing goals and working toward their accomplishment keeps the proactive hygienist on the path of career development.

A career is a lifelong endeavor that provides professional and personal development. When growth no longer occurs, practitioners need to revise their career plans to reflect current roles, values, and priorities. The existing position's compatibility with the new career plan is then evaluated. When the present practice is no longer compatible, the employment search begins. The revised career plan is used to evaluate the compatibility of practices that are interviewed. Just as with many processes in life, career development is dynamic. The career plan and employment need to reflect the dynamic nature of career development. Professional and personal growth are necessary for retention of dental hygienists in private practices and in their chosen careers.

## Summary

As health care professionals recognize that a career is a lifelong endeavor, careful planning is necessary for career development. Before a job search is initiated, practitioners should develop a career plan that reflects their professional and personal roles, values and priorities. The job search, cover letter development, resume writing, and interviewing strategies will focus on the identified professional and personal priorities. Most likely, these pri-

orities will focus on providing NSPT to insurers of oral health care. After the interview, practice compatibility with the career plan is determined. The career plan can be modified to reflect changes in an individual's professional or personal life. Updating the career plan can help maintain the health care professional on the path of career development.

# Case Studies

**Case Study One:** A dental hygienist has been employed full-time in a practice for three years, is recently married, and decides to return to college to work toward a higher degree. What modifications in the career plan would reflect these changes?

**Case Study Two:** Eva Reich has developed a career plan that includes professional and personal roles, values, and priorities. After interviewing at Practice A and Practice B, Eva has computed a total score of 75 for each practice. Both practices have offered employment to Eva. What should she consider when making an employment decision?

**Case Study Three:** The following advertisement was found in the "Want Ads" in the local newspaper:

> **Dental Hyg wanted** for a fast-paced, quality-oriented practice. Must have experience. Respond to Box 656, Llewellyn, PA 17944.

How would a dental hygienist design a cover letter to match this advertisement?

**Case Study Four:** An employer offers employment to Becky Recla in her private practice and compensation on a per hour salary basis. The employer asks Becky if she would like to be considered an independent contractor. What should Becky consider before responding?

**Case Study Five:** During the discussion of compensation, the employer offers John Hopp (who could be a dental hygienist or dentist) a salary that is $5.00 lower than the rate for the geographic region and his compensation needs as defined by the career plan. The benefits being offered are paid vacation, dental care, and cash bonuses. What should John do?

# Case Study Discussions

**Discussion—Case Study One:** The dental hygienist needs to carefully assess the changes in his/her personal and professional roles. The family member role becomes more complex as a person is in a married relationship and has more responsibilities. This change in role may necessitate new values being written for the family member role, such as financial considerations. Wages and/or benefits can increase more or decrease less than the previous level. A new role, "Student", can be added to the career plan and values associated with it are determined. The personal values should be reprioritized including the change in the family member and "Student" values. Other personal values may have less priority than before. A change in the "Employer Support" value can be important if the hygienist has to enroll in classes during normal working hours.

**Discussion—Case Study Two:** Eva should follow the decision-making process by first determining a realistic view of the facts. Both practices have equal scores of 75 and are fairly compatible with the career plan. Another fact is that both practices have offered employment. The second step is to list the alternative decision choices and their consequences. Eva could review the career plan and determine which practice met the values with the highest priority in the professional and personal categories. If she selected the practice that met the higher rated values, it may or may not meet the other values on the career plan. Another choice is to request another interview with each practice to renegotiate the values that scored low on the career plan. If both practices agreed, the renegotiation may or may not change the total score on the career plan. If one practice agrees to the renegotiation and the other does not, then the total scores may or may not change. If both practices disagree to renegotiate, Eva can decline employment at both practices and wait for other employment opportunities.

**Discussion—Case Study Three:** The advertisement does not list an employer's name, therefore the letter begins with "Dear Doctor". The first paragraph should contain the message that the letter is in response to the advertisement for a dental hygiene position found in the *Record* on Sunday, May 5th. The second paragraph of the cover letter should be developed to match the conditions listed in the advertisement. The hygienist has to convince the employer that he is qualified to work in a fast-paced office by his previous experience. Convincing the employer that the hygienist can provide quality care is also necessary. In order to show that the practitioner is experienced, the number of years that the hygienist has been practicing can be mentioned along with other career highlights. The enclosed resume is mentioned for further specifics about experience. The third paragraph has to be written from the standpoint that the hygienist cannot contact the employer to arrange an interview. When this situation occurs, the hygienist should identify when he can be contacted by telephone and be available for an interview. This contract should occur at the home residence if the present employer is not aware that the hygienist is seeking employment elsewhere.

**Discussion—Case Study Four:** Becky should consider whether employment is an employer/employee or independent contractor relationship. If the working relationship is a typical practice setting, Becky is probably an employee. Consideration of the factors associated with this relationship can be studied by securing a copy of the IRS Publication 937, the employer filing Form SS-8 with an IRS District Director or consulting a certified public accountant.

**Discussion—Case Study Five:** John should try to renegotiate a higher salary, to a rate that is consistent with the geographic region and his career plan. More information about the cash bonus needs to be secured. Questions about the frequency of the bonus payment and method of computation need to be asked to assess whether accepting the job at a lower salary is feasible. The practitioner also needs to know how often performance is reviewed and the amount of salary increase that can be expected. The criteria that will be used to evaluate performance should also be identified. If salary negotiation efforts are impossible, John could negotiate the addition of more benefits such as paid continuing education, professional dues and liability insurance, sick days, and health insurance. If more benefits could be negotiated, then John's budget expenses could be decreased and accepting the lower salary might be feasible.

## REFERENCES

Bader, J. D. & Sams, D. H. (1992). Factors associated with job and career satisfaction among dental hygienists. *Journal of Public Health, 52*, 43–51.

Beatty, R. H. (1991). *The resume kit* (2nd ed.). New York: John Wiley & Sons, Inc.

Benicewicz, D. & Metzger, C. (1989). Supervision and practice of dental hygienists: Report of ADHA survey. *Journal of Dental Hygiene, 63*, 173–180.

Boyer, E. M. (1994). Factors related to career retention among dental hygienists. *Journal of Dental Hygiene, 68*, 68–74.

Boyer, E. M. & Gupta, G. C. (1990). Dentist involvement in care provided by the dental hygienist. *Journal of Dental Hygiene, 64*, 273–277.

Boyer, E. M. & Gupta, G. C. (1992). Clinical dental hygienists' perceptions of quality dental hygiene care. *Journal of Dental Hygiene, 66*, 216–219.

Burt, P. D. (1993a). 1993 RDH wages and benefits survey results. *RDH, 13*(7), 24–26, 28.

Burt, P. D. (1993b). A regional analysis. *RDH, 13*(7), 32, 34, 38.

Burt, P. D. (1993c). Where do benefits fit the picture? *RDH, 13*(7), 40.

Calley, K. H., Darby, M. L., Bowen, D. M., & Miller, D. L. (1996). Factors influencing dental hygiene retention in private practice. *Journal of Dental Hygiene, 70*, 151–160.

Carney, C. G. & Wells, C. F. (1987). *Career planning: Skills to build your future.* Monterey, CA: Brooks/Cole Publishing Company.

Companies are offering flexibility in paid time off. *Personnel Journal, 73*(11), 16–17.

Covey, S. R. (1989). *The 7 habits of highly effective people.* New York: Simon & Schuster.

Coxford, L. M. (1995). *Resume writing made easy* (5th ed.). Scottsdale, AZ: Gorsuch Scarisbrick Publishers.

Darby, M. L. (1983). Collaborative practice model: The future of dental hygiene. *Journal of Dental Education, 47*, 589–593.

de St. Georges, J. M. (1991). The future is now: Seven steps for making it happen. *Canadian Dental Association Journal, 57*, 856–857.

DeCenzo, D. A. & Holoviak, S. J. (1990). *Employee benefits.* Englewood Cliffs, NJ: Prentice Hall, Inc.

Drafke, M. W. (1994). *Working in healthcare: What you need to know to succeed.* Philadelphia, PA: F.A. Davis Co..

Fry, R. W. (1991). *Healthcare career directory.* Hawthorne, NJ: The Career Press.

Good, C. E. & Fitzpatrick, W. G. (1993). *Does your resume wear blue jeans?* Rocklin, CA: Prima Publishing.

Guralnik, D. B. (1976). *Webster's New World Dictionary,* William Collins and World Publishing Co., Inc.

Kaplan, R. M. (1990). *Sure-hire resumes* (2nd ed.). New York: American Management Association.

Kennedy, J. L. & Laramore, D. (1990). *Joyce Lain Kennedy's career book.* Lincolnwood, IL: National Textbook Company Publishing Group.

Lakin, L. B. (1988). Winning strategies. *RDH, 8*(3), 30–32, 35.

Le Bel, L. A. (1992). What issues should be considered when negotiating an employment contract? Employment contracts for CRNAs: Protecting yourself amid the new economic realities. *Nurse Anesthesia, 3*(1), 25–30.

Linden, R. C. & Parsons, C. K. (1989). Understanding interpersonal behavior in the employment interview: A reciprocal interaction analysis. In R. W. Eder & G. R. Ferris (Eds.), *The employment interview: Theory, research and practice* (pp. 219–232). Newbury Park, CA: Sage Publications, Inc.

Loiacono, C. (1989). Manager's guide to reducing dental hygiene turnover. *Journal of Dental Hygiene, 63*, 328–334.

Manji, I. (1991). Mobilizing your workforce. *Journal of the Canadian Dental Association, 57*, 779–780.

Miller, D. L. (1990). Manpower issues related to nonpracticing dental hygienists. *Journal of Dental Hygiene, 64*, 226–234.

Miller, D. L. (1991). An investigation into attrition of dental hygienists from the workforce. *Journal of Dental Hygiene, 65*, 25–31.

Pollack, R. (1991). Team approaches to periodontal care. *Dental Teamwork, 4*(5), 19–20.

Pollack, R. (1992, January/February). How to motivate the team: It takes more than money. *Dental Teamwork, 5*(1), 10–12.

Pride, J. R. (1993). Dental hygiene: Adding value to your practice. *Journal of the American Dental Association, 124*, 251–253.

Pritzel, S. J. & Green, T. G. (1990). Working relationship between dentists and dental hygienists: Their perceptions. *Journal of Dental Hygiene, 64*, 269–272.

Sack, S. M. (1995). *From hiring to firing: The legal survival guide for employers in the 90s.* New York: Legal Strategies, Inc.

U.S. Department of the Treasury. (1993). *Employment taxes and information returns.* Washington, DC: U.S. Government Printing Office.

Uldricks, J. M., Hicks, H. L., Whitacre, H. L., Anderson, J., & Moeschberger, M. L. (1993). Dental hygienists' utilization of periodontal assessment skills and perceived collaboration with dentist/employer. *Journal of Dental Hygiene, 67*, 22–29.

Willis, D. O. & Butters, J. M. (1992). How does family status affect staff's view of employee benefits? *Journal of the American Dental Association, 123*(8), 82, 84, 86, 88.

Willis, D. O. & Butters, J. M. (1993). Money isn't everything . . . or is it? *RDH, 13*(7), 42, 44, 46, 58.

# CHAPTER 19

# Implementing Nonsurgical Periodontal Therapy into General Practice

## Key Terms

cotherapist
informed consent
material needs assessment
performance evaluations
periodontal client percentage
personnel needs assessment

prebooked system
production goal
program
standard of care
team concept

## INTRODUCTION

The successful implementation of nonsurgical periodontal therapy (NSPT) into a general practice is dependent on multiple factors ranging from the recognition of periodontal diseases to the development of an NSPT program. Ultimately, the success of the program requires the collaboration of the dentist/employer, dental hygienist, dental assistant, office personnel and the periodontist. It is imperative that every member of an oral health team understands the phases of periodontal therapy and shares responsibility for the periodontal health of clients. The term **program** is used throughout the text; however, it does not imply a single approach to therapy for all clients. Instead, the term refers to the way in which NSPT is implemented in an individual office setting. A program designed for one office might differ from another office, yet both programs meet the basic goals of providing NSPT to its clients.

The goals of NSPT may differ according to the phase of therapy, the client response, and the clinician's ability. The *ultimate goal* is to sustain teeth in a state of health. The *immediate goal* of therapy is to prevent, arrest, control, or alleviate periodontal disease. The *ideal goal* would be to achieve healing through regeneration of lost form, function, esthetics, and comfort. Sometimes the ideal cannot be achieved and a compromise in therapy must occur. The compromise, or *pragmatic goal*, is to repair damage resulting from periodontal disease activity. The clinician's role in achieving these goals is to provide therapy incorporating professional knowledge, skill,

and experience, while considering the host response (AAP, 1989a).

This chapter will review a plan for developing an NSPT program which includes a practice assessment, communication recommendations for the team, an implementation phase, and continual evaluation. The benefits of the NSPT program to the client, the employer, and the dental hygienist will be discussed. It is hoped that readers who are initiating a program, or enhancing an existing program, will discover some useful concepts for their practice. Even though this chapter focuses on nonsurgical care delivered in the traditional office practice setting, the concepts within are applicable to alternative and contemporary practice settings.

## DEVELOPMENT OF A NONSURGICAL PERIODONTAL THERAPY PROGRAM

Development of an NSPT program requires an understanding of the program as a whole, as well as of the individual clients who will participate and benefit from NSPT. Recommendations included herein are similar to those suggested for planning a community health program; and, thus, should be somewhat familiar to the student and practicing dental hygienist. The planning process for the initiation of an NSPT program requires a systematic approach as seen in Figure 19-1. The components of the planning process will be discussed in detail. They include the development of a practice philosophy, which will in turn lead to a practice assessment, and the

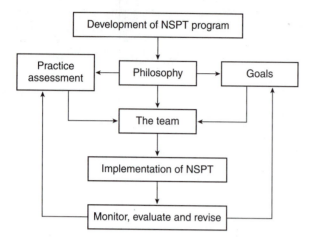

**Figure 19-1** Nonsurgical periodontal therapy planning process.

establishment of goals. The support of team members is vital in the planning process and the role of each must be defined. Implementation of the program requires putting the plan into operation. The planning process, as well as implementation, should be flexible and responsive to any new developments or technological advances (Mann, 1988). Upon implementation, the success of the program will be determined by continual monitoring and evaluation.

## Philosophy

Initially, the dentist and dental hygienist need to collaborate and agree upon a philosophy for the treatment of clients in the practice who are diagnosed with gingivitis and periodontitis. It is vital for the success of any new program in the office to have the full support of all personnel. This is especially true with the institution of an NSPT program because it requires an understanding of not simply procedures and fees, but often a new direction in office philosophy. Strategic planning ensures that each member of the team contributes and believes in the philosophy and goals of the program (Barr, 1993). The NSPT practice philosophy should be included in the office manual, along with a written explanation of the program's elements. This philosophy statement is available to new employees and is used to continually evaluate the implementation of nonsurgical therapy. Below is an example of how an existing practice philosophy statement is modified.

An existing practice philosophy reads:

*To provide excellence in family dentistry with an emphasis on prevention.*

New philosophy might read:

*To provide excellence in restorative and oral hygiene care with an emphasis on prevention and nonsurgical intervention for periodontal diseases.*

## Practice Assessment

The first phase in the planning stage requires an assessment of the practice needs, which in the case of NSPT begins with an awareness of the number of clients with periodontitis, the number of personnel needed to support client care, as well as the materials and supplies needed. Recent studies have focused on the advanced stages of periodontal disease and results show that even though the risk of periodontal disease increases with age, the severity of the disease is more limited than once thought (AAP, 1993; Miller, Brunelle, Carlos, Brown, & Löe, 1987; Ramfjord, 1993). In other words, numbers of clients with advanced bone loss are limited; however, many clients manifest signs of periodontitis with early or moderate bone loss. Consideration must be given to the multitude of factors (bone loss, furcations, mobility, loss of attachment) considered in historical studies assessing periodontal diseases and the changes in classifications of disease over time. The differences in methodology between these studies may actually account for an underestimation of the prevalence of the disease in the general population (Papapanou, 1994).

Keeping in mind the diverse nature of periodontal diseases and the various clients cared for in a general practice, it is likely that a vast majority of clients will exhibit stages of periodontitis treatable with NSPT (Ramfjord, 1993). Thus, it would be beneficial to determine the percentage of clients with periodontitis, termed the **periodontal client percentage**. While persons with gingivitis should not be overlooked due to the possibility of disease progression to periodontitis, they are not considered in the periodontal client percentage. Determination of this percentage requires careful assessment and monitoring. The first step in determining such a percentage is the recognition and diagnosis of periodontitis by means of a thorough, systematic periodontal assessment (see Chapter 3) performed on all new and established clients. Individuals with chronic adult periodontitis in the early stages of the disease process should be considered in the assessment, as well as clients with advancing stages or aggressive forms of the disease. Using the periodontal disease classification system established by the American Academy of Periodontology (see Chapter 1) aids practitioners in applying accurate diagnoses to client care and client renumeration for care by insurance carriers. Once assessment skills are mastered, the practice is monitored for several months to determine the total number of clients with periodontitis who require some form of NSPT. Comparing this number with the total number of clients seen during the monitoring period will yield the periodontal client percentage.

An example of a periodontal client percentage monitoring sheet is seen in Figure 19-2. This form could be computerized or customized depending on office needs. For example, a separate tally could be employed for new clients versus those clients requiring periodontal maintenance procedures (PMP). A column could be added if

| MONTH | January | | | | | |
|---|---|---|---|---|---|---|
| Classification | Health | Gingivitis | Adult EP | Adult MP | Adult AP | Aggressive Forms |
| NUMBER OF CLIENTS SEEN | 卌 | 卌 卌 卌 ⫼ | 卌 卌 卌 卌 卌 卌 ⫼ | 卌 卌 卌 ⫼ | 卌 卌 | ⫼ |
| TOTAL NUMBER OF CLIENTS | 5 | 18 | 32 | 17 | 10 | 2 |

Clients with Periodontitis     = 61   (Add last 4 columns)
Total Clients     = 84   (Add all columns)
Periodontal Client Percentage = 73%

**Figure 19-2** Periodontal client percentage monitoring sheet.

an oral health care team member desired to know how many clients were referred to a periodontist for further treatment. The establishment of a periodontal client percentage leads to an increased awareness of the practice's need for NSPT, which better enables the hygienist and dentist to meet the total oral health needs of each client.

A practice assessment also considers the number of personnel necessary to establish and implement a successful program, referred to as the **personnel needs assessment**. The need for additional hygienists and/or dental hygiene assistant(s) might be a consideration in a new or established program and is determined by evaluating the number of new clients per month, as well as the number of clients returning for maintenance therapy. The responsibilities and availability of the hygienist(s) and assistant(s) is then adjusted to meet the needs of the practice. The roles of each oral health team member in NSPT will be discussed in further detail later in this chapter. A **material needs assessment** determines additional instruments and equipment that are necessary materials considered or desired for implementing NSPT. The materials include the type and brand of periodontal self-care aids (see Chapter 6), the manufacture and volume of hand-activated and ultrasonic/sonic inserts needed, the type of mechanized device used for debridement (see Chapter 12), and the materials needed to provide supportive treatment (see Chapter 14). Details involved in the material needs assessment are discussed in the implementation stage of the planning process.

## Goals

Establishing goals for client care, as well as expectations for the practice begins with the dentist and dental hygienist, and ultimately involves the entire team. Ownership of the program by all oral health care members is essential in establishing quality and pride in the NSPT services rendered. Team members need to understand how their function affects the whole program, so it becomes necessary that the overall goal of NSPT is understood. The overall goal in developing a program might include increasing the periodontal services delivered by oral health professionals, in addition to diagnosing and treating clients in the earliest phases of the disease process. Just as there is a growing demand for periodontal services, there is an ever increasing demand on a practice to identify patients with periodontal problems (Levin, 1991). Studies have found that many dental practices fail to recognize and inform clients of early periodontal disease, as well as to perform comprehensive assessments (Brady, 1984; Hicks, Uldricks, Whitacre, Anderson, & Moeschberger, 1993). An increase in the utilization of the staff might be an additional goal to be considered. Delegation of procedures, including appointment scheduling, assistance in assessment, and oral self-care education will increase involvement of all personnel.

Current literature on various aspects of NSPT can be reviewed prior to the establishment of goals. All aspects of treatment including assessment, education, preventive and nonsurgical periodontal therapy, reevaluation, and maintenance procedures must be considered in establishing realistic production goals. A hygiene **production goal** should be established that is reasonable and attainable. It is important for the hygienist to know the hourly production goal. In an established practice the production goal is assessed by reviewing the previous years average production by dental hygienists, and the number of days worked. From that assessment, one can determine the average hygiene production per day and per hour and establish a goal to increase that production. In a dental practice that is just initiating a periodontal program, a goal must be established at the outset and monitored throughout the first year to assure that the production goal per day and per hour is realistically attainable. Overhead factors such as instruments and supplies will affect the production goal. The salaries of the hygienists are additional factors to consider, as well as the salaries of hygiene assistants, when applicable. Courses in practice management offer guidelines regarding aspects of dental hygiene care that can be included in dental hygiene production figures. These courses offer average ranges of acceptable hygiene production and avenues for increasing production by establishing realistic goals. Table 19-1 outlines broad practice goals for nonsurgical care that can be used to develop specific goals applicable to each oral care setting.

## COMMUNICATION

Communication of the importance of each oral health team member's role will help in development and transition of NSPT programs. The foundation of the **team concept** depends on the overall goal of therapy being understood, and the individual's recognition of how

**Table 19-1 Nonsurgical Periodontal Therapy Program Goals**

| Component of Care | Goals |
|---|---|
| Assessment | 1. Provide client-centered periodontal assessment focusing on gingival inflammation, bleeding on probing, periodontal pocket depth, and loss of attachment.<br>2. Recognize when further periodontal assessment is needed to determine furcations, mobility, and suppuration.<br>3. Include additional diagnostic testing as it becomes accessible, practical, and useful.<br>4. Select and expose appropriate radiographs for periodontal evaluation (vertical bitewings). |
| Diagnosis | 1. Render a presumptive diagnosis for each client differentiating between health, gingivitis, and periodontitis.<br>2. Incorporate the presumptive periodontal diagnosis in each assessment and care plan.<br>3. Include the presumptive periodontal diagnosis within the dental hygiene diagnosis.<br>4. Focus on two areas: the detection of early stages of periodontitis and aggressive forms. |
| Care Planning | 1. Build the nonsurgical periodontal therapy into the total care plan.<br>2. Ensure that adequate appointment time is scheduled and its need explained to the client.<br>3. Discuss reevaluation as an essential component of care.<br>4. Thoroughly explain the case presentation.<br>5. Prioritize the need for informal consent for each client's therapy. |
| Implementation | 1. Strive to deliver quality periodontal instrumentation incorporating the most recent technology available.<br>2. Recognize the vital role client self-care plays in achieving periodontal health or stability.<br>3. Devote adequate time to discuss client-centered self-care education including both disease theory and skill assessment.<br>4. Deliver appropriate and timely supportive therapy as needed (i.e., overhang removal, desensitization, periodontal fiber therapy, etc.). |
| Evaluation | 1. Continually evaluate care at each appointment during initial therapy.<br>2. Recognize that evaluation includes self-care education as well as the quality of the technical skills delivered. |
| Periodontal Maintenance | 1. Strive to motivate clients to accept the need for carefully monitored and timely maintenance therapy.<br>2. Discuss with clients the relationship of professional therapy and self-care practices.<br>3. Explain the system for notifying clients about maintenance intervals.<br>4. Involve the client in decisions regarding maintenance. |
| Finances | 1. Include the client's responsibility for fees rendered for nonsurgical care in the case presentation.<br>2. Explain the role of the insurance carrier in fee reimbursement.<br>3. Evaluate fees for NSPT on a yearly basis.<br>4. Meet quarterly to standardize fees assessed for care by dental hygiene therapists.<br>5. Strive to meet and evaluate the dental hygiene production figures. |
| Knowledge | 1. Commit to reading and evaluating professional literature related to nonsurgical care.<br>2. Share knowledge and literature with other team members.<br>3. Attend at least two continuing education seminars regarding NSPT per year.<br>4. Participate in dental hygiene staff meetings that discuss and standardize the nonsurgical care provided for the well-being of the client. |

his/her function affects the goals. An all-office staff meeting is an effective way for the dentist and hygienist to be able to explain the goals for improving the health of the clients. Sharing the periodontal client percentage and communicating the standard of care will increase staff motivation. Staff meetings can incorporate clinical education and in-services if necessary. For example, the dentist and hygienist might standardize probe measurements by performing periodontal probing on the same client, in a specific quadrant. The chairside assistants could also practice the charting associated with the periodontal probing. Inservices on new technology or information gained from continuing education courses can be shared with the entire team, which will lead to discussion on whether or not changes will benefit the clients and the practice.

It may be helpful to implement additional staff meetings or short reviews of the NSPT program with progress-to-date information as implementation advances. Time should be allotted for the team members to discuss their perception of the barriers to success, vent their own frustrations with the changes, and, above all, to make suggestions for improvement. Clients are more inclined to accept periodontal and restorative care from an informed, motivated staff (Kutnick, 1991), that is enhanced by regular staff meetings that encourage open and frequent communication.

### Dentist/Employer

Once the employer/dentist and hygienist have agreed upon goals for NSPT, the dentist's role involves support for the program. The staff must believe that the dentist wants the NSPT program for the benefit of clients and the practice. The dentist needs to express as much enthusiasm for the program as the dental hygienist(s) and be willing to help the other team members through any "resistance to change." When there is more than one dentist in the practice they all might be involved in NSPT, or one dentist/employer might assume the administrative role for the program. The dentist must also support the hygienist's professional role and expertise in providing nonsurgical therapy. The dentist's confidence in the hygienist's clinical ability as well as the ability to implement the program into the practice should be evident to the other staff members. In order for the employer to be able to offer this support, the dental hygienist must have already proven clinical expertise and gained the respect of the dentist in the role of **cotherapist**. Wilkins (1994) defines a cotherapist as "a term used to describe the relationships between the patient, dentist, and dental hygienist when coordinating the efforts to attain and maintain the oral health of the patient" (p. 4). The hygienist should exhibit a desire to share the responsibility for the client's care with the dentist. The dentist must be able to trust not only the clinical skills, but the commitment level of the hygienist, not just to the client but to the dental practice as well. The dentist is being asked to invest

money, time, energy, credibility, and his reputation in this program; therefore, the hygienist should be worthy of this trust. It is also important for the dentist to communicate support for the dental hygienist to each client. It is vital that the client believes that the dentist and dental hygienist agree that the nonsurgical therapy being recommended is the proper course of treatment. The client must feel that the dentist has total confidence in the dental hygienist's clinical skills and ability to make client-centered decisions as therapy progresses. When clients know that they have two very competent professionals concerned with their oral health care, it is very reassuring.

The dentist and hygienist must have parallel philosophies about appointment time needed for NSPT and associated fees for services to prevent confusion when discussing therapy with the clients. These two practitioners should also determine which facets of treatment each will present. For the client new to the practice, some dentists prefer to do all data gathering and case presentation prior to any dental hygiene visit. Others might meet the client and visit briefly, but rely on the dental hygienist for data gathering, prior to dental hygiene prognosis and case presentation. Information about fees, number of appointments, and insurance coverage is often the responsibility of the hygienist. The periodontal maintenance visit may be less formal. Information on disease and possible treatment at this visit might be presented by either practitioner depending upon whether the dentist sees the client before, during, or after dental hygiene treatment.

### Dental Hygiene Assistant

Just as the title implies, the dental assistant's role centers around using one's abilities to help someone else perform their job effectively. The dental assistant is utilized to assist the hygienist in performing NSPT in the operatory and to help educate clients about effective oral self-care. Many of the duties the assistant performs for the dentist will be the same when assisting the dental hygienist, which is referred to as four-handed dental hygiene. Exposing and developing radiographs, setting up and cleaning the operatory, sterilizing instruments, and assisting during client therapy should be routine. Unfortunately, many dental hygiene operatories are not designed for fourhanded procedures and the dental assistant may not have the ideal amount of space in which to work. The dental hygienist can utilize the assistant effectively during data collection, especially for periodontal charting. In addition to recording, the assistant aids in the discussion of assessment findings, if appropriate. There is an increased potential for client involvement during the discussion of bleeding points, recession, furcations, and pocket depth (Boyer, 1990). Depending on state practice acts, the dental assistant may also perform coronal polishing, if indicated, and fluoride treatments allowing the hygienist time to perform other oral health care.

The certified dental assistant can also be effective in

patient self-care education after the dentist and/or dental hygienist spend adequate time to ensure that the assistant understands the etiology and treatment of periodontal diseases. It is vital that correct and patient-centered information be given when the assistant answers a patient's questions. The assistant must have thorough knowledge about the different aids that might be prescribed, how and why they are used, and must possess proficiency at demonstrating their use in a patient's oral cavity. Observing the hygienist during oral self-care education and reading professional literature enhances the assistant's skills and confidence.

Choosing a dental assistant for the hygienist is often a challenging task. Unfortunately, some assistants might have the perception that assisting the hygienist is a somewhat less important position than working with the dentist. Great care should be taken to make this team member feel that the role of dental hygiene assistant is a vital link providing quality NSPT for clients. Increased responsibility for the client's education along with verbal appreciation from both the dentist and hygienist can encourage the assistant to be creative and enjoy the job. Sometimes it is necessary to hire an assistant new to the practice for this position. Ideally, this person should be a "people person" and practice effective communication with peers and clients. Most often, the clinically-oriented skills can be easily taught and learned.

Remember that many hygienists perform NSPT without the help of their own assistant. However, the use of an assistant simply enables the hygienist to accomplish more undelegable tasks efficiently and effectively (McCullough, 1993).

## Additional Dental Hygienists

Many practices employ more than one dental hygienist in a variety of full-time and part-time combinations. These dental hygiene professionals should agree on the concept of NSPT to ease implementation of the program. Obviously, it is best to have unity among those with whom the major weight for success or failure of the program rests. It is beneficial to schedule dental hygiene staff meetings periodically to assess current procedures, standardize care and to stay informed of new developments.

Collaborating about the fundamental elements of the program can be an exciting and stimulating challenge. It is advisable to decide whether clients should be scheduled with the same hygienist for each reappointment or whether alternating treatment between hygienists is acceptable. Having a colleague to act as a "sounding board" or to work out dental hygiene diagnosis and care planning can be very encouraging, especially if one hygienist has less experience.

It is possible that not all hygienists will share the same enthusiasm for implementation of NSPT into the practice. It is important to have open and effective communication about the program with one another. Each

dental hygienist must be treated as a professional and comments and opinions should be handled diplomatically so as to not cause judgment or division. Remember, change can be very intimidating. Stepping out of one's comfort zone into untested waters can be viewed as a challenge to some and a threat to others. Try to identify the real barriers to agreement. Sometimes it is helpful to first point out the shortcomings of the present system not only for the client but for the hygienist as well. Some dental hygienists may not have established the confidence in either their clinical or communication skills to participate immediately. Continuing education classes directed at both theory and clinical skills can enhance confidence. Enthusiasm for the program may develop many months after implementation when the problems have been solved and the benefits become apparent. Discouragement over the lack of improvement in a client's oral health, fatigue, and boredom can all be changed through participating in a valued NSPT program.

## Front Office Personnel

Front office personnel perform many roles including receptionist, schedule/office coordinator, insurance secretary, financial coordinator, and office manager. The responsibilities performed by this individual coordinate all phases of the NSPT program with one another. This person often controls the appointment book, which in turn controls the clinician's day. It cannot be stressed enough that this individual must understand the goals of NSPT and why creative scheduling may be necessary. The front office staff must accept the idea that the NSPT program is what the dentist wants and that the benefits to the client and the practice are tangible. The front office personnel must be as committed as other team members to the success of the NSPT program. Their job is every bit as demanding as that of the hygienist. The schedule can and often does change several times in one day, and the dynamics of keeping the clinician booked for optimum client care, production, and limited stress is a formidable skill. Details of scheduling will be discussed in a subsequent section.

The front office person may be involved in quoting or collecting fees for professional care. Here again, time is well-spent in educating this team member as to the level of difficulty of the therapy appointments, and how the therapy might be used to help preserve the entire dentition. Front office personnel must be as comfortable as the hygienist and dentist when discussing fees with clients. It is important that persons who are covered by dental insurance know that their policy is an individual plan chosen and purchased by their employer. The extent of coverage depends on the amount of money the employer has chosen to spend. Inadequate coverage should not have any bearing on the diagnosis of the periodontal condition or the treatment indicated and delivered. Not all companies accept or pay for services even though the procedure is identified by American Dental Association (ADA) codes. An effective communicator at the front desk can clarify this concept and encourage clients to accept responsibility for fees not covered by the insurance carrier. A subsection of this chapter addresses insurance coverage and codes.

## Periodontist

It is inevitable that some clients will need surgical intervention after the nonsurgical phase of treatment. A harmonious working relationship with the periodontist is an advantage for the general practice "in rendering comprehensive care that is the patient's right to receive and the dentist's responsibility to deliver" (Fisher, 1990, p. 456). The dentist must decide whether he/she has the required skills to treat the client or if referral to a specialist is indicated. After informing the client of the need for specialized care, the dentist is obliged in assisting the client to make a prudent choice and to explain the consequence of not following through with the referral (Hall, 1994). If there are several periodontists to choose from in the geographical area, it is suggested that the dentist and dental hygienist take time to discuss philosophy and treatment options with each professional. Establishing common ground between the dentist, dental hygienist, and periodontist about the general course of therapy is important. It is beneficial to have one or two specialists to whom the general dentist can comfortably refer, and with whom communication is effective. Topics to discuss with the periodontist include referral guidelines, new client consultation, surgical criteria, transferring of client information between offices, and maintenance procedures. A list of questions to consider asking the periodontist follows.

1. At what point should the client be referred?
2. What takes place during a new client consultation appointment?
3. What radiographs and other records are desired?
4. In what way will the periodontist communicate with the referring office as to the client's status?
5. What is the criteria for surgery?
6. Are periodontal maintenance procedures performed in the specialist's office, the general office, or perhaps alternated between the two?
7. What adjunct aids (automated/sonic toothbrush or oral irrigator) might be suggested for oral self-care and for which client conditions are they recommended?

The topic of communication between offices or professionals is very important. Some general dentists have been reluctant to refer, feeling that the client might be lost by the referring office when maintained in the specialist's office. The dentist and periodontist might agree that the client be referred back to the general practice for yearly or biyearly assessment and caries examination. This coordination of client care allays the fear of "losing" the client to the periodontist. The general dentist should continue to be the primary provider of restorative care (AAP, 1989b). When acceptable, alternating the three-month periodontal maintenance appointment can help professionals share responsibility for the client's care. The AAP (1989c) offers suggestions as to when alternating between offices is acceptable. It is stated that the periodontist ultimately decides in which office the periodontal maintenance procedures should occur. Also, "patients treated for advanced periodontal diseases or with residual compromise defects should be maintained by the periodontist" (AAP, 1989c, pp. 1x-27). It is appropriate for clients with moderate periodontal problems to alternate between the referring dentist and the periodontist.

One tool the hygienist can employ to enhance communication between offices is the use of a referral form (see Figure 19-3). This form provides the periodontist with much more information than is customary. This example includes the periodontal classification of the case, what records are accompanying the referral, what client services have been performed, and what procedures are planned in the future, including restorative needs. The referral form also has a place for inclusion of home care regimens as well as clinician observations about the client's motivation, or any other considerations that could help the specialist in formulating the care plan. If the client has another appointment scheduled in the general office, it might be wise to include that information for prompt return of records from the specialist. Providing the periodontist with pertinent information before the client's appointment will serve to illustrate a commitment to comprehensive care and should stimulate facilitative communication in return. When designing a form to fit the individual office, inquire of the periodontist as to what information would be of assistance and tailor it to meet the needs of any and all offices used in the referral process. The periodontist might also be willing to share preferred forms for duplication and use by the referring office (Simonds, 1991).

Ideally, the periodontist should have confidence in the professional's skill in diagnosing and treating the case prior to referral. If referral for surgical intervention is necessary, the periodontist should be confident that proper periodontal instrumentation and supportive treatment has been performed and that the sites designated are ready for surgery without further preparation. Further communication takes place either by telephone or mail, keeping both offices well apprised of the client's progress. The periodontist is a ready resource for questions regarding difficult cases or systemic complications and is a vital member of the NSPT team. The result of this team approach is greater consistency of care between all treating professionals and increased confidence for the patient (Simonds, 1991).

Dear Dr. _____   .   Date _____

Regarding our client _____

We are referring this client to you for periodontal consultation.

Enclosed please find:

☐   BWX                                              ☐   FMX
☐   Panographic film                                 ☐   Periodontal charting

**INITIAL DIAGNOSIS**

☐   Gingivitis                                        ☐   Bruxism
☐   Early adult periodontitis                         ☐   Occlusal trauma
☐   Moderate adult periodontitis                      ☐   Other _____
☐   Advanced adult periodontitis
☐   Aggessive periodontitis _____

**TOTAL CARE PLAN**

☐   Extractions _____                       ☐   Crown/bridge _____
☐   Restorations _____                      ☐   Debridement/scaling/root planing
☐   Occlusal therapy _____                      _____
☐   Endodontics _____                       ☐   Other _____

**CARE COMPLETED TO DATE**

☐   Examination and radiographs                       ☐   Tetracycline fiber therapy
☐   Periodontal assessment                            ☐   Desensitization
☐   Bacterial evaluation                              ☐   Irrigation
☐   Debridement/scaling/root planing                  ☐   Other _____
☐   Periodontal maintenance procedures

**HOME CARE IN PLACE AT THIS TIME**

_____

**COMMENTS:**




Client's next appointment is scheduled _____

If you have any questions, please feel free to call.


_____            _____
        (signature of RDH)                              (signature of DDS)

**Figure 19-3**  Periodontal referral form.

# IMPLEMENTATION OF NONSURGICAL PERIODONTAL THERAPY

The implementation process, like the developmental phase of planning, requires the collaboration of each member of the dental team. Initially, the implementation process will include preparatory steps that need to be addressed prior to activating the plan. These preparatory steps include identifying any physical limitations and acquiring needed supplies, materials, and equipment. After the preparatory steps have been completed, other factors such as scheduling, fees, and insurance can be dealt with. Communication concerning how the program will run and the responsibility of each team member will be ongoing in the implementation of NSPT.

## Physical Limitations

Often the practice's physical arrangement limits the implementation of NSPT. The most common roadblock is lack of operatory space. Obviously, if operatory space is not available, clients cannot be added to the practice. Each office will need to arrive at its own best solutions to physical problems. The key term is "creativity." One solution is to utilize one of the dentist's operatories one day a week for dental hygiene care. The dentist can be scheduled for maximized production in fewer operatories, and an additional hygienist scheduled for the available operatory. Depending on the individual state's practice acts, the dental hygienist may be able to treat clients without the dentist present. If the law allows general supervision, periodontal maintenance appointments for clients not requiring examinations by the dentist might be scheduled on these days.

In some geographical locations, it is difficult to find dental hygienists to add to the practice. It has been shown that hygienists leave the profession due to frustrations arising from lack of utilization and environments where collaboration between the hygienist and dentist are not encouraged (Miller, 1991). Offices that offer hygienists the chance to increase their knowledge and skills, and then put that knowledge into practice rarely are the ones that have trouble recruiting. Hygienists who are fully utilized and treated as cotherapists by the dentist reap the benefits of positively impacting their clients' health and generally remain not only in the profession, but in those practices (Hamman, 1992).

## Supplies

The first step in the actual implementation of NSPT is to complete the material needs assessment. Together, the dentist and dental hygienist must select the necessary equipment and instruments and prioritize those items that are essential from the outset of the program. The use of ultrasonic instrumentation, subgingival irrigation, and the availability of advanced diagnostic procedures will have a place in needs assessment. Consideration should be given to the periodontal client percentage, the number of dental hygienists practicing at a given time, and the frequency of sterilization procedures. In an office with an existing NSPT program, there will be times that instruments and/or equipment will need to be updated or augmented. By staying abreast of research and new developments in instrument technique and design, the dentist and hygienist can make knowledgeable decisions as to what instruments and equipment will best suit the needs of their practice. A system of replacing worn, ineffective instruments can be established by developing a "want list." This practice facilitates monitoring of supplies and planning for future needs of the NSPT program. It allows the dentist and hygienist to formulate a plan for replacing or ordering additional instruments at certain intervals without placing too much strain on overhead in any given time period.

In addition to instrument and equipment considerations, the dental hygienist must assess the need for other supplies such as equipment for subgingival irrigation, fiber therapy, fluoride therapy, desensitizing agents, and pastes for coronal polishing. Providing the client with oral hygiene aids to facilitate home care and promote continued maintenance will enhance an NSPT program. Decisions must be made as to what types and brands of aids will be recommended and what will be provided as part of the service. Educational materials can be valuable tools to augment assessment and treatment planning and to facilitate patient understanding of periodontal disease (McCullough, 1993). These materials may range from illustrations of proper home care techniques for prevention and/or maintenance of periodontal disease to information concerning the progressive stages of periodontitis. Literature is available from sources such as the ADA or directly from product companies. If information from product companies is utilized, evaluation of the content is necessary to ensure that the information is factual and that bias for the company's product is not the main topic. Reviewing the literature will enable the dental hygienist to select those materials that best reflect the practice's philosophy concerning NSPT.

## Records

The utilization of appropriate records for documentation of periodontal conditions and therapy is a critical aspect of NSPT. There are many forms and systems available and there is no one accepted standard format for periodontal record keeping. Many practitioners utilize existing forms as models and then customize these forms to fit the needs of their particular practice. It should be remembered to acknowledge the copyright of existing material in the development of such forms. There can be a tremendous number of forms in a client's permanent files; however, it is best to have more information recorded than to not have enough information to provide quality care. Multiple forms serve to categorize information in order to help practitioners focus on the different components of therapy and standardize delivery of care. Most offices have the following records: a client personal data form, a health history, an oral examination form, a restorative and/or periodontal examination form, a care plan(s), bacterial plaque or deposit evaluation systems, oral self-care information, and a record of the services rendered. Each of these records is addressed in detail in previous chapters except for the record of services, which is discussed later in this chapter.

The purpose of the periodontal examination should be considered when utilizing an existing chart or formatting an original form. The charting system should accommodate the recording of all information gathered during the assessment (McCullough, 1993). This form should have adequate room for reevaluation appointments and subsequent PMP. The periodontal charting should be easy to read and understand so that clinicians can evaluate the success of previous NSPT at a glance. If the office uses marketed systems, such as the Periodontal Screening and Recording System or automated probing devices, special forms will be incorporated into client care. The dental hygienist might choose to formulate other forms to facilitate the implementation of NSPT, to standardize oral health care teams with more than one dental hygienist, or to maintain consistency from client to client. An example is an NSPT care plan that includes therapy regimes, as well as self-care education (see Chapter 6) and supportive care (see Chapter 14).

Use of periodontal and oral hygiene indices to track client progress and standardize care will require unique forms and systems. Offices will sometimes choose to develop a periodontal assessment/charting form that includes spaces for recording bacterial plaque, gingivitis, and calculus index numbers, and self-care practices. Many practitioners note the extent of deposits in general terms based on location (supra- or subgingival, localized or generalized) or amount (light, moderate, or heavy). It is important that the systems chosen to quantify deposits allow oral health care team members to compare extent of deposits at subsequent maintenance appointments to the previous appointment, thus assisting in motivating the client toward self-care and an appropriate interval for maintenance. The extent of deposits by no means should serve as the sole indicator in assessment and reevaluation. Risk indicators (see Chapter 1), extent of periodontitis (see Chapter 5), and self-care practices (see Chapters 6 and 8) also must be considered.

## Scheduling

Managing the appointment book can be one of the most frustrating tasks in the dental office. There are certainly many systems that are effective and it is each team's choice as to which method suits their practice the best. The person, or persons, responsible for scheduling must be detail-oriented, persistent, and an effective communicator. In smaller practices, it may be that one person in the front office has the enormous responsibility of making appointments not only for the dentist, but also for the hygienist. This task becomes challenging as the practice grows and there are multiple rooms in which the dentist and hygienist(s) work. In some cases, one person simply can not engineer the schedule to maximize both productivity and the clinical personnel's energy level. The solution can be the addition of another front office person whose only responsibility is scheduling for the hygienist(s). This individual has adequate time to "work" the scheduling system and to create time needed for the longer procedures required for NSPT.

Time requirements for different phases of treatment and maintenance procedures should be considered. It must be kept in mind that there is a broad range of therapy in NSPT, and the establishment of time requirements can only serve as guidelines for providing services. The treatment approach itself must be individualized to fulfill the specific needs of each case (AAP, 1993) (see Chapter 6).

**Recare Scheduling Systems.** Initial NSPT will require a series of long therapy appointments followed by PMP. The consistent and careful maintenance for NSPT is vital to the continued stability of the periodontium once it has been achieved. Therefore, the scheduling system used by the office must achieve this goal. In order to address these scheduling needs, a brief discussion of the common recare systems is necessary. The intent of this discussion is not to comment in depth on a particular type of system, but to discuss only those elements of each system that affect the implementation of NSPT.

There are many variations of two main scheduling systems. First, clients can be appointed at the time the care is needed, which is referred to as nonprebooked systems. Secondly appointment for the next recare visit can occur, which is called a **prebooked system**. Both systems require an efficient schedule coordinator for maximum effectiveness. In an office where clients are not prebooked, the appointment book is only full a few weeks in advance and NSPT clients who telephone for an appointment can be accommodated fairly easily. However, the disadvantages of the nonprebooked system include the potential loss of clients through poor follow-up, inconsistent client compliance, and the overwhelming number of hours required by the schedule coordinator to manage this system. The nonprebooked system requires office-initiated contact with the client and client response to that contact. If the contact is by reminder postcard, which is common, the client must take the initiative to respond by telephoning the office. Many clients delay or forget to call, resulting in the need for another office-initiated contact. Many hours must be spent by the schedule coordinator to persistently follow-up on those individuals who do not respond. Without efficient back-up systems for tracking unscheduled clients, clients are lost or maintained at erratic and ineffective intervals.

With the prebooked system, the client, upon completion of initial therapy, is scheduled at the appropriate interval before leaving the office. This scheduling is completed by the dental hygienist, hygiene assistant, or schedule coordinator. Some dental hygienists prefer to prebook their clients themselves because they are able to disperse difficult appointments among easier ones and thereby control the dynamics of each day. Dental hygienists who accept responsibility for prebooking need to ensure that adequate appointment time is allotted to discuss scheduling with the client. Practitioners realize that making appointments with clients is sometimes a time-consuming responsibility. The client can be scheduled for PMP appointments from one month to six months in advance and a reminder card is sent two to three weeks ahead of the appointment. The front office personnel should still be responsible for appointments needed in the current ninety days, as these are the appointments most subject to change. The initial therapy appointments for NSPT, as well as any evaluation appointments and appointments for individuals new to the practice, will usually be scheduled by the front office personnel. A small number of clients might choose not to prebook due to unpredictable work schedules or travel plans. These clients are placed on a "pending" list and follow-up of some kind, either by postcard or telephone, will be required in order to schedule PMP.

Advantages of the prebooked system include retention of clients, less front office time spent tracking clients and "filling" the schedule, and increased client compliance to the recommended recare interval. One disadvantage of the prebooked system is that the current month's schedule might be prebooked so full that it does not easily accommodate the insertion of initial NSPT appointments. It is frustrating to have educated the client in the need for NSPT and obtained case acceptance, only to find that there is no time available in the upcoming weeks to initiate treatment. One way to combat this lack of appointment availability is to designate blocks of time for initial therapy in advance and then exercise discipline to ensure the time remains open for use by the schedule coordinator in the current month. The team might start by designating a two-hour block one morning and one afternoon per week. These blocks of time are not used for any prebooking of PMP. The amount of designated time can be adjusted to meet the specific needs of the practice. Standard recare postcards are available that inform the client that it is time for an examination. Because standardized formats do not address nonsurgical periodontal therapy, oral health care team members might choose to design a PMP card (see Figure 19-4). This reminder card can be used with either type of scheduling system. It is sent to confirm the prebooked appointment time or to request that the client telephone to arrange an appointment.

**Troubleshooting.** It is challenging to implement NSPT into a busy practice, because time must be accessible in the dental appointment book for long appointments. If operatory space and an assistant are both available, the

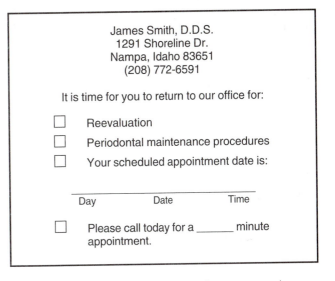

**Figure 19-4** Periodontal maintenance therapy recare/reminder card.

hygienist may be able to "double-book" clients who do not require long time blocks (see Figure 19-5). By utilizing two operatories, the hygienist can care for more clients in the day, freeing up time in the appointment book and increasing production (Hutchinson, 1993). This method requires that the dental hygienist perform only those tasks that cannot be delegated to the dental assistant, and that the assistant's use is maximized. All support tasks such as blood pressure monitoring, exposing and developing radiographs, preliminary oral self-care education, appointment scheduling, room turnover, and sterilization can and should be completed by the assistant. Time is reserved at the beginning of each appointment for the assistant to accomplish the necessary support tasks prior to the hygienist entering the operatory. The schedule in Figure 19-5 shows overlapping times when the dental assistant is with one client in one operatory and the dental hygienist is with another client in another operatory. The client benefits because the entire appointment is spent with an oral health care team member. The hygienist can remain punctual, and even if running late, knows that the client is receiving attention, thereby reducing stress for both the hygienist and the client (Blitz, 1994). While the hygienist is performing treatment, the assistant is free to assist with the dental examinations, dismiss the client, perform sterilization procedures, and to clean and set up the operatory for the next client. The assistant is also available to assist the hygienist with periodontal charting and other NSPT procedures.

There is a need for pertinent information gathered by the hygienist during the periodontal maintenance visit to be communicated to the dentist. This is easily accomplished during the examination when the hygienist and dentist are both present and can confer. When double-booking is employed, some dental hygienists are

| APPOINTMENT TIME | | CHAIR 1 | CHAIR 2 |
|---|---|---|---|
| | 0 | *Seat Pt #1 | |
| | 10 | **HYG TX** = 40 min | |
| **1:00** | 20 | | |
| | 30 | | |
| | 40 | | *Seat Pt #2 |
| | 50 | *Dismiss Pt #1 | **HYG TX** = 40 min |
| | 0 | | |
| | 10 | | |
| **2:00** | 20 | *Seat Pt #3 | |
| | 30 | **HYG TX** = 30 min | *Dismiss Pt #2 |
| | 40 | | |
| | 50 | | *Seat Pt #4 |
| | 0 | *Dismiss Pt #3 | **HYG TX** = 30 min |
| | 10 | | |
| **3:00** | 20 | *Seat Pt #5 | |
| | 30 | **HYG TX** = 40 min | *Dismiss Pt #4 |
| | 40 | | |
| | 50 | | |
| | 0 | | *Seat Pt #6 |
| | 10 | *Dismiss Pt #5 | **HYG TX** = 40 min |
| **4:00** | 20 | | |
| | 30 | | |
| | 40 | | |
| | 50 | | *Dismiss Pt #6 |

*ASSISTANT – those set in italics: Duties include seating/dismissing, blood pressure, appropriate radiographs, fluoride treatment, examination with dentist, preliminary oral self-care education, assisting with periodontal probing, cleanup, setup, and sterilization

**HYGIENIST (HYG)** – those set in boldface: Duties include all dental hygiene treatment that by law cannot be delegated to the dental assistant, oral self-care education, and treatment records

**Figure 19-5** Double-booking.

reluctant to delegate the communication of this important data to the dental assistant. Effective record keeping, chart notations, and verbal communication between the hygienist and assistant can give the hygienist the freedom to move to the next client, and the confidence that the necessary information will be received by the dentist.

Another way to gain some appointment time is to add another hygienist to the team. If operatory space is available, even adding dental hygiene care for one day a week provides ample appointments to begin implementing NSPT. If there is more than one hygienist and available space, an accelerated schedule might include one hygienist using two operatories for PMP or routine recare, and a second hygienist providing active NSPT or caring for clients new to the practice (see Figure 19-6). Both hygienists could share an assistant. When the practice can support this type of scheduling, there must be an extremely accomplished and dedicated front office person responsible for the appointment book.

Increasing the number of clients in a day also potentially increases the number of examinations for the dentist. Dentists and hygienists alike express concern that there is not enough time in an accelerated schedule to perform an examination on all clients. To alleviate the

| APPOINTMENT TIME | | CHAIR 1 | CHAIR 2 | CHAIR 3 |
|---|---|---|---|---|
| | | Dental Hygienist #1 | | Dental Hygienist #2 |
| | 0 | **Jack Jones** | | **Ray Johnson** |
| | 10 | PMP/3 mos. | | NSPT |
| **8:00** | 20 | Exam | | DE/SC/RP/Anes. |
| | 30 | | | Max./Mand. Rt. |
| | 40 | | | |
| | 50 | | **Ellen Rich** | |
| | 0 | | PMP/3 mos. | |
| | 10 | | No exam | |
| **9:00** | 20 | | | |
| | 30 | | | **Janice Gonzales** |
| | 40 | **James Smith** | | Reeval., probe |
| | 50 | Routine maintenance | | Selective polish |
| | 0 | BWX | | **Kay Anderson** |
| | 10 | Exam | | NP |
| **10:00** | 20 | | **Mabel Wright** | Exam |
| | 30 | | PMP/4 mos. | FMX |
| | 40 | | No Exam | |
| | 50 | | | |
| | 0 | **Carrie Lewis** | | |
| | 10 | Child | | |
| **11:00** | 20 | Exam | | **Frank Morton** |
| | 30 | | **Joshua Lewis** | Reeval., probe |
| | 40 | | Child | Selective polish |
| | 50 | | BWX/Exam | |

Accelerated Schedule – Two dental hygienists and one assistant

Dental Hygienist #1 – Two operatories for PMP or routine recare

Dental Hygienist #2 – Longer appointments for NSPT and clients new to the practice. Reevaluation appointments are also scheduled.

Dental Hygiene Assistant – Responsibilities would include those duties listed on Figure19-5.

**Figure 19-6** Accelerated schedule.

stress of multiple examinations, and at the same time meet the needs of the client, a schedule for restorative examination based on the recare interval can be established. Most NSPT clients will need frequent maintenance intervals of three months (Greenwell, Bissada, & Willwer, 1990), but might only need an examination by the dentist every six months. Other clients, having achieved a low caries rate and periodontal stability, might be seen by the hygienist every three months and have an examination with the dentist only once a year.

Another tool for gaining availability of time in the schedule is to use ten minute increments rather than the traditional fifteen minutes (McKenzie, 1993). If the office is currently using a fifteen-minute incremental schedule, then appointments are automatically set in thirty-, forty-five-, or sixty-minute lengths. Switching to an appointment sheet printed in ten-minute intervals provides more flexibility for all appointments, not just NSPT. Clients might require 40 minutes rather than 30, or 50 minutes rather than 60. Focus for care should be moved from a standard for all clients to individual treatment based on assessed needs (Kraemer & Gurenlian, 1989). This type of flexible scheduling allows the hygienist to precisely tailor the appointment time. Short appointments for reevaluation should be scheduled around longer appointments.

If the practice finds that the appointment book is congested with children's appointments, especially in the afternoons, one option is to incorporate a "kid's day." These days are best scheduled around a holiday or on days when schools are closed. All operatories are scheduled for children's appointments and each is staffed with a dental hygienist. The option of "double-booking" works well if one hygienist per operatory is not available. Four operatories scheduled with two hygienists, each utilizing an assistant, can provide care for many children in one day. It is best not to schedule the dentist with any operative procedures on this day because of the number of examinations required. Three or four of these days a year are usually sufficient to meet client demands. Offices might consider a theme or special client rewards to help make this extremely busy day enjoyable.

One last idea for gaining time in the appointment book is to evaluate the recare intervals at which clients are being seen. With careful assessment, intervals can and should be individualized. The dental hygiene profession should not feel bound by the standard six-month interval. Clients should be treated at intervals that allow their health to be maintained. This time period may prove to be nine months or even one year for those individuals with good periodontal health (Ramfjord, 1993). Look for those clients whose maintenance schedule can be lengthened. As the number of NSPT clients increases, more time will be needed for the recommended three-month interval for PMP.

## Fee Schedule

Factors that need to be considered in the development of a fee schedule include the following:

1. Competitiveness with other fees in the area.
2. Quality of services rendered.
3. Comprehensiveness of care provided.
4. Office production standards.
5. Inflation.

To assess competitiveness of fees, inquiry telephone calls concerning price ranges, rather than exact fees, are useful. Attendance at local professional meetings serves as another avenue to discuss these issues. Meeting with the periodontists to whom the practice will refer clients might provide some insight into their practice's fees. Customarily, charges in general practices are slightly lower than fees assessed in the periodontist's office. All professionals strive to provide quality care; however, fees might be adjusted according to what is possible to render at the initiation of the program. With time and experience, it is natural and it is hoped that the quality of care improves. In an established practice that has not previously had an NSPT program, there will be returning clients in need of NSPT who have been charged fees for oral prophylaxis that are lower than fees for initial NSPT and maintenance. The hygienist plays a key role in educating and informing the client of the difference between a routine prophylaxis and the definitive treatment necessary for NSPT. An established practice might consider raising NSPT fees *gradually* to enhance rapport with clients of record.

Nonsurgical programs will be comprehensive; however, over time, services become more comprehensive and predictable. Usually the fee for intraoral and extraoral assessment requires a charge separate from the therapy rendered. Due to the varying factors involved in NSPT, the fee schedule might be established as a range based on the classification of periodontal disease and the extent of dental hygiene care planned. The fee will be dependent on the severity of the case and/or the amount of time needed to provide the individual care plan. The fee can be determined and presented to the client per service rendered (e.g., per quadrant of scaling/root planing/debridement) or as a total package without breaking down the fee for each component of therapy. The hygienist must include fees for supportive therapy such as nitrous oxide analgesia and/or local anesthesia, systemic antibiotic therapy, fiber therapy, overhang removal, desensitization, or subgingival irrigation. The fee for the reevaluation appointment must also be considered. Periodontal fiber therapy has a corresponding insurance code and a significant fee for this service is charged. This supportive care is customarily charged as a separate fee from scaling/root planing/debridement therapy. On the other hand, overhang removal, per se, is not covered by insurance and is part of scaling/root planing/debridement therapy; therefore, the fee for margination is considered within the fee charged for scaling/root planing/debridement.

The hygienist also considers recommendations for client self-care in the fee for care. The incorporation of an oral irrigator or automated toothbrush can be an essential part of maintenance and serve as a motivational factor for the client. The client might purchase the recommended aid, requiring that the clinician follow-up on compliance. This follow-up necessitates that the aid be brought to the office for instructions in use and care, as well as observation of use to assure effective bacterial plaque removal without damaging the periodontium. Another option for incorporating a home care device would be to supply the client with the recommended aid during the in-office therapy affording immediate instruction in its use and care. In this case, the fee for the aid is either included in the total fee for NSPT or the aid is given to the client upon completion of treatment as an added incentive.

Office production standards have previously been discussed and involve the team philosophy and goals, the number of personnel used to deliver NSPT, and overhead factors. Inflation will affect reassignment of fees. It is the decision of each practice or employer to determine how often fees should be raised. One suggestion is to consider adjustments yearly and to base the increase on the inflation rate as well as enhancements incorporated into the NSPT program. Increasing fees annually makes the increment, from the client's standpoint, justifiable as compared to larger fee increases determined every three to five years.

## Insurance

The availability of dental benefit plans plays an important role in the financial considerations associated with NSPT and involves the collaboration of the dental hygienist and the front office personnel handling insurance. In the course of educating the client and presenting the proposed therapy for NSPT, the hygienist may be the first source of information concerning insurance coverage for periodontal services. In the previous discussion on fee scheduling, customary and usual insurance fees were not included as a factor in establishing fees. Although it would be naive to assume that they have no role in helping to establish fees in the area, it would be nonproductive to let maximum insurance fees determine the charges. When a practice's fees parallel customary and usual insurance fees and methods of payment of different plans, clients are charged differently for the same quality and comprehensiveness of nonsurgical care. This approach seems unethical if not unprofessional. The AAP maintains the philosophy that the development of a care plan should be according to professional standards rather than according to the provisions of the insurance contract (AAP, 1995a).

An insurance system has been established for classifications of periodontal disease (see Chapter 1). The client must be informed of the differences between a routine prophylaxis (normal periodontal health), scaling in the presence of gingival inflammation (Case Type 1), and the definitive treatment necessary for the maintenance of periodontal disease (Case Type II, III, IV, V). As an incentive for prevention, many insurance companies in the United States will provide better coverage for a routine prophylaxis than for periodontal procedures. In addition to the differences in coverage between procedures, dental benefit plans vary as to the allowable interval for maintenance in a given year. Some plans provide coverage for appointments scheduled six months apart, while others may limit the coverage to once per year. If the coverage is intended for twice per year, it is advisable to determine if the appointments *must* be at six month intervals. Many insurance carriers will not provide coverage if the client is scheduled for an appointment prior to the six month

date. An insurance carrier might provide more frequent coverage for PMP upon receiving documentation of the periodontal condition from the dentist and hygienist, along with the rationale for more frequent care (see Chapter 16). If the carrier does not provide coverage at three- or four-month intervals, the client assumes responsibility for payment of PMP fees. The hygienist plays a key role in educating and motivating the client to accepting responsibility for the long-term benefits of periodontal health.

Variations may exist between dental benefit plans as to the use of certain codes for particular procedures, the frequency in which the codes may be used, and the amount that may be charged for each code. If questions arise concerning specific benefit plans, the front office personnel communicates with the carrier before treatment begins. This procedure ensures accurate reporting of periodontal services and provides the best possible coverage for the client and the practice. Definitions and explanations of procedures exist to promote accurate reporting and to aid in consistent interpretation of periodontal services provided under dental benefit programs. The most frequently used codes for NSPT are listed in Table 19-2 (AAP, 1995a; AAP, 1995b).

When submitting a claim form, the front office personnel must include a written diagnosis, the AAP case type, the proper code number with the listing of the treatment to be performed or already completed, and the estimated or actual fee charged for each service (AAP, 1995a). The AAP makes the following recommendations when submitting claims for periodontal maintenance (04910) (AAP, 1995b):

1. Code 00120 (periodic oral examination) may be used for assessment in conjunction with 04910 (periodontal maintenance procedures).
2. Documentation of prior active therapy may be requested. Writing "previous active therapy" on the claim form will ensure proper benefits.
3. Claims should not alternate between 01110 (adult prophylaxis) and 04910. Code 04910 should be used as many times as it is actually performed.
4. If the fee is lower due to missing teeth in a quadrant, note "partial quadrant" on the claim form with a brief description.

Examples of claim forms completed for nonsurgical services are shown in Figure 19-7. All supporting documentation such as the diagnosis, periodontal charting, and radiographs should be included with insurance billing to alleviate time delays.

This discussion concerning insurance has been presented in an attempt to help practitioners plan a program and understand some basic principles of insurance policies and carriers. The AAP reviews insurance codes and procedures every few years; therefore, codes presented in Table 19-2 are subject to change. It is imperative that the hygienist and the front office personnel update infor-

**Table 19-2  Insurance Codes for Nonsurgical/Adjunctive Services**

| Code | Procedure | Definition |
|------|-----------|------------|
| *00120 | Periodic oral examination | Performed on a patient of record who has had previous comprehensive or periodic examination. |
| *00150 | Comprehensive oral examination | Typically includes the evaluation and recording of periodontal conditions. |
| 01110 | Adult prophylaxis | Scaling/polishing for patients with normal or good periodontal health. May require more than one appointment or one extended appointment. |
| 01310 | Nutritional counseling for the control of dental disease | Counseling on dietary habits as part of the treatment and control of periodontal disease. |
| 01320 | Tobacco counseling for the control of oral disease | Reduce patient risks of developing tobacco-related oral diseases. Improves prognosis for certain dental therapies. |
| 01330 | Oral hygiene instructions | May include instructions for self-care, including the use of special oral hygiene aids. |
| 04341 | Periodontal scaling and root planing, per quadrant | Therapeutic procedure performed on patients with periodontal disease. May be definitive treatment or a presurgical procedure. |
| 04355 | Full-mouth debridement to enable comprehensive periodontal evaluation and diagnosis | Preliminary procedure to remove subgingival and/or supragingival plaque. Does not preclude the need for other procedures. |
| 04381 | Localized delivery of chemotherapeutic agents, per tooth, by report | Short-term use of a controlled time-release therapeutic agent. Does not replace conventional or surgical therapy. |
| 04910 | Periodontal maintenance procedures (following active therapy) | Periodic maintenance treatment following periodontal therapy (exclusive of 04355). Not synonymous with prophylaxis. |
| 09630 | Other drugs and/or medicaments, by report | Includes, but is not limited to, oral antibiotics, oral analgesics, oral sedatives, and topical fluoride dispensed in the office for home use. |
| 09910 | Application of desensitizing medicaments | Includes in-office treatment for root sensitivity. |

*See Chapter 3 for further discussion.

(Data from American Academy of Periodontology, Insurance reporting update, Department of Scientific , Clinical, and Educational Affairs, Chicago, 1995b)

mation when necessary and be knowledgeable in the use of the codes for nonsurgical and adjunctive services. A printed office fee schedule with AAP classifications, codes, number of appointments estimated, and a range of fees for services is useful for enhanced communication and standardization between the dental hygienist, schedule coordinator, and the person responsible for insurance. It requires occasional updating, but provides an effective means of sharing responsibility in NSPT.

## Legal Documentation

In general, the **standard of care** in dentistry requires dentists and/or dental hygienists to provide the same level of care as provided by other practitioners, under similar circumstances (Morris, 1995; Palat, 1989; Zarkowski, 1990). State laws vary concerning the definition, but traditionally the "same community" standard of care pro-

vides that the practitioner must practice with the same skill and knowledge as other members of the profession in the same community. This definition has been expanded to the "same or similar localities" in many legal decisions, which allows a locality to set the standard of practice (Morris, 1995). A more progressive view of the standard of care is the "state of the art" concept which holds all practitioners to the same standard, regardless of where they practice (Morris, 1995). Another factor that could be considered in determining appropriate standard of care is the "prudent practice" guideline that includes methods taught in dental schools, continuing education courses, and/or covered in textbooks or articles (Zinman, 1990). In the case of NSPT, courts have been proven to expect thorough diagnosis and treatment consistent with the standards of a specialist, if the patient is not referred (Ebersold, 1989). The standard of care concerning the performance of a dental hygienist

EXAMPLE: STATEMENT OF ACTUAL SERVICES

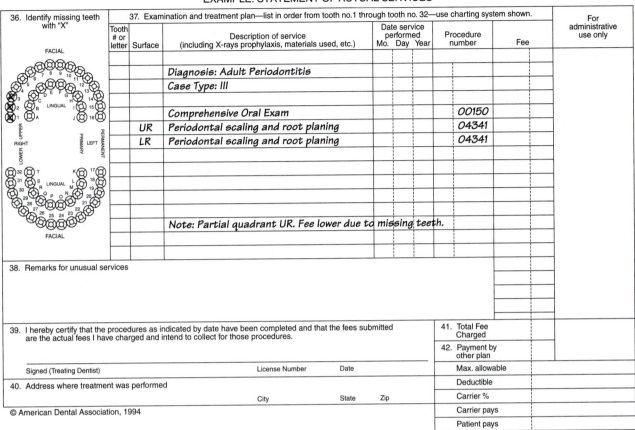

| 36. Identify missing teeth with "X" | 37. Examination and treatment plan—list in order from tooth no.1 through tooth no. 32—use charting system shown. | | | | | | For administrative use only |
|---|---|---|---|---|---|---|---|
| | Tooth # or letter | Surface | Description of service (including X-rays prophylaxis, materials used, etc.) | Date service performed Mo. Day Year | Procedure number | Fee | |
| | | | Diagnosis: Adult Periodontitis | | | | |
| | | | Case Type: III | | | | |
| | | | Comprehensive Oral Exam | | 00150 | | |
| | UR | | Periodontal scaling and root planing | | 04341 | | |
| | LR | | Periodontal scaling and root planing | | 04341 | | |
| | | | Note: Partial quadrant UR. Fee lower due to missing teeth. | | | | |

38. Remarks for unusual services

| 39. I hereby certify that the procedures as indicated by date have been completed and that the fees submitted are the actual fees I have charged and intend to collect for those procedures. | 41. Total Fee Charged | |
|---|---|---|
| | 42. Payment by other plan | |
| Signed (Treating Dentist)        License Number        Date | Max. allowable | |
| 40. Address where treatment was performed | Deductible | |
| City        State        Zip | Carrier % | |
| © American Dental Association, 1994 | Carrier pays | |
| | Patient pays | |

EXAMPLE: PERIODONTAL MAINTENANCE PROCEDURES

| 36. Identify missing teeth with "X" | 37. Examination and treatment plan—list in order from tooth no.1 through tooth no. 32—use charting system shown. | | | | | | For administrative use only |
|---|---|---|---|---|---|---|---|
| | Tooth # or letter | Surface | Description of service (including X-rays prophylaxis, materials used, etc.) | Date service performed Mo. Day Year | Procedure number | Fee | |
| | | | Periodic Oral Exam | | 00120 | | |
| | | | Periodontal Maintenance Procedures | | 04910 | | |
| | | | Note: Previous active therapy – treatment completed xx/xx/xx | | | | |

38. Remarks for unusual services

| 39. I hereby certify that the procedures as indicated by date have been completed and that the fees submitted are the actual fees I have charged and intend to collect for those procedures. | 41. Total Fee Charged | |
|---|---|---|
| | 42. Payment by other plan | |
| Signed (Treating Dentist)        License Number        Date | Max. allowable | |
| 40. Address where treatment was performed | Deductible | |
| City        State        Zip | Carrier % | |
| © American Dental Association, 1994 | Carrier pays | |
| | Patient pays | |

**Figure 19-7** Insurance claim form. (Courtesy of the American Dental Association, 1994)

has not been tested at this point in time (Morris, 1995). As consumers of dental hygiene care become increasingly aware of dental hygiene practice and changes occur in supervisory laws, hygienists will be held to a greater degree of accountability for their actions (DeVore, 1993).

The standard of care in NSPT requires first the recognition of periodontal disease and then the gathering of information necessary for diagnosis, followed by actual treatment and maintenance. Documentation is necessary not only for the treatment phase of periodontal disease, but becomes the legal proof of the diagnosis and subsequent care provided. The most commonly unrecorded disease entity in dentistry is periodontal disease (Ebersold, 1989). The findings of a 1988 study published in the Journal of Periodontology, showed that out of 2,488 records chosen at random in thirty-six dental practices, only 16 percent were complete or adequate in regard to periodontal information (McCullough, 1993; McFall & Bader, 1988). It is essential for the dental hygienist involved in NSPT to be aware of what constitutes acceptable record keeping. Refer to Table 19-3 for a review of basic components of the dental record recommended by the American Dental Association (ADA, 1987).

Failure to diagnose and inform patients of periodontal disease resulted in 62 percent of all dental malpractice lawsuits in 1990 (McCullough, 1993). Because claims have been made against dentists for failure to detect and properly treat periodontal disease more than any other single disease of the mouth (Morris, 1995), it is in the best interest of practitioners to record detailed progress notes (Item 8, Table 19-3). The record of services should include chronological documentation of treatment provided as well as all contacts with the

**Table 19-3 Basic Components of the Dental Record**

|  | Description |
| --- | --- |
| 1. Identification Data | Personal information, insurance information, emergency information |
| 2. Medical History | Comprehensive evaluation of general health |
| 3. Dental History | Chief complaint, past dental experiences, family history |
| 4. Clinical Examination | Assessment, radiographs |
| 5. Diagnosis | Clearly written in record |
| 6. Treatment Plan | Preferred plan, options for treatment and referrals |
| 7. Informed Consent | Written, verbal, or both |
| 8. Progress Notes | Chronological record of services provided |
| 9. Completion Notes | Termination of care by the dentist, or at the request of the patient |

client. Table 19-6 lists items to consider including in the record of services to thoroughly document progress in treatment.

**Informed consent** (see Chapter 8) is a critical component of NSPT and the record of services. The client must be informed of all aspects of treatment including specific fees, optional plans, potential risks, and consequences of not pursuing treatment on a level the client understands. Given this information, the individual then has the choice of continuing with, or declining, the proposed treatment. The client must be given the opportunity to ask questions. If the client declines treatment, the reasons should be documented in the permanent record. Acceptance of treatment may be indicated by either verbal agreement, which must be documented in the record, or by written, signed consent. Properly performed informed consent involves the active participation of the client, and reduces the likelihood of malpractice litigation (Bressman, 1993).

Preceding chapters have included aspects of NSPT that must be included in the permanent record of services for legal documentation. The dentist and hygienist must keep in mind general guidelines to ensure quality record keeping and maintain consistency in the practice. Dental records should be in legible handwriting, typewritten, or computerized. If abbreviations are used, they should be readily understood, or a key provided. The record should be dated, completed in pen, and signed or initialed by the provider of the service. If dental records contain omissions or errors, it might lead to misinterpretations (Burns & Haun, 1989). Likewise, additions that are crowded in the margins, or between lines, may be misconstrued. Every attempt should be made to utilize the space provided and not skip lines between entries. If an error is made, a single line should be drawn through the entry, and the correction made, including the reason(s) for the correction. All changes or additions to the record of services should be made within a reasonable length of time. The entry should be initialed and dated using the date in which the changes are made, with a note that the information was not included on the original date (Zarkowski, 1990). Signs of erasures or the use of a whiting agent should not be present in the record. All information obtained during the assessment, diagnosis and treatment of the client, including health history information, should be considered confidential and should be released only with the client's written consent (DeVore, 1995).

Depending on the statute of limitations within a state, litigation can occur years after the client is treated in a dental practice, further reenforcing the need for thorough documentation (Zarkowski, 1991). Records should be kept for at least the period of the statute of limitations in the local jurisdiction. This period varies from state to state. Prior to discarding records, the practitioner should be aware of the length of the statute of limitations and any related laws unique to the state. The best advice is to retain records indefinitely. Records should

**Table 19-4 Specific Progress Notes**

| Item | Example |
|---|---|
| 1. Significant health history findings and precautions | • Antibiotic prophylactic regime for rheumatic heart disease<br>• Diabetes (type and necessary precautions) |
| 2. Significant assessment findings | • Lesions and descriptions<br>• Localized vertical bony defect |
| 3. Significant statements (communication) from the client concerning any phase of treatment | • "I will never floss."<br>• "I know you think radiographs are valuable, but I do not want them." |
| 4. Diagnosis of the extent of periodontal disease including dental hygiene diagnosis | • Record the periodontal classification<br>• Stable/deteriorating |
| 5. Oral self-care education presented including chief complaint, conditions, theories, aids, and client skill level | • Conditions: pockets, bleeding sites, LOA, furcations, etc.<br>• Aids: soft toothbrush or automated brush; interdental brush<br>• Skill: performs Bass technique well. |
| 6. Compliance or lack of compliance with self-care recommendations | • Brushing twice daily with soft brush, Bass method<br>• Not using the interdental brush |
| 7. Informed consent | • Consented to treatment except for in-office and home fluoride |
| 8. Consultation with physicians, specialists, or other health professionals | • Antibiotic coverage indicated for prosthetic hip per Dr. _____'s instructions.   Rx: _____ |
| 9. Referral to physicians, specialists, or other health professional | • To periodontist to evaluate extensive loss of attached gingiva<br>• To specialist for implant |
| 10. Prescriptions written with pertinent details | • Type of antibiotic coverage and regime<br>• Chlorhexidine and regime |
| 11. Administration of medicine or drugs | • Local anesthesia<br>• Nitrous oxide-oxygen analgesia |
| 12. Treatment rendered, including basic component of care and detailed information about the therapy and location | • Debridement performed mandibular right<br>• Ultrasonic devices and hand instruments<br>• Marginations #14 M, #12 D<br>• Placement of periodontal fiber #14, #15 |
| 13. Reactions to treatment rendered | • Hematoma<br>• Topical anesthetic caused significant tissue sloughing and pain |
| 14. Significant factors about the care plan including important notations for the next appointment | • Recheck lesion<br>• Reprobe<br>• Reevaluate plaque removal #4 and #5 |
| 15. Prognosis of care | • Retaining #2 and #3 is doubtful; client chooses not to be referred to a periodontist |
| 16. Cancellations, no-shows, late arrivals, or appointment changes | • Cancellation for initial NSPT 30 minutes prior to appointment<br>• Arrived 30 minutes late for one-hour dental hygiene appointment |
| 17. Periodontal maintenance procedure interval and compliance | • Three-month or four-month<br>• Has not scheduled PMP for one year |

contain, at the minimum, all relevant clinical data (including radiographs), all diagnoses (classification of periodontal disease), and a chronological record of all treatment provided (Ebersold, 1989). Just as documentation provides the legal proof of the care provided in NSPT, failure to document might be viewed as a failure to provide treatment (Bressman, 1993; Burns & Haun, 1989). If in doubt about what to record, it is probably wis-est to include all pertinent information rather than omit something that could be useful in the future. In establishing an NSPT program, oral health professionals are challenged to stay informed of new developments and research, to provide the client with the established standard of care, and to maintain well-documented records for the benefit of the practice, the individuals delivering care, and above all, for the client.

## MONITORING AND EVALUATION

Once an NSPT program has been implemented, monitoring of each phase of the program is necessary to ensure continued success. The office team should determine if established goals are being met, how well individual team members are performing their jobs, and how well the resources involved in the implementation phase meet the needs of the practice. Continual monitoring of these factors provides an opportunity to "fine-tune" the existing program or make necessary adjustments and/or revisions before problems occur. An example of a monitoring checklist is presented in Table 19-5. Each team member involved in the NSPT program should assess the goals and aspects of implementation. A column for comments could be added to the check-list to identify improvements, suggestions, or areas of concern to address at future staff meetings. This type of check-list puts the entire program in perspective and is a viable component of the evaluation process. Evaluation of a program consists of measuring the progress and effectiveness of each phase, identifying problems, and planning revisions and modifications (Mann, 1988). The evaluation of an NSPT program might consist of an evaluation of the program as a whole as discussed above, an evaluation of the performance of each team member, and an evaluation of therapy provided to each individual.

**Performance evaluations**, or appraisals, provide a way to communicate expectations to each member of the dental team, identify ways to improve technical skills or behavior, and serve as a basis for salary adjustments or additional compensation (Barr, 1993). The emphasis of

**Table 19-5  Nonsurgical Periodontal Therapy Monitoring Sheet**

| Phase | Questions | Yes (Y) or No (N) | Comments |
|---|---|---|---|
| Development | 1. Has there been an increase in periodontal therapy? (Refer to periodontal client percentage.) | Y | There was a significant increase in initial therapy and supportive care this month. |
| | 2. Are there personnel needs and is the staff well-utilized? | Y | Dental hygienists need more assistance with periodontal charting. |
| | 3. Has there been an increase in dental hygiene production? | Y | A 20% increase occurred in one month out of the last three months evaluated. |
| Implementation | 1. Are enough operatories available? | Y | |
| | 2. Are the supplies adequate? | N | Two ultrasonic scaling devices and four sets of subgingival precision-thin inserts are needed. Specific interdental aids need to be selected and ordered. Order educational information on periodontal disease from ADA. |
| | 3. Are the forms current and useful? | N | Consider developing another periodontal assessment chart form that includes recording of *all* disease entities. It should be easy to compare data from appointment to appointment. |
| | 4. Is dental hygiene scheduling adequate? | N | Time is needed for 1-hour to 1½-hour PMP appointments. Consider an accelerated schedule. |
| | 5. Are the fees charged reasonable/appropriate? | Y | |
| | 6. Is insurance well-explained and processed? | Y | A study of appropriate codes is necessary. Dental hygiene assistants are aiding in explanations. |
| | 7. Is documentation on clients' records thorough and consistent? | Y | The standardization meeting for hygienists and assistants was successful. |
| | 8. Other *Discuss a specific monitoring system using client data.* | Y | Schedule a staff meeting in one month to discuss monitoring. Be prepared with written suggestions. |

performance appraisal systems has evolved from being personality-based to being criteria-based and the focus is on performance rather than on the person (McConnell, 1993). An important consideration in the development or selection of a performance evaluation system is that it is objective, meaning that the job and the expected performance must be clearly defined (Rotty, 1994). Variations in performance are customarily evaluated through the use of a rating scale (see Chapter 18). A behavioral-based system is just one of many objective systems used to measure performance. This type of system is based on employee behaviors and is easily adapted to a dental practice. The performance evaluation can focus on specific clinical skills, such as the ability to perform accurate assessments, take diagnostic radiographs, or perform periodontal instrumentation in an efficient manner, in addition to nonclinical skills, such as communication with clients or willingness to help team members (Rotty, 1994). Regardless of which appraisal system is utilized, the development and use of a performance evaluation will result in a motivated, productive team, which will further strengthen an NSPT program.

Evaluation of the effectiveness of NSPT for each client is an ongoing process. The dental hygienist will play a major role in evaluation, which occurs in three stages: as care is being rendered, at the reevaluation appointment after performance of initial or active NSPT, and as part of the continuing care provided by PMP (DeVore,

Hicks, & Claman, 1989). Evaluation will include assessment of the procedures performed during therapy such as periodontal instrumentation, as well as assessment of the periodontal status to determine the presence or absence of disease. Clinical measures such as attachment loss, identification of bleeding sites, mobility, and furcation involvement must be supplemented periodically by radiographic evaluation. The effectiveness of self-care procedures and the presence of risk factors are additional points to consider in the evaluation of each client's periodontal status. Long-term maintenance requires comparing periodontal assessments at regular intervals and conclusions will help determine the effectiveness of the NSPT program for each client. At this point in time, the clinician must determine if the client should continue with the recommended periodontal maintenance schedule or if modifications are in order such as more frequent PMP, or possibly a return to active NSPT. It is beneficial to periodically assess the overall success rate of NSPT for the clients in the practice by randomly selecting charts to review stability of periodontal probing, attachment loss, and bleeding sites. This random assessment can be categorized and tallied much like the periodontal client percentage previously presented (see Figure 19-2). The overall goal of stopping the progression of disease must be considered when trying to determine those factors that indicate success of NSPT.

## Summary

An NSPT program benefits the client, the employer/dentist, and the dental hygienist. The team concept is critical in planning and carrying out the established goals for NSPT that will have a direct correlation to the benefits derived from successful implementation. Each member of the team will experience satisfaction from a program that emphasizes quality care and the team concept. The benefits discussed herein for the dental hygienist may be applied to all members of the dental team involved in NSPT. Raising the client's awareness of periodontal health and involving the client in all aspects of care leads to a higher acceptance of care planning recommendations, resulting in a more motivated client. In most instances, it is beneficial to complete nonsurgical periodontal therapy to establish a healthy environment before initiating further treatment such as final restorations and reconstruction. In the presence of a healthy environment, the client is more likely to opt for comprehensive and/or cosmetic dentistry, which benefits the client as well as the practice. The long-term benefits of PMP allow most clients to experience improved oral health without surgery. If the individual is compliant with self-

care recommendations and frequent PMP visits, the chances of needing more aggressive treatment are reduced.

The implementation of an NSPT program ensures that oral health care professionals are treating clients according to the standard of care. The delegation of duties to trained, educated employees will lead to a higher level of commitment, which is rewarding for all concerned. The prevention and treatment of periodontal disease is not only a service that is in demand, but one that can be productive for the practice (Levin, 1991). In addition to the production gained from periodontal services, the restorative needs stimulated by periodontal therapy will help increase a dental practice's volume (Christensen, 1991). Involvement in an NSPT program creates an opportunity for the dental hygienist to enhance education. Sharing responsibility for the practice's periodontal health by participating in the development and implementation of an NSPT program will give the dental hygienist an opportunity for upward mobility and presents the type of challenge and motivation that leads to longevity in the profession or in a given practice.

# Case Studies

**Case Study One:** A dental hygienist has worked for three years in a relatively new practice that does not have an established NSPT program. The hygienist has attended continuing education courses on NSPT and would like to implement a program in the practice. The dentist/employer does not feel that the practice has enough clients with periodontitis to warrant implementation of a new program. What steps could the hygienist take to determine the need?

**Case Study Two:** Susan Jones, a dental hygienist experienced in NSPT, begins working in an established practice that has traditionally scheduled all clients at six-month intervals. The practice policy is to routinely refer clients with "active periodontal disease" to the periodontist for all aspects of periodontal care. Susan notes that many of the returning clients have periodontal probe readings of 4 to 6 mm, mild to moderate gingival inflammation, and attachment loss. The front office person has been with the practice ten years and handles all the scheduling. The dentist has been in practice for twenty-three years and does not perform periodontal therapy. What communication will be effective for the implementation of NSPT into this practice?

**Case Study Three:** This practice has two full-time hygienists and a busy dentist. The prebooked dental hygiene schedule uses fifteen-minute intervals and the appointment book is full for eight weeks. How can time be created for routine oral prophylaxis appointments and long NSPT appointments?

**Case Study Four:** Bill Evans, a 42-year-old construction worker, has not had dental hygiene care in ten years and presents himself for a routine prophylaxis and examination. He is in excellent health. Plaque and calculus deposits are heavy. Examination findings include generalized gingival inflammation with probing depths of 5 to 6 mm on posterior proximal surfaces. Radiographic evaluation reveals moderate bone loss. The presumptive periodontal diagnosis is moderate adult periodontitis and moderate bone loss. Bill does not have a chief complaint but has just acquired dental insurance that covers "100% of preventive services." What should the hygienist consider in determining the fee for service and what might the role of the front office personnel be in fee presentation?

**Case Study Five:** Jane Adams, a 24-year-old secretary, is a new client to the practice and mentions "bleeding gums," which is her chief complaint. Health history findings indicate that she is in good health. Jane indicates that she is "nervous to receive dental treatment." The periodontal assessment reveals the following:

1. Generalized severe gingival inflammation.
2. Generalized moderate to heavy plaque and calculus deposits.
3. Gingival recession in posterior regions with accompanying sensitivity.
4. Pocket depths of 4 to 5 mm in posterior regions with generalized bleeding upon probing.
5. A full-mouth series of radiographs showing early bone loss.

Jane is informed of the assessment findings and the need for definitive treatment for periodontal instrumentation, followed by a reevaluation appointment. Local anesthesia and desensitization are recommended, but Jane refuses anesthesia. Jane has had nitrous oxide analgesia in the past and would like nitrous oxide again. Jane states that she brushes twice a day, but does not floss. Self-care education is given that includes modifications in brushing technique. Prior to dismissal, Jane is appointed for three, one-hour appointments for debridement. Based on the above information, write a description of the services provided for the record of services.

# Case Study Discussions

**Discussion—Case Study One:** The dental hygienist determines the periodontal needs of the practice by figuring the periodontal client percentage as follows:

1. Refine assessment skills to identify those clients with periodontal disease, utilizing the American Academy of Periodontology's classification system. The hygienist should consider individuals with early stages of periodontitis, as well as clients with advancing stages and aggressive disease.
2. Select the number of months to be used for a monitoring period.
3. During the specified monitoring period, track the total number of clients seen for dental hygiene services and the total number of clients who would benefit from NSPT. The total number of clients might range from those requiring debridement with subsequent maintenance appointments, to those who require referral for surgical evaluation.
4. Compare the total number of clients seen, to the total number requiring NSPT to yield the periodontal client percentage.

**Discussion—Case Study Two:** Because Susan is a new employee, it is wise not to try to change the practice too quickly. Some time will be needed to learn opinions and attitudes of the staff and dentist. Susan should first share concerns with the dentist and express the desire to treat clients earlier in the disease process to possibly prevent the need for referral in the future. All data gathered during assessment should be presented to the dentist during examinations so that proper diagnosis can be made. Once the dentist lends support to NSPT and goals are established, proceeding one case at a time might ease the front office person into the scheduling requirements. In staff meetings, sharing goals for meeting individual needs of the clients and expectations for the practice in general will involve and motivate the entire staff.

**Discussion—Case Study Three:** The following options should be considered:

1. Change the appointment book to ten-minute intervals and carefully monitor the time needed for each procedure.
2. Eliminate some examinations. Clients who return frequently, or at three-month intervals, might not need an examination by the dentist at each visit.
3. If general supervision is allowed, consider providing dental hygiene care when the dentist is out of the office.
4. Consider adding a dental hygiene assistant to accomplish all tasks that can be delegated; thus allowing hygienists to care for more clients.
5. If operatory space and/or a dental assistant is available, double-book clients by using two operatories per hygienist, each utilizing an assistant.

**Discussion—Case Study Four:** The dental hygienist must first determine the need for supportive therapy. Consider whether local anesthesia and desensitization are necessary. A reevaluation appointment is indicated. These services could be included in the fee for periodontal instrumentation. Bill must be educated and informed of the differences between a routine prophylaxis and the definitive treatment necessary for moderate adult periodontitis. Due to the length of time since Bill's last dental hygiene appointment, the amount of deposits, and the periodontal diagnosis, several appointments will be needed for dental hygiene care and reevaluation. The front office personnel handling insurance will want to establish the percentage that Bill's dental benefit plan covers for periodontal procedures in order to give Bill an estimate of his share of the total fee. Bill must be informed of all aspects of care including specific fees, optional plans, potential risks, and consequences of not pursuing NSPT prior to continuing other treatment.

**Discussion—Case Study Five:** New client: oral exam, restorative exam and periodontal assessment. Chief complaint: "bleeding gums." Discussed periodontal disease progression and related to gingival inflammation—bleeding—pocket depths. Adult periodontitis with early bone loss. Discussed recession/loss of attachment and sensitivity; recommended in-office desensitization. Informed client of need for debridement and recommended local anesthesia. Received informed consent for all aspects of care *except* local anesthesia. Client requests nitrous oxide. Reviewed brushing technique and modified to Bass technique to promote gingival stimulation; client demonstrated technique well. Does not floss due to a management discrepancy. Flossing technique appeared adequate. Focus on interproximal cleansing as periodontal instrumentation progresses. Reappointed for three one-hour appointments. Reevaluation appointment necessary. Next appointment: nitrous oxide for debridement in mandibular R, begin maxillary R—desensitization—evaluate brushing—recommend saline rinse. FMX (16 PA's 4 BWX) 15/90 12 imp.

Note: Abbreviations can be used if they are readily understood, or a key is provided on the record of services form. The entry must be signed, or initialed, by the provider of the service.

## REFERENCES

American Academy of Periodontology. (1989a). Consensus Report, Discussion Section II. *Proceedings of the world workshop in clinical periodontics* (pp. II-13). Chicago: American Academy of Periodontology.

American Academy of Periodontology. (1989b). Consensus Report, Discussion Section IX. *Proceedings of the world workshop in clinical periodontics* (pp. IX 24-26). Chicago: American Academy of Periodontology.

American Academy of Periodontology. (1989c). Consensus Report, Summary of Plenary Session. *Proceedings of the world workshop in clinical periodontics* (pp. IX-27). Chicago: American Academy of Periodontology.

American Academy of Periodontology. (1993, June). *Guidelines for periodontal therapy.* Chicago: American Academy of Periodontology, Department of Scientific, Clinical, and Educational Affairs, 1-5.

American Academy of Periodontology. (1995a). *Current procedural terminology for periodontics and insurance reporting manual* (7th ed.). Chicago: American Academy of Periodontology.

American Academy of Periodontology. (1995b). *Insurance reporting update.* Chicago: American Academy of Periodontology, Department of Scientific, Clinical, and Educational Affairs.

American Dental Association. (1987). *The dental patient record: Structure and function guidelines.* Chicago, 1–12.

Barr, E. S. (1993). Enhancing staff performance through a customized evaluation form. *Journal of the American Dental Association, 124,* 51–53.

Blitz, P. (1994). It takes two. *RDH, 14*(9), 18–25.

Boyer, E. M. (1990). The roles of other dental personnel in the patient care provided by dental hygienists in traditional and non-traditional settings. *Journal of Dental Hygiene, 64*(2), 86–89.

Brady, W. F. (1984). Periodontal disease awareness. *Journal of the American Dental Association, 109,* 706–710.

Bressman, J. K. (1993). Risk management for the 90's. *Journal of the American Dental Association, 124,* 64–67.

Burns, S. & Haun, J. (1989). The "5-R's" for nonsurgical periodontal treatment in the general practice. *Seminars in Dental Hygiene, 1*(2), 1–5.

Christensen, G. J. (1992). Why do most GP's shun periodontics? *Journal of the American Dental Association, 123,* 75–76.

DeVore, C. H., Hicks, M. J., & Claman, L. (1989). A system for insuring success of long-term supportive periodontal therapy. *Journal of Dental Hygiene, 63*(5), 214–220.

DeVore, C. H. (1993). Professional liability. *RDH, 13*(8), 12–14.

DeVore, C. H. (1995). Keep it under locks. *RDH, 15*(2), 31–32.

Ebersold, L. A. (1989). Periodontal malpractice: Current standards and record keeping requirements. *Journal of the Michigan Dental Association, 71*(9), 483–486.

Fisher, E. (1990). General dentist and periodontist working together. *Compendium, 11*(7), 454–456.

Greenwell, H., Bissada, N., & Willwer, J. (1990). Periodontics in general practice: Professional plaque control. *Journal of the American Dental Association, 121,* 642–644.

Hamman, K. (1992). *Factors influencing dental hygiene job retention in the private practice setting.* Unpublished master's thesis, Old Dominion University, Norfolk, VA.

Hall, W. B. & Sumner, C. F. (1994). Referral to a periodontist. In Hall, Roberts, & LaBarre (Eds.), *Decision making in dental treatment planning.* St. Louis: Mosby-Year Book, Inc.

Hicks, M. J., Uldricks, J. M., Whitacre, H. L., Anderson, J., & Moeschberger, M. L. (1993). A national study of periodontal assessment by dental hygienists. *Journal of Dental Hygiene, 67*(2), 82–91.

Hutchinson, L. (1993). Enhancing dental hygiene productivity. *Dental Hygiene News, 6*(4), 21–22.

Kraemer, L. & Gurenlian, J. (1989). An educational model for preparing dental hygiene students in the treatment of periodontal diseases. *Journal of Dental Hygiene, 63*(5), 232–236.

Kutnick, J. D. (1991). A knowledgeable staff is the best marketing tool a dentist can have. *Dental Office, 10*(8), 7.

Levin, R. P. (1991). Periodontal services growing. *Dental Economics, 81*(12), 43.

Mann, M. L. (1988). Planning for community programs. In A. W. Jong (Ed.), *Community dental health* (2nd ed.). (Appraisal.) St. Louis: Mosby-Year Book, Inc.

McConnell, C. R. (1993). *The health care manager's guide to performance evaluations.* Gaithersburg, MD: Aspen Publishers.

McCullough, C. (1993). Essential elements of the periodontal examination. *Access, 7*(2), 24–26.

McFall, W. T. & Bader, J. D. (1988). Presence of periodontal data in patient records of general practitioners. *Journal of Periodontology, 59*(7), 445–449.

McKenzie, S. A. (1993). Is your hygiene department healthy? *Dental Teamwork, 6*(5), 28–29.

Miller, A. J., Brunelle, J. A., Carlos, J. P., Brown, L. J., & Löe, H. (1987). *Oral health of United States adults* (NIH Publication No. 97-2868). Bethesda, MD: National Institute of Dental Research.

Miller, D. L. (1991). An investigation into attrition of dental hygienists from the workforce. *Journal of Dental Hygiene, 65,* 25–31.

Morris, W. O. (1995). *The dentist's legal advisor.* St. Louis: Mosby-Year Book, Inc.

Palat, M. (1989). Failure to timely diagnose periodontal disease—The legal standard of care. *Journal of Law & Ethics in Dentistry, 2*(3 & 4), 160–167.

Papapanou, P. J. (1994). Epidemiology and natural history of periodontal disease. In N. P. Lang & T. Karring, T. (Eds.), *Proceedings of the 1st european workshop on periodontology.* London: Quintessence Publishing Co., Ltd.

Ramfjord, S. P. (1993). Maintenance care and supportive periodontal therapy. *Quintessence International, 24*(7), 465–471.

Rotty, R. W. (1994). Performance evaluations in the oral health care setting. *Access, 8*(4), 60–64.

Simonds, J. A. (1991). The general dentist/periodontist team—An unrecognized synergy? *Journal of the California Dental Association, 19*(12), 32–34.

Wilkins, E. M. (1994). *Clinical practice of the dental hygienist* (7th ed.). Baltimore: Williams & Wilkins.

Zarkowski, P. (1991). Legal considerations in periodontal therapy. *Dental Hygiene News, 4*(4), 4–5.

Zarkowski, P. (1990). Legal issues in the practice of dental hygiene. *Seminars in Dental Hygiene, II*(1), 1–7.

Zinman, E. J. (1990). Legal considerations. In M. G. Newman & K. S. Kornman (Eds.), *Antibiotic/antimicrobial use in dental practice.* Chicago: Quintessence Publishing Co., Inc.

# Glossary

**abrasion**—The wearing away of a surface through friction. The abrasive in a polishing agent is a substance consisting of particles of sufficient hardness and sharpness to groove or scratch a softer substance when drawn across its surface.

**active listening skills**—In the dental hygiene setting, being attentive to what the client is saying and the nonverbals being portrayed.

**active therapy**—A treatment planning approach that can include nonsurgical periodontal therapy, periodontal surgery, or both.

**allografts**—Processed human cadaver bone, which is usually freeze-dried and demineralized. Freeze-drying greatly reduces the antigenicity of the graft material, while demineralization results in enhancing the ostogenic potential by exposing the bone-inducing agent bone-morphogenic protein.

**amplitude**—Controls the distance the tip of an ultrasonic instrument travels in one single vibration; referred to as **tip displacement**. The greater the amplitude, the further the distance the tip travels in the vibration. The power setting on the ultrasonic unit affects the amplitude of the vibration.

**analgesia**—A decreased ability or inability for the client to perceive pain. Nitrous oxide is classified as a mildly potent general anesthetic. It is mixed with oxygen in dental inhalation sedation units and administered to obtain analgesia.

**antimicrobial therapy**—The use of specific agents for the control or destruction of microorganisms, either systematically or at specific sites. Commonly, antimicrobials refer to mouthrinses.

**antiseptic**—Any agent used for chemical plaque control that inhibits growth and development of microorganisms.

**area-specific curets**—Curets that were developed to adapt to deep and nonaccessible periodontal pockets without traumatic distention of the gingiva. Area-specific refers to instruments made to adapt to specific areas or surfaces of the dentition.

**assessment strokes**—This type of stroke employs the lightest grasp and lateral pressure possible to evaluate the root surface for the presence of deposits, irregularities, anatomy, or any other plaque-retentive factors. Also commonly called the "exploratory stroke" because it is seeking information about the root surface.

**autografts**—Bone grafts obtained from the same patient; usually harvested from the surgical sight (cortical shavings or osseous coagulum) or from another intraoral site (such as cortical or cancellous bone from the tuberosity or an edentulous ridge).

**autotuned unit**—An ultrasonic unit with a preset frequency within the device that automatically tunes the cycles per second to maximum efficiency for each insert within the handpiece. This feature minimizes the clinician's choice to decrease energy output to reduce the tip movement.

**bacterial endocarditis**—Inflammation of the inner lining of the heart due to a bacterial infection.

**ball-type flow meter**—The most common machine used in dentistry for nitrous oxide-oxygen analgesia that indicates the amount of gas being administered for inhalation sedation. Two knobs are used to regulate the amount of nitrous oxide and oxygen flow and as more gas is used a ball floats in the nitrous oxide or oxygen glass tubing to indicate how much gas is being dispensed. (See Figure 9-1).

**base salary plus commission**—A combination of salary and commission. Salary is paid until the gross receipts for dental hygiene services reaches a specified amount, then the hygienist receives commission on the receipts above that amount.

**Brannstrom's hydrodynamic theory**—According to this theory, a stimulus such as cold, applied at the dentinal surfaces causes fluid within the dentinal tubules to move toward the pulp. This fluid movement displaces or disturbs the pulpal nerve endings causing pain. Brannstrom's hydrodynamic theory is the most widely accepted theory describing the mechanism of pain production associated with dentinal hypersensitivity.

**bruxism**—The repetitive grinding of maxillary and mandibular teeth against each other. The teeth involved may be as few as one from each arch or all teeth in both arches. Bruxism also includes clenching of the teeth.

**calculus removal working strokes**—This type of stroke is employed with instruments that have cutting edges (curets, sickles, and files) to remove calculus and associated bacterial plaque, as well as overhanging restorative margins.

**care plan**—A "blueprint" or guide to determine how many appointments are needed and what care procedures will be performed at each appointment session. It is the result of the planning phase of the dental hygiene process of care.

**career development**—Continual growth in both the professional and personal dimensions over time. The result of continued career development should be success in the professional and personal dimensions, and, thus career satisfaction.

**career**—A profession/occupation that one prepares for and pursues as lifework.

**carpal tunnel syndrome**—The most commonly identified cumulative trauma disorder. It is characterized by pain, numbness, and tingling in the area of distribution of the median nerve in the hand due to compression as the nerve passes through the tunnel. Early symptoms also include an intolerance to cold and sometimes a burning sensation.

**category of disease progression, Case Type**—Categories or case types are based on disease progression at the time of examination and evaluation. After practitioners determine the quantity of bone loss as early, moderate, or advanced, and recognize patterns and distribution of loss, the appropriate category or case type is determined for insurance reporting.

**cavitation**—A phenomenon that occurs when water flows to the end of an ultrasonic insert and contacts the moving tip. When water passes over the intense vibration of the oscillating tip, a spray results and rapid formation and destruction of small air cavities occur at maximum vibrating points along the working end.

**cavity preparation**—The removal of caries-altered tooth structure to render it capable of receiving a dental restoration.

**cervix**—The junction of the root and crown. Roots are widest at the cervix, near the cementoenamel junction (CEJ), and gradually taper and become narrower as they ascend to the apex. The cervix is typically constricted or concave in relation to the clinical crown.

**channeling**—Channeling, or removing the mineralized calculus deposit piece by piece, is the result of short (1 to 3 mm) powerful, controlled wrist rocks while rolling and pivoting the dental instrument to keep the terminal portion adapted. On the proximal surfaces, the goal is to channel calculus by advancing to the contact area in a constant upward movement while maintaining proper adaptation.

**chronological resume**—Lists abilities and accomplishments under headings that present information in reverse chronological order, beginning with the most recent experience.

**cleansing**—In coronal or traditional polishing, cleansing is the first of two steps. An abrasive, such as flour of pumice, is applied to all tooth surfaces to remove acquired pellicle, bacterial plaque, materia alba, and extrinsic stain. See also **final polishing**.

**clinical attachment level**—The relative probing depth corresponding to the distance from the cementoenamel junction (CEJ) to the location of the periodontal probe tip against the epithelial attachment.

**clinical or objective factors**—Factors that influence treatment decisions and care planning including assessment findings and information about instrumentation, polishing, supportive treatment, and self-care education.

**collaboration**—Dentists and hygienists working together in an environment of respect and trust, and cooperating and being responsible for the care they provide to the client, to achieve the mutual goal of oral health.

**combination resume**—Uses both the chronological and functional format combined into one resume. The combination resume follows the traditional chronological style that employers are familiar with and emphasizes functional skills that provide depth to the resume. Generally, used by an experienced clinician.

**commission**—The wages that a hygienist is paid as a percentage of the gross receipts for services that the hygienist provides. The commission varies between geographic regions and ranges between 40 to 60 percent.

**communication**—A giving or exchanging of information, signals, or messages by talk, gesture, or writing.

**conscious sedation**—A minimally depressed level of consciousness that can be produced by pharmacological means (such as nitrous oxide), by nonpharmacologic methods, or a combination of both.

**continuing care**—Synonymous with recare. A term suggested to replace recall.

**contributing or subjective factors**—Factors that influence treatment decisions and care planning including the chief concern(s), client motivation, the provider's ability/experience, financial resources, time, intuition, and ethical/legal concerns.

**coronal polishing**—The use of an abrasive agent on all accessible tooth surfaces (exposed root and crown or anatomic crown depending on philosophy) to remove bacterial plaque and

stain. Coronal or traditional polishing is a two-step procedure: **cleansing** and **final polishing**.

**cotherapist**—A term used to describe the relationships between the patient, dentist, and dental hygienist when coordinating oral health care to attain and maintain the health of the patient.

**cumulative trauma disorders (CTD) or repetitive strain injuries (RSI)**—Musculoskeletal and nerve impairments caused by repetitive work activities, especially when performed forcefully and/or in awkward postures. Common CTDs include **carpal tunnel syndrome (CTS)**, ulnar nerve compression at the elbow, ulnar nerve entrapment at the wrist, thoracic outlet syndrome, Raynaud's syndrome, tenosynovitis, tendinitis, and lateral epicondylitis.

**debridement work strokes**—These strokes employ the use of very light lateral pressure and are multidirectional. Their purpose is to remove residual calculus remaining after calculus removal work strokes, and to remove or dislodge bacterial plaque and its endotoxins. Debridement strokes are automatically performed with calculus removal working strokes and independently performed in the presence of gingival inflammation, bleeding on probing, and/or pocket depth where calculus is not detected.

**decision making**—The judgment or conclusion made as a result of the critical thinking process. This procedure is a crucial and integral part of the dental hygiene process, for without it, implementation and evaluation of care can be haphazard and unsuccessful.

**deductive reasoning**—Deriving of a conclusion by reasoning or inference in which the conclusion follows from the premise.

**Dental Hygiene Human Needs Conceptual Model**—Dental hygiene theorists have recently developed this model to assist clinicians in providing care that is scientific, humanistic, and holistic, thereby guaranteeing that treatment is more client-oriented rather than task-oriented. Based on human needs theory.

**dental hygiene diagnosis**—A formal statement or statements of the dental hygienist's decision regarding the actual or potential oral health problems of a patient that are amenable to treatment through the dental hygiene process of care.

**dental hypersensitivity**—Pain arising from exposed dentin, typically in response to thermal, mechanical, chemical, or osmotic stimuli that can not be explained as arising from any other form of dental defect or pathology.

**dental restoration**—Any material or prosthesis that replaces lost tooth structure, teeth or oral tissues. Dental restorations are classified as either **intracoronal** or **extracoronal**.

**dentinopulpal complex**—Integrates the concepts that dentin is the mature end-product of the odontoblast cells of the pulp and that the dentin contains protoplasmic extensions of the odontoplasts called odontoplastic processes. Because of this relationship, the dentin and pulp can be considered as one compound tissue.

**deplaquing**—Removal or disruption of bacterial plaque and its toxins subgingivally, following the completion of supragingival and subgingival debridement. It is performed at reevaluation and maintenance appointments using curets or ultrasonic instrumentation.

**developmental depressions**—Cratered, valleylike shapes in the root of a tooth. Depressions are beneficial because they provide more attachment area increasing periodontal support. Synonymous with concavities.

**developmental grooves**—The result of the union of portions of the crown or root. Narrow and deep, they usually appear within depressions proximally or in maxillary incisors along the palatogingival groove.

**digital subtraction radiography**—A filmless method using sensors; used for longitudinal assessment of slight changes in periodontal structures making it possible to quantify and objectively assess an area.

**direct restorations**—Dental restorations that are fabricated within the confines of the preparation and are typically composed of materials that harden or polymerize after placement in the preparation. Contrast **indirect restorations**.

**disease activity**—Bone or attachment loss that is ongoing at the time of the clinical examination. It refers to periods of "quiescence" and "exacerbation."

**disease severity**—A measure of all the destruction and healing that has taken place prior to the examination. It is established after clinical assessment that includes visual inspection, palpation, periodontal probing, and radiographs.

**disease theory**—Knowledge shared with the client about (periodontal) diseases. Theory is related to the cognitive domain and includes, but is not limited to, the causes, classification, and stage of bone loss.

**electronic dental anesthesia (EDA)**—An effective noninvasive method of achieving oral anesthesia for pain control in dentistry. A needle is not required to achieve anesthesia with EDA. Electrode pads are placed bilaterally in the vestibule next to the teeth being treated. The client is in control of the amount of anesthesia used by increasing the intensity of electrical stimulation from a handheld control unit.

**emergence angle or profile**—Indicated by the angle or outline between the natural tooth structure and the restoration at their juncture.

**employee**—As an employee, the employer withholds income, social security, and Medicare tax from the employee's wages. The employer also pays federal unemployment insurance, and a share of the social security and Medicare tax. The state may require that the employer carry workmen's compensation and disability insurance for the employee.

**endosseous implants**—Placed directly in the bone and are the most popular type of implant in use today. Endosseous implants are subclassified into two main forms: blade and root (cylinder) forms.

**endotoxin**—Currently renamed lipo-oligosaccharide (LOS), is a toxin or poisonous substance that is found in the outer cell wall of gram-negative bacteria; therefore it is found in high concentrations in periodontal pockets. Endotoxin is highly toxic, penetrates gingival epithelium, is released when cells die, and may also be released from viable cells.

**ergonomics**—A discipline that studies workers and their relationship to their occupational environment. It is an applied science that interfaces the design of work devices, systems, and physical working conditions with the requirements and capacities of the worker. For dental professionals, ergonomics includes concepts such as positioning themselves and their clients, how they perform their tasks and procedures, how they utilize their equipment, and the impact of these concepts and actions on their musculoskeletal health.

**expression of body**—Nonverbal behaviors such as body orientation, posture, facial expressions, gestures, touch, and distance/space. Also see **expression of tone of voice**.

**expression of tone of voice**—Nonverbal behaviors such as hesitation, loudness, intonation, or inflection of the word or "noise" that is heard. Also see **expression of body**.

**extended shank curets**—Area-specific curets that have a terminal shank that is 3 mm longer than the standard area-specific design, which are intended to negotiate periodontal pockets of 5 mm or greater.

**external motivational strategies**—How the professional encourages or instills behavioral changes in another. Individual clinicians have different approaches designed to encourage oral self-care depending on each practitioner's style, skill, and experience.

**external motivation**—An individual's reliance on others' opinions or belief systems to guide them. Contrast **internal motivation**.

**extracoronal restorations**—Dental restorations located outside or external to the crown portion of a natural tooth. Extracoronal restorations include artificial crowns made of porcelain, porcelain fused to metal, gold or other metal alloys, and veneers for facial surfaces of teeth made of porcelain or composite. Contrast **intracoronal restorations**.

**extrinsic stain**—A discoloration located on the tooth surface or within soft (acquired pellicle, plaque) or hard (calculus) deposit. Contrast **intrinsic stain**.

**facilitative communication**—Describes the interaction between the health care provider and the helpee. In the dental hygiene setting, the ease with which the clinician and the client receiving nonsurgical periodontal therapy cooperatively communicate. The dental hygienist acts as the facilitator in the NSPT and works in harmony with the client to successfully achieve common goals set by both parties.

**fail-safe system**—A system that provides additional safety measures during inhalation sedation. The fail-safe system is designed so that the nitrous oxide will automatically turn off when oxygen is depleted before the $N_2O$ tank is empty. An audible alarm also sounds to alert the clinician that the client is no longer receiving $N_2O$-$O_2$.

**final polishing**—In coronal or traditional polishing, final polishing is the second of two steps. After **cleansing**, final polishing is accomplished by applying a fine abrasive, such as whiting, to the tooth surface to produce a smooth, lustrous surface. With the advent of commercially prepared pastes, clinicians select a single paste to perform both cleansing and polishing functions.

**finger activation**—Technique where the finger(s) and thumb move back and forth to push and pull the dental instrument. Pulling constantly will tire the fingers even though finger activation results in deposit removal.

**free graft**—One type of surgical procedure to treat or correct anatomic gingival defects, specifically, inadequate zones of masticatory mucosa/attached gingiva, or mucogingival involvement. In the case of narrow zones of attached gingiva or the presence of recession, it needs to be determined if the patient is able to keep the area free of inflammation. The ability to keep the area in question inflammation free or the lack of progression of recession usually obviates the need for **gingival augmentation**.

**frequency**—The number of cycles per second that affects the speed of movement of the insert tip of the ultrasonic unit.

**functional resume**—Organizes abilities and accomplishments under headings that describe broad skill or ability areas. Dates are not included and this can negatively impact an employer. The functional resume is an acceptable style of listing abilities and accomplishments, especially for people who are reentering the workforce, or for practitioners who have been employed for a long period of time and have varied experiences or increased responsibility within the practice.

**functional shank**—Overall distance from the working end to the handle of an instrument.

**gingival augmentation**—A type of surgical procedure to treat or correct anatomic gingival defects, specifically, inadequate zones of mucosa/attached gingiva or mucogingival involvement. If a patient is unable to keep the existing zone of gingiva healthy, or if the recession is progressive, gingival grafting is often needed to correct the problem.

**gingival crevicular fluid**—An exudate that flows from the gingival sulcus or pocket. In a strictly healthy gingiva, little or no fluid can be detected. It increases in quantity during inflammation and its presence reflects the nature of the inflammation within the pocket wall.

**gingivectomy**—Excision of the soft tissue wall of the periodontal pocket by removal of a collar of marginal gingiva.

**grit or particle size**—The various grades of abrasive agents such as extrafine, fine, medium, coarse, and plus. Clinicians rely on the manufacturer's labeling of commercial pastes, which indicate grit or particle size.

**health history**—A set of questions, either written or verbal, used by oral health professionals to acquire information concerning their clients' health statuses. Used interchangeably with **medical history**.

**horizontal angulation**—Radiographs where the horizontal angulation is directed perpendicular to the contact areas of the teeth in order to prevent overlapping the crowns of the teeth and surrounding tissues.

**horizontal bone loss**—The uniform loss of interproximal bone, where the crest of bone is still evident in a horizontal plane parallel with an imaginary line extending between the cementoenamel junctions of adjacent teeth and perpendicular to the long axes of those teeth. Contrast **vertical angular bone** loss.

**implant system**—The manufacturer or brand of an implant. Implant systems include not only the implant itself, but also the special surgical and restorative equipment necessary for their placement. Selection of one system over another is based on reliability, ease of use, and manufacturer support.

**independent contractor**—As an independent contractor, the contracted practitioner is self-employed and responsible for paying all income, social security, and Medicare taxes. The accounting and paperwork associated with self-employment are also the hygienist's responsibility.

**indirect restorations**—Dental restorations that are formed partially or wholly outside the tooth preparation, often from an impression and subsequent cast of the preparation. Contrast **direct restorations**.

**inflammation**—A defense reaction of the body that occurs in response to injury. Inflammatory cells migrate to an area of irritation through chemotaxis, a chemical process that causes them to become mobile and travel to the localized area of injury.

**informed consent**—The process by which a client agrees to proposed treatment following a complete case presentation.

**initial therapy**—The first phase of treatment of periodontal disease (nonsurgical periodontal therapy is the first phase of treatment in the majority of cases). Sometimes referred to as initial preparation or anti-infective therapy.

**insert**—The part of the ultrasonic instrument that is interchangeable and is designed for various root/tooth surfaces and functions. See **transducer** for it's function. The insert parts are described in Figure 12-1.

**interdependence**—The highest level of relationships where individuals work together by combining their abilities to create something better than could be accomplished alone.

**internal motivation**—An individual's existing desire or willingness to alter behavior, and the ability to attempt behavior change. Contrast **external motivation**.

**interventions**—The individual client's treatment regimen for meeting assessed needs.

**intracoronal restorations**—Dental restorations located within the confines of the cusps and normal proximal axial contour. Intracoronal restorations are classified by the surfaces involved in the cavity preparation (Class I–VI). Contrast **extracoronal restorations**.

**intrinsic stain**—A discoloration incorporated within the tooth structure. Contrast **extrinsic stain**.

**job "burnout"**—The negative psychological reaction to one's work and the workplace environment when one is not able to manage stress or solve problems.

**kilovolt peak (kVp)**—Dental radiographs are generally taken at either low kilovolt setting (65 to 70 kVp), or at a high kVp setting (90 kVp). The kilovoltage is related to the energy of the x-ray beam; the higher the kVp the greater the energy or penetrating power of the beam.

**language**—Used in communication; needs to be straightforward and delivered in a nonthreatening manner. The words spoken are selected carefully for a particular client. Verbal behaviors include language, active listening, and paraphrasing.

**lateral pressure**—The force exerted against the tooth surface or deposit with the cutting edge of the sickle, curet, or file. Lateral pressure is achieved by the following: 1) using the ring finger, the finger rest, to firmly stabilize the stroke; 2) lightly pressing the finger rest (ring finger) into the tooth surface; and 3) slightly flexing the index finger and thumb to exert pressure on the instrument.

**Learning Ladder Continuum**—An approach to assessing a client's readiness to learn based on the concept that learning occurs in a progressive series of steps or intervals.

**local anesthesia**—The elimination of sensations, especially pain, in part of the body by the topical application or regional injection of a drug.

**magnetostrictive unit**—A type of ultrasonic unit with an insert that is either a stack of metal (nickel-cobalt) strips or a ferromagnetic rod attached to the working end. Inside the handpiece is a coil of copper wire in which, when the current is turned on and the insert is in place, the core becomes magnetized and demagnetized. When magnetized, the core contracts altering the electromagnetic field and causing the working end of the insert to vibrate in an elliptical or orbital motion. Unlike the **piezoelectric units**, the working end can be used on all sides, enhancing its adaptability to tooth surfaces.

**maintenance sharpening**—Performed for all instruments at a routine time, not in the presence of a client. For example, students learning sharpening procedures often schedule a time period each week to examine and sharpen instruments in preparation for the next week's clinical experiences.

**maintenance**—A state of being maintained or a means of upkeep in a desirable condition. Dental patients need to be maintained even if they have never had periodontitis.

**management discrepancy**—A situation that exists when the client possesses the know-how and psychomotor ability, but does not perform self-care regularly or adequately. See also **skill discrepancy**.

**manual tuned unit**—An ultrasonic unit with a frequency that can be adjusted by the professional via a frequency control or tuning knob. The clinician's ability to control the frequency or energy being used is a decisive advantage of manual tuned units. This control permits adjustment of the speed of movement of the tip when needed for certain oral and client conditions.

**margination**—overhang removal procedures.

**Maslow's Needs Hierarchy**—A familiar model used by professionals to determine a client's needs. This needs theory utilizes human nature to explain the motivational process. Five needs are arranged to show that as one need is satisfied, an individual is then motivated to satisfy the next need, or level, in the hierarchy.

**material needs assessment**—Determines additional instruments and equipment that are necessary materials considered or desired for implementing nonsurgical periodontal therapy. The materials include the type and brand of periodontal self-care aids, the manufacture and number of hand-activated and ultrasonic/sonic inserts needed, the type of mechanized device used for debridement, and the materials needed to provide supportive treatment.

**maximum safe dosage (MSD)**— Dosage of anesthetic agents that are established according to milligrams of drug per pound of body weight. Absolute MSDs are based on 150-pound healthy adult clients who respond to anesthetic in "an average" manner or within the middle of the normal distribution curve (see Table 9-7).

**medical history**—A set of questions, either written or verbal, used by oral health professionals to acquire information concerning their clients' health statuses. Used interchangeably with **health history**.

**microbial assessment**—Microbial sampling used to monitor the effects of therapy as well as determine if antibiotics should be prescribed.

**microleakage**—The leakage of oral fluids often from a microscopically imperfect junction at the margin of direct restorations.

**mini-bladed curets**—Combines the features of the area-specific extended shank curets with a 50 percent reduction in blade length as compared to the area-specific extended shank or standard designs. Mini-bladed curets offer better adaption to narrow facial and lingual surfaces of anterior teeth, furcations, and root surfaces in narrow and deep periodontal pockets.

**networking**—Establishing an organized system of relationships with contacts from common skills, backgrounds, or interests. The network is built on the idea of a mutual exchange of information between contacts about employment opportunities, practice environment, and ranges of wages and benefits.

**neuromusculoskeletal disorder**—Injuries to the nerves related to tendons and tendon sheaths. A specific musculoskeletal disorder. Musculoskeletal pain in dental and dental hygiene practitioners has been most frequently documented in the upper and lower back, neck, shoulders, arms and legs; however, it may occur in any part of the body.

**neutral wrist position**—When the arm and wrist are in a continuum (see Figure 15-2E). The most mechanically efficient position for the wrist is an extension of approximately 30° with fingers that are flexed slightly. Prolonged use of the wrist in ulnar deviation, or cocked medially toward the midline of the arm, has been shown to contribute to both CTS and DeQuervain's tenosynovitis. A full-arm stroke that employs the muscles of the entire arm, not only reduces wrist strokes and potential for nerve impairment, but also maintains a neutral wrist position and provides more power.

**neutral, balanced body position**—A position in which all the muscles are centered and no muscle or muscle group is overworking; the total musculoskeletal structure is in balance.

**nonsurgical periodontal therapy (NSPT)**—Includes plaque removal and its control, supra- and subgingival scaling, root planing, and use of chemical agents. Nonsurgical periodontal therapy requires a thorough periodontal assessment and evaluation of risk factors prior to therapy and careful reevaluation following therapy.

**occupational exposure**—"Reasonably anticipated skin, eye, mucous membrane, or parenteral contact with blood or other potentially infectious materials that may result from the performance of an employee's duties," (Occupational Safety and Health Act of 1970).

**occupational hazard**—Exposure or potential for exposure to injury or disease within the workplace environment. Being able to recognize existing hazards or identify potential hazards is critical to effective prevention and maintenance of occupational hazards for the dental health care worker.

**occupational stress**—A condition that exists when there is disharmony between the individual and the work environment. Sources of stress, or **stressors**, can exist from factors within ourselves, from factors outside of ourselves, and from factors in the environment. Factors within ourselves include beliefs, values, responsibilities, coworkers, family members, and friends. Stressors from the environment include equipment, layout of an office, and scheduling.

**oral prophylaxis**—Oral prophylaxis is performed when supragingival and subgingival scaling are combined with selective coronal polishing of the teeth to remove plaque, calculus, and stains.

**oral self-care**—Client removal or reduction of bacterial plaque both supragingivally and subgingivally (1 to 3 mm) to help resolve periodontal inflammation. Similar terms include oral hygiene measures, plaque control, and mechanical plaque removal.

**organic heart murmur**—Pathologic atypical sound of the heart that requires antibiotic prophylaxis for NSPT and other oral health care.

**osseointegration**—A direct structural and functional connection between ordered and living bone and the surface of a load-carrying implant. (See Figure 14-9).

**ostectomy**—Removal of supporting bundle bone that becomes necessary if the desired result cannot be achieved by reshaping the bone alone (as in the case of certain vertical and circumferential defects).

**osteoplasty**—Reshaping of existing bone without exposure of additional tooth structure. Osteoplasty allows the surgeon to modify the existing crestal profile (in the case of irregularities) or remove bony impediments (thickened crestal ledges or tori) that would interfere with the soft tissues healing normally around the teeth, which results in a reduction in pocketing.

**osteoradionecrosis**—Bone necrosis due to irradiation. Ongoing periodontal disease is a contributing factor in osteoradionecrosis.

**pain and anxiety control**—The use of various physical, chemical, and psychological modalities to prevent or treat preoperative, operative, or postoperative patient apprehension and pain.

**palliative**—Part of a European approach to describing continuing care. A type of treatment that is designed to prevent, slow down, or arrest disease progression in clients who can not receive appropriate treatment because of medical conditions, poor oral hygiene, or lack of compliance. Palliative treatment is the optimal treatment given these circumstances.

**paralleling technique**—A preferred radiographic technique for periapical films that involves placing the x-ray film parallel to the long axis of the teeth, with the central ray of the x-ray beam directed at right angles to both the film and the teeth. Also called the right-angle technique or long-cone technique.

**paraphrasing**—An avenue for the listener to repeat what was seen or heard. Paraphrasing corrects any misconceptions and allows for a free flowing interaction including feelings and thoughts. Also referred to as reflecting, a perception check, or feedback.

**performance evaluations**—Are appraisals completed by employers that provide a way to communicate expectations to each member of the oral health care team, identify ways to improve technical skills or behavior, and serve as a basis for salary adjustments or additional compensation.

**periimplant gingivitis**—Inflammation of the marginal tissues surrounding implants. Periimplant gingivitis is histochemically and clinically similar to gingivitis.

**periimplantitis**—The inflammatory process resulting from microbial insult to implants that closely resembles periodontitis. The microflora associated with stable and failing implants closely resembles the microflora associated with healthy and diseased teeth, respectively.

**periodontal client percentage**—Percentage of clients with periodontitis. Determination of this percentage requires careful assessment and monitoring.

**periodontal debridement**—Removal of all subgingival plaque and its by-products (as evidenced by clinical signs of inflammation), clinically detectable plaque-retentive factors (calculus, overhangs), and detectable calculus-embedded cementum to finish the root surface during periodontal instrumentation while preserving as much of the tooth surface as possible.

**periodontal disease activity**—The stage(s) of the disease characterized by loss of periodontal attachment.

**periodontal disease**—A group of diseases that adversely affect the tissues of the periodontium. These diseases are classified as types of gingivitis when effects are confined to the gingiva, and as periodontitis when destruction extends into the supporting structures of the teeth.

**periodontal maintenance procedures (PMP)**—An extension of periodontal therapy that involves continuing periodic assessment and preventive treatment of the periodontal structures to allow for early detection and treatment of new or recurring periodontal disease. Also previously referred to as maintenance therapy or supportive periodontal therapy (SPT).

**personnel needs assessment**— Within a general practice or clinical setting, the number of personnel necessary to establish and implement a successful NSPT program.

**piezoelectric unit**—A type of ultrasonic unit that houses a crystal transducer. The source of vibration occurs when alternating electrical currents are applied to the crystal transducer creating a dimensional change that is transmitted to the tip in the form of a vibration. The movement of this vibration is in a linear pattern. Only two sides of the working tip are activated, limiting the tip's ability to adapt to the topography of the tooth surface on all sides. Contrast **magnetostrictive unit**.

**pivoting**—The movement of the hand, wrist and forearm in an arc within the same plane or across planes. If pivoting can be achieved while the hand, wrist, and forearm are in a neutral position, then less strain occurs decreasing predisposure to musculoskeletal disorders. Both pivoting and rocking motions require movement on the finger rest to negotiate tooth structure topography.

**pocket elimination**—Posttreatment sulci of 1 to 3 mm.

**pocket reduction**—A decrease in probe depth with an absence of bleeding.

**powered toothbrush**—Recommended and useful for cases where the manual brush is not achieving the desired result.

**prebooked system**—One of two main continuing care scheduling systems. First, clients can be appointed at the time the care is needed, which is referred to as a **nonprebooked system**. Second, an appointment for the next recare visit can occur, which is called a prebooked system. With the prebooked system, the client, upon completion of initial therapy, is scheduled at the appropriate interval before leaving the office.

**precision-thin inserts**—New ultrasonic insert designs, referred to as precision-thin inserts. These newly designed inserts are thinner in diameter than the original, standard inserts; their narrow design facilitates adaptation subgingivally and in hard-to-reach areas such as furcations and narrow periodontal pockets. Other terms for the precision-thin insert are modified tips or microultrasonics.

**predictive value**—A clinical test that has both high sensitivity and specificity; that is, the test can be used to accurately identify active disease and predict future disease.

**presumptive diagnosis**—The result of the clinical examination during initial therapy. It is preliminary in nature.

**primary occlusal traumatism**—Situations where abnormal forces (either in direction or quantity) acting on relatively sound periodontal structures produce signs or symptoms of pathosis. Occlusal trauma is classified as either primary or secondary.

**primary prevention**—Part of a European approach to describing continuing care. For those who are healthy or those who have gingivitis, the focus of treatment is to prevent gingivitis from becoming periodontitis. Also see **secondary prevention**.

**proactive**—Taking the initiative and responsibility to make things happen in one's own life. Proactive individuals assume the responsibility and initiative for their career development and do not let circumstances, events, or persons control their future.

**probing depth**—The distance between the gingival margin and the location of the periodontal probe tip against the epithelial attachment.

**productive goal**—A reasonable and attainable monetary goal usually based on hourly production. In an established practice, the production goal is assessed by reviewing the previous year's average production by dental hygienists and the number of days worked. From that assessment, one can determine the average hygiene production per day and per hour and establish a goal to increase that production.

**program**—This term does not imply a single approach to therapy for all clients. Instead, it refers to the way in which NSPT is implemented in an individual office setting.

**psychosomatic methods**—Nonpharmacologic pain control methods used to alleviate the client's dental fear or anxiety. Examples include facilitative communication, behavior therapy, distraction techniques, creative imagery, counseling, hypnosis, biofeedback, or progressive relaxation.

**readiness**—A term used to describe the client's position or attitude toward changing behavior. Factors used to assess readiness include willingness to attempt change and ability to change at a given time.

**recall system**—A method an office or clinic uses to track intervals and notify clients about continuing care.

**recall**—The process of requesting that a client return for care at a specified interval. **Recare** or **continuing care** have recently been suggested as more appropriate terms.

**recare**—The term, suggested to replace recall, is used to represent appropriately timed maintenance where the client assumes responsibility to track compliance with continuing care.

**reevaluation**—A formal process of care planning that occurs four to six weeks after the completion of initial or active therapy for the purpose of evaluating the response to initial care and make further treatment recommendations, if indicated.

**regenerative techniques**—Surgical method that offers the surgeon the opportunity to stimulate new periodontal ligament, bundle bone, and root cementum in areas where it was previously lost due to disease. The benefit of performing regenerative surgery is that pocket reduction is achieved through regrowth of the lost attachment versus removal of attachment through resection. See also **resection**.

**resective techniques**—Osseous surgery that involves modification and reshaping of the alveolar bone to create a more physiologic crestal architecture, thus yielding **pocket reduction**. See also regenerative techniques.

**retipping**—When an instrument is improperly contoured, the clinician must decide if enough metal remains to warrant recontouring or if the instrument should be replaced or retipped. Retipping is no longer supported because it compromises the constructional integrity creating a risk for clients and practitioners. Reduced quality may lead to tip loss, cracks in the handle, lack of balance, and undue wearing due to inferior steel.

**retrograde implantitis**—Retrograde implant failure due to bone microfractures caused by premature implant loading, over-loading, trauma, or occlusal factors. It is suspected when bone loss is seen radiographically that does not accompany gingival inflammation.

**rheumatic heart disease**—Damage to the heart muscle and/or valves caused by the occurrence of rheumatic fever.

**rocking**—The up and down motion creating by moving the wrist from left to right. Rocking allows the clinician to move the instrument from the epithelial attachment to portions of the root and crown positioned coronally. Both rocking and pivoting motions require movement on the finger rest to negotiate tooth structure topography.

**rolling**—Rolling the dental instrument in between the thumb and index finger is an essential movement that facilitates tactile sensation, adaptation, activation, and client and therapist comfort during debridement, and if these fingers touch, this movement is negatively affected.

**root planing**—A definitive procedure that removes cementum and dentin that is rough, permeated by calculus, or contaminated with toxins or microorganisms.

**salary**—The wages that a hygienist is paid either on an hourly, daily, weekly, monthly, or yearly basis.

**scaling**—Instrumentation of the teeth to remove plaque and calculus. Employed only in areas where calculus deposits exist, without intentional removal of tooth surface.

**secondary prevention**—Part of a European approach to describing continuing care. The phase of care after completion of active therapy for clients with periodontal diseases. Also see **primary prevention**.

**self-administered written questionnaire**—Used by oral health professionals to acquire a client's medical or health history. Currently, the self-administered questionnaire is the most commonly used format because of the risk of dental malpractice claims and the need for written documentation.

**self-exploration**—Clients discuss with the dental hygienist what dental needs are important to them, what self-care aids they are willing to use, how many times a day they are willing to use these aids, and their commitment to the total treatment plan. Empathy, respect, and warmth are important for the health care provider because they are vital for client self-exploration.

**sensitivity** (of a diagnostic test)—The ability of a clinical and supplemental diagnostic test to detect disease when it is there.

**sensitivity** (of a medical history)—The need for broad-based questions on a medical history. The questions included on the health history should allow for a mix of **sensitivity** and **specificity**.

**skill discrepancy**—A situation that exists when the client does not have the knowledge and psychomotor ability to perform self-care. See also **management discrepancy**.

**skill enhancement**—The teaching of brushing, interdental aids, and other self-care devices or practices (oral rinsing, irrigation) to enhance plaque removal. It involves analysis of the psychomotor domain.

**soft tissue curettage**—Debriding the soft tissue wall of a periodontal pocket. It has been determined that new connective tissue attachment as a result of soft tissue curettage is precluded by the formation of a long junctional epithelium. Pocket reduction achieved following soft tissue curettage alone is accomplished by tissue shrinkage and reattachment of junctional epithelium rather than by new connective tissue attachment.

**specificity** (of a health history)——A question that has the ability to trigger another set of questions from the professional conducting a health history interview. The questions included on the health history should allow for a mix of **specificity** and **sensitivity**.

**specificity** (of a diagnostic test)——The ability of a clinical and supplemental diagnostic test to rule out disease when it is absent.

**standard of care**—Requires dentists and/or dental hygienists to provide the same level of care as provided by other practitioners, under similar circumstances.

**stressors**—Sources of stress. Stressors can exist from factors within ourselves, from factors outside of ourselves, and from factors in the environment. Factors within ourselves include beliefs, values, responsibilities, and health. Factors outside of ourselves encompass clients, employers, coworkers, family members, and friends. Stressors from the environment include equipment, layout of an office, and scheduling.

**subgingival ultrasonic periodontal debridement**—Removal of bacterial plaque and retentive factors from the crown and root surface via ultrasonic instrumentation to promote health of the gingiva and periodontal tissues.

**substantivity**—The ability of an antimicrobial agent to be retained in the oral cavity for extended periods with subsequent slow and sustained release of the active ingredient at effective levels. Substantive agents are effective in both laboratory and clinical testing.

**supportive treatment procedures**—Therapeutic interventions that augment debridement for the control of periodontal diseases and the maintenance of periodontal health. The procedures include the use of chemical agents and different methods of delivery, desensitization, overhang removal, and special considerations for the care of dental implants.

**surgical crown lengthening**—The exposure of sound root structure apical to deep carious lesions or fractures. In these situations, intentional removal of bone must be completed in order to reestablish the biologic width of the dentogingival complex as well as to allow for fabrication of a properly sealed restoration.

**team concept**—The foundation of the team concept depends on the overall goal of therapy being understood, and the individual's recognition of how his/her function affects the goals.

**terminal shank**—Extends between the working end and the first bend in a shank of an instrument.

**tip displacement**—The distance the tip of an ultrasonic instrument travels in one single vibration. See **Amplitude**.

**topical anesthetics**—Used to decrease discomfort associated with the initial penetration of a needle. They also can be used to reduce discomfort during scaling and root planing by applying the topical directly on the adjacent gingival tissue. Topical anesthetics are only effective on abraded skin or mucous membranes.

**total compensation package**—The number of hours worked per week and compensation that can be accepted for employment, including wages and benefits.

**transducer**—In an ultrasonic instrument, a transducer converts the electrical energy to mechanical energy which, in turn, causes the working end to vibrate. Synonymous with **insert**.

**transmission radiographs**—Comparisons of radiographic examinations made over time. Comparative or transmission radiographs should always be correlated with corresponding clinical evaluations.

**triangulation**—A wedge-shaped radiolucent area formed between the crestal proximal bone and the tooth surface. It appears in radiographs as an inverted triangle with the apex pointing apically.

**trituration techniques**—In inhalation sedation, trituration techniques allow for gradual increases in the concentration of $N_2O$ delivered to the client. This technique permits the total flow of gases to remain constant if so desired.

**ultrasonics**—A range of acoustical vibrations that cannot be heard by the human ear. In the application of dentistry, ultrasonic frequencies range from approximately 20,000 vibrations per second to 50,000 vibrations per second. These ultrasonic vibrations are a unit of frequency often referred to as cycles per second (cps) or hertz (Hz).

**universal characteristics**—All explorers, regardless of design, have universal characteristics, meaning that both sides of the tip can be adapted to all surfaces on the buccal or lingual by alternating the side of the tip. For example, the buccal surfaces of teeth #31 to 28 can be explored with the same end. The distal surfaces are explored with one side of the tip and the buccal and mesial surfaces are explored with the other side of the tip. When the opposing surfaces (linguals) are assessed, the other end is used.

**universal curets**—Curets that are able to adjust to mesial and distal surfaces by alternating the dual cutting edges, adjusting fulcrum placement and positioning, and changing operator and client positioning.

**vasoconstrictors**—Agent that increases the duration of local anesthesia, provides hemostases, and helps prevent toxicity related to high levels of the local anesthetic agent. By slowing the absorption of the drug into the bloodstream, anesthetic blood levels are lower and the potential for overdose is decreased.

**vertical (angular) bone loss**—Appears as a V-shaped defect along the proximal side of the root. Bone is not parallel to the two corresponding cementoenamel junctions, nor perpendicular to the long axes of those teeth. Vertical bone loss occurs because the base of the infrabony periodontal pocket is apical to the crest of the alveolar bone.

**vertical angulation**—The major problem influencing the sensitivity of periapical films in diagnosis, where elongation or foreshortening can appear to either increase or decrease bony support when no actual change has occurred.

**vertical bitewing radiographs**—Allows the clinician to view a maximum of osseous tissue in both arches simultaneously. When exposing this type of bitewing, the film is placed in either the posterior or anterior region of the mouth with the long axis of the film positioned vertically. Preferred, instead of horizontal bitewings, when periodontal disease has advanced beyond the early stages.

**working end**—The part of the instrument from the terminal shank to the point of an explorer or the toe of a curet.

# Index

Abrasion, 354–358
  abrasive agents, 355–357
  clinical technique, 357–358
  tooth surface integrity, 358
Activation, 303–304
Active listening skills, 187
Active therapy, 6
AIDS (acquired immune deficiency syndrome), 42, 45
Air-powder abrasive polishing, 351–353
  compared with rubber cup polishing, 353–354
Allografts, 464
Alveolar bone, 9–10
  diseased, 127–129
    patterns and distribution of bone loss, 128–129
    quantification of bone loss, 128
  normal, 125, 127
Amplitude, 323
Analgesia, 228
Angulation, in instrumentation, 303
Antimicrobial rinses, 369–376
  product evaluation and regulation, 369–370
  substantive and nonsubstantive agents, 370–376
    chlorhexidine, 371, 373
    future agents, 376
    multilevel marketing, 375–376
    other agents, 375
    phenolic compounds, 373–374
    quaternary ammonium compounds, 374–375
    sanquinarine, 375
    stannous fluoride, 373
Antimicrobial therapy, 367
APF. *See* Apically positioned flap
Apically positioned flap (APF), 462
  healing, 462
  procedure, 462
Appointment planning and scheduling, 55–56
Area-specific curets, 277
Asepsis, 143
Assessment strokes, 304
Attachment loss, 445–446
Autografts, 463
Autotuned ultrasonic unit, 323

Bacterial endocarditis, 36
Bacterial plaque, 63–64
  formation, 264–266
  and self-care, 197
Ball-type flow meters, 229
Base salary plus commission, 500–501
Behavior types, 190, 191
Benefits, 501–504
Biocompatibility of dental material, 93–94
Biological basis for periodontal therapy, 19–23
  histopathology of periodontal disease, 20–23
Biological hazards, 428
Bitewing surveys, 120–122

Bleeding disorders, 39–40
Bleeding on probing, 62–63, 446
Bone grafts, 463–464
Bone loss
  patterns and distribution of, 128–129
  quantification of, 128
Brannstrom's hydrodynamic theory, 391
Bruxism, 97
Burnout, 427

Calculus, 64–65
  formation, 266–268
Calculus removal working strokes, 304
Cancer treatment, 40–41
Cardiovascular disease and stress, 43–44
Career development, 479–506
  career plan description, 479–487
    personal values and priorities, 485–486
    practice rating and scoring, 486–487
    professional and personal roles, 480–481
    professional values and priorities, 481–485
  compensation, 495, 499–504
    benefits, 501–504
    methods, 499–500
    wages, 500–501
  employment search, 487–495
    cover letter preparation, 491–492
    creating a resume, 488–491
    interviewing strategies, 492–495
  future career development, 504
Care plan, 153
Care planning, 97–98, 155–162
  care plan documentation, 159–162
  considerations in, 98
  evaluation, 158–159
  goals, 156
  interventions for NSPT, 156–158
    aggressive disease states, 156, 158
    chronic disease states, 156
  priorities, 155–156
Carpal tunnel syndrome (CTS), 414
Case presentation, 217–223
  client consent for care, 221–222
  documentation, 223
  of need for local anesthesia, 244, 247
  purpose, 217, 219
  recommendations, 219–221
"Case Type," 129
Cast metal alloys, 95–96
Category of disease progression, 129
Cavitation, 322
  cavitational activity, 330
Cavity preparation, 90
Cementum, 9
Ceramics, 95
Cervix, of tooth, 257

Channeling, in instrumentation, 305
Chemical hazards, 428–429
Chemotherapy, 367–369, 449
    overview of, 367–369
        agents, 368
        method of delivery, 368–369
Chlorhexidine, 371, 373
Chronological resume, 488
Cleansing of tooth, 345
Client compliance, 197–198, 450–451
    barriers to, 201, 203–204
Client consent for care, 221–222
Clinical assessment, 56–67
    bleeding on probing, 62–63
    deposits, 63–65
    exudate, 63
    furcation involvement, 66–67
    gingival examination, 57–59
    loss of attachment, 60, 62
    mobility, 65–66
    pocket depths, 59–60, 61
Clinical attachment level, 62
Clinical factors, 153
Collaboration, 483
Combination resume, 490
Commission, 500
Communication, 183, 510–514
    additional dental hygienists, 512
    dental hygiene assistant, 511–512
    dentist/employer, 511
    front office personnel, 512–513
    periodontist, 513–514
Communication skills, applying to therapy, 183–195
    documenting communication, 190, 192–193
    forms of communication, 185–191
        building confidence and trust, 188–190
        interpersonal, 185–188
        intrapersonal, 185
        six behavior types and suggestions for coping with them, 190, 191
    improving communication skills, 193
    principles of communication, 183–185
Compensation, 495, 499–504
    benefits, 501–504
    methods, 499–500
    wages, 500–501
Composite resins, 94–95
Composite restorations, 102
Computed tomography, magnetic resonance imaging, and nuclear medicine bone scanning, 142–143
Computer-assisted radiography, 140
Connective nerve compression, 416–417
Conscious sedation, 228
Continuing care, 439
Contributing factors, 153
Control factors affecting periodontal interpretation, 123–124
Controlled-release devices, 380–384
    future directions, 382–384
    tetracycline fiber therapy, 381–382
Coronal polishing, 345
Cotherapist, 511
Cover letter preparation, 491–492
Cumulative trauma disorders (CTD), 413

Curets, 277–280, 292–297, 309–311
    recontouring, 297
    sharpening, 292–297
        armamentarium, 296–297
        evaluating sharpness, 295–296
    techniques for, 309–311

Debridement, 4–5, 256, 320
Debridement work strokes, 305
Decision-making process, 154–155
Dental history, 56, 444
Dental hygiene assistant, 512
Dental hygiene diagnosis, 156
Dental Hygiene Human Needs Conceptual Model, 200
Dental hygienist, 512
Dental implants, 394–400
    assessment, 398–399
    maintenance, 399–400
    microbiology, 397–398
    selection considerations, 394–395
    structure and function, 396–397
    types, 395–396
Dental restoration, 90
Dentinal hypersensitivity, 389–394
    current perspectives on treatment of, 391–394
        client therapies, 393–394
        professional therapies, 391–393
    prevalence and etiology, 390–391
Dentinopulpal complex, 91
Dentist/employer, 511
Deplaquing, 4
Deposit accumulation, 447
Deposits, 63–65, 264–268
    bacterial plaque, 63–64, 264–266
    calculus, 64–65, 266–268
    stain, 65
Developmental depressions, 256–257
Developmental grooves, 257
Diabetes mellitus and stress, 44
Diagnostic tests, supplemental, 73–78
    biochemical assessments, 75–76
    decision making, 76–78
    immunological assessments, 76
    microbiological assessment, 73–75
    physical assessment tests, 73
Digital radiography, 140
Digital subtraction radiography, 141
Direct restorations, 90
Direct restorative materials, 99–103
    composite restorations, 102
    glass ionomers, 103
    silver amalgam alloy, 99–102
Disease activity, 55
Disease severity, 54
Diseases of the periodontium, 15–19
    gingivitis, 15–17
    periodontitis, 17–19
Disease theory, 197, 206, 208–210
Documentation
    administration of local anesthesia, 247
    case presentation and client consent, 223
    communication, 190, 192–193
    instrumentation techniques, 312

instruments, 282
oral self-care, 217
periodontal findings, 82
periodontal maintenance procedures, 452
polishing, 361
radiographic interpretation and exposure, 143–145
supportive treatment procedures, 400–401

Education, process of, 206–210
closure, 210
disease theory, 206, 208–210
initiation, 206
skill enhancement, 210
Electronic dental anesthesia (EDA), 248–249
Emergence angle or profile, 91
Employee, 499
Employment search, 487–495
cover letter preparation, 491–492
creating a resume, 488–491
interviewing strategies, 492–495
Endosseous implants, 395
Ergonomic hazards, 413–424
contributing risk factors and prevention, 417–421
force, 420
mechanical stresses, 420–421
posture, 417–420
repetitiveness, 417
temperature, 421
vibration, 421
musculoskeletal and nerve impairment disorders, 413–417
connective nerve compression, 416–417
nerve impairments, 414–416
vascular compression, 416
proposed ergonomic standard, 421, 423–424
Ergonomics, 413
Etiology of periodontal diseases, 10–12
Excessive root exposure and furcation involvement, 107
Explorers, 273–274, 307–309
techniques for, 307–309
Exposure, protocol for, 137–140
considerations, 137–140
implants, 140
Expression of body, 185
Extended-shank curets, 280
Externally motivated individual, 199
External motivational strategies, 199
Extracoronal restorations, 90
Extraoral examination, 444
Extrinsic stain, 361
Exudate, 63

Facilitative communication, 188
Fail-safe system, dental analgesic units, 230
Federal regulations regarding occupational health, 430–431
Fees, 449–450
Fee schedule, 520–521
Files, 276–277
sharpening, 297–298
techniques for, 311
Film speed, 123
Final polishing, 345
Finger activation, 305
Force, as ergonomic hazard, 420

Free gingival grafting, 466
healing, 466
procedure, 466
Free graft, 460
Frequency (cycles per second), 323
Front office personnel, 512–513
Functional resume, 490
Functional shank, 269
Furcation involvement, 66–67, 107, 261–263, 447
and excessive root exposure, 107
Furcation management, 464–465
hemisection, 464
root resection, 464–465
Future career development, 504

Gingiva, 6–8
Gingival augmentation, 460
Gingival conditions, 445
Gingival contour and tone, 264
Gingival crevicular fluid, 63
Gingival curettage, 386–387
Gingival examination, 57–59
Gingivectomy, 461
Gingivitis, 15–17, 54
associated with systemic diseases, 17
chronic, 15
necrotizing ulcerative, 15–17
Glass ionomers, 95, 103
Goals, 509–510
Grit, or particle size, of commercial pastes, 355
Guide tissue regeneration, 463

Hand-activated instrumentation, 289–319
documentation, 312–313
endpoint of instrumentation, 311–312
geometric terms, 289–290
instrumentation principles, 298–311
adaptation, 302–306
activation, 303–304
fundamentals, 298–302
techniques, 306–311
instrument sequencing, 312
instrument sharpening, 290–298
file sharpening, 297–298
objectives, 291–292
recontouring curets, 297
technique recommendations for curets, 292–297
Health history, 29
Hemisection, 464
Histopathology of periodontal disease, 20–23
advanced stage: periodontitis, 21
stages of gingivitis, 20–21
wound healing in periodontal disease, 21–23
HIV (human immunodeficient virus), 42, 45
Horizontal angulation, 121
Horizontal bone loss, 128

Immunosuppression, 45–46
Implants, 140
Implant system, 396
Impressions and temporization, 96
Independent contractor, 499
Indices used in periodontal assessment, 67–72

Indirect restorations, 90, 103–106
Infectious diseases, 42
Inflammation, 19
Informed consent, 221, 524
Initial therapy, 6
Inserts, ultrasonic, 321, 324–327
    design, 325–326
    maintenance of, 339
    relationship to energy, 324–325
    research with modified inserts, 326–327
Insurance, 521–522, 523
Instrumentation, 448–449. *See also* Hand-activated
    instrumentation
Instrumentation principles, 298–311
    adaptation, 302–306
        activation, 303–304
        angulation, 303
        insertion, 302
        stroke directions, 305–306
        terminal position of working end, 302–303
        three types of strokes, 304–305
        working end selection, 302
    fundamentals, 298–302
        fulcrum, 299–300
        grasp, 298–299
        mirror use, 300–302
        positioning, 298
    techniques, 306–311
        curets, 309–311
        explorers, 307–309
        files, 311
        manual periodontal probes, 306–307
Instrument selection, 253–288
    anatomical considerations, 256–264
        furcation involvement, 261–263
        gingival contour and tone, 264
        pocket topography, 263–264
        root anatomy, 256–261
        root surface irregularities, 261
    deposit characteristics, 264–268
        bacterial plaque formation, 264–266
        calculus formation, 266–268
    documentation, 282
    efficacy of scaling and root planing, 253–255
    instrument selection considerations, 268–280
        curets, 277–280
        explorers, 273–274
        files, 276–277
        instrument description, 268–269
        instrument identification, 268
        probes, 269–273
        sickles, 277
        ultrasonic inserts, 274–276
    nonsurgical and surgical interventions, 255
    philosophy, 255–256
    selection strategies, 280–281
Interdental cleaning devices, 165–168
Interdependence, 481
Internal motivation, 198
Interpersonal communication, 185–188
    nonverbal behaviors, 185–186
    verbal behaviors, 187–188
Interventions, 155, 255

Interviewing strategies, 492–495
Intracoronal restorations, 90
Intraoral examination, 444
Intrapersonal communication, 185
Intrinsic stain, 361
Irrigation, 376–380
    marginal, 379
    subgingival, 379–380
    supragingival, 378–379

Job and career satisfaction, 427–428
Job "burnout," 424

Kilovolt peak (kVp), 123

Language, and communication, 187
Lateral pressure, 304
Learning Ladder Continuum, 204–205
Legal documentation, 522, 524–525
Local anesthesia in nonsurgical periodontal therapy, 235–247
    background information, 235–236
    case presentation and documentation, 244, 247
    factors to consider when determining the need for local
        anesthesia, 236
    selection of injections, 241–243
    selection of local anesthetic agents, 236–241
    technique, 243–244
Loss of attachment, 60, 62

Magnetostrictive unit, 322
Maintenance in NSPT, 439
Maintenance sharpening, 295
Management discrepancy, 204
Manual tuned ultrasonic unit, 323
Marginal irrigation, 379
Margination, 108–110, 387
Margin location, 93
Margin quality, 92–93
Maslow's Needs Hierarchy, 199–200
Material needs assessment, 509
Maximum safe dosage (MSD), 240
Mechanical stresses, 420–421
Medical history, 29, 444
Medical history evaluation and alterations for care, 29–52
    medical history evaluation, 30–36
        verbal questioning, 31, 33–34
        written health history, 30–31
    physician consultations, 34–36
    posttreatment considerations, 47
    pretreatment alterations, 36–43
    treatment concerns, 43–47
Medications, and pretreatment alterations, 41–42
Microflora, effects of, 329–330
Microleakage, 90
Mini-bladed curet, 280
Mirror use, 300–302
Mobility, 65–66, 447
Modified Widman flap (MWF), 467
    healing, 462
    procedure, 462
Monitoring and evaluation, 526–527
Mucogingival reconstruction, 466
    free gingival grafting, 466

Musculoskeletal and nerve impairment disorders, 413–417
MWF. *See* Modified Widman flap

Nerve impairments, 414–416
Networking, 487
Neuromusculoskeletal disorder, 413
Neutral, balanced body position, 419
Neutral wrist position, 420
Nitrous oxide-oxygen analgesia, used for conscious sedation,
    228–235
   armamentarium, 229–231
   occupational exposure to nitrous oxide, 234–235
   patient evaluation, indications and contraindications,
    228–229
   technique, 231–234
Nonverbal behavior, 185–186
Nonsurgical periodontal therapy, implementing into general
    practice, 543
   communication, 510–514
    additional dental hygienists, 512
    dental hygiene assistant, 511–512
    dentist/employer, 511
    front office personnel, 512–513
    periodontist, 513–514
   development of a nonsurgical periodontal therapy
    program, 507–510
    goals, 509–510
    philosophy, 508
    practice assessment, 508–509
   implementation of nonsurgical periodontal therapy,
    515–525
    fee schedule, 520–521
    insurance, 521–522, 523
    legal documentation, 522, 524–525
    physical limitations, 515
    records, 515–516
    scheduling, 516–520
    supplies, 515
   monitoring and evaluation, 526–527
Nonsurgical periodontal therapy (NSPT), introduction to,
    3–28
   biological basis for periodontal therapy, 19–23
   definitions related to NSPT, 4–6
   disease of the periodontium, 15–19
   etiology and associated risk factors in periodontal diseases,
    10–15
   review of the periodontium, 6–10
Nonsurgical periodontal therapy, relationship of polishing
    to, 358–361

Objective factors in care planning, 153
Occlusion and occlusal traumatism, 96–97
   functional and parafunctional occlusal forces, 97
   occlusal therapy, 97
   occlusal traumatism, 96–97
Occupational exposure, 428
Occupational hazards, 412–436
   ergonomic hazards, 413–424
   federal regulations regarding occupational health,
    430–431
   historical perspective, 412–413
   other hazards, 428–430
    biological, 428

    chemical, 428–429
    physical, 430
   psychosocial hazards, 424–428
Occupational stress, 424
Oral prophylaxis, 4
Oral self-care education and case presentation, 196–226
   case presentation, 217–223
   oral self-care, 196–217
   *See also* Case presentation; Oral self-care
Oral self-care, 196–217
   bacterial plaque and self-care, 197
   barriers to compliance, 201, 203–204
   client compliance, 197–198
   documentation, 217
   effective teaching, 210–217
   learning, 204–205
   motivation and needs, 198–201
   process of education, 206–210
Oral self-care devices, selection of, 163–168
   interdental cleaning devices, 165–168
   toothbrushes, 163–165
Organic heart murmur, 37
Osseointegration, 396
Osseous regeneration, 463–464
   bone grafts, 463–464
   guided tissue regeneration, 463
Osseous resective surgery, 462–463
Ostectomy, 463
Osteoplasty, 463
Overhang removal, 387–389
   procedure for removal, 387–389
   relationship to periodontal disease, 387

Pain and anxiety control, 227
Pain control modalities, use of, 227–252
   alternative methods, 247–249
   local anesthesia in nonsurgical periodontal therapy,
    235–247
   nitrous oxide-oxygen analgesia for conscious sedation,
    228–235
Palliative SPC, 440
Panoramic films, 122–123
Paralleling technique, 120
Paraphrasing, 187
Performance evaluations, 526
Periapical radiographs, 119–120
Periimplant gingivitis, 397
Periimplantitis, 397
Periodontal assessment, 53–87
   appointment planning and scheduling, 55–56
   background information, 53–55
    existing disease, 54–55
    gingivitis, 54
    periodontitis, 54
    value of a test, 55
   clinical assessment, 56–67
   components of a comprehensive periodontal assessment,
    55
   dental and personal histories, 56
   documentation, 82
   identification of risk factors, 78–82
   indices, 67–72
   supplemental diagnostic tests, 73–78

Periodontal client percentage, 508
Periodontal debridement, 5
Periodontal diagnosis and care planning, 153–179
    application of planning to nonsurgical care, 168–175
    components of care planning, 155–162
    decision-making process, 154–155
    phases of care, 153–154
    selection of mechanical oral self-care devices, 163–168
Periodontal disease activity, 17
Periodontal disease, etiology and associated risk factors in, 10–15
    current perspective on role of bacterial plaque, 12
    historical perspective on bacterial plaque, 10–12
    risk factors in periodontal diseases, 12–15
Periodontal evaluation, 444–445
Periodontal ligament, 8–9
Periodontal maintenance procedures (PMP), 5–6, 439–457
    client compliance, 450–451
    components of a PMP appointment, 442–447
        assessment, 442–447
        deposit accumulation, 447
        radiographic assessment, 447
    diagnosis, 447–448
    documentation, 452
    effectiveness of maintenance, 440–442
        combined self-care and professional care, 440–442
    implementation, 448–449
        chemotherapy, 449
        instrumentation, 448–449
        self-care education, 448
    objectives maintenance, 439–440
    planning, 448
    recare intervals, 450
    referral to periodontist, 451–452
    scheduling and fees, 449–450
Periodontal-restorative interactions, 88–117
    care planning, 97–98
    occlusion and occlusal traumatism, 96–97
    overview of restorative dentistry, 88–96
    periodontally relevant restorative dentistry, 98–110
    team approach to restorative dentistry, 110–113
Periodontal Screening and Recording™ (PSR)™, 60, 61
Periodontist, 451–452, 513–514
    referral to, 451–452
Periodontitis, 17–19, 54
    adult, 18
    associated with systemic diseases, 18–19
    early-onset, 18
    refractory, 18
Periodontium, 6–10
    alveolar bone, 9–10
    cementum, 9
    gingiva, 6–8
    periodontal ligament, 8–9
Personal history, 56
Personal values and priorities, 485–486
Personal needs assessment, 509
Phenolic compounds, 373–374
Physical hazards, 430
Physical limits of office space, 515
Physician consultations, 34–36
Piezoelectric ultrasonic unit, 321
Pivoting an instrument, 300

PMP. *See* Periodontal maintenance procedures
Pocket depths, 59–60
    automated probing, 60
    manual probing, 59–60
    Periodontal Screening and Recording™ (PSR)™, 60, 61
Pocket elimination, 459
Pocket reduction, 459
Pocket topography, 263–264
Polishing, clinical applications for, 345–366
    abrasion, 354–358
        abrasive agents, 355–357
        clinician technique, 357–358
        tooth surface integrity, 358
    documentation, 361
    methods, 349–354
        air-powder abrasive polishing, 351–353
        comparing rubber cup and air polishing, 353–354
        rubber cup polishing, 350–351
    philosophies, 345–349
        professional mechanical tooth-cleaning, 348–349
        selective polishing, 346–348
        therapeutic polishing, 349
        traditional polishing, 345–346
    relationship of polishing to nonsurgical periodontal therapy, 358–361
Positioning, and treatment concerns, 47
Posttreatment considerations, 47
Posture, 417–420
Powered toothbrush, 163
Practice assessment, 508–509
Practice rating and scoring, 486–487
Prebooked system, 516
Precision-thin inserts, 320
Predictive value, 55
Predisposing factors, 135–137
Presumptive diagnosis, 55
Pretreatment alterations, 36–43
    bleeding disorders, 39–40
    cancer treatment, 40–41
    infectious diseases, 42
    medications, 41–42
    prophylactic antibiotics, 36–39
    vital signs, 42–43
Primary occlusal traumatism, 96
Primary prevention, 440
Proactive individuals, 479
Probing depth, 59, 445
Probes, 269–273, 306–307
    force, 270
    force-controlled probes, 270–271
    gingival condition, 270
    manual probes, 271–273
    probe diameter, 270
    techniques for manual periodontal probes, 306–307
Production goal, 509
Professional and personal roles, 480–481
Professional mechanical tooth-cleaning, 348–349
Professional values and priorities, 481–485
Program, nonsurgical periodontal therapy, 507
Prophylactic antibiotics, 36–39
Psychosocial hazards, 424–428
    burnout, 427

job and career satisfaction, 427–428
stress, 424–427
Psychosomatic methods of pain control, 247

Quality assurance, and periodontal interpretation, 124
Quaternary ammonium compounds, 374–375

Radiographs, recommendations for, 118–149
additional images, 140–143
computed tomography, magnetic resonance imaging, and nuclear medicine bone scanning, 142–143
computer-assisted radiography, 140
asepsis, 143
correlating radiographic and clinical findings, 129–135
documentation, 143–145
interpretation of periodontal diseases, 124–129
diseased alveolar bone, 127–129
normal alveolar bone, 125, 127
predisposing factors, 135–137
protocol for exposure, 137–140
considerations, 137–140
implants, 140
selection of conventional radiographs for periodontal evaluation, 118–123
bitewing surveys, 120–122
panoramic films, 122–123
periapical radiographs, 119–120
technical factors affecting periodontal interpretation, 123–124
control factors, 123–124
film speed, 123
quality assurance, 124
Readiness, of client, 204
Recall, 439
Recall system, 439
Recare, 439
Recare intervals, 450
Recare scheduling systems, 516–517
Recording forms, 78–82
Records in periodontal assessment, 515–516
Reevaluation, 158
Referral to a periodontist, 451–452
Regenerative techniques, 458
Repetitiveness, 417
Repetitive strain injuries (RSI), 413
Resective techniques, 458
Respiratory and other stress-induced problems, 45
Restoration morphology, 91–92
Restorative dentistry
overview of, 88–96
background information, 90–91
characteristics of restorative materials, 94–96
restoration to tissue interface, 91–94
periodontally relevant, 98–110
direct restorative materials, 99–103
indirect restorations, 103–106
maintenance of restorative materials, 107–108
margination, 108–110
team approach to, 110–113
assessment, 110, 112
combining restorative and periodontal treatment appointments, 113

education, 112
maintenance of dental restorations, 113
restorative placement, 113
Restorative examination, 444
Restorative materials, maintenance of, 107–108
Restorative placement, by dental hygienist, 113
Resume, creating, 488–491
Retipping instruments, 297
Retrograde implantitis, 398
Rheumatic heart disease, 36
Risk factors in periodontal disease, identification of, 78–82
recording forms, 78–82
Risk factors in periodontal diseases, 12–15
assessing, and predicting disease progression, 15
changing subject-related factors, 14–15
dentally-related, 13
unchanging, subject-related factors, 14
Rocking an instrument, 300
Rolling an instrument, 298
Root anatomy, 256–261
Root planing, 4, 328–329
Root surface caries, 106
Root surface irregularities, 261
Root resection, 464–465
Rubber cup polishing, 350–351
compared with air polishing methods, 353–354

Salary, 500
Sanquinarine, 375
Scaling, 4
Scheduling, 449–450, 516–520
recare scheduling systems, 516–517
troubleshooting, 517–520
Secondary prevention, 440
Selective polishing, 346–348
Self-administered written questionnaire, 30
Self-care education, 448
Self-exploration, 188
Sensitivity, 55
Sickles, 277
Silver amalgam alloys, 94, 99–102
Skill discrepancy, 204
Skill enhancement, 197, 210
Soft tissue curettage, 386
SPC. *See* Supportive periodontal care
Specificity, 55
Stain, 65, 361
extrinsic, 361
intrinsic, 361
Standard of care, 522
Stannous fluoride, 373
Stress, 43–45, 424–427
cardiovascular disease, 43–44
diabetes mellitus, 44
respiratory and other stress-induced problems, 45
Stressors, 424
Strokes in instrumentation
direction of, 305–306
types of, 304–305
Subgingival irrigation, 379–380
Subgingival ultrasonic periodontal debridement, 320
Subjective factors, 153
Subperiosteal implants, 395

Substantivity, 370
Supplies, 515
Supportive periodontal care (SPC), 440
　　palliative SPC, 440
Supportive treatment procedures
　　antimicrobial rinses, 369–376
　　controlled-release devices, 380–384
　　dental implants, 394–400
　　dentinal hypersensitivity, 389–394
　　documentation, 400–401
　　gingival curettage, 386–387
　　irrigation, 376–380
　　overhang removal, 387–389
　　overview of chemotherapy, 367–369
　　　　agents, 368
　　　　method of delivery, 368–369
　　systemic antibiotics, 384–386
Suppuration, 447
Supragingival irrigation, 378–379
Surgical crown lengthening, 463
Surgical intervention, 458–475
　　case preparation, 460–461
　　mucogingival reconstruction, 466
　　　　free gingival grafting, 466
　　periodontal flaps and alveolar bone management, 461–465
　　　　apically positioned flap, 462
　　　　furcation management, 464–465
　　　　modified Widman flap, 462
　　　　osseous regeneration, 463–464
　　　　osseous resective surgery, 462–463
　　　　postoperative care for flap surgery, 465
　　principles of surgery, 458–460
　　surgical evaluation, 461
Systemic antibiotics, 384–386

Teaching that is effective, 210–217
Team approach to restorative dentistry, 110–113
　　assessment, 110, 112
　　combining restorative and periodontal treatment
　　　　appointments, 113
　　education, 112
　　maintenance of dental restorations, 113
　　restorative placement, 113
Team concept, 510
Temperature, as ergonomic hazard, 421
Terminal shank, 269
Tetracycline fiber therapy, 381–382
　　clinical application, 381–382
　　research findings, 381
Therapeutic polishing, 349
Tip displacement, 323
Tobacco smoking, 46–47
Tone of voice, 185
Toothbrushes, 163–165
Topical anesthetics, 247–248
Total compensation package, 486
Traditional polishing, 345–346

Transducer, 321
Transmission radiographs, 122
Transosteal implants, 395
Treatment concerns, 43–47
　　immunosuppression, 45–46
　　local anesthesia, 47
　　positioning, 47
　　stress, 43–45
　　tobacco smoking, 46–47
Triangulation, 131
Troubleshooting, 517–520

Ultrasonic inserts, 274–276
Ultrasonic periodontal debridement, 320–344
　　background information, 327–331
　　　　antimicrobial irrigation during ultrasonic debridement,
　　　　　　330
　　　　calculus removal, 328
　　　　cavitational activity, 330
　　　　clinical parameters, 329
　　　　effects of microflora, 329–330
　　　　effects on restorations, 330–331
　　　　root planing, 328–329
　　case selection, 331–332
　　current trends in ultrasonic equipment, 322–327
　　　　inserts, 324–327
　　　　units, 323–324
　　history of ultrasonic scaling devices, 320–321
　　instrumentation recommendations, 332–338
　　　　adaptation and activation, 336–337
　　　　infection control, 334
　　　　insert selection, 335
　　　　positioning, 334–335
　　　　sequencing, 336
　　　　special situations, 337–338
　　　　tuning the unit, 335–336
　　maintenance of inserts, 339
　　principles of ultrasonic instruments, 321–322
Ultrasonics, 322
Universal characteristics of explorers, 307
Universal curets, 277

Vascular compression, 416
Vasoconstrictors, 240
Verbal behaviors, 187–188
Vertical (angular) bone loss, 128
Vertical angulation, 119
Vertical bitewing radiographs, 120
Vibration as a contributing factor in development of nerve
　　　　neuropathies, 421
Vital signs, 42–43

Wages, 500–501
Working end of instrument, 269, 302–303
　　selection, 302
　　terminal, position of, 302–303